Diseases of the Horse, Part 2/II

Diseases of the Horse

A Handbook for Science and Practice

Part 2/II

Edited by

Prof. Dr. sc. med. vet. Olof Dietz, Berlin

Prof. Dr. sc. med. vet. Ekkehard Wiesner, Berlin

English translation edited by

Dr. A. S. Turner, Fort Collins, Colo.

205 figures (partly in color), 11 tables, 1984

KARGER

S. Karger · Basel · München · Paris · London · New York · Tokyo · Sydney

Translated from the original German edition by TERRY C. TELGER, Marina, Calif.

National Library of Medicine. Cataloging in Publication

Handbuch der Pferdekrankheiten für Wissenschaft und Praxis. English.
Diseases of the horse: a handbook for science and practice / edited by Olof Dietz, Ekkehard Wiesner; English translation edited by A. S. Turner. Basel; New York: Karger, 1984. Translation of: Handbuch der Pferdekrankheiten für Wissenschaft und Praxis.
1. Horse Diseases I. Dietz, Olof II. Turner, A. Simon III. Wiesner, Ekkehard
ISBN 3-8055-3497-3
SF 951 H 236

Printed in the German Democratic Republic
ISBN 3-8055-3497-3

Contents of the Present Volume

Contents of the Complete Work

Part 2/II Special Part (Continuation)

2.1.18. Diseases of the Forelimbs

2.1.18.1. Diseases of the Shoulder and Upper Arm, Shoulder Lameness

Definition. 'Shoulder lameness' is a collective term applied to locomotor disturbances referable to pathologic processes in the shoulder region. More specifically, it includes the various forms of omarthritis, osteochondritis dissecans of the shoulder joint, and intertuberal bursitis. Shoulder lameness is characterized chiefly a swinging-leg lameness. Symptoms of mixed lameness may also develop in some cases. The anterior phase of the stride is shortened, and the animal has difficulty lifting the foot from the ground. As a result, the hoof tends to drag the ground even when the animal is backing. The lameness is exacerbated on soft ground and when the animal is walked uphill. The same is true when the animal is walked in a circle with the affected limb outermost.

With bursitis of the shoulder joint, there is a lateral movement or circumduction of the limb when the horse is walking, and the limb is abducted while the animal is standing.

Shoulder lamenesses are rare compared to diseases involving the more distal parts of the limb. Pathologic changes of the distal limb should first be excluded before the cause of a lameness is localized to the shoulder region.

2.1.18.1.1. Diseases of the Shoulder Joint (Omarthritis, Omarthrosis, Osteochondritis dissecans)

Definition and Occurrence. There are four basic forms of shoulder joint disease, which differ in their course and pathogenesis:

— acute aseptic omarthritis
— suppurative omarthritis
— chronic degenerative omarthritis (omarthrosis)
— osteochondritis dissecans.

While the first two forms can occur as serous, aseptic, pyogenic or serofibrinous inflammations in all horses, omarthrosis occurs mainly in heavy draft horses and rarely affects riding horses. It takes an insidious course, and some time passes before overt symptoms appear. The primary lesions are confined to the cartilage and joint capsule, the most common sites of occurrence being the medial half of the humeral head, the glenoid cavity of the scapula and the peripheral portions of the shoulder joint. Osteochondritis dissecans is usually a disease of young horses.

Acute Omarthritis and Suppurative Omarthritis

Etiology. Contusions and sprains caused by collisions with solid objects, entanglement in fences, etc. cause damage to the shoulder joint capsule and articular cartilage. This results in a serous or serofibrinous omarthritis. Purulent omarthritis is a common sequel to perforating joint wounds caused by a kick, wood splinter, barbed wire, etc. It may take the form of a pyogenic, serous, fibrinous or suppurative omarthritis, joint empyema, capsular cellulitis or suppurative panarthritis. The character of the inflammation is determined by the nature of the infecting organism, the route of infection and the infectious process.

Metastatic suppurative omarthritis occurs as a sequel to septicemia in foals. The organisms most commonly involved are streptococci, *Corynebacterium equi* and organisms of foal septicemia *(Actinobacillus equuli)*.

Symptoms. The initial sign is a lameness of sudden onset that worsens during exercise. Passive extension, flexion and rotation of the limb at the shoulder are strongly resented by the animal and cause obvious pain. Examination of the joint reveals local heat, tenderness and distension of the capsule.

With open joint wounds, severe lameness develops 2—3 days after the injury. Purulent synovial fluid leaks from the wound opening, and a hot painful swelling appears in the shoulder region. If allowed to progress, this suppurative joint inflammation will lead to necrosis and erosion of articular cartilage. Movement of the limb provokes a gelatinous, purulent discharge from the wound, and crepitant sounds may be audible. A febrile systemic reaction is usually present.

Differential Diagnosis. The attitude of the limbs and manner of weight-bearing while standing may cause the examiner to mistake aseptic omarthritis for a subluxation of the humerus, cubital arthritis (inflammation of the elbow joint), radial nerve paralysis or ulnar fracture. Suppurative omarthritis is similar in appearance to bursitis of the shoulder joint.

Diagnosis. Symptomatic relief following intra-articular anesthesia of the shoulder joint establishes the diagnosis of aseptic omarthritis. Wounds in proximity to the joint that are associated with discharge of purulent synovial fluid and local symptoms in the shoulder region (heat, tenderness, distension of joint capsule) suggest a diagnosis of acute pyogenic omarthritis. Moderate to severe shoulder lameness and fever are also common in such cases. Metastatic omarthritis is a feature of septicemia in foals. Traumatic chip fractures or osteochondral fragments like those seen in osteochondritis dissecans can be visualized by radiography.

Treatment. Closed contusions and sprains are treated with immediate rest and cold application (cooling ointments or poultices, ice bags). After about 48 hours, moist heat and rubefacient drugs are applied to hasten the absorption of effusion and promote healing. Ointments containing heparin and heparinoids (mainly mucopolysaccharide sulfuric acid esters) inhibit inflammatory processes while stimulating blood flow and the absorption of inflammatory products. The oral or parenteral administration of phenylbutazone and its derivatives, and certain glucocorticoids has proved a beneficial adjunct to topical treatment. In addition, single or multiple intra-articular injections of glucocorticoids often bring rapid improvement.

If the swelling of periarticular tissues cannot ensure adequate closure of a joint wound, the wound must be surgically debrided and closed by suture. The joint capsule should be sutured only in areas where the sutures can be placed without tension. Restoration of the periarticular tissue investment and good skin closure are important aspects of the procedure.

Dirty joint wounds must be mechanically cleansed. Irrigations and the local application of chemotherapeutic agents can cause irreversible harm to the articular cartilage and so must be used with caution. The joint is flushed with aqueous antibiotic solutions (1—2 million I.U. per injection). For systemic therapy, 5—10 million I.U. penicillin are injected intramuscularly for 5—7 days. Hyperemia is stimulated in the area surrounding the wound.

Chronic Degenerative Omarthritis, Omarthrosis

Etiology. This disease may supervene on acute omarthritis if adequate rest is not ensured, or if there is severe preexisting capsular or cartilaginous injury. In other cases the disease may take an insidious course from the outset. This can occur in shoulder joints that are subjected to recurrent shocks associated with rapid gaits on hard surfaces. In riding horses, unequal loads on the forequarters and frequent abrupt turns can cause such a lameness.

Predisposing factors are base-wide and base-narrow conformation, and an unsually wide or narrow chest (increased loads on one joint half and poor angulation of the shoulder).

Symptoms. The horse manifests a chronic lameness that is exacerbated when the animal is ridden, and especially when sharp turns are executed. In contrast to acute omarthritis, local inflammatory changes are absent. The contour of the shoulder joint is unusually prominent due to atrophy of the shoulder muscles. In long-standing cases, palpation reveals hypertrophic new bone growth around the periphery of the joint ('lipping') with associated joint enlargement. As in acute omarthritis, pain is produced by manipulation. The lameness may show temporary improvement after rest.

The lesions correspond to those of degenerative joint disease. The end-result of the pathologic process is a flattening, erosion and enlargement of the articular surface. Proliferation of chondrocytes occurs in the periphery of the articular cartilage. The ground substance of the cartilage swells and softens. Later the cartilage cells degenerate, forming cavities that collapse leaving cartilaginous defects on the articular surfaces. Knobby or spurlike exostoses form at the joint margins. Ankylosis may develop as the disease progesses. The capsular ligament is thickened, and the synovial villi are hyperplastic. Loose bodies are rarely found.

Differential Diagnosis. The atrophy of the infra- and supraspinatus muscles and accentuated contour of the shoulder joint may cause confusion with suprascapular nerve paralysis. The 'dropping' of the shoulder during weight-bearing is absent in omarthrosis, however.

Diagnosis. The insidious clinical course, the mixed lameness that worsens during exercise, the pain on manipulation, and the local changes in the shoulder joint are characteristic of chronic degenerative omarthritis. A diagnostic injection of local anesthetic into the shoulder joint will relieve the lameness only in the early stage of the disease, before mechanical obstructions have formed. Transthoracic and medio-lateral radiographs will demonstrate intra-articular and periarticular changes.

Treatment. A complete recovery cannot be expected if degenerative changes have developed. Thus, the goal of treatment is to restore a maximum degree of function.

Enforced rest for 3—4 months is recommended. Classical treatment methods include the vigorous use of rubefacient drugs or cauterization by firing followed by the application of a blister. When such methods are used, care must be taken that the joint region is not altered, and that ointments are not licked from the skin. Formerly, beneficial results were sometimes achieved by the introduction of setons (fig. 2.1.18. — 1). The subcutaneous injection of terpentine oil in the joint region is not advised, because it predisposes to cellulitis and fascial necrosis. The impaired nutritive function of the synovial fluid resulting from the disturbance of intra-articular metabolism can be improved by the replacement of deficient intercellular substances (Arteparon) or through enzyme inhibition (aprotinin).

One or two intra-articular injections of glucocorticoids can be of value in acute cases. Surgery is indicated for the removal of loose bodies within the joint that could cause irritation of the synovial membrane. Supportive measures may be beneficial. Corrective shoeing, dietary restrictions for weight reduction, and modification of use should be employed as needed to assist recovery.

Prognosis. Experience has shown that omarthrosis following on acute aseptic omarthritis has a more favorable prognosis than primary chronic forms caused by recurrent microtrauma. In the latter case the articular changes are usually too far advanced to respond to therapy. It is worthwhile to attempt treatment in the case of breeding horses, but we do not recommend it for racing or draft horses.

1

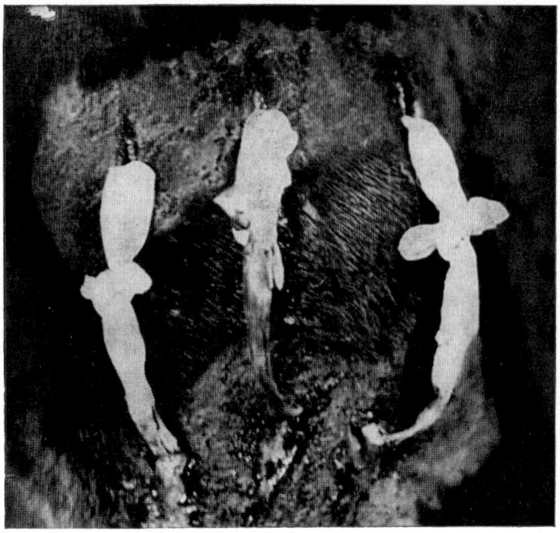

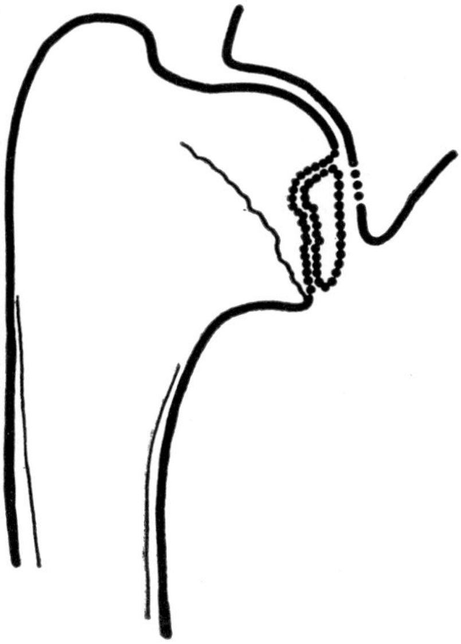

2

Fig. 2.1.18. — 1. Setons passed through shoulder region as a treatment for chronic degenerative omarthritis (antiquated treatment method).

Fig. 2.1.18. — 2. Osteochondritis dissecans: stage of cartilage flanking.

Osteochondritis dissecans of the Shoulder Joint in Foals

Occurrence and Etiology. Osteochondritis dissecans or aseptic necrosis of the head of the humerus affects fast-growing, active horses between the ages of 7 and 12 months. The caudal half of the articular surface of the humeral head is most commonly affected, as it is subjected to the greatest static and dynamic loads.

The cause is unknown. A circulatory disturbance that develops at the conclusion of longitudinal growth, at which time the vascular regions of the epiphysis and metaphysis are still separated by the epiphyseal plate, may be the cause. The associated blood-flow deficiencies lead to circumscribed areas of aseptic necrosis with subsequent splitting of the overlying cartilage under physiologic loads.

This assumption is supported by the observation that the necrosis heals only after blood-flow conditions improve as a result of epiphyseal closure.

Symptoms. Tearing of the articular cartilage is marked by the sudden appearance of a moderate to severe lameness. This may improve over a period of 2—3 weeks but tends to recur when the animal is exercised. Pain is evident when the shoulder is palpated or manipulated. Crepitation can sometimes be detected in the shoulder joint.

Differential Diagnosis. Traumatic chip fractures of the shoulder joint and aseptic omarthritis must be excluded. Chip fractures cause an acute, severe swinging-leg lameness. Radiographs are diagnostic.

Diagnosis. Radiographic examination reveals the nature of the changes in the epiphysis and joint (fig. 2.1.18. — 2).

Only a flattening or indentation of the humeral head or atrophy of cancellous bone areas is demonstrable in the early stage. Later a reactive medullary fibrosis and reparative cancellous bone sclerosis are observed. Pieces of articular cartilage separate to form loose bodies which, after mineralization, can also be demonstrated by x-ray. Radiographs are made with the animal anesthetized and dorsally recumbent [Meagher et al., 1975].

Treatment. A functional recovery can be achieved following a prolonged period of restricted motion, provided the joint changes precipitated by the aseptic necrosis have not progressed too far.

Schebitz [1965] states that severe secondary degenerative changes can be prevented by surgical curettage of the osteochondral defect. The loose, pale-blue cartilage, which appears wrinkled in the case of larger defects, is surgically removed at the earliest opportunity, and the exposed cartilage is curetted. Return of function should be noted several weeks postoperatively.

Prognosis. In mild cases the foal can recover to functional soundness with minor secondary degenerative joint changes. Prompt surgical revision of the osteochondral defect prevents severe joint disease and thus improves the prognosis.

Luxations and Subluxations of the Humerus

Occurrence and Etiology. Luxations and subluxations of the humerus occasionally occur in racing and riding horses that sustain a blow to the shoulder during a fall on a hard surface. If the upper arm is in abduction or adduction at the time of the injury, it can pry the humeral head out of the shallow glenoid cavity. This invariably causes tears of the joint capsule and intra-articular hemorrhage, and may be associated with cartilage damage or chip fractures of the humerus or scapula.

Symptoms. The injury is followed by an immediate, severe swinging-leg lameness, and weight is borne on the toe of the foot while standing. All joints are held in flexion. If the dislocation is severe, the limb appears shortened. Passive movement and extension are difficult and extremely painful. If crepitation is heard during such manipulations, a fracture or comminution of the articular surface is indicated. There is deformity of the shoulder joint in accordance with the direction of the luxation, and either the glenoid cavity or the humeral head may be more accessible to palpation. Marked atrophy of the shoulder muscles develops within a few days. With a subluxation of the humerus, the affected limb can bear weight during walking. However, the leg is advanced with hesitation and circumduction and bears weight only momentarily. Tenderness and deformation of the joint are less pronounced.

Diagnosis. The clinical signs of a complete luxation are unmistakable. Subluxations can be reliably distinguished from acute omarthritis, radial paralysis, ulnar fractures and cubital arthritis only by radiography. Films are made in the medio-lateral projection with the limb pulled forward. Luxations in the medial or lateral direction are radiographed in the PA projection with the cassette held in front of the shoulder joint. The radiograph will also demonstrate any chip fractures or defects in the joint surface that may be present.

Treatment. Reduction should be attempted as soon as possible. However, reduction is worthwhile only in valuable horses that are suitable for breeding use. Under deep anesthesia and muscle relaxation, the head of the humerus is returned to the glenoid cavity by strong traction on the limb and pressure on the humeral head, thereby reducing the luxation along the same path that it occurred. Complete stall rest aids in healing.

Prognosis. The end-result may be uncertain, because damage to the joint capsule, cartilage or bone may be so severe that it precludes a permanent reduction. It is not unusual for secondary degenerative changes to develop in the injured joint.

2.1.18.1.2. Traumatic Myositis of the Shoulder Muscles

Occurrence and Etiology. Inflammation of the shoulder muscles in the horse is most commonly caused by trauma due to running or bumping into solid objects, ill-fitting tack, or kicks from other horses. Strains due to slipping or falling are less common. Allergic diseases were once thought to have significance, but this theory has not withstood scientific testing.

Trauma causes contusions of the muscles and leads to hematoma formation. These lesions most commonly affect the brachiocephalic muscle in its inferior portion anterior to the shoulder joint, as well as the biceps brachii muscle (fig. 2.1.18. — 3).

Symptoms. Besides a typical swinging-leg lameness, a circumscribed, painful, hot swelling is found in the region of the affected muscles. There may be fluctuation as a sign of hematoma formation, or a defect in the course of the muscles indicating a muscular tear. Passive flexion and backward traction on the limb cause pain. The serum enzymes of muscular origin, CPK and ALD, as well as nonspecific enzymes such as ASAT and LDH show increased activities within 24 hours after the trauma. These elevations are smaller than those associated with tying-up syndromes.

Differential Diagnosis. Traumatic myositis of the brachiocephalic muscle must be differentiated from botryomycosis of the pectoral or shoulder region. However, the latter develops very gradually, and weeks or months pass before a swelling appears lateral and anterior to the shoulder. The ventral cervical lymph nodes are always involved.

Diagnosis. A circumscribed, tender, sometimes pulsatile swelling appears suddenly in the region of the shoulder muscles, and a typical swinging-leg lameness develops. The serum muscle enzymes are markedly elevated within 24 hours after the trauma.

Treatment and Prognosis. Traumatic myositis of the shoulder muscles heals spontaneously within 1—2 weeks. The affected part should be rested by confining the horse to a well-padded box stall.

Local and systemic measures are indicated for the first few days to reduce inflammation, hemorrhage and pain (Aciterran, Hepathromb ointment, phenylbutazone injections). Afterward, absorption-promoting agents are employed (camphor or iodine ointments, local massage).

In cases where fibrous scar-tissue formation is inadequate, Fraser [1961] reports good results with Faradic current treatments given 3—4 times weekly. The myopathy may also respond favorably to the administration of vitamin E-selenium preparations. Muscular contusions and tears require 2—4 weeks to heal.

The application of blistering ointments is necessary only in long-standing cases that are associated with much tissue degeneration or fibrosis of a hematoma. Weight-bearing should be resumed in such a manner that the scar tissue is able to adapt functionally. If weight is borne too early, too late or to excess, there may be injury to the replacement tissue leading to a recurrence.

2.1.18.1.3. Bicipital Bursitis, Intertuberal Bursitis

Definition and Occurrence. The bicipital bursa in the horse lies between the tendon of origin of the biceps brachii muscle and the bicipital groove of the humerus, where it is exposed to various forms of trauma. An acute aseptic, pyogenic or chronic aseptic bursitis can result.

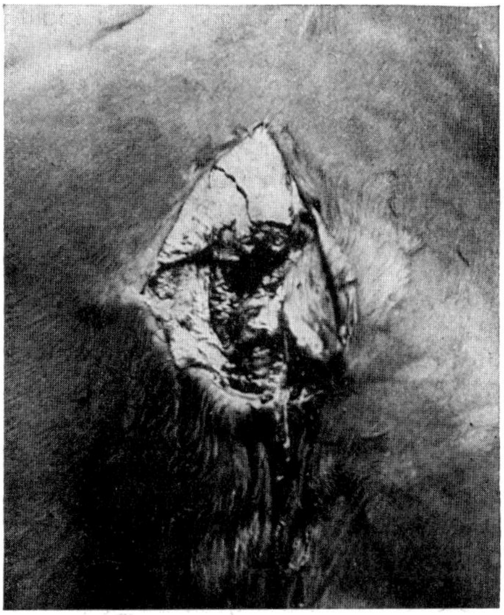

3

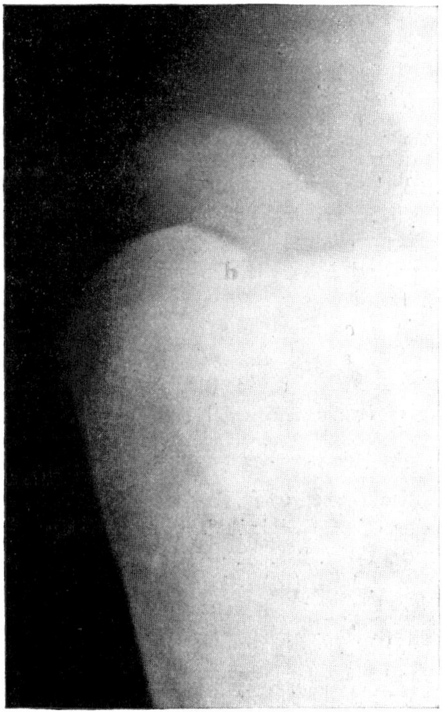

4

Fig. 2.1.18. — 3. Muscular wound of the shoulder.

Fig. 2.1.18. — 4. Ossification in the area of the bicipital bursa.

Etiology and Symptoms

a) Acute aseptic bursitis is the most common form and may occur as a serous or serofibrinous inflammation. The causes are excessive stresses associated with rapid gaits and unphysiologic movements (circus horses, equestrian gymnastics), contusions from falls, blows or collisions, etc. Often, however, the condition represents the response to repeated trauma caused by age-related disturbances of muscular coordination and locomotor sequences.

Symptoms in the early stage are subtle. At the trot, the animal exhibits an unsteady, somewhat stumbling gait, a delay in the advance of the affected limb, and a shortening of the stride. Later a mixed lameness develops that is most pronounced in the swinging-leg phase. Sometimes the horse ceases to put any weight on the affected limb and holds it caudal to the normal position while standing. During backing, the foot is dragged flat along the ground with the carpal and digital joints extended.

A slight, tender, edematous swelling is found in the area of the bicipital groove. The bursa itself is distended with fluid, and the overlying biceps brachii tendon is under increased tension. Pain is produced by pulling the limb backward, which will cause the horse to rear or step away from the examiner.

b) Pyogenic bursitis is most commonly the result of perforating wounds. Isolated cases may result from a blood- or lymph-borne infection, brucellosis, etc. Purulent bursitis usually produces a swinging-leg lameness of rapid onset. A painful, phlegmonous swelling is found in the area of the bursa, and a purulent exudate drains from the wound. A febrile systemic reaction is present.

c) Chronic aseptic bursitis is frequently observed in draft horses that must do heavy work at a rapid pace. It may be bilateral. The symptoms differ from those of acute aseptic bursitis only in degree. Acute inflammatory symptoms are absent, and there is less distension of the bursa.

Differential diagnosis must be made from omarthritis. The limb carriage and manner of weight-bearing while standing may cause confusion with ulnar fractures, distal radial nerve paralysis and cubital arthritis.

Diagnosis. The typical symptoms of bicipital bursitis, besides the local changes, are the manner of dragging the foot while backing and evidence of pain when the limb is pulled backward. In doubtful cases omarthritis can be differentiated from bicipital bursitis by response to intra-articular anesthesia of the shoulder joint. The extent of the changes can only be evaluated at necropsy.

The lesions affect not only the bursa but also the biceps tendon and the bony and cartilaginous tissues of the articular surface of the humerus.

In many cases the wall of the bursa is thickened and covered with granulation tissue.

The cavity of the bursa is filled with a serous, serofibrinous or purulent fluid. The tendon shows areas of fibrillation, necrosis and ossification. Exostoses are found at the border of the bicipital groove, and cartilage defects on the articular surfaces of the humerus (fig. 2.1.18. — 4).

Treatment. The horse is placed in a large, well-padded stall, and rest is enforced for 6—12 weeks. In aseptic cases, local heat and rubefacient drugs are indicated. The local use of glucocorticoids is usually of only temporary benefit. Wounds of the bursa and suppurative bursitis are managed in the same way as a pyogenic arthritis or tendovaginitis.

Prognosis. Chronic bursitis, especially when bilateral, and acute cases with marked symptoms are frequently refractory to treatment. Many horses become recumbent and die from associated complications, such as decubitus or pneumonia.

Comments. Chronically affected horses are useful only for breeding, and recovered cases are sound only for light work at a moderate pace. Even in mild cases, recovery can take months.

2.1.18.1.4. Bursitis of the Infraspinatus Muscle

Occurrence and Etiology. A bursa is present beneath the tendon of the infraspinatus muscle where it attaches to the lateral tuberosity of the humerus. This bursa may become contused, and subsequently inflamed, as a result of falls, blows, slips or heavy loading. The tendon is also involved in most cases.

Symptoms. Pressure on the tendon is painful. This results in a peculiar form of shoulder lameness in which the affected limb is advanced somewhat reluctantly in an almost semicircular outward arc. The foot is held in abduction during standing.

A painful swelling is evident in the area of the lateral tuberosity, and a soft crepitation is sometimes audible.

Diagnosis. The lameness is relieved by local anesthesia of the bursa or surrounding tissues. Chip fractures of the scapula or humerus are demonstrable by radiography.

Treatment. Treatment consists of moist heat application, massage, and the use of topical irritants or cautery and blisters; 4—8 weeks are required for healing.

Prognosis. Excluding chip fractures of the lateral tuberosity of the humerus, the prognosis is good.

2.1.18.1.5. *Subcutaneous Bursitis of the Shoulder*

In young harness horses, unaccustomed pressure from tack can cause the inflammation of subcutaneous bursae in the region of the scapular spine several fingerwidths below the tuber spinae. It is manifested by a painful swelling about the size of a hen's egg. Surgical ablation is indicated and should even enable the horse to wear a harness collar if a strong surgical scar is formed.

2.1.18.1.6. *Luxation of the Biceps Brachii Tendon*

In rare cases the tendon of the biceps brachii muscle can become dislocated laterally by an unfavorable levering action. A severe swinging-leg lameness results. The limb is extended and trails behind the other legs during progression. During standing there is an acute angulation in the shoulder joint, and the contours of the joint appear unusually prominent. Later a diffuse swelling appears in the shoulder region. The condition is incurable.

2.1.18.1.7. *Fractures of the Scapula*

Occurence and Etiology. Scapular fractures may be caused by blunt trauma, falls, jumps, running into obstacles, abrupt reining, turns, kicks, etc. Often they are associated with a concomitant severe sprain of the shoulder joint, brachial plexus paralysis or luxation of the humerus. Most are closed comminuted fractures with involvement of the glenoid cavity. Open fractures and injuries of the scapular cartilage are rare. Scapular fractures may be divided into those involving the body of the scapula (including the glenoid, neck, and anterior and posterior angles) and those involving its processes (scapular spine, coracoid process, tuber scapulae). Bilateral scapular fractures are seen in racehorses and jumpers.

Symptoms. The severity of clinical manifestations varies with the nature of the fracture and associated complications (sprain of shoulder joint, brachial plexus paralysis, luxation of humerus).

Fractures of the glenoid, neck and base, as well as comminuted fractures, result in an immediate, swinging- and supporting-limb lameness. The affected limb does not bear weight and drags the ground during movement. Marked swelling of the shoulder region is seen following the injury. This makes it difficult to palpate the area, and it is seldom possible to detect displacements of individual bone fragments or crepitation. With fractures through the neck of the scapula, abnormal mobility of the limb will be evident.

The remaining types of scapular fracture present less characteristic symptoms. Weight is borne on the limb during standing. However, a severe swinging-leg lameness is present during movement in the early stage of the disease. Crepitation cannot be detected. With open fractures, wound infection leads to the development of cartilage and bone necrosis and fistulous tracts with the discharge of a foul-smelling pus.

Differential Diagnosis. Fractures of the proximal humerus and luxations and subluxations of the humerus should be excluded in the presence of scapular neck and glenoid fractures.

Diagnosis. The sudden occurrence of a severe swinging-leg lameness and a local, painful swelling in the scapular area, with otherwise negative findings in the remainder of the limb, suggest a diagnosis of scapular fracture. The diagnosis is confirmed by

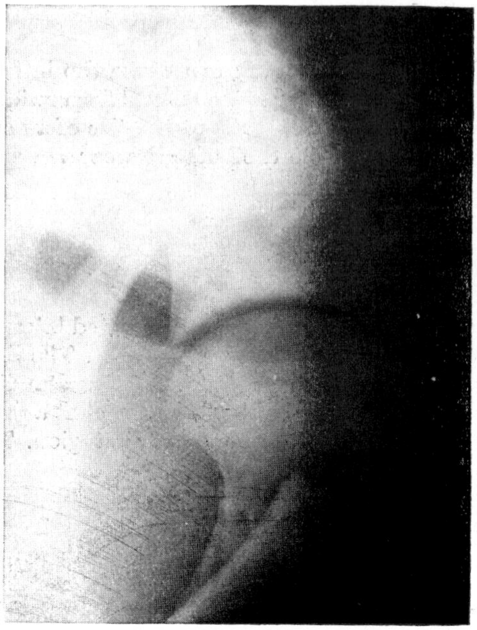
5

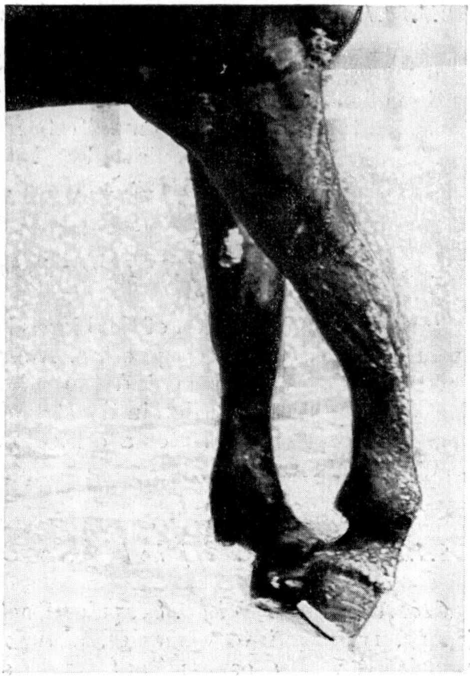
6

Fig. 2.1.18. — 5. Oblique fracture of the shaft of the humerus.
Fig. 2.1.18. — 6. Fracture of the humerus: typical limb carriage.

the presence of crepitation, displaced bone fragments or corresponding radiographic findings.

Radiographs provide information on the location and course of the fracture line. They are obtained with the animal cast onto the affected side. The affected limb is pulled well forward, and the healthy limb is pulled backward to separate the scapular shadows on the radiograph.

Fractures of the scapular neck can also be demonstrated in the standing animal by means of an oblique PA view.

Treatment. In open fractures, the wound is explored, bone fragments are removed, drainage is established, and closure is carried out. In some cases fistulous tracts will develop as a result of sequestered bone fragments or cartilage damage. These must be probed, opened and resected. With perforation of the scapula, a burr hole must be made in order to reach the base of the fistula. It is not unusual for new fistulous openings to appear later, and these are managed in the same way.

Prognosis. Fractures of the scapular neck, glenoid cavity and base are generally untreatable, especially if associated with brachial plexus paralysis and vascular tears. Severe muscular atrophy, general emaciation, extensive callus formation, progressive necrosis and pseudarthrosis of the shoulder joint lead to permanent lameness. In mares, recovery is sometimes sufficient to restore breeding soundness. Fractures involving the scapular processes will eventually heal if the bone fragments have been sloughed or surgically removed.

2.1.18.1.8. Fractures of the Humerus

Occurrence and Etiology. Fractures of the humerus, like scapular fractures, occur as a result of external violence. Spontaneous fractures associated with other diseases such as bone tumors, osteomalacia, osteomyelitis and tuberculous osteitis are relatively uncommon.

Fractures of the humerus may involve the shaft, epiphysis or condyles (fig. 2.1.18. — 5). Fractures of the shaft are the most common in mature horses, while foals are more prone to epiphyseal fractures. Avulsion fractures of the areas of attachment of the infraspinatus and supraspinatus muscles (lateral and medial tuberosities) are less common.

Symptoms. The clinical signs of a humeral fracture include marked lameness, increased mobility, crepitation, swelling, and sometimes an apparent shortening of the limb (fig. 2.1.18. — 6). In chip fractures, the fragment is usually displaced by muscular traction, with the result that crepitation and abnormal motion cannot always be detected.

The diagnosis is established by the foregoing symptoms and by the radiographic examination.

Radiographs are obtained in two planes and provide accurate information on the form and course of the fracture line. This is especially important in the case of chip fractures and fissure fractures; otherwise the latter will go unnoticed until they develop into complete fractures.

Treatment. Closed fractures of the humeral shaft in foals weighing up to about 250 kg will heal completely in 3—4 months with confined rest in a small box stall. In mature horses, these fractures are frequently incurable, especially if comminution is present.

Internal fixation by means of compression plating may be tried in valuable horses.

Closed chip fractures of the lateral tuberosity will generally heal with enforced rest. Open fractures can heal only if loose bone fragments are surgically removed.

The operative treatment of fractures is carried out under general anesthesia, which will also provide adequate muscle relaxation. Antibiotic lavage of the medullary cavity and fracture line is also important. A 5- to 10-day course of parenteral antibiotics (8—10 million I.U.) is indicated postoperatively. In this way primary healing can be achieved in open or infected fractures. Screws and cerclage wire are usually well tolerated for long periods.

A frequent cause of failure in mature horses is the development of a 'stress' laminitis in the healthy limb, or recumbency and subsequent death from emaciation, decubitus, pneumonia or a general pyogenic infection.

2.1.18.1.9. Thrombosis of the Axillary Artery and Brachial Artery

Occurrence and Etiology. Occlusion of the axillary or brachial artery can occur as a result of endarteritis or migrating strongyle larvae and embolism.

Symptoms. Clinical signs first appear following vigorous exercise, when the blood supply is inadequate to meet the increased oxygen demand. A lameness appears which, as in paralysis of the axillary plexus, is manifested by an unsteady gait, shortened stride and tentative weight-bearing. Following frequent stumbling and toe dragging, the fetlock and carpal joints finally give way, and the leg goes limp.

Sometimes the horse will paw the ground with the affected leg. There are usually marked systemic reactions such as sweating, tremor, rapid pulse and dyspnea. Total collapse is rare. The affected limb feels cold and insensitive. Pulsation of the metacarpal artery is weak or absent, depending on the degree of occlusion. Symptoms regress spontaneously with 15—20 minutes of rest.

While at rest, the blood flow through the narrowed vascular lumen or collateral circulation is generally adequate to enable the limb to bear weight.

Diagnosis. The diagnosis is based on the presence of intermittent lameness symptoms. Paresthesia, anesthesia and hyperesthesia are rare. The chance of recovery depends on the degree of thrombosis that has occurred.

Treatment and Prognosis. Improvement and occasional cures have been achieved with the i.v. administration of fibrolysin, heparin, calcium thiosulfate or sodium gluconate for several months. The therapeutic efficacy in such cases derives from canalization of the thrombus, collateral vasodilation and new blood vessel formation. The patient's progress can be favorably influenced by repeated, temporary vasodilation through stellate ganglion blockade and moderate exercise. In mild cases, light exercise is beneficial. If an adequate collateral supply is not established, or satisfactory canalization of the thrombus is not achieved, the prognosis is poor due to a lack of alternate treatment methods.

2.1.18.1.10. Neoplasms in the Region of the Scapula and Humerus

Occurrence. Soft-tissue tumors such as papillomas, fibromas, rhabdomyomas and sarcomas occasionally develop in the region of the shoulder joint, scapula and humerus, especially in older horses, and can be a source of lameness. The incidence of such neoplasms in horses is low (2 % according to Überreiter [1965]).

Symptoms. Benign tumors of the skin, subcutis, fatty tissue and muscles are round or spheroidal, as are tumors of the mixed variety. They vary in size, may be superficial or deeply-situated, and can be moved relative to underlying tissues. Superficial tumors with a broad area of attachment and more deeply-situated tumors that are poorly delineated relative to surrounding tissues are malignant soft-tissue neoplasms (sarcomas, malignant mixed tumors).

The skin over such tumors tends to be glossy, often hairless, cornified, fissured, and is prone to degeneration. Neoplasms in this region of the limb may be single or multiple. Their consistency ranges from hard to soft and pliable. Pain generally is evident only when the lesion is subjected to external irritation from tack or other causes. If metastatic lesions develop in the regional lymph nodes (superficial cervical or axillary nodes), lameness generally results. Bone tumors (osteoma, osteosarcoma) affecting the humerus or scapula may be incidental findings in the horse. They are characterized by a constantly-growing, hard swelling with progressive lameness. Systemic signs or emaciation are suggestive of metastatic spread.

Osteomas often cease growing and undergo consolidation.

Differential diagnosis must be made from deep-seated abscesses, organized hematomas and fungal granulomas.

Diagnosis. The diagnosis is established by histologic examination following a biopsy or total exstirpation. The radiographic visualization of neoplasms depends largely on their size and density and on the tissues that lie in the path of the x-ray beam. The absence of demonstrable change does not necessarily mean that a tumor is absent. By the same token, when changes suggestive of a neoplasm are demonstrated, it is not always possible to determine the etiology. The most informative and best-tolerated diagnostic procedure is the isotope scan. It can serve as a supplement to the radiographic examination. Most neoplasms in the horse are papillomas, fibromas and melanosarcomas.

Prognosis and Treatment. The response to treatment depends on the nature and development of the neoplasm. Benign tumors may be surgically removed if they impair the animal's usefulness. In the case of malignancies, extirpation of the tumor and associated lymph nodes should suffice to prevent a recurrence for some months. The prognosis for bone tumors is poor.

If the patient is a valuable breeding horse, irradiation therapy may be tried. Soft-tissue tumors should receive a total dose of 619—929 mC/kg (2,400—3,600 r) delivered in individual doses of 62—77 mC/kg (240—300 r) through 0.5—1 mm Cu^{-+} 1 Al, allowing 2-day intervals between irradiations.

In the case of primary tumors, radiation is administered following the extirpation. Bone tumors receive 10—15 individual doses.

Considerably higher doses are usually administered by the implantation of radio-isotopes (1,290—2,580 mC/kg = 5,000—10,000 r).

The tumors may regress under this therapy. No experience is available on the use of other treatment methods in the horse (e.g., immunotherapy, chemotherapy, hormones, cryosurgery).

2.1.18.1.11. Suprascapular Nerve Paralysis

See Sec. 2.1.14.2.4.

References

Cardeihac, P. I.: Recent approaches to the treatment of neoplastic diseases in animals. J. Amer. vet. med. Assoc. *156:* 355 (1970).

Dixon, R. T.: Radiation therapy in horses. Austral. vet. J. *43:* 508 (1967).

Dixon, R. T.: Results of radon 322 gamma radiation therapy in an equine practice. Austral. vet. J. *48:* 279 (1972).

Eisenmenger, E.: Experimenteller Beitrag zur intraartikulären Injektion von Mukopolysaccharid-polyschwefelsäureester (Eleparon). Berliner Münchener tierärztl. Wschr. *81:* 386 (1968).

Eisenmenger, E.: Gelenkpunktion für Diagnostik und Therapie. Nutzen und Risiko. tierärztl. praxis *2:* 401 (1974).

Fawwaz, R. A.: Potential early diagnosis of cancer with radioactive compounds. Recent Advances in Nuclear Medicine. (Lawrence, Grune and Stratton, New York 1971).

Fraser, A. C.: The treatment of lameness in horses by faradism, a report of one hundred cases. Vet. Rec. *73:* 94 (1961).

Kralj, J.: Rijedak slučaj obostranog prijeloma lopatice kod konja dijagnosticiran rendgenom. Veterinaria, Sarajewo *14:* 553 (1965).

Kubitza, G.: Zur Therapie degenerativer Gelenkerkrankungen bei Pferden und Hunden. Tierärztl. Umschau *21:* 402, 407 (1966).

Lundvall, R. L.: Observations on the treatment of fractures of the long bones in large animals. J. Amer. vet. med. Assoc. *137:* 308 (1960).

Meagher, D. M.; Pool, R. P.; O'Brien, T. R.: Osteochondritis of the shoulder joint in horses. Proc. 19th Annual Convention Amer. Assoc. Equine Pract., p. 247 (1975).

Morgan, J. P.: Radiographic diagnosis of bone and joint diseases in the horse. Cornell Vet., suppl. 58, p. 28 (1968).

Schebitz, H.: Degenerative Arthritis of the shoulder joint following aseptic necrosis of the humoral head in foals. Proc. 11th Annual Convention Amer. Assoc. Equine Pract., p. 359 (1965).

Schebitz, H.; Wilkens, H.: Zur röntgenologischen Untersuchung des Schultergelenkes beim Pferd. Tierärztl. Umschau *20:* 486 (1965).

Schmidt, G. B.; Dueland, R.; Vaughan, J. T.: Osteochondrosis dissecans of the equine shoulder joint. Vet. Med. and Small Animal Clinician *70:* 542 (1975).

SZELIGOWSKI, E.: Ein Beitrag zur Ätiologie der Bursitis intertubercularis des Pferdes mit besonderer Berücksichtigung der funktionellen Aufgaben des M. biceps brachialis. Wiener tierärztl. Mschr. *49:* 499 (1962).
THRONICKE, R.: Zur Tomanol-Therapie bei Bewegungsstörungen des Pferdes. Tierärztl. Umschau *24:* 188 (1969).
ÜBERREITER, O.: Über das Vorkommen und Behandlungserfolge von Neubildungen bei Tieren (Hund, Katze, Pferd). Zbl. Vet.-Med. R. A *12:* 711 (1965).
WINTZER, H.-J.; GLASENAPP, H. VON: Über eine lokale Myopathie bei Trabrennpferden. Berliner Münchener tierärztl. Wschr. *86:* 221 (1973).

2.1.18.2. Diseases of the Elbow and Forearm

2.1.18.2.1. Paralysis of the Triceps Brachii Muscle (Anconeal Paralysis)

Definition and Etiology. The triceps brachii muscle serves as the extensor of the elbow joint. It presents as a bulge ('torus anconeus') in the angle between the scapula and point of the elbow and stands out clearly against the tendinous surface of the torso.

Rhabdomyolysis and muscular strains can lead to dysfunction of the triceps brachii muscle. Heavy breeds are especially prone to this condition.

Symptoms. The animal has great difficulty in fixing the elbow joint during movement, and there is a compulsory flexion of the carpus each time weight is supported. During standing, weight is frequently shifted off the affected limb. Atrophy of the triceps brachii gradually develops.

Differential Diagnosis. In contrast to proximal radial nerve paralysis, extension of the digit is possible with paralysis of the triceps brachii.

Diagnosis. A history of prior rhabdomyolysis or severe muscular strain should prompt suspicion of triceps brachii paralysis. At necropsy microscopic signs of a waxy, hyaline degeneration are visible in the affected muscle (pallor, friable consistency, granular turbidity, loss of cross striations).

Treatment corresponds to that for myositis of the shoulder muscles.

Multiple blockades of the stellate ganglion can promote healing by stimulating blood flow through the region. Injections of vitamin E-selenium combinations are also beneficial.

The *prognosis* is guarded. If marked muscle atrophy has developed, treatment is of little value. In the absence of such atrophy, improvement can be achieved over a period of weeks or months.

2.1.18.2.2. Olecranon Bursitis and Parabursitis (Capped Elbow, Shoe Boil)

Definition. The term 'shoe boil' or 'capped elbow' is applied to any enlargement at the point of the elbow. It may be unilateral or bilateral and is due to trauma caused by the foot of the affected limb pressing against the point of the elbow during recumbency on a hard floor, especially when the horse is wearing shoes with calks or overlong branches. It is particularly common in narrow stalls where movement is unduly restricted. In high-gaited trotting horses, deep wounds can be inflicted to the olecranon region by the ipsilateral hind limb. This occurs during the winter when calked shoes are worn for racing.

Inflammatory changes may be present in the skin, subcutis or olecranon bursa, depending on the nature and severity of the trauma. A purulent infection can develop as a result of superficial or perforating wounds. A distinction is made, therefore, between the aseptic and purulent form of this disease.

Symptoms. The aseptic form is manifested acutely by a circumscribed, doughy, warm, painful and sometimes fluctuant swelling. This swelling appears suddenly and may reach the size of an apple or fist. Vascular damage leads to hematoma formation or a hemorrhagic, serous infiltration. Lameness is observed only in severe cases. The swelling may regress completely after the cause is eliminated and suitable treatment is instituted. If the cause persists, a hygroma or chronic fibrous bursitis will gradually develop. In this case the bursa undergoes a cystlike thickening with fibrosis of its wall. In addition, the skin over the shoe boil frequently undergoes a callous thickening and sclerotic degeneration.

The purulent form is manifested by an acute, phlegmonous, diffuse swelling over the point of the elbow. A mild to moderate swinging-leg lameness is evident even during walking. During standing, the affected limb is favored and often bears weight only on the toe. Systemic signs (fever, anorexia) generally are present initially. A seropurulent exudate is discharged from any existing wounds or abscess openings. Abscessation may be accompanied by necrosis of the skin and subsequent demarcation, with the appearance of granulation tissue beneath the sloughed skin.

Differential diagnosis is made from fractures of the ulna or olecranon process.

Diagnosis. If clinical findings are inconclusive, radiographs should be obtained in the latero-medial projection to exclude bony injuries.

Treatment. It is imperative that the cause of the condition be eliminated. Calks and shoes with overlong branches are removed. The horse is placed into a roomy stall with ample soft bedding. For Standardbred horses with the condition, an elbow protector should be temporarily incorporated into the harness.

With an acute aseptic inflammation involving mainly the skin and subcutaneous tissue, treatment with moist heat, absorption-promoting or anti-inflammatory ointments (Jokamvasol, camphor ointment or ointments with a heparin or gluccocorticoid base) is recommended. Aseptic bursitis often can be cured completely by repeated intrabursal injections of glucocorticoids.

Sclerosing injections with tincture of iodine or 5% copper sulfate solution is an old treatment method that still has its place. Eight to 10 days later the necrotic synovial membrane is incised and removed. Simple puncture or incision without prior sclerosing is useless and leads to fistulization.

Surgical removal of the bursa is often the most expedient way of achieving the desired goal. In this procedure a curved incision is made over the side of the swelling, and the bursa is shelled out *in toto*. Care is taken to spare the skin so that the suture will not come under excessive tension during movement. For this reason the horse should be cross-tied for 8—10 days so that it cannot lie down.

Purulent shoe boils are extirpated (suture, drainage) after the swelling due to cellulitis has regressed. Fresh superficial and perforating wounds are managed according to surgical principles.

Prognosis. Older shoe boils often create cosmetic defects that do not impair the animal's usefulness. Nevertheless, acute cases should be treated without delay, for this will maximize the chance of a complete recovery. Prevention is important. Roomy, well-padded stalls, long tie chains, and the use of short, base-narrow-rimmed shoes and rounded shoe branches without calks are useful in preventing the disease. In horses that are predisposed to capped elbow as a result of age or recumbency habits, additional protection can be provided with leather or rubber pads.

2.1.18.2.3. *Cubital Arthritis (Inflammation of the Elbow Joint)*

Occurrence and Etiology. Acute aseptic inflammations of the elbow joint are rare in the horse. They are usually traumatic in origin. Occasionally a chronic degenerative arthritis will supervene. On the other hand, pyogenic arthritis resulting from injuries due to kicks or pitchfork wounds to the lateral aspect of the joint are fairly common in horses.

Symptoms. Acute aseptic arthritis produces a moderate to severe lameness. The carriage of the limb during standing resembles that associated with radial paralysis or ulnar fractures. The carpal joint is held in slight flexion with only the toe of the foot touching the ground. The area around the joint is swollen and painful.

Perforating wounds lead to a copious discharge of purulent synovial fluid. If the joint has not been opened, it takes about 8—10 days for these clinical signs to appear. This results from erosion of the joint capsule by infection in the region of the lateral tuberosity of the radius, which has little or no muscular covering.

The result is a joint infection with capsular cellulitis. Pitchfork injuries take a similar course.

Chronic degenerative arthritis and hygromas of the elbow joint are very rare. In chronic cubital arthritis, lameness develops very gradually. The lateral side of the joint feels hard and is enlarged.

Differential diagnosis must be made from radial paralysis and ulnar fractures. The latter are excluded by radiography.

Diagnosis. The diagnosis is made on the basis of local findings and the typical limb carriage. In chronic degenerative inflammation, radiography and diagnostic intra-articular anesthesia of the joint are useful.

Treatment. Acute aseptic cubital arthritis is treated with rest and topical rubefacients. The intra-articular injection of glucocorticoids can be beneficial in the early stage.

The acute or subacute stages of the inflammation also respond favorably to the i.v. or i.m. administration of an analgesic combined with prednisolone. Acute serous pyogenic inflammations are treated with local and systemic antibiotics. In some cases a chronic degenerative arthritis develops leading to stiffness of the joint and permanent disability.

Prognosis. All wounds of the lateral side of the elbow joint have a guarded prognosis. If the horse has no potential breeding value, euthanasia should be contemplated.

2.1.18.2.4. *Luxation of the Radius and Ulna (Antebrachial Dislocation, Dislocation of the Elbow Joint)*

Definition and Occurrence. Dislocation of the elbow joint is uncommon in the horse and is due to violent trauma. Complete luxations, as opposed to subluxations, are invariably associated with tears of the joint capsule, ligamentous ruptures, and sometimes with fractures of the bones that comprise the elbow joint.

The luxation may take various forms depending on the nature and direction of the dislocation of the radius and ulna:

1. Luxations of both the radius and ulna:

— lateral luxation,
— medial luxation,
— caudal luxation,
— cranial luxation.

2. Isolated luxation of the radius or ulna.

Symptoms. With lateral and medial luxations, the limb is held in flexion. The articular cross-section is broadened, and the limb axis is deviated to one side. The mobility of the limb is severely restricted, and only lateral passive movement is possible. With a medial luxation, coexisting chip fractures are frequently present at the joint margins. With a caudal luxation, the proximal parts of the radius and ulna are displaced behind the humerus. This causes the limb to appear shortened. The leg is held in extension, and the sagittal joint diameter is enlarged. A dorsal or cranial luxation is almost always accompanied by a fracture of the ulna, usually a transverse fracture of the olecranon.

Weight is not placed on the affected limb. The horse stands with the foot somewhat ahead of the opposite forefoot, with the elbow joint flexed. The joint is enlarged, and a marked discontinuity is palpable. Isolated luxations of the radius or ulna are uncommon and usually occur only in connection with fractures of these bones.

Diagnosis. Reduction should be attempted only with the animal recumbent and under general anesthesia, for any manipulation of the joint causes pain and subsequent struggling. Muscle relaxants may facilitate the reduction. A medial luxation is reduced by hyperextending the joint and applying lateral pressure. Lateral luxations are more difficult to reduce. The humerus is placed in apposition to the olecranon process in such a way that the latter can serve as a fulcrum. Then the joint is extended and the luxation reduced by applying pressure to the lateral aspect of the forearm and medial condyle of the humerus.

A cranial luxation is reduced by pulling on the limb while simultaneously applying pressure to the olecranon. Luxations with associated fractures can sometimes be surgically reduced, using internal fixation to stabilize the bone fragments. The joint should be immobilized for about 8 days following the reduction. This is best done by confining the animal to a relatively small box stall. Careful exercise and massage are started after that period.

Prognosis. Even with successful reduction, there is little chance of a complete recovery. Capsular or ligamentous ruptures and chip fractures of the joint margins usually lead to a chronic degenerative arthritis that results in restricted joint movement.

2.1.18.2.5. Fractures of the Radius and Ulna

Occurrence and Forms. Closed fractures of the distal radial shaft are the most common. Not infrequently, complete and incomplete subperiosteal fractures are also found. Kicks from other horses can cause spiral or comminuted fractures of the radius. Fractures of the olecranon are usually closed. The distal, narrow part of the ulna may also be involved, in which case the fracture line extends into the interosseous space.

Symptoms. With a fracture of the radius, all the typical signs of a fracture are apparent. Ulnar fractures are additionally characterized by a typical limb carriage during standing, the elbow and carpal joints being held in flexion. The digital joints are extended, and weight is borne only on the toe.

Differential diagnosis is made from radial nerve paralysis and acute aseptic cubital arthritis.

Diagnosis. The foregoing symptoms and radiographs in the latero-medial projection are sufficient to make a diagnosis. Incomplete fractures of the radius are often recognized as a painful line or by a swelling confined to the periosteum. In foals,

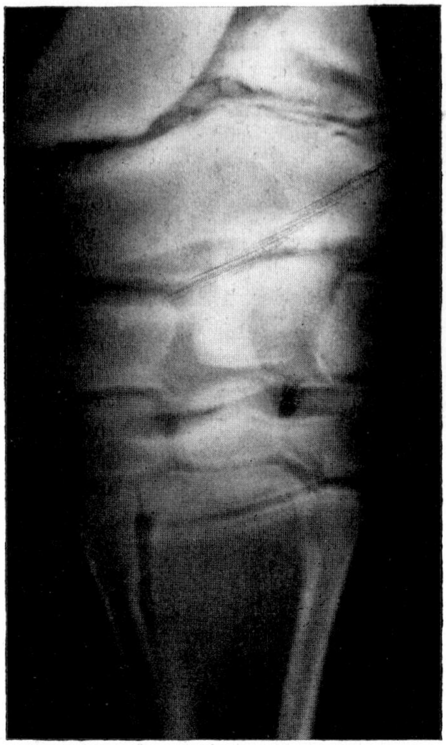

Fig. 2.1.18. — 7. Fracture of the distal radial epiphysis.

radiographs in the cranial medial oblique or caudal lateral oblique projection may reveal an oblique line on the distal epiphysis of the radius. This represents the line of fusion between the radius and ulna and generally closes during the 1st month of life. It should not be mistaken for a fracture line (fig. 2.1.18. — 7).

Treatment. Distal *radial fractures*, especially in foals, may be treated with a plaster or fiberglass cast that extends from the hoof to the elbow joint.

Ulnar fractures sometimes heal with 10—12 weeks of absolute stall rest. Good results have been achieved in ponies with intramedullary nails inserted from the olecranon process to the radius. Other authors attach a bone plate of the caudal aspect of the ulna with screws. Good vascularization and callus formation are obtained with this method. Intramedullary nailing has an adverse effect on endosteal callus formation. To minimize surgical trauma and prevent postoperative suture dehiscence, a curvilinear incision is made through the skin and fascia. Special attention should be given to the tension side of the bone and to the location of blood vessels, nerves and muscles. Kopf and Rettenbacher [1981] employ 'tension band' fixation so that forces tending to produce distraction of the fragments are transmitted to the radial shaft. The longitudinal axis is stabilized with a Küntscher nail.

In *fractures of the radial shaft*, percutaneous fixation (transfixation) in association with the various external fixator devices is suitable in some cases. However, the end-result is hampered in many cases by reactive periostitis, purulent osteomyelitis, cellulitis or breakage of the pins. Better results have been achieved with compression plates using AO/ASIF internal-fixation techniques and equipment.

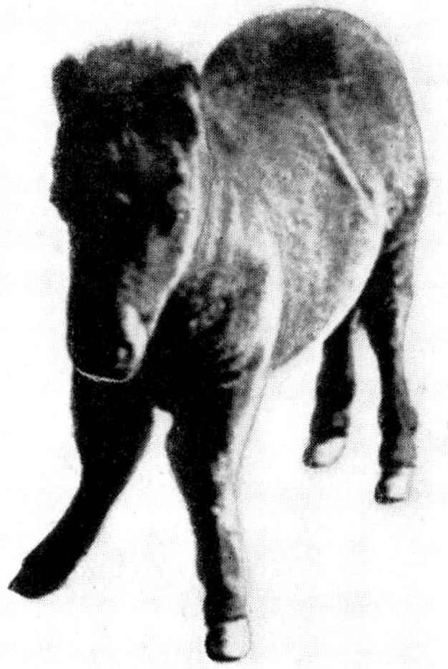

8

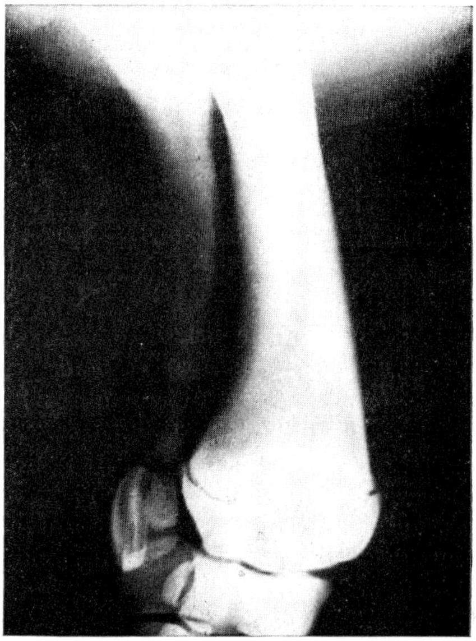

9

Fig. 2.1.18. — 8. Medial deviation of the carpal joints in a pony foal.
Fig. 2.1.18. — 9. Radiograph of animal in fig. 2.1.18. — 8: deviation with persistence of the ulna (styloid process).

Prognosis. Radial fractures have an unfavorable prognosis. Treatment may be attempted in ponies, foals or valuable breeding stock. Ulnar fractures, even in adults, including those with joint involvement, are usually amenable to surgical treatment.

2.1.18.2.6. Medial Deviation of the Carpus

Definition and Occurrence. Medial deviation of the carpus is a congenital abnormality of conformation that most commonly affects the thoracic limbs. It occurs in all breeds (fig. 2.1.18. — 8).

The deviation is variable in degree and may affect one or both limbs. The conformation may be normal initially, or the condition may be present at birth and then either improve or worsen with age.

Etiology. Radiographic examination reveals that the condition has its seat in the distal growth plate (physis) of the radius (or tibia if the pelvic limb is affected) (fig. 2.1.18. — 9). No further changes are found above or below this level. If longitudinal growth is retarded on one side of the distal epiphysis, the epiphysis will appear wedge-shaped on x-rays. When the apex of the resulting epiphyseal triangle is directed laterally, an outward angulation of the limb will result. Inherited or metabolic factors are assumed to be the cause of the congenital form. Adams [1966] states that nutritional deficiencies in the form of a ricketts-like syndrome may be a factor in acquired cases.

Symptoms. The symptoms are obvious: The feet assume a base-wide, toe-out conformation, while the carpal (or tarsal) joints are in close proximity or even direct contact ('knock knees'), depending on the degree of the deviation.

Diagnosis. The diagnosis is easily made on the basis of signs. The etiology, however, may be difficult to establish. All cases should be closely checked for nutrition, and blood samples should be analyzed although they are frequently normal. A high incidence of the condition in certain mare and stallion lines suggests an hereditary etiology.

Treatment. Treatment should begin at an early age, preferably at about 3 weeks. In most cases a splint is applied over a plaster cast to correct the deviation, the limb having been straightened under anesthesia. The cast should be well padded, especially over pressure points, to avoid rubbing sores. The cast is left on for 3 weeks and is reapplied as often as necessary to correct the deformity. An interval of 2—3 weeks is recommended between cast applications to minimize disuse atrophy of the muscles. ADAMS [1966] reports that good results are achieved with hinged braces applied over a stable, well-padded leg wrap. These braces require daily checking and resetting. HEINZE [1966] recommends operative treatment in which a staple is driven into the metaphysis and epiphysis for the purpose of preventing further longitudinal growth on the convex side of the epiphysis. The staple is left in place until the limb is straightened. Healing is most rapid if the stapling is done before the age of 5 months. Corrective hoof trimming is an important adjunct.

Prognosis. The prognosis depends on the degree of the deviation. When a plaster cast is applied, complications in the form of rubbing sores can easily arise and interfere with the recovery. Surgical treatment with epiphyseal staples has proved particularly effective.

2.1.18.2.7. Diseases of the Distal Epiphysis of the Radius

Definition and Occurrence. In 2- and 3-year-old racehorses that are undergoing rigorous training, circumscribed, osteophyte-like changes can develop in the area of the epiphyseal line on the mediocaudal and occasionally the laterocaudal aspect of the distal epiphysis of the radius. This causes a pronounced widening of the epiphyseal line. Focal areas of osteoporosis are found in proximity to this line [GARNER et al., 1966].

Symptoms. The earliest symptom is a characteristic shortening of the stride. Later a mild to moderate supporting-leg lameness develops, depending on the severity of the disease. A more or less pronounced, hard swelling appears proximal to the carpal joint. With the leg raised, local pain is produced by digital pressure on the posterior part of the epiphysis.

Etiology. GARNER et al. [1966] suggest that the changes in the distal radial epiphysis of the racehorse are attributable to forced training procedures that place excessive stress on the growing, still-immature bone at the sites of ligamentous attachment.

Differential Diagnosis. Slab and chip fractures of the carpal bones and chronic forms of carpitis must be excluded.

Diagnosis. Besides the characteristic shortening of the stride and abnormalities upon palpation, radiographs are important in making a definitive diagnosis.

Treatment. A training break of at least 8 weeks is recommended. Phenylbutazone may be given for temporary symptom relief. Vitamin D may be beneficial.

Prognosis. With adequate rest, a full recovery may be expected.

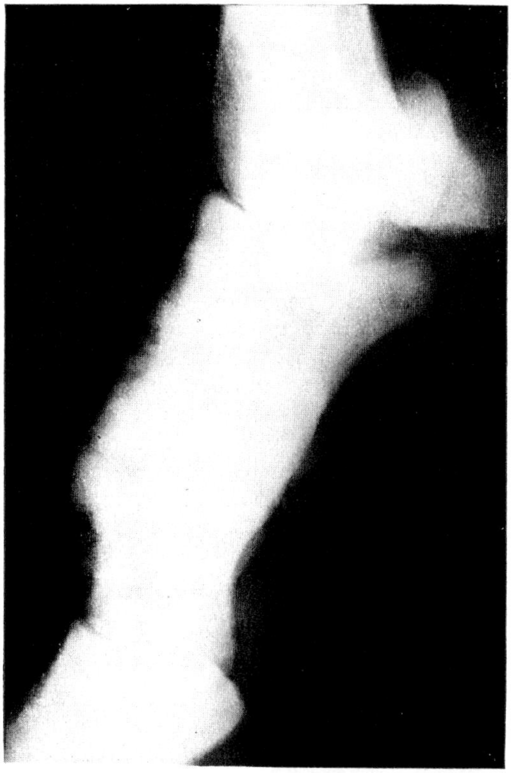

10

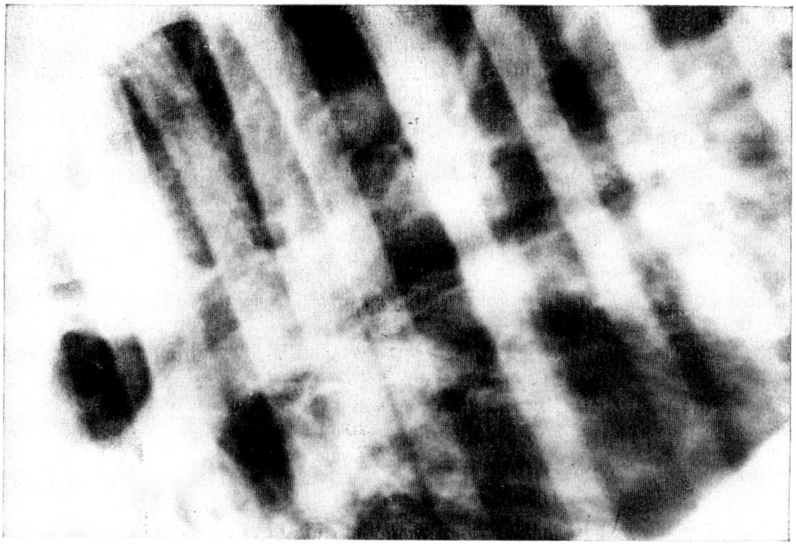

11

Fig. 2.1.18. — 10. Digital bones in acropachy (hypertrophic osteodystrophy).
Fig. 2.1.18. — 11. Same patient as in fig. 2.1.18. — 10: bronchopneumonia.

2.1.18.2.8. Neoplasms of the Radius and Ulna

Neoplasms of the equine forearm are rare. When they are encountered, their diagnosis, treatment and prognosis are the same as described for tumors of the shoulder region.

2.1.18.3. Acropachy (Hypertrophic Pulmonary Osteopathy, Hypertrophic Osteodystrophy)

The phalangeal bones of the horse can be affected by primary changes that later progress to an extensive periostitis and ossification that may involve the radius, ulna, tibia, metacarpal and metatarsal bones. Affected bones are covered with jagged or cauliflowerlike, verrucous bony excresences that cause an overall thickening of the bone (fig. 2.1.18. — 10). Lameness is not usually present. The condition is considered to be a result of chronic, internal organic disease (pulmonary diseases [fig. 2.1.18. — 11], urticaria, cachexia). Presumably the bony changes are caused by the action of toxic metabolic products. Radiography is diagnostic in doubtful cases. No treatment is available.

References

Adams, O. R.: Lameness in horses; 2nd ed. (Lea & Febiger, Philadelphia 1966).

Arnbjerg, J.: Fracture of ulna in the horse with case reports on three ponies. Nord. Vet.-Med. *21:* 389 (1969).

Blevins, W.: Bone vascularisation and its effect on fracture healing. Iowa State Univ. Vet. *30:* 41 (1972).

Carlson, R. L.; Lohse, C. L.; Eld, L. A.; Hughbanks, F. G.: Correction of angular limb deformities by physical stapling. Mod. vet. Prac. *53:* 41 (1972).

Chochlow, A. L.: Rentgenodiagnostika i klassifikacija, perelomow falang. Veterinarija, Moskva *42 (2):* 84.

Daniels, H.: Grundlagen der AO-Synthese bei Gross- und Kleintieren. Prakt. Tierarzt *53:* 473 (1972).

Dingwall, J. S.; Duncan, D. B.; Horney, F. D.: Compression plating in large animal orthopedics. J. Amer. vet. med. Assoc. *159:* 1651 (1971).

Ebert, E. F.: Reducing an equine luxation. Vet. Med. and Small Animal Clinician *64:* 1288 (1969).

Garner, H. E.; Clair, L. E. St.; Hardenbrook, H. J.: Clinical and radiographic studies of the distal portion of the radius in race horses. J. Amer. vet. med. Assoc. *149:* 1536 (1966).

Gertsen, K. E.; Brinker, W. O.: Fracture repair in ponies using bone plates. J. Amer. vet. med. Assoc. *154:* 900 (1969).

Hallström, M.: Experiments with two methods of forming pins for transfixing fractures of the long bones in large animals. Acta vet. scand *7:* 157 (1966).

Hanselke, D. V.; Boyd, C. L.; Joyce, J. R.: External fixation of a large animal fracture with a resin-bonded fibre glass cast. Vet. Med. and Small Animal Clinician *67:* 519 (1972).

Heinze, C. D.: Epiphyseal stapling in the horse. Mod. vet. Pract. *47:* 40 (1966).

Hurtienne, H.; Jörn, J.: Ein Beitrag zur Fraktur des Processus olecrani. Dtsch. tierärztl. Wschr. *74:* 560 (1967).

Huskamp, B.: Möglichkeiten und Grenzen der operativen Knochenbehandlung beim Pferd. Prakt. Tierarzt *53:* 469, 472 (1972).

Johnson, J. H.; Gutler, H. G.: The tension-band principle in fixation of an equine ulnar fracture. Vet. Med. and Small Animal Clinician *66:* 552 (1977).

Kopf, N.; Rettenbacher, G.: Die Zuggurtung der Olekranonfraktur. IV. Tag. Pferdekrankheiten. Equitana (1981), Essen.

LINGARD, D. R.: Strain of the superior check ligament of the horse. J. Amer. vet. med. Assoc. *148:* 364 (1966).
LUNDVALL, R. L.: Observations on the treatment of fractures of the long bones in large animals. J. Amer. vet. med. Assoc. *137:* 308 (1960).
MASON, T. A.; BOURKE, J. M.: Closure of the distal radial epiphysis and its relationship to unsoundness in two year old thoroughbreeds. Aust. vet. J. *49:* 222 (1973).
MILNE, D. W.; TURNER, A. S.; GABEL, A. A.: Surgical approaches to certain long bones of the horse for application of tension band plates. J. Amer. vet. med. Assoc. *168:* 48 (1976).
PAATSAMA, S.; JURSILA, J.; ALITALO, J.: Changes in the distal epiphysis, the epiphyseal plate and the metaphysis of the radius as a cause of lameness in finish-bred horses. Equine vet. J. *2:* 308 (1970).
PETTERSSON, H.: Die konservative und chirurgische Versorgung der Ulnafraktur. IV. Tag. Pferdekrankheiten. Equitana (1981), Essen.
RAKER, C. W.; EVANS, L. H.: Volare Suprakarpalexostosen beim Vollblutpferd. Wiener tierärztl. Mschr. *58:* 150 (1971).
WEST, W. R. G.: The application of resin-bonded fibre glass for the immobilisation of fractured or damaged equine and bovine limbs. Vet. Rec. *75:* 424 (1963).

2.1.18.4. Diseases of the Carpal Joint

2.1.18.4.1. Injuries of the Skin and Tendon Sheaths of the Carpus

Occurrence and Etiology. The anterior surface of the carpus has little protection and is highly vulnerable to many forms of trauma. Skin wounds, contusions, wounds of the tendons and tendon sheaths, cellulitis, abscesses and exuberant granulation tissue can all occur in the carpal area as a direct or indirect result of trauma. Most wounds and closed injuries are caused by falls onto the carpus. Injuries from barbed wire generally take the form of lacerations and flap-shaped wounds. Pitchfork wounds are also common and frequently lead to cellulitus, abscessation and purulent tendovaginitis.

In Standardbred horses, subcutaneous hematomas very often develop on the medial aspect of the carpus when this area is struck by the adjacent hoof as a result of an irregular gait.

In foals, an idiopathic, acute, infectious tendovaginitis involving mainly the carpal tendon sheaths frequently develops as a complication of metastatic infectious polyarthritis. In other cases polytendovaginitis may first appear several weeks after birth, due to the transport of pathogenic organisms from the bowel into the arterial system by strongyle larvae [VAN PELT, 1969].

Symptoms. Skin abrasions of varying extent represent the mildest form of injury. Generally motion is limited only if the abrasion is complicated by edema or subcutaneous hematoma. Subcutaneous cellulitis and abscessation can then supervene as a result of pyogenic infection. This is manifested by a moderate to severe lameness and marked local tenderness, especially to flexion of the carpus. Systemic signs are usually present.

Extensive areas of necrosis with sloughing and the formation of granulating, suppurating wound surfaces are uncommon. Smooth incised wounds and flap-shaped wounds are much more frequent. These usually disrupt not just the skin but also the superficial and deep carpal fascia. Tension associated with movement causes the wound edges to gape widely within a short time. Thus, with improper care, injuries of this type are highly susceptible to the development of exuberant granulation

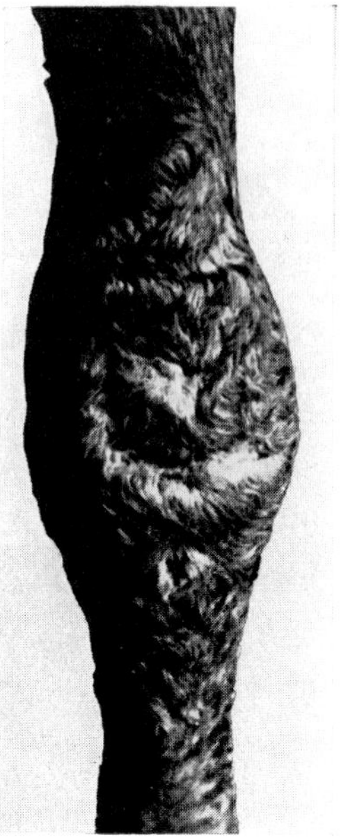
12

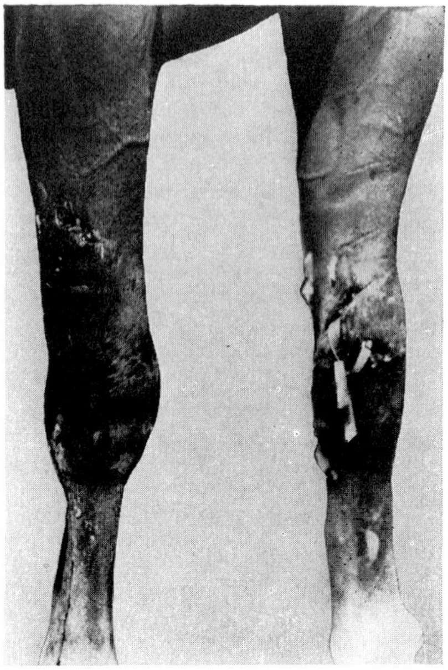
13

Fig. 2.1.18. — 12—13. Cutaneous and tendon-sheath wounds of the carpus.

tissue ('proud flesh') (figs. 2.1.18. — 12 and — 13). Deeper wounds may cause opening of the tendon sheaths that course through the carpal region. Incised wounds can completely sever one or more tendon sheaths, whose stumps are visible during passive flexion of the joint. The open tendon sheaths are susceptible to pyogenic infection. This is manifested by a moderate to severe lameness, hot and painful swelling, and an initially serous, later seropurulent, frothy wound discharge. The result is a purulent tendovaginitis with partial tendon necrosis.

Differential Diagnosis. Hygromas of the tendon sheaths are painless and do not cause lameness. Carpitis and pericarpitis are distinguished by a typical hard, spindle-shaped swelling of the carpus. Gradual lameness always develops. Fractures of the carpal bones are excluded by radiography.

Treatment for skin abrasions consists in cleansing the wound and surrounding skin and applying a water-soluble, disinfectant ointment or spray.

Small hematomas are treated with heparin-containing ointments or with stronger irritants. If the effusion is not absorbed, or if the hematomas are too large, they are incised at their lowest point after 8—10 days to permit drainage.

Abscesses are brought to a point with 20—25 % ichthammol ointment or are incised. If pocketing has occurred, ventral drainage must be established. The wound cavity is flushed with antiseptic solutions and bandaged. Cellulitis is best treated with warm, moist antiseptic dressings and parenteral sulfonamides or antibiotics, possibly combined with glucocorticoids.

Wounds with areas of superficial necrosis are surgically reconstructed, and epithelialization is promoted. The wound is kept under bandage until a crust is formed. Exuberant granulation tissue is removed. In favorable cases the wound will close with an eschar. Wounds of this type may be subsequently treated with a dessicative powder (e.g.: Müller's mixture) and will heal well in time without a bandage if they are not too extensive. In the presence of a large defect, epithelialization can be hastened by applying a skin graft after healthy granulation tissue has formed. Fresh incised and flap-shaped wounds are sutured and immobilized under a bandage. For fresh puncture wounds, we recommend applying a caustic agent around the wound opening. In the presence of tendon sheath infection, antibiotics are administered intratendovaginally and parenterally for several days. With purulent tendovaginitis, usually the only recourse is to open the sheath and irrigate it with antiseptic drugs. Afterward the sheath is filled with solutions or emulsions of sulfonamides or antibiotics. For tendon sheath cellulitis, we additionally recommend rubefacient therapy with warm, moist dressings or ointment dressings. However, it is not unusual in such cases for a periarticular, ossifying arthritis to develop leading to restricted joint motion. Johnson and Ryan [1975] described a case in which permanent lameness resulted from a synovial fistula following a tendon sheath injury of the lateral digital extensor with an open carpal joint.

Tendon sheath cellulitis on the flexor surface of the carpal joint is accompanied by severe lameness and marked swelling of surrounding tissues. Multiple abscess formation with necrosis of the skin and fascia is common in such cases. Following stimulation of hyperemia, the tendon sheath is incised medially for a length of about 50 cm at the carpal attachment of the suspensory ligament of the deep flexor tendon. About 3 months are required for healing. Heavy horses often contract stress laminitis in the sound leg during the protracted convalescence and die from attendant complications.

Prognosis. Skin abrasions, hematomas, subcutaneous abscesses and cellulitis usually heal without complications. Skin necrosis and large incised and flap-shaped wounds often are very slow to heal due to the difficulty of adequately immobilizing the wound. Exuberant granulation tissue may make treatment uneconomical. Often scarring is left behind which permanently limits carpal joint mobility. The same is true for wounds of the tendons and tendon sheaths. Tendon sheath cellulitis on the flexor surface of the carpal joint usually has an unfavorable prognosis. Recovery depends upon prompt, expert care. The value of treatment under a bandage must be recognized.

In Standardbred horses that are susceptible to carpal injuries due to irregularities of gait, temporary 'knee protectors' or knee wraps are recommended. Corrective shoeing can also be helpful (shorter, narrower branches and rounded toe).

2.1.18.4.2. Precarpal Bursitis (Capped Knee)

Definition. 'Capped knee' refers to any swelling over the anterior aspect of the carpus. This may be a thickening of the skin, an acute or chronic inflammation of the subcutaneous bursa, a bursal hygroma, or an organized hematoma.

Etiology. The swelling over the carpus is caused by falls onto the carpal joint or by recurrent contusion that occurs when the animal lies down on hard, rough ground.

Symptoms. A painless swelling gradually develops on the anterior surface of the carpus. The swelling is usually firm but may be soft and fluctuating and may reach a considerable size (figs. 2.1.18. — 14 and — 15). Swellings of this type are associated with a slight degree of pain and restricted motion, especially when the limb is flexed and advanced. In some cases large, firm, painless swellings appear that are associated with cutaneous thickening and local hair loss. These swellings are loculated and show little fluctuation.

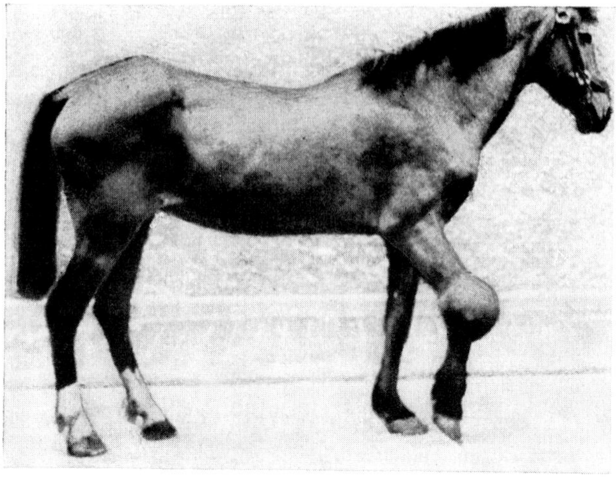

14

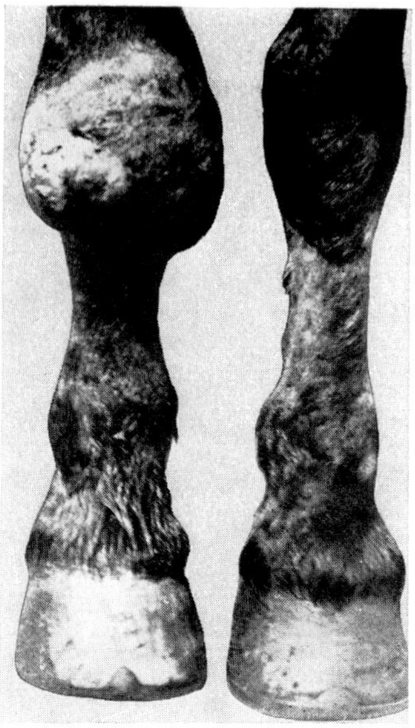

15

Fig. 2.1.18. — 14. Precarpal bursitis.
Fig. 2.1.18. — 15. Chronic precarpal bursitis.

Differential diagnosis must be made from acute contusion, circumscribed cellulitis, abscesses, tendovaginitis, tendon sheath hygromas and, in riding horses, tendon sheath hygroma of the extensor carpi radialis muscle.

Diagnosis. Thickenings develop gradually and are not warm or painful. Subcutaneous hematomas and acute carpal bursitis, on the other hand, appear suddenly and produce a soft, painful, fluctuating enlargement that is accompanied by lameness. Chronic serofibrinous bursitis, bursal hygroma and organized, encapsulated hematomas are rare and develop gradually. In doubtful cases, aspiration will assist in making the diagnosis. Periosteal new bone growth around the carpal joint is demonstrated by radiography.

Treatment. Factors that could cause or perpetuate the swelling must be removed. This is done by placing the animal in a roomy stall with soft bedding. The treatment of subcutaneous hematomas was described in Sec. 2.1.18.4.1. Acute bursitis responds well to the topical application of absorption-promoting drugs. Aspirations and single or multiple injections of corticosteroids may be beneficial in some cases. With bursal hygroma or serofibrinous precarpal bursitis, this is not always the case. Sometimes good results are achieved with injections of a sclerosing agent such as 20—100 ml tincture of iodine or 100—500 ml of 5 % copper sulfate solution, after first aspirating all fluid from the bursal sac. Eight to 10 days later the necrotic capsule is incised on the lateral side and removed by curettage. This therapy is somewhat antiquated and not without risks.

Loculated hygromas can be surgically removed. A curved skin incision is made distal to the enlargement in a lateromedial direction, and the bursa is dissected out bluntly. The skin is closed with a double row of sutures, and the wound cavity is packed. The wound is kept under bandage for 3—4 weeks postoperatively and should heal completely during this time.

Prognosis. Swellings over the carpus that do not cause disability should be treated only in advanced cases. Treatment may be ineffectual in the case of marked thickening, and is of only limited value in the case of bursal hygromas, organized hematomas and chronic serofibrinous bursitis. Subcutaneous hematomas and acute bursitides usually resolve completely.

2.1.18.4.3. Hygroma of the Tendon Sheaths at the Carpus

Occurrence and Etiology. This fluid collection within the tendon sheath causes marked swelling but does not produce pain or lameness. Both the flexor and extensor tendon sheaths at the carpus are affected. The condition may be secondary to an acute or chronic inflammation or may be congenital.

Symptoms. A localized, painless swelling appears whose location corresponds to that of the tendon sheath hygroma.

The contents of the sheath are displaceable during palpation.

a) Hygroma of the extensor carpi radialis tendon sheath is a fluctuating, sharply-circumscribed, sausage-shaped to arm-size swelling on the dorsal surface of the carpus that may extend proximally to the radius.

b) Hygroma of the common digital extensor tendon sheath is less common, is situated somewhat more laterally, and affects a more extensive area.

c) Hygroma of the lateral digital extensor tendon sheath occurs only sporadically and presents as a round or sausage-shaped swelling low on the lateral surface of the carpus.

d) Hygroma of the abductor pollicis longus tendon sheath has a similar appearance. It is equally uncommon and courses obliquely in a lateromedial direction over the dorsal surface of the carpal joint.

e) Hygromas of the common, large tendon sheath of the superficial and deep flexor tendons (flexor digitalis superficialis and flexor digitalis profundus muscles) on the palmar side of the carpus can reach a considerable size and extend below the carpal joint on each side of the deep flexor tendon.

Differential Diagnosis. Tendon sheath hygromas are distinguished from acute and chronic tendovaginitis by the absence of pain and lameness. Precarpal bursitis and hematomas also must be differentiated.

Diagnosis. Aspirated synovial fluid is usually clear, watery and contains few cells. Cytologic evaluation of the synovial fluid is diagnostic in doubtful cases.

Treatment and Prognosis. Because tendon sheath hygromas generally are not disabling, treatment is undertaken only if the owner requests it. An improvement or cure can be effected by single or multiple injections of corticosteroids into the tendon sheath (having previously aspirated the fluid), followed by the application of a well-applied pressure bandage. In exceptional cases one may attempt a surgical size reduction of the tendon sheath by partial extirpation of the sheath wall.

2.1.18.4.4. Hygroma of the Carpal Joint

Hygroma of the carpal joint presents as a fluctuating, transverse swelling over the dorsal surface of the carpus that is constricted by the overlying extensor tendon. A rounded, goose-egg-size swelling also appears immediately behind the radius proximal to the accessory carpal bone. The capsule of the radiocarpal joint is affected. The swelling represents a cosmetic defect only and can be eliminated by the intra-articular injection of corticosteroids.

2.1.18.4.5. Acute Serous and Chronic Aseptic Tendovaginitis of the Extensor Carpi Radialis Muscle

Occurrence and Etiology. Acute to chronic aseptic tendovaginitis of the extensor carpi radialis muscle occurs in riding horses that strike the distal part of the radius against a solid object during a jump or fall. It can also result from strains of the tendon following overexertion.

Symptoms and Diagnosis. No weight is borne on the limb during standing. During walking, the leg is carefully advanced without flexing the carpus, and the toe is dragged on the ground. A patchy, sausage-shaped, fluctuating, warm and painful swelling is found extending along the dorsal surface of the limb from the mid-forearm to the carpus. Aspiration yields a bloody, serous synovial fluid.

Differential Diagnosis. Hygromas of the extensor tendon sheath at the carpus cause no pain or disability. Precarpal bursitis occurs more distally on the dorsal surface of the carpus.

Prognosis and Treatment. Recovery should follow 3—4 weeks after immobilization and the application of moist, cooling bandages, followed later by topical rubefacients. The injection of corticosteroids also achieves good results.

WALLACE [1972] reports on the successful operative treatment of a tendovaginitis of the extensor carpi radialis that had not responded to previous steroid therapy. In this procedure the tendon sheath was opened, areas of necrosis were excised, and adhesions between the tendon and tendon-sheath wall were broken down.

Residual hygroma of the tendon sheath is sometimes observed but does not affect the animal's soundness.

2.1.18.4.6. Carpal Tunnel Syndrome

Definition and Occurrence. The carpal tunnel is formed by the medial surface of the radius above the carpal joint, which is separated from the carpus by the palmar carpal fascia and is bounded caudally and medially by the posterior annular ligament of the carpus. The carpal tunnel contains nerves, blood vessels, and the carpal tendon sheath with the deep and superficial flexor tendons.

The carpal tunnel may become narrowed as a result of fibrous or bony tissue proliferation or inflammatory processes, causing pressure to be exerted on the nerves and vessels within it. The changes may result from a fracture of the accessory bone, a tendovaginitis of the proximal flexor tendon sheath, or a sprain of the superior check ligament (proximal accessory ligament) [LINGARD, 1966].

Symptoms. A painful swelling is palpable in the region of the carpal joint. The animal is apt to resent the examination, especially if the carpus is flexed suddenly. No pathologic changes are evident on the dorsal surface of the carpus.

Lesions. Varying degrees of carpitis or periostitis can be found at ligamentous attachments on the caudal surface of the radius.

Diagnosis. The limb is flexed and bears no weight during standing. Pain and struggling in response to sudden flexion of the carpal joint and a painful swelling on the distal, mediocaudal surface of the radius are suggestive of carpal tunnel syndrome. Clinical findings are supplemented by radiographs, which may reveal exostoses on the carpus and radius.

Treatment and Prognosis. Marked inflammatory distension of the flexor tendon sheath can be relieved by repeated corticosteroid injections.

If this fails to produce definite improvement, the lameness can be corrected surgically by the freeing of adhesions [MACKAY-SMITH et al., 1972].

2.1.18.4.7. Carpitis

Definition and Occurrence. There are three joints in the carpus: the radiocarpal joint, the intercarpal joint and the carpometacarpal joint. The intercarpal and carpometacarpal joints communicate. One or more of these joints may undergo inflammatory change, usually as a result of external trauma. A distinction is made between purulent carpitis, acute aseptic carpitis, and chronic degenerative carpitis. Acute aseptic carpitis is frequently observed in 2-year-old Thoroughbreds that are worked too hard during training, as skeletal growth in these horses is not yet complete. Chronic degenerative carpitis may develop from the acute form and often goes unrecognized for some time owing to its insidious course. Carpitis is usually confined to one limb, although bilateral cases can develop in riding, Standardbred, and heavy draft horses. The medial areas of the joint are predominantly affected. In suppurative forms of the disease, all stages of the purulent joint inflammation may be observed. Frequently, the inflammation is complicated by fractures of the carpal bones.

Acute Suppurative Carpitis

Etiology. This disease occurs as a complication of perforating joint wounds due to falls, pitchfork injuries, lacerations and contusions.

Symptoms. A moderate to severe swinging- and supporting-limb (mixed) lameness is present. The limb is advanced by dragging the toe on the ground, avoiding flexion of the carpus, and weight is placed on the limb only momentarily. Passive movement of the joint is difficult and produces pain. The joint contours are indistinct, and usually the entire joint shows some swelling. A clear synovial fluid is discharged from the wound in acute cases. Later the fluid becomes purulent and contains yellow fibrin flakes. A systemic reaction is usually present. Heavy horses often develop a stress laminitis in the sound limb and become recumbent. With large incised wounds, the tendon sheaths on the anterior side of the carpus are usually opened and infected.

Diagnosis. In questionable cases the diagnosis is established by aspiration of joint fluid under aseptic conditions, with the joint held in flexion. Suspected fractures are confirmed by radiography.

Treatment. The horse is placed in a large stall with soft bedding. Fresh flap-shaped carpal joint wounds are sutured immediately. With a puncture wound, an ointment is applied around the wound, and appropriate antibiotics are administered intra-articularly and systemically for several days. The radiocarpal joint is accessible from the lateral aspect through the groove between the radius and extensor carpi ulnaris muscle, and the intercarpal and carpometacarpal joints from the anterior aspect with the carpus flexed. The joint is immobilized with a bandage.

Prognosis. Infections of the radiocarpal joint have an unfavorable prognosis, especially in heavy draft horses and cases complicated by open fractures of the carpal bones. In such cases the horse should be euthanized. The prognosis is good for suppurative inflammation of the carpometacarpal joint, and guarded when the intercarpal joint is also involved.

Acute Aseptic Carpitis, Chronic Degenerative Carpitis

Etiology. In many cases the inflammation takes an insidious course as a result of trauma to the small carpal bones associated with chronic hyperextension of the joint (‘stress osteitis’).

This occurs in racehorses that are exercised on hard ground or deep sand, but may also result from frequent, abrupt reining, sharp turns, jumps, and the premature training of young horses whose skeletal growth is not yet complete. In addition, the

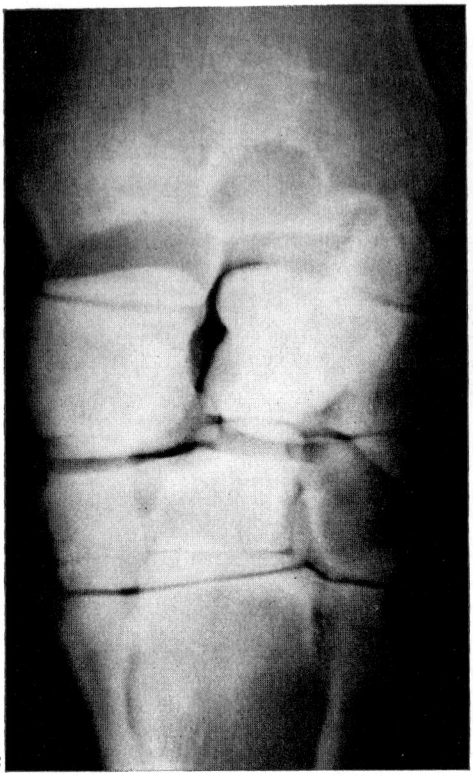

16

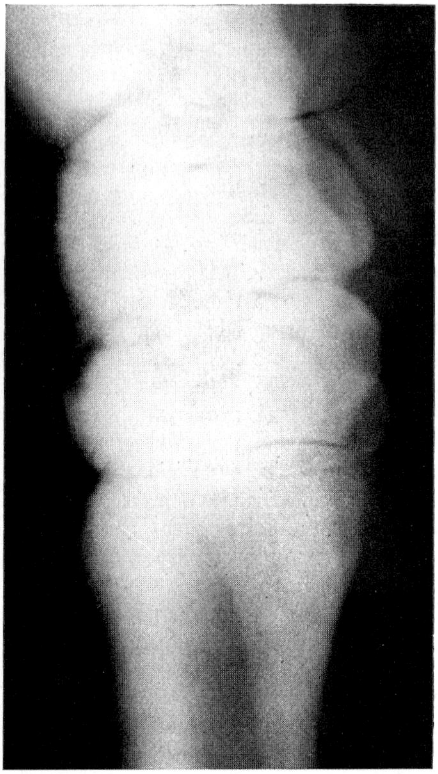

17

Fig. 2.1.18. — *16*—*17*. Pericarpitis.

high action of the carpal joint in certain Standardbred horses apparently can predispose to chronic carpitis. The medial aspect of the joint is the side most prone to such forces and so is the most severely affected [RAKER, 1968].

It is reported that narrow 'constricted' joints, a steep shoulder slope and short forearm predispose to the disease. Faults of limb conformation (cranial, caudal, medial or lateral deviations) can also be contributing factors. In addition, inflammatory processes in proximity to the carpus (precarpal bursitis, tendovaginitis, periostitis, etc.) may spread to involve the joint.

Luxations and subluxations, sprains, ligament ruptures, acute aseptic and purulent arthritides, carpal bone fractures, wounds, tendon sheath cellulitis, chip fractures, etc. are common primary causes. In these cases the bony lesions are not confined to the dorsal and medial joint surfaces.

Symptoms. The disease begins with a serofibrinous arthritis of the radiocarpal joint. The joint appears distended, and a type of crepitus (grating sound) is elicited by pressing inward on the joint capsule with the carpus flexed.

Later a supporting- and swinging-leg lameness gradually develops that is exacerbated by strenuous exercise. Often the lameness is observed only at the start of exercise. It may improve or disappear completely after a prolonged rest. If both forelimbs are affected, the gait becomes stiff and stilted. Intra- and periarticular osteophytes in the region of the less mobile carpometacarpal joint usually do not cause lameness.

The lameness is increased by flexion of the carpal joint (flexion test). Considerable exostosis formation, especially on the anteromedial side of the joint capsule, produces large, nontender swellings that later may involve the dorsal and lateral joint surfaces. This causes passive joint movement to become painful and restricted. Often the carpus shows a cranial deviation, and the muscles of the shoulder and forearm atrophy. The joint contours become boxy or spindle-shaped. The hoof acquires a blunted shape due to excessive wear of the anterior wall.

Necropsy reveals articular (chronic degenerative arthritis) as well as periarticular lesions (periarthritis). The changes correspond in essence and origin to those of spavin, ringbone and chronic omarthritis.

Differential Diagnosis. Hygromas and excessive scarring must not be confused with a pericarpitis.

Diagnosis. A positive flexion test, combined with visible and palpatory findings, suggests a diagnosis of chronic carpitis. In the early stage, continuous lameness can be temporarily relieved by intra-articular anesthesia of the carpal joint (injection of local anesthetic into the radiocarpal joint or radiocarpal and intercarpal joints). In all cases the joint should be radiographed in two planes, possibly supplemented by a tangential view, to evaluate the extent, size and form of the boney changes. Areas of increased density or lucency are also frequently observed in the structure of the bone (figs. 2.1.18. — 16 and — 17).

Treatment. Early cases can be cured by intra-articular corticosteroid injections into the radiocarpal joint and then resting the horse for 3—4 months. Better results have been reported with the combined use of hyaluronic acid and prednisolone or hyaluronic acid alone [Rydell et al., 1970]. At the onset of chronic pericarpitis and carpitis, blistering combined with complete rest for 2—3 months can restore soundness even for racing. Good results have also been reported with radiation therapy [Clapp et al., 1963; Dixon, 1967, 1972].

A combined neurectomy of the median and ulnar nerves is an old treatment method that may be tried as a last resort in draft horses.

Prognosis. The prognosis is poor in the presence of joint contracture and stiffness. The milder the changes and the more distal their location, the better the prognosis.

2.1.18.4.8. Fractures of the Carpal Bones

Definition, Occurrence and Etiology. The carpus of the horse is comprised of 7 and in some cases 8 polyhedral bones that are arranged in a proximal and distal row. Slab fractures or chip fractures can affect one or more of the carpal bones and are especially common in racehorses. The radial, ulnar, 3rd, 4th and accessory carpal bones are the bones most commonly fractured.

Symptoms. There is a moderate to severe supporting- and swinging-leg lameness of sudden onset. The toe drags the ground as the limb is advanced. Initially, local tenderness is usually present on the medial or lateral side of the proximal or distal row of carpal bones. Later the symptoms of an acute arthritis supervene. Open fractures, especially of the proximal carpal bones, usually lead to pyogenic arthritis and systemic infection within 4—5 days.

The *diagnosis* is established by radiographs taken in various planes. An accurate record should be made of the nature, form and exact location of the fracture for later reference during treatment. Five views are obtained: latero-medial, dorso-palmar, 45° medio-lateral, 30° latero-medial and 60° latero-medial [Dixon].

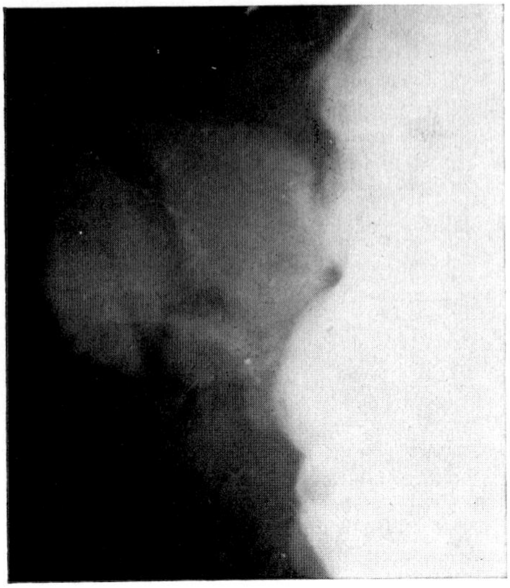

Fig. 2.1.18. — 18. Fracture of the accessory carpal bone.

In some circumstances arthroscopy can be used for accurate localization. It can reveal joint changes that are inaccessible to radiography. Using aseptic technique, the arthroscope is introduced into the joint of the recumbent animal, the joint having previously been filled with sterile saline [HALL and KEERAN, 1975].

Prognosis and Treatment. Many chip fractures, especially those of the radial, ulnar, 2nd and 4th carpal bones, will heal well in 3—4 months if the horse is confined to a large, well-padded stall and the affected area is treated with warm, moist dressings and immobilized. Often, however, chronic degenerative arthritis will develop resulting in permanent lameness. Early surgical removal of the chip fragments is the procedure of choice. This is best done in the absence of chronic joint changes, and if the animal has not received local corticosteroid therapy during the past 3 months. The fragment to be removed is approached by the most direct route available. The wound is closed in three layers, the joint capsule being sutured with silk or chromic catgut. A well-padded bandage is applied, and a 10-day course of antibiotics is administered to prevent complications during healing. Complete recovery will require at least 6 months. WYBURN and GOULDEN [1974] recommend internal fixation for slab fractures and larger chip fractures, using lag screws. In valuable breeding horses with simple or comminuted fractures, the affected carpal bone can in some cases be extracted and replaced with a prosthetic bone modeled from acrylic resin [WINSTANLEY and GLEESON, 1974]. This establishes an ankylosed joint that will give the animal a mobility sufficient for breeding purposes. Open fractures complicated by suppurative arthritis have a poor prognosis.

Fracture of the Accessory Carpal Bone

Occurrence. This fracture is commonly observed in racehorses and horses involved in jumping. Most are complete fractures; small chip fractures are rare.

Symptoms. Lameness first appears following exercise and increases to the point where the toe drags on the ground during walking. During standing the carpus is held in a characteristic flexed position, and the distal joints are also flexed. Swelling is evident on the flexor surface of the carpus, and flexion produces pain. The fragments are readily displaceable, and crepitation is present. The swelling subsides in about 2 weeks; lameness at the walk disappears in about 4 weeks.

Etiology. The accessory bone may be fractured by being compressed between the radius and metacarpus during a fall onto the flexed carpus.

Diagnosis. The diagnosis is suggested by the history, local changes, and radiographs in the latero-medial view (fig. 2.1.18. — 18).

Treatment. Fracture healing is supported in the early stage by warm, moist dressings and later by rubefacient ointments. Immobilizing bandages are not indicated. Internal fixation with screws or wire sutures may be possible [Larson and Dixon, 1970; Wyburn and Goulden, 1974].

Prognosis. Function usually returns after 3—4 months' rest, although racehorses may not be returned to their original performance level.

Bucked Knees (Knee Sprung)

Contracture of the flexor carpi radialis and ulnaris muscles results in a constant partial flexion of the carpal joint that is known as 'bucked knees' or 'knee sprung'. It occurs mainly in older horses but may also be present at birth. The cause is a weakness of the extensor muscles resulting from premature stress or constant strain. The condition is seldom curable, although improvement can sometimes be achieved in younger horses by pasturing and rest. Vitamin D and calcium supplementation have also been used. In most cases the working capacity of the horse is not affected. Many good jumping and military horses are 'knee sprung'.

2.1.18.4.9. Luxation of the Carpal Bones

Occurrence and Etiology. Luxations in the carpal joint are rare owing to the strong inelastic ligaments that stabilize the joint. Unilateral or bilateral subluxations are occasionally seen in foals [Lewandowski, 1965]. They are caused by falls onto the flexed carpus or by running into obstacles.

Symptoms. The limb axis is deviated cranially or caudally, depending on the direction of the luxation. In fresh cases a 'step' is palpable in this area. Later a large, diffuse, painful swelling develops that makes examination difficult.

Diagnosis and Prognosis. Radiographs in two planes confirm the diagnosis and will reveal any fractures that may be present. The prognosis is guarded. If multiple fractures are present, the animal should be euthanized.

2.1.18.4.10. Luxation of the Lateral Digital Extensor

In rare cases, trauma produces a lateral dislocation of the tendon of the lateral digital extensor muscle. This is manifested by a sudden, severe supporting-leg lameness and lateral displacement of the tendon at the distal end of the radius. Usually the dislocation can be successfully reduced with the animal recumbent and anesthetized or sedated. Point firing followed by the application of irritating solutions can contribute to reattachment by stimulating scar tissue formation.

References

Brown, M. P.; Meagher, D. M.: Equine carpal fracture (A case report). Vet. Med. and Small Animal Clinician *70:* 963 (1975).

Clapp, N. K.; Carlson, W. D.; Morgan, J. P.: Radiation therapy for lameness in horses. J. Amer. vet. med. Assoc. *143:* 277 (1963).

DIXON, R. T.: Radiation therapy in horses. Austral. vet. J. *43:* 508 (1967).
DIXON, R. T.: Radiography of the equine carpus. Austral. vet. J. *45:* 171 (1969).
DIXON, R. T.: Results of radon 222 gamma radiation therapy in the equine practice. Austral. vet. J. *48:* 279 (1972).
DUBS, B.; QUASTEL, T.: Hauttransplantation beim Pferd. tierärztl. praxis, München *3:* 57 (1975).
FLIPOT, J. L.; CHAMBLY, CH.; SAINT HUBÆRT, P. Q.: Les fractures carpiènnes chez le cheval de sport. Rec. Méd. vét. *144:* 927 (1968).
FRANKLAND, A. L.; MORRIS, P. G. D.; SPREULL, J. S. A.: Free, autologous, skin transplantation in the horse. Vet. Rec. *98:* 105 (1976).
FRYE, F. FL.; FAWWAZ, R. A.: A practical disposable dermal trephine made from discarded materials. Vet. Med. and Small Animal Clinician *69:* 1419 (1974).
HALL, M. E.; KEERAN, R. J.: Use of the arthroscope in the horse. Vet. Med. and Small Animal Clinician *70:* 705 (1975).
HOUDESHELL, J. W.; BLOOMFIELD, N. J.: Field trials of a new longacting corticosteroid in the treatment of equine arthropathies. Vet. Med. and Small Animal Clinician *64:* 782 (1969).
JOHNSON, J. E.; RYAN, G. D.: Intersynovial fistula in the carpus of a horse. Cornell Vet. *65:* 84 (1975).
JOHNSTON, G.: Equine joint surgery in the standing position. Vet. Med. and Small Animal Clinician *70:* 1293 (1975).
JOICE, J. R.: Cryosurgery for removal of equine sarcoids. Vet. Med. and Small Animal Clinician *70:* 200, 202 (1975).
LARSEN, L. H.; DIXON, R. T.: Management of carpal injuries in the fastgaited horse. Austral. vet. J. *46:* 33 (1970).
LEWANDOWSKI, M.: Subluxatio obu stawów nadgarskowych o niezmanej etiologii. Med. weteryn. *21:* 419 (1965).
LINGARD, D. R.: Strain of superior check ligament of the horse. J. Amer. vet. med. Assoc. *148:* 364 (1966).
MACKAY-SMITH, M. P.; CUSHING, L. S.; LESLIE, J. M.: 'Carpal canal' syndrome in horses. J. Amer. vet. med. Assoc. *160:* 7 (1972).
MONTGOMERY, T.: Leg problems in race horses. Vet. Med. and Small Animal Clinician *60:* 1106 (1965).
MORGAN, J. P.: Radiographic diagnosis of bone and joint diseases in the horse. Cornell Vet., suppl. 58, p. 28 (1968).
O'BRIEN, T. R.; MORGAN, J. P.; PARK, R. D.; LEBEL, J. L.: Radiography in equine carpale lameness. Cornell Vet. *61:* 646 (1971).
PARK, R. D.; MORGAN, J. P.; O'BRIEN, T. R.: Chip fractures in the carpus of the horse. A radiographic study of the incidence and localisation. J. Amer. vet. med. Assoc. *157:* 1305 (1970).
PELT, R. W. VAN: Idiopathic tendosynovitis in foals. J. Amer. vet. med. Assoc. *155:* 510 (1969).
PELT, R. W. VAN; TILLOTSON, P. J.; GERTSEN, K. E.: Intraarticular injection of betamethasone in arthritis in horses. J. Amer. vet. med. Assoc. *156:* 1589 (1970).
PELT, R. W. VAN; TILLOTSON, P. J.; GERTSEN, K. E.; GALLAGHER, K. F.: Effects of intraarticular injection of fluomethasone suspension in joint diseases in horses. J. Amer. vet. med. Assoc. *159:* 739 (1971).
RYDELL, N. W.; BUTLER, J.; BALAZS, E.: Hyaluronic acid in synovial fluid. VI. Effect of intraarticular injection of hyaluronic acid on the clinical symptoms of arthritis in track horses. Acta vet. scand. *11:* 139 (1970).
STIHL, H. G.: Frakturen als orthopädisches Problem beim Sportpferd. Schweiz. Arch. Tierheilk. *110:* 309 (1968).
THRALL, D. E.; LEBEL, J. L.; O'BRIEN, T. R.: A five-year survey of the incidence and localisation of equine carpal chip fractures. J. Amer. vet. med. Assoc. *158:* 1366 (1971).
WALLACE, CH. E.: Chronic tendosynovitis of the extensor carpi radialis tendon in the horse. Austral. vet. J. *48:* 585 (1972).
WINSTANLEY, E. W.; GLEESON, L. N.: Prothetic radial carpal bone in a mare. J. Amer. vet. med. Assoc. *165:* 87 (1974).
WYBURN, L. R. S.; GOULDEN, B. E.: Fractures of the equine carpus: a report on 57 cases. New Zealand vet. .J *22:* 135 (1974).

2.1.19. Diseases of the Hind Limbs

2.1.19.1. Diseases of the Thigh

2.1.19.1.1. Wounds and Wound Infections

Definition and Occurrence. Wounds of the thigh region may take the form of puncture wounds, lacerations, contusions or incised wounds. Unless these wounds are given prompt surgical treatment, infection with pyogenic, or anaerobic organisms (Clostridia) is likely. Such infections are especially common with wounds of the quadriceps, biceps, semitendinosus, semimembranosus and gluteal muscles. The wounds can vary greatly in depth and extent. Besides the skin and fascia, they may cause serious damage to deeper tissues, including blood vessels, nerves, muscles, tendons and bone.

Symptoms. Besides the local changes, which are characteristic of the particular wound type, there may be functional disability associated with damage to deeper tissues. In addition, systemic signs may be observed as a result of wound infection (figs. 2.1.19. — 1 through — 3).

Specific injuries are often associated with typical functional disturbances. With division of the quadriceps femoris muscle, for example, a severe supporting-leg lameness develops in the early stage, and the stifle collapses in jack-knife fashion when extension of this joint is attempted (fig. 2.1.19. — 4). Wounds in the area of the tensor fasciae latae muscle produce a severe swinging-leg lameness. During movement, the horse advances the affected limb only to the level of the healthy supporting leg. This functional disturbance is similar to that associated with chip fractures of the tuber coxae. Severe swinging-leg lameness can also result from divisions of the biceps, semitendinosus or semimembranosus muscle. If motor nerves have become severed in complicated wounds of the thigh, losses of function will be apparent during standing or walking that are characteristic of the corresponding nerve paralysis. Most such wounds occur at the junction of the thigh and gaskin, especially in the vicinity of the popliteal fossa. Muscle wounds of this type are frequently accompanied by extensive tissue loss. Also, the muscle stumps have a tendency to retract immediately after the injury. The division of major arteries is rare and is characterized by an immediate, profuse hemorrhage. The popliteal artery may be severed in wounds involving the popliteal fossa. The remaining large blood vessels course along the medial surface of the thigh and so are relatively well protected from injury. Inflammatory edema quickly develops in the tissues surrounding the wound and may spread to the gaskin or even the inguinal region. If pyogenic organisms have been introduced into the wound, a septic subcutaneous, subfascial or intermuscular cellulitis will probably develop within 2—3 days (fig. 2.1.19. — 5). As this occurs, the lameness becomes progressively more severe, and more or less marked systemic signs appear. The subcutaneous fascia becomes very tense, as does the overlying skin. Subfascial fluid collections may spread toward the popliteal fossa. The infection takes a peracute course if, besides pyogenic organisms, the wound becomes contaminated with clostridial organisms or other gas-producing organisms. The area surrounding the wound and perhaps the entire thigh and gaskin region swells to 2—3 times its normal size within 1—2 days. The horse no longer bears any weight on the limb. A liquid, grayish-brown, malodorous, bubbly or frothy wound discharge is present. In the presence of gas gangrene infection, the affected muscle becomes friable and can easily be plucked apart with a forceps. Crepitation is evident on palpation of the wound area. In the absence of immediate, vigorous general and surgical therapy, the condition will progress to a fatal septicemia or toxemia.

1 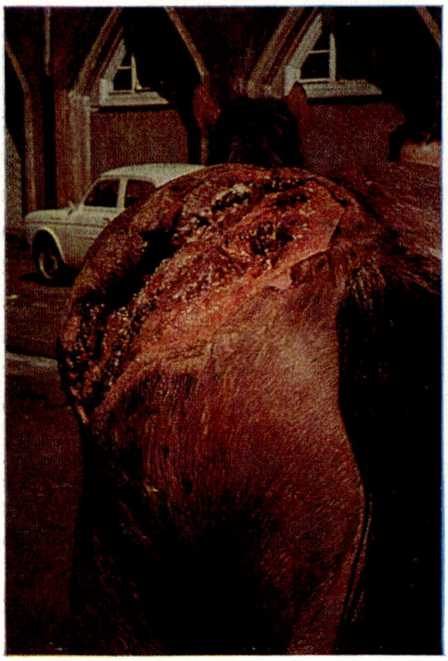

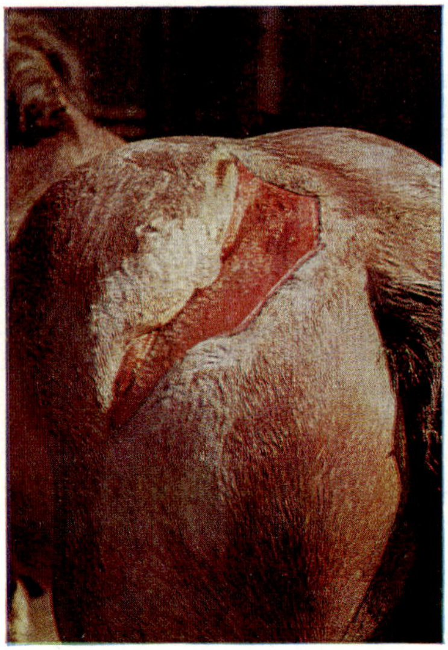 2

Fig. 2.1.19. — 1. Fresh muscle laceration on the croup.
Fig. 2.1.19. — 2. Same horse as in fig. 2.1.19. — 1 four weeks later: normal granulation healing.

Etiology. Muscle lacerations, with or without subsequent infection, are caused by kicks from other horses, pitchfork wounds, traffic accidents, or may occur when a bolting horse runs into a wooden fence, barbed wire or other obstacle. In wounds inflicted by wooden objects, plowshares or falls onto tilling equipment, it must always be assumed that the wound is infected with pus-forming or clostridial organism species.

Differential diagnosis must be made from trauma-related subcutaneous emphysema and infected hematomas of the thigh region.

Diagnosis. The diagnosis is made by the characteristics of the wound. The nature of a wound infection can be inferred with some confidence from the clinical course and from the consistency, color and odor of wound discharges. With severe, deep wounds, an attempt should be made to culture organisms from the wound and determine their drug sensitivity. In most cases, however, such diagnostic measures are usually too late to be of therapeutic value.

Treatment. Fresh skin, fascial and muscle wounds are managed according to general surgical rules, i.e., the wound edges are excised, and the wound is sutured. If there is pocketing of the wound, it is useful to make a counterincision to establish drainage. Foreign bodies, such as wooden splinters and hairs, or avulsed pieces of muscle or fascia that could act as foreign bodies must be removed. Macerated and devitalized tissues also are removed. If a wound of the thigh is already several days old, swelling and involvement of surrounding tissues usually will have progressed too far to permit excision of the wound edges. Nevertheless, an attempt should be made to suture at least a portion of large incised and flap-shaped wounds, as this can significantly shorten the healing time. If second-intention healing is the goal, then the wound should be irrigated with H_2O_2, acridine dye or potassium permanganate solutions. Treating the wound with antibiotics or sulfonamide solutions is effective only if healthy granulation has not yet formed. This should be preceded by treatment with agents such as chloramine solutions or Dakin's fluid. If a clinically manifest

3 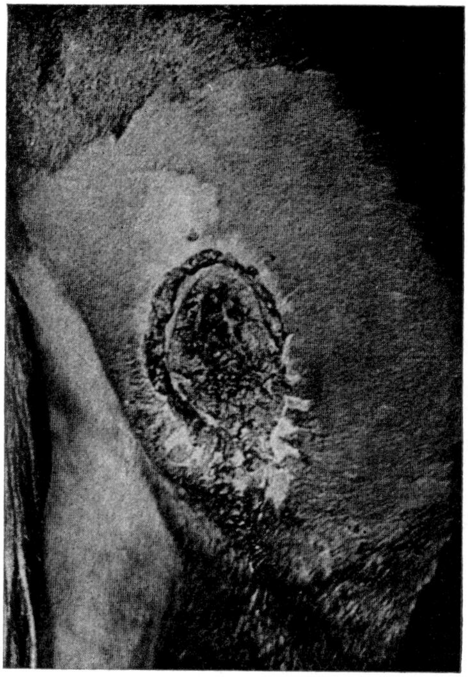

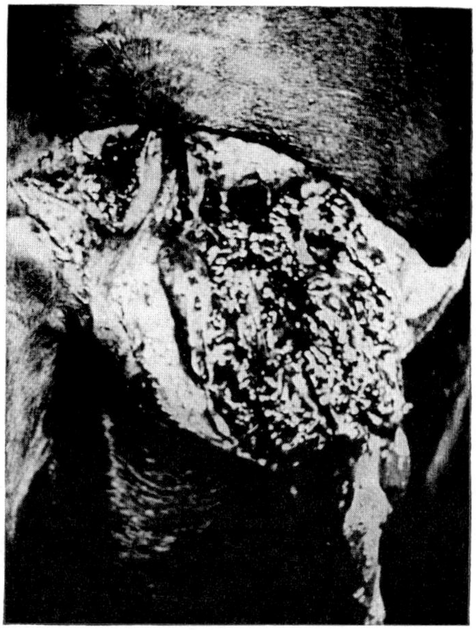 4

Fig. 2.1.19. — 3. Decubitus in the thigh region.
Fig. 2.1.19. — 4. Muscle laceration at the knee.

gas gangrene infection is already present, treatment follows recognized guidelines for such infections: these include deep incisions, irrigations with oxygen-liberating drugs, and local applications of sulfonamides or antibiotics that are active against anaerobes.

In the presence of subfascial cellulitis with abscessation, the popliteal area should be incised and drained immediately. If a fistula forms during the healing of a thigh wound, the tract is incised and a search made for foreign bodies. Bone sequestra often do not become visibly demarcated until 4—6 weeks after the injury. Systemic signs may arise in association with pyogenic wound infection. When this occurs, large doses of systemic antibiotics are administered for 5 to 8 days. Systemic treatment must be instituted immediately in the presence of a gas gangrene infection. Sulfonamides or antibiotics are administered that are active against anaerobic bacteria. Systemic treatment with caffeine, strophanthin (a cardiac stimulant) glucose and essential amino acids is also indicated to arrest degeneration in parenchymal tissues by stimulation of blood supply to the areas.

With all recent wounds of the thigh region, tetanus prophylaxis is indicated for the nonimmunized animal. With deep muscle wounds, polyvalent clostridial antiserum (50 ml for small horses, 100 ml for large horses) should always be administered before overt signs of infection appear.

Prognosis. The prognosis for recent wounds is always favorable, regardless of wound size. The earlier general surgical treatment is instituted, the shorter the healing time. Even in anaerobic infections, healing often can be achieved with appropriate treatment. However, with the extensive involvement and general loss of condition that accompany such infections it is likely that at least 4—8 weeks will be required for

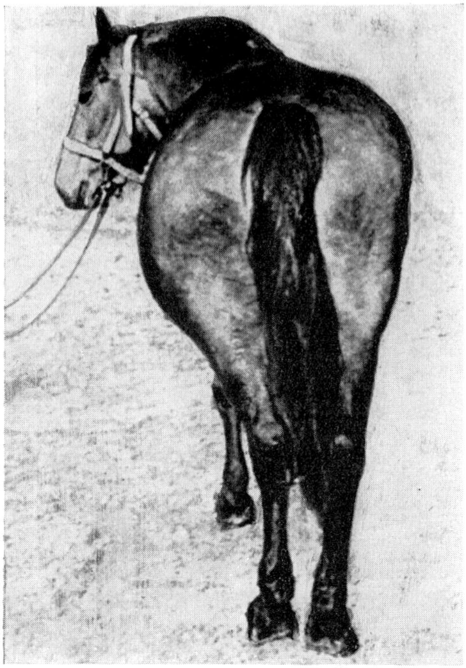

Fig. 2.1.19. — 5. Subfascial cellulitis of the croup and thigh.

healing. Anaerobic infections may however take a peracute course that terminates fatally within a matter of days.

Comments. With proper treatment primary healing can be achieved in most thigh wounds within 8—10 days. Special attention should be given to the prevention and treatment of wound infection, for the involved tissues are highly susceptible to infection by anaerobic bacteria.

2.1.19.1.2. Paralytic Myoglobinuria (Equine Paralytic Myoglobinuria, Azoturia)

Definition and Occurrence. Paralytic myoglobinuria (azoturia) in the horse is a paralysis-like locomotor disorder that occurs acutely during exercise. It is characterized by muscular degeneration with the liberation of myoglobin from the muscle fibers, which escapes in the urine.

Myoglobinuria is chiefly a disease of younger draft horses of the heavy breeds, although it is not uncommon in light horses. Outbreaks are sporadic and usually are observed in cool weather soon after the beginning of exercise following a rest period of several days (Monday morning disease). A similar but milder syndrome, called 'tying up' or 'cording up', is encountered in trotters and Thoroughbreds (see Sec. 2.1.19. 1.3.).

Symptoms. Typically, the affected horse has been put back to work following a rest period of 1 or 2 days, and has been kept on full rations during that period.

Fifteen minutes to one hour after the start of exercise, the horse begins to sweat profusely, even though it is being worked at a usual level of exertion. First the gait becomes stiff, then muscular tremors appear, and if exercise or movement is continued, the hind limbs will give way and the animal will collapse.

If the disease affects only the muscles of one hind limb, or occasionaly one forelimb, severe lameness is usually present.

The affected muscles, usually of the femoral and gluteal groups, often appear swollen and rigid initially. By the next day they generally will feel soft and relaxed when palpated. Marked fever is rarely present. In most cases the rectal temperature is only slightly elevated (up to 39 °C) or normal. Abnormalities of the activity of the heart may be noted, depending on the severity of the attack. In mild cases the pulse rate is only moderately elevated, while severe cases may show pronounced tachycardia with premature beats and atrial fibrillation. Marked changes are evident in the ECG. The respiratory rate is also increased.

A particularly salient feature of the disease is the dark brown or blackish discoloration of the urine ('coffee-colored urine'). Often the animal is unable to urinate, however, and so catheterization must be employed to collect a sample. The urine contains a large amount of myoglobin, as well as protein and crystalline and organic components such as renal epithelial cells, casts, and isolated red and white cells. Renal failure, which may be transitory, is manifested by elevations of the blood urea level (uremia).

Blood studies show that the erythrocyte count is increased by 2 to 3 10^{12}/l, with an associated increase in the hemoglobin level. Elevations are also seen in the blood levels of glucose, pyruvic acid and lactic acid. The parameters of the acid-base balance may show a metabolic acidosis. Hyperphosphatemia (to more than 3.23 mmol/l) and hyperkalemia are also detected in the early stage.

The tying-up syndrome in racehorses, which some authors assign to this disease complex, generally runs a milder course (see Sec. 2.1.19.1.3.).

Etiology and Pathogenesis. The actual cause or causal factor remains unclear, despite the fact that the disease has been known and described for some 100 years. A constitutional predisposition is assumed to play a role. On the other hand, the factors that actually precipitate attacks or promote their occurrence are fairly well known. CARLSTRÖM [1931, 1932] is credited with having made the first comprehensive, experimental study of the cause and pathogenesis of the disease. Even in the light of more recent research, his explanations continue to have validity. An important factor in the pathogenesis of paralytic myoglobinuria is the relatively high glycogen content of the equine musculature, which can be further increased by a carbohydrate-rich diet. Given the relatively large proportion of white muscle fibers, muscular exertion triggers an immediate and intense glycogenolysis. Under these circumstances a relative deficiency of blood flow due to cold, muscle fatigue or other stress factors will create a hypoxic situation in the muscle tissues with a predominance of anaerobic lactic acid formation. At the same time, oxidative energy production and the resynthesis of glycogen and ATP are deficient. A coexisting insufficiency of the pancreatic islet system has been postulated by various authors, but this has not been definitely confirmed.

The accumulation of acid metabolites (lactic and pyruvic acid) causes damage to the muscle fibers with the destruction of muscle protein and the liberation of myoglobin. These degenerative, acidosis-induced changes affect mainly the large muscle groups of the croup and lumbar region but may also affect the psoas muscles and other muscles of the hind limbs and occasionally the forelimbs. Involvement of the myocardium is also usually present. Degenerative changes are found in the parenchymatous organs (liver, kidneys), and a discolored urine is found in the bladder.

Differential Diagnosis. The main disease to be differentiated is *enzootic myoglobinuria*, which is observed with increasing frequency. According to FORENBACHER et al. [1957, 1976], this form of myopathy is tied to certain geographic regions, where occasional outbreaks occur and mainly affect foals. The lesions are confined mainly to the lingual muscles, the muscles of mastication and deglutition, and the muscles of the shoulder girdle and forelimbs. The course may be subacute to chronic.

Tetanus causes a rigidity of gait similar to that of paralytic myoglobinuria. However, tetanus also produces trismus, prolapse of the nictating membrane, rigidity of all head and neck muscles, and hyperexcitability — signs that serve to distinguish it from myoglobinuria. In laminitis, the major symptoms occur in the forelimbs. In doubtful cases, serum enzyme studies will enable a differentiation to be made. According to Lugowski [1971], serum transaminase activities may rise to 2—3.5 times normal in laminitis, as compared to at least a 10-fold increase in paralytic myoglobinuria.

Diseases of the spine, spinal cord and joints of the hind limbs may also have to be differentiated. Hemoglobinuria is excluded by urinalysis. Because myoglobin has a very low renal threshold, the blood serum shows little or no discoloration in the presence of muscular disease. Spectrophotometry is necessary for accurate differentiation of the pigments.

Diagnosis. The immediate diagnosis is made from the history and clinical signs. The detection of myoglobin in the urine confirms the diagnosis. Serious cases are not difficult to recognize. Mild attacks, on the other hand, can be diagnosed with confidence only by serum enzyme studies, especially if myoglobinuria is no longer present. Various enzyme activities should be determined: CPK, ASAT (SGOT), GPT, ALD and AP.

The activity of creatine phosphokinase (CPK) increases 30- to 60-fold within a few hours, peaks in 3—6 hours and returns to normal in 1—3 days. ASAT, GPT and ALD activities are demonstrable only after 18—24 hours but persist for a longer time. The response of ASAT is the most pronounced. In no other disease are ASAT levels so elevated as in paralytic myoglobinuria, and they remain elevated for 2—4 weeks. Alkaline phosphate (AP) remains within physiologic limits, which enables the myopathy to be differentiated from hepatic disease.

Cardinet et al. [1967] point out that in the tying-up syndrome, as opposed to typical myoglobinuria, the ASAT (SGOT) activity is already elevated at the onset of the disease and even for some time prior to the appearance of symptoms.

Determinations of the glucose, lactic acid, pyruvic acid and inorganic phosphorus levels in the blood can also contribute to the diagnosis.

Prognosis. The prognosis depends largely on the degree and duration of the disease, and on whether or not exercise was stopped immediately when symptoms first appeared, and whether the animal itself causes exacerbation as a result of severe motor unrest.

For this reason the rate of recovery varies widely between 30 and 70 %. We personally obtained a 61.5 % cure rate in a series of 78 clinical patients.

An important prognostic criterion is the animal's ability or inability to remain standing after an attack. If the horse stays on its feet, symptoms may regress completely within 12—24 hours in mild cases. Even if the animal is lying quietly and is able to stand with help by the 2nd or 3rd day, the prognosis is still favorable. If the animal is unable to stand by the 3rd day, there is usually little hope of recovery.

Caution is advised when making a prognosis, for recovery is not always complete. Frequently an acute attack will be followed by muscle atrophy and permanent lameness. Our experience shows that this is most probable when the changes are unilateral and are localized to the forelimb.

Treatment. It is imperative that all exercise be stopped immediately when the first signs of the disease appear. The animal should remain where it is until it is completely calm. Blanketing is helpful during this time. Only when the horse is quiet and warm may it be transported home by low-level trailer or walked slowly back to its stall. Local heat and massage of the affected muscle groups are helpful in stimulating blood flow and improving the oxygen supply.

FORENBACHER [1956] states that vitamin B_1, when administered promptly by intravenous injection in a dose of 0.5—2.0 g, leads to a rapid normalization of the blood glucose level and a reduction of pyruvic acid levels. Relaxation of the muscles and stimulation of diuresis are additional benefits of this therapy.

GŽICKIJ et al. [1957] recommend insulin injections (100 I.U. s.c.). This will lower the blood glucose and inorganic phosphorus, thus effecting an improvement in carbohydrate metabolism and general condition.

Sodium bicarbonate is given to correct the acidosis if present. 300—400 g may be dissolved in water and given orally, or 100 g may be administered i.v. in the form of a 5% solution.

Various 'classical' therapies are of dubious value and can no longer be recommended. These include the infusion of calcium solutions, and the administration of methylene blue solutions.

The use of glucocorticoids is described by various authors. However, as FORENBACHER [1956] has pointed out, the secretion of glucocorticoids is already elevated in affected animals. Increases in the abnormalities of carbohydrate metabolism, especially hyperglycemia, have been reported following experimental injections of additional glucocorticoids. According to observations by LINDHOLM [1974], 37% of Thoroughbreds treated with dexamethasone or prednisolone developed tying-up symptoms within 3—5 days.

Animals that show marked restlessness or pain should be given an analgesic, such as sodium noramidopyrine methane sulfonate (e.g., metapyrine, 40—60 ml), or a neuroplegic such as chlorpromazine (20—25 ml) or tranquilizer. Recumbent animals should be provided with soft bedding and turned onto the opposite side every 4—6 hours. Every 12 hours, an attempt should be made to get the horse to its feet. Slinging may be helpful in some cases, but the sling should be removed as soon as the horse is steady on its feet.

Prevention. The cornerstone of prevention is the provision of a ration that is commensurate with the amount of work the animal is doing. Above all, the feeding of concentrated rations must be avoided during periods of inactivity. It is not always easy to adhere to a low-carbohydrate dietary regimen, however, and so regular daily exercise is recommended as an alternative to layoff periods.

In problem animals, periodic serum enzyme determinations may be made during the training period so that muscle damage can be detected early. Animals that have frequent attacks should be withdrawn from competitive racing.

2.1.19.1.3. Tying-Up Syndrome (Cording-Up Syndrome)

Definition. The tying-up syndrome is a myopathy that closely resembles paralytic myoglobinuria but affects racehorses almost exclusively. It occurs immediately after a race or strenuous workout and tends to affect the long back muscles such as the longissimus dorsi and the iliopsoas group. The quadriceps and gluteals may be involved in severe cases.

Symptoms. The disease tends to occur after strenuous training or at the conclusion of a race. However, nervous horses may manifest similar symptoms or early signs of tying-up even at the beginning of work. In some cases a prolonged rest period may precede an attack. Stiffness is apparent in the movement of the hindquarters. At the trot, the hind legs do not flex normally, and a shuffling gait may be exhibited. The back is rigid and may even be arched slightly. Pain is elicited by palpating the long back muscles, especially in the lumbar region. It can also be produced by palpating the iliopsoas group of muscles during rectal exploration. The affected muscles feel hard to the touch. In some severe cases the muscular involvement may extend to the gluteals and the quadriceps. Most horses with tying-up syndrome do not lie down. Recumbent animals can usually get to their feet without assistance. Serologic studies show pathologic increases in the activities of ASAT (SGOT), LDH and CPK.

Some horses with the syndrome show a mild myoglobinuria. If the horse is walked for a time, the clinical symptoms usually improve.

Etiology. It has often been suggested that the tying-up syndrome is a mild form of the paralytic myoglobinuria seen in heavy horses. In both syndromes there is an increase of lactic acid formation in the affected muscles, although in tying-up, the accumulation of lactic acid is not sufficient to cause muscular degeneration.

Tying-up always occurs in highly conditioned horses, in which lactic acid formation is a slow process. The disease bears some relation to nervous temperament. Highly sensitive horses are more susceptible to attacks than even-tempered animals. Thus, the condition may be seen following transportation by car or airplane or following temperamental outbursts when the horse is broken to saddle. Reportedly, tying-up is more common in mares than in stallions. Horses once affected with the condition seem to be subject to a recurrence at any time. A chronic condition develops in many animals that are not treated promptly after an attack.

Adams [1974] explains the pathogenesis of the tying-up syndrome as follows: Energy is produced in the body by two means: anaerobic and aerobic. The anaerobic or glycolytic pathway utilizes carbohydrates exclusively for the breakdown of glycogen and glucose, with a subsequent production of lactic acid. No oxygen is consumed in these processes. Energy consumption by the muscles can be estimated from the postexercise oxygen debt that is incurred, or from the difference between pre- and postexercise lactic acid concentrations.

There is a direct relationship between oxygen debt and the rise in the lactic acid level. The aerobic or oxidative pathway utilizes carbohydrates, fat and protein and yields energy by the combustion of these substances. The extent to which this pathway is utilized can be measured from the oxygen consumption during exercise. Anaerobic energy production is of primary interest in the racehorse, for this pathway is used during physical exertion under 3 minutes' duration. Through glycolysis, lactic acid is formed by anaerobic oxidation. If blood flow through the muscles is adequate to meet the oxygen demand, lactic acid buildup is not a problem. Adams [1974] states that in the tying-up syndrome, there apparently is a decreased blood flow in the affected muscles caused by a spasm of the arterioles. This results in decreased blood flow at a time when a good supply is needed. Too much lactic acid is formed because of the increased anaerobic conditions, and too little is removed because of the decreased circulation. The accumulation of lactic acid in the muscles and blood is the most common limiting factor of muscular activity and apparently results in cramping of the affected muscles, causing the firmness that is felt on palpation. Horses that are improperly conditioned will create a larger oxygen debt than those that are properly trained. Presumably there are inherited differences between horses that influence the size of the oxygen debt.

Various authors have also pointed to a deficiency of vitamin E and selenium as contributing to the etiology of the syndrome.

Diagnosis. In racehorses the diagnosis is based on the history and clinical signs. The characteristic feature of tying-up is its appearance within minutes after strenuous exertion, i.e., after racing or heavy training. In rare cases signs will be exhibited soon after work begins. Hand pressure over the longissimus muscles in the region of the lumbosacral junction will invariably produce pain. A rectal examination should always be performed to complete the diagnosis, for palpation of the iliopsoas group of muscles also elicits pain. The gait is stiff in both hind limbs. In more severe cases pain also will be evident in the area of the gluteal and quadriceps muscles.

Differential Diagnosis. The most difficult differentiation is from paralytic myoglobinuria. In this syndrome clinical symptoms appear immediately after work is begun, while in tying-up the symptoms generally do not appear until after the completion of vigorous exercise. Serologic studies with determinations of the ASAT, LDH and CPK activities do not contribute to the differential diagnosis, because elevations are characteristic of both syndromes.

Treatment. The horse is walked for 30—40 minutes. Affected muscles are massaged with alcohol liniments. As in azoturia, sodium bicarbonate solutions and calcium gluconate are administered i.v. Selenium-vitamin E combinations, thiamine and low doses of chlorpromazine have also proved beneficial. Vitamin E-selenium combinations are given i.v. in a dose of 1 ml/100 kg BW. The injections may be repeated at weekly intervals. According to ADAMS [1974], the i.v. administration of 30—50 g sodium bicarbonate prior to work may prevent the syndrome.

Prognosis. The prognosis for recovery is generally good, although recurrences cannot be excluded. Following the 2nd or 3rd recurrence, atrophy and fibrosis can develop in the affected muscles.

Comments. Horses that have recovered from an attack are subject to recurrences. For these animals, daily prophylactic doses of 60—120 g sodium bicarbonate are recommended.

References

CARDINET, C. H.; FOWLER, M. E.; TYLER, W. S.: Effects of training, excercise and tying-up on serum transaminase. Amer. J. vet. Res. *24:* 102, 980 (1963).

CARDINET, C. H.; LITTRELL, J. F.; FREELAND, R. A.: Comparative investigations of serum creatine phosphokinase and glutamic-oxaloacetic transaminase activities in equine paralytic myoglobinuria. Res. vet. Sci. *8:* 219 (1967).

CARLSTRÖM, B.: Über die Ätiologie und Pathogenese der Kreuzlähme des Pferdes (Haemoglobinaemia paralytica). Skand. Arch. Physiol. *62:* 1 (1931).

CARLSTRÖM, B.: Über die Ätiologie und Pathogenese der Kreuzlähme des Pferdes. Skand. Arch. Physiol. *63:* 164 (1932).

FERRIOT, M.: Treatment of myoglobinuria. Bull. Soc. Vet. Pract. *45:* 214 (1961).

ENGELHARDT, W. v.; HÖRNICKE, H.; EHRLEIN, H.-J.; SCHMIDT, E.: Lactat, Pyruvat, Glucose und Wasserstoffionen im venösen Blut bei Reitpferden in unterschiedlichem Trainingszustand. Zbl. Vet.-Med. R. A. *20:* 173 (1973).

FORENBACHER, S.: Istraživanja o paralitičnoj mioglobinemiji konja. III. Mliječna kiselina u krvi. Vet. Arhiv, Zagreb *25:* 275 (1955).

FORENBACHER, S.: Istraživanja o paralitičnoj mioglobinemiji konja. IV. Utjecaj adenozintrifosforne kiseline na gliokolizu u krvi. Vet. Arhiv, Zagreb *25:* 355 (1955).

FORENBACHER, S.: Vitamin B_1 kod paralitične mioglobinurije konja. Vet. Arhiv, Zagreb *26:* 229 (1956).

FORENBACHER, S.: Über die Rolle der neuro-hormonalen Regulation bei der Entstehung der paralytischen Myoglobinurie des Pferdes. Zbl. Vet.-Med. *3:* 613 (1956).

FORENBACHER, S.; MALTAR, J.; MARZAN, B.: O pojavi t. zv. enzootičke mioglobinurije konja kod nas. Vet. Arhiv, Zagreb *27:* 1 (1957).

FORENBACHER, S.; MIHALJEVIĆ, K.: Vitamin E i selen kod enzooticne miglobinurije konja (Prethodno saopcenje). Vet. Arhiv, Zagreb *46:* 95 (1976).

FORENBACHER, S.; RODE, B.: Investigations on the role played by the insular apparatus in the pathogenesis of paralytic myoglobinuria in the horse. I. Changes in the structure and function of the insular apparatus in the healthy horse under the effect of Cobalt chloride, Alloxan and Glucose. Zbl. Vet.-Med. *8:* 1 (1961).

FRIES, J. H.: Treatment of the tying-up-syndrome. Proc. 7th Ann. A. AEP (1961).

GEISER, D. R.: The azoturia tying-up syndrome. Vet. Med. and Small Animal Clinician *70:* 10 (1975).

GERBER, H.: Aktivitätsbestimmungen von Serumenzymen in der Veterinärmedizin. Schweiz. Arch. Tierheilkd. *106:* 85 (1964).

GERBER, H.: Enzymdiagnostik bei inneren Krankheiten des Pferdes. Zbl. Vet.-Med. R. A. *11:* 135 (1964).

GERBER, H.: Aktivitätsbestimmungen von Serumenzymen in der Veterinärmedizin. III. E. Serum-Enzymmuster bei paralytischer Myoglobinämie des Pferdes. Schweiz. Arch. Tierheilkd. *107:* 685 (1965).

GERBER, H.: The clinical significance of serum enzyme activities with particular reference to myoglobinuria. Proc. AAEP. (1968), p. 81.

GERBER, H.; MARTIG, J.; STRAUB, R.: Enzymuntersuchungen im Serum von Grosstieren im Hinblick auf Diagnose und Prognose. tierärztl. praxis *1:* 5 (1973).

GLASENAPP, H. v.: Über die Brauchbarkeit der Aktivitätsbestimmung spezifischer Serumenzyme für die Diagnostik von muskelbedingten Bewegungsstörungen bei Pferden — insbesondere bei Trabrennpferden. Vet.-med. Diss., Berlin-Dahlem (1972).

GRODZKI, K.: Elektrokardiogram w miesniochwacie porazennym koni. Polsk. Arch. Weteryn. *8:* 505 (1964).

GÜRTLER, H.: Die diagnostische Bedeutung einiger Serumfermente. Zbl. Vet.-Med. *7:* 160 (1960).

GŽICKIJ, S. Z.; GERMANJUK, JA. L.; GOLOVACKIJ, I. D.: Primenenie gljukoinsulinovoj terapii, adenosin-trifosfornoj i glujutaminovoj kislot pro zabolevanijach s.-ch. životnych s rezkim narušeniem obmena veščestv. Trudy Moskovsk. veterin. akad. *21:* 157 (1957).

HILL, H. E.: Selenium-Vitamin E treatment of tying-up horses. Mod. Vet. Pract. *43:* 66 (1962).

LAPPAS, M.: Les myosites du cheval de Sport. Bull Soc. Sci. vétérin. Med. comp. *77:* 259 (1975).

LINDHOLM, A.: 'Tying-up' and serum enzymes in standardbred trotters. Svensk. Vet.-Tidn. *24:* 871 (1972).

LINDHOLM, A.; JOHANSSON, H.-E.; KJAERSCAARD, P.: Acute rhabdomyolysis ('Tying-up') in standardbred horses. A morphological and biochemical study. Acta vet. scand. *15:* 325 (1974).

LINDHOLM, A.; PIEHL, K.: Fibre composition, enzyme activity and concentrations of metabolites and electrolytes in muscles of standardbred horses. Acta vet. scand. *15:* 287 (1974).

LINDHOLM, A.; SALTIN, B.: The physiological and biochemical response of standardbred horses to exercise of varying speed and duration. Acta vet. scand. *15:* 310 (1974).

LUGOWSKI, T.: Aktywność aminotransferazy asparginianowej (AspAT) i alaninowej (ALAT) w surowicy koni chorych na ochwat kopytowy i miesniochwat porazenny. Ann. Univ. Mariae Curie-Skłodowska, Lublin, Section DD *26:* 183 (1971).

MCLEAN, J. G.: Equine paralytic myoglobinuria ('Azoturia'). A review. Austral. vet. J. *49:* 41 (1973).

MEGINNIS, P.: Myositis (Tying-up) in race horses. J. Amer. veterin. med. Assoc. *167:* 237 (1975).

MILLER, W. C.: Atypical myoglobinuria. Irish Vet. J. *15:* 154 (1961).

Panel Report: Azoturia in the horse. Mod. Vet. Pract. *41* (5): 45 (1960).

PINKIEWICZ, E.; ZIMOWSKI, A.: Aktywność enzymow AspAT, ALAT, ALD, PHI, AP w surowiey koni chorych na mieśniochwat porazenny. Ann. Univ. Mariae Curie-Skłodowska, Lublin, Section DD *24:* 199 (1969).

RICO, A. G.; GODFRAIN, J.-C.; BRAUN, J.-P.; BENARD, P.; BURGAT-SACAZE, V.: Dosages enzymatiques seriques en clinique equine. Rev. Méd. vét. *37* (125): 781 (1974).

SANDERSLEBEN, J. v.; SCHLOTKE, B.: Die Muskeldystrophie (Weißmuskelkrankheit) bei Fohlen, eine offensichtlich im Zunehmen begriffene Erkrankung. Dtsch. tierärztl. Wschr. *84:* 105 (1977).

SCHLOTKE, B.: Muskeldystrophie bei Fohlen. Berliner Münchener Tierärztl. Wschr. *87:* 84 (1974).
SMYTHE, R. H.: Azoturia. Proc. Brit. Equine Vet. Assoc., p. 37 (1964).
STEEL, J. D.: Abnormalities of gait in the racehorse referred to as tying-up syndromes. Austral. vet. J. *45:* 162 (1969).
VERMA, B. B.; PRASAD, B.: Equine paralytic myoglobinuria — a case report. Indian Vet. J. *44:* 896 (1967).
VICARD, A.; STARON, TH.: Au sujet de la myoglobinurie paroxystique du cheval. Bull. Acad. vét. France *47:* 25 (1974).
WILLENBERG, S.: Über erfolgreiche Behandlung der Myoglobinaemia paralytica equi (Lumbago) mit dem Neuroplegicum Chlorpromazin. Mh. Vet.-Med. *22:* 59 (1967).
WINTZER, H.-J.; GLASENAPP, H. v.: Über eine lokale Myopathie bei Trabrennpferden. Berliner Münchener Tierärztl. Wschr. *86:* 221 (1973).

2.1.19.1.4. Paralysis of the Quadriceps Muscle

Definition. Quadriceps paralysis involves a loss of function in the muscle that extends the stifle joint.

Symptoms. No systemic signs are present. Examination of the limb distal to and including the stifle shows no abnormalities when the animal is standing. However, a large depression is seen proximal to the stifle in the area of the quadriceps femoris muscle. This causes the stifle joint and patella to appear unusually prominent relative to surrounding tissues. No heat or pain is evident in the stifle and quadriceps region. A moderate to severe supporting-leg lameness, generally unilateral, is evident during standing and walking. Thus, the animal stands with the toe of the affected limb resting on the ground, and when weight is placed on the affected leg, the limb gives way at the stifle and hock joints, and a slight knuckling of the fetlock may occur. At this time fascia-like cords are visible in and beneath the skin of the quadriceps region. If the horse is forced to move, the lameness will become worse and the stride will shorten.

Etiology. The cause may be a primary disease of the muscle or the femoral nerve. Myogenic paralysis is caused by a fibrosing myositis resulting from azoturia. If the symptoms of the azoturia do not disappear in 8—14 days, then the quadriceps muscle will become severely atrophied and replaced with a fascia-like tissue. Concomitant atrophy of the gluteals is sometimes present.

Neurogenic paralysis is caused by a contusion, rupture or inflammation of the femoral nerve. In years past, femoral nerve paralysis was a fairly common sequel to dourine.

Differential Diagnosis. Lateral luxation of the patella should be considered. In this condition the patella is displaced over the lateral condyle of the femur, and atrophy of the quadriceps muscle is absent. Quadriceps atrophy is likewise absent in motor paralysis of the tibial nerve; this fact, plus the history, distinguish it from quadriceps paralysis.

Diagnosis. The history (e.g., azoturia) and typical clinical symptoms provide sufficient grounds for making the diagnosis.

A waxy hyaline (Zenker's) degeneration of the muscle is seen at necropsy. Even with myogenic paralysis, degenerative changes are evident in the femoral nerve.

Prognosis. It is guarded in cases of unilateral quadriceps paralysis and unfavorable when the paralysis is bilateral. Horses with bilateral quadriceps paralysis are unable to stand and succumb to decubitus and systemic pyogenic infection within days or weeks. The more rapid the quadriceps atrophy, the less favorable the prognosis. With rupture of the femoral nerve, there is little or no chance of functional recovery.

Treatment. An effort is made to improve circulation in the affected muscle. This can be achieved with repeated lumbar sympathetic blockades at 3- to 4-day intervals. Local massage, blistering, shortwave and microwave therapy have also proved beneficial. Vitamin E and selenium should be given intravenously every 8 days. Neurogenic cases respond favorably to large doses of Vitamin B_{12} or B-complex vitamins.

Comments. Treatment should be continued only if function improves and the progress of muscle atrophy is halted during the first few days of therapy. In rare cases functional recovery may follow several months of rest and treatment, but this is recommended only in the case of valuable breeding stock.

2.1.19.1.5. Acute Coxitis

Occurrence. The hip joint of the horse is covered by a powerful muscle mass, and so acute aseptic inflammation of this joint is very rare.

Symptoms. A sudden, mild to moderate, mixed or sometimes swinging-leg lameness appears. It is typical for the horse to move diagonally when walking, as many normal dogs do. Pain is elicited by any passive movement of the limb at the coxofemoral joint. The spavin test (flexion test) exacerbates the lameness. The equine hip joint is poorly accessible to palpation.

Etiology. Acute aseptic coxitis in the horse is caused by trauma to the hip joint resulting from a slip or fall. The resulting contusion, or sprain if the leg becomes caught, leads to acute coxitis. If the hind limb slips laterally on a smooth floor, the hip joint capsule will become stretched in its ventral portion and contused in its dorsal portion. This results in joint effusion and consequent acute aseptic arthritis. Coxofemoral sprains and contusions may be accompanied by small chip fractures of the acetabular lip.

Differential Diagnosis. Swinging-leg and mixed lamenesses are also characteristic of gonitis. In both gonitis and coxitis, lameness is exacerbated by movement. With bone spavin, the horse tends to 'warm out' of the lameness after exercising a short time. Separation of the proximal femoral epiphysis should be considered in foals.

Diagnosis. In racing horses, a presumptive diagnosis of coxitis often can be made from the history. The pathology can be localized to the hip region by exclusion, i.e., by working upward from the foot at the start of the clinical examination. Anesthesia of the plantar nerve may be used if necessary to aid in localizing the seat of the lameness. In any case, disease of the hock and stifle joints must be excluded. A diagnostic injection of the hip joint may be helpful. The needle, which should be 10 to 12 cm long, is passed into the joint through the notch located just cranial to the greater trochanter, and 10—15 ml of a concentrated anesthetic solution is injected. Aseptic precautions are taken during the injection, and a small dose of penicillin is administered concurrently for prophylaxis.

Treatment and Prognosis. The horse is placed in a large box stall. Treatment with topical rubefacients is more symptomatic than beneficial. Healing time can be significantly shortened by adding 200 mg of prednisolone to the diagnostic injection. In addition, 20 ml phenylbutazone is injected i.v. daily for the next 4—5 days, and 200 mg prednisolone/day is administered at intervals of 6—7 days. If no improvement is seen in 8—10 days under this regimen, a rupture of the round ligament or chip fracture of the acetabular lip should be suspected. These conditions lead to the gradual development of a chronic degenerative coxarthritis or coxarthrosis. Cases of this type are incurable.

Comments. If lameness is not gone in 2—3 weeks, the muscles of the croup and hip will become severely atrophic, and chronicity will result. Breeding animals may be preserved with anti-inflammatory therapy and, if necessary, corrective shoeing.

2.1.19.1.6. Dysplasia of the Hip Joint

Definition. This is a structural abnormality characterized by progressive changes in the hip joint. The most common change is a flattening of both acetabula, which may precipitate reactive changes in the joint capsule, round ligament, and head and neck of the femur.

Occurrence. We have observed flattened acetabula in 12- to 15-month-old foals that had very straight hocks. Proliferative changes had already developed in the head and neck of the femur. Animals with this condition are unsound for athletic use.

Symptoms. Affected foals show faults of gait, and a shuffling action may be seen in the hind limbs. There is very little angulation of the hock, and a 'coon-footed' break is evident in the pastern and foot axis.

Etiology. In the horse as in the dog, there is little question that the etiology is hereditary.

Differential Diagnosis. Bilateral separation of the proximal femoral epiphysis should be considered in foals.

Diagnosis. A ventro-dorsal radiograph is made with the animal under general anesthesia. For this examination the hind limbs are placed in extreme flexion and rotated medially, or both hind limbs are well extended and abducted.

Treatment and Prognosis. The condition is incurable, and destruction is necessary. Rehabilitative treatments of the type used in dogs have not yet been tested in the horse.

2.1.19.1.7. Coxarthrosis

Definition and Occurrence. Coxarthrosis is a degenerative disease of aged horses occurring as a result of wear in the coxofemoral joint. Both the acetabulum and the femoral head develop extensive cartilage defects, cartilage fractures, a thickened synovial membrane, and fibrin deposits within the joint capsule. Coxarthrosis is especially common in heavy draft horses that have spent their lives pulling heavy loads.

Symptoms. As in degenerative spondylosis, horses affected with coxarthrosis have difficulty standing up. At the walk the gait is stiff and clumsy, and the animal tires rapidly. In typical cases the feet of both hind limbs are advanced with the heels rotated laterally. A characteristic swinging-leg lameness is apparent. Sometimes crepitant sounds can be heard during passive manipulation of the hind limbs.

Etiology. The basic cause is attrition, and usually the immediate precipitating causes cannot be identified. Horses affected with coxarthrosis may also have degenerative changes in the hock joint.

Diagnosis. It is possible only to make a presumptive diagnosis by exclusion. The animal resents lifting of the affected limb. The lameness is not alleviated by plantar anesthesia. Transrectal or transvaginal radiographs sometimes show reactive changes on the acetabular lip. It may also be possible to obtain ventro-dorsal views in lighter horses.

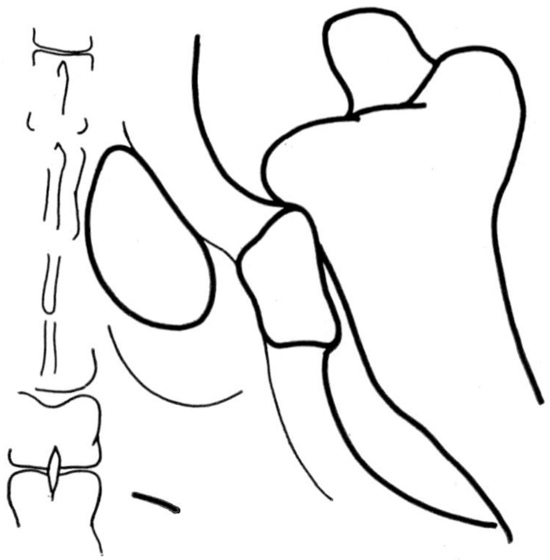

Fig. 2.1.19. — 6. Luxation of the femur.

Differential Diagnosis. Degenerative spondylosis and a luxation or subluxation of the sacroiliac joint should be excluded.

Prognosis. Coxarthrosis is incurable.

Treatment and Comments. Treatment is useless, and destruction is generally necessary, although some mares may still be fit for breeding.

2.1.19.1.8. Luxation of the Femur

Definition. Violence can cause the head of the femur to dislocate from the acetabulum, accompanied by rupture of the round ligament and joint capsule. Muscular traction fixes the femoral head in its luxated position.

Symptoms. The horse is severely lame and may hobble on three legs. The affected limb appears shortened. When the animal is viewed from behind, an asymmetry is evident about the hip joint on the affected side. If the affected limb is placed behind the sound opposite limb, the horse will be unable to lift the affected limb or even advance it. Passive movement, especially rotation and flexion/extension of the stifle and hock joints, produces crepitant sounds over the hip joint.

Etiology. Luxation of the femur is occasionally observed in 1- to 2-year-old colts and fillies. The immediate history shows that the animal has been playing at pasture or in a large stall.

Differential diagnosis must be made from traumatic separation of the proximal femoral epiphysis.

Diagnosis. A presumptive diagnosis can be made with confidence from the shortening of the limb and palpable projection of the femoral head past the acetabular lip. The clinical diagnosis is easily confirmed by radiography (fig. 2.1.19. — 6).

Prognosis and Treatment. Femoral luxation in the horse is always supraglenoidal. While it is possible to return the femoral head to the acetabulum, it is not possible to restore tension and stability. For this reason, horses with a luxated femur should be destroyed.

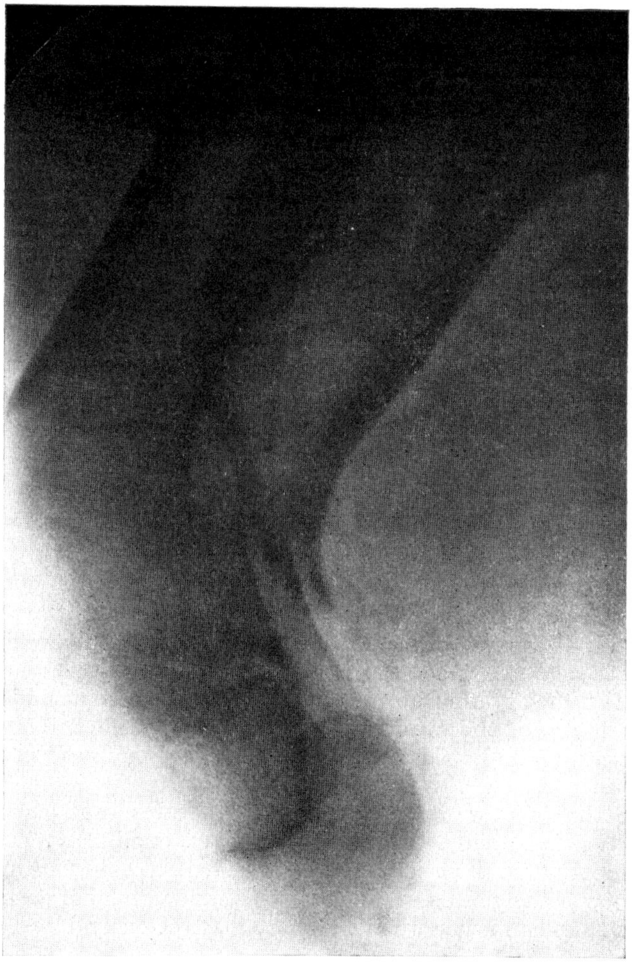

Fig. 2.1.19. — 7. Fracture of the femoral shaft.

2.1.19.1.9. Fracture of the Femur

Definition and Occurrence. Fractures of the femoral shaft are most common in adult horses. Fractures of the neck are very rare [Mackay-Smith, 1964], and supracondylar fractures are occasionally seen in foals. Shaft fractures are usually spiral or oblique; comminuted shaft fractures are uncommon (figs. 2.1.19. — 7 through — 9).

Symptoms. There is sudden severe lameness, abnormal mobility of the part, and a very rapid swelling in the thigh region due to massive hematoma formation (especially with shaft fractures). Adult horses become anxious and break out in a heavy sweat. Many animals collapse at the time of the injury and are unable to rise. In the standing animal, marked crepitant sounds are elicited by manipulation of the limb.

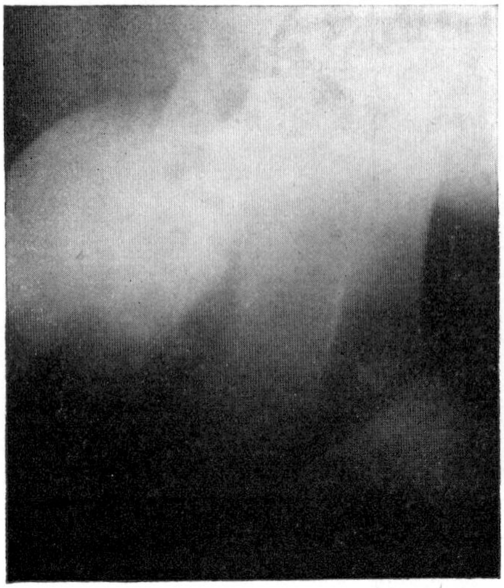

Fig. 2.1.19. — 8. Supracondylar fracture of the femur.

Chip fractures can occur at the greater trochanter. As in trochanteric bursitis, this causes a sudden, severe swinging-leg lameness, and a circumscribed, painful swelling is palpable over the hip joint.

Supracondylar fractures and condylar chip fractures in foals also produce a sudden, severe lameness, which tends to be of the swinging-leg type. When the animal is standing, the entire anterior wall of the hoof is in contact with the ground [Pettit and Wheat, 1961].

Etiology. Chip fractures of the greater trochanter, shaft fractures, and supracondylar fractures are caused by falls, slips, or forcible casting. Very rarely, shaft fractures occur as a result of inadequate relaxation and anesthesia. Most chip fractures of the greater trochanter are caused by falls onto the hip. Supracondylar fractures and condylar chip fractures in foals can occur when the mare inadvertently steps on the recumbent foal or intentionally kicks it.

Differential Diagnosis. Separation of the proximal epiphysis should be considered in foals.

Diagnosis. Fractures of the femur are typified by such classic fracture symptoms as abnormal mobility, crepitation, pain and rapid swelling. A sudden, severe lameness accompanies these symptoms. Radiographic examination has become a fairly routine procedure in equine medicine, and it is essential for making a prognosis and for planning and conducting internal fixation. It is also indispensible for the differential diagnosis of epiphyseal plate separations in foals and of the very rare femoral dislocations.

Prognosis. In large, mature horses, fractures of the femoral shaft are usually incurable. In young horses and in very light horses that are able to rise without assistance, spiral fractures of the femoral shaft will usually heal spontaneously in 12—16 weeks. Intramedullary nailing has not proved effective in the adult horse. If the horse is not too heavy, and if the instrumentation is available, internal fixation with compression plates may be attempted. The prognosis following such a procedure depends on whether the horse is able to stand soon after the operation and can bear weight on the operated limb.

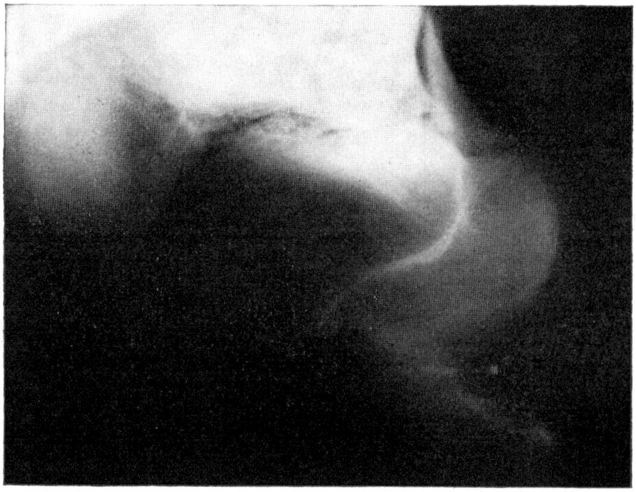

Fig. 2.1.19. — 9. Incomplete fracture at the distal femoral epiphysis.

Treatment. The animal is placed in a large stall with soft bedding (especially foals). If open reduction and fixation is proposed in a mature horse, the animal should be cast onto its healthy side no later than 2—3 days following the injury. The operation is performed under halothane anesthesia. With a femoral shaft fracture, the quadriceps muscle is divided parallel to the direction of its fibers in order to expose the fracture hematoma and the fracture itself from the lateral side. Reduction of the fracture is followed by compression plating, preferably with plates approximately 30 cm long. We have obtained good healing of condylar chip fractures even without surgery, and with no residual lameness. Every internal fixation should be followed by a 10- to 12-day course of prophylactic antibiotics. This will reduce the danger of osteomyelitis.

Comments. Treatment should be attempted in foals. Screw fixation is especially well suited for this age group. In mature horses, internal fixation is worthwhile if the animal has potential breeding value.

2.1.19.1.10. Separation of the Proximal Femoral Epiphysis

Definition and Occurrence. This is a separation at the epiphyseal plate that is accompanied by degeneration and remodeling of the proximal epiphysis of the femur. The condition is especially common in foals of the heavy breeds. We have also encountered it in young Thoroughbreds and trotters (fig. 2.1.19. — 10).

Symptoms. The foal suddenly develops a severe swinging-leg lameness. The affected limb is not advanced past the level of the sound supporting leg. In the standing position the affected leg is held in slight flexion and bears weight only on the anterior hoof wall. It also is deviated medially toward the diagonally opposite forelimb. Palpation of the hip joint elicits pain. In addition, grating or crepitant sounds are audible during passive movement. An asymmetry of the pelvic region is evident when the foal is viewed from behind. If the condition has existed for several days,

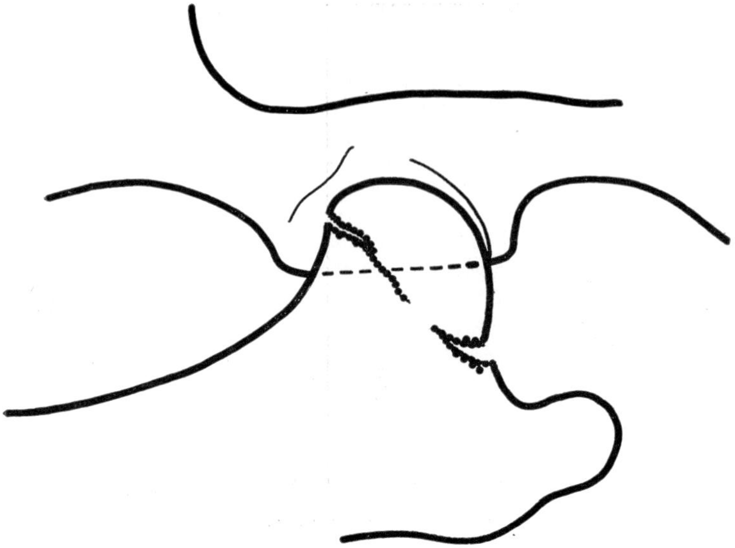

Fig. 2.1.19. — 10. Partial separation of the proximal femoral epiphysis.

there will be atrophy of the gluteal muscles and unusual prominence of the greater trochanter. In bilateral cases the foal is barely able to bear weight with the hind-quarters.

Etiology. Traumatic separation of the epiphysis appears to be extremely rare in foals. It may result from falls onto the hip joint or from being trampled or kicked by another horse.

As in other domestic animals, most notably swine, idiopathic separation of the proximal femoral epiphysis in foals may belong to the osteochondrosis syndrome. Primary changes involve the epiphyseal plate, and osteoporotic changes in the epiphysis itself develop secondarily. The ossification of osteoid tissue becomes deficient on both sides of the epiphyseal plate. The eventual result is separation of the femoral head from the shaft. Foals of the heavy breeds and foals that are undergoing growth spurts are predisposed. Thus, separation of the proximal femoral epiphysis can be assigned both etiologically and pathogenically to the osteochondrosis-arthrosis complex.

Differential Diagnosis. Gonotrochleosis (degenerative disease of the femoropatellar joint) should be considered in foals. Luxation of the femur is relatively rare.

Diagnosis. The sudden, severe lameness, combined with the patient's history and age, are suggestive of the diagnosis. Crepitant sounds at the hip joint on passive manipulation of the limb enable a separation of the proximal femoral epiphysis to be diagnosed with reasonable confidence. Confirmation is easily obtained by radiography.

Prognosis. The prognosis is poor in idiopathic cases.

Treatment. In the rare cases of traumatic origin, internal fixation with a lag screw or stack pinning may be attempted.

2.1.19.1.11. Trochanteric Bursitis (Gluteal Bursitis)

Definition. This is an aseptic, usually acute but sometimes chronic inflammation of the bursa situated between the greater trochanter of the femur and the tendon of the middle gluteal muscle.

Symptoms. A circumscribed, painful, tense swelling is found about a hand's width above the hip joint. The swelling feels like an egg-size tumor when palpated. If the bursitis is of long standing, crepitation may be detected on palpation. The lameness is characteristic. The anterior phase of the stride is shortened, and the affected limb contacts the ground well below the abdomen, bearing weight only on the inside of the foot. As a result, the hind feet are carried away from the affected side, causing the horse to travel like a dog.

Etiology. Trochanteric bursitis is the result of single or repeated contusion. Typically the horse has lost its footing on slippery flooring and fallen onto the hip.

Differential Diagnosis. Because the disease affects adult horses almost exclusively, chronic coxitis should be considered in the differential diagnosis.

Diagnosis. Trochanteric bursitis is typified by the presence of a tense, fluctuating swelling above the hip joint and the resulting 'crooked walk'.

Prognosis and Treatment. If the same site is subjected to repeated contusion, it is imperative that the cause be removed. Local treatment with solvents or alcohol liniments is of little or no value. We recommend the injection of glucocorticoid solutions into the bursa, e.g., 100—200 mg prednisolone. The injection may be repeated in 6—8 days if necessary. In addition, phenylbutazone can be administered i.v. for a period of 5—6 days. The prognosis is generally good if treatment is rendered during the acute stage.

Comments. When an acute bursitis proves refractory to treatment and becomes chronic, exostoses will develop on the greater trochanter and lead to permanent lameness.

2.1.19.1.12. Thrombosis of the Posterior Aorta and its Branches (Iliac, Femoral and Hypogastric Arteries), Intermittent Claudication

Definition. With thrombosis of the terminal segment of the aorta, insufficient blood is supplied to the pelvic limbs, resulting in an intermittent lameness that generally is precipitated by exercise.

Symptoms. Thrombosis of the posterior aorta (fig. 2.1.19. — 11) or one of its branches is characterized by an intermittent lameness that appears with exercise and disappears with rest (intermittent claudication). If the vascular occlusion is great, pulsations may be absent in the metatarsal arteries of one or both hind limbs even when the animal is resting. With sustained exercise, a lameness very quickly develops that may be unilateral or bilateral and may be of the supporting-leg, swinging-leg or mixed variety depending on the location and size of the thrombus. As the lameness appears, the horse begins to advance the affected limb in a shuffling fashion. If exercise is stopped at this point, the animal will stand on the anterior wall of the hoof or even on the flexed fetlock. Horses with unilateral thrombosis pull up shortly after exercise begins and stand with the affected limb in flexion. Horses with severe thrombosis of the posterior aorta or bilateral thrombosis of its branches quickly give way in the hindquarters, first assuming a dog-sitting posture and then falling to one side. The recumbent animal shows a greatly elevated heart rate, increased respiration, cyanosis of the mucosae, strong muscle tremors, and profuse sweating everywhere

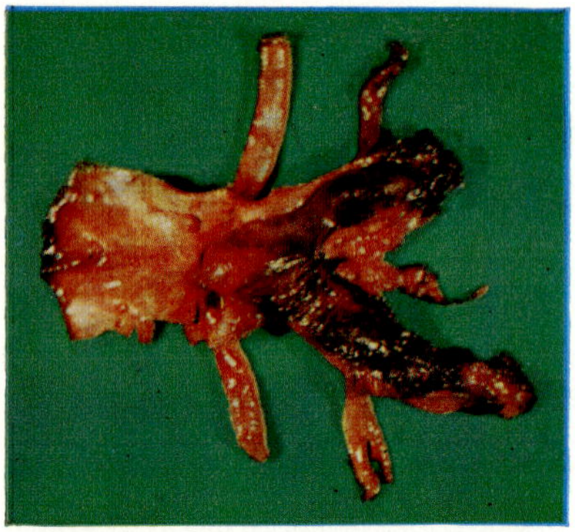

Fig. 2.1.19. — 11. Thrombosis of the iliac division of the aorta (specimen photo).

except on the hind limb(s) whose blood supply is occluded. If only one hind limb is affected, normal pulsation can be felt in the metatarsal artery of the sound limb, while no such pulsation is detectable in the affected limb. Horses that collapse with unilateral thrombosis tend to recover relatively quickly and are able to stand within minutes. With rest, the lameness will disappear and often the horse can be walked back to its stall without difficulty. However, the symptoms will return quickly if vigorous exercise is resumed. When the animal is recumbent and sweating, the veins on the affected limb(s) will be entirely collapsed, while the veins on the normal limb will stand out. Even at rest the affected member will always feel cooler than the opposite limb.

Etiology. Partial or complete occlusion of the posterior aorta or one of its branches is due to irritation of the intima, especially that caused by migrating larval forms of *Strongylus vulgaris*. The associated vascular damage leads to fibrin formation and the subsequent formation of a thrombus. Vascular damage caused by bacterial, traumatic or pharmacologic irritants is not a cause at this location.

Diagnosis. The diagnosis is based upon clinical symptoms, i.e., the collapse of one or both hind limbs following exercise. The diagnosis is confirmed by rectal examination. The posterior aorta is readily palpated in the horse, and so there should be no difficulty in detecting an absence or decrease of arterial pulsations, be it unilateral, bilateral, or affecting the posterior aorta itself. Pulsations in the metatarsal arteries are also absent or greatly diminished. Partial thromboses of the terminal branches of the aorta are manifested by firm, unilateral or bilateral enlargements in which pulsations are absent or a fremitus is felt. Pulsations in the peripheral vessels should always be compared with those in the forelimbs. In most cases cutaneous sensation is not disturbed on the affected limb. However, this may occur in extreme cases where occlusion of the vessels is sufficient to produce gangrenous changes. Many horses with intermittent claudication also have myocardial damage and suffer from pulmonary emphysema or pulmonary edema.

Differential Diagnosis. Myoglobinemia and the tying-up syndrome must be excluded. Pelvic fractures also should be excluded during the rectal examination.

Prognosis. Thromboses of the posterior aorta have an unfavorable prognosis. If the animal is rested for a month in a large stall, the vessels may be able to establish a collateral circulation that will prevent claudication during light exercise. Moreover, the thrombus may become canalized in time, resulting in improved circulation. Even in the best of circumstances, the prognosis for high-performance horses is poor.

Treatment. Treatment should be attempted in valuable horses. At one time large doses of fibrinolytic enzymes were administered intravenously. More recently, heparin has also been used. Results have not been conclusive, however. Limited movement in a large stall is helpful in promoting the development of a collateral circulation Lumbar sympathetic blockades produce dilatation of the collateral vessels for hours. while supplementary gluccorticoid injections promote the breakdown of the thrombus, Some authors [Tillotson, 1966; Branscomb, 1968; Schneider, 1976] have reported good results with the slow intravenous infusion of sodium gluconate. 500—600 mg/kg BW are administered in a 20 % solution by continuous drip infusion of 2 to $2^1/_2$ hours' duration. The infusion is discontinued at once if shock symptoms appear. In addition, the horse should be wormed with thiabendazole given at a rate of 4 g/50 kg BW once weekly for 3 weeks. This treatment may be effective in destroying migrating *Strongylus vulgaris* larvae. We have achieved good results in breeding stallions treated with a combination of coumarin and heparin.

Comments. Our own results with sodium gluconate are encouraging but require further testing. A large percentage of horses with thrombosis of the posterior aorta were sound only for breeding. Other horses had to be destroyed.

2.1.19.1.13. Hematomas of the Thigh and Croup Region

Definition. These are fist- to breadloaf-size hemorrhagic effusions that form subcutaneously or intramuscularly as a result of blunt trauma.

Symptoms. A swelling of variable size appears suddenly over the anterior stifle, posterior thigh or sometimes the medial thigh (fig. 2.1.19. — 12). It may extend to involve the muscles of the croup. Palpation reveals fluctuation as well as pain initially, but the latter decreases or disappears entirely in 8—10 days. Hematomas of the thigh and croup region usually result in a stiff, cautious gait, rather than marked lameness. However, if there is an associated rupture of one or more hindquarter muscles, a lameness will develop that is characteristic of a rupture or inflammation of the affected muscle. If the hematoma is several days old, it will have lost much of its tension, and the overlying skin will be plicated or wavy. Fluctuation rarely persists for longer than about 2 weeks, due to fibrin formation and loculation within the hematoma. The inferior portions show a greater degree of protrusion, while the superior portions appear sunken.

Etiology. Hematomas of the thigh and croup region are caused by kicks from other horses, those of the inner thigh by the straddling of sidebars in stocks, and those of the posterior thigh by contusions from the rear of stocks or by traffic accidents.

Diagnosis. The sudden appearance of a tense, fluid-containing swelling with little pain suggests the diagnosis. In doubtful cases an aspiration may be done under aseptic precautions in order to differentiate the mass from an abscess. Hematomas over the anterior stifle are easily confused with abdominal hernias. Differentiation is established by rectal examination and, if necessary, aspiration. Hematomas resulting from a femoral fracture are always accompanied by severe lameness and other characteristic fracture symptoms. Confusion with subcutaneous or subfascial abscesses or cellulitis is unlikely, as such lesions are invariably accompanied by marked lameness and systemic signs.

The *prognosis* is always favorable.

Treatment. Very large hematomas are incised at their lowest point, preferably in two places, after 8—10 days to permit spontaneous drainage. It is not unusual for several liters of serum and large amounts of blood clot to escape when large hemato-

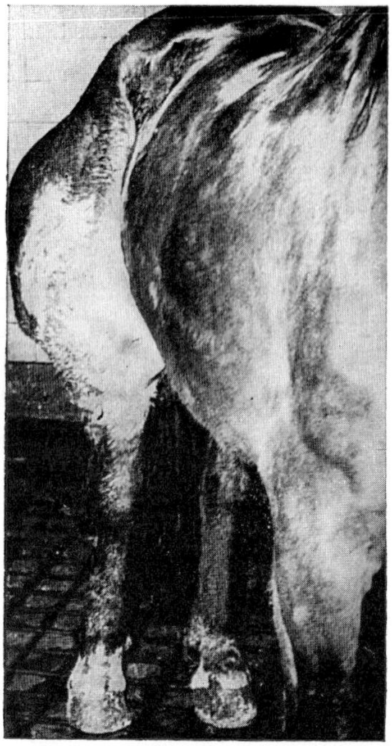

Fig. 2.1.19. — 12. Hematoma of the thigh.

mas are incised. The 'evacuation' of the incised hematoma is contraindicated. Three to four days later the hematoma cavity may be carefully flushed with antiseptic solutions such as 3 % H_2O_2, chloramine solution or acridine dye solution. The incision is treated as an open wound until resolution of the hematoma is complete. With very small hematomas, dissipation and absorption can often be achieved with nonsurgical measures, such as the application of iodine or camphor ointment.

Comments. Hematomas of the thigh and croup region should always be treated in the horse, because the organization of such hematomas results in a permanent, hard and always disfiguring enlargement that lessens the animal's value.

2.1.19.1.14. Neoplasms of the Thigh and Croup Region

Occurrence. Blastomas are relatively rare in the thigh and croup region of the horse, except in grays, which occasionally develop melanomas.

Symptoms. Masses of varying size and shape are found in the skin or subcutaneous tissue, and very rarely between the muscles. Most neoplasms are well delineated with respect to surrounding tissues. Myomas, papillomas and fibromas are most common. Blastomas of the skin or subcutaneous tissue may present a crusted, nodulated surface and bleed easily when traumatized. Lameness is extremely rare.

Diagnosis. The clinical examination enables only a presumptive diagnosis to be made. Histologic examination is necessary for definitive diagnosis.

Differential Diagnosis. Benign neoplasms that have their seat in the skin or subcutaneous tissue should not be confused with exuberant granulation or muscle hernias following major wounds of the skin or fascia. Irritations during secondary wound healing can cause tumorlike granulomas to form about the thigh and croup that may mislead the examiner.

Treatment and Prognosis. Soft-tissue tumors are extirpated in toto, and the wound is closed with sutures. Neoplasms in grays are left alone, even if they create a cosmetic blemish.

2.1.19.2. Diseases of the Stifle Joint

2.1.19.2.1. Acute Gonitis

Definition. Acute arthritis of the stifle joint may take the form of an aseptic, serous inflammation or a suppurative arthritis caused by the action of bacterial organisms. It may involve the medial or lateral half of the femorotibial joint, the femoropatellar joint, or several of these areas concurrently.

Symptoms. With acute serous gonitis, no systemic reaction occurs. When standing, the horse places little weight on the affected limb or holds the leg in a typical flexed position. When moving, the animal manifests a swinging-leg lameness. The anterior phase of the stride is shortened, weight is borne only on the toe, and full extension of the stifle and hock joints is avoided. If exercise is prolonged, the lameness will increase in severity. Conversely, the lameness will appear to improve with several days' rest. If the acute serous inflammation enters a subacute or chronic stage, atrophy will develop in the quadriceps and croup muscles. Distension is present in the affected portion(s) of the joint. This is best demonstrated by comparison with the healthy side, with the examiner standing behind the horse and alternately placing the hands around the anterior side of each stifle. Accompanying the distension are heat, pain, and possibly fluctuation. Often the lateral, middle and medial patellar ligaments are difficult to palpate in such cases.

In acute purulent gonitis caused by bacterial infection, systemic signs appear no later than 24—48 hours after the onset of the disease. The temperature rises to 39.0—39.5 °C. A moderate to severe lameness appears within 2—3 days. In the standing position the animal places little or no weight on the affected limb. If forced to move, the horse will hobble on three legs for the first few steps, then bear weight very gingerly on the affected leg. The entire stifle region is affected with phlegmonous swelling or inflammatory edema. In most cases a perforating wound can be found in the lateral part of the femorotibial joint, or sometimes in the area of the femoropatellar joint. The surrounding skin is soiled with a dried, purulent discharge. If the perforating joint wound is very recent, a flocculent synovial fluid will drip or spurt from the wound when the joint is moved. Horses that have had a suppurative gonitis for a week or so may go down and be unable to rise. Unless prompt care is rendered, a suppurative panarthritis will develop, leading to fatal septicemia.

In severe cases of acute aseptic gonitis, slight movement between the femur and tibia or mild crepitation may be detected when the femur is fixed and the tibia is moved in a cranial or lateral direction. This laxness or crepitation signifies damage to a meniscus or a tear of the anterior cruciate, posterior cruciate or medial collateral ligament.

Etiology. Acute serous aseptic gonitis is the result of a single severe contusion or mild, recurrent contusions about the stifle. When this occurs, the menisci, cruciate ligaments or collateral ligaments may become stretched or torn as a result of direct or indirect trauma.

Suppurative gonitis is generally caused by perforating wounds or blows that create a portal for infection. Metastatic cases can develop as a result of joint ill (septicemia) in foals. Finally, cellulitic abscesses of the thigh can break through into

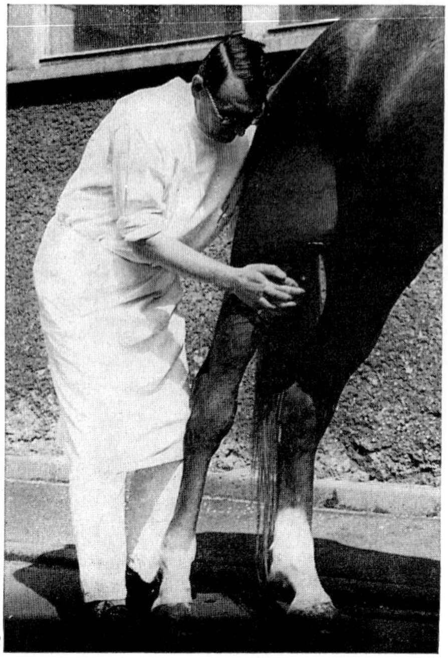

13

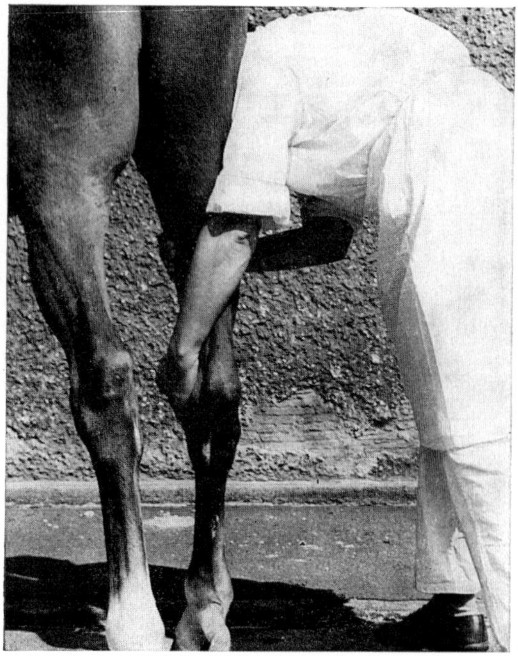

14

Fig. 2.1.19. — 13. Testing for rupture of the cruciate ligaments.
Fig. 2.1.19. — 14. Testing for rupture of a collateral ligament.

the stifle joint, usually from the popliteal fossa. Horses with brucellosis infection can contract an allergic hypersensitivity type of gonitis.

Differential Diagnosis. It is necessary to exclude supracondylar femoral fractures, patellar fractures, and fractures of the upper tibia, for periarticular fractures of this type are always associated with joint effusion. Therefore, radiographs of the stifle joint should always be obtained if possible, and should be taken in two planes to facilitate recognition of meniscus lesions and ligamentous tears.

Diagnosis. An absence of systemic signs, a swinging-leg lameness that worsens with exercise, distension of one or more parts of the joint capsule, and localized tenderness are characteristic of acute serous aseptic gonitis. The stifle is examined for lesions of the cruciate ligaments as follows: The examiner stands with his shoulder pressed against the tuber ischii, locks his hands around the anterior face of the upper tibia, and, with his knee behind the point of the hock, attempts to move the tibia posteriorally (fig. 2.1.19. — 13). Any laxness or crepitation felt during this maneuver signifies a rupture of the anterior, or rarely the posterior, cruciate ligament. This test is always negative in the normal horse.

To test for injury of the medial collateral ligament, the examiner stands next to the horse, places one hand on the inside of the hock and the other on the medial aspect of the stifle joint, and presses his shoulder against the thigh. Any lateral movement of the stifle joint indicates rupture of the medial collateral ligament. Mobility in the stifle joint is especially well palpated on the medial aspect of the joint (fig. 2.1.19. — 14).

In mild cases of acute serous aseptic gonitis, lameness will increase if the spavin test is performed. This is especially true if there are associated meniscus or ligamentous injuries. Aspiration of the joint yields a clear, red-tinged synovia. Anesthetic injections can be utilized diagnostically but are unnecessary in the presence of definite clinical signs. With arthroscopy, which can be done as a supplementary study in the recumbent, anesthetized horse, it is possible to demonstrate sites of cartilage wear, free-floating cartilage fragments, or a torn meniscus.

With suppurative gonitis, a turbid or purulent synovial fluid is discharged from the perforating joint wound. The horse is severely lame and develops systemic signs. If metastatic gonitis is suspected, aspiration is necessary to establish the diagnosis.

Prognosis. The prognosis of acute aseptic serous gonitis is good in the absence of coexisting ligamentous ruptures or meniscus injuries. If such injuries are present, the inflammation will progress to a chronic degenerative gonitis. Acute suppurative gonitis occurring as a complication of perforating joint wounds has a good prognosis if treatment is carried out within 2—3 days after the wound is sustained. Otherwise a chronic degenerative gonitis is inevitable. In addition, animals that are severely lame for a prolonged period tend to develop stress laminitis of the sound hind limb, leading to recumbency.

Treatment. Acute serous aseptic gonitis is treated with immediate rest, preferably in a large stall with soft bedding. In the absence of symptoms referable to a damaged meniscus or torn ligament, mild cases of gonitis usually respond to moist heat or topical irritants such as iodine or camphor ointment. If lameness disappears in 10 to 14 days under this regimen, rest should still be enforced for at least 4 weeks. In acute serous gonitis with more pronounced lameness, the intra-articular injection of corticosteroid solutions combined with prophylactic antibiotics may be tried. However, this treatment is contraindicated in the presence of meniscus or ligamentous tears. For very severe lameness, phenylbutazone may be given intravenously for several consecutive days. If a meniscus or ligamentous tear is present, absolute rest for 3—4 months is required. This confinement may be sufficient to return the horse to soundness.

In the presence of fresh joint wounds, sutures are placed as needed to effect closure of the wound and capsule. With a puncture wound, 10—20 % biiodate ointment is applied to the surrounding skin. If the perforating joint wound is already 2 or 3 days old, the joint is punctured in its unaffected portion, and 2—3 million I.U. of aqueous penicillin solution are injected. In addition, large doses of antibiotics should be given systemically for up to a week whenever a perforating joint wound is sustained.

Comments. If horses with acute serous aseptic gonitis are treated too late, or if meniscus or ligamentous tears are present, chronic degenerative gonitis will gradually develop. This is a serious disease that may render the animal unsound for all uses but breeding. If suppurative panarthrosis is already present, destruction of the animal should be considered.

2.1.19.2.2. Gonarthrosis (Chronic Degenerative Gonitis, Degenerative Disease of the Stifle Joint)

Definition. Gonarthrosis is a degenerative disease of the stifle joint that occurs in older horses and very often progresses to a chronic gonitis or is associated with it.

Symptoms. The early stage of a gonarthrosis or chronic degenerative gonitis usually goes unnoticed by the owner or attendant. Following strenuous work or racing, a mild lameness is observed that disappears with rest, but gradually becomes more pro-

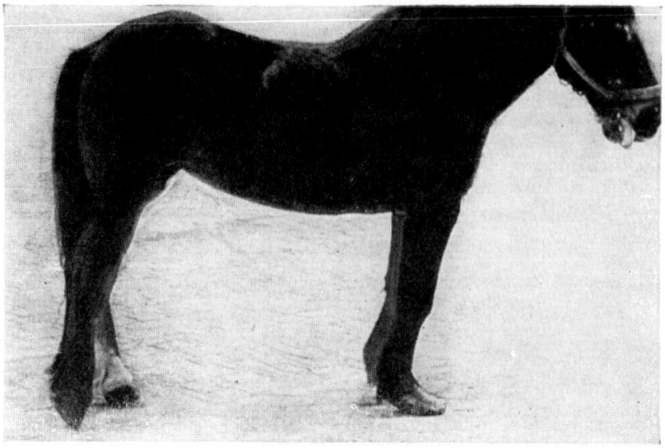

Fig. 2.1.19. — 15. Typical limb carriage in gonarthrosis.

nounced over a period of weeks or months. The lameness is of the mixed type but is most apparent in the swinging-leg phase. This causes increased stress and wear to the anterior hoof wall, especially at the start of exercise. The forward motion of the limb is delayed and somewhat stiff, and the anterior phase of the stride is shortened. As in acute gonitis, the horse attempts to take weight off the affected limb when standing by keeping the leg in slight flexion and holding the foot off the ground (fig. 2.1.19. — 15). The toe of the shoe is excessively worn, as in spavin. The spavin test is positive, especially if it is combined with a simultaneous rotation of the stifle. As the degenerative changes in the femorotibial joint surfaces progress, irregular-shaped areas of reactive new bone growth appear on the medial aspect of the upper tibia, causing a narrowing of the palpable joint space. The quadriceps and gluteal muscles gradually become atrophic. As time passes, the disease spreads to involve the femoropatellar joint, which shows marked fluid distension.

In heavy draft horses that have spent years working on uneven ground, it is not unusual for a gonarthrosis or chronic degenerative gonarthritis to develop in both the stifle joints. In such cases the hind limbs move in short steps with a 'tiptoe' gait and straight hocks. The animal falls easily on hard pavement and has great difficulty getting back on its feet. Many such horses refuse to lie down and gradually become emaciated. When standing, the animal tends to hold the affected limb off the ground and will bear weight only momentarily on the anterior hoof wall.

Palpation of the affected limb reveals slight distension of the medial and later the lateral joint half. This is sufficient to hinder palpation of the three patellar ligaments. Percussion with a hammer produces mild pain. The diameter of the stifle joint appears enlarged when viewed from the side. If the animal is forced to do work, the lameness will become noticeably worse.

Etiology. Gonarthrosis or chronic degenerative gonitis is a disease of attrition. The most common cause is prolonged, excessive mechanical stress on the stifle joint. The continual pulling of heavy loads, fast checks by a rider, and repeated quick turns like those executed in the show ring can all lead to degenerative changes in the stifle joint. Similar changes are produced by severe sprains or contusions with associated meniscus and ligamentous damage, faults of conformation, and improper shoeing. Signs of wear develop initially in the articular cartilage and joint capsule and later involve the bone. Degenerative joint disease of the stifle is becoming increasingly common in horses used for serum production.

Differential Diagnosis. The less common hip joint diseases, spavin, chronic diseases of the hock joint and sesamoiditis must be excluded. Gonarthrosis or chronic degenerative gonarthritis must not be confused with gonotrochleosis or osteochondrosis of the femoropatellar joint occurring in foals.

Diagnosis. The history is significant. Palpation and percussion of the stifle joint region elicits only mild pain. The affected portions of the joint usually show slight distension, though this is not always present. The spavin test (flexion test) is always positive. Horses with gonarthrosis generally have a milder reaction to this test than do horses with true spavin lameness. If the disease has been present for some months, marked lipping is palpable at the joint margins. Diagnostic injections can be used to accurately localize the affected portion or portions of the joint. The first injection should be made into the medial half of the femorotibial joint. If the lameness is not alleviated by the injection of about 40 ml of a concentrated anesthetic solution, the lateral half of the joint should also be injected. Radiographs taken in two planes can also contribute to the diagnosis even in the early stage of the disease. In longstanding cases, exostoses can be demonstrated at the attachment of the joint capsule, together with areas of cartilage wear and separation. Detached cartilage fragments may also be found as free-floating loose bodies within the joint. Aspiration yields a largely acellular synovial fluid with a slight reddish discoloration. If necessary, arthroscopy may be used to visualize meniscus lesions, cartilage wear, cartilage defects, loose bodies, and thickened, elongated synovial villi.

Prognosis. The prognosis is poor. Due to the presence of primary degenerative changes in the joint, only several months of confinement combined with cartilage-regenerating drug therapy offers a chance of improvement.

Treatment. The horse is confined to a large box stall. Intra-articular injections of an hyaluronic acid preparation may be tried once weekly for 6—8 weeks. Recently, good results have been reported with intra-articular injections of hyaluronic acid. Because primary degenerative changes are involved, the injection of glucocorticoid preparations into the stifle joint can be of only temporary benefit. In any case, such treatment is contraindicated because it enables the animal to place undue stress on the diseased joint, causing further damage. The use of cautery or counterirritants in animals with gonarthrosis remains controversial. This includes the application of blistering agents, most notably red biiodate ointment. Corrective shoeing is also indicated. Shoes with calks and means for toe alignment should be used to improve the flight of the foot at the walk. Shoeing of this type is effective only on hard ground, however. Even after firing and blistering, the horse should have a least 4—6 months' enforced rest in a large stall.

Comments. It may be possible to keep broodmares with gonarthrosis or chronic degenerative gonitis in breeding condition by implementing the therapeutic measures recommended above. In all other cases, destruction should be considered.

2.1.19.2.3. Chronic Gonitis due to Ossification of the Menisci

Definition. This is an ossifying process affecting mainly the medial meniscus of the stifle joint and leading gradually to the clinical picture of chronic gonitis. The disease has been diagnosed by Huskamp and Verharr [1977], by Valdez and Adams [1978] and by us, in 1978 and 1979, in several clinical patients.

Symptoms. This form of gonitis appears to affect show horses, military horses and jumpers. The animals present with a history of gradually progressive lameness in one of the hind limbs that is most pronounced after exercise. So far, we have always

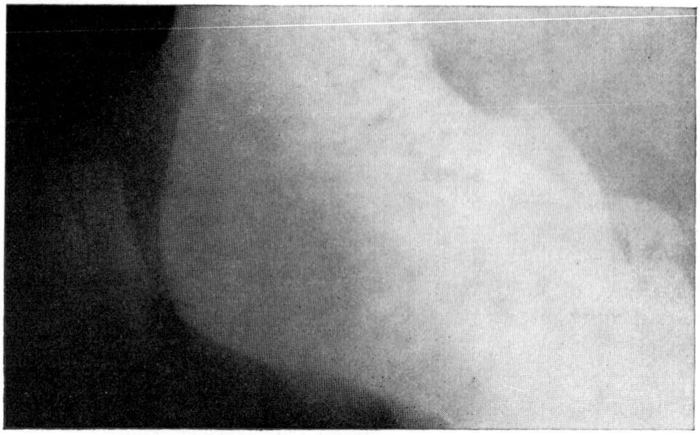

Fig. 2.1.19. — 16. Ossification of the medial meniscus, preoperative x-ray (oblique view).

been able to exclude the hock joint and distal limb as the seat of the lameness by means of diagnostic anesthesia. Anesthesia of the medial part of the stifle joint always improves the lameness but does not relieve it completely.

Etiology. It is known that the menisci, by their interposition between the femur and tibia, create a 'functional congruity' between these bones that would otherwise be lacking between the physically incongruent articular surfaces. The medial meniscus, like other medial joint structures, is subjected to greater stresses than the lateral meniscus. Apparently this predisposes the elastic cartilage of this meniscus to premature ossification, especially in animals that have led a life of strenuous physical exertion (fig. 2.1.19. — 16). The result is a gradual loss of the shock-absorbing capability of the meniscus, and a kind of ankylosis develops in the medial and posterior parts of the joint. The ligaments that anchor the meniscus to the femur and tibia gradually become involved in the ossifying process.

Diagnosis. Besides diagnostic injections of local anesthetic into the medial part of the femorotibial joint, radiographic examination in the latero-medial view enables a definitive diagnosis to be made.

Treatment and Prognosis. HUSKAMP and VERHAAR [1977] and VALDEZ and ADAMS [1978] have proposed a partial or complete meniscectomy to treat the condition. HUSKAMP and VERHAAR [1977] perform a partial meniscectomy by opening the joint caudal to the medial collateral ligament and resecting the ossified meniscus. VALDEZ and ADAMS [1978] recommend a complete medial meniscectomy. They open the stifle joint from the medial side by making one incision through the skin and joint capsule directly posterior to the medial patellar ligament, and a second, parallel incision caudal to the medial capsular ligament. First the ligaments anchoring the meniscus to the femoral condyles and tibia are divided through these two incisions. When the meniscus is freed from its sites of attachment, it is removed through the posterior incision. The arthrotomy wound should heal without complications, as confirmed by our own limited experience with this procedure. The effect of a partial or complete meniscectomy on the animal's athletic performance is difficult to predict. Some patients will be able to return to racing, while others will be fit only for use as pleasure or breeding stock.

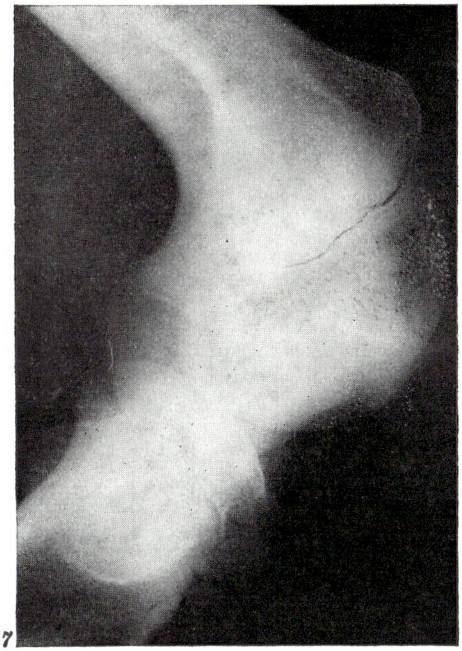

17

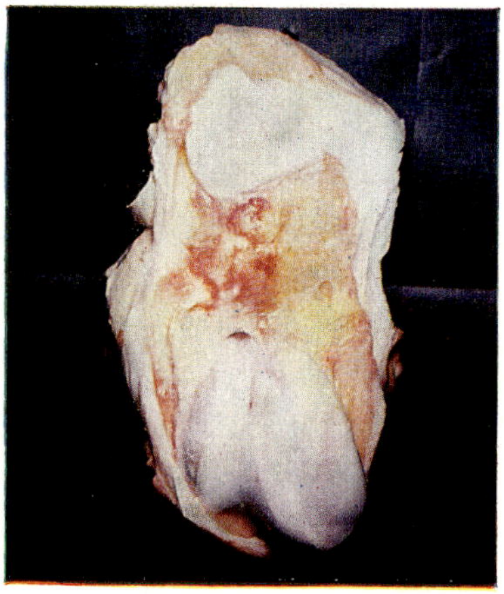

18

Fig. 2.1.19. — 17. Gonotrochleosis: articular defects.
Fig. 2.1.19. — 18. Gonotrochleosis (specimen photo).

2.1.19.2.4. Gonotrochleosis (Arthrosis of the Femoropatellar Joint, Osteochondrosis of the Femoropatellar Joint)

Definition. This is a very severe degenerative disease of the femoropatellar joint that develops as a sequel to osteochondritis dissecans. Cartilage defects occur mainly on the lateral femoral condyle and articular surface of the patella (figs. 2. 1. 19. — 17 through — 19). The disease is accompanied by a loss of depth in the trochlear groove and a dysplastic remodeling of the lateral femoral condyle. Detached cartilage fragments may enter the joint as loose bodies or remain adherent to the synovial membrane (fig. 2.1.19. — 20).

Symptoms. The earliest symptoms may appear at the age of 5—6 months, though the disease is also observed up to 3 years of age. At one time it was assumed that only foals of the cold-blooded breeds were affected, but in recent years the disease has been described in foals of all breeds. The onset of the disease usualy goes unnoticed by the owner or breeder. In most cases, distension is noticed in one or both stifle joints purely by chance. This is accompanied by an unsteady gait with a shortened stride. A moderate to severe mixed lameness usually appears several weeks or months afterwards. When standing, the foal holds the limb in slight flexion with only the toe or front of the hoof touching the ground. When moving, the animal avoids extending the joints and does not contact the ground squarely with the foot. Atrophy of the croup and thigh muscles develops in long-standing cases. Because weight is borne only on the toe, the heels grow long, leading to the development of

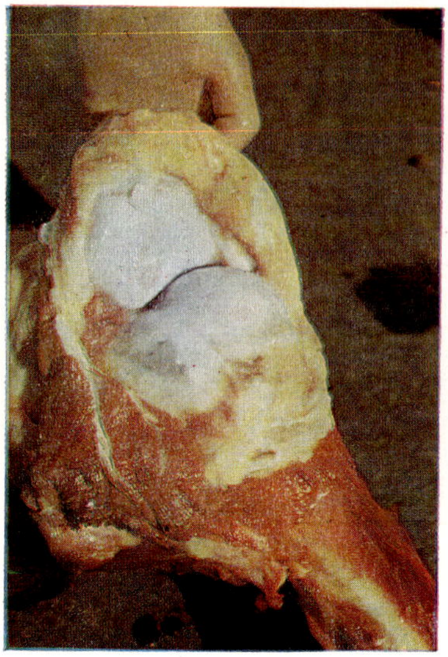

19

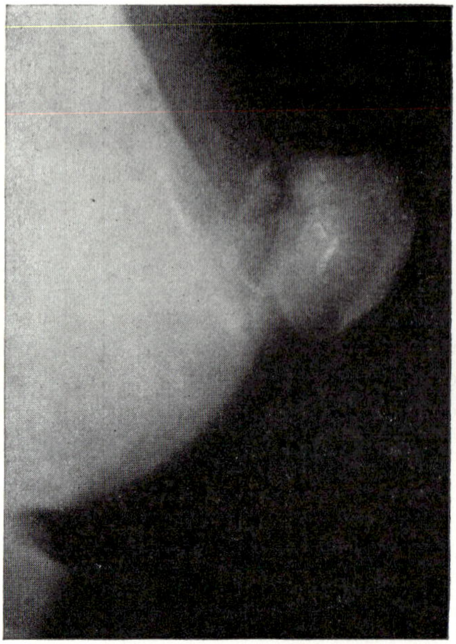

20

Fig. 2.1.19. — 19. Osteochondrosis: articular defects on the femoral condyles and patella.
Fig. 2.1.19. — 20. Cartilage fragment (loose body) in the femoropatellar joint.

a club foot that may simulate knuckling due to tendon disease. Local findings include distention of the femoropatellar joint, which in long-standing cases can spread to involve both the medial and lateral portions of the femorotibial joint. There is no local heat or pain. The cartilage wear on the lateral condyle and flattening of the intercondylar groove are accompanied by a stretching and loosening of the straight patellar ligaments that is characteristic of gonotrochleosis.

The dysplastic changes in the lateral condyle, distension of the femoropatellar joint and stretching of the patellar ligaments create a situation in which the patella can easily dislocate over the flattened lateral femoral condyle. This abnormal patellar mobility may be evident with each stride and is easily palpated by placing the hand onto the stifle joint while the animal is walking. In the standing animal, the patella can easily be pushed laterally out of the trochlear groove, and this will be accompanied by a snapping or crepitus-like sound. Usually the patella will slip back into place spontaneously when released. If the condition is bilateral, the animal goes on its toes in a somewhat stiff, semicrouched stance.

Etiology. The actual cause of the disease is unknown. It affects well-nourished, rapidly-growing foals. Often the juvenile cartilage is not mature enough to withstand the stresses placed upon it. Accordingly we might ascribe the disease to disturbances of epiphyseal maturation, as in dogs and swine, later leading to osteochondritis dissecans and ultimately to degenerative changes in the femoropatellar joint. The increased incidence in certain lines is consistent with the theory that the disease is inherited as a recessive trait. In cold-blooded foals, the left femoropatellar joint is more commonly affected.

Differential Diagnosis. The absence of systemic signs in gonotrochleosis serves to differentiate this condition from infectious diseases complicated by polyarthritis (e.g., foal septicemia). The disease is most commonly mistaken for a sustained or intermittent upward or lateral luxation of the patella. In patellar luxations, however, effusion is absent, the patellar ligaments are tense, and the femoral condyles and intercondylar groove are well formed.

Diagnosis. Three stages can be distinguished in gonotrochleosis of the foal:

1. The first symptom is distension of the femoropatellar joint unaccompanied by lameness. It is generally caused by osteochondritis dissecans, which produces distension by irritating the synovial membrane, as in osteochondritis dissecans of the hock joint.
2. The cartilage fragments, whether adherent to the synovial membrane or floating freely in the joint as loose bodies, lead to chronic irritation of the synovial membrane and to increased wear of the articular surfaces of the femur and patella. This in turn leads to lameness with a characteristic limb carriage during standing and weight-bearing on the toe during progression.
3. The final stage of the disease is characterized by stretching of the patellar ligaments, dysplastic changes in the lateral condyle with severe cartilage wear, and a moderate to severe lameness. The clinical picture is typical of advanced degenerative joint disease. This, combined with the abnormal patellar mobility, enables a clinical diagnosis to be made. Radiographs should also be taken in two planes, as they have an important bearing on the prognosis. They will reveal articular defects, detached osteochondral fragments, subchondral osteoporosis and other subcartilaginous structural changes, as well as a flattened lateral femoral condyle and shallow intercondylar groove. Diagnostic injections of the affected joints are usually unnecessary. The history, clinical picture and radiographic findings enable a definitive diagnosis to be made.

Necropsy Findings. A large amount of red-tinged synovial fluid is found in the femoropatellar and femorotibial joints. The synovial villi show proliferation and may be several millimeters long. Marked degenerative changes are noted on the articular surface of the patella and on the lateral femoral condyle, and reactive changes may be evident at the attachment of the joint capsule. Facet-like wear spots are frequently found on the lateral femoral condyle.

Prognosis. The prognosis is poor, unless the foal has received appropriate treatment in the early stage of the disease, and the clinical symptoms are referable entirely to osteochondritis dissecans, with no patellar dislocation. Sometimes improvement is seen following months of pasturing. Even if soundness is restored, however, the foal has no future as a performance horse.

Treatment. Because osteochondritis dissecans constitutes the early stage of the disease, an arthrotomy should be undertaken if osteochondral fragments are present in the joint as loose bodies, or if radiographs suggest that such fragments are adherent to the synovial membrane. If distension has developed as a result of irritation, it is still possible to relieve functional disability by surgical removal of the cartilage fragments.

In the early stage of the disease, it may be useful to follow removal of the cartilage fragments with an intra-articular injection of hyaluronic acid preparations. The intramuscular administration of anabolics is also performed by some.

The intra-articular use of glucocorticoids is dangerous and contraindicated. Firing and blistering are equally hazardous and are also contraindicated.

Comments. The surgical treatment of gonotrochleosis is indicated only in the early stage of the disease. In advanced cases, destruction is necessary once a diagnosis has been made.

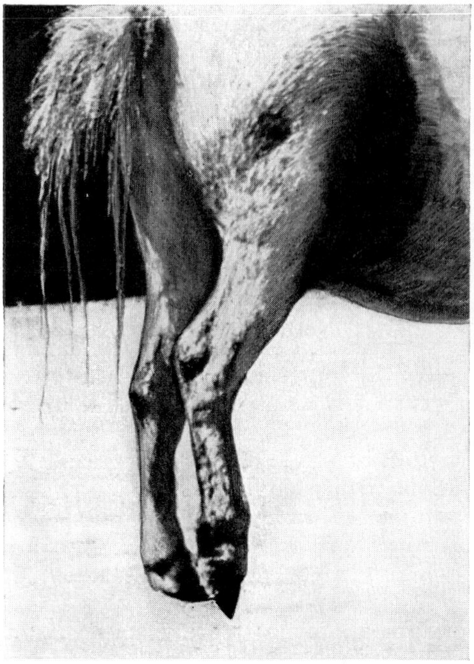

21

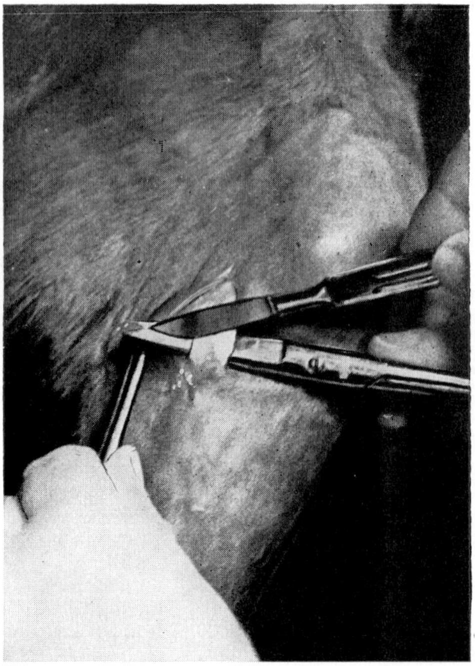

22

Fig. 2.1.19. — 21. Upward fixation of the patella, clinical picture.
Fig. 2.1.19. — 22. Upward fixation of the patella: desmotomy of the medial patellar ligament.

2.1.19.2.5. Luxation of the Patella

Definition. This is a sustained or recurrent luxation in which the patella becomes positioned on top of the medial femoral condyle or dislocates laterally out of the trochlear groove. Medial luxation of the patella is extremely rare in the horse.

Symptoms. With *upward* luxation of the patella, known also as *upward fixation*, the patella glides upward during maximal extension of the limb and catches over the medial condyle of the femur. This causes the stifle and hock joints to become locked in an extended position (figs. 2.1.19. — 21 and — 22). This in turn leads to a simultaneous flexion of the fetlock, pastern and coffin joints, so that the anterior wall of the hoof rests on the ground. If now the horse steps slightly to the side or if it is driven forward with a whip, the patella may go back into place with an audible snap. This process can occur spontaneously and repeatedly during further progression, creating a condition of recurrent luxation (intermittent upward fixation). In other cases the patella may remain locked in upward fixation. If the horse is forced to walk in this condition, with the stifle and hock joints extended and the digital joints flexed, the limb is advanced in an outward arc with the front of the hoof dragging the ground. While the limb is locked, the patella can be palpated on the medial femoral condyle, together with the tightly-stretched patellar ligaments.

Lateral luxation of the patella tends to be sustained and is characterized by flexion of the stifle and hock joints when weight is placed on the affected limb (figs. 2.1.19. – 23 and — 24). This effect is so pronounced that the limb appears to collapse at the moment weight is borne. Frequently the quadriceps muscle appears atrophied. On

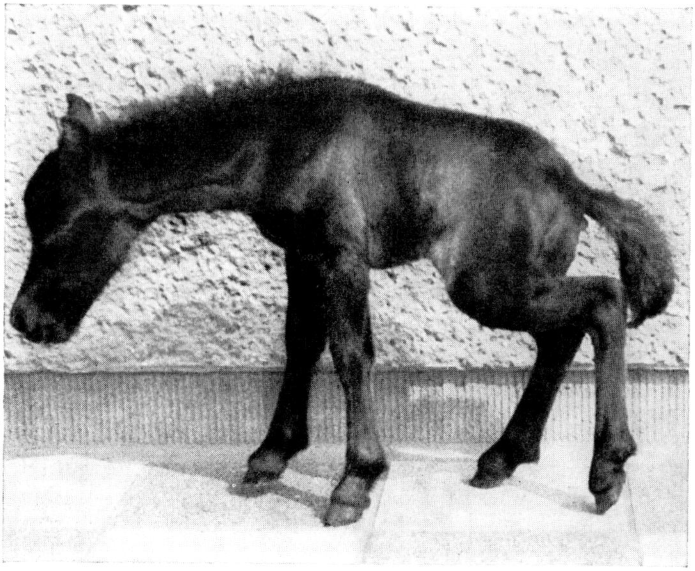

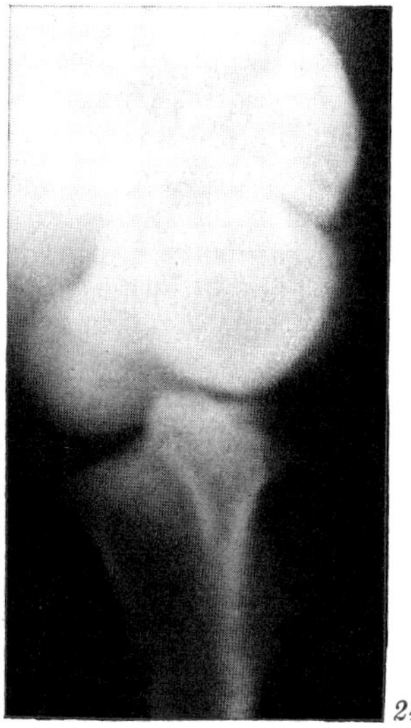

24

23

Fig. 2.1.19. — 23. Congenital lateral luxation of the patella.
Fig. 2.1.19. — 24. Radiograph of stifle joint in fig. 2.1.19. — 23.

palpation of the stifle, the patella can be felt in its abnormal position over the lateral femoral condyle. Recurrent lateral luxation may occur in ponies, especially Shetlands. In this case the patella slips laterally out of the trochlear groove and glides up onto the lateral condyle, then slips back into place a few moments later. When the horse is standing, the patella can be manually dislocated laterally out of the trochlear groove. Often this is possible in both stifle joints of ponies.

Occasionally a congenital lateral patellar luxation is seen in foals. Affected foals walk with a 'creeping' action in the hindquarters and are unable to extend the stifle and hock.

Etiology. Intermittent upward fixation of the patella is frequently congenital but usually does not become clinically manifest until the animal is 2 or 3 years old. Traumatic cases result from excessive contraction of the quadriceps muscle during hyperextension of the limb. This may occur when the animal stands, slips, jumps, kicks violently with the hind limbs, or is forcibly pulled out of stocks from behind. Obstetric manipulations can also cause upward fixation of the patella through traction on the fetal hind limbs during a breech delivery.

Sustained lateral luxation of the patella is caused by extreme stretching or rupture of the medial patellar ligament. The condition is congenital in ponies and is associated with a flattening of the trochlear groove and lateral femoral condyle.

Diagnosis. The diagnosis is made from the clinical picture and findings on palpation and can be confirmed by radiography, especially in cases of lateral luxation.

Differential Diagnosis. Lateral patellar luxation in young horses and ponies should not be mistaken for gonotrochleosis or osteochondritis dissecans of the femoropatellar joint. In contrast to gonotrochleosis, distension of the femoropatellar joint is rarely present in acquired patellar luxations. Radiography can also be used to make the differentiation. Acquired lateral patellar luxations produce clinical signs that are very similar to quadriceps or femoral nerve paralysis. In quadriceps paralysis, however, the patella remains seated with the trochlear groove.

Prognosis. In sustained or recurrent upward fixation of the patella, the prognosis for functional recovery is good. With lateral luxations of the patella due to traumatic causes, the prognosis is poor in large horses, but is favorable in small horses due to the possibility of surgical correction.

Treatment. Upward fixation of the patella may reduce spontaneously with an audible and palpable snap. When this occurs, all clinical symptoms disappear immediately; most notably, the stifle and hock joints are no longer locked in extension. This reduction may be permanent. Sometimes the patella can be released by walking the horse several steps backward, preferably on a slight downslope. Backing out of a horse trailer, for example, will generally disengage the patella. If a reduction cannot be obtained in this way, the limb should be pulled forward and slightly upward with the aid of a rope passed over the animal's neck and around the fetlock. The horse is forced to step forward, and at the same time the patella is pushed medially and downward until it slips back into the trochlear groove. If this also fails, we recommend anesthetizing the horse and administering muscle relaxants, and then attempting the reduction with the animal cast onto the healthy side. Usually reduction can also be achieved by restraining the animal with barbiturate injections or with central- or peripheral-acting muscle relaxants. Finally, a sustained upward fixation can be relieved by performing a desmotomy of the medial patellar ligament. This may be done either under general anesthesia with the animal recumbent, or under local anesthesia with the animal standing.

Intermittent catching of the patella may occur when the animal is standing up, turning, backing, or during the first few steps of walking. This causes a 'hitching' gait in which movement is periodically interrupted by brief extension of the limb each time the patella catches, followed by an audible snap as the patella slips back into place. As in recurrent upward fixation of the patella, the treatment of choice is desmotomy of the medial patellar ligament. The procedure is done under infiltration anesthesia with the animal standing. The medial patellar ligament is severed just above its tibial attachment. In quiet animals the skin incision may be dispensed with, and a sharp-pointed desmotone may be inserted directly through the skin. The ligament is then severed using control by palpation. Hickman and Walker suggested in 1964 that medial patellar desmotomy for recurrent upward fixation be dispensed with in favor of a resection of the fibrous accessory cartilage, a finger-thick structure that passes in hook fashion from the medial ligament to the patella. The procedure is done with the animal recumbent. The accessory cartilage is exposed and resected, taking care not to damage the medial patellar ligament. Reportedly this operation prevents the recurrences that are occasionally observed following a medial patellar desmotomy.

With sustained lateral patellar luxation, point firing and blistering may be the only means available for stabilizing the stifle ligaments. Results are uncertain.

Singh Rathor and Numans [1971] have tested and recommended surgical treatment for recurrent *lateral* patellar luxation. The idea is to eliminate all lateral forces exerted on the patella by fascia, muscles and ligaments. The skin incision extends from the lower third of the femur to the upper third of the tibia on the lateral aspect of the stifle joint. The fascia lata is incised, and the biceps femoris and vastus lateralis muscles are exposed. The tendinous portion of the cranial part of the biceps femoris muscle is divided at its lateral insertion on the patella. The vastus lateralis is likewise divided at its patellar attachment. Following reduction of the patella, the stifle joint is extended. If this again causes the patella to dislocate, additional tissues attaching laterally to the patella must be severed. The procedure concludes by placing a reefing (imbricating) suture on the medial surface of the stifle.

Comments. Horses with sustained upward patellar fixation should return to full soundness, regardless of therapy. Horses with recurrent upward fixation may never be sound for high-performance work. Horses with sustained lateral patellar luxation are at best fit for breeding use. In ponies with recurrent lateral patellar luxation, surgical treatment should be attempted and in many cases will restore the animal to soundness. However, it must be considered that the condition is hereditary in some instances.

2.1.19.2.6. Fracture of the Patella

Definition. Patellar fractures may be closed or open, single or multiple. Because the patella is embedded in the tendon of the quadriceps muscle and also limits the stifle joint and femoropatellar joint anteriorally, the majority of patellar fractures that are not of the chip variety represent intra-articular fractures, with the fracture line extending into the joint. Patellar fractures may also be characterized as horizontal (transverse) or vertical (longitudinal).

Symptoms. With nearly all patellar fractures, a severe mixed lameness develops within hours after the injury, or weight is not supported on the affected limb. If weight-bearing is attempted, the limb will probably give way at the stifle joint, especially when a horizontal fracture is present, because fixation of the joint is impossible or at least very painful. Swelling is apparent and is most pronounced in the anterior part of the joint. The presence of effusion and associated distension of the femorotibial or femoropatellar joint is a sure sign of articular involvement in the fracture. Crepitation usually cannot be detected. With open and infected fractures, it may be possible to detect a fragment by probing. With closed horizontal and vertical fractures and with chip fractures, the lameness and signs of periarticular inflammation may be somewhat less pronounced.

Etiology. The etiology is trauma. Kicks from other horses are usually responsible.

Diagnosis is established by the functional disturbances, findings on palpation and radiographic examination.

Differential diagnosis must be made from acute gonitis, distal infrapatellar or prepatellar bursitis, lateral patellar luxation and quadriceps paralysis.

Treatment. Closed patellar fractures in the horse are treated conservatively. With chip fractures, the surgical removal of small fragments should be considered. The prognosis is always guarded.

Comments. Chronic degenerative disease of the femoropatellar joint is a probable sequel to all types of patellar fracture in the horse.

2.1.19.2.7. Bursitides of the Stifle Joint (Subpatellar Bursitis, Prepatellar Bursitis)

Definition. The subpatellar bursa is a cherry- to plum-size bursa located at the tibial attachment of the middle patellar ligament. The prepatellar bursa is a subcutaneous pad located on the cranial surface of the patella. Aseptic or pyogenic processes may be involved in inflammation of these bursae.

Symptoms. Subpatellar bursitis is manifested by a round, fluctuating, approximately plum-size subcutaneous swelling on the anterior side of the tibia about a hand's width below the patella. Heat and pain are usually present. If the bursa is open, flocculent synovial fluid will drain intermittently from the wound. A mucoid coating or crust is found on the skin around and especially below the wound. If the bursa is infected, a parabursal cellulitis will also be present. With prepatellar bursitis, similar symptoms are evident on the anterior surface of the patella. Both aseptic and pyogenic cases are usually accompanied by a mild to moderate mixed lameness. If untreated, aseptic bursitides will undergo organization and develop a cystlike loculation.

Etiology. Both bursae can be contused by blunt trauma, and this is the cause of aseptic forms. Perforating wounds of the bursae are caused by kicks and pitchfork injuries.

Diagnosis is made from local findings.

Differential Diagnosis. The aseptic forms of this inflammation should not be confused with gonotrochleosis in young animals or with aseptic gonitis or gonarthrosis in older horses.

Treatment. In acute cases of aseptic prepatellar bursitis, iodine- or camphor-containing ointments can be applied to promote dissipation and absorption of effusions. However, clinical symptoms are relieved more rapidly by aspiration of the bursa followed by the injection of a glucocorticoid solution (up to 200 mg prednisolone or 40—60 mg dexamethasone). Sclerosing infections of tincture of iodine into an aseptically inflamed bursa are not without risk. The femorotibial or femoropatellar joint may become opened and infected as a result of such treatment. Fresh, small bursal wounds are closed immediately by suture; a blister is applied around puncture wounds.

Organized, older bursitides or bursal hygromas represent cosmetic defects. The only remedy is complete extirpation.

2.1.19.3. Diseases of the Gaskin

2.1.19.3.1. Wounds and Wound Infection

Definition and Occurrence. The medial side of the gaskin is not heavily muscled like the lateral and anterior sides, and so wounds of the skin, periosteum and bone can occur in this area. The anterior and lateral sides of the gaskin can sustain wounds of the muscles, fascia, tendons and tendon sheaths. Such wounds are susceptible to infection by pyogenic or bacterial organisms, leading to subcutaneous, subfascial or even intermuscular cellulitis, fascial necrosis, and purulent tendovaginitis near the hock joint. Bony wounds on the medial side of the gaskin are susceptible to bacterial infection resulting in purulent periostitis, ostitis, or even purulent osteomyelitis in the case of fractures.

Symptoms. Recent lacerations, puncture wounds and contusions of the skin, underlying fascia and tibial muscles are characterized by symptoms typical of a fresh wound, and may produce no other symptoms in the absence of complete muscle ruptures (fig. 2.1.19. — 25). Injuries of the medial surface (planum cutaneum) cause contusions and wounds of the periosteum and sometimes of the bone. Such wounds are very painful and therefore cause an immediate moderate to severe lameness.

Within a few hours after the injury, a warm, very painful swelling arising from the medial surface of the gaskin is detected on palpation. By the 2nd or 3rd day the inflammatory swelling has spread to involve the entire gaskin region. At this point lameness is severe, and systemic signs appear such as fever and signs of systemic pyogenic infection. Symptoms of septicemia will also be present if bacterial organisms

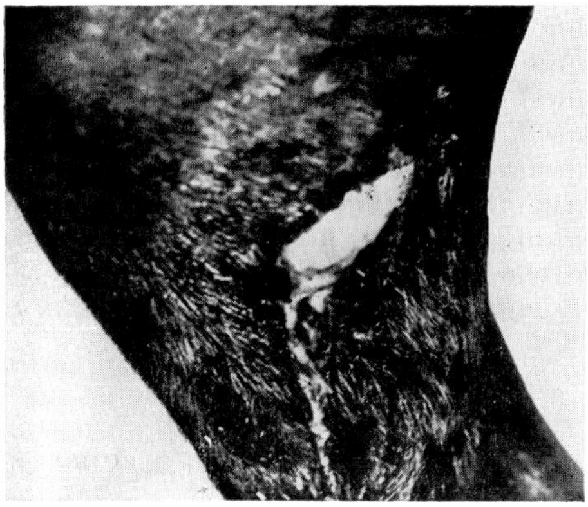

25

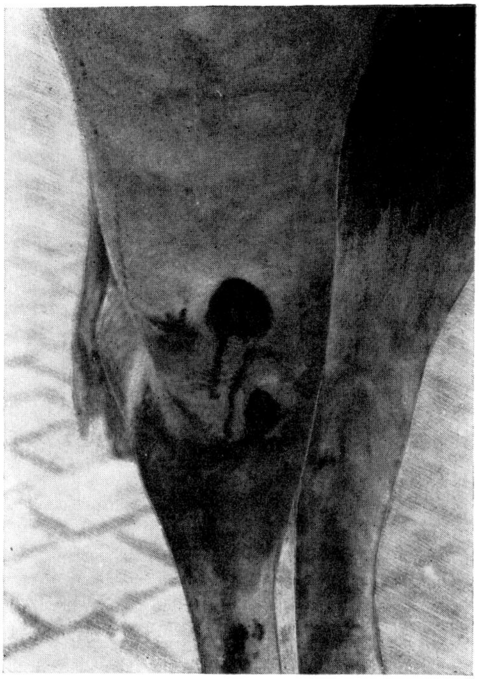

26

Fig. 2.1.19. — *25.* Laceration of the gaskin.
Fig. 2.1.19. — *26.* Cellulitic abscessation in the gaskin region.

have infected the wound. A yellowish, mucoid exudate is discharged from the wound and will be permeated with gas bubbles in the presence of aerobic or anaerobic bacteria. If small periosteal and osseous wounds on the medial side of the tibia are several weeks old, fistula-like wound openings will be evident, together with small areas of exuberant granulation. Fibrous induration is also found in the area surrounding these openings.

Perforating wounds of various tendon sheaths that course through the gaskin region, such as the extensor digitalis longus and tibialis cranialis tendon sheaths, cause circumscribed swellings to appear. These are found either lateral to and below the stifle joint or directly on the anterior surface of the gaskin above the hock joint. In both cases there may be painful fluctuation and tension. These tendon-sheath infections have a tendency to spread. Thus, a purulent tendovaginitis of the long digital extensor on the lateral side of the stifle can easily invade the lateral part of the femorotibial joint, giving rise to a suppurative gonitis. With purulent tendovaginitis of the tibialis cranialis muscle, a diffuse, subfascial cellulitis can develop leading rapidly to a systemic pyogenic infection. In both cases the animal is severely lame and usually places no weight on the affected limb.

Etiology. Lacerations of the gaskin region are caused by barbed wire. Lacerations and contusions of the medial side of the gaskin are caused by kicks, and a fissure fracture of the tibia should always be suspected if this history is given. Suture dehiscence following a neurectomy of the tibial nerve or deep fibular nerve can lead to subcutaneous and subfascial cellulitis. Streptococci are the principal infectious organisms of most gaskin wounds.

Differential Diagnosis. Fissured and depressed fractures of the tibia should be considered and can be excluded if necessary by radiography. Moreover, it should be remembered that a fissure fracture can easily be converted to a complete fracture by the simple act of lying down or standing up. Purulent tendovaginitis of the long digital extensor may be confused with an acute suppurative gonitis. Purulent tendovaginitis of the tibialis cranialis muscle should not be mistaken for a suppurative inflammation of the hock joint.

Diagnosis. A diffuse, hot, painful swelling in the gaskin region associated with mild lameness and few if any systemic signs is suggestive of subcutaneous cellulitis. However, a tense, possibly fluctuant swelling extending to the popliteal fossa associated with severe lameness and a marked systemic reaction indicates a subfascial cellulitis that is undergoing abscessation (fig. 2.1.19. — 26). Wounds that damage the periosteum on the medial aspect of the tibia, or that expose the cortical bone, lead within days to a suppurative, ossifying periostitis, purulent osteitis and osteomyelitis. A highly purulent exudate is discharged from such wounds. A probe when inserted may encounter rough bony tissue or may even enter the medullary cavity of the tibia in the presence of a depressed fracture. Older cases, as mentioned, show typical bony fistulae and exuberant granulation tissue. During radiographic examination, it may be possible to insert a probe into the fistulous tract and thus obtain further information on the extent of a purulent osteitis or osteomyelitis and on any bone sequestra that may be present. Complete and incomplete fractures can be excluded by the radiographic examination. With purulent tendovaginitis of the common digital extensor, the fluctuation is localized on the lateral side of the hock joint a short distance below the stifle.

Treatment and Prognosis. Fresh wounds of the skin, fascia and muscle are managed according to general surgical principles: debridement, suturing, and, if necessary, antibiotic and tetanus prophylaxis. If a wound has been inflicted by a dirty object, rotted wood or rusty metal, the injection of a polyvalent clostridial antiserum is indicated. With subcutaneous cellulitis, the prognosis for recovery is good. Hyperemia is stimulated with moist or dry heat, and absorption-promoting ointments are applied. In the absence of fever, mild exercise may be used to promote absorption. With subfascial cellulitis that is undergoing abscessation, spontaneous rupture is often a very slow process, and so an incision should be made at the lowest point of the tense fluctuation, or sometimes in the popliteal fossa. This should be done at the earliest opportunity; otherwise the suppurative process will invariably break through into the tendon sheaths at the hock joint or even into the hock joint itself. The incision is followed by antiseptic irrigation. In some circumstances a counterincision must be placed and a drain inserted. Necrosis of the fasciae and portions of the tendons and muscles sometimes occurs. Long-acting antibiotics or sulfonamides should be administered intramuscularly or intravenously, respectively, until fever is gone. This treatment should be continued for 6—8 days. In the presence of cellulitic abscessation, the patient should not be moved until fever has subsided. The prognosis is guarded. With purulent osteitis and osteomyelitis, and in cases where fistulae have formed on the inside of the gaskin, the focus in the bone must be surgically exposed and excavated. Sequestra must be removed. If the medullary cavity is opened during the operation, it should be curetted over a circumscribed area and filled at regular intervals with antibiotic solutions and ointments. Postoperative treatment should be administered under a bandage, if possible, and should be continued until healthy, dry, pink granulation tissue has formed. This is accompanied by systemic treatment with antibiotics and sulfonamides until fever is gone. The prognosis is guarded. Suppurative lesions of the bone sometimes take a very protracted course. They may be complicated in 4—6 weeks by tibial fractures if undue stress is placed on the limb.

For purulent tendovaginitis of the long digital extensor, an incision is made in the lower part of the gaskin. If the suppuration does not yet involve the stifle joint,

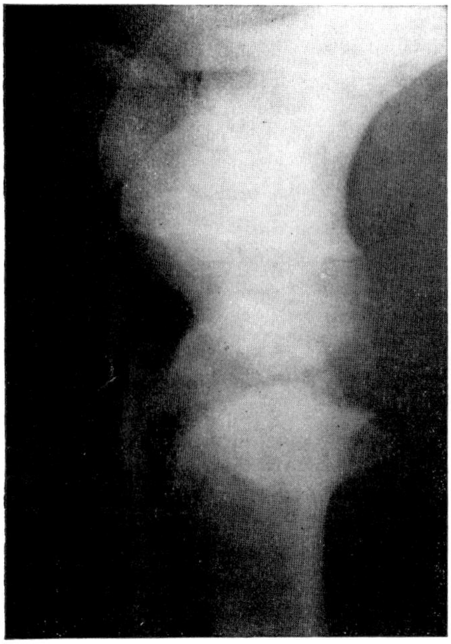

27

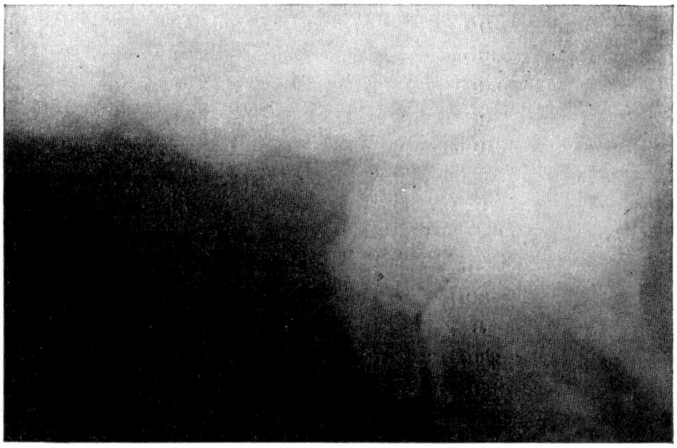

28

Fig. 2.1.19. — 27—28. Traumatic separation of the tibial crest and proximal tibial epiphysis.

the lameness will improve rapidly, and the prognosis is good. Open wound treatment is maintained until healing occurs. If the stifle joint is already involved, the prognosis is poor. Lameness becomes severe, and the entire stifle region shows a diffuse swelling.

For a purulent tendovaginitis of the tibialis cranialis muscle, the procedure is the same as for a subfascial cellulitis. The tendon sheath is incised, and open wound care is administered. The prognosis is guarded.

Comments. Wounds of the gaskin region should be managed promptly according to general surgical rules, as this offers the best chance of complete anatomic and functional recovery. In cases that are not seen until subfascial cellulitis, suppurative periostitis, osteitis and osteomyelitis have supervened, treatment may be uneconomical and of little value.

2.1.19.3.2. Separation of the Tibial Crest in the Young, Growing Horse (Osgood-Schlatter Disease, Osteochondrosis of the Tibial Tuberosity)

Definition. This condition involves a separation of the tibial crest in the young, growing horse with associated displacement, deformity and resorption. Osgood-Schlatter disease and osteochondrosis of the tibial tuberosity are names applied to similar conditions in dogs and man. The ossification center in the distal part of the tibial crest is mainly affected, leading to disturbances of ossification in the form of gaps and irregular areas of density in the radiographic shadow, multiple fragmented areas and separations (figs. 2.1.19. — 27 and — 28).

Symptoms. A slight, painful swelling appears at the tibial crest in young horses that are undergoing rigorous training. If the condition is bilateral, the horse will trot like a dog. The anterior wall of the hoof may touch the ground.

In other cases that are the result of direct trauma, a mild to moderate lameness is present. On palpation, marked tenderness is noted in the tibial crest, or the crest may be movable and produce crepitation. If the separation is complete, effusion will be observed in the stifle joint, and the patella may become displaced upward. No systemic signs occur.

Etiology. The disease is almost always the result of direct or indirect trauma. The tibial tuberosity can suffer direct trauma, for example, in a jumping horse that strikes an obstacle with the trailing leg. Indirect trauma can occur during the training of young horses as a result of sustained traction on the immature tibial tubercle from the three tendons of the quadriceps femoris muscle.

Diagnosis. The diagnosis is made by obtaining a history of a single severe trauma to the tibial crest or of recurrent trauma during the training of 1- to 3-year-old horses. Local findings and the latero-medial radiograph also contribute to the diagnosis. Radiographs should be taken of both hind limbs for comparison purposes, although ossification of the tibial crest may vary. Examination may show a partial separation of the tibial crest, a widening of the epiphyseal line of the tibial crest, evidence of bone resorption, or, in extreme cases, a nearly perpendicular upward displacement of the tuberosity.

Prognosis. The prognosis is generally good. If adequate rest is provided, i.e., if strenuous work is avoided, spontaneous recovery will ensue.

Differential diagnosis is made from tibial fractures and gonitis.

Treatment. Stall rest is indicated. Subcutaneous injection of Lugol's solution over the affected area may hasten recovery. Corticosteroids are contraindicated. If there is much displacement of the tibial crest, fixation with a cortical compression screw may be attempted in some circumstances.

Comments. Generally, all locomotor disability will regress following the conclusion of growth.

2.1.19.3.3. Fracture of the Tibia

Definition. Most tibial fractures in the horse are oblique or spiral fractures of the shaft. Tibial fractures in the horse rank third in frequency behind fractures of the proximal phalanx and pelvis.

Symptoms. Weight is not borne on the fractured limb. If the horse is made to move, it will hobble forward on three legs. Abnormal mobility is evident above the hock joint whenever the distal part of the limb is passively moved. If the horse is examined shortly after the fracture occurs, crepitation is audible and can even be felt by placing the hand on the medial surface of the tibia. Several hours later, the development of a fracture hematoma will produce a very severe swelling that usually is visible over the midportion of the tibia. Thus, the fracture line can usually be discerned only for the first few hours following the injury, and by the 2nd or 3rd day it can no longer be detected. Any palpation or manipulation of the limb produces severe pain. Small chip fractures cause only a mild to moderate lameness, local pain and circumscribed swelling; classic fracture symptoms are absent.

A fissure fracture of the tibia is often the precursor of a complete fracture. The trauma producing the incomplete fracture is followed initially by a mild to moderate supporting-leg lameness. However, local pain and swelling can be demonstrated on the inside of the gaskin. With fractures of this type, the mild to moderate lameness persists for some time, as do the pain and swelling. If absolute rest is enforced, healing will ensue in 12—16 weeks. In many cases, however, the fissure fracture becomes

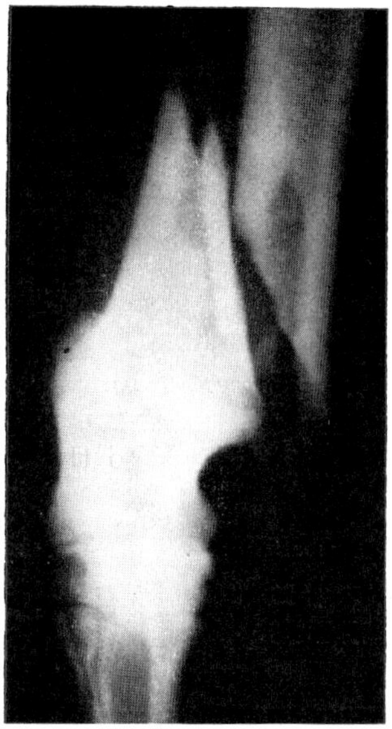

Fig. 2.1.19. — 29. Fracture of the tibia.

complete under the stress of weight bearing — even that associated with such simple acts as getting up and down.

Etiology. The anterior, lateral and posterior aspects of the tibia are relatively well padded by muscles and a strong tendon system. For this reason, most tibial fractures in the horse result from violence to the inside of the gaskin due to kicks from other animals, falls, running into obstacles, or entanglement of the limb.

Differential Diagnosis. The abnormal mobility in the gaskin region may cause a tibial fracture to be confused at first sight with a rupture of the peroneus tertius muscle. In the latter case, however, the weight-bearing ability of the limb is not impaired.

Diagnosis. Typical fracture symptoms such as abnormal motion, crepitation, hematoma and severe disability enable a complete tibial fracture to be diagnosed with confidence even without radiography. However, a fissure fracture or subperiosteal fracture can be diagnosed with certainty only on the basis of radiographic findings. With all fractures, radiographs will provide information on the shape of the fracture line and on the position and displacement of the fragments (fig. 2.1.19. — 29).

Prognosis. Union of the fracture can be achieved in horses but depends upon whether the fragments can be completely immobilized, regardless of the treatment method employed, and upon whether the horse is able to lie down and get up without difficulty during the healing period. With weeks of non-weight-bearing on the affected limb, there is a risk that stress laminitis will develop in the sound limb, causing recumbency, decubitus and finally septicemia.

Even with fissure fractures of the tibia, the prognosis is always guarded. This is due to the fact that a fissure fracture can progress to a complete fracture at any time.

Treatment. If it is decided to undertake treatment in a large adult horse, the animal should be sedated immediately after occurrence of the fracture and confined to a stall with soft bedding until the time of operation. Slinging is contraindicated. Treatment depends largely on available instrumentation and may involve percutaneous fixation with an external fixator, or the use of Rush pins in small horses and ponies. Internal compression plating should by all means be attempted if suitable plates and screws are available, as it may provide the only means of achieving fracture union. However, this method is suitable only for transverse fractures and short spiral fractures. For closed tibial fractures in foals of all breeds, conservative treatment with casts and/or modified Thomas splints may be tried.

Whenever a tibial fracture is managed operatively, the horse should receive at least 10 million units of penicillin per day for a period of 10—14 days.

Chip fractures located anywhere on the tibia will lead to bone necrosis with the consequent formation of sequestra. Thus, in the presence of fistulization and sequestration, a sequestrotomy should be performed without delay. At this time any areas of osteomyelitis are treated vigorously with local antibiotics following curettage of the focus. The patient should be handled as gently as possible so that the lesion will not progress to a complete fracture.

Comments. Tibial fractures in large adult horses should be treated only at the express wish of the owner, because success can never be guaranteed, and serious complications may arise at any time during the healing period.

2.1.19.3.4. Fracture of the Fibula

Definition. Violent breaks in the continuity of the fibula are extremely rare owing to the powerful muscles that surround and protect this rudimentary bone. Fractures should not be confused with the formation of *gaps* in the bone as a result of developmental defects. In many horses epiphyseal closure may be delayed until the age of 15 or may never occur at all.

Symptoms. Isolated fractures of the rudimentary fibula are always associated with local pain or the presence of a hematoma or wound on the lateral side of the leg below the stifle joint. Some degree of lameness will be present.

Defects in the union of the fibula do *not* produce clinical signs. Often this condition is an incidental finding during radiography of the hind limb.

Diagnosis. If evidence suggests a true fibular fracture of traumatic origin, then a radiographic examination should be made to establish the diagnosis.

If local clinical signs are absent, and radiographs of the tibial region incidentally show a defect in the fibula, then a radiograph should also be taken of the opposite fibula. In about two-thirds of cases (60—70 %), a defect will be found there, too.

Etiology. Fibular fractures are caused by external violence (kicks, etc.). With regard to defects of union, epiphyseal closure is normally complete in the fibula by the time growth is concluded. In many horses, however, ossification in this bone may by delayed until the age of 15 or may never occur. Statistical studies show that fibular ossification is complete by age 5 in about 37 % of horses, by age 6—10 in 24 %, and by age 11—15 in another 6 %. In about 33 % of horses, complete ossification is never achieved. Defects of this type may be unilateral or bilateral, and multiple defects may be present in the same bone. They are located either between the head and shaft of the fibula or within the shaft itself. The defect runs at right angles to the long axis of the fibula, and there is an associated club-like thickening of the ends of the bone. The defect ranges from a few millimeters to several centimeters in width. This condition may be interpreted as a phylogenic retrogression of the bone.

Prognosis and Treatment. Open fractures of the fibula are exposed, and loose bone fragments are removed. The prognosis is good. Defects in the union of the fibula have no clinical significance and do not require treatment.

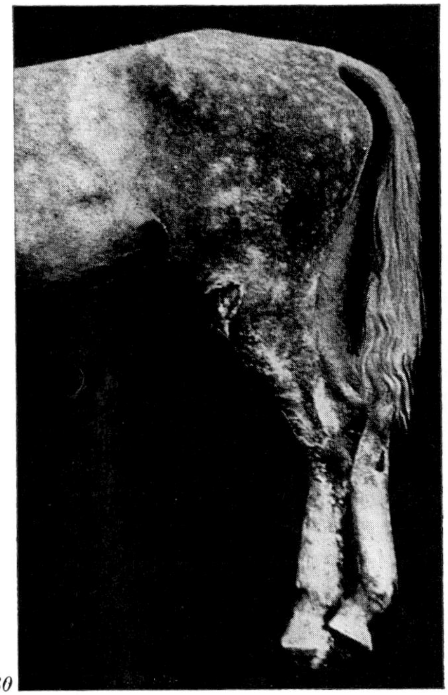

30

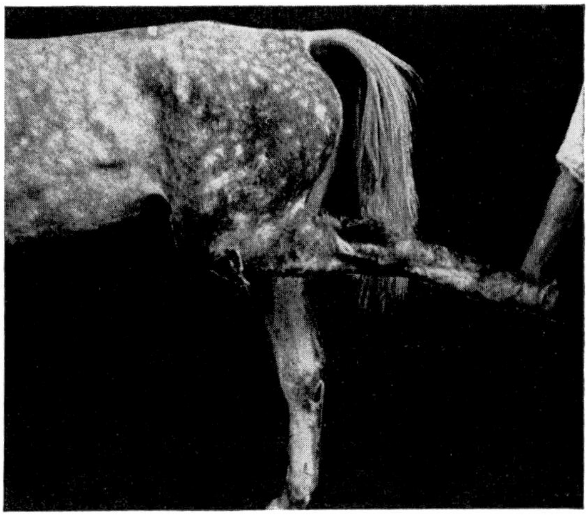

31

Fig. 2.1.19. — 30—31. Rupture of the peroneus tertius muscle.

2.1.19.3.5. Rupture of the Peroneus Tertius

Definition. This is a rupture of the narrow peroneus tertius muscle or its tendon on the anterior surface of the tibia (fig. 2.1.19. — 30). The peroneus tertius muscle is tendinous in the horse. It originates in common with the long digital extensor from the extensor fossa of the femur. At the upper tibia the peroneus tertius muscle separates from the long digital extensor and passes down over the hock joint to terminate in a strong, broad tendon. The muscle is innervated by the fibular nerve. In the horse it is superficially located and is easily palpated through the skin. The muscle may rupture at its tendon of origin in the extensor fossa or at the narrow muscle belly. Ruptures at the tendon of insertion are very rare.

Symptoms. The signs of peroneus tertius rupture are characteristic. The animal is unable to flex the hock joint, and the hock appears abnormally straight when the animal is standing. Further straightening occurs when the limb is lifted from the ground. In the swinging-leg phase, i.e., at the start of progression, the portion of the limb below the hock hangs limp, accompanied by a dimpling of the antagonistic Achilles tendon complex, comprised of the gastrocnemius, soleus, accessory and superficial flexor tendons. When the limb is passively lifted from the ground while the animal is standing, it is possible to extend the hock fully without resistance, even though the stifle is flexed. If the rupture is very recent, a gap in the muscle, a small hematoma, or an area of circumscribed pain may be detected below the stifle. If the lesion is several days old, such local changes will be absent. Systemic signs are not present.

Etiology. Rupture of the peroneus tertius results from overextension of the hock joint. This may occur when the animal kicks back violently or struggles violently to free an entrapped leg or break out of stocks.

Diagnosis. A clinical diagnosis is easily made from the typical symptoms that appear when the animal is standing or being walked, such as the straight hock, limp lower leg, and dimpling of the Achilles tendon when the leg is lifted (fig. 2.1.19. — 31).

Differential Diagnosis. Fractures of the tibia must be excluded.

Prognosis and Treatment. The prognosis is generally good. Ruptures in the area of the muscle belly will heal in 8—10 weeks without treatment. If the tendon is torn from its origin in the extensor fossa of the femur, the prognosis is still good for eventual recovery of limb function. Topical rubefacients can be applied to reduce healing time. The value of direct drug injections for stimulating granulation- and fibrous-tissue growth is of doubtful value.

Comments. Prolonged stall rest is always beneficial in racing animals. At the very least, horses with peroneus tertius ruptures are fit for breeding service.

2.1.19.3.6. Partial or Complete Rupture of the Achilles Tendon

Definition and Anatomy. The Achilles tendon is a collective term for the flexor tendons above the hock. It is an antagonist of the peroneus tertius. The structures that comprise the Achilles tendon are the gastrocnemius tendon, soleus tendon, accessory tendon and plantar portion of the superficial flexor tendon. The peroneus tertius and Achilles tendon system, especially the superficial flexor tendon, act in concert to produce reciprocal movement of the hock and stifle joints. This functional unit is called the reciprocal apparatus. Its function is partly or completely abolished when the continuity of the Achilles tendon is disrupted, or when the tendon becomes detached from the calcaneus.

Symptoms. With a partial disruption of the Achilles tendon (fig. 2.1.19. — 32), a functional disturbance is evident in the hock joint at the moment weight is supported. With a complete disruption of the tendon, the hock collapses when weight is borne. The degree of the functional disturbance is a guide to the portion or portions of the Achilles tendon that are involved. The disturbance of hock action is mild when the gastrocnemius tendon alone is ruptured above its site of union with the soleus tendon. The same applies to isolated divisions of the superficial flexor tendon or soleus tendon. All these lesions cause only a slight dropping of the hock during weight bearing. With a concomitant rupture of the superficial flexor tendon and gastrocnemius tendon, there will be a greater angulation of the hock when weight is supported. If the limb is lifted forward as for the spavin test, some resistance to hock flexion will still be encountered. If the superficial flexor tendon, gastrocnemius tendon and soleus or accessory tendon are all ruptured, the limb will be unable to support weight, and the hock will collapse if it is attempted. When this occurs, the metatarsus becomes nearly horizontal, and the fetlock joint is flexed at a right angle. When the limb is picked up while the animal is standing, the distal portion will swing forward and backward as a sign of the tension loss. Similar disturbances are seen in avulsion fractures of the calcaneus.

When the Achilles tendon is partially or completely severed due to a sharp trauma, the aforementioned functional disturbances will be accompanied by skin and tendon wounds that tend to be contaminated and infected. If such wounds are several days old, there will be necrosis of the tendon stumps and swelling of the area around the wound.

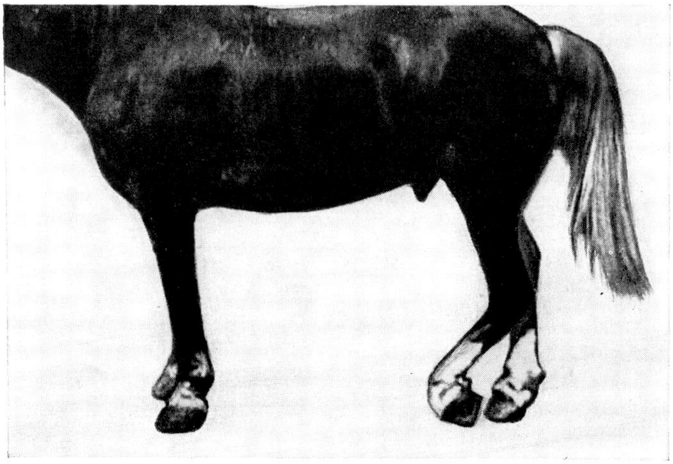

Fig. 2.1.19. — 32. Partial rupture of the Achilles tendon.

Closed ruptures of the Achilles tendon are characterized by firm, painful swellings over the calcaneus. Generally it is possible to identify the individual components of the tendon. Chip fractures of the tuber calcis provoke inflammatory edema of the surrounding area. Distension of the superficial flexor tendon sheath is always present in such cases. With a recent avulsion fracture of the calcaneus, crepitation can be elicited by passive movement of the hock joint. This crepitation is no longer detected by the 2nd or 3rd day, however, because the superior fragment is quickly retracted by muscle tension. Systemic signs are initially absent in the presence of fresh tendon ruptures or divisions.

Etiology. Partial or complete ruptures of the Achilles tendon can result from slips, overstretching of the Achilles tendon, falls onto the flexed hock, and kicks from other horses. It is less common for the tendon to become severed by sharp objects, as may occur when the animal backs into a barbed wire fence.

Differential Diagnosis. The functional disturbance caused by tibial nerve paralysis closely resembles that associated with partial rupture of the Achilles tendon. The latter, however, is distinguished by local changes in the tuber calcis or course of the Achilles tendon.

Diagnosis. Divisions of all or part of the Achilles tendon associated with lacerated and incised wounds are not difficult to diagnose. With closed complete or partial ruptures, the affected portion of the Achilles tendon usually can be identified by digital palpation. The diagnosis is facilitated by the subcutaneous insufflation of air followed by radiographic examination. In addition, avulsion fractures of the calcaneus are well demonstrated by radiographs in the latero-medial projection.

Prognosis and Treatment. Complete ruptures or divisions have a poor prognosis, and euthanasia is required. With partial ruptures or divisions, treatment may be attempted. Wounds are managed according to general surgical principles. Tendon sutures are usually unsuccessful in the horse. An attempt should be made to obtain complete immobilization of the lower limb from the stifle to the hoof by applying a cast. If the cast permits the animal to walk for a healing period of 8—10 weeks, thus preventing stress laminitis of the sound hind limb and consequent recumbency, a functional recovery may be expected. If instability is still excessive at the end of that period, the area around the tuber calcis is sometimes fired or blistered in an effort to stimulate fibrosis. Avulsion fractures of the calcaneus have an equally unfavorable prognosis.

Comments. Treatment should be attempted only in partial ruptures or divisions of the Achilles tendon. Even if treatment is successful, the athletic future of the horse is still questionable.

2.1.19.3.7. Stringhalt

Definition. Stringhalt is a spasmodic flexion of one or both hind limbs that is most pronounced when the animal is walking or when a forward movement is first made. It may be so marked that the flexed fetlock actually strikes the ventral surface of the abdomen. The limb is also brought back down with exaggerated force, often creating the appearance of the step of a parade horse.

Symptoms. True stringhalt usually develops suddenly, and in most cases no prior cause can be ascertained. Mild cases are usually bilateral, while severe cases tend to be unilateral. The spasmodic flexion affects the hock, stifle and fetlock joints. The extension of the limb that follows this flexion is also very abrupt, causing the foot to strike the ground flat and with force. In bilateral cases the limbs are not usually raised to the level of the abdomen, and the animal moves forward with a choppy, stabbing gait.

Etiology. The cause of idiopathic or true stringhalt is not known. The onset is usually sudden but may be gradual. Some cases show a history of subcutaneous cellulitis or myositis of the affected limb weeks or months prior to the attack. It has often been suggested that inflammation of peripheral nerves of the hind limbs (femoral, peroneal or tibial) is responsible. It is also reported that lesions of the internuncial neurons (interneurons) of the spinal cord can produce signs of stringhalt. It has also been suggested, but not confirmed, that stringhalt is due to a shortening of the fascia of the thigh, tensor fasciae latae or lateral digital extensor secondary to inflammatory conditions of the thigh and gaskin.

Differential Diagnosis. This idiopathic form of stringhalt must be differentiated from symptomatic forms. Thus, symptoms similar to stringhalt may be associated with spavin, recurrent patellar luxation, and sometimes with corns.

Diagnosis. Following the exclusion of other causes, the diagnosis is made on the basis of characteristic functional disturbances.

Prognosis and Treatment. Idiopathic stringhalt in the horse cannot be cured with certainty. In many cases the signs of stringhalt will disappear with 5—10 minutes of exercise. In other cases a month's rest may be needed before symptoms disappear.

Various methods of surgical correction have been recommended, but none is 100 % successful. One such method is a partial tenectomy of the lateral digital extensor tendon. In this procedure the skin and fascia are incised on the lateral side of the metatarsus about a hand's width distal to the hock joint. The tendon is exposed before its union with the deep flexor tendon, and a segment about 5 cm long is excised from its terminal portion.

Adams [1974] recommends a complete resection of the lateral digital extensor tendon. In this method an incision through the skin and fascia is made above the hock joint at the tendinous junction of the lateral extensor muscle, level with the upper border of the calcaneus. A second incision is made over the distal portion of the tendon just before it joins the long extensor (about a hand's width below the hock). After the distal portion has been severed, traction is exerted on the proximal stump to free any adhesions that might be present within the tendon sheath. The tendon is pulled out of the sheath, sectioned at its junction with the muscle belly, and removed from the proximal wound.

Both procedures may be carried out using local anesthesia and sedation or with the animal cast and under general anesthesia. A desmotomy of the medial patellar ligament will give relief only in cases of symptomatic stringhalt due to upward fixation of the patella.

We have obtained very good results with single or repeated lumbar sympathetic blockades in the treatment of idiopathic stringhalt. Vitamin B_2 and B_{12} injections are useful adjuncts to this therapy.

Dixon and Stewart [1969] have had success with the administration of centrally-acting muscle relaxants. This would confirm the theory that stringhalt results from the irritation of internuncial neurons in the spinal cord. Further study is needed before definite conclusions can be drawn.

Comments. Experience in recent years with sympathetic blockades and the intravenous administration of centrally-acting muscle relaxants is sufficient to recommend them as a first-line treatment for idiopathic stringhalt. A tenectomy should be done only if the response to drug therapy is poor.

References

Adams, O. R.: Lameness in horses; 3rd ed. (Lea and Febiger, Philadelphia 1974).

Azzie, M. A. J.: Aortic iliac thrombosis of thoroughbred horses. Equine vet. J. *1:* 113 (1969).

Baker, R. H.: Osteochondrosis of the tibial tuberosity of the horse. J. Amer. vet. med. Assoc. *137:* 354 (1960).

Banks, W. C.; Schultz, C. W.: Additional studies of fibular defects in horses. J. Amer. vet. med. Assoc. *133:* 422 (1958).

Branscomb, B. L.: Treatment of arterial thrombosis in a horse with sodium gluconate. J. Amer. vet. med. Assoc. *152:* 1643 (1968).

Carter, E. I.; Horney, F. D.; Pennock, P. W.: Distal tibial fractures in the horse. Mod. vet. Pract. *53:* 41 (1972).

Davison, D. J.: A case of coxo-femoral subluxation in a Welsh-pony. Vet. Rec. *80:* 441 (1967).

Delahanty, D. D.: Defects — not fractures — of the fibulae in horses. J. Amer. vet. med. Assoc. *133:* 258 (1958).

Delahanty, D. D.: Medial patellar desmotomy in a pony. Sci. Proc. Amer. vet. med. Assoc., p. 81 (1963).

Dietz, O.; Rechenberg, R.: Betrachtungen zu Osgood-Schlatterschen Erkrankungen bei Pferd, Hund und Katze. Mh. Vet.-Med. *17:* 868 (1962).

Dixon, R. T.; Stewart, G. A.: Clinical and pharmalogical observations in the care of equine stringhalt. Austral. Vet. J. *45:* 127 (1969).

Finocchio, E. J.; Guffy, M. M.: Congenital patellar ectopia in a foal. J. Amer. vet. med. Assoc. *156:* 222 (1970).

Hickman, J.; Walker, R. G.: Upward retention of the patella in the horse. Vet. Rec. *76:* 1198 (1964).

Huskamp, B.; Verhaar, W. M.: Partielle Meniscektomie beim Pferd. Prakt. Tierarzt *9:* 627 (1977).

Kaneko, M.; Kiryu, K.; Oikawa, M.; Kanemaru, T.; Satoh, H.: Discontinous condition in the fibulae in the light horse. Exp. Res. Equine Health Lab. *12:* 1 (1975).

Lundvall, R. L.: Fracture of the fibula in the horse. J. Amer. vet. med. Assoc. *129:* 10 (1956).

Lundvall, R. L.: Lameness of the upper hind leg. Iowa State Univ. Veterinarian *24:* 7 (1961/62).

Lush, N. D.; Rosborough, J. P.: Fibular fracture in a filly. J. Amer. vet. med. Assoc. *130:* 4 (1957).

Mackay-Smith, M. P.: Management of fracture and luxation of femoral head in two ponies. J. Amer. vet. med. Assoc. *145:* 248 (1964).

Mackay-Smith, M. P.; Raker, C. W.: Mechanical defects of the equine stifle: Diagnosis and treatment. Sci. Proc. 100th Meet. Amer. vet. med. Assoc. (1964).
Miller, R. M.: Thrombophlebitis of the external iliac vein in a horse. Vet. Med. and Small Animal Clinician *65:* 153 (1970).
Paatsama, S.: Diagnostik, Therapie und Prognose bei Kniegelenkslahmheiten beim Pferd. tierärztl. praxis *3:* 445 (1975).
Pattison, M.: Progressive hind limb weakness in a pony associated with a lesion in the thoracic spinal cord. Vet. Rec. *85:* 11 (1969).
Pelt, R. W. van: Intra-articular injection of the equine stifle for therapeutic and diagnostic purposes. J. Amer. vet. med. Assoc. *147:* 490 (1965).
Pelt, R. W. van: Stifle disease (gonitis) in horses: Clinicopathologic findings and intra-articular therapy. J. Amer. vet. med. Assoc. *157:* 1173 (1970).
Pettit, G. D.; Wheat, J. D.: Distal epiphyseal fracture of the femur in a Shetland pony. J. Amer. vet. med. Assoc. *138:* 13 (1961).
Rao, S. V.: Hey-Grove's knife for patellar desmotomy in the bovine. Nord. Vet.-Med. *17:* 172 (1965).
Rooney, J. R.; Raker, C. W.; Harmany, K. J.: Congenital lateral luxation of the patella in the horse. Cornell Vet. *61:* 670 (1971).
Rothenbacher, H.; Hokanson, J. F.: Coxofemoral joint luxation in a quarter horse. J. Amer. vet. med. Assoc. *147:* 148 (1965).
Seddon, H. D.: Sudden case of stringhalt in a horse. Austral. Vet. J. *45:* 127 (1963).
Singh Rathor, S.; Numans, S. R.: Lateral patellar luxation and its operative treatment in Shetland ponies. Indian vet. J. *48:* 861, 969 (1971).
Springstead, B. K.: Fracture of the tibia in a horse. J. Amer. vet. med. Assoc. *155:* 1370 (1969).
Schützler, H.: Ein Beitrag zur Hüftgelenklahmheit beim Pferd. Berliner und Münchener tierärztl. Wschr. *72:* 104 (1959).
Szabuniewicz, M.; Titus, R. S.: Rupture of the peronaeus tertius in the horse. Vet. Med. and Small Animal Clinician *62:* 993 (1967).
Tillotson, P. J.; Kopper, P. H.: Treatment of aortic thrombosis in a horse. J. Amer. vet. med. Assoc. *149:* 766 (1966).
Valdez, H., Adams, O. R.: Surgical approach for medial meniscetomy in the horse. J. Amer. vet. med. Assoc. *173:* 766 (1978).
White, N. A., Wheat, J. D.: An expansion and compression technique for reducing and stabilizing proximal epiphyseal fractures of the tibia in foals. J. Amer. vet. med. Assoc. *167:* 733 (1975).
Žežkov, F.: A study of discontinuity of the fibula in the horse. Amer. J. Vet. Res. *78:* 852 (1959).
Žežkov, B., Marolt, J., Vukelic, E., Dolinar, Ž.: Fracture or congenital discontinuity of the fibular in the horse. Brit. vet. J. *114:* 145 (1958).

2.1.19.4. Diseases of the Hock Joint

2.1.19.4.1. Tarsal Osteoarthritis (Spavin)
(Chronic, Local Periarthritis and Arthrosis of the Small Tarsal Joints)

Definition and Occurrence. Spavin is a disease of the hock joint that has been known for centuries and is among the most common causes of lameness in horses. According to Grande [1972] and Müller [1972], spavin can affect horses of any age whose gait or conformation imposes unphysiologic stress on the medial aspect of the hock joint (occupational disease). This is especially true in the Standardbred [Richter, 1975].

It is difficult to find a comprehensive definition for spavin which takes into account its etiology. Customarily, spavin is considered to be a bony enlargement on the inner aspect of the hock, associated with a characteristic lameness that improves with exercise. However, in a great many horses with spavin lameness there is little or no demonstrable enlargement on the medial surface of the hock. Conversely, a horse may exhibit no lameness yet show considerable spavin exostosis.

Excluding all other diseases of the tarsus, such as arthritis, hydrarthrosis, cunean tendon bursitis, tendovaginitis, osteochondritis dissecans, etc., spavin may be regarded as a unilateral or bilateral, local, chronic periarthritis and osteoarthrosis involving the medial aspect of the small less moveable tarsal joints [Bolz et al., 1975].

Symptoms. The initial clinical symptom is pain when weight is placed on the affected limb, leading to a locomotor disturbance or lameness. Later, exostosis may develop causing a hard, painless enlargement of variable size that can be seen and palpated on the lower third of the inner aspect of the hock. Thus, spavin lameness (or 'spavin gait') and spavin exostosis are the typical manifestations of this disease. Each can exist independently of the other.

— *Spavin lameness* usually develops gradually but may have a sudden onset in isolated cases. In mature horses it is most pronounced during the change from a slow gait (walk) to a faster gait (trot). In such cases a mild to moderate mixed lameness or predominantly supporting-leg lameness frequently appears during the first few strides. In advanced cases the animal places no weight at all on the affected limb when first exercised, and then bears weight cautiously after the first few steps. The lameness improves or disappears entirely as exercise is continued. Standardbreds with bilateral, equal involvement of the hind limbs exhibit a stilted gait (paddling or stabbing) and are apt to break into a gallop to lessen stress on the affected joints. Signs of spavin lameness are difficult to detect at the gallop.

The tendency to bear weight on the toe causes excessive wear to the toe of the hoof wall or of the shoe. However, this change is obvious only if the disease is unilateral or if the disease process is at different stages in the two hind limbs. The excessive toe wear and the atrophy of the extensor muscles frequently described in horses with spavin are not very pronounced in the Standardbred. In advanced cases the horse may flex the hock in a spasmodic manner (stringhalt).

When standing, the horse favors the affected limb and may stand with the leg partially flexed and the foot anterior and medial. It may even rest the affected leg on the foot of the opposite limb.

Spavin is also seen in young horses, especially those with a base-narrow, toe-out conformation. Müller [1972] has described this condition. Affected horses tend to drag the foot on the ground causing excessive toe wear. This form of spavin lameness can be 'ridden away' by a good rider. The initial symptoms are manifested less by locomotor disturbances of the hind limbs than by an abnormal rigidity of the back.

— *Spavin exostoses* appear as hard, painless enlargements of variable size in the lower third of the medial aspect of the hock. They are of only minor importance in the diagnosis of spavin in older horses, for, as Wamberg [1953] points out, 80—90% of horses with functionally sound hock joints show pathologic changes in the small tarsal bones. Hence, these alterations must be considered a product of physiologic remodeling processes that are promoted by age, activity or conformation.

Exostoses on the central, second and third tarsal bones, and occasionally on the metatarsus and proximal end of the medial splint bone, are regularly encountered in spavin. Initially they are often difficult to detect, however, because they develop only as the disease progresses (occult spavin).

In the standing horse, spavin exostosis is easily recognized by comparing the two hocks from behind (fig. 2.1.19. — 33). The shape and location of the exostoses are variable. They most commonly occur in the area of the central and third tarsal bones, but may be situated farther proximally, distally, cranially or caudally. They

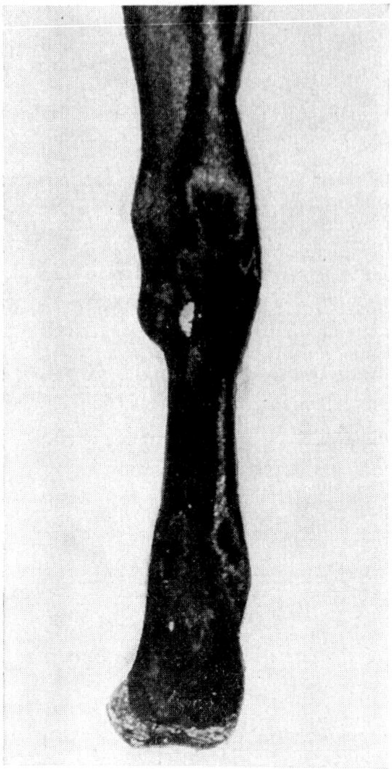

Fig. 2.1.19. — 33. Spavin exostosis.

may be flat or protuberant, but they are always firmly adherent to the underlying bone. No heat or tenderness is present.

Etiology. Both direct and indirect causal factors act in concert to produce the disease [Bolz et al., 1975]:

1. The internal, indirect or predisposing causes encompass not only a general constitutional weakness, but also defects in the fine structure of the tarsal bones. Andreewa [1960] has shown that spavin affects only those tarsal joints in which the nutrient artery has extensive connections with the blood vessels accompanying the cutaneous nerves of the medial gaskin and with the skin. This pattern of neurovascular anastomosis is seen with a primitive mode of union among the tarsal bones. Additional predisposing factors are abnormalities of conformation (sickle hocks, cow hocks, bow legs, coon-footed, camped behind, etc.), abnormalities of gross hock joint structure (flat, narrow, constricted hock), and the angulation of the tarsus. Young, spirited horses are also thought to be predisposed. The inheritance of spavin is disputed, but a genetically-linked predisposition for the disease is believed to be possible.

Significance is also attached to dietary mineral deficiencies. According to Krook [1968], an imbalance in the calcium : phosphorus ratio gives rise to a generalized osteopathy that predisposes to various diseases of the musculoskeletal system, including spavin.

Rooney [1968] points to asynchronous movements among the tarsal bones as a cause of spavin. He states that the complex etiology and pathogenesis of spavin can be understood only by analyzing the micro-movements and simultaneous macro-movements that take place in the joint.

Many authors argue that the hock joint shows a tendency toward simplification through ankylosis during the course of its phylogenic development. Viewed in these terms, spavin is not a disease entity, but an inherited transitional form that is independent of mechanical influences [JOLY, 1898].

Interestingly, LUTZ and GABEL [1969] found inflammation of the cunean bursa in a large proportion of predominantly young horses with lameness of the hock joint.

2. The direct, external cause relates mainly to the cumulative effect of repeated microtrauma to the medial aspect of the hock joint, chiefly in the form of very slight contusions and other injuries. A single trauma can also lead to spavin, however.

Owing to the discovery that horses with highly sloping foot and pastern axes have a greater reach than horses with steeper foot axes, the heels of Standardbred horses are often trimmed very low to encourage this action. It is believed that this practice also predisposes to spavin.

Necropsy Findings. In the early stage the tarsal bones have an abnormally soft consistency, and the cut surface shows a spotty or uniform redness (rarefying osteitis, osteoporosis,osteoclasia). Hard new bone tissue later forms in the soft inflammatory foci (condensing osteitis, osteosclerosis). The articular cartilage is dull and shows bluish-red discoloration, superficial fibrillation, deep clefts, and wear spots of variable shape and extent. Small, white calcificied spots appear on the cartilage surface, followed later by hypertrophic new bone growth (cartilage wear, osteoarthrosis, arthritis sicca, chronic degenerative arthritis). As the disease progresses, adhesions and areas of direct fusion appear between the individual tarsal bones, sometimes involving the tarsometatarsal joint. The disease process, which initially is confined to the area of the central, second and third tarsal bones, may spread to involve the metatarsus (third metatarsal), the medial splint bone and other tarsal bones (first and second tarsal bones and tibial tarsal bone). Chronic degenerative arthritis and periarthritis of the entire hock joint may result [SILBERSIEPE et al., 1976].

Differential diagnosis must be made from chronic diseases of the hip, stifle and talocrural joints, osteochondritis dissecans of the hock joint, sesamoiditis, cunean tendon bursitis, idiopathic stringhalt and, in some circumstances, from sprains and ringbone of the digital joints. If necessary, diagnostic anesthesia may be used as an aid to differentiation. Spavin exostosis should not be confused with scar tissue and periosteal new bone growth.

Diagnosis. The recognition of spavin is difficult and requires experience. Repeated examinations may be necessary before a diagnosis can be reached. When examining the standing horse, special attention should be given to the conformation of the limbs, the structure and contour of the hock joint, the foot conformation, the wear to the anterior hoof wall or shoe, the carriage of the limb, and any atrophy that may have developed in the muscles of the croup. When palpating the plantomedial surface of the hock joint, experience is necessary to detect distension of the cunean bursa or the presence of small spavin exostoses. The examiner should have a thorough knowledge of the topography of the hock region. In addition, all findings should be compared with the opposite side, bearing in mind that the sound limb may show pathologic changes of the hock joint.

Next the animal is examined from behind and from the side while in motion. This examination starts by having the horse move about in its stall and continues as the animal is led from the stall. At the walk, special note is taken of any shortening of the forward flight of the limb. This is followed by trotting the horse on hard and soft ground.

While lameness is easily detected in more severe cases of spavin, there may be no irregularities of gait in mild cases, especially in trotters that are exercised along

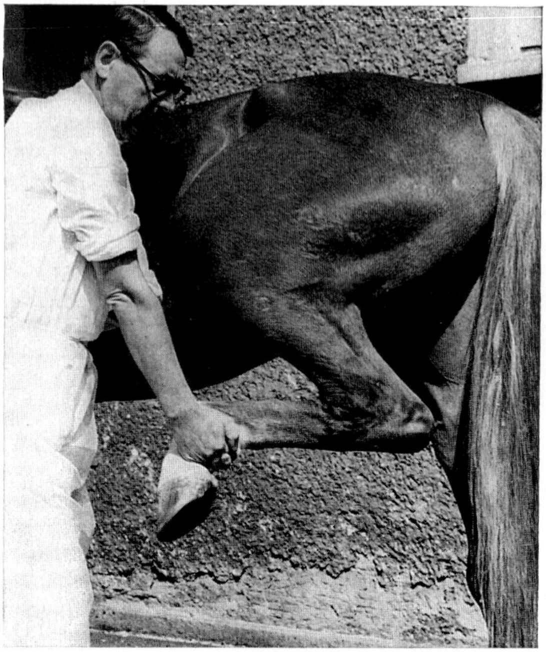

34

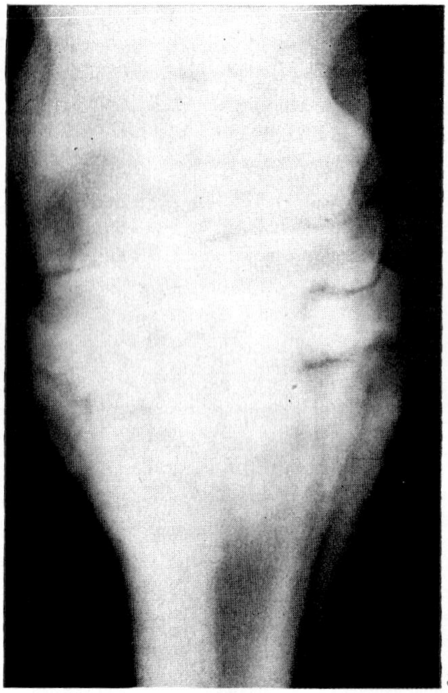

3

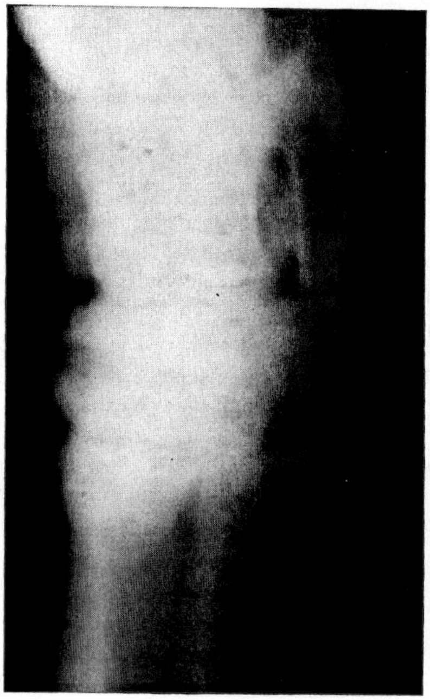

36

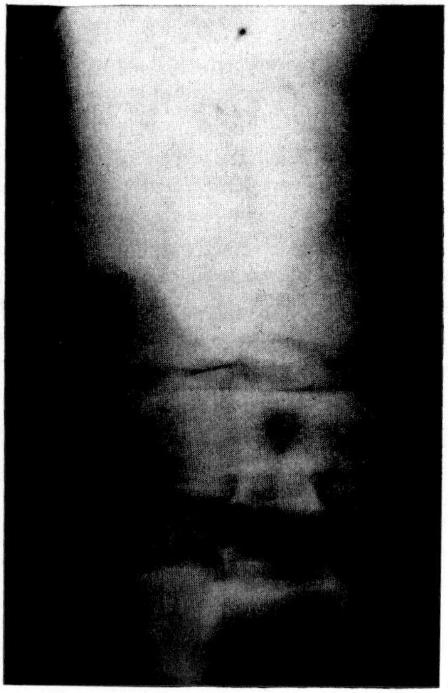

37

Fig. 2.1.19. — 34. The spavin test.
Fig. 2.1.19. — 35. Periarticular changes in spavin.
Fig. 2.1.19. — 36. Intertarsal osteochondrotic changes (internal spavin).
Fig. 2.1.19. — 37. Cystlike changes in the central tarsal bone.

a straight path or in horses that have rested in their stall for some time prior to the examination. In these cases the horse should be exercised at a fast trot or longed in deep sand. Schebitz and Wilkens [1967] as well as Zeller [1968] contend that typical 'spavin lameness' does not exist in Standardbred horses.

The lameness is often of the mixed variety, although a pure supporting- or swinging-leg lameness may be present depending on the location and extent of the pathologic process. The lameness is accentuated by the spavin test. This test consists of flexing the hock for 3 minutes and then putting the horse into a trot. In positive cases the animal will show more lameness than before, especially during the first few steps. However, it must be understood that diseases of the hip and stifle joints can produce a similar reaction to this test (fig. 2.1.19. — 34).

Another diagnostic aid is subcutaneous infiltration anesthesia by the method of Berge [1934], in which 30—50 ml of a concentrated local anesthetic solution are injected in rhomboid fashion about the spavin exostosis or spavin area. The patient should not be moved for about 5—15 minutes to allow the anesthetic to take effect. If the horse goes sound and the spavin test is negative following the anesthesia, the diagnosis is considered to be established. If the lameness persists, then normal joint motion may be impaired due to mechanical reasons or perhaps the local anesthetic used was not effectively distributed. A negative Berge injection therefore does not necessarily exclude spavin. Schebitz and Wilkens [1967] state that the efficacy of the anesthesia can be enhanced by supplementary anesthesia of the hock joint, owing to the presence of a communication between the proximal intertarsal joint and the tibiotarsal joint. If there is mild involvement of the opposite limb, then lameness will become apparent in this limb when the first leg is anesthetized. Subcutaneous infiltration anesthesia is of little value for diagnosing spavin in young horses.

Lutz and Gabel [1969] state that a diagnosis of cunean tendon bursitis, which is especially common in horses that advance the ipsilateral limbs together, can be confirmed by injecting anesthetic into the bursa. This bursa is situated between the medial tendon of the tibialis cranialis muscle and the medial collateral ligament of the hock joint.

Finally, a radiographic examination is made. The radiographic technique is of prime importance. Besides dorso-plantar and lateral views, oblique projections are of considerable value [Saschek, 1964; Zeller, 1968] (figs. 2.1.19. — 35 through — 37). As a rule, spavin cannot be demonstrated until there are exostoses, changes in the course of the osteochondral boundaries, and narrowing of the joint spaces. Hartung [1977] found that these changes were already present in 50 % of young, untrained Standardbred horses. This led him to conclude that radiographic examination alone is not diagnostic for spavin, although it is a useful adjunct for confirming the clinical diagnosis.

Treatment. Treatment is directed mainly toward alleviating lameness both by hastening ankylosis of the joint and by systemic or local pain relief. Prophylaxis consists of assuring an optimum mineral supply, especially during early growth. The following treatment methods are used at the present time:

1. Corrective trimming and shoeing. Besides the use of a spavin shoe (rolled toe and raised branch), Müller [1972] recommends Nyffenegger's [1956] shoeing technique for spavin in young horses (branch widened where hoof is subjected to greatest loads). If lameness improves, a program of exercise therapy is instituted.

Mild cases of spavin lameness can be completely cured through corrective shoeing.

2. In the early stage of spavin, Creswell and Smythe [1963] recommend that corrective shoeing be supplemented with heat treatment over a one-month period

(mild rubefacient drugs) and enforced rest until the lameness is gone. This complete rest does not apply to racehorses that already are well conditioned. In these animals, analgesic and anti-inflammatory drugs [Houdeshell and Bloomfield, 1969] are given so that the animal can be put on a regular work schedule to maintain condition. The loss of condition resulting from a prolonged training break would place too great a stress on the affected limb and jeopardize the success of treatment.

3. On similar grounds, a peripheral neurectomy using the Wamberg [1953] technique (periosteotomy) is recommended for horses in full training. In this procedure a subcutaneous rhomboid-type incision is made through all tissues around the exostoses or spavin area. A double-edged spavin knife is used, and the cut is made through all tissues (ligaments, joint capsule) down to the bone, regardless of the structures that are divided. The theory is that this diamond-shaped cut will ensure that all peripheral nerve fibers are severed. Before the wound is sutured, the detached tissues are massaged to force the blood out through the incision. A firm adhesive bandage is applied.

Postoperative care forms an important part of this treatment method. The horse is exercised daily starting on postoperative day 1 with 15 minutes of walking twice daily. The duration and intensity of the exercise are gradually increased until, after 10—14 days, the animal is performing 50- to 100-meter dashes. The object of the exercise is to adapt the scar tissue to movement of the hock joint. Rest or static exercise could lead to the formation of scarring that would stretch and tear during later exertion with a recurrence of lameness.

4. Equally good results are achieved with a tenotomy or tenectomy of the medial tendon of the tibialis cranialis muscle. The animal can be returned to work 4 weeks after the operation [Grande, 1972].

5. The spavin operation of Peters [1938] is a periostomy. Starting distal to the spavin area, three subcutaneous incisions that diverge in a fanwise manner are made with a narrow, curved, wide-backed knife through the fascia, ligaments, bursae, etc. down to the bone.

In addition to analgesia, this causes a tissue irritation which hastens ankylosis of the intertarsal and/or tarsometatarsal joints. This procedure may be combined with Wamberg's [1953] operation.

6. Double neurectomy of the tibial and deep peroneal nerves is considered a 'last ditch' effort to cure lameness in working horses that are to be used for a predetermined period. Postoperative complications limit the success of this procedure, especially if it is carelessly used.

7. The rationale for surgical destruction of the affected joint surfaces (arthrodesis) is based on the observation that spavin lameness persists until ankylosis develops in the affected joint or joints. At least 60 % of the articular cartilage must be destroyed in this method. The arthrodesis is carried out on both the distal intertarsal and the tarsometatarsal joints [Adams, 1970].

8. Soennichsen [1977] makes a drill opening in the cortical tissue of the affected bone (fenestration). The theory is that the resulting pressure relief will relieve pain and restore function.

9. Blisters (e.g., mercury biiodate ointment) do not always produce the desired result, even with prolonged stall rest. They are contraindicated for spavin in young horses.

10. Firing (intracutaneous point or line firing) is still widely used in the treatment of spavin. In this method 30 points or diagonal lines are fired into the medial surface of the hock, followed by blistering.

Schebitz and Wilkens [1967] state that better results are obtained by driving the firing point directly into the exostoses. The danger of opening the joint is one disadvantage of this method, however. Firing is followed by 2 months' stall rest, or 3—4 months' rest in the case of Standardbreds. Silbersiepe et al. [1976], consider it necessary to fire both hind limbs simultaneously in Standardbreds.

11. Based on the etiology of the spavin diseases, acid mucopolysaccharides (e.g., arumalon) have recently been used [Schneider, 1972] with the object of promoting the synthesis of sulfated mucopolysaccharides, counteracting autolytic cartilage destruction, and stimulating the regeneration of joint cartilage. Arumalon is injected intramuscularly at 2-day intervals for a period of 6—8 weeks.

Prognosis. The prognosis is poor in terms of achieving a complete recovery. The goal of treatment, therefore, must be to restore the horse to working soundness. The treatment of choice will depend on the intended use of the patient. While a clean trotting action will be desired in show horses or standardbreds, less stringent demands are placed upon jumpers, draft animals or speed horses. Wamberg [1953] claims that with his operation, he can return 90 % of trotting horses to their former working capacity. With other treatment methods as well, the prognosis for a functional recovery is good. Spontaneous recoveries may occur in isolated cases but require a convalescence of 1 to 2 years.

Comments. Many authors share the view that there is a tendency in the phylogenic development of the hock toward simplification through the fusion and ankylosis of its joints. If true, this would mean that spavin is not a disease at all, but an inherited transitional form that is independent of mechanical influences [Joly, 1898].

References

Adams, O. R.: Surgical arthrodesis for treatment of bone spavin. J. Amer. Vet. Med. Assoc. *157:* 1180 (1970).

Andreewa, S. P.: Besonderheiten des anatomischen Baues des Tarsalgelenkes, welche die Entstehung der Spatkrankheit begünstigen. Wien. tierärztl. Mschr., Festschrift *15:* (1960).

Berge, E.: Zur Diagnose des Spat beim Pferd. Berliner tierärztl. Wschr. *36:* 593 (1934).

Bolz, W., Dietz, O., Schleiter, H., Teuscher, R.: Lehrbuch der Speziellen Veterinärchirurgie; 2. Aufl. (VEB Gustav Fischer Verlag, Jena 1975).

Cohrs, P., Messow, C.: Gelenke; in Joest: Handbuch der speziellen pathologischen Anatomie der Haustiere, 3. Aufl., Bd. 1 (Parey, Berlin 1962).

Creswell, H., Smythe, R. H.: Lameness of the hindlimb. Equine Medicine and Surgery (Amer. Vet. Public. Inc., 1963).

Dietz, O.; Mill, J.; Richter, W.: Beurteilung des Therapieerfolges beim Spat des Traberpferdes mit Hilfe von Leistungskriterien. Mh. Vet.-Med. *24:* 579 (1969).

Grande, E. M.: The surgical treatment of bone spavin. Wamberg's spavin operation and tenectomy of the medial branch of the anterior tibial muscle. A comparison of the results of surgical treatment in trotting horses. Nord. Vet.-Med. *74:* 388 (1972).

Hartung, K.: Röntgenologische Veränderungen am Sprunggelenk und ihre Bedeutung. Prakt. Tierarzt *58:* 13 (1977).

Houdeshell, J. W.; Bloomfield, N. J.: Field trials of a new longacting corticosteroid in the treatment of equine arthropathies. Vet. Med. Small Animal Clinician *64:* 782 (1969).

Joly, G.: Fortschritte in der Einzehigkeit der Einhufer. Ann. méd. vét. *47:* 49 (1898).

Krook, L.: Dietary calcium-phosphorus and lameness in the horses. Cornell Vet., suppl. 58, p. 59 (1968).

Lutz, W. H.; Gabel, A.: Spavin in standardbred race horses. Mod. Vet. Pract. *50:* 38 (1969).

Mackay, R. C. J.; Lidell, W. A.: Arthrodesis in the treatment of bone spavin. Equine Vet. *4:* 34 (1972).

MÜLLER, H.: Diagnostik und Therapie einiger wichtiger Lahmheiten des Reitpferdes. Prakt. Tierarzt *53:* 477, 484 (1972).
NYFFENEGGER, A.; LÖHRER, J.: Ein neues Spezialeisen zur Behandlung der Spatlahmheit. Schweiz. Arch. Tierheilk. *98:* 505 (1956).
PETERS, H.: Orthopädie an den Extremitäten der Fohlen. Dtsch. tierärztl. Wschr. *22:* 337 (1938).
RICHTER, W.: Erhebungen über belastungsbedingte Gliedmaßenerkrankungen des juvenilen und adulten Sportpferdes. Vet.-med. Diss. (B), Berlin (1975).
RONNEY, J. R.: Biomechanics of equine lameness. Cornell. Vet., suppl. 58, p. 49 (1968).
SASCHEK, M.: Röntgenanatomische Studien zum Spat des Pferdes. Vet.-med. Diss., Hannover (1964).
SCHEBITZ, H.; WILKENS, H.: Zum Spat des Pferdes — Untersuchung u. Therapie. Berliner Münchener tierärztl. Wschr. *80:* 385 (1967).
SCHNEIDER, W.: Weitere Untersuchungen über die Wirksamkeit von Arumalon ad us. vet. bei degenerativen Gelenkerkrankungen der Pferde. Tierärztl. Umschau *27:* 132 (1972).
SILBERSIEPE, E.; BERGE, E.; MÜLLER, H.: Lehrbuch der speziellen Chirurgie (Enke, Stuttgart 1976).
SOENNICHSEN, H. V.: personal commun. (1977).
WAMBERG, K.: Eine neue Behandlungsmethode bei Spat. Kongressbericht, Stockholm, p. 957 (1953).
ZELLER, R.: Zur Therapie des Spat. Bericht über 104 Spatoperationen nach Wamberg. Berliner Münchner tierärztl. Wschr. *81:* 382 (1968).

2.1.19.4.2. Osteochondritis dissecans (OCD) of the Hock Joint

(OCD of the Shoulder Joint in Foals, see 2.1.18.1.1.; Gonotrochleosis, see 2.1.19.2.4.)

Occurrence. Osteochondritis dissecans is a disease that is common in man as well as in cattle, swine, dogs and horses. However, its occurrence in horses frequently goes unrecognized. BIRKELAND and HAAKENSTAD [1968] described 7 cases of 'intracapsular bone fragments' from the distal tibia in horses. No doubt osteochondritis dissecans was present in some of these cases. In 1970 VAN PELT recorded sporadic cases of OCD in the stifle joint of the horse.

Since the publications of DE MOOR et al. [1971, 1972], this disease has become a subject of greater interest, and much has been learned about its prevalence [ADAMS, 1974; BOLZ et al., 1975; HAAKENSTAD and BIRKELAND, 1974; SCHEBITZ et al., 1975). OCD of the hock joint is most often seen in Standardbreds and in trotters and is less common in Thoroughbreds, riding horses and draft horses. In Thoroughbreds and Standardbreds, OCD affects the stifle joint more frequently than the hock [STRÖMBERG and REJNÖ, 1978]. The disease is very rare in ponies. It is most commonly diagnosed in 1- to 2-years-olds. The changes usually develop at the age of 3—6 months, during a period of rapid bone growth. However, a typical bilateral osteochondrosis has been observed in a 3-day-old trotter foal [REJNÖ and STRÖMBERG, 1978]. The disease is somewhat more common in males than females. It is bilateral in 80 % of cases. With unilateral OCD of the hock joint, the left tibiotarsal joint is affected more frequently than the right. Osteochondritic lesions are most common of the intermediate ridge of the distal end of the tibia, but they also occur on the medial malleolus or the ridges of the tibial tarsal bone. In some cases more than one part of the joint is affected. In the femoropatellar joint, lesions occur mainly on the lateral edge of the femoral trochlea [O'BRIEN, 1973]. The fibers of the extensor digitalis longus tendon are usually frayed near their site of origin [STRÖMBERG, 1973], and this is a site of predilection for the occurrence of bilateral OCD. Sometimes the disease affects the patella or one of the femoral condyles. The humeral head may also be affected [MASON and MCLEAN, 1977].

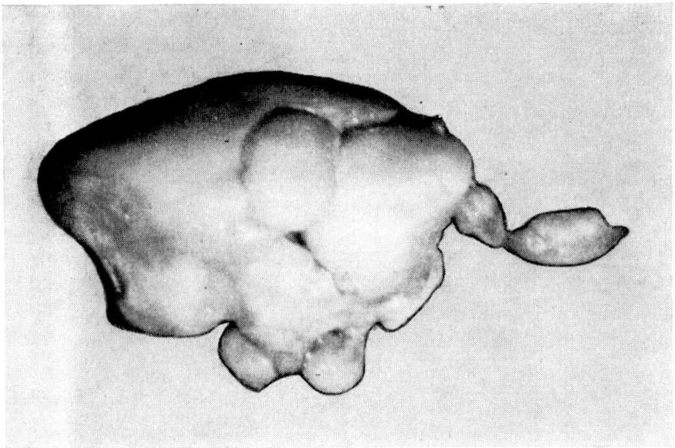

Fig. 2.1.19. — 38. Osteochondritis dissecans of the hock joint: multiple fragments at the distal end of the tibia.

Definition. In man, OCD is characterized by the idiopathic separation of a subchondral bone fragment and overlying cartilage at the level of a convex joint surface. This definition holds to some extent for OCD in horses, although multiple fragments are more common in this species (fig. 2.1.19. — 38).

Symptoms. In most cases the volume of joint fluid is increased, sometimes markedly. The synovial fluid looks almost normal on gross examination. Analysis of the fluid reveals an increase in all LDH fractions. If severe cartilage lesions are present, there is a particularly marked increase in the LDH-5 fraction, which is located almost exclusively in the cartilage [Rejnö, 1976].

Approximately 25 % of horses with OCD of the hock manifest a lameness with reduced flexion of the tibiotarsal joint, go stiffly at the trot, or have difficulty turning. Patients with small fragments usually show no clinical symptoms, and their condition is discovered incidentally during radiographie examination. Some animals present with an acute lameness caused by the separation of a large fragment from its bed. The spavin test is positive in less than half of cases. OCD of the stifle joint is characterized by a positive spavin test and a mild to moderate lameness. Lateral luxation of the patella is often present [Strömberg, 1976].

Etiology and Pathogenesis. The etiology of osteochondritis dissecans is not fully understood. The ischemic theory, which involves an interruption of the blood supply to an area of subchondral bone, is difficult to explain without assuming a concomitant fracture or multiple thrombi in the subchondral bone. However this bone is devoid of terminal blood vessels. Some authors [Aichroth, 1971; Bandi, 1951; Schebitz et al., 1975] suggest that the condition is due to an acute subchondral fracture. In many cases, however, no history of trauma can be elicited.

The disease tends to be bilateral both in man and in horses. Based upon experimental studies, Langenskiöld [1955] and Tallquist [1962] suggest that OCD could be the result of cartilage fractures in which a bony nucleus subsequently developed. While this theory may be correct in the dog, it cannot account for the deep defects in the subchondral bone that are found in man and the horse. Aichroth [1971] showed in the rabbit that experimental osteochondral fractures of the medial femoral condyle progress to a pseudarthrosis when there is movement at the level of the fracture. Radiographic

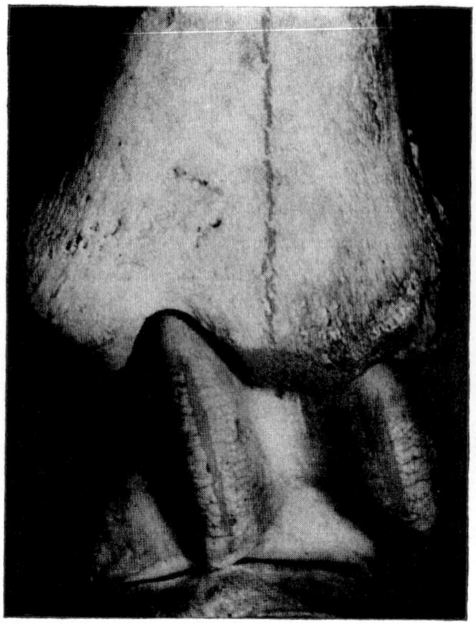

39

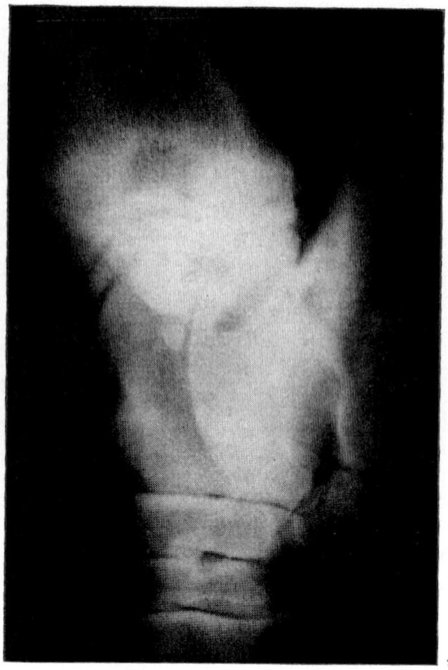

40

Fig. 2.1.19. — 39. Osteochondritis dissecans of the hock joint: angle between tibia and tibial tarsal bone.

Fig. 2.1.19. — 40. Osteochondritis dissecans of the intermediate ridge of the distal tibia (craniolateral-to-caudomedial view).

and histologic studies show much similarity between these osteochondral fragments and osteochondritis dissecans in the human knee. Smillie [1960] believed that OCD might be due to the separation of a fragment from an ossification center, with necrosis ensuing due to the lack of a blood supply. In the horse, however, there is no special ossification center in the part of the distal tibia where typical lesions are found. Other authors state that the bone necrosis is the result of repeated microtrauma at a site where abnormal stresses are imposed due to defects of conformation, weak articular ligaments, incongruent joint surfaces or deficient blood flow. An abnormal angle between the tibia and the tibial tarsal bone may also be a contributing factor in the horse (fig. 2.1.19. — 39). During extreme flexion of the hock joint, the dorsal ridge of the distal tibia engages against the dorsal surface of the central tarsal bone. During flexion of the stifle joint, the patella exerts pressure on the lateral edge of the femoral trochlea. The theory holds that these 'stress sites' are predisposed to the development of vasomotor disturbances, capillary ruptures or microfractures, leading to necrosis in a portion of the bone. As a result of this necrosis, a plane of cleavage develops between the necrotic fragments and surrounding bone, creating a fibrous and fibrocartilaginous pseudarthrosis that interferes with healing. In favorable cases where the limb is kept relatively immobile, the fragment may become reattached to its bed through bony union. The fragment that is held in its bed only by cartilage and connective tissue can be dislodged by trauma and become a loose body (joint mouse). In most cases the surface of the defect becomes covered with a thin layer of fibrocartilaginous tissue. The theory of recurrent microtrauma at predisposed sites is consistent with the observation of a predisposition for the disease. This predisposition may take various forms and may involve defects of anatomy, tissue quality

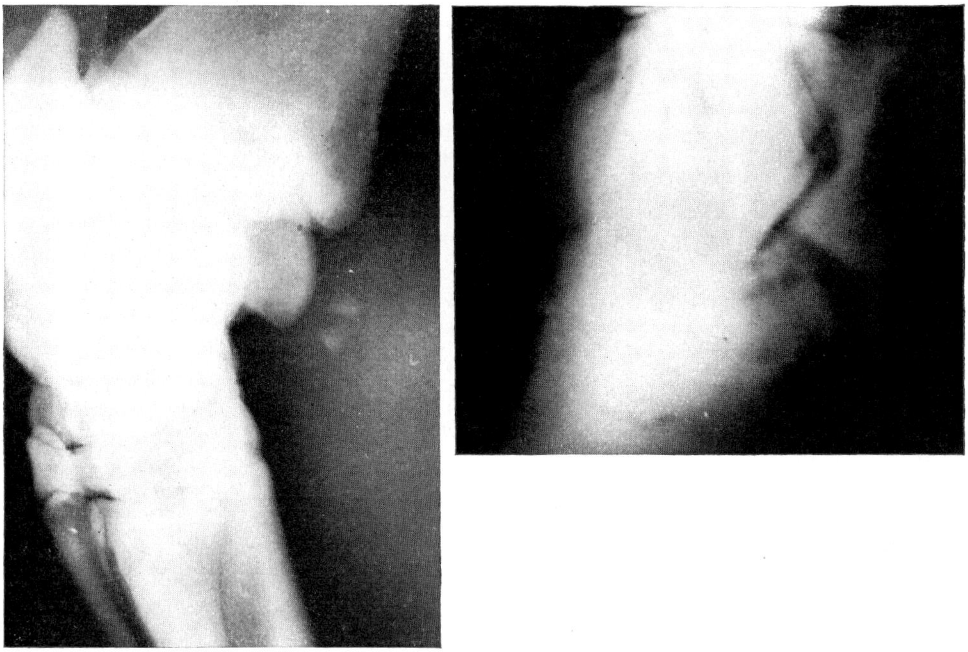

Fig. 2.1.19. — 41. Osteochondritis dissecans of the intermediate ridge of the distal tibia (caudo-ateral-to-craniomedial view).

or blood flow. The frequent bilateral occurrence of OCD could perhaps be the result of bilateral constitutional defects. A familial incidence has often been described in man. In horses, we have discovered a number of 'familial cases' among Standardbreds.

The occurrence of the disease in young, growing animals might be due to weakness of the epiphyses, since strong subchondral bone has not yet had time to form.

Osteochondritis dissecans may also be a manifestation of a systemic osteochondrosis. This is described as a primary cartilaginous disease with cartilage thickening, a disturbance of endochondral ossification, and a degeneration and necrosis of the cartilage [Rejnö and Strömberg, 1978]. Constant pressure and excessive stress cause fissures to develop in the basal layers of the thickened cartilage. The fissure may extend from the deep layer to the cartilage surface. The metaphyseal growth cartilage may also become involved — this at a time when the growth zone is in a period of increased activity. There is an hereditary predisposition for the disease. It is associated with rapid growth and the consumption of high-energy feeds [Strömberg, 1979].

Diagnosis. Radiographs are necessary for a definitive diagnosis, and bilateral films are recommended. Usually 2—4 radiographs are taken of each joint. The hock joint is best demonstrated with craniolateral-to-caudomedial (70°) and caudolateral-to-craniomedial (115°) views (figs. 2.1.19. — 40 and — 41).

The radiographs reveal a crater-like zone of decalcification with an associated separation of one or more subchondral bone fragments. Sometimes loose bodies are seen, or other changes may be evident such as degenerative joint disease of the intertarsal or tarsometatarsal joints (in about 20% of cases), tibial subchondral bone cysts, or intra-articular fractures. It is unclear whether a connection exists between

42
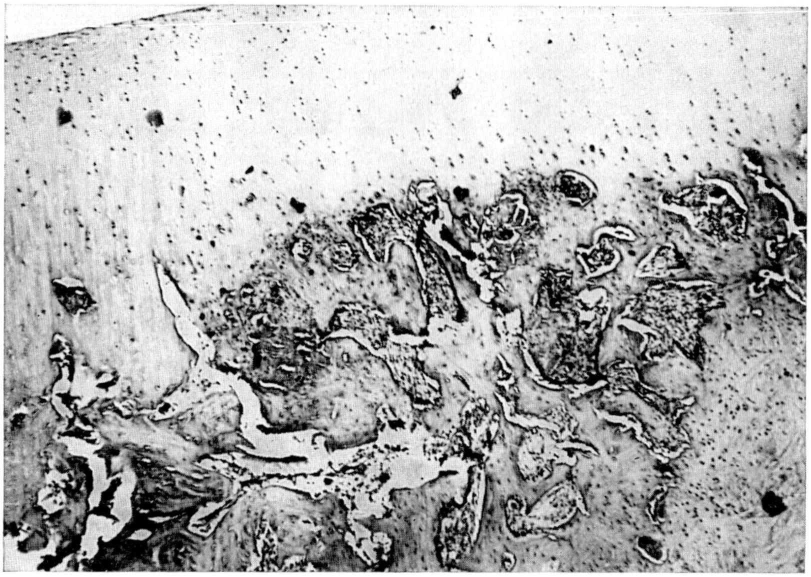

43
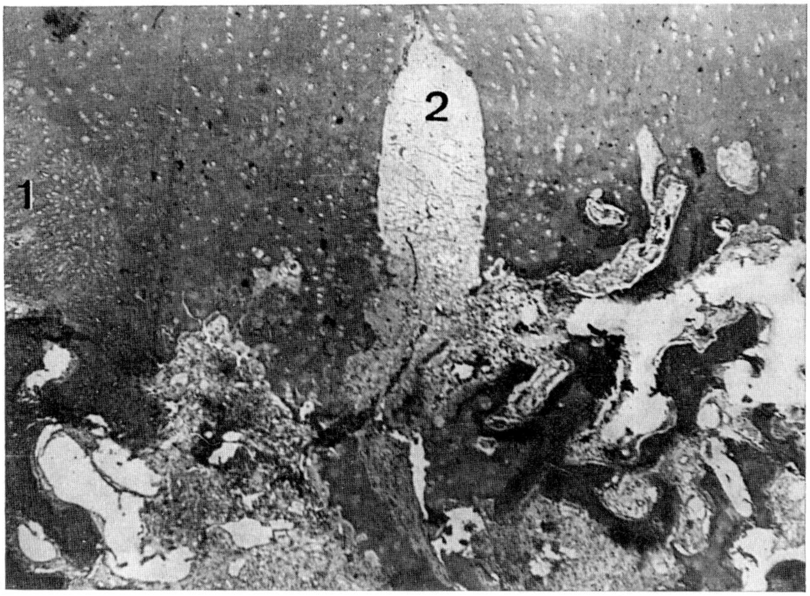

Fig. 2.1.19. — 42. Osteochondritis dissecans: bone fragment with three different tissues: cartilage, bone, collagenous connective tissue.

Fig. 2.1.19. — 43. Osteochondritis dissecans: local regressive cartilage changes. 1 = fibrillation; 2 = cleft formation due to hemorrhage.

OCD and degenerative joint disease of the intertarsal or tarsometatarsal joints. Osteochondritis dissecans of the lateral edge of the femoral trochlea is best demonstrated in the lateral-to-medial view. This will show defects with irregularities in the subchondral bone and often will reveal loose bodies. Xeroradiography shows the lesions very clearly.

Lesions. Histologically the fragments are composed of 3 tissue types: cartilage, bone, and connective tissue.

The cartilage has roughly the appearance of normal articular cartilage with a columnar chondrocyte architecture (fig. 2.1.19. — 42). Each fragment contains a zone of calcification that is often irregular. The cartilage shows such degenerative changes as vacuolization, fibrillation and fissuring due to hemorrhage (fig. 2.1.19. — 43).

The bone usually has a lamellar arrangement and shows various hemorrhagic foci. Necrosis is uncommon and is limited to areas surrounding the hemorrhagic foci. Schebitz et al. [1975] were unable to detect ischemia-induced necrosis of medullary and bony tissues or any vascular lesions that could produce such changes. Numerous foci of fibrous cartilage with young fibroblasts are found in the bone. Fibrillation and fibrosis of adjacent bone marrow are generally present. Fluorescence has been demonstrated in the bone tissue of animals injected with oxytetracycline, indicating that this tissue is not necrotic.

Electron microscopic examination reveals hyperplasia, degeneration and inflammation of the synovial cell layers.

Both grossly and microscopically, the fragments show a greater similarity to OCD in man than to OCD in dogs. Necrotic bone changes are much less pronounced than in man, however.

Prognosis. The prognosis depends mainly on the degree of functional disability and thus on the extent and number of fragments and their degree of attachment with their beds. Equally important is the unilateral or bilateral occurrence of the disease, and the presence or absence of arthrotic changes and wear lines on the articular surfaces of the distal tibia and the tibial tarsal bone. When the stifle joint is affected, the prognosis is guarded, regardless of whether or not surgical intervention is attempted (Strömberg and Rejnö, 1978].

Treatment. Cases with little or no joint distension, no functional disability and small-size fragments will usually heal without treatment. Overfeeding should be avoided. These animals can sometimes be restored to a very good performance level. Of course, there is always a danger that the fragment or fragments will separate to become loose bodies. In animals with pronounced hydarthrosis and locomotor disability, conservative treatment with intra-articular injections of long-acting glucocorticosteroids and rest is useless and will at best serve to temporarily check the accumulation of joint fluid.

Intra-articular injections of hyaluronic acid or chondroitin sulfuric acid appear to be more beneficial than corticosteroids. Surgical intervention is indicated only if large fragments or loose bodies are present, there is an extreme accumulation of synovial fluid, or significant locomotor disability exists. If the function of only one joint is impaired in bilateral cases of OCD, only unilateral surgery is necessary.

Surgical treatment will have little chance of success, however, if degenerative joint disease or other changes have developed in the hock joint or other parts of the limb.

Haakenstad and Birkeland [1974] achieved good results, especially in animals under 4 years of age, with the following surgical method: The horse is placed in lateral recumbency under halothane anesthesia, and the affected limb is positioned with the hock joint slightly flexed. The skin is incised parallel and lateral to the

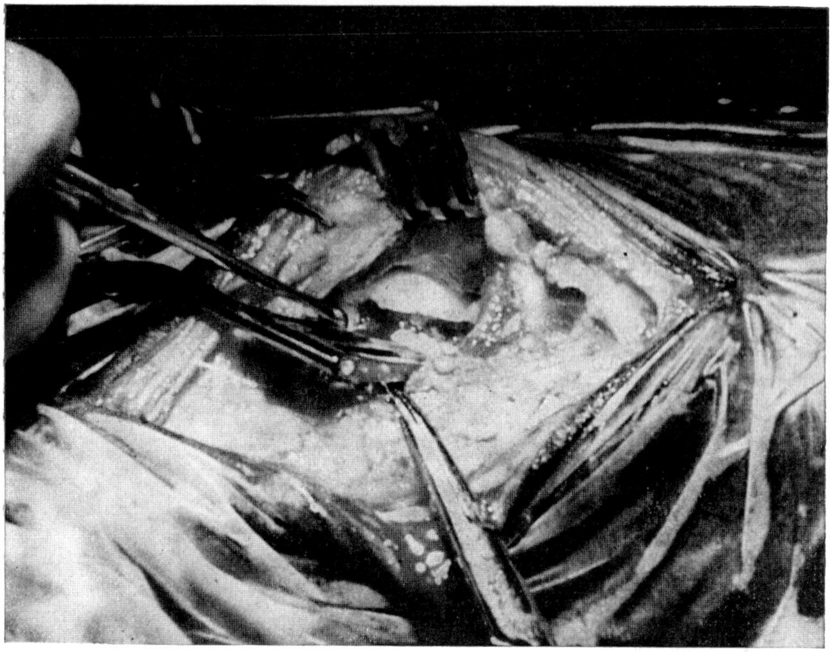

Fig. 2.1.19. — 44. Osteochondritis dissecans of the lateral ridge of the tibial tarsal bone: curettage down to healthy, bleeding bone.

tendon of the long digital extensor muscle, the incision extending from 3 cm above the malleolus to 5 cm below it. If the volume of synovial fluid is increased, a bulge will appear at this site when pressure is applied to the large dorsomedial articular sac.

The superficial and deep fibers are divided, taking care to spare the superficial peroneal nerve. The anterior tibial vein is dissected free, and small lateral branches are ligated.

At this stage it is usually possible to palpate the fragment or fragments through the joint capsule. The capsule is opened with a 2-cm-long incision placed slightly lateral to the fragment. In many cases hypertrophic synovial villi will immediately protrude from the wound.

The fragment is carefully freed with a periosteal elevator or meniscotome and removed with a forceps. It the fragment is already loose, this is easily done. If it is firmly adherent to cartilage, connective tissue or a ligament, it must be carefully detached with a small chisel.

If the fragment is situated on the intermediate ridge of the distal tibia, curettage is unnecessary. If it is on one of the ridges of the tibial tarsal bone, it is best to curet down to healthy, bleeding bone in order to promote cartilage regeneration (fig. 2.1.19. — 44). If the animal has been treated with intra-articular injections of glucocorticoids, the arthrotomy should be deferred until 6—8 weeks after the last injection.

Detached fragments are removed from the joint. Sometimes this is difficult due to the extensor tendon, which hinders surgery on the medial side. The joint is irrigated with physiologic saline and antibiotics and sutured in two layers. The synovial layer is closed with interrupted mattress sutures of 3/0 silk, and the fibrous layer with a continuous suture, also of 3/0 silk.

After the deep fascia, subcutaneous connective tissue and skin have been sutured, the joint is protected with cotton and an elastic bandage. On the 8th postoperative day the bandage is changed, the wound is inspected, and any excess synovial fluid is aspirated. The joint is kept under a bandage for 3 weeks. Six months' postoperative rest is recommended.

The results of the operation are favorable if no additional lesions are present. The clinical symptoms of osteochondritis dissecans of the stifle and shoulder joints are usually improved by surgical treatment, However, in most cases there is little chance that the animal will recover to full soundness.

References

ADAMS, O. R.: Lameness in horses (Lea & Febiger, Philadelphia 1974).

AICHROTH, P. M.: Osteochondritis dissecans of the knee. A clinical study. J. Bone & Joint Surg. (1971), 53-B, 440, 448.

BANDI, W.: Über die Ätiologie des Osteochondritis dissecans. Helvet. Chirurg. Acta *18:* 221 (1951).

BIRKELAND, R.; HAAKENSTAD, L. E.: Intracapsular body fragments of the distal tibia of the horse. J. Amer. vet. med. Assoc. *152:* 1526 (1968).

BOLZ, W.; DIETZ, O.; SCHLEITER, H.; TEUSCHER, R.: Lehrbuch der Speziellen Veterinärchirurgie, 2. Aufl. (VEB Gustav Fischer Verlag, Jena 1975).

BURROWS, H. J.: Osteochondritis juvenilis. J. Bone & Joint Surg. (1959), 41-B, 455.

DE MOOR, A.; VERSCHOOTEN, F.; HOORENS, J.: Osteochondritis dissecans of the tibiotarsal joint in the horse. Proc. XIXth World Veterin. Congr., Mexico City, 1971, Vol. 1, p. 378.

DE MOOR, A.; VERSCHOOTEN, F.; DESMET, P.; STEENHAUT, M.; HOORENS, J.; WOLF, G.: Osteochondritis dissecans of the tibio-tarsal joint in the horse. Equine Vet. J. *4:* 139 (1972).

HAAKENSTAD, L. H.; BIRKELAND, R.: Osteochondritis dissecans i hasseleddet hos hest. Kirurgisk og konservativ behandling. Proc. 12th Nordisk Vet. Congr., Reykjavik, 1974, p. 34.

JOHANSSON, H.; REJNÖ, S.: Light and electron microscopic examination of equine synovial membrane. A comparison between healthy joints and joints with intraarticular fractures and osteochondrosis dissecans. Acta vet. scand. *17:* 153 (1976).

LANGENSKIÖLD, A.: Can osteochondritis dissecans arise as a sequel of cartilage fracture in early childhood? Acta Chirurg. Scand *109:* 206 (1955).

MASON, T.; MCLEAN, A.: Osteochondrosis dissecans of the head of the humerus in two foals. Equine Vet. J. *9:* 189 (1977).

MOORE, J.; MCILWRAITH, W.: Osteochondrosis of the equine stifle. Vet. Rec. *100:* 133 (1977).

O'BRIEN, T.: Radiology of the equine stifle. Proc. 19th Ann. Conv. Amer. Assoc. Equine Pract., p. 271 (1973).

PELT, R. W. VAN; RIILEY, W. F.; TILLOTSON, P. J.: Stifle disease (gonitis) in horses: clinicopathologic findings and intra-articular therapy. J. Amer. vet. med. Assoc. *157:* 1173 (1970).

REJNÖ, S.: LDH and LDH iso-enzymes of synovial fluid in the horse. Acta vet. scand. *17:* 178 (1976).

REJNÖ, S.; STRÖMBERG, B.: Osteochondrosis in the horse. II. Pathology. Acta Radiol., Stockholm, suppl. 358, 153 (1978).

SAMY, M.: Osteochondrosis dissecans bei Mensch, Hund und Pferd. Vet.-med. Diss., Hannover (1977).

SCHEBITZ, H.; DÄMMRICH, K.; WAIBL, H.: Intraartikuläre Absprengungsfrakturen im Articulus talocruralis beim Pferd. Berliner Münchener Tierärztl. Wschr. *88:* 309 (1975).

SMILLIE, I. S.: Osteochondritis dissecans (Livingstone, Edinburgh 1960).

STRÖMBERG, B.: Osteochondrosis dissecans of the knee joint. A clinical, radiographic and pathologic study. J. Amer. Vet. Rad. Soc. *14:* 83 (1973).

STRÖMBERG, B.: Osteochondrosis dissecans of the stifle joint in the horse: A clinical, radiographic and pathologic study. J. Amer. Vet. Rad. Soc. *17:* 117 (1976).

Strömberg, B.: A review of the salient features of osteochondrosis in the horse. Equine Vet. J. *11:* 211 (1979).
Strömberg, B.; Rejnö, S.: Osteochondrosis in the horse. I. A clinical and radiologic investigation of osteochondritis dissecans of the knee and hock joint. Acta Radiol., Stockholm, suppl. 358, 139 (1978).
Tallquist, G.: The reaction to mechanical trauma in growing articular cartilage. Acta Orthop. Scand., suppl. 53 (1962).
Wyburn, R. S.: A degenerative joint disease in the horse. New Zealand Vet. J. *25:* 321 (1977).

2.1.19.4.3. Hock Splints

Definition and Occurrence. A 'hock splint' is a hard, usually painless enlargement occurring on the lateral aspect of the hock. The term encompasses different processes of varying etiology:

1. a spavin-like chronic inflammation in the area of the fourth tarsal bone ('spavin splint');
2. an ossifying periostitis in the lateral, distal portion of the tarsus, which may spread to involve the third metatarsal or proximal end of the fourth metatarsal;
3. a chronic inflammation of the lateral capsular ligament (periarthritis) or of the tendon and tendon sheath of the lateral digital extensor;
4. abnormal enlargement of the proximal end of the fourth metatarsal or fourth tarsal, causing unusual prominence of the lateral contour of the hock ('congenital hock splint').

Etiology. Spavin splint has a pathogenesis similar to that of bone spavin. Ossifying periostitis and chronic periarthritis are usually the result of a single, forceful trauma or of subcutaneous injuries, tendon sheath wounds or local abscessation.

Diagnosis. A hard, painless enlargement on the lateral aspect of the tarsus readily differentiates hock splints from other conditions. Spavin splints may cause a moderate lameness that improves with exercise.

Radiographs may be taken in order to localize the change and ascertain its specific nature.

Treatment and Prognosis. Acquired spavin splints have been treated with firing followed by blistering and corrective shoeing. Congenital hock splints require no treatment and are important only in terms of differential diagnosis.

2.1.19.4.4. Arthritis of the Hock Joint, Tarsitis

Definition and Occurrence. The hock joint is comprised of the tibiotarsal, intertarsal, and tarsometatarsal joints. The proximal intertarsal joint communicates with the tibiotarsal joint. Besides spavin, the following inflammatory diseases can occur in this region:

— acute or chronic, aseptic arthritis;
— chronic degenerative arthritis and periarthritis, a diffuse, usually unilateral inflammation involving the entire hock joint and occurring at any age. Idiopathic, infectious tarsitis is seen in foals with metastatic pyogenic polyarthritis;
— suppurative arthritis resulting from perforating injuries or the extension of suppurative inflammatory processes from surrounding tissues.

2.1.19.4.5. Acute Tarsitis, Chronic Tarsitis

Etiology. Aseptic acute and chronic tarsitis are caused by single or repeated contusions or sprains of the hock joint. Less frequently they are the result of closed fractures or luxations of the tarsal bones.

Symptoms. There is a fluctuating, painful distension of the hock, especially in the area of the tibiotarsal joint. A mild to moderate mixed lameness is present. No systemic reaction occurs.

Differential diagnosis is made chiefly from edema of the joint capsule or tendon sheaths (absence of pain and lameness) and from spavin.

Peritarsitis is distinguished by a hard, periarticular swelling with little pain. When a sudden, severe lameness develops in the hock joint, a luxation or fracture of one of the tarsal bones should be suspected. Radiographic findings will enable a differentiation to be made.

Diagnosis. The clinical symptoms and course of the disease will identify the tarsitis as being chronic or acute. The diagnosis can be established by aspirating the joint and analyzing the synovial fluid and by radiographic examination.

Treatment. Acute aseptic tarsitis can be managed by single or repeated intra-articular injections of glucocorticoid preparations, with or without hyaluronic acid [Rydell et al., 1970]. Good results are also achieved with moist heat and mild rubefacients or dimethylsulfoxide. A rest period of at least 4 weeks is necessary in both cases.

With chronic arthritis, blistering and point firing followed by 6—8 weeks' rest may be indicated. Often, however, this treatment will only worsen the animal's condition, especially in cases where degenerative processes are already present. The parenteral or oral administration of phenylbutazone and glucocorticoids can favorably influence healing.

Prognosis. Recurrences are possible in chronic cases. Therefore, affected horses should remain on a light work schedule for some time following treatment. Corrective shoeing with a spavin shoe is also helpful in relieving stress on the tarsus.

2.1.19.4.6. Wounds and Wound Infections of the Hock Joint (Acute Traumatic Suppurative Arthritis of the Tibiotarsal, Intertarsal and Tarsometatarsal Joints)

Definition and Etiology. Various forms and degrees of trauma (kicks, pitchfork and barbed wire injuries, etc.) can cause superficial or perforating wounds of the hock, especially in its less protected portions. These wounds can lead to pyogenic joint infection with all the stages of suppurative joint inflammation, acute pyogenic serous or serofibrinous arthritis, acute suppurative synovitis, capsular cellulitis and purulent panarthritis (fig. 2.1.19. — 45).

Symptoms. Fresh wounds that penetrate the joint are marked by the discharge of a clear or blood-tinged, slightly frothy synovial fluid. Lameness is not present initially. Only after 1—2 days does the hock joint acquire a spindle-shape contour, the synovial fluid becoming cloudy and flocculent. A mild to severe lameness appears and is usually accompanied by a febrile systemic reaction. The lameness and joint distension become progressively worse during subsequent days. In the stage of acute suppurative synovitis (joint empyema), recumbency may develop if stress laminitis of the sound limb complicates the disease process.

Diagnosis. Escaping synovial fluid, painful joint distension and moderate to severe lameness are symptomatic of joint infection. Aspiration is necessary only in doubtful

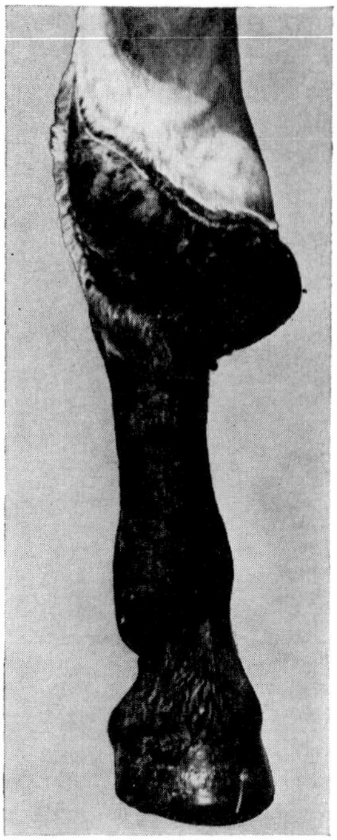

45

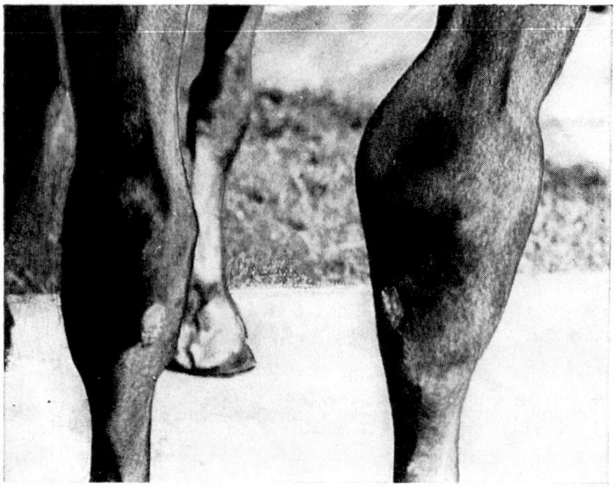

46

Fig. 2.1.19. — 45. Old lacerated wound of the hock.
Fig. 2.1.19. — 46. Bog spavin.

cases, using strict aseptic technic. Identification of the infectious organism may be of therapeutic and prognostic value.

Treatment. Fresh joint wounds are treated with antibiotics and closed. Large wounds, however, must be sutured in several layers to obtain a secure closure; the joint capsule is also closed if possible. Antibiotics are administered intra-articularly (2 to 3 million I.U.) and systemically (4—8 million I.U. penicillin daily). The wound is immobilized and protected with a well-fitting, padded bandage (danger of decubitus over tuber calcis). Intra-articular injections of antibiotic are made between the calcaneus and tibia, at a distance from the wound. In older cases, large doses of local and systemic antibiotics are repeatedly administered until fever has subsided.

Prognosis. The sooner treatment is instituted, the better the chance of recovery. In the stage of empyema and abscess-forming panarthritis, recovery is no longer possible without destruction of the joint. Perforating wounds of the intertarsal or tarsometatarsal joints have a more favorable prognosis than wounds of the tibiotarsal joint.

2.1.19.4.7. Chronic Degenerative Tarsitis and Peritarsitis

Etiology. This may be a primary condition caused by injuries, fractures or sprains, or may develop secondarily due to the spread of inflammatory processes from neighboring tissues. Thus, a chronic degenerative inflammation involving the entire tarsus can develop gradually as a result of spavin, curb, tendovaginitis, chronic arthritis of the tibiotarsal joint and cellulitis.

Symptoms. The most characteristic finding is a diffuse, hard, usually spindle-shaped swelling of the entire hock joint that shows little heat and has been preceded by a painful inflammatory condition. Ankylosis may develop, restricting or prohibiting movement in the joint. Lameness may be absent or may develop suddenly following a fall. Sometimes the lameness disappears with exercise. Horses with chronic degenerative tarsitis may be reluctant to lie down and, once recumbent, have great difficulty rising. Following renewed trauma, the process may flare up causing sudden lameness. Systemic signs are absent.

Differential diagnosis must be made from all acute pathologic processes in the hock region.

Diagnosis. A diffuse, hard swelling of the entire hock, together with the nature of the lameness and absence of systemic signs, suggests a diagnosis of chronic degenerative tarsitis and peritarsitis.

Diagnostic anesthesia can be used to ascertain the extent of any ankylosis that may have developed. Radiographs in the latero-medial and dorso-plantar projection provide information on the degree of changes within the joint. In severe cases the ossifying processes may spread to the tibia and the metatarsal bones.

Treatment. Mild cases respond best to rubefacient therapy (rest, moist heat, microwave therapy, iodine and camphor ointments). Intra- and periarticular glucocorticoid injections are of little value. Corrective shoeing with a spavin shoe will reduce stress on the hock joint. Good results have been reported with the use of acid mucopolysaccharides (arumalon, arteparon) [SCHNEIDER, 1972; KUBITZA, 1966]. In some cases function can be temporarily restored with repeated oral or parenteral doses of phenylbutazone and glucocorticoids. Point firing and blistering frequently make the condition worse. Finally, a permanent lameness can be corrected by a double neurectomy of the tibial and deep peroneal nerve. This method is antiquated, however, and should be used only as a last resort due to the loss of sensation in the distal part of the limb.

Prognosis. An anatomic restoration cannot be achieved.

Comments. When lameness is relieved, the horse is still serviceable for light work or breeding.

2.1.19.4.8. Bog Spavin

Definition and Occurrence. Bog spavin is a distension of the tibiotarsal joint capsule that is unassociated with inflammatory symptoms. It may be unilateral or bilateral.

Etiology. A distinction is made between congenital and acquired bog spavin. In many horses the condition appears between 1 and 2 years of age, possibly as the result of vitamin and mineral deficiency. Acquired bog spavin occurs secondarily to acute or chronic joint inflammation.

Symptoms. Lameness is absent. The swellings are round to oval in shape, soft and fluctuating, and are neither warm nor painful. Generally there are 2, or less frequently 3, characteristic swellings that appear at different points about the hock:

— a lateral swelling, located on the upper posterolateral aspect of the hock near the end of the tibia (fig. 2.1.19. — 46);
— a larger medial swelling, located on the lower anteromedial aspect of the hock anterior to the medial collateral ligament.

Besides these two swellings, there may also be a simple lateral or anterior swelling, or the swelling may extend about the circumference of the hock. These forms are less common.

Differential diagnosis must be made from osteochondritis dissecans of the hock joint. Exclusion is made by radiography.

Diagnosis. Distension of the tibiotarsal joint unaccompanied by inflammatory changes, and lameness are features of bog spavin. In congenital cases aspiration yields a thin, clear, watery, largely acellular synovial fluid. In acquired cases the fluid may be viscous, stringy, dark yellow and permeated with flakes. The cell count is within normal limits [GÄNGEL, 1970].

The synovial villi are proliferated and thickened, like the fibrous wall layer of the joint capsule. Strands and septae are sometimes present in the joint cavity.

Treatment. Acquired bog spavin responds well to single or repeated intra-articular glucocorticoid injections [VAN PELT, 1968]. Chronic bog spavin with joint capsule thickening may cause lameness and has been treated with blistering or firing. Mucopolysaccharide therapy may be tried in congenital cases.

Prognosis. Congenital and acquired bogs often represent simple cosmetic blemishes. However, an acute or chronic arthritis can develop at any time when stresses are imposed on the joint. Horses with congenital bog spavin are considered unfit for breeding.

2.1.19.4.9. Wounds and Inflammation of the Tendon Sheaths of the Hock Joint (Tendovaginitis at the Tarsal Joint)

Wounds and Inflammations of the Common Tendon Sheath of the Flexor Hallucis Longus and Tibialis Caudalis Muscles

Definition and Occurrence. The tendons of the flexor hallucis longus and tibialis caudalis muscles possess a common tendon sheath as they traverse the medial side of the tarsus. Injuries can cause various forms of inflammation with pronounced swelling, because distally the very long mesotenon of this sheath is constricted in annular fashion by the tarsal ligament. Intratendovaginal inflammation or pus can spread to involve the tendon and can lead to partial necrosis.

Serous, serofibrinous and metastatic inflammation as a result of strains and pyogenic polyarthritides is rare. The tarsal joint may also be inflamed in some cases.

Etiology. The causes are perforating wounds of the medial aspect of the hock joint resulting from pitchfork injuries, kicks, and lacerations sustained when jumping over hurdles. Infection can occur either primarily from an open wound of the tendon sheath, or secondarily through the extension of pyogenic processes from adjacent tissues. In rare cases fibrillary tendon tears due to excessive strain can be a cause of aseptic inflammation.

Symptoms. Acute pyogenic tendovaginitis always produces a febrile systemic reaction. During rest the limb is held in flexion and bears no weight. During progression the foot is slow to break over the center of the toe, and the horse goes on its heels. A similar 'plodding' gait is seen with tendon ruptures. In advanced cases, weight is no longer borne on the affected limb. Locally there is a very painful, warm swelling extending from the chestnut to a hand's width above the calcaneus, parallel to the Achilles tendon. This swelling is soft initially but later becomes more firm. If cellulitis has developed, the medial aspect of the hock joint will be enlarged. Wounds are marked by the discharge of an initially clear, later turbid, grayish-yellow synovial fluid or a thick, creamy pus. With an acute aseptic tendovaginitis, clinical symptoms are less pronounced, and lameness may be slight.

Differential diagnosis must be made from acute inflammation of the tibiotarsal joint. This is difficult only if pronounced peritendovaginal cellulitis is present.

Diagnosis. The localization of the changes and the typical visual findings on palpation establish the diagnosis. Small wounds often are already healed at the time of examination, while larger wounds may show early granulation. A gelatinous, purulent exudate is discharged from the wound opening. In doubtful cases a synovial fluid analysis can be done to evaluate for tendon sheath infection.

Treatment. Fresh wounds are immediately closed after first treating the tendon sheath with antibiotics. In older cases where an infectious tendovaginitis has been demonstrated, a 40- to 50-mm incision is made at the lowest point of the swelling, the sheath is irrigated with antiseptic agents, and antibiotics are instilled. The tendon sheath may also be opened at both ends and drained. Better results are obtained in old and severe cases by a complete resection of both tendons contained within the sheath. In this procedure both muscles are sectioned transversely with a blunt bistoury at their musculotendinous junctions. Then the tendon is freed, either digitally or with instruments, through a second incision at the distal recess. The isolated tendon stump is exteriorized and severed at its site of attachment with the long digital flexor tendon. Because this tendon forms the main component of the deep flexor tendon, the effect of the operation is similar to that of a tendon rupture, i.e., there is hyperextension of the third phalanx, which is corrected by means of a shoe with extended heels. In about 3 months a connective-tissue band will form that will partially assume the function of the resected tendon.

Applying warm dressings moistened with antiseptic solutions, confining the patient to a large stall with soft bedding, and giving systemic sulfonamides and antibiotics until fever has subsided will also aid recovery. Aseptic inflammations respond favorably to topical rubefacients, or intratendovaginal glucocorticoid injections [van Pelt, 1969]. Either the swelling will recede, or a fibrous-tissue thickening will remain.

Prognosis. In heavy horses with purulent tendovaginitis, the prognosis is unfavorable. Light horses that are treated surgically (tenectomy) for this condition are sound for working at slow gaits. In cases of aseptic inflammation, even race horses can recover to full working capacity.

Wounds and Inflammation of the Tendon Sheath of the Lateral Digital Extensor

Occurrence and Etiology. The tendon of the lateral digital extensor runs over the lateral aspect of the hock joint. It is provided with only a short synovial sheath that may become opened and infected as a result of trauma, especially pitchfork injuries.

Symptoms. An elongated, fluctuating, painful swelling is evident on the lateral aspect of the hock. The associated locomotor disturbance is slight.

Prognosis and Treatment. Perforating puncture wounds heal well when treated with topical agents and antibiotic injections.

2.1.19.4.10. Scar Tissue on the Flexor Surface of the Hock

Definition and Occurrence. Perforating cutaneous wounds of the hock region may lead to the occurrence of an enlargement on the flexor surface of the hock joint or, less commonly, on its lateral aspect. This is often a consequence of improper wound care. In time connective tissue develops that is either devoid of epithelium or has some epithelium that is prone to keratinization.

Etiology and Symptoms. Usually there is a history of an old wound to the flexor surface of the hock. Lameness is present only if repeated wound infection causes cellulitis to supervene. A firm growth, usually surrounded by a narrow epithelial margin, is seen on the flexor surface of the hock joint or slightly lateral to it. At its center the tissue is grayish-white in color, shows fissures, sinuses and ulceration, and may be covered with scales or crusts. The scar tissue shows fibrous thickening at its periphery, and keratinized zones are sometimes seen at junctions with epithelium.

Exuberant granulation usually develops following lacerations, incised wounds and contusions. A large wound surface appears within a short time as a result of wound swelling and skin retraction. Sutures placed in the wound are often torn by the strong tension in the hollow of the hock joint and by the development of infection.

Healing is by second intention even when immediate and expert wound care is administered. Exuberant granulation tissue is the product of constant irritation due to joint movement, rubbing, scraping, licking, dirt contamination, and irritation by parasites. Foreign bodies and demarcated necrotic tissue (tendon necrosis, sequestra) also play a role, in that they predispose to fistula formation.

Treatment and Prognosis. Exuberant fibrous tissue is surgically removed down to below skin level, taking care to spare the marginal epithelium. Any foreign bodies, necrotic tendinous tissue and bone sequestra are also removed at this time.

Smaller wound surfaces become crusted and will heal under a pressure dressing in 4—6 weeks. When a more extensive wound surface is left by removal of the keloid, a skin graft is recommended to hasten epithelialization. This may consist of a tunnel graft by the method of McLennon-Obel (Bolz et al., 1970), in which skin strips are pulled through the keloid at the level of the surrounding skin. Scar tissue projecting above this level is removed after 10—14 days. Following removal of the granulation tissue and the formation of a more healthy, dry, bright-red type of tissue, small skin flaps or plugs are implanted (skin graft of Brown, Reverdin, Ammann). The wound is protected with a well-fitting bandage.

Flaps employing the principle of the Thiersch graft are also finding increasing use [Dubs and Quastel, 1975; Frankland et al., 1976].

Comments. Treatment may prove uneconomical due to the many months of therapy that are often required.

2.1.19.4.11. Fractures of the Tarsal Bones

The tarsus consists of six bones arranged in three rows. The proximal row is formed by the tibial tarsal bone (talus) and the fibular tarsal bone (calcaneus), and the distal row by the first, second, third and fourth tarsal bones. The first and second tarsals are fused into a single bone. The central tarsal bone is interposed between the proximal and distal rows. The laterally situated calcaneus forms a lever for the muscles that extend the hock joint. All fractures of the tarsal bones are intra-articular and hence are always associated with arthritis. They may be closed or open and infected.

Etiology. Fractures of the tibial, fibular and central tarsal bones are caused by sharp turns or by kicks from other horses. They may also occur spontaneously following tibial and peroneal neurectomies.

Symptoms. With fractures or sprain-fractures of the calcaneus, the Achilles tendon becomes lax. The detached bone fragment is displaced by muscle traction. The animal exhibits a severe supporting-leg lameness and collapses when weight-bearing is attempted. Swelling, pain and heat are evident. When the limb is extended, crepitation is sometimes detected in the area of the tuber calcis. Fractures of the tibial tarsal bone, central tarsal bone, and bones of the distal row produce symptoms of a severe, acute arthritis. The entire joint is swollen and painful, and the horse ceases to bear weight on the affected limb. With open fractures, synovial fluid is discharged. A severe, febrile systemic reaction develops in 2—3 days as a result of pyogenic infection, leading to recumbency and decubital ulcers. Chip fractures at the margins of the tibiotarsal joint usually produce clinical symptoms only if the fragment has become interposed in the joint space. Otherwise distension is the only symptom [SCHEBITZ et al., 1975].

Differential Diagnosis. Paralysis of the motor branches of the tibial nerve causes a lameness that resembles a calcaneus fracture but lacks the characteristic local signs. With other tarsal fractures, an acute arthritis of the hock joint must be differentiated.

Diagnosis. A sudden, severe lameness, combined with the local findings described above, is suggestive of a fracture. The diagnosis is verified by radiographs taken in two or more planes.

Treatment and Prognosis. Fractures of the tarsal bones have an unfavorable prognosis. Only valuable broodmares should be candidates for treatment. Internal fixation may be attempted in such cases. Dynamic compression plates are indicated for calcaneus fractures.

With other tarsal fractures, ankylosis usually results. For chip fractures at the margin of the tibiotarsal joint, surgical removal of the bone fragment may be indicated. The chance of recovery is good. The operation is identical to that for osteochondritis dissecans (cf. Sec. 2.1.19.4.2.).

2.1.19.4.12. Luxation of the Tarsal Bones

Definition. In exceptional cases the tibial tarsal bone may become dislocated in a posterior or medial direction.

Symptoms. Besides a sudden severe lameness, posterior luxation of the tibial tarsal bone produces an increase in the antero-posterior joint diameter, because the distal tibial epiphysis comes to lie anterior to the talus. With a medial luxation of the tibial tarsal bone, the joint diameter is increased in the latero-medial direction. In all cases the joint is very painful and its passive mobility is restricted.

Diagnosis. The clinical findings and radiographs in two planes establish the diagnosis. They can also provide evidence of distal tibial fractures or chip fractures of the lateral or medial malleolus that may have accompanied the luxation.

Treatment and Prognosis. The prognosis is poor. Reduction may be successful in foals. General anesthesia and a high degree of muscle relaxation are required for this maneuver.

2.1.19.4.13. Fluid Accumulation and Hygroma of the Tarsal Tendon Sheaths

Definition and Occurrence. Fluid distension of the tarsal tendon sheaths with swelling of individual sheaths are common in the horse. They mainly affect the sheaths of the flexor hallucis longus (long digital flexor) and tibialis caudalis tendons, the superficial digital flexor tendon or bursa, the lateral digital extensor tendon, and in some cases the long digital extensor tendon. The distension may be congenital or develop secondarily to a tendovaginitis.

Symptoms. (a) Hygroma of the long digital flexor and tibialis caudalis tendon sheath, known also as thoroughpin or soft curb, presents as an oval, fluctuating, painless swelling on the lateral and medial side of the hock. It may reach considerable size and may extend distally to the chestnut. (b) Fluid accumulation in the bursa of the superficial digital flexor produces a fluctuating, egg-size bulge over the calcaneus on both sides of the Achilles tendon. (c) Hygroma of the lateral digital extensor tendon sheath produces an approximately walnut-size swelling on the lower lateral aspect of the hock. (d) Hygroma of the long digital extensor tendon sheath is approximately thumb-size and occurs sporadically at the center of the flexor surface of the hock.

All these hygromas contain a clear, watery, largely acellular synovial fluid. There is no inflammatory reaction or lameness.

Diagnosis. The diagnosis is suggested by a fluctuating, subcutaneous swelling occurring at a characteristic location and unassociated with inflammatory symptoms and lameness.

Treatment and Prognosis. Tendon sheath hygromas seldom if ever cause functional disturbances and so do not necessarily require treatment. Occasionally, trauma can lead to an acute tendovaginitis that causes lameness.

In foals, especially of the heavy breeds, these hygromas sometimes regress spontaneously with age. This may be promoted by supplementing the feed with vitamin D_2 and minerals. In many cases a size reduction or complete absorption of the hygroma can be achieved by aspirating the hygroma and then injecting it repeatedly with glucocorticoids. A well-padded bandage is essential to the success of treatment. Any subsequent inflammatory reaction that occurs will subside without treatment in a short time. Injections of a tannic acid-alcohol solution at 3—4 week intervals have also proved beneficial. In foals with congenital tendon sheath hygroma, an inherited predisposition must be assumed, and so these animals should not be bred.

2.1.19.4.14. Luxation of the Superficial Flexor Tendon

Definition and Etiology. The superficial flexor tendon that runs downward over the tuber calcis may slip laterally or medially off the point of the hock, either spontaneously or as a result of trauma. This usually happens during the pulling of very heavy loads, during excessive leg action, during jumps over hurdles, or when the animal struggles to free a leg that has been secured for shoeing.

The luxation tends to be unilateral in working horses but sometimes affects both hind limbs in racehorses.

Symptoms. The lesion is manifested by an unsteady, staggering gait in which the toe drags the ground. Locally, a painful swelling is found above and lateral to the calcaneus. A constant lateral or medial dislocation of the superficial flexor tendon is evident. The bursa that surrounds the tendon in this area is inflamed and markedly enlarged. Knuckling of the fetlock joint is accentuated. The normal angulation of the hock joint is lost in most cases.

Differential diagnosis is made from rupture of the peroneus tertius muscle or rupture of the superficial flexor tendon. The absence of local symptoms about the point of the hock distinguishes these lesions from a luxation.

Treatment and Prognosis. A permanent reduction is not possible. Blistering or point firing has been done to stabilize the tuber calcis through connective tissue formation, thereby restoring an affected working horse to soundness. Riding and racing horses are suitable only for breeding.

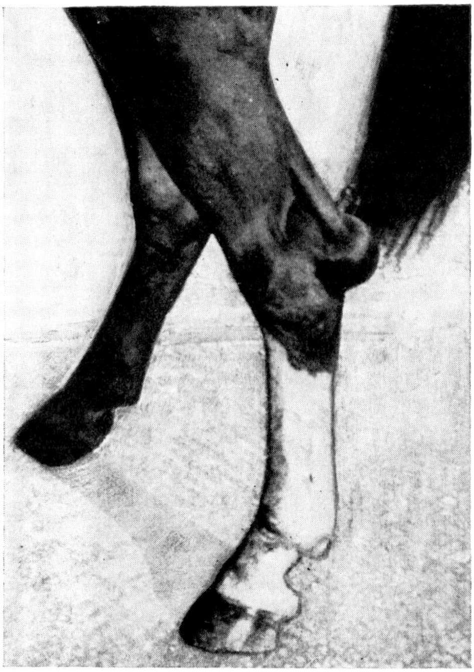

47

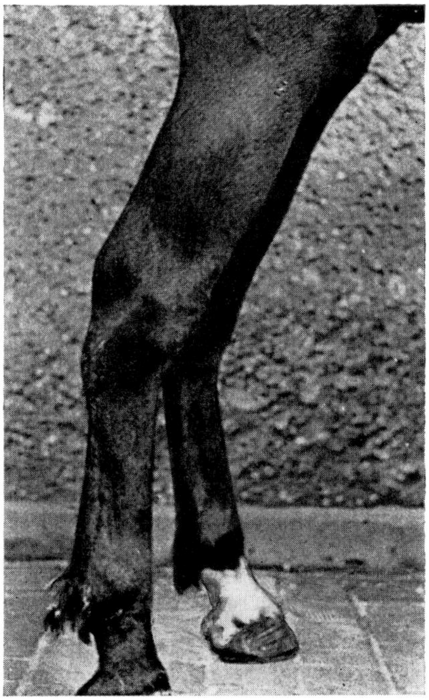

48

Fig. 2.1.19. — 47. Capped hock.
Fig. 2.1.19. — 48. Curb.

2.1.19.4.15. Chronic Aseptic and Suppurative Inflammation of the Subcutaneous Calcanean Bursa and Subtendinous Calcanean Bursa (Capped Hock)

Definition and Etiology. The term 'capped hock' refers to any swelling over the point of the hock. It may be unilateral or bilateral. It is caused by trauma induced when the horse kicks against a fence, the wall of a stall or crate, or the tailgate of a trailer.

Various lesions may occur, depending on the nature and degree of the trauma:

a) contusions of the skin and subcutaneous tissue (1st and 2nd degree contusions, dermatitis, hematoma, thickened skin, cellulitis);

b) contusions of the cap of the superficial digital flexor or subtendinous calcanean bursa (tendinitis, acute and chronic bursitis);

c) complete and incomplete fractures of the calcaneus (ossifying periostitis).

In general, the lesions of capped hock are aseptic, although pyogenic infection can result from open wounds.

Symptoms. Capped hock may develop very rapidly and appear as a soft, fluctuating, pressure-sensitive swelling over the point of the hock. A mild to moderate lameness is usually present. Trauma to the subtendinous calcanean bursa causes fluctuating, egg-size swellings to develop next to the cap of the superficial digital flexor (fig. 2.1.19. — 47).

Circumscribed, painful swellings with excoriation or scabbing indicate a contusion of the skin and subcutaneous tissue. A thickening of the skin with hair loss and pigmentary infiltration occurs following repeated contusions of the skin. If the horse goes suddenly lame and is unable to bear weight on the affected limb, a calcaneus fracture should be suspected. Exostoses on the tuber calcis cause a small, hard, painless swelling that may be accompanied by slight lameness.

Diagnosis. The localization of the change and the findings on palpation together with any evidence of lameness that may be present, enable a diagnosis of capped hock to be made. Complete or incomplete fractures, exostoses, or an ossifying periostitis can be detected by radiography.

Treatment. All acute inflammatory changes are treated with moist antiseptic or anti-inflammatory dressings or poultices (ethacridine lactate, Burow's mixture, Aciterran, glucocorticoid ointments) or later with topical rubefacients (camphor, iodoform, ichthammol or carbol-mercury ointment). Older skin thickenings respond favorably to stronger absorption-promoting ointments or liniments (blisters). A similar therapeutic approach may be taken with chronic bursitides, bursal hygromas and exostoses on the calcaneus. The result is not always good, however. Repeated intra-articular injections of glucocorticoids rarely produce good results in subtendinous calcaneal bursitis, and usually lead to poor results in subcutaneous calcanean bursitis [van Pelt and Riley, 1968]. In cases of purulent bursitis and peribursal cellulitic abscessation, a cure can sometimes be effected with rubefacient therapy and the use of sulfonamides and antibiotics. Finally, hygroma of the subcutaneous bursa and bursitis with abscessation can be treated by surgical removal of the bursa. In this procedure either a lateral or medial skin incision is used. The sutured wound is protected with a bandage. It is important that the animal be kept standing with cross ties for 8—10 days postoperatively in order to prevent suture dehiscence. If second-intention healing occurs, exuberant granulation will form that is very difficult to control. Extensive granulation tissue formation is common in such cases.

Prognosis. If the swelling does not hamper the animal's usefulness, treatment is unnecessary. Acute bursitides, contusions of the skin and subcutaneous tissue, hematomas and phlegmons can usually be cured completely. With exostoses of the tuber calcis, permanent lameness often results.

Open, suppurating lesions have a guarded prognosis.

2.1.19.4.16. *Curb*

Definition. Curb is a term applied to various conditions affecting the posterior aspect of the calcaneus or hock joint. All are characterized by a curved or semicircular enlargement in the lower plantar area of the hock, which is most obvious when the limb is viewed from the side. Curb may be congenital or acquired. Congenital curb is a peculiar hereditary trait of many Thoroughbred lines. In acquired curb, a distinction is made between bone curb and tendon curb (common in Standardbreds), depending on the nature of the lesions.

Etiology. Tendon curb is caused by interstitial tendon tears, which can occur during riding and jumping at fast gaits. In bone curb, trauma is often the exciting cause (lying on hard ground).

Symptoms. Tendon curb is characterized by a circumscribed, painful tickening of the deep flexor tendon and especially of its check ligament (tendinitis), or a softer swelling with slight fluctuation and pain (bursitis; fig. 2.1.19. — 48) in the area of the tarsometatarsal joint. Bone curb is recognized by a largely painless bony enlargement which gives a curved contour to the posterior aspect of the calcaneus.

In both diseases, the horse is unable to extend the hock joint fully. A mild to moderate supporting-leg lameness is present.

Diagnosis. The diagnosis is made from local findings and lameness symptoms. In bone curb, radiographs will show evidence of an ossifying periostitis.

Treatment and Prognosis. Stall rest for 4—8 weeks, combined with topical anti-inflammatory agents will usually ensure a complete recovery in animals with tendon curb. Chronic cases and bone curb have been treated with firing and blistering. A spavin shoe is applied, and stall rest is enforced for 6—8 weeks. It is imperative that soft bedding be provided. Even racehorses should recover to full soundness following treatment.

References

Dixon, R. T.: Results of radon 222 gamma radiation therapy in an equine practice. Austral. vet. J. *48:* 279 (1972).

Dubs, B.; Quastel, T.: Hauttransplantation beim Pferd. tierärztl. praxis *3:* 57 (1975).

Frankland, A. L.; Morris, P. G. D.; Spreull, J. S. A.: Free autologous skin transplantation in the horse. Vet. Rec. *98:* 105 (1976).

Frye, F. Fl.; Fawwaz, R. A.: A practical disposable dermal trephine made from discarded materials. Vet. Med. and Small Animal Clinician *69:* 1419 (1974).

Gängel, H.: Diagnostische Aspekte der Synovialzytologie bei Pferd und Rind. Habil.-Schrift, Humboldt-Univ., Berlin (1970).

Heinze, C. D.: Equine orthopaedic surgery. Mod. vet. Pract. *47:* 63 (1966).

Houdeshell, J. W.; Bloomfield, N. J.: Field trials of a new long-acting corticosteroid in the treatment of equine arthropathies. Vet. Med. and Small Animal Clinician *64:* 782 (1969).

Kroney, J. R.: Bog spavin and tibiotarsal joint lesions in the horse. Mod. vet. Pract. *54:* 43 (1973).

Kubitza, G.: Zur Therapie degenerativer Gelenkerkrankungen bei Pferden und Hunden. Tierärztl. Umschau *21:* 402 (1966).

Morgan, J. P.: Necrosis of the third tarsal bone of the horse. J. Amer. vet. med. Assoc. *151:* 1334 (1967).

Morgan, J. P.: Radiographic diagnosis of bone and joint diseases in the horse. Cornell Vet. *58:* suppl. 28 (1968).

Pelt, R. W. van: Arthrocentesis and injection of the equine tarsus. J. Amer. vet. med. Assoc. *148:* 367 (1966).

Pelt, R. W. van: Intraarticular injection of 6-α-methyl-17-α-hydroxyprogesteronacetat into the tarsal joint of the horse. J. Amer. vet. med. Assoc. *151:* 1159 (1967).

Pelt, R. W. van: Tarsal hydarthrosis (bog spavin) in the horse. Amer. J. vet. Res. *29:* 569 (1968).

Pelt, R. W. van: Idiopathic subcutaneus calcaneal bursitis (Capped hock) in the horse. J. Amer. vet. med. Assoc. *155:* 510 (1969).

Pelt, R. W. van: Tendosynovitis in the horse. J. Amer. vet. med. Assoc. *154:* 1022 (1969).

Pelt, R. W. van: Inflammation of the tarsal synovial sheath (thoroughpin) in horses. J. Amer. vet. med. Assoc. *155:* 1481 (1969).

Pelt, R. W. van; Rilley, W. F., jr.: Therapeutic management of tarsal hydarthrosis (bog spavin) in the horse by intraarticular injection of prednisolone. J. Amer. vet. med. Assoc. *151:* 328 (1967).

Pelt, R. W. van; Rilley, W. F., jr.: Traumatic subcutaneus calcaneal bursitis (Capped hock) in the horse. J. Amer. vet. med. Assoc. *153:* 1176 (1968).

Pelt, R. W. van; Tillotson, P. J.; Gertsen, K. E.: Intraarticular injection of beta-methasone in arthritis in horses. J. Amer. vet. med. Assoc. *156:* 1589 (1970).

Pelt, R. W. van; Tillotson, P. J.; Gertsen, K. E.; Gallagher, K. F.: Effects of intraarticular injection of fluomethasone suspension in joint diseases in horses. J. Amer. vet. med. Assoc. *159:* 739 (1971).

Raker, C. W.: Clinical observations of bone and joint lesions in the horses. Cornell Vet. *58:* suppl. 15 (1968).

Rydell, N. W.; Butler, J.; Balazs, E.: Hyaluronic acid in synovial fluid. VI. Effect of intraarticular injection of hyaluronic acid on the clinical symptoms of arthritis in track horses. Acta vet. scand. *11:* 139 (1970).

SCHEBITZ, H.; DÄMMRICH, K.; WAIBL, H.: Intraartikuläre Absprengungsfrakturen im Articulus talocruralis beim Pferd. Berliner Münchener tierärztl. Wschr. *88:* 309 (1975).

SCHNEIDER, W.: Weitere Untersuchungen über die Wirksamkeit von Arumalon ad us. vet. bei degenerativen Gelenkerkrankungen der Pferde. Tierärztl. Umschau *27:* 132 (1972).

TRONICKE, R.: Zur Tomanol-Therapie bei Bewegungsstörungen des Pferdes. Tierärztl. Umschau *24:* 188 (1969).

VIDDA, P. D.; QUEIROLO, L. E.: Synovitis tarsica zu toros. Gac. Vet., Buenos Aires *33:* 303 (1971).

WHEAT, J. D.; RHODE, E. A.: Luxation and fractures of the hock of the horse. J. Amer. vet. med. Assoc. *145:* 341 (1964).

2.1.20. Diseases of the Metacarpus, Metatarsus and Digit

2.1.20.1. Diseases of the Metacarpus and Metatarsus

2.1.20.1.1. Wounds of the Metacarpus and Metatarsus

Occurence, Forms and Etiology. Wounds of the metacarpus are usually caused by falls or running into obstacles, whereas wounds of the metatarsus are generally lacerations or incised wounds inflicted by barbed wire or other sharp objects (fig. 2.1.20. — 1).

In racehorses, deep wounds are commonly inflicted to the plantar aspect of the metatarsus during races by hoof strikes from trailing horses. In addition, interfering causes a variety of self-inflicted wounds to the medial aspect of the metacarpus and metatarsus.

Areas of skin necrosis can develop as a result of deficient blood flow due to faulty bandaging.

Symptoms and Diagnosis. Simple skin wounds seldom cause lameness and produce systemic signs only if infected with pyogenic organisms. However, if damage occurs to the tendons, ligaments or periosteum, pronounced and often typical lameness symptoms can arise. The lamenesses produced by tendon divisions, for example, are well known. In such cases the severed, grayish-white tendon stumps will be visible in the wound. Puncture wounds usually cannot be seen until after the hair is clipped.

All wounds of the cannon region are prone to exuberant granulation tissue formation unless proper wound care is administered. These may reach huge proportions (figs. 2.1.20. — 2 through — 4) if chronic irritation is produced by tendon necrosis, bone sequestra (figs. 2.1.20. — 5 and — 6), foreign bodies or exogenous influences.

Bony injuries are detected by radiographs taken in multiple planes.

Treatment. Fresh wounds are managed according to general surgical principles. If possible, the wound is closed by suture. A well-padded bandage should always be applied and should extend from the hock to below the fetlock. If the wound shows a poor healing tendency, heavy discharge or even fistula formation in the granulation tissue, the cause is probably tendon necrosis or bone sequestrum that must be removed. Granulation tissue is removed with great care taken to spare the surrounding skin and epithelial margin. The wound edges are approximated with sutures. If this is not possible, then an eschar (scab) is produced, and the wound is allowed to heal under the eschar. Smaller skin defects will heal well if not irritated by rubbing or gnawing by the horse. Larger wounds should be protected with a well-padded bandage. Even large wounds benefit from moderate exposure to air and sunshine. The epithelialization of large skin defects can be hastened by means of skin grafting. Tunnel grafting, the implantation of small skin flaps or plugs, or other flap techniques may be used for this purpose [DUBS and QUASTEL, 1975].

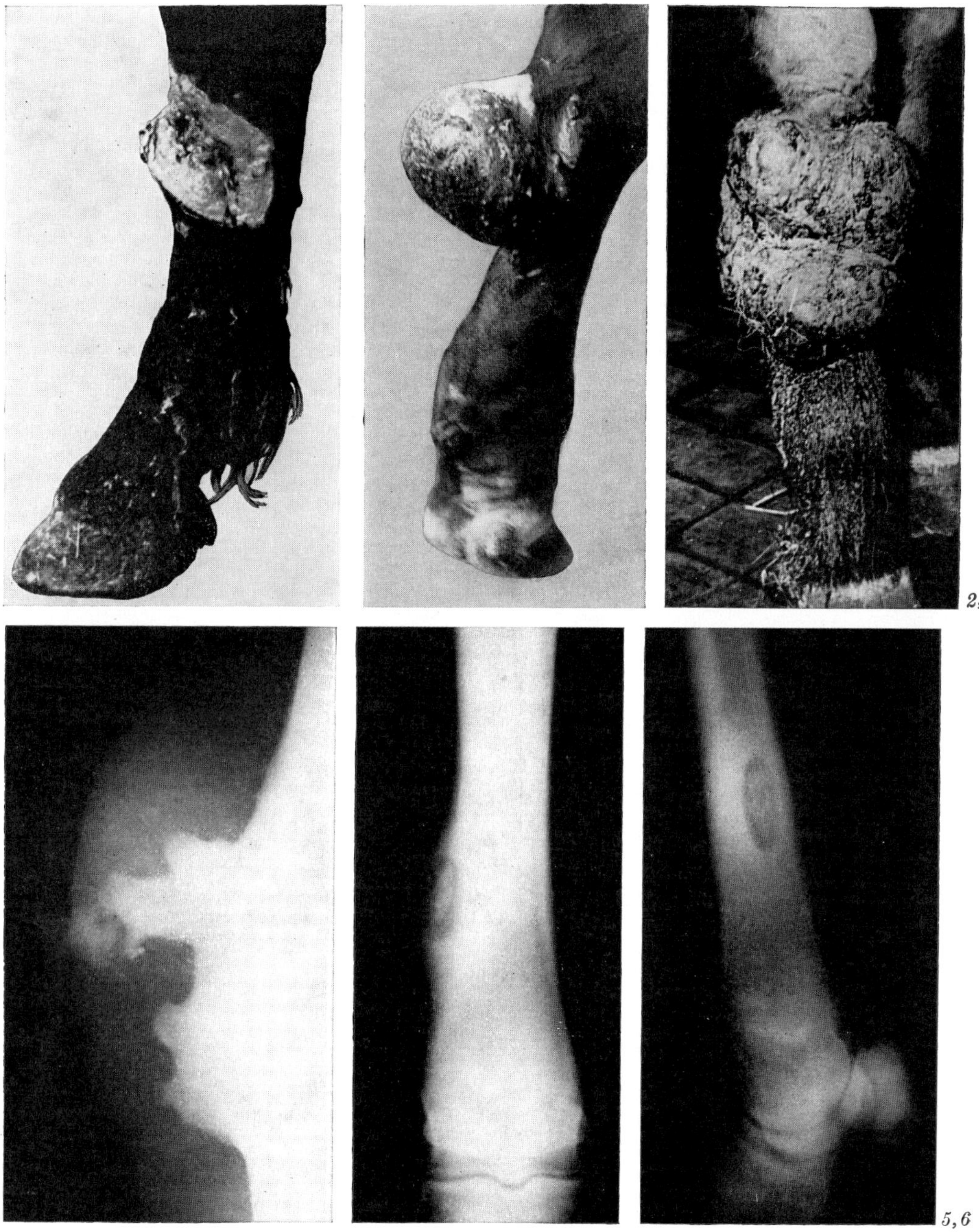

Fig. 2.1.20. — *1.* Laceration of the metatarsus.
Fig. 2.1.20. — *2—3.* Granulation tissue on the cannon region.
Fig. 2.1.20. — *4.* Exostoses and periosteal injuries on the cannon bone, with granulation tissue.
Fig. 2.1.20. — *5—6.* Osteomyelitis with embedded sequestrum.

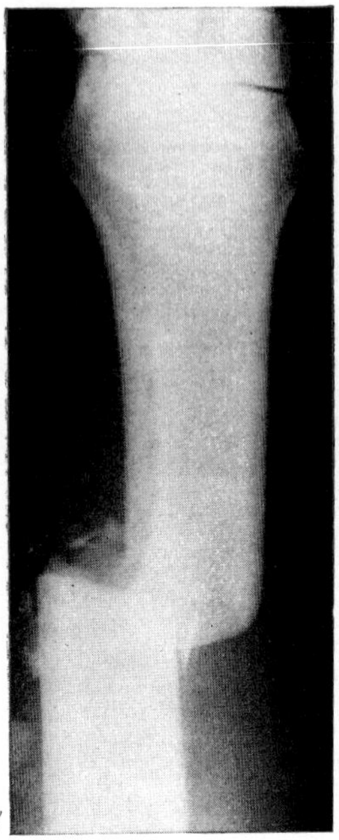
7

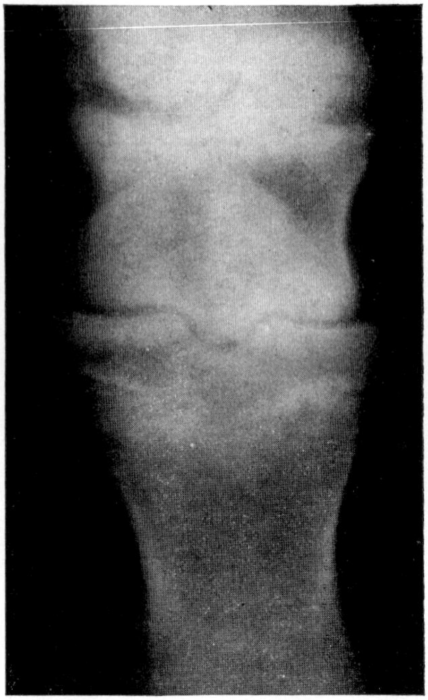
8

Fig. 2.1.20. — 7. Transverse fracture of the cannon bone.
Fig. 2.1.20. — 8. Distal epiphyseal separation of the cannon bone due to metabolic bone disease.

Prognosis. Fresh skin wounds will undergo first-intention healing with proper treatment. With tendon and bone wounds, there is always a tendency toward exuberant granulation which greatly prolongs healing time.

2.1.20.1.2. Fractures of the Metacarpus or Metatarsus (Cannon Fractures)

Occurrence, Forms and Etiology. Complete or incomplete fractures of the cannon bone most commonly occur in racehorses as a result of external violence. Most are open or closed sagittal or oblique fractures. One or both splint bones may also be involved (figs. 2.1.20. — 7 and — 8).

Fissure fractures and longitudinal fractures of the distal condyles occur frequently in racehorses that are in training. They occur when, during hyperextension at high speed, the lateral condyle of the cannon bone engages against the lateral proximal surface of the proximal phalanx. Occasionally, subperiosteal fissure fractures are found in the metacarpus of 2-year-old Thoroughbreds that have undergone hard training.

In addition, suckling foals often sustain cannon fractures as a result of being stepped on by their dam.

Symptoms. An immediate, severe lameness develops. The forelimb is slightly flexed and anterior, while the hind limb just touches the ground with the tip of the toe. The fracture hematoma soon produces swelling of the entire cannon region. Crepitation can usually be detected. Marked pain is also elicited and often serves to localize the fissure or fracture line. If pronounced lameness follows trauma to the cannon region in the absence of obvious lesions, the possibility of subperiosteal fissure fractures should be considered.

Diagnosis. Radiographs are taken to exclude partial and complete ruptures of the flexor tendons, which also cause considerable pain and swelling. Cracking sounds on passive movement of the cannon at the tarsal joint (pseudocrepitation) may be a source of confusion. Radiographs in several planes are often necessary for the detection of hairline fractures.

Treatment. Immediate rest and confinement to a large box stall with soft bedding are indicated. After swelling has subsided following a simple oblique or sagittal cannon fracture, an unpadded bandage of zinc gelatin, splinted or unsplinted plaster, fiberglass or polyurethane foam may be applied. Various internal fixation methods have been used to advantage in many cases. Metacarpal fractures in ponies and foals have been treated by intramedullary fixation with a Jonas pin. To stimulate callus formation, bone denuded of periosteum can be taken from the rib of a donor animal and grafted into the fracture defect. Huskamp [1972] uses a Steinmann pin driven transversely into the radius in combination with a tension-band plate. Increasingly, good results are being reported with the use of bone plates and screws, including dynamic compression plates. Comminuted fractures in ponies and older foals have healed well with the aid of these devices.

In a valuable broodmare, Koger et al. [1970] amputated the right foreleg at the carpometacarpal joint on account of a comminuted fracture. The amputated portion of the limb was replaced with an aluminium prosthesis, which enabled the animal to walk almost normally and continue its life as a broodmare.

A period of 6—12 weeks is required for fracture healing in the horse.

Prognosis. Incomplete fractures have a favorable prognosis even when treated on an outpatient basis. With complete fractures, on the other hand, the prognosis for recovery in large, adult horses is still guarded. Compound and comminuted fractures have a poor prognosis. In foals and ponies, good results can usually be achieved with modern internal fixation methods (ASIF, AO techniques).

Comments. Even with successful internal fixation, adult horses cannot be restored to their original soundness due to residual deformation of the metacarpal or metatarsal bones which hampers tendon function.

2.1.20.1.3. Splint Bone Fractures

Definition and Occurrence. The splint bones, known also as the second and fourth metacarpal or metatarsal bones, are situated medially and laterally behind the third metacarpus or metatarsus. Fractures of these bones are observed in both the fore and hind limbs. A distinction is made between:

— open or closed proximal splint fractures (fig. 2.1.20. — 9) and
— closed distal splint fractures (figs. 2.1.20. — 10 and — 11).

Fractures of the first type occur in all horses, while those of the second type tend to be an 'occupational disease' mainly of older Standardbreds. However, they also occur in Thoroughbreds and other performance horses.

Etiology. Open and closed proximal splint fractures are caused by external trauma. The distal closed fractures have a different, more complex etiology. During the normal process of ossification, the splint bone starts to become ossified at the age of 2 years, and a synostotic union begins to form between this bone and the large metacarpal or metatarsal bone. When this process is complete, union is achieved that prevents

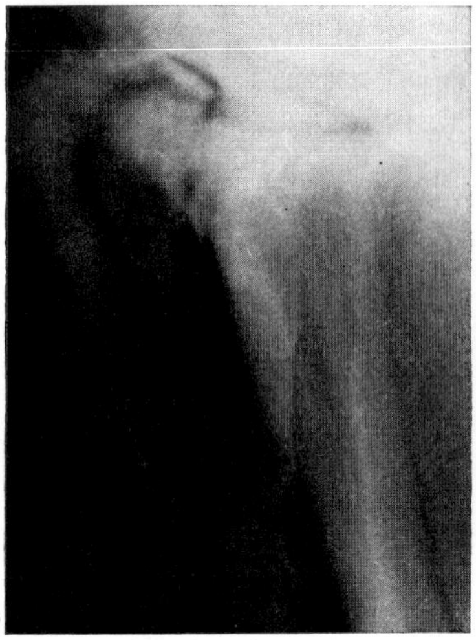

9

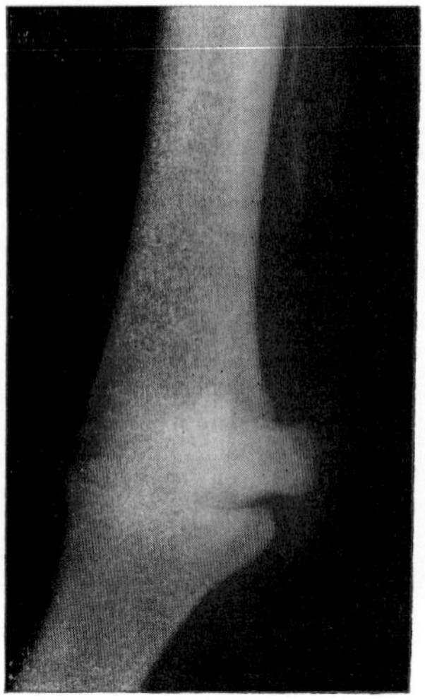

10

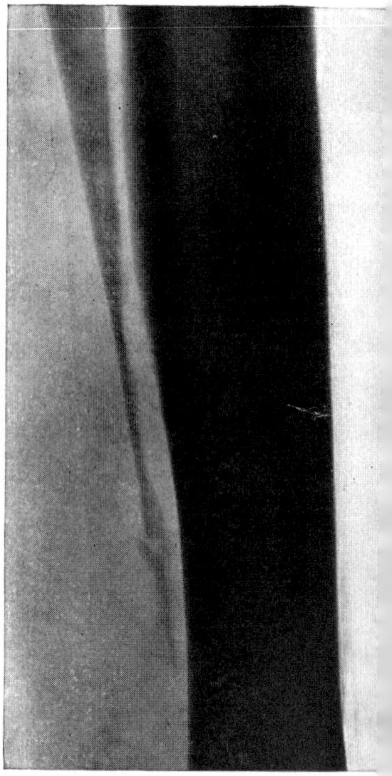

Fig. 2.1.20. — 9. Proximal splint fracture due to trauma.

Fig. 2.1.20. — 10. Closed distal splint fracture with displaced fragment; proximal sesamoid fracture discovered at operation.

Fig. 2.1.20. — 11. Closed distal splint fracture.

constant lateral and medial movement of the free ends of the splint bones by the action of the adjacent branches of the suspensory ligament during strenuous exercise at high speed. This situation creates a site of least resistance in the area of the partially ossified epiphyseal plate that, while stable against bending, is vulnerable to kinking and twisting forces.

Predisposing factors include abnormal remodeling processes such as periostitis and osteitis, which are viewed as a reaction to the continual irritation of training. In these cases a 'fatigue fracture' is said to be present.

Symptoms. Proximal splint fractures are manifested by a mild to moderate supporting-leg lameness and a painful inflammatory edema of this region.

In the case of open fractures, pyogenic wound infection can lead to the development of an osteitis and suppurative osteomyelitis with the formation of sequestra. The process may invade the distal, rigid portion of the carpal or tarsal joint, causing infection and subsequent ankylosis in that area.

Healing of this fracture is accompanied by extensive exostosis formation, leading to the development of splints in the area of the suspensory ligament and check ligament of the deep flexor tendon. This can result in permanent lameness.

With closed distal splint fractures, the animal may have a long history of gait imperfection or a recurring, mild to moderate supporting-leg lameness. Accompanying these symptoms are painful, inflammatory edematous or nodular swellings about the branch of the suspensory that is adjacent to the distal end of the splint bone. There may be abnormal mobility at the distal extremity of the splint bone, asymmetry, or marked tenderness to pressure. Simple length disparities of the splint bones should not be interpreted as evidence of a fracture, however.

Differential Diagnosis. Aseptic inflammations of the suspensory ligament and cellulitis in this area must be excluded. In horses under 2 years of age, which are rarely affected, radiolucent epiphyseal lines on the radiograph are apt to be mistaken for splint fractures. However, these smooth-edged 'discontinuities' lack the adjacent zones of remodeling that are characteristic of true fractures.

Diagnosis. Radiographic findings confirm the diagnosis. If a distal closed splint fracture is suspected, it is best to obtain separate oblique views of each splint bone. Diagnostic anesthesia of the deep ulnar or fibular nerve may also be useful.

Treatment. Compound proximal fractures are treated surgically (wound therapy, removal of chip fragments or sequestra). When ankylosis has developed in the distal portions of the carpal or tarsal joint, point firing or fibular neurectomy can be used to restore working capacity. This therapy is contraindicated in racing animals.

Conservative treatment for closed distal fractures, involving rest and rubefacient drugs or firing, has not proved satisfactory. Heavy callus formation or poor healing of the distal fragment leads to constant irritation of the suspensory ligament and thus to a recurrence of lameness. Therefore, removal of the distal fragment combined with a partial resection of the remainder of the splint bone somewhat proximal to the fracture line is the recommended treatment.

The procedure is done under general anesthesia. The skin is incised along the anterior border of the affected splint bone from its distal extremity to a point above the fracture line. The free end of the splint bone is dissected free, taking care not to open the fetlock joint. Then the distal fragment is removed, and a portion of bone above the fracture line is resected. Any exostoses that have formed are also removed. Following a thorough hemostasis, the fascia and skin are sutured. Postoperative bleeding and wound infection are avoided by applying a compression bandage until healing is complete. Training can begin after 4 weeks' stall rest and 4 weeks' pasturing or light exercise. In cases where severe, chronic, inflammatory changes have already developed in the adjacent branch of the suspensory ligament, additional cauterization of this area is indicated after the surgical wound has healed.

Prognosis and Comments. While open or closed proximal splint fractures have a guarded prognosis, running horses with closed distal splint fractures usually recover to full soundness.

2.1.20.1.4. Splints

Definition. Changes in the contour of bones are known variously as osteophytes, exostoses or hyperostoses. When such changes involve the metacarpal or metatarsal bones, they are called splints.

Occurrence and Classification. Splints are mainly a disease of young horses. The forelimb is most often affected in riding horses, but the metatarsus may develop splints in Standardbreds and show horses. One or more limbs may be affected. Splints can be classified by etiology as traumatic or spontaneous. They may also be classified by location as:

a) intermetacarpal splints,
b) postmetacarpal splints or
c) low metacarpal splints.

Symptoms and Etiology. Traumatic splints are caused by interfering, overreaching, or striking an obstacle with the leg. They are rare and are not usually associated with lameness. In acute cases with active periostitis, the symptoms of an acute inflammation are exhibited. However, Pajtle [1963] was able to produce a periostitis experimentally only if there was irritation to the bone tissue as well as the periosteum, or if an infection with pathogenic organisms supervened.

The etiology of spontaneous splints is based in part on the tension-compression syndrome. However, the etiology is complex and also relates to such factors as endocrine abnormalities, malnutrition (disturbances of bone metabolism) and neglected foot care.

a) Lateral intermetacarpal splints develop as a result of irritation to the periosteum at the sites of insertion of the suspensory ligament. In particular, static compression and tension cause a state of irritation that leads to chronic periostitis of the metacarpal bones. Tension from above has an adverse effect in animals with a toe-out conformation, and this problem is exacerbated by horseshoes with an inside branch that is too narrow.

These splints are usually bean- to walnut-size and cause only a supporting-leg lameness if they develop rapidly ('remount disease') or lead to carpal joint inflammation.

b) Posterior metacarpal splints begin at the attachment of the outer layer of the carpal fascia. In connection with tension from the suspensory ligament, a chronic inflammation of the periosteum develops. Lameness occurs when the exostoses constrict the suspensory ligament or the inferior check ligament of the deep flexor tendon. The splint usually has a fissured surface and can be demonstrated radiographically as well as by palpation when the foot is lifted and the flexor tendons are relaxed. According to Vasall [1968], radiographs show evidence of change before palpatory evidence appears.

c) The low metacarpal splint is located at the insertion of the suspensory ligament and the inferior check ligament tendon and causes a chronic lameness that is refractory to treatment. The localization of this splint makes it difficult to detect.

The *differential diagnosis and diagnosis* are based upon the foregoing symptoms. An existing lameness can be temporarily relieved by infiltration anesthesia in the splint area. Lameness caused by a low metacarpal splint is temporarily relieved by anesthesia of the ulnar nerve.

Diagnosis and Treatment. Acute or subacute periostitis like that associated with traumatic splints will respond to rest and moist heat initially, followed later by iodine-containing ointments or liniments. Local glucocorticoid injections are also recommended owing to their anti-inflammatory effect. Vrigasoff [1956] reports good results with iodine iontophoresis.

Lameness from intermetacarpal splints disappears spontaneously with the completion of ossification between the cannon bone and splint bones. This process can be hastened by point firing (perforating if necessary) or the application of caustic ointments (red blister). Krook [1968] is opposed to firing in any form. He considers it more advisable to analyze the horse's diet and correct any deficiencies that exist, especially in remount disease.

Any defects of limb conformation that predispose to splints should be eliminated with corrective shoeing. Shoes with widened inside branches to support the more heavily-loaded inner hoof wall in horses with base-wide or toe-out conformations should be used with caution due to the increased danger of interference.

The treatment of postmetacarpal and low metacarpal splints is seldom effective. Local injections of glucocorticoids may be tried. An ulnar neurectomy may also be tried as a means of correcting the associated lameness.

Higginbotham [1974] achieved a complete regression of exostoses in 80% of cases by injecting 2.5—5 ml sodium oleate subperiosteally or directly into the interosseous ligament or interspace. This therapy should be deferred until 4—6 weeks after the last steroid injection.

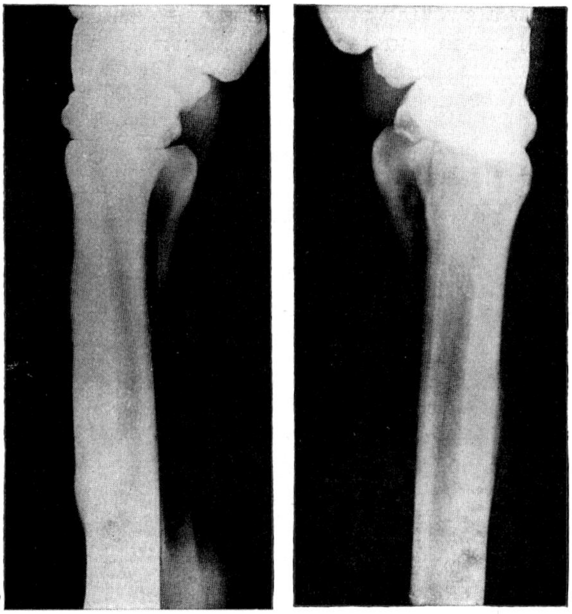

12 13

Fig. 2.1.20. — 12—13. Peri- and endostosis in bucked shins.

2.1.20.1.5. Bucked Shins (Metacarpal Periostosis of Thoroughbreds)

Definition and Occurrence. 'Bucked shins' or 'sore shins' is a painful, firm swelling occurring at the junction of the upper and middle thirds of the dorsal surface of the third metacarpal bone. The anatomically imprecise name of the disease relates to the fact that the metacarpus is often called the 'shin' in breeding and racing circles. This condition is seen almost exclusively in 2-year-old Thoroughbreds, and occasionally in 3-year-olds. The metatarsus may also be affected in Standardbreds.

Etiology. Bucked shins represents a reactive periostitis with consequent hyperostosis. It is seen mainly in the metacarpus, because the extreme flexion and subsequent rapid extension of the joints at the gallop imposes a very great stress on the dorsal cortex of this bone. If the ground is soft and elastic, much of the bending pressure is absorbed, and the bone is acted upon primarily by a bending mode. If the ground is hard, then the bending pressure is increased and acts more abruptly on the bone.

A bone that is not sturdy enough to withstand these stresses will attempt to adapt through transformation or hypertrophy, i.e., by strengthening the stressed zones. The cause of this inadequate stress resistance of the bone is believed to be a generalized osteopathy resulting from a deficient nutrient supply to the bone prior to the conclusion of skeletal growth (Ca : P ratio, protein intake). Therefore, this disease is mainly seen in 2-year-old Thoroughbreds following strenuous workouts or racing on hard ground.

Symptoms and Diagnosis. A firm, painful, swelling is present on the dorsal surface of the third metacarpus. Supporting-leg lameness, if present, is usually mild and increases with exercise. In bilateral cases the anterior phase of the stride is shortened (stiff or choppy gait).

Radiographs in the early stage show a swelling of the periosteum. As the disease progresses, osteophytes become visible. The end result is a partly circumscribed, partly diffuse thickening of the subperiosteal cortical bone that tends to be permanent. Radiographic changes often can be demonstrated before clinical symptoms appear (figs. 2.1.20. — 12 and — 13).

Treatment and Prognosis. The primary goal of treatment is to relieve the local reaction. This can be done with anti-inflammatory and rubefacient drugs. We prefer iodine-containing medicaments, which relieve both swelling and pain with repeated use.

Pronounced or recurrent 'sore shins' do not respond to these mild agents and must be treated with more caustic drugs. These must be used with caution, however, because they often cause skin damage that results in unsightly scars. Anti-inflammatory and anesthetic drugs are of only temporary benefit. In mild cases the animal may be returned to light work, while in severe cases rest is essential to reduce stress and minimize bone transformation. Because sodium oleate is assumed to hasten osteogenesis, Genovese [1974] has injected this drug in doses of 0.125—0.25 ml in several vertically-arranged depots on or beneath the affected periosteum, and has achieved good results with this therapy. The longest break from training and work was 21 days.

Comments. Prophylaxis is an important consideration. A well-balanced nutrient content of the ration and regular exercise throughout adolescence, avoiding hard training before skeletal growth is complete (24—28 months in Thoroughbreds), are particularly emphasized.

2.1.20.1.6. Tendon Injuries

Tendinitis, Tendinosis, Bowed Tendons

Definition and Occurrence. Tendinitis generally refers to a tendon inflammation that is accompanied by new tissue formation. It results from a fibrillary or fascicular tear or partial or complete rupture of the tendon. According to Soennichsen [1966, 1975], lesions may involve only the paratenon, in which case a 'paratendinitis' is present. Because degeneration of tendon cells due to impaired blood flow begins before an acute lesion develops, it might be more accurate to characterize the disease as a tendinosis, rather than a tendinitis. The following tendons are affected in the metacarpus or metatarsus:

— the superficial digital flexor tendon (with possible involvement of its check ligament; fig. 2.1.10. — 14),
— the deep digital flexor tendon (with its check ligament),
— the suspensory ligament, (superior sesamoidean ligament),
— the extensor tendon (tendon of the long digital extensor or common digital extensor). This tendon is rarely affected.

Tendinitis of the superficial flexor tendon and suspensory ligament is one of the most common injuries affecting the riding and racing horse. In working horses, the deep flexor tendon and its check ligament come under the greatest stress when the foot is pushing off. While the flexor tendons of the forelimbs are almost exclusively affected in riding and running horses, the hind limbs may also be affected in draft horses and trotters.

The tendinitis may be acute or chronic.

Etiology. Disruptions in the continuity of tendons are mainly the result of overstretching and are rarely caused by external trauma. This overstretching leads to a loosening of the fibrils and fascicles in the interfibrillary or interfascicular connective tissue, and thus to a loss of elasticity. Elasticity is ensured through the

14
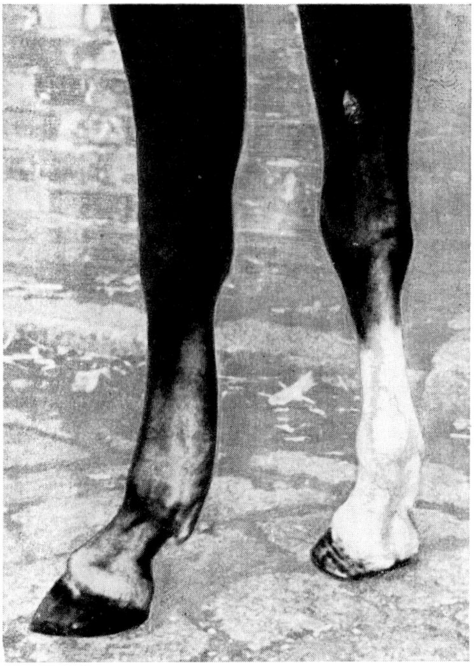
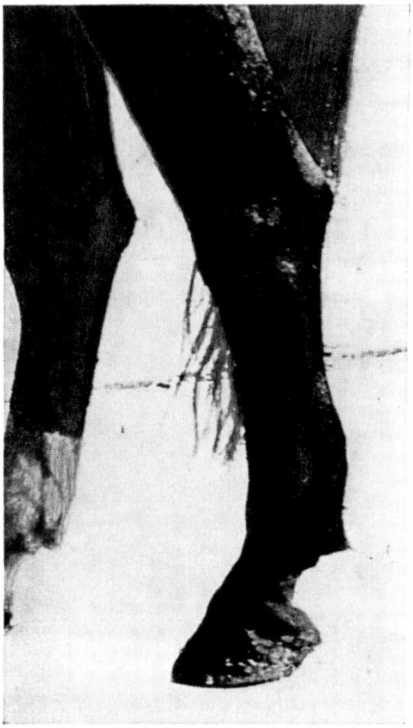
15

Fig. 2.1.20. — 14. Tendinitis of both superficial flexor tendons of the forelimbs.
Fig. 2.1.20. — 15. Tendinitis (low bowed tendon) of the hind limb.

transmission of muscular contractility. If the muscle is fatigued or in poor condition, excessive loads associated with falls, jumps, quick reining, stumbles, sustained heavy work, etc. can cause undue stress to be imposed on the tendon. Horses with weak tendons or long, weak, upright pasterns are predisposed. Defects of conformation as well as abnormally short horseshoes like those frequently worn by athletic horses can also be contributing factors.

Soennichsen [1966, 1975] assigns a special pathogenic importance to the blood supply that arises from the peritenon and runs parallel to the tendon, stating that this supply is greatly diminished during tensile stress owing to the anatomic arrangement of the vessels and their spiral course. As a result, local hypoxemia occurs at the moment when oxygen demand is greatest, causing reduced metabolic activity in the tendinous tissue. This in turn leads to aseptic necrosis of the fibrils.

In the Balkan states and the Soviet Union, infections with *Onchocerca reticulata*, possibly followed by arteriosclerosis, are a significant cause of diminished blood flow to the tendons and ligaments [Marolt et al., 1966].

Willi [1951] showed experimentally that the suspensory ligament of cold-blooded horses contains less connective tissue, and is less dense, than that of the pure breeds. In cold-bloods the rupture strength of this tendon is 4—11 times the resting stress.

Some 60 % of experimentally-produced tears ran through the branches of the suspensory ligament, and the remainder through the body. In rats conditioned by running for varying times and at varying speeds, an increase was found in the diameter and tensile strength of the Achilles tendon [Tittel and Otto, 1970].

This is considered evidence that tendinous tissue is capable of being conditioned, and thus that blood-flow conditions in such tissue can be improved.

Various other mechanisms of tendon injury are possible. Thus, spontaneous or pathologic tendon ruptures can occur in connection with calcium-phosphorus imbalances, or tendons can become severed as a result of open injuries, necrosis following pyogenic infection, and as a complication of neurectomies. Diseases of the extensor tendons occur almost exclusively in the hind legs of jumpers and result from trauma inflicted from contact with hurdles. The subtendinous bursa of the fetlock joint is also involved in most cases.

Symptoms. In acute tendinitis there is always a moderate to severe supporting-leg lameness that often improves after a few steps are taken. Pulsation in the metacarpal or metatarsal arteries may be somewhat increased. Findings on palpation and inspection depend on the specific tendon affected and the severity of the lesion. The major findings are local swelling, heat, tenderness to pressure, a loss of sharp contours, and a decrease in the normal firm consistency of the tendon.

When the flexor tendons are affected within their common tendon sheath, this sheath is distended with fluid and also shows inflammatory change.

In acute cases one may refer to a 'high' or 'low' bowed tendon, depending on the level at which the swelling, or where the bow is located (fig. 2.1.20. — 15) (the terms 'high calf' and 'low calf' are sometimes colloquially applied). Minor defects (paratendinitis) producing a state of 'tendon fatigue' are sometimes manifested by a slight temperature rise that is difficult to detect on palpation.

Chronic tendinitis can develop gradually from recurrent, subclinical fibrillary tendon tears or from an acute tendinitis in horses that are put to work too early or worked too hard.

Supporting-leg lameness is mild or absent. A nodular or uniform swelling is noted in the affected tendon. The scar tissue in the tendon is tender to pressure. Lifting and hyperextending the digit is strongly resented.

With inflammation of the deep digital flexor, in which the inferior check ligament is almost always involved, a circumscribed swelling is visible on the palmar surface in the proximal third of the metacarpal region. This swelling is warm, hard, knobby and tender to pressure. The horse exhibits a supporting-leg lameness that usually progresses in severity, and stands abnormally straight in the fetlock joint. With bilateral involvement the gait becomes stilted.

Chronic tendinitis of the deep flexor tendon and its inferior check ligament may progress to an acquired knuckling of the fetlock in working horses.

The necropsy findings of acute tendinitis vary with the degree of degeneration that has occurred. The subcutaneous tissue is suffused with blood and serous fluid. The paratenon is edematous and loosened. Hemorrhages extend into the tendon, which shows varying degrees of swelling and a pale-red discoloration.

Striate or more diffuse hemorrhages are visible among degenerated or necrotic fibers and fiber bundles, which show considerable tearing and tortuosity. In cases of peritendinitis, changes are confined to the peritenon. In chronic tendinitis the tendon is surrounded by firm strips of connective tissue. Pink, rigid connective tissue has formed between the torn fibers and unites the fiber stumps. Overall, the tendon has the appearance of a hard, thickened cord.

Histologically, torn and separate fibrils are found during the early stage of tendon healing. The tears tend to run vertically. Later, cell proliferation is evident in the widened interfibrillary tissue.

Under functional loading, newly-formed connective-tissue fibrils become incorporated into the longitudinal alignment of the tendon fibers. They differ from true tendon tissue by their lack of luster, their greater abundance of cells, and their shorter fiber length.

When the rupture occurs within the tendon sheath, healing time is delayed and the healing process is deficient.

The demonstrable pathologic changes in tendinitis of the suspensory ligament are located in the area behind the fetlock joint between the cannon bone and the superficial and deep flexor tendon. The initially diffuse, warm, painful swelling later becomes a nodular, sinewy thickening.

When the suspensory ligament is involved, radiographs sometimes reveal the presence of bony islets (ossifying tendinitis). Lameness is often present.

Tendinitis of the common extensor tendon is manifested by an elongated, sausage-shaped, initially spongy, often fluctuating swelling on the anterior surface of the metacarpus or metatarsus that extends from the fetlock to a hand's width below the carpal or tarsal joint. Later the swelling becomes firmer. No lameness is apparent. The changes usually regress without treatment.

Sometimes a connective-tissue thickening remains. Adhesions between tendons are extremely rare.

Differential Diagnosis and Diagnosis. The diagnosis is based upon visual findings, which in mild cases should be supplemented by careful palpation of the entire course of the tendon with the foot raised. In exceptional cases a radiographic examination using subcutaneous air insufflation and skin thermometry should be done to supplement visual findings.

Oblique radiographs are especially useful for demonstrating closed, distal splint fractures, which have an important bearing on the therapy of tendinitis of the suspensory ligament.

High proximal palmar or plantar anesthesia will often relieve the lameness. The inferior check ligament and the suspensory ligament are supplied by the ulnar nerve. Nerve blocks of this type are seldom needed to make a diagnosis, however.

Treatment. Complete recovery is at present a very difficult goal due to poor vascularity of the tendon tissue. A more realistic goal is to improve circulation in an effort to obtain a fibrillary cicatricial repair tissue that is capable of withstanding functional stresses on a long-term basis.

Acute tendinitis is treated with rest, cold, moist dressings, poultices (Burow's mixture, Aciterran, Pyrantin) or continuous hydrotherapy. After 2—3 days moist heat is applied to promote absorption of hematoma and serous exudation.

Following the regression of acute inflammatory symptoms (absorption of effusion and relief of pain), elastic bandages are applied.

Zinc gelatin bandages have proved to be of particular advantage. They fit snugly but elastically against the tendon, and during movement they provide a continuous massage by constantly changing the limb diameter in the metacarpal region, thereby stimulating blood flow to the tendon. These bandages are especially useful during the convalescent period. In healthy horses they may be applied prophylactically prior to strenuous work (e.g., flat harness races or hurdle races, three-day-event trials).

If absorption is proceeding too slowly, it can be hastened with topical rubefacients (Jokamvasol, camphor ointment, camphor spirit) and by applying a firm cotton or foam bandage.

During this time the horse is confined to a box stall or walked for brief periods. Corrective shoeing is recommended to relieve stress on the deep flexor tendon (shoe with rolled toe and thickened branches or calks).

Inflammatory reactions (pain, edema) can be relieved by the local use of DMSO and glucocorticoids.

In many cases symptoms will recur due to an inadequacy of repair processes or premature loading. With proper treatment, a functional recovery should be possible in mild to moderate cases.

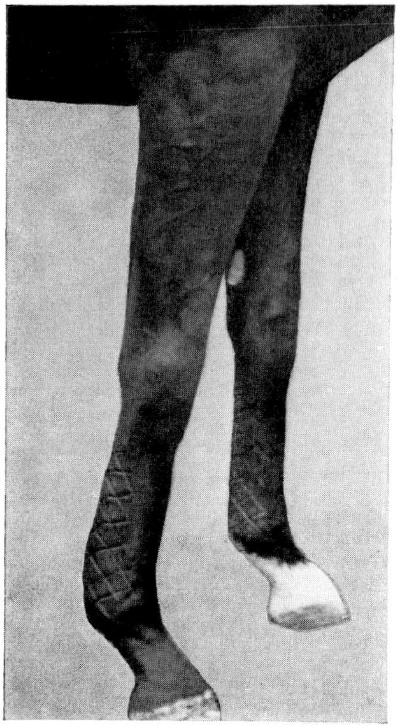

Fig. 2.1.20. — 16. Grid firing for tendinitis.

If signs of tendinitis reappear when work is resumed, more caustic topical agents are often applied. Red blister is most commonly used for this purpose (unguentum hydrargyri rubrum, 4—20 %), which is rubbed for 2—10 minutes into the previously clipped skin. Cantharidin tincture is also used. In addition, various ready-to-use preparations with similar actions are available commercially. After the blister has been rubbed in, an absorbent bandage is applied and left on for 2—4 weeks; this bandage will harden through the drying of exudates.

If this treatment is unsuccessful, or if the tissue disruptions are too extensive to respond to such therapy, then the metacarpus or metatarsus is often fired and then blistered. A grid firing pattern is generally used when lesions are extensive (fig. 2.1.20. — 16), and point firing when changes are more circumscribed. In many cases the procedure can be done with the horse standing after analgesics have been given. Afterward an absorbent bandage is applied and left on for 14 days if no local or system disturbances arise. It is customary to treat both sides so that the fired limb will not be favored. After 6—8 weeks the horse may be walked, and after an additional 4 weeks it may be placed in a paddock. Training is resumed 6—8 weeks thereafter.

Other treatment methods, less frequently used, include local injections of caustic agents [Milne, 1961; Stihl and Leuthold, 1964] or sclerosing agents [Robinson, 1968] into the affected tendon, the use of UV light, shortwaves and microwaves [Gold, 1952], and in rare cases radiation therapy [Dixon, 1972].

Inconsistent results have prompted efforts to develop other operative treatments for the condition. For example, Asheim [1964] has described a procedure in which the tendon is incised longitudinally and altered tendon tissue is excised in wedge-shaped fashion, with the object of improving vascularization and thus increasing the ability of the tendon to heal. After the paratenon and skin have been sutured, a well-padded elastic bandage is applied. The horse is rested for 2 months, whereupon light training is resumed.

Racehorses can return to racing after 9 months.

Angiographic and histologic studies following tendon-splitting operations in which the tendon was incised laterally and split from the top downward demonstrate excellent vascularization and regeneration of the affected tissue [Norberg et al., 1967]. The operation may be performed under local anesthesia with the animal standing [Maxwell, 1971]. 70—75 % success has been reported in horses with tendinitis of the suspensory ligament [Nilsson, 1970, 1971]. Fackelmann [1973] achieved good results by implanting an autologous graft in the diseased tendon.

Inflammation of the inferior check ligament in draft horses is treated by applying a corrective extended-toe shoe. These animals should be used for work on softer surfaces.

Residual lameness left by disease of one branch of the suspensory ligament has been relieved by a unilateral high neurectomy of the palmar or plantar nerve.

Prognosis. Mild cases of acute tendinitis (peritendinitis) can recover well with immediate rest. The return of full function depends on the extent of the changes. The successful treatment of chronic tendinitis requires an adequate rest period followed by an optimum training program that takes into account the tendon pathology and loss of condition. In general, at least 12 months are needed before the animal will be able to resume racing or other types of competition. Zinc gelatin bandages may be applied prophylactically prior to strenuous work.

Comments. Given its pathogenesis, tendinitis invariably lessens the value of a performance animal and constitutes a serious training problem. Tendon, like other tissues, must be adapted gradually to increased stresses and an increased oxygen capacity.

Tendon Ruptures

Definition and Occurrence. A tendon rupture is a complete disruption in the continuity of a tendon and generally affects only the flexor tendon. 'Breakdown' in racing and riding horses is the result of a sudden rupture of the superficial digital flexor tendon or suspensory ligament (figs. 2.1.20. — 17 and — 18).

Symptoms. Most ruptures of the superficial digital flexor tendon occur at the level of the cannon bone. They are manifested by a severe supporting-leg lameness with a dropping of the fetlock joint. A defect forms at the rupture site and quickly fills with blood. Pronounced dropping of the fetlock is also characteristic of suspensory ligament ruptures, depending on whether the body is ruptured or there is a uni- or bilateral tear of its branches. The suspensory ligament may also be torn from its sites of insertion on the sesamoid bones. A very violent trauma can rupture both the superficial flexor tendon and the suspensory ligament.

The deep digital flexor tendon usually ruptures over the navicular bone or separates from its attachment on the third phalanx. The toe tips upward, and the horse stands on the heels or bulbs of the heels. During walking the hoof is advanced in a flailing fashion and lands on the walls of the heel or heel of the horseshoe.

Differential diagnosis must be made from fractures of the sesamoids and phalanges as well as luxations of the interphalangeal joints.

Diagnosis. Typical lameness symptoms, palpatory findings and a negative radiograph suggest a rupture of the flexor tendons. The diagnosis can sometimes be difficult, especially if the animal is excited (e.g., following competition).

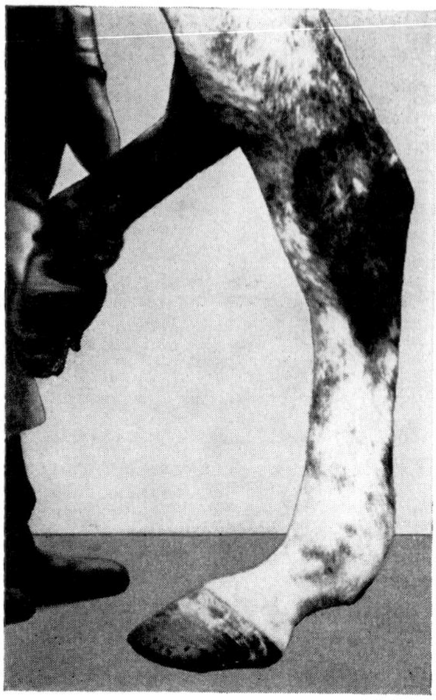
17

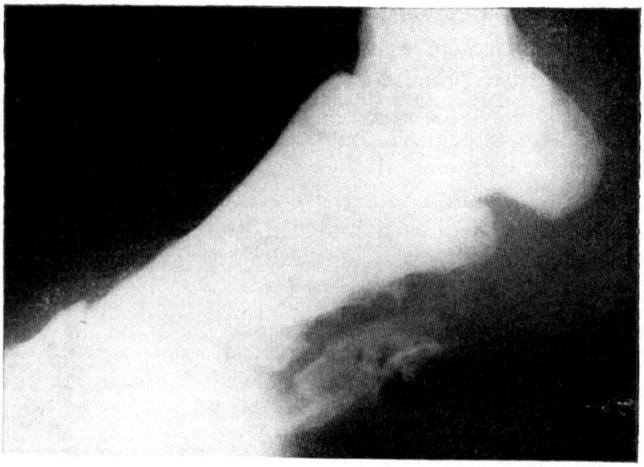
18

Fig. 2.1.20. — 17. Rupture of both flexor tendons.

Fig. 2.1.20. — 18. Same patient as in fig. 2.1.10. — 17 with ossifying processes in the deep digital flexor tendon.

Treatment. The horse is placed in a large box stall with soft bedding and, when acute inflammation subsides, an immobilizing bandage is applied (zinc gelatin, fiberglass, polyurethane foam). To support the fetlock, the foot is shod with an extended-heel bar shoe.

Prognosis. Ruptures of the deep digital flexor tendon, the suspensory ligament or both of its branches have a poor prognosis. Breeding soundness can be restored in some cases. With ruptures of the superficial digital flexor tendon or one branch of the suspensory ligament, recovery is often possible.

Comments. Horses with tendon ruptures are best used for breeding only.

Tendon Wounds

Occurrence and Etiology. Wounds of the flexor and extensor tendons occur mainly in the hind limbs. The angled position of the metatarsus predisposes to extensor tendon injuries during the negotiation of wire fences and makes it difficult to free an entangled leg. Flexor tendon injuries may occur as a result of abrasion, backing into sharp objects, being struck from behind by a wagon with bad brakes, or being cut down in a race by a horse coming up from behind. Flexor tendon wounds of the forelimb can be self-inflicted as a result of overreaching.

Symptoms. A large, flap-shaped wound is usually present on the limb. Separation of the tendon stumps is visible in the depths of the wound during flexion and extension of the digit. If the presence of foreign bodies is suspected, the examination may be supplemented with radiographs. With wounds of the extensor tendon, the digit will flail during the swinging-leg phase. With flexor tendon wounds, sagging of the fetlock joint is frequently present.

Diagnosis. Careful examination of the wound will identify the affected tendon and reveal the degree of disruption or displacement that has occurred.

Treatment. With fresh tendon wounds, suturing should be attempted if the tendon stumps can be apposed. A horseshoe with extended branches and a bar attached with screw calks will aid in approximating the tendon stumps and reducing stresses on them. As healing progresses, the bar of the shoe is progressively thinned. Finally it may be replaced with a spavin shoe or a shoe with thickened heels.

If a tendon suture is not necessary or possible, antibiotics are administered, and only the skin is sutured. In treating an open tendon sheath, it is best to close the synovial sheath, fibrous sheath and skin if at all possible. A well-padded bandage is applied and, if bacterial infection is suspected, is repeatedly moistened with hot antiseptic solutions (ethacridine lactate).

Unless removed, foreign bodies in the wound (necrotic tendon tissue, bone sequestra, hairs, etc.) will irritate the wound and lead to the formation of exuberant granulation tissue and fistulae.

Thickened areas that remain in the course of the flexor tendons are sometimes fired after a period of 6—8 weeks.

Prognosis. Extensor tendon wounds have a favorable prognosis for healing, as do wounds of the superficial flexor tendon. However, the development of exuberant granulation can greatly delay healing.

Divisions of both flexor tendons are considered incurable.

2.1.20.1.7. Tendovaginitis of the Distal Common Flexor Tendon Sheath

Occurrence and Classification. The most common disease affecting the equine tendon sheath is inflammation of the common distal flexor sheath. In all cases the tendovaginitis is characterized by a marked bulge of the affected sheath due to the presence of excessive synovial fluid. The inflammation may be septic or aseptic, acute or chronic. The hind limbs are more commonly affected.

Acute Aseptic Tendovaginitis

Symptoms. A mild to moderate supporting-leg lameness is present. Systemic signs are absent during the 2nd stage.

An elongated, circumscribed, warm, tender, and markedly fluctuating, occasionalle tense swelling appears proximal to the fetlock joint and lateral and medial to tht digital flexors. Swelling is also evident beneath the proximal digital annular ligament on the volar side of the pastern. A bowing of the flexor tendon sheath is visible ar sites where the sheath is subcutaneous. Following contusions, the entire flexos tendon region may appear thickened. Pain is elicited by pressing on the flexor tendon and by extending the fetlock joint. An acute aseptic tendovaginitis may be characterized as serous or serofibrinous, depending on the nature of the exudate. In the serous form the exudate is yellow to yellow-red in color and has a stringy consistency. The catarrhal form leads to a mild swelling of the synovial sheath. The presence of fibrin flakes characterizes the serofibrinous form of tendovaginitis. There is also a hemorrhagic form, characterized by a hemorrhagic exudate.

Histologically, acute tendosynovitis is marked by increased capillary filling and a leukocytic and histiocytic infiltration, especially perivascularly. These reactions are the least pronounced in acute serous synovitis, and are most pronounced in the serofibrinous form. A similar relationship applies to the leukocyte content of the exudate.

Etiology. Acute aseptic tendovaginitis of the distal common flexor tendon sheath is a result of mechanical influences (stretching, compression). Sesamoid lameness is also associated with distension of the flexor tendon sheath.

The etiologic significance of primary tendon sheath disease is unclear. There is much evidence to show that the primary disorder is a tendinitis that leads secondarily to inflammation of the sheath.

Differential diagnosis is made from arthritis of the fetlock joint and all other forms of tendovaginitis (by aspiration), as well as from pododermatitis.

Diagnosis. By aspirating the tendon sheath it is possible to evaluate the general character of the inflammation. Relief of lameness following the injection of a concentrated local anesthetic containing 200,000—400,000 I.U. penicillin is diagnostic of an acute aseptic tendovaginitis.

Treatment. For the shod horse, immediate corrective shoeing is indicated to relieve stress on the tendon sheath. In the hind limbs this is accomplished by applying a spavin shoe, and in the forelimbs by elevating the heels with leather wedges or screw calks. Warm, moist dressings with astringents are beneficial for the first few days. After a week, zinc gelatin bandages or mild topical rubefacients may be applied. Good results are obtained by resting the animal for 2—3 weeks while repeatedly injecting glucocorticoids into the affected sheath. Intravenous phenylbutazone is a useful adjunct.

Prognosis. A complete recovery may be expected if rest is enforced. A coexisting tendinitis adversely affects the prognosis.

Chronic Aseptic Tendovaginitis

Symptoms. A lameness of variable degree appears following prolonged, vigorous exertion. The tendon sheath is distended, sometimes presenting a fist-size bulge, and shows palpable thickening. Often an abnormal firmness of the sheath is also palpable (chronic fibrous tendovaginitis).

In chronic serous synovitis, the thickened synovial tissue acquires a villus-like texture. The majority of infiltrating cells consist of lymphocytes; the proportion of unclassified mononuclear and plasma cells is variable. Often these cells are clumped together to form small nodules on the surface of the synovial villi. These changes are nonspecific, however.

Etiology. Chronic tendovaginitis is very often the result of a previous acute inflammation or a large, unabsorbed hematoma. It may also develop gradually, unaccompanied by clinical signs of acute inflammation.

Differential Diagnosis. Diseases of the sesamoid bones must be excluded by radiography.

Diagnosis. An existing lameness cannot always be completely relieved by diagnostic intratendovaginal anesthesia, for in chronic tendovaginitis the tendon sheath is sometimes heavily loculated. Adhesions between the flexor tendons and sheath wall can be well demonstrated radiographically by means of air contrast filling. Calcifications can also be detected in this way (chronic ossifying tendovaginitis).

Treatment. In chronic serous aseptic tendovaginitis, distension is relieved and function is restored by the intratendovaginal injection of glucocorticoids. Sometimes a residual fibrous thickening persists. Blistering or firing is sometimes recommended to stimulate hyperemia. Corrective shoeing is also indicated. Often microwave therapy and paraffin camphor packs are used successfully.

Prognosis. A complete recovery is rare, although many horses are still fit for light work on soft ground.

Tendon Sheath Hygroma

A tendon sheath hygroma is a fluid distension of the tendon sheath that is unaccompanied by inflammation or lameness. It can be classified etiologically as follows:

— congenital hygroma,
— hygroma of insidious onset,
— recurrent synovitis.

Cytologically, tendon sheath hygroma is marked by a low cell count and a low percentage of granulocytes. Higher cell counts are found in hygromas that occur as a sequel to inflammation. Treatment is indicated only if the owner requests it, for hygromas are cosmetic blemishes that cause no functional disability. Treatment consists in repeated glucocorticoid injections, after first evacuating most of the synovial fluid from the sheath. This should be followed by the application of a firm bandage and stall rest. Complete remissions have also been reported following the injection of 30—60 ml of a 1% epinephrine solution into the tendon sheath; the animal is put back to work 2 days after the injection.

Spontaneous recoveries are sometimes reported in young animals.

Infectious Tendovaginitis

Symptoms. A generalized pyogenic infection with marked systemic effects is usually present. Food is refused, and emaciation follows. Affected horses stand with the body drawn up and bear no weight on the affected limb. Recumbency may develop in older horses.

The limb is diffusely swollen, warm and painful from the carpal or tarsal joint downward. In the early stage the distended tendon sheath appears unusually prominent relative to surrounding tissues. If a wound is present, a turbid synovial fluid that contains fibrin flakes is discharged initially. Later the discharge becomes reddish-brown or dark brown.

Etiology. Infections of the common distal flexor tendon sheath may be primary as a result of perforating wounds, or secondary as a result of blood- or lymph-borne infection from other tissues. Any of a number of bacteria may be responsible. Direct causes of perforating wounds are pitchfork injuries, indriven foreign bodies, and injuries from wire or sharp-edged objects. Small puncture wounds close rapidly and are no longer detectable after a few days. With puncture wounds of the foot, there may be an immediate perforation of the tendon sheath, or an infection may develop in connection with a suppurative cellulitis. When wounds are extensive, concomitant injury of the flexor tendon is usually present.

Blood-borne infections of the flexor tendon sheath occur in newborn foals as a result of metastatic pyogenic polyarthritis caused by *Actinobacillus equuli*, *Escherichia coli*, streptococci, *Corynebacterium equi* or *Salmonella enteritidis*.

The infection may be delayed for some weeks in cases where actinobacilli are carried into the arterial system by strongyles migrating from the bowel.

In mature horses, hematogenous infections occur in connection with pneumonia, strangles, and in sensitized serum horses.

Differential Diagnosis. Infectious tendovaginitis, unlike the aseptic form, is generally accompanied by systemic signs. A cytologic examination of the synovial fluid is rewarding in doubtful cases, for the infectious inflammation is associated with an increase in polymorphonuclear leukocytes.

Cellulitis also must be differentiated, unless it is related to the development of the tendovaginitis.

Diagnosis. Fluid collected from the tendon sheath is a useful aid to diagnosis. A large-gauge needle should be used for this purpose. Often the pus is so thick that it cannot flow from the sheath spontaneously, and therefore must be aspirated or expressed by insufflating air into the sheath. In many cases, however, the amount contained in the needle will be sufficient for cytologic and microbiologic examination.

Treatment. The animal is placed in a box stall with soft bedding to avoid decubital lesions and stress laminitis. Fresh wounds are managed according to general surgical rules, and the tendon sheath cavity is flushed with an antibiotic. Purulent tendovaginitis is treated by the intrasynovial injection of antibiotics or sulfonamides and the application of hot antiseptic dressings. In addition, sulfonamides or antibiotics and analgesic drugs are given parenterally. With tendon sheath empyema or abscessation, drainage can be established by opening the sheath at its proximal and distal ends.

Prognosis. In general, horses with purulent tendovaginitis of the flexor tendon sheath will regain use of the limb only if prompt treatment is rendered. Later, the development of adhesions between the flexor tendons and sheath wall will lead to permanent lameness.

References

ALEXANDER, J. T.: The application of a fiberglass cast to the equine forelimb. Proc. 17th Ann. Conv. Amer. Assoc. Equine Pract., p. 269 (1971).

ANTEPLEPLIOGLU, H.: Results of the treatment of tendinitis in race horses. Ankara Univ. Vet. Fak. *20:* 2/3 (1974).

ASHEIM, A.: Surgical treatment of tendcn injuries in the horse. J. Amer. Vet. Med. Assoc. *140:* 447 (1964).

ASHEIM, A.; KUNDSEN, O.: Percutaneous tendon splitting. Amer. Assoc. of Equine Pract., p. 255 (1967).

BECKER, E.: Über die Versorgung von Knochenbrüchen durch perkutane Osteosynthese. Prakt. Tierarzt *55:* 253 (1974).

CORNELL, M. R.: Healing in repair of bone fractures in large animals. Vet. Med. and Small Animal Clinician *69:* 631 (1974).

DANIELI, Y.; MAESTRO, M.: Calcification of the superficial digital flexor tendon in a mule. Refuah Vet. *23:* 53 (1966).

DIETZ, O.; MILL, J.; RICHTER, W.; WILSDORF, G.: Zur Problematik der sog. Schienbeinerkrankung des Vollblutpferdes. Mh. Vet.-Med. *26:* 703 (1971).

DIETZ, O.; NAGEL, E.; KOCH, T.; BERG, R.; STERBA, O.: Zur Entstehung und zur Klinik der sog. gedeckten, distalen Griffelbeinfrakturen. Schweiz. Arch. Tierheilk. *105:* 87 (1963).

DIETZ, O.; NAGEL, E.; RECHENBERG, R.: Beitrag zur Gliedmaßenchirurgie bei Vollblutgalopp- und Vollbluttraberpferden. Mh. Vet.-Med. *18:* Sonderheft 1, 5 (1963).

DIETZ, O.; RICHTER, W.: Zur Tendinitis bei Sportpferden. Mh. Vet.-Med. *20:* 476 (1965).

DINGWALL, J. S.; DUNCAN, D. B.; HORNLY, F. D.: Compression plating in large animal orthopedics. J. Amer. vet. med. Assoc. *159:* 1651 (1971).

DIXON, R. T.: Results of radon 222 gamma radiation therapy in an equine practice. Austral. Vet. J. *48:* 279 (1972).

DIXON, R. T., BELLENGER, C. R.: Fissurfraktur des Metakarpus und Metatarsus beim Pferd. J. Amer. vet. med. Assoc. *153:* 1289 (1968).

DOIMO, J. C.: Des nouvelles perspectives dans la prophylaxie et le traitement des tendinitis chez les chevaux des course. Vet.-med. Diss., Toulouse (1972).

DUBS, B.; QUASTEL, T.: Hauttransplantation beim Pferd. tierärztl. praxis *3:* 57 (1975).

EY, G.: Untersuchungen über die Verwendungsfähigkeit von Polyurethanschaum zur Gliedmaßenfixation bei Haustieren. Vet.-med. Diss., Hannover (1971).

FACKELMANN, G. E.: The nature of tendon damage and its repair. Equine Vet. J. *5:* 141 (1973).

FACKELMANN, G. E.: Autologous tendon transplantation in the horse. The technic and its histology. Schweiz. Arch. Tierheilk. *115:* 231 (1973).

FRÖLICH, D.: Versuche zur intramedullären Osteosynthese des Metakarpus beim Pferd. Vet.-med. Diss., Zürich (1973).

GENOVESE, R. L.: The use of sodium oleate in splints and bucked shins. Proc. 20th Ann. Conv. Amer. Assoc. Equine Pract., p. 237 (1974).

GERLACH, CH.: Verbände in der Veterinärmedizin unter Verwendung von Kunststoffen. Vet.-med. Diss., Berlin-Dahlem (1967).

GERTSEN, K. E.; BRINKER, W. O.: Fracture repair in ponies using bone plates. J. Amer. vet. med. Assoc. *154:* 900 (1969).

GOLD, T. N.: The technical and practical application of electrotherapy in equines. Vet. Rec. *64:* 681 (1952).

GUFFY, M. M.: Knochensequester und nicht heilende Wunden bei Pferden. J. Amer. vet. med. Assoc. *152:* 1638 (1968).

HALLSTRÖM, M.: Versuche mit zwei verschiedenen Formen der Stifte bei Transfixierung von Röhrenknochenfrakturen größerer Haustiere. Acta vet. scand. *7:* 157 (1966).

HANSELKE, D. V.; BOYD, C. L.; JOYCE, J. R.: External fixation of a large animal fracture with a resin-bonded fiberglass cast. Vet. Med. and Small Animal Clinician *67:* 519 (1972).

HEINZE, C. D.: Equine orthopedic surgery. Med. vet. Pract. *47:* 63 (1966).

HIGGENBOTHAM, R. L.: The use of sodium oleate for splint lameness in the standardbred. Proc. 20th Ann. Conv. Amer. Assoc. Equine Pract., p. 235 (1974).

KOGER, L. M.; MCILHATTAN, J.; SCHLADETZKY, R.: Prothesis for partielly amputated foreleg in a horse. J. Amer. vet. med. Assoc. *156:* 1600 (1970).

KUNDSEN, O.; ASHEIM, A.: Perkutane Operation von Sehnen und Fesselband beim Pferd. Svensk. Veterin. Tidskr. *22:* 576 (1970).

LEUTHOLD, A.: Die Griffelbeinfraktur beim Pferd. Schweiz. Arch. Tierheilk. *108:* 681 (1966).

LINGARD, D. R.: Fissure fracture of the equine metatarsus. Vet. Med. and Small Animal Clinician *64:* 895 (1969).

MAROLT, J.; ZUKOVIC, M.; MOLNAR, M.: Die Onchocercosis beim Pferd. Dtsch. tierärztl. Wschr. *73:* 130 (1966).

MARTIENSEN, G.: Knochenfissuren als Lahmheitsursache beim Pferd. Dtsch. tierärztl. Wschr. *74:* 554 (1967).

MAXWELL, J. A. L.: Treatment of tendosynovitis in the horse by the tendon splitting operation. Austral. vet. J. *47:* 192 (1971).

MILNE, F. J.: Thought and observations on counterirritation in the horse. Zbl. Vet.-Med. *8:* 1095 (1961).

MILNE, D. W.; TURNER, A. S.; GABEL, A. A.: Surgical approaches to certain long bones of the horse for application of tension band plates. J. Amer. vet. med. Assoc. *168:* 48 (1976).

NILSSON, G.: A survey of the results of the tendon splitting operation for chronic tendinitis in the horse. Equine Vet. J. *2:* 111 (1970).

NILSSON, G.: Tendon splitting for chronic tendinitis in horses. Mod. vet. Pract. *52:* 56 (1971).

NILSSON, G.; BÖRLK, G.: Surgical treatment of chronic tendinitis in the horse. J. Amer. vet. med. Assoc. *155:* 920 (1969).

NORBERG, A. J.; RAKER, C. W.; DODD, D.: Equine tendinitis — an angiographic and histologic study. Proc. 13th Ann. Conv. Amer. Assoc. Equine Pract., New Orleans 1967, p. 243.

PAATSAMA, S.; RISSANEN, P.; ROKKANEN, P.: Effect of androgen, estrogen, cortisone, growth hormone, and parathyroid and thyrotropic hormone on tendinous tissue. A experimental investigation in young dogs. Nord. Vet.-Med. *21:* 41 (1969).

PAJTLE, M.: Die Aktivität der alkalischen Phosphatase bei experimentell hervorgerufener Periostotis beim Pferd. Ber. XVII. Welttierärztekongreß, Hannover 1963, p. 1223.

PELT, R. W. VAN: Tendosynovitis in the horse. J. Amer. vet. med. Assoc. *154:* 1022 (1969).

PELT, R. W. VAN: Idiopathic tendosynovitis in foals. J. Amer. vet. med. Assoc. *155:* 510 (1969).

RICHTER, W.: Erhebungen über belastungsbedingte Gliedmaßenerkrankungen des juvenilen und adulten Sportpferdes. Vet.-med. Diss. (B), Berlin (1975).

ROBINSON, R. C.: The use of sclerosing agents in tendon repair of racehorses. Austral. vet. J. *44:* 200 (1968).

RONNEY, J. R.: Distal condylar fractures of the cannon bone in the horse. Med. vet. Pract. *55:* 113 (1974).

RONNEY, J. R.; PRICKETT, M. E.; LEXINGTON, K.: Foreleg splints in horses. Cornell Vet. *56:* 259 (1966).

SOENNICHSEN, H. V.: Tendinitis chronica. 6th Congress European Soc. of Vet. Surg., Helsinki 1966.

SOENNICHSEN, H. V.: The primary site of damage in bowed tendon of the horse. Mod. vet. Pract. *54:* 58 (1975).
SOENNICHSEN, H. V.: Tendinitis des Pferdes. Definition, Therapie und Prognose. tierärztl. praxis *3:* 315 (1975).
SOUBAGNE, J. M.: La thermometrie des tendons chez le cheval de course. Diss. École Nat. Vét., Toulouse (1969).
STIHL, H. G.: Frakturen als orthopädisches Problem beim Sportpferd. Schweiz. Arch. Tierheilk. *110:* 309 (1968).
STIHL, H. G.; LEUTHOLD, A.: Zur subkutanen Jodtherapie der Tendinitis chronica beim Pferd. Schweiz. Arch. Tierheilk. *106:* 216 (1964).
STROMBERG, B.: The normal and diseased superficial flexor tendon in race horses. A morphological and physiological investigation. Vet.-med. Diss., Stockholm (1971).
TITTEL, K.; OTTO, H.: Der Einfluß eines Lauftrainings unterschiedlicher Dauer und Intensität auf die Hyperthrophie, Zugfestigkeit und Dehnungsfähigkeit des straffen, kollagenen Bindegewebes (am Beispiel der Achillessehne). Medizin und Sport *10:* 308 (1970).
ÜBERREITER, O.: Die spontane Griffelbeinfraktur bei Sportpferden. Wiener tierärztl. Wschr. *53:* 404 (1966).
VASALL, H.: Beitrag zur klinischen Untersuchung von Sportpferden. Vet.-med. Diss., Berlin-Dahlem (1968).
VRIGASOFF, A.: Ein Beitrag zur Behandlung der ossifizierenden Periostiden der Osteoarthrosen. Zschr. Forschungsinst. Landw. Ministerium Sofia (1956), p. 204.
WILSDORF, G.: Beitrag zur Biomechanik der Vorderextremität des Galopprennpferdes und deren Beziehung zur sog. Schienbeinerkrankung. Mh. Vet.-Med. *26:* 939 (1971).
WILLI, W.: Versuche über die Elastizität und Festigkeit der Beugesehnen des Pferdes unter spezieller Berücksichtigung des Tendo interosseus. Vet.-med. Diss., Zürich (1951).
WHEAT, J. D.: Bilateral fractures of the third metacarpal bone of a thoroughbred. J. Amer. vet. med. Assoc. *140:* 815 (1962).
WHITFORD, E. L.: A case report fracture of metatarsus in a pinto stallion. J. Amer. vet. med. Assoc. *137:* 58 (1960).

2.1.20.2. Diseases of the Fetlock Joint and Pastern

2.1.20.2.1. Metacarpophalangeal Arthritis (Inflammation of the Fetlock Joint)

Occurrence and Classification. The fetlock joint is a ginglymus joint which, like all phalangeal joints, is subjected to varying stresses at varying sites owing to the angulation and break of the digital axis. As a result, diseases of the fetlock joint are fairly common in the athletic horse. Inflammation may be classified as follows according to their etiology and course:
— acute aseptic arthritis,
— infectious arthritis,
— chronic degenerative arthritis and periarthritis,
— chronic serous arthritis and fluid distention of the metacarpophalangeal joint.

Etiology. Acute aseptic metacarpophalangeal arthritis is caused by sprains and contusions (fig. 2.1.20. — 19). These may result from a misstep, slip, fall, entrapment of the foot, sharp turn, sudden change of gait. It may also occur when the animal is rising or when it lands after a jump on the overextended digit. Faults of conformation, especially 'weak pasterns', and improper shoeing can also predispose to the disease. In Standardbreds and running horses, the 'inside' fetlock joint can come under increased stress if the turns on the track are not adequately banked. Perforating wounds or suppurative processes that have spread from nearby tissues can lead to a pyogenic or infectious arthritis.

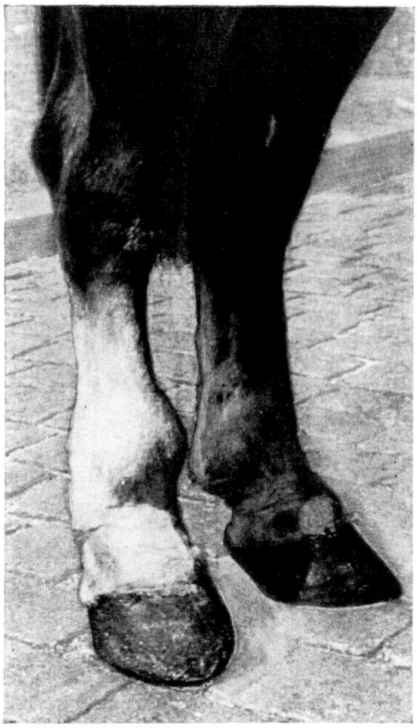

19

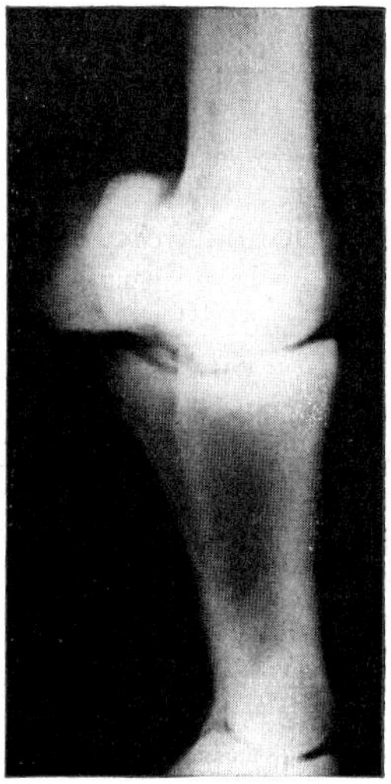

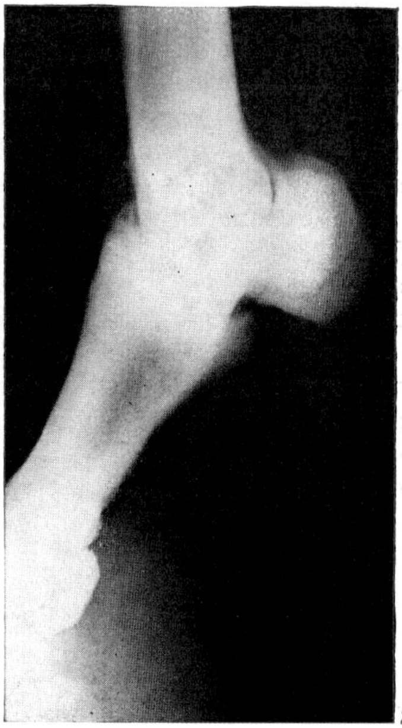

20, 21

Fig. 2.1.20. — 19. Subtendinous bursitis at the dorsum of the fetlock following trauma.
Fig. 2.1.20. — 20. Osteochondritis dissecans of the metacarpal portion of the fetlock joint.
Fig. 2.1.20. — 21. Loose body (fragment) on the dorsal surface of the fetlock joint.

Both types of inflammation, like fractures that involve the joint surfaces, can result in chronic inflammation leading to degenerative change. Chronic degenerative arthritis can also develop from a gradual erosion of the fetlock joint caused by the sustained action of tensile and compressive forces during movement.

2.1.20.2.2. Acute Aseptic Arthritis

Symptoms. Acute aseptic metacarpophalangeal arthritis is manifested by a moderate swelling of the fetlock joint of sudden onset. Additional signs are an upright pastern, and incomplete dorsiflexion and occasional knuckling of the fetlock. In more serious cases the distended joint capsule protrudes laterally and medially behind the distal ends of the splint bones. Other findings vary with the nature of the pathologic changes (rupture of joint capsule and collateral ligaments, hemarthrosis and contusion of joint cartilage; figs. 2.1.20. — 20 and — 21).

Diagnosis. The diagnosis is based on clinical signs. The synovial fluid may be examined to obtain more information on the severity of the disease. Radiographs in at least two planes are necessary for differentiating chip fractures of the joint margins and fractures of the cannon or pastern bone.

Treatment. Rest and soft, deep bedding will assist healing. Cooling bandages (Aciterran, Burow's mixture) are indicated for the first 2—3 days. Then warm, moist compresses are applied to promote absorption. Shoeing with raised heels (calks or shims) reduces stress on the fetlock joint.

Good results have been obtained with single or repeated intra-articular injections of glucocorticoids and hyaluronic acid. However, this must be followed by complete rest for 4—6 weeks. Some cases of intractable lameness respond favorably to anesthesia of the joint or palmar (plantar) nerves using a depot anesthetic.

Absorption-promoting and anti-inflammatory drugs are also effective (dimethylsulfoxide, hepathromb ointment, mobilat, etc.).

With coexisting chip fractures, the lameness is severe. Fragments chipped from the joint margin must be surgically removed. Most fractures of this type occur at the anterior border of the 1st phalanx or on the palmar (plantar) surface below the sesamoids. Fragments that are not removed lead to chronic degenerative joint disease.

Prognosis. Lameness due to mild sprains or contusions will regress in a few days with proper treatment. In all other cases the prognosis is guarded in terms of anatomic and functional recovery, especially if there is a coexisting fissure fracture encroaching on the joint space. The disease may take an insidious course, leading to a chronic degenerative joint disease or fluid accumulation.

2.1.20.2.3. Infectious Arthritis

Symptoms and Diagnosis. In the stage of purulent synovitis, a turbid, flaky but nonviscous synovial fluid is discharged from the joint wound. Initially this is accompanied by a mild to moderate supporting-leg lameness. Stasis of the purulent synovial fluid leads to joint empyema and later to capsular cellulitis. Pain is severe, and weight is no longer borne on the affected limb. The pus that accumulates in the joint becomes viscous and will no longer flow spontaneously during arthrocentesis. A febrile systemic reaction is usually present.

Treatment. The joint is immobilized with a moist, antiseptic bandage, having first been flushed with physiologic saline and filled with penicillin. With larger wounds, it is recommended that the antibiotic be applied to the joint in the form of an ointment or suspension. In addition, large doses of sulfonamides or antibiotics should be given systemically. This treatment is continued until an improvement of general condition and lameness is noted.

Prognosis. The earlier treatment is instituted, the better the chance of recovery. Very often a purulent arthritis will progress to a chronic degenerative condition with internal or external ankylosis and permanent lameness.

2.1.20.2.4. Chronic Degenerative Joint Disease and Periarthritis

Symptoms. A prominent swelling that is neither warm nor painful appears in the region of the fetlock joint. The limb is held slightly anterior and bears no weight. In racehorses, edematous swellings are sometimes observed following strenuous work. The degree of lameness depends on the location and extent of the lesions. Often lameness is absent, or a supporting-leg lameness appears only after exercise.

Diagnosis. Radiographs show periarticular bony changes that are mainly localized at the insertions of the collateral ligaments and lateral digital extensor, and distal to that site.

There is a narrowing of the joint space as a result of cartilage erosion. Lameness, if present, will only be relieved by diagnostic anesthesia if mechanical obstruction has not produced ankylosis.

Treatment. Warm, moist compresses are indicated in the early stage, followed later by iodine-containing ointments, several daily applications of dimethylsulfoxide, or the intra-articular or systemic administration of mucopolysaccharides (arteparon, arumalon).

The intra-articular injection of glucocorticoids is rarely successful in the presence of degenerative change. Such treatment may be supported by parenteral or oral analgesics (phenylbutazone, tomanol).

If bony changes are severe, improvement can sometimes be achieved by radiation therapy. 60—70 % success has been reported [Clapp et al., 1963].

If diagnostic anesthesia of the palmar or plantar nerves is positive, a functional cure can be effected by neurectomy of these nerves (prohibited in some countries including the U.S.).

Prognosis. The prognosis for an anatomic and functional recovery is guarded due to the irreversible bony and cartilage changes that occur.

Comments. In advanced cases of chronic degenerative joint disease and periarthritis with stiffening of the joint *arthrodesis* of the fetlock joint can restore a degree of function that is sufficient for breeding purposes.

2.1.20.2.5. Chronic Serous Arthritis, Hydrarthrosis of the Fetlock Joint

Chronic irritation can cause an acute aseptic inflammation to progress to a chronic serous arthritis. If lameness is absent but joint distension persists, a condition of hydrarthrosis (hydrops articuli) is said to exist. It is characterized by an excessive filling of the joint which produces a lateral and medial bulge between the suspensory ligament branches and the cannon bone (windpuffs). Inflammatory signs are absent.

Repeated intra-articular glucocorticoid injections followed by bandaging will cure many cases. Recurrences are possible, however.

2.1.20.2.6. Constriction of the Palmar or Plantar Annular Ligaments

Definition. The palmar (volar) or plantar annular ligament of the fetlock joint is a tendinous sheet formed by a thickening of the deep fascia and contiguous with the common flexor tendon sheath. It blends with the intersesamoidean ligament, the sesamoid bones, and in some places with the surface of the superficial flexor tendon. Farther distally it unites with a second tendinous sheet, the proximal digital annular ligament, which attaches the two branches of the superficial flexor tendon to each other and to the proximal phalanx.

The palmar annular ligament acts to prevent displacement of the superficial flexor tendon, which would destroy its mechanical efficiency. Traumatic or infectious conditions of the tendon or annular ligament can lead to a constriction of this ligament, resulting in ischemia and necrosis of the enclosed tendon. The consequences of this are scar tissue formation and the development of adhesions with the tendon sheath, which seriously hamper tendon function and cause lameness.

Symptoms. In nearly all cases there is distension of the common tendon sheath of the superficial and deep flexor tendons proximal to the annular ligament. The superficial flexor tendon is often thickened in this area. This may lead to the mistaken assumption that the primary problem is a low bowed tendon.

Viewing the fetlock from the side, one can always see a 'notch' on the proximal side of the annular ligament. This is caused by constriction of the annular ligament with an associated accumulation of synovial fluid in the tendon sheath (fig. 2.1.20. – 22).

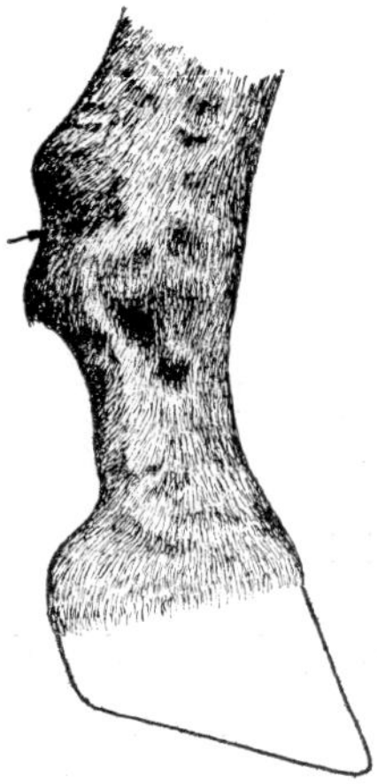

Fig. 2.1.20. — 22. Constriction of the annular ligament of the fetlock joint; arrow indicates site of incision.

A persistent supporting-leg lameness is always present and usually becomes more pronounced with exercise. The lameness increases as the inflammation and constriction progress.

The growing pressure impairs blood flow through the flexor tendon and leads to necrotic changes. Careful palpation will reveal thickening and fibrosis at the junction of the superficial flexor tendon with the annular ligament, indicating involvement of the ligament.

Etiology. Constriction of the palmar or plantar annular ligament may result from a primary inflammation of the annular ligament due, for example, to an incised or puncture wound. In the healing process, scar tissue forms leading to a stricture that exerts pressure on the superficial flexor tendon. Because the annular ligament itself is not elastic, swellings of the superficial digital flexor caused by tendovaginitis can also cause the same signs as constriction of the annular ligament. Often, however, inflammatory processes associated with tendinitis lead to direct involvement of the annular ligament due to the partial anatomic fusion between the ligament and superficial flexor tendon [Boyes].

Differential diagnosis must be made from all forms of tendovaginitis by palpation and diagnostic tendon-sheath anesthesia. With a constriction of the annular ligament, anesthesia may improve the lameness but will never relieve it completely. In tendovaginitis, moreover, there is no fibrous thickening at the junction of the annular ligament and superficial flexor tendon.

Inflammatory changes of the flexor tendons also must be excluded. Most bowed tendons will eventually become sound with rest, at least at the walk and trot. Whenever there is tendinitis of the superficial flexor tendon in its distal portion (low bowed tendon), it should be ascertained whether a primary constriction of the annular ligament is involved, or whether an enlargement of the tendon has led to these symptoms owing to the inelasticity of the annular ligament.

Diagnosis. Persistent lameness accompanied by a notching in the proximal part of the palmar or plantar annular ligament of the fetlock, together with palpatory evidence of fibrous tissue formation at the junction of the annular ligament and superficial flexor tendon, is the basis for diagnosis. Even after weeks or months, the lameness shows no tendency toward improvement.

Treatment. ADAMS [1974] states that surgical incision of the palmar or plantar annular ligament is the only effective treatment. Under general anesthesia, and after proper surgical preparation of the area, an incision is made on the lateral edge of the superficial flexor tendon, behind the digital vessels and nerves. The incision continues through the annular ligament and into the tendon sheath. If inflammation has been present for some time, the ligament and tendon sheath cannot be separated on account of fibrous adhesions. After the palmar or plantar ligament has been completely severed, the subcutaneous tissues are sutured with an absorbable suture and the skin with a noncapillary, nonabsorbable suture. The wound is protected with a snug-fitting bandage. Exercise is begun in three days, hand-walking the horse in a gradually increasing regimen so that adhesions will not reunite the divided ligament. Antibiotics should be administered for several days and tetanus prophylaxis provided.

Prognosis. If the primary cause is a constriction of the palmar or plantar annular ligament that is not accompanied by extensive changes in the superficial flexor tendon, the prognosis is favorable in terms of functional recovery. In almost all cases, the horse is free of lameness following incision of the affected annular ligament.

2.1.20.2.7. Luxation of the Proximal Phalanx

Classification and Etiology. Excessive flexion and extension can lead to stretching and tearing of the joint capsule and collateral ligaments, with consequent luxation of the proximal phalanx. This can occur during falls and stumbles on rough ground or when the animal steps into a hole or gets a foot caught between rails, etc.

In a complete luxation, the portions of the cannon and proximal phalanx that form the fetlock joint are widely displaced; with a subluxation, the articular surfaces of these bones are still touching (fig. 2.1.20. — 23). The lameness is less severe than with a complete luxation, and there is no abnormal motion in the joint.

Symptoms. In racehorses, an anterior luxation is observed following rupture of the flexor tendons and suspensory apparatus. In this case the distal end of the cannon bone becomes displaced and causes an unusual hyperextension at the fetlock. Posterior luxation is very rare and can happen only if the collateral ligaments of the sesamoid apparatus are torn. In both cases the joint diameter is enlarged, a 'step' is formed, and a severe supporting-leg lameness is present in the early stage.

Differential Diagnosis. Subluxations must not be confused with knuckling of the fetlock, which is due mainly to stretching of the ligaments of the hind limb. Anesthesia of the tibial nerve is also accompanied by a pronounced knuckling of the fetlock.

Treatment and Prognosis. With a complete luxation, treatment is worthwhile only in valuable breeding stock. The luxation is reduced under general anesthesia, whereupon the joint is immobilized with a bandage of rigid zinc gelatin, plaster or fiberglass. A subluxation is treated in similar fashion and has a more favorable prognosis.

2.1.20.2.8. Fracture of the Proximal Sesamoid Bones

Occurrence and Classification. Sesamoid fractures usually occur in the hind limbs of Standardbreds and draft horses, while in riding horses, especially racehorses and jumpers, they are most common in the forelimb. The fractures may be closed or open and may involve one or both sesamoids of the same limb. Most sesamoid fractures occur in horses between 2 and 4 years of age.

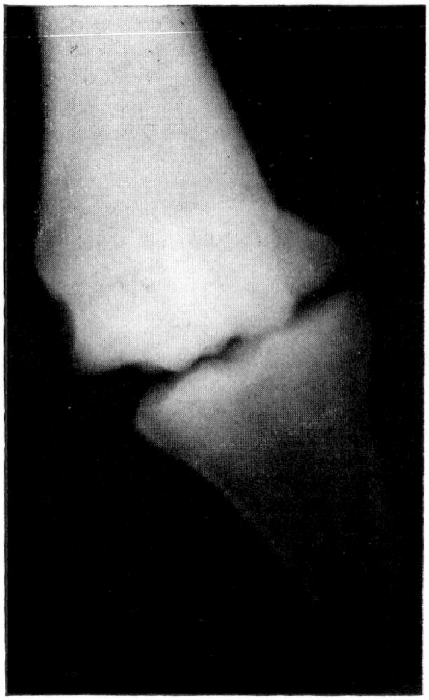

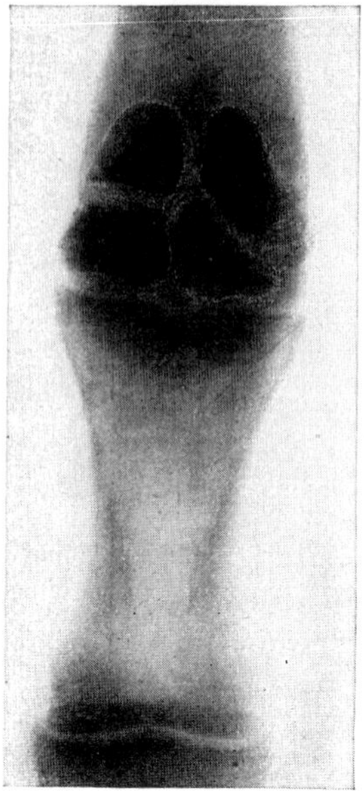

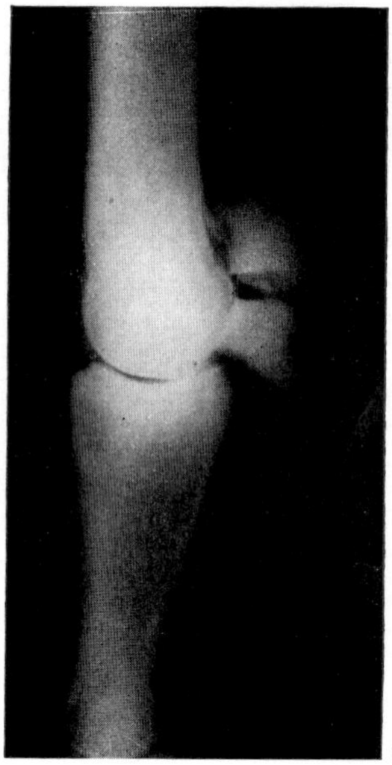

25

23, 24

Fig. 2.1.20. — 23. Luxation of the proximal phalanx.

Fig. 2.1.20. — 24. Horizontal fracture of both sesamoid bones with approximately equal-size fragments (dorso-palmar projection).

Fig. 2.1.20. — 25. Horizontal fracture of both sesamoid bones with approximately equal-size fragments (latero-medial projection).

Two basic types of sesamoid fracture according to the localization of the fracture line occur (some fractures may exhibit features of both types):

— Horizontal fractures with equal-size fragments. This form almost always affects both the lateral and medial sesamoids and mainly occurs in the front limbs of jumpers or horses that run flat races. The ligaments surrounding the sesamoids may show varying degrees of concomitant injury.

— Avulsion fractures or transverse fractures of a single sesamoid bone with unequal-size fragments, a form occurring mainly in the hind limbs of Standardbreds and forelimbs of running horses. Posterior displacement of the sesamoids may occur if there is a complete rupture of the distal sesamoidean ligaments. Five subclasses of this fracture type are recognized from a therapeutic standpoint [Dietz et al., 1981].

Symptoms. The clinical manifestations of the first fracture type are dramatic. The injury is followed by an immediate, severe supporting-leg lameness. There is a pronounced dropping of the fetlock joint when weight is borne on the limb. In the acute stage before swelling appears, a defect is palpable in the sesamoid bone when the fetlock joint is flexed. Pain is evident in the sesamoid area and is accompanied in most cases by crepitation and abnormal mobility.

With fractures of the second type, the avulsion usually occurs at the pyramid-like apex of the sesamoid bone; basal fractures are less common. In both cases there is considerable displacement of the bone fragment owing to the function of the sesamoids

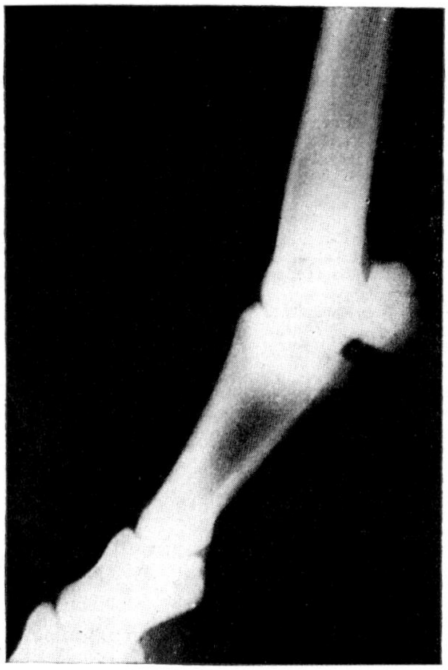

26

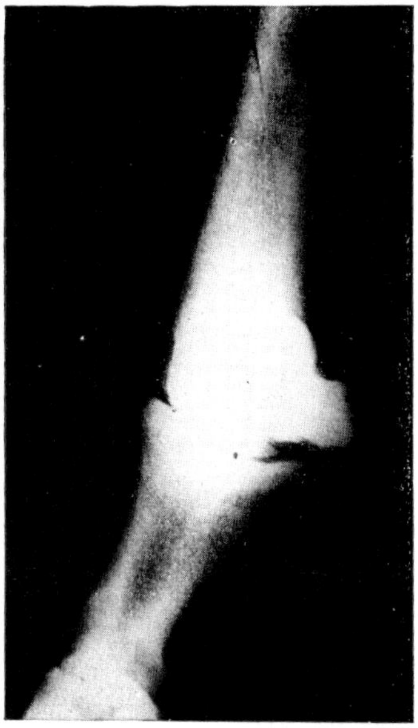

27

Fig. 2.1.20. — 26. Proximal fracture of a sesamoid bone, before operation.
Fig. 2.1.20. — 27. Proximal fracture of a sesamoid bone, after operation.

in the suspensory apparatus. The clinical symptoms of these fractures differ from those of the first type. There is usually a gradually progressive lameness, combined with swelling and tenderness. The animal favors the limb and bears weight gingerly, avoiding pressure on the toe. Crepitation cannot be demonstrated. Chronic cases show symptoms of sesamoid lameness.

Etiology. Closed sesamoid fractures result from a sudden, extreme stress such as may occur during racing or jumping, or, in draft animals, from external trauma. Osteoporotic changes predispose to such fractures. Open fractures are usually seen in connection with wounds occurring when a racehorse is struck by a another horse coming up from behind. Often the common tendon sheath or fetlock joint is also opened in such cases.

Differential Diagnosis. Ruptures of the suspensory ligament and its branches, tears of the superficial flexor tendon, and fissure fractures of the proximal phalanx or cannon bone produce similar symptoms and can be ruled out by palpation or radiography.

Diagnosis. Radiographs are necessary to establish the diagnosis. Views in three planes are needed and should demonstrate each sesamoid bone separately. In this way the course of the fracture line can be ascertained and any further complications identified (luxation, subluxation; figs. 2.1.20. — 24 through — 27).

Treatment. The sesamoid fragments have little tendency to undergo bony union owing to the strong pull of the attached ligaments. Fibrous tissue replacement is incapable of withstanding the rigors of training, and this will inevitably lead to redisplacement when work is resumed.

In the acute stage, warm, moist dressings are applied to promote absorption of effusion. Further treatment depends on the type of fracture that is present. For horizontal fractures with equal-size fragments in both sesamoids, 9 months' stall rest is recommended if the animal is to be used only for breeding or light work. For distal chip fractures and fractures involving a third or more of the bone, Sevelius and Tufvesson [1963] recommend a tenotomy of the associated branch of the suspensory ligament, while Bessignana [1967] recommends a lateral or medial plantar or palmar neurectomy.

Six to nine months are required for healing. Operative removal of the fragment is indicated if the fragment is no larger than $^1/_3$ of the entire sesamoid bone [Churchill, 1956]. Removal may also be undertaken for basal chip fractures [Wheat and Rhode, 1958; Heinze, 1966]. The procedure is done under general anesthesia. A tourniquet is applied to obtain a bloodless field, and an incision about 8—10 cm long is made over the posterior surface of the cannon bone approximately 5 mm cranial to the palmar nerve and parallel to it. The subcutaneous tissue is divided down to the collateral sesamoidean ligament and suspensory ligament and carefully separated from underlying structures in a palmar direction. Dietz et al. [1963] state that the tendon sheath can be spared by incising down to the bone between the sheath and the metacarpus, and from that point separating the ligamentous attachments from the sesamoid fragment using small, scraping motions of the scalpel. After the palmar side has been dissected free, the fragment can be immobilized with forceps and separated from its short ligamentous attachments in the direction of the joint. Antibiotic is injected into the joint and joint capsule, and the subcutaneous tissue and skin are sutured. A snug-fitting bandage is applied.

Internal fixation by the method of McKibbin and Armstrong and the method of Pettersson [1981] using compression screws is indicated for fractures with equal-size fragments.

Prognosis. Open or closed horizontal fractures of both sesamoid bones have an unfavorable prognosis. Recovery is possible in the case of chip fractures and horizontal fractures of one sesamoid.

2.1.20.2.9. Sesamoid Lameness

Definition. Sesamoid lameness (sesamoiditis, sesamoidosis) is a collective term applied to all primary degenerative and chronic diseases of the sesamoid bones themselves, the sesamoidean ligaments, and the deep digital flexor tendon at the site where these structures pass over the sesamoid bones. The common deep flexor tendon sheath may also be involved.

Riding horses are usually affected in the forelimbs, while work horses of the heavy breeds are mainly affected in the hind limbs. Nemeth [1973, 1974] states that even very young horses are susceptible to sesamoid lameness.

Symptoms. In riding horses the onset of sesamoid lameness in the forelimbs is rarely observed. Lameness, or a stilted gait with a shortened stride, gradually appears. As the disease progresses, a supporting-leg lameness becomes apparent. Usually both forelimbs are affected, one more severely than the other. In the standing position, weight is frequently taken off the more severely affected forelimb, and the limb is held slightly forward with only the toe of the foot touching the ground. In heavy work horses with sesamoid lameness of a hind limb, the animal holds the limb slightly forward while standing, bears weight only on the toe, or may hold the foot off the ground in severe cases.

During walking, the horse will not allow the fetlock to descend to a normal level. The pastern is abnormally upright. In the second supporting-leg phase, the fetlock may knuckle over for brief periods. Many riding horses with sesamoid lameness of both forelimbs have a tendency to stumble.

Athletic (fast-gaited) horses with sesamoiditis of the forelimbs usually show no distension of the common flexor tendon sheath. In working horses with sesamoiditis of the hind limbs, there is often a more or less tense swelling of the common flexor tendon sheath. Pain may be produced when the limb is lifted and the fetlock joint is passively extended. Continuous pressure on the sesamoids or deep flexor tendon sheath at the level of the sesamoids elicits pain. Both branches of the suspensory ligament may be tender and show nodular thickening. Percussion with a hammer may reveal the painful sesamoid bone or bones. When the limb is lifted, changes may also be palpable in the intersesamoidean ligaments and the oblique distal sesamoidean ligaments.

Etiology. Sesamoid lameness is caused by repeated strains of the sesamoid ligaments or sustained concussion of the forelimbs with subsequent degenerative changes in the sesamoid apparatus. It is most common in race horses, hunters and jumpers that perform at fast gaits on rough terrain or run and jump under a heavy rider. In draft horses, it can result from planting the hind limbs to pull against heavy loads. This causes very small tears to develop in the sesamoid ligaments, leading to blood flow disturbances, cartilage defects, and chronic disease of the tendons, ligaments and sesamoid bones themselves. Thus, a condition similar to tendinitis develops that involves both branches of the suspensory ligament, the intersesamoidean ligament, the straight and oblique sesamoidean ligaments, the lateral and medial sesamoidean ligaments, and the short and cruciate sesamoidean ligaments. The changes in the deep flexor tendon are similar. Here, too, reactive processes following partial tears or microruptures lead to nodular thickening, partial ossification and ultimately to shortening of the ligaments. Nemeth [1973, 1974] considers sesamoid lameness to be a part of the arthrosis syndrome. In racehorses and jumpers, it is believed that sesamoiditis is closely related to navicular disease. In many cases, an insufficiency can be demonstrated in the blood supply of the sesamoid apparatus, even in young horses, leading to arteriosclerosis and thrombosis. Finally, it has been shown that filariasis may be a precipitating cause of sesamoid lameness in some animals. Radiographs reveal osteoporotic changes in the sesamoid bones themselves. The nutrient foramina may be considerably enlarged, and exostoses can later be demonstrated on the proximopalmar or proximoplantar margin. Ossification of the intersesamoidean ligament is not unusual. High-spirited horses that have a correspondingly high limb action may be predisposed. Another predisposing factor is faulty trimming of the hoof with excessive shortening of the heels or inadequate shortening of the toe, resulting in a broken foot and pastern axis.

Differential Diagnosis. In cases where both forelimbs are involved, navicular disease should be considered. With recent sesamoid fractures, lameness appears suddenly and is usually more pronounced in one limb than the other. In heavy draft horses, chronic degenerative gonitis, spavin and degenerative tarsitis must be excluded by radiographic examination and diagnostic anesthesia.

Diagnosis. Diagnostic anesthesia should be used to localize the cause of the lameness to the sesamoid area. Anesthesia of the palmar nerve at the fetlock will not completely alleviate lameness due to chronic changes in and on the sesamoid bones themselves, the intersesamoidean ligament or the suspensory ligament branches. A proximal or high palmar nerve block will nearly always relieve the lameness, provided there is no significant suspensory ligament disease. Anesthesia of the common flexor tendon sheath with 40—60 ml of a concentrated local anesthetic solution is especially useful when there is distension of this synovial space.

After the lameness has been localized to the sesamoid region, radiographs of the sesamoids should be taken. These will reveal any ossification of the sesamoid liga-

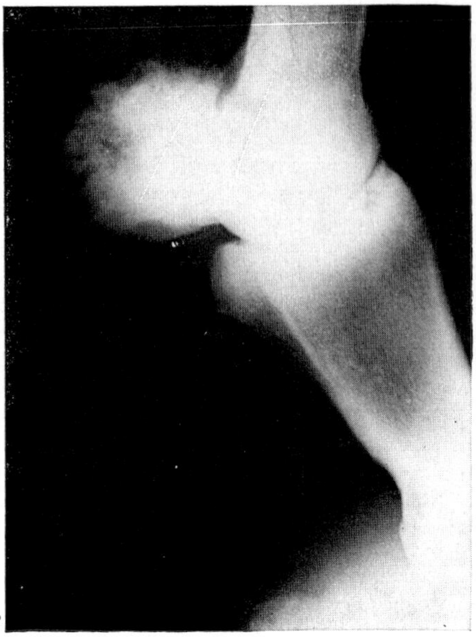
28

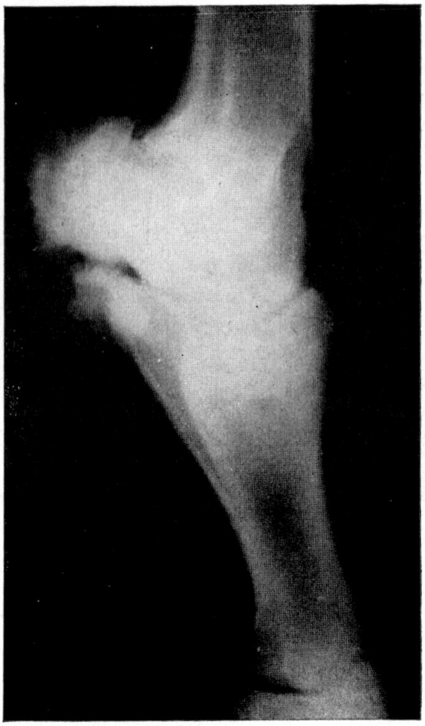
29

Fig. 2.1.20. — 28—29. Sesamoid bone changes in sesamoid lameness.

ments, osteoporotic foci and exostoses in and on the sesamoid bones. Oblique films are taken to visualize each sesamoid bone individually. Defects of the articular surfaces are particularly well demonstrated with this method (figs. 2.1.20. — 28 and — 29).

Prognosis. In view of the chronic nature of the disease, the prognosis is unfavorable. MAROLT et al. [1966] and NEMETH [1973, 1974] state that because the osteoporotic changes in the sesamoid bones themselves are the result of arteriosclerosis of the sesamoid vessels, and the presumed primary cause of this arteriosclerosis is infestation with filariae or Onchocerca, these pathologic changes do not respond to conventional treatment methods.

Treatment. Treatment may be attempted by removing the animal from work and applying moist heat, massage and counterirritants. Cutaneous line or point firing and subsequent blistering are still the most widely-used therapy in Europe. The affected limb is shod with a roller-motion shoe. If the foot and pastern axis is broken and the heels are low, a leather wedge or plastic insert can be used to elevate the heels slightly. Draft horses with sesamoiditis of the hind limbs are shod with calked and roller-motion shoes.

Given an etiology and pathogenesis similar to that of navicular disease, good results may be expected in sesamoiditis with the use of anticoagulants in the form of coumarin derivatives, analogous to the treatment proposed by COLLES [1979].

In Europe a high palmar neurectomy has often been employed in athletic horses with sesamoiditis of the forelimbs. Show horses have been used for up to 6 years without lameness following such a procedure. Work horses with sesamoid lameness

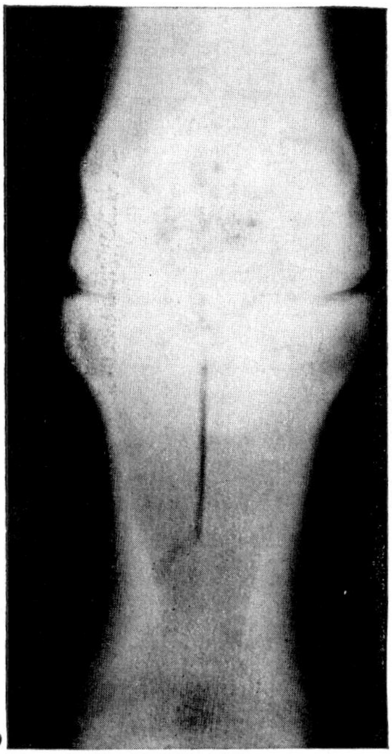

30

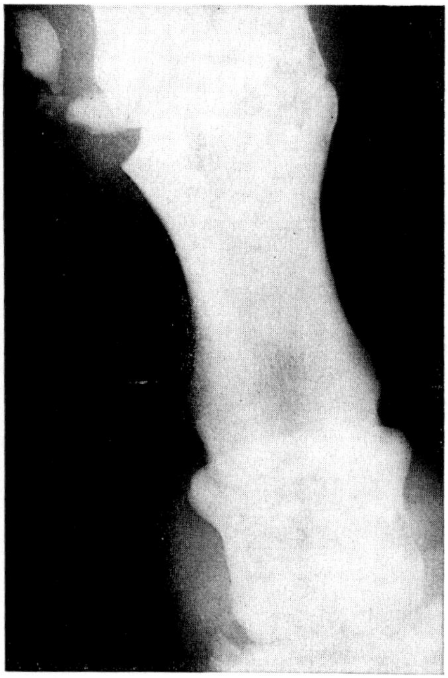

31

Fig. 2.1.20. — 30. Sagittal fracture of the proximal phalanx.
Fig. 2.1.20. — 31. Proximal chip fracture of the proximal phalanx.

of the hind limbs can be made sound for years by a tibial neurectomy, provided the animal is worked only at a walking pace, and any injuries of the neurectomized portion of the limb are given immediate treatment.

Comments. The value of athletic horses with sesamoid lameness of the forelimbs is greatly diminished. If the suggested treatment measures do not restore functional soundness, the animal will still be sound for breeding.

2.1.20.2.10. Fracture of the Proximal Phalanx

Occurrence, Classification and Etiology. Fractures of the proximal phalanx P1 (pastern bone) can take various forms:

1. sagittal fractures (fig. 2.1.20. — 30),
2. segmental or transverse fractures (fig. 2.1.20. — 32),
3. chip fractures (figs. 2.1.20. — 31 and — 33).

Comminuted fractures are classified either as sagittal or segmental, depending on the configuration of the fracture lines.

The most frequent type of P1 fracture is the sagittal fracture, which is most commonly caused by a misstep or sharp turn. The mechanism of its occurrence is the 'chisel effect' of the ridge of the cannon bone on the articular surface of P1. Most fractures of this type are closed. Open fractures are rare and are caused by kicks from other horses, traffic accidents, etc. A special form of the sagittal fracture is the Y-shaped fracture. In this case the fracture line initially runs in a sagittal direction

32, 33

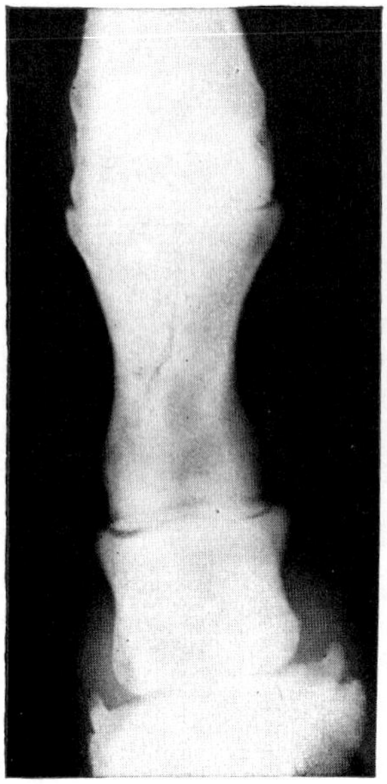

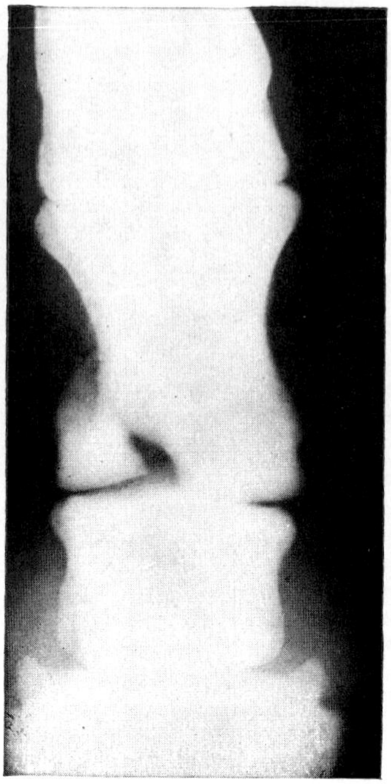

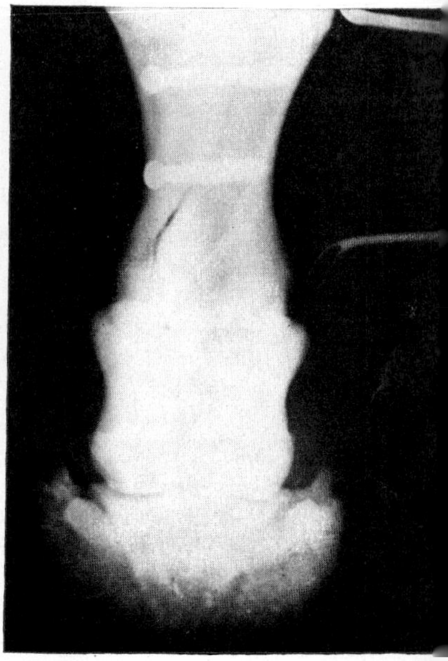

Fig. 2.1.20. — 32. Segmental and transverse fracture of the proximal phalanx.
Fig. 2.1.20. — 33. Distal chip fracture of the proximal phalanx.
Fig. 2.1.20. – 34. Sagittal fracture repaired by screw fixation.

but then splits in Y-shape fashion near the midportion of the bone. Fractures of P1, of the forelimb are more common in athletic horses due to the greater stresses to which the forelimbs are exposed.

Symptoms. A sudden, severe supporting-leg lameness appears in the early stage, unaccompanied by systemic signs. Usually no weight is placed on the affected leg. When standing, the horse holds the limb in a slightly cranial position. After about 2 hours, swelling and increased pulsation develops in the pastern region. If the bone is fractured into the joint, passive movements are extremely painful. Crepitation and displacement are detected only with a comminuted fracture. Another clinical sign is the presence of a 'line of tenderness' that is discovered on digital palpation. First the anterior surface of P1 is palpated without exerting pressure on the back of the pastern. A line of tenderness in such cases usually indicates a sagittal fracture. A segmental fracture can be detected during palpation of the lateral and medial ligaments. Rotation of P1 should be avoided if possible.

Diagnosis. The diagnosis is made from the foregoing clinical symptoms.

Differential diagnosis must be made from all severe supporting-leg lamenesses of sudden onset. These may be due to other phalangeal fractures, sprains, contusions, luxations, and puncture wounds of the foot.

The symptoms of a fissure fracture of the pastern bone differ from those of a complete fracture only in degree. In this case radiographs are necessary to classify the fracture. Dorsopalmar and lateromedial views should be obtained.

The progress of clinical signs provides an important clue as to whether a complete or incomplete fracture is present. With a fissure fracture, the clinical manifestations quickly subside after the injury. If radiographs are inconclusive, repeating the examination in 30—40 days should disclose the presence of a callus and thus confirm the diagnosis. In no case should local anesthetics or sedatives be used to make a diagnosis, because they may encourage use of the limb that would convert an incomplete fracture to a complete one.

Treatment. Initially, a firm bandage is applied to the limb as an emergency measure to control fracture hematoma and limit displacement. Then the horse is confined to a large box stall with soft bedding. Further treatment may be conservative, or surgical (internal fixation).

With fissure fractures and sagittal fractures, it is often sufficient to apply a warm, moist bandage for 8—10 days. The horse should be confined to its stall for at least 8 weeks. However, immobilizing bandages of zinc gelatin or plaster, preferably reinforced with splints, are recommended to prevent displacement of the fragments. If required, traction and reduction are carried out while the horse is under general anesthesia.

Plaster casts have certain disadvantages: they are heavy, may break, and can cause pressure necrosis. Hence, resin-bound fiberglass casts are preferred. With conservative treatment, there is always a danger that the fragments will become displaced before healing is complete. A wide fracture defect remains, and the resulting callus that forms on the articular surface can lead to chronic degenerative joint disease. The best way to avoid this situation is to stabilize the fracture surgically by internal fixation. To minimize wound infection, this should be done under antibiotic protection.

Several methods are available for the operative repair of P1 fractures in the horse. Berubé [1963] treated a comminuted fracture of the first phalanx with a special apparatus consisting of a metal footplate fitted with two braces extending from the heels to the level of the metacarpus. The braces were anchored to the limb with two screws driven horizontally into the metacarpus, one above the other. Afterward the footplate was screwed under tension to the bearing surface of the hoof, and a plaster cast was applied to the pastern bone. This relieved stress on the fracture site while providing a stable immobilization, and the fracture went on to successful healing. Huskamp [1972] achieves this effect with a Steinmann pin that is driven horizontally into the metacarpus or metatarsus and is combined with a tension-band plate.

This method was originally introduced by the Association for the Study of Internal Fixation (ASIF). Fissure fractures and sagittal fractures of the pastern bone can also be accurately stabilized with ASIF cortical bone screws (Breuer, 1972; fig. 2.1.20. — 34).

Prognosis. Fissure fractures have a favorable prognosis with prompt treatment. Intra-articular fractures can restrict movement of the pastern or fetlock joint as a result of callus formation. Even in racing animals with comminuted fractures, however, complete functional recoveries have been achieved.

At least 10 weeks' rest is indicated in the case of fissure fractures, and 4 months' rest for complete fractures. Premature weight-bearing can bring on a recurrence.

2.1.20.2.11. Chronic Ossifying Periostitis of the Proximal Phalanx (P1)

Definition and Occurrence. Ossifying periostitis is a new bone growth (exostosis or hyperostosis) occurring at sites of ligamentous attachment on the P1. It mainly affects the forelimbs of heavy draft horses (fig. 2.1.20. — 35), though the front and

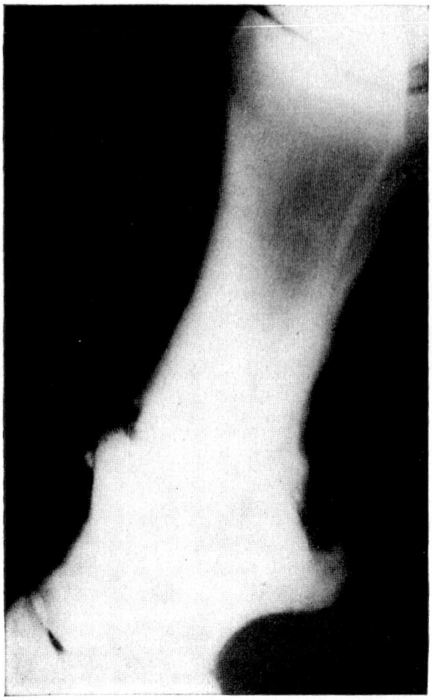

Fig. 2.1.20. — 35. Exostosis of the proximal phalanx and periarthritis of the pastern joint.

hind limbs may be affected simultaneously. According to WITTMANN [1934], the following parts of P1 may be involved:

— The midportion of the lateral border.
Exostoses surrounded by fibrous, thickened ligamentous masses appear at the attachments of the lateral palmar (or plantar) ligaments of the pastern joint. The exostoses rarely spread to the dorsal and palmar aspects of the P1 but can lead to adhesions with surrounding ligaments.

— The distal third of the lateral border.
Distal to the attachments of the lateral palmar ligaments is the insertion of the band from the P1 to the digital cushion. The exostoses that form here are smaller and more ridge-shaped. They may extend distally to the ligamentous eminences of P1.

— The distal lateral end in the region of the ligamentous eminences.
The exostoses form at the attachments of collateral ligaments of the pastern joint and may lead to ringbone of this joint.

— The palmar (plantar) surface.
This exostosis at the common attachments of the oblique sesamoidean ligaments and palmar ligaments has the oblique, distally-convergent shape that is typical of proximal phalangeal exostoses. The already rough trigonum of P1 becomes covered with osteophytes.

Etiology. The exostosis is caused by a continual pull exerted on the ligamentous attachments to P1. The insertions of the oblique sesamoidean ligaments are mainly affected in show and racing horses, while the pastern joint ligaments, and band to the digital cushion, are affected in draft horses.

In Standardbreds that use toe-weight shoes, the palmar ligaments tend to be affected.

Predisposing factors include defects of limb conformation, a broken pastern axis, an upright pastern, and heavy draft work.

Finally, exostosis can develop from the periostitis that accompanies acute and chronic aseptic or infectious inflammation of adjacent tissues.

Symptoms and Diagnosis. Generally the exostoses do not cause lameness. In advanced cases a stiffness of gait will be apparent on hard surfaces. On palpation and visual inspection, the lesions present as round, thickened ligamentous masses on the lateral border of P1. These masses enclose the bony exostoses.

Palmar exostoses are detected by lifting the foot, grasping the pastern with both hands, and running the thumbs from the dorsal aspect of the pastern around the lateral and medial borders to the palmar surface. Radiographs are necessary for confirming the diagnosis. Often exostoses of P1 are discovered incidentally during radiography. Their significance should not be overemphasized during examinations for purchasing.

Treatment. In the past, moist heat, blistering and firing have been used in an attempt to arrest the process. A padded shoe was also applied (rubber, plastic, felt or leather).

In Europe a palmar or plantar neurectomy is recommended as a last resort but is effective only if no mechanical obstruction has formed (joint ankylosis).

2.1.20.2.12. Knuckling

Definition. 'Knuckling' is used to denote both an abnormal erectness of the pastern and the more severe condition in which the fetlock is completely knuckled forward. A distinction is made between congenital knuckling in the newborn foal, acquired knuckling of the forelimbs in older foals, and acquired knuckling in mature horses, usually involving the forelimbs. Lysholt and Soennichsen [1969] differentiate between cases with contraction of the deep flexor tendon in foals, and contraction of the superficial flexor tendon in yearlings.

Congenital Knuckling in the Foal

Symptoms. Foals with congenital knuckling exhibit a strong palmar flexion of all digital joints that appears either immediately after birth or during the first days of life. Often there is some degree of permanent carpal joint flexion, in which case the term 'bucked knees' or 'sprung knees' may be applied (fig. 2.1.20. — 36). During progression, the animal often places weight only on the toe of the foot, and it may stand on the dorsum of the fetlock. A large part of the body weight is borne by the hind limbs, which, like in laminitis, are carried well below the body. Active or passive extension of the digital and carpal joints is extremely difficult. Often the horse is hardly able to walk unaided and cannot even feed itself without human assistance. Malnutrition, systemic infection from decubitus sores at pressure points, and pneumonia frequently complicate the condition and lead to death. Initially mild forms may become more severe during the first days of life.

Etiology. Congenital knuckling is believed to be due to a weakness of the extensor muscles, a disproportion between bone and tendon growth, and an unfavorable intrauterine position.

A dietary mineral and vitamin deficiency in the pregnant mare may also play a role. An hereditary transmission of the defect cannot be excluded.

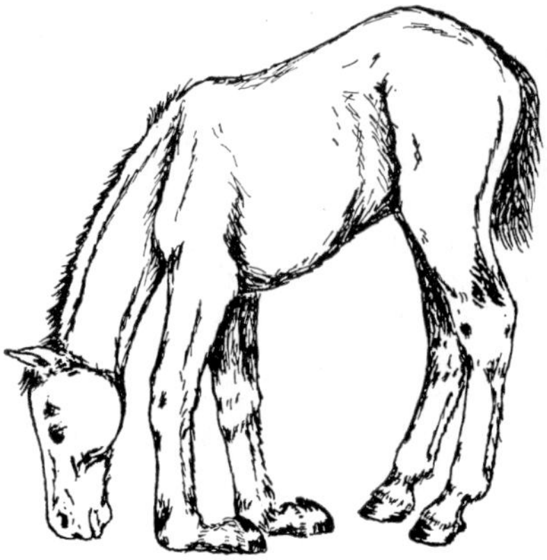

36

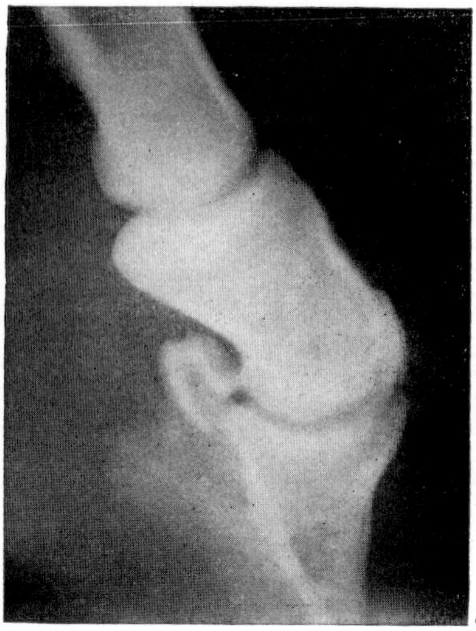

37

Fig. 2.1.20. — 36. Congenital knuckling in a foal.
Fig. 2.1.20. — 37. Radiograph of the digit of a foal with congenital knuckling.

Diagnosis. The diagnosis is made from the characteristic changes and their time of occurrence (fig. 2.1.20. — 37).

Treatment. Mild knuckling often can be relieved simply by ensuring a proper mineral and vitamin intake during the first 4—6 weeks of life. More pronounced cases can be corrected through orthopedic measures. Before treatment is begun, the involved joints should be protected and supported with bandages to prevent injury. In severe cases this is insufficient, and supportive plaster or plastic bandages must be applied with the animal recumbent and well restrained. A Cramer wire splint or rods made of aluminum or poplar wood can be incorporated to stabilize the limb. The bandage includes the carpal joint and is changed every 10 days. The development of decubitus ulcers at pressure points is a disadvantage of this method. Healing is supported by placing the foot in a shoe with a wide toe extension. Later this can be replaced with a semicircular tip shoe when the fetlock no longer 'knuckles over'. If these orthopedic measures are unsuccessful, surgical treatment may be tried. This consists in a tenotomy of the ulnaris lateralis and flexor carpi ulnaris tendons, or tenotomy of the deep flexor tendon on the back of the pastern. Selective vitamin and mineral supplementation may also be useful.

Prognosis. If treatment is prompt and there is no deformity of the carpal bones, a complete recovery may be expected. If general condition is impaired and decubitus sores are already present, treatment is not advised. Some tenotomized foals will later be fit for doing limited work.

Comments. Because the predisposition to knuckling may be inheritable, affected animals are considered unfit for breeding.

Acquired Knuckling in the Foal

Symptoms. During the 1st to 3rd year of life, the phalanges may acquire an abnormal conformation over a period of days or weeks, accompanied by a forward or backward break in the digital axis. One or both forelimbs may be involved (figs.

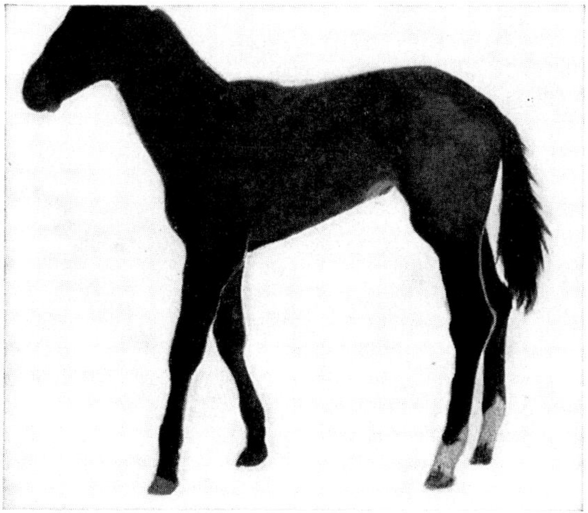

38

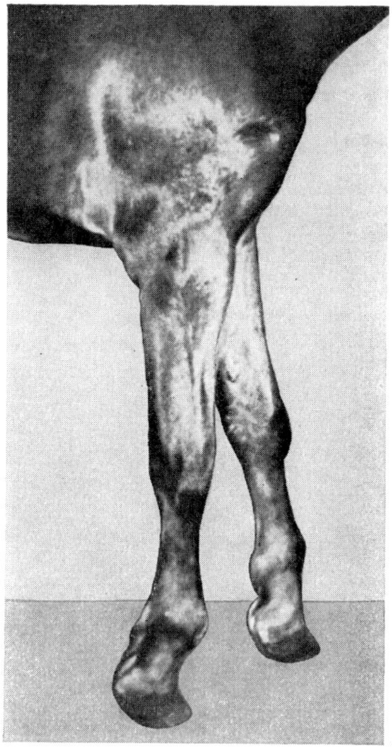

39

Fig. 2.1.20. — 38—39. Acquired knuckling in a foal.

2.1.20. — 38 and — 39). Peters [1938] distinguishes two forms. In the first form, only the hoof wall is upright (going on the toes, high heels); 'acquired clubfoot' is the term applied to this condition. In the second form, the hoof axis may be normal or even show an excessive slope ('cocked ankles'). In most cases, however, it is slightly elevated at the heels. The pastern is vertical. To compensate, the digital axis is broken backward at the pastern joint and possibly at the coffin joint as well.

Etiology. Deficiencies of vitamin and mineral nutrition are presumed to underlie the development of acquired knuckling in foals. The condition of the ground can also play a role. Thus, it is frequently seen in foals that are pastured during dry years, when the ground is hard and grass growth is slight. This results in excessive wear to the toe. On the other hand, acquired upright pastern can also develop on moist pasture, when the sinking-in of the toe compels an upright digital axis. A similar effect occurs in foals that are kept stalled continuously on soft bedding.

Diagnosis. The history combined with visual and palpatory findings suggest the diagnosis. Luxations of P1 and exostoses of the fetlock joint can be excluded if necessary by radiographic examination.

Treatment. The treatment of acquired knuckling in foals begins with corrective shoeing. In the process, the heels are gradually shortened. The foot is placed in an extended-toe shoe. The lengthened toe or extension can be shortened as dorsiflexion of the fetlock joint improves. A disadvantage of this methos is that the toe wall can easily become damaged if the animal stumbles. This shoe is also useful if surgical correction is employed. Exercise several times daily on firm ground is essential to a successful recovery. If the condition cannot be corrected by shoeing, a tenotomy of the deep digital flexor tendon may be tried as a last resort. In acquired cases with

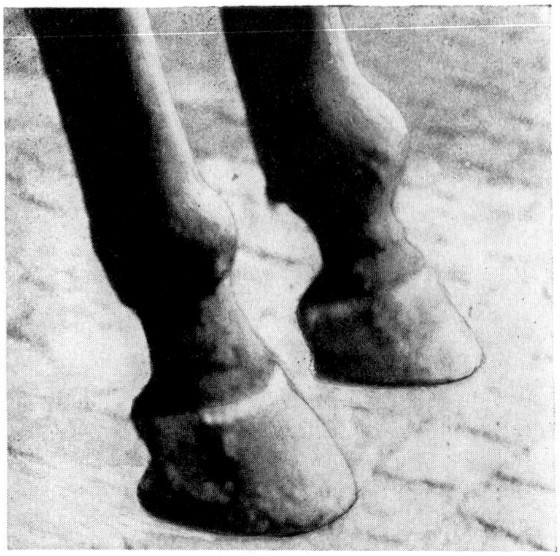

Fig. 2.1.20. — 40. Knuckling in a mature horse.

palmar flexion of the pastern and coffin joints, the deep flexor tendon is severed on the back of the pastern, or the inferior check ligament is divided. Following surgery, the foot is placed in an extended-toe or calked shoe. The level is continually changed until a normal pastern angle is obtained. FORSELL [1952] recommends tenotomy of the superficial flexor tendon when the fetlock is knuckled forward, because this is more effective in dropping the fetlock to the desired degree. The tendon is severed in the middle of the metacarpus in a diagonal or zigzag fashion, rather than transversely. LEWANDOWSKI [1967] as well as LYSHOLT and SOENNICHSEN [1969] advise a desmotomy of the inferior check ligament of the deep flexor tendon and an extended-toe shoe of spring steel. They also recommend that the feed ration be checked and modified as needed.

Knuckling in the Mature Horse

Classification and Etiology. Knuckling in adult horses can be classified on the basis of etiology: i.e., due to tendon or joint problems. Both forms may affect either the front or hind limbs. Knuckling due to tendon problems develops as a result of chronic tendinitis of the deep flexor tendor or inferior check ligament. Knuckling due to joint problems occurs secondary to fractures of the phalanges as well as to arthritis of the phalangeal joints.

Symptoms. The salient feature is the erect position of the phalanges. In very pronounced cases weight is borne only on the toe (fig. 2.1.20. — 40), and there is no position in which the foot appears stable. On the dorsal side of the cannon bone, the normally indistinct extendor tendon appears as a prominent, rigid cord. In cases due to tendon problems where the fetlock is knuckled over, the pastern axis tends to be broken backward; in cases due to joint problems it is usually broken forward.

Differential Diagnosis and Diagnosis. Because the etiology has an important bearing on treatment and prognosis, it is necessary to differentiate if the cause is secondary to joint or tendon problems. Chronic tendinitis with contraction of the flexor tendon is diagnosed by inspection and palpation, and chronic arthritis by palpation and radiographic examination.

Treatment. Blistering and firing has been used in the past. A suitable corrective shoe is applied. This may be of the type used for base-wide correction or an extended-toe shoe, depending on the degree of change. Screw calks are also used to support the damaged tendon, and these are shortened or removed entirely as improvement occurs. With chronic inflammation and contraction of the deep flexor check ligament, a tenotomy of the deep digital flexor tendon in the middle of the metacarpus may also be indicated. Knuckling due to joint pathology is usually refractory to treatment. Ankylosis is often present, and so a functional recovery is no longer possible, even with a neurectomy.

Prognosis. A poor prognosis is indicated. Most mature horses can be restored only to limited usefulness. The treatment of older horses is therefore not advised. Tenotomized horses are suitable only for light draft work.

2.1.20.2.13. Hyperextension of the Flexor Tendons

Definition. This condition is the opposite of knuckling and is characterized by a hyperextension of the fetlock joint, and usually of the pastern and coffin joints as well. The horse may bear weight on the bulbs of the heels or even on the palmar surface of the pastern, depending on the severity of the condition. All legs may show the condition, though the forelimbs are most commonly affected.

Symptoms. The most prominent sign is a dropping of the fetlock joint. Weight is borne on the wall of the heel or the bulbs, and the fetlock may even hit the ground. The toe is tipped upward, so that the sole is visible from the front.

Etiology. The hyperextension may represent a congenital weakness of the flexor tendons. In foals with long pasterns that are stalled much of the time, a disproportion can develop between horn production and horn wear. The result is a stretching of the digital flexors. Fackelmann and Clodius [1972] consider a disproportion between skeletal growth and soft-tissue development to be the major cause.

Differential Diagnosis. Partial or complete ruptures of the flexor tendons must be excluded. In coon-footed horses, the toe remains in contact with the ground.

Treatment. Severe cases can be corrected with the aid of splints and plaster casts. Less severe cases often respond well to corrective shoeing with a bar and extended heels. Secure fixation of the shoe is necessary when such an arrangement is employed.

For orthopedic treatment to be effective, the animal must be exercised regularly on firm ground so that it can adapt to the altered conditions of weight bearing. The shoe should be changed every 3—4 weeks, during which time the hooves are trimmed and the shoe configuration is changed in accordance with the degree of flexor tendon shortening that has occurred (figs. 2.1.20. — 41 and — 42). The condition can be prevented or corrected through regular foot care and orthopedic shoeing (fig. 2.1.20. — 43).

Fackelmann and Clodius [1972] describe an operative method in which the superficial and deep flexor tendons are divided longitudinally and transversely, a segment of predetermined length is excised, and the stumps are reunited.

The tendons are reattached with wire sutures, each of the 4 stumps being treated as a separate unit. Finally a fiberglass cast is applied. In all cases the horses regained full, normal use of the limb within 12 weeks after the procedure.

Prognosis. The chance of recovery with conservative treatment is usually good, barring pressure necrosis at the fetlock joint. The tendon-shortening procedure described above is costly but appears to have a good prognosis.

41
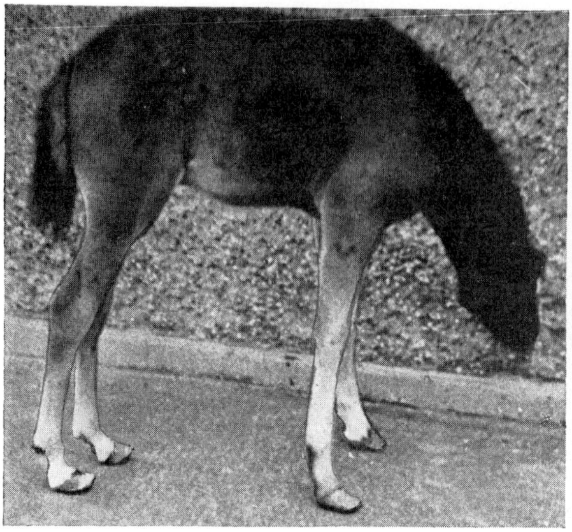

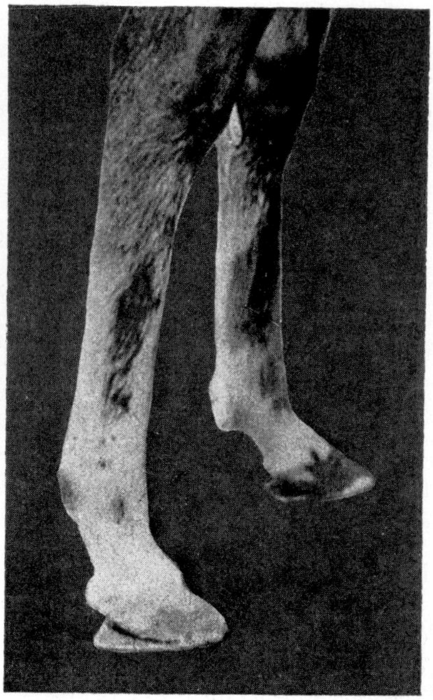
42

Fig. 2.1.20. — 41. Hyperextension of the flexor tendons before shoeing.
Fig. 2.1.20. — 42. Hyperextension of the flexor tendons after shoeing.

2.1.20.2.14. Coon-Footed

Definition, Occurrence and Etiology. In horses with weak pasterns, P_1 and P_2 bone can assume an almost horizontal position, while P_3 is erect. As a result, the foot axis becomes steeper than the pastern axis: 'coon-footed'. It is a congenital condition.

Symptoms. The condition is most apparent when weight is placed on the limb. The pastern bone may assume a horizontal position or, if the foot axis slopes markedly, may even slant upward from back to front. The ergot approaches the ground. The angle of the hoof axis varies but is always broken noticeably toward the front.

Differential Diagnosis. Hyperextension of the flexor tendons must be excluded in foals. It is characterized by weight bearing on the heels.

Prognosis and Treatment. No treatment is necessary in mild to moderate cases. Extreme cases in which the fetlock touches the ground can be corrected with orthopedic shoeing (heels raised with calks). The calks should be just high enough to keep the animal from landing too heavily on the heels.

2.1.20.2.15. Polydactyly

See Sec. 2.8.7.2.

2.1.20.2.16. Dermatitis verrucosa

See Sec. 2.11.3.1.

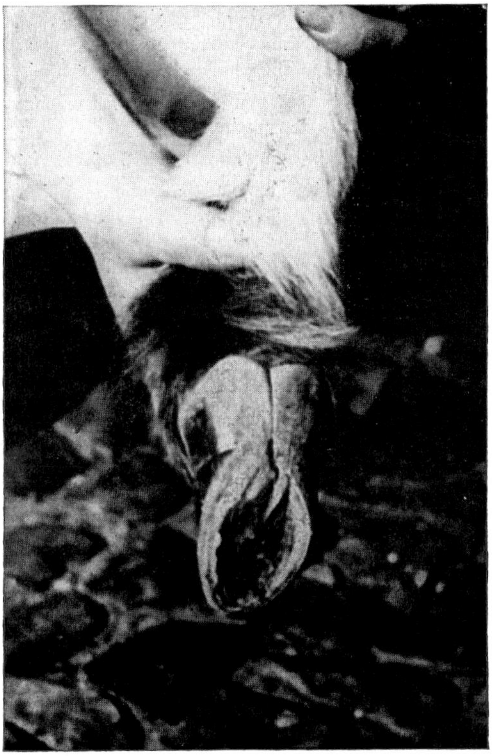

Fig. 2.1.20. — 43. Microhoof in hyperextension of the flexor tendons.

2.1.20.2.17. Interfering

Definition. Interfering is a fault of gait in which the supporting foot is struck by the opposite foot, as it passes by, during locomotion.

Occurrence. Interfering can occur at any age, may involve the front and hind limbs, and may be permanent or temporary.

Symptoms. Evidence of interfering may consist of hair loss, excoriation, severe abrasions or wounds occurring on the horny wall, coronet, fetlock joint, cannon bone, or even the carpal or tarsal joint. Wounds from interfering are prone to infection, and tetanus is also a problem. The appearance, extent and depth of the wounds depend on the site responsible for the injury (edge of shoe, projecting nails, calks, projecting medial clip).

In horses that interfere repeatedly or chronically, thickened masses develop on the skin, especially on unusually prominent fetlock joints. A periosteal reaction can often be detected under these lesions.

Etiology. The causes of interfering are:

1. Faults of limb conformation: With a base-wide conformation, the foot 'wings' to the inside when advanced and frequently causes interference with the opposite supporting limb. Knock knees (forelimb) and cow hocks (hind limb) also predispose to interfering.

2. Faults of digital conformation: A toe-out conformation is a major cause of interfering, as it, too, causes the foot to advance in an inside arc. Defects of limb and digital conformation can in some cases cancel out, resulting in a straight foot path (e.g., base-wide, toe-in conformation). However, one defect will usually predominate, and the foot will advance in an inside arc, with interfering, or an outside arc.

3. Breaks in the digital axis: The foot axis deviates from the pastern axis when viewed from the front. In other words, there is a lateral or medial break in the digital axis. A break in either direction can sometimes lead to interfering, even with a normal limb and digital conformation. Interfering is especially likely if the broken axis is combined with defects of limb or digital conformation.

4. Improper trimming of the hoof can cause any of the conformation faults described above, thus leading to interference. A neglected, untrimmed, frayed, broken horny wall can also predispose.

5. Improper shoeing: an inside branch with base-wide correction, inward-slanting calks, clips on the inside branch, excessive roller motion, exposed or projecting nails, etc. Occasionally a loose shoe can cause interfering in cases where a the horse has gone too long between shoeings.

6. Interfering can also result from limb weariness, even with proper trimming, balancing and shoeing.

7. Improper harnessing and bridling.

8. Lameness and locomotor disturbances.

Differential diagnosis must be made from incidental wounds and injuries from overreaching. The latter commonly occur near the hock in Standardbreds.

Diagnosis. The offending site is usually worn smooth and may be covered with blood. If interfering is suspected but cannot be seen, chalk may be placed on the presumed offending site. The contact will leave a chalk mark on the limb that is struck, while the offending site will be free of chalk.

Bone changes (periostitis) can be demonstrated by radiography.

Prognosis. The prognosis is favorable if the cause of the interfering can be eliminated.

Treatment. The correction of conformation defects and axial faults should begin in the foal. Foals cannot be expected to 'grow out of it'. A certain percentage of the defects are hereditary and therefore should be eradicated through strict selection of breeding stock.

Expert farriers that work hand-in-hand with the veterinarian and have a knowledge of orthopedics are invaluable in improving or correcting faults of conformation, or keeping the horse in serviceable condition despite the presence of such faults.

The Viennese School employs a corrective program that emphasizes physiology and gradual changes. In the immature horse (less than 5 years old), faults of limb and digital conformation and breaks in the digital axes are treated initially by corrective trimming that is guided *not* by the pattern of foot or shoe wear, but from the standpoint of achieving a correct conformation, and thus a faultless gait. If trimming does not achieve the desired result, *corrective shoeing* is employed: half shoes, three-quarter shoes, thinned branches, weighted shoes, etc. (fig. 2.1.20. — 44). This must be combined with an optimum program of exercise, nutrition (vitamins, minerals) and use, which preferably is deferred until the age of 5 years, when full maturity is reached.

In the mature horse, on the other hand, trimming and shoeing are guided mainly by the pattern of shoe wear. In every case, the object of trimming and shoeing is to make the foot land flat, thus achieving 'level shoe wear'. This principle is based

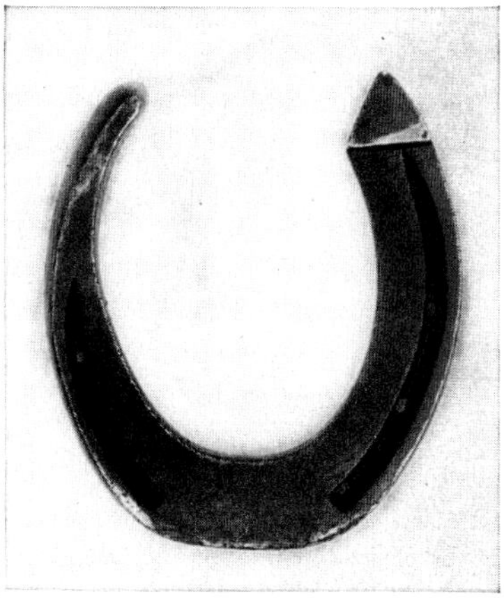

44

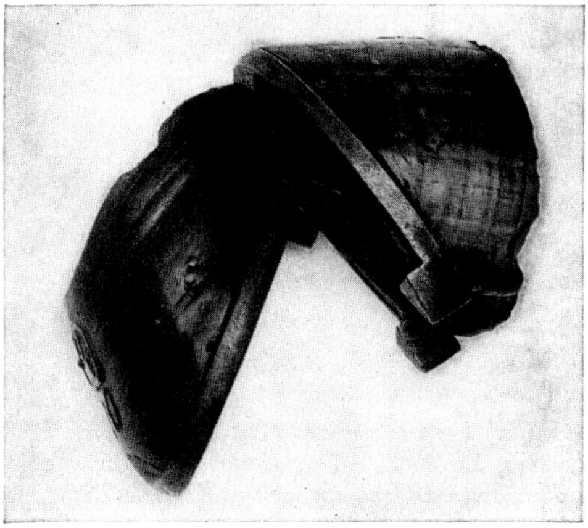

45

Fig. 2.1.20. — 44. Corrective shoe for interfering, with calks and thinned branch.
Fig. 2.1.20. — 45. Overreaching. The toe of the hind shoe catches on the heel of the front shoe.

on the assumption that faults of limb and digital conformation generally can no longer be improved in the fully mature horse, whereas breaks in the digital axis often are amenable to correction.

The harness should be carefully checked. Traces should be of equal lengths. The thickened skin lesions caused by interfering are often difficult to remove and should be watched for when purchasing a horse.

Athletic horses (Standardbreds, three-day-event horses) are given special shoes and suitable protective leg gear (bell boots, caps, bandages, boots, etc.

Injuries are managed according to general rules, with attention given to tetanus prophylaxis.

Prevention. Broodstock should be selected for sound limb and foot conformation. Proper conditions of care, exercise and feeding should be adhered to, and work should be deferred until full maturity is reached.

2.1.20.2.18. Overreaching

Definition. 'Overreaching' is a fault of gait in which the hind foot strikes the forefoot, usually on the same side (fig. 2.1.20. — 45).

Symptoms. The hind foot may strike the ground surface of the front shoe, the heel of the shoe, the heel bulbs, or less frequently the posterior surface of the metacarpus. This can occur at a fast trot, at the gallop, during jumps, and even at the walk. Trotters exhibit a special form of overreaching in which the mediodistal area of the hock ('spavin region') strikes the diagonally opposite forefoot (cross-firing). If the shoes collide, a metallic clang is heard, which accounts for the term 'forging' as applied to this condition.

The front shoe often appears as if it has been struck repeatedly with a hammer at the heel or edge. Similar damage is evident on the toe or toe clips of the hind shoe. In neglected cases, the wall epidermis (matrix) of the rear hoof may become exposed in the distal part of the anterior wall unless prompt measures are taken to correct the fault. Not infrequently, the coronet of the overreaching hind foot also shows

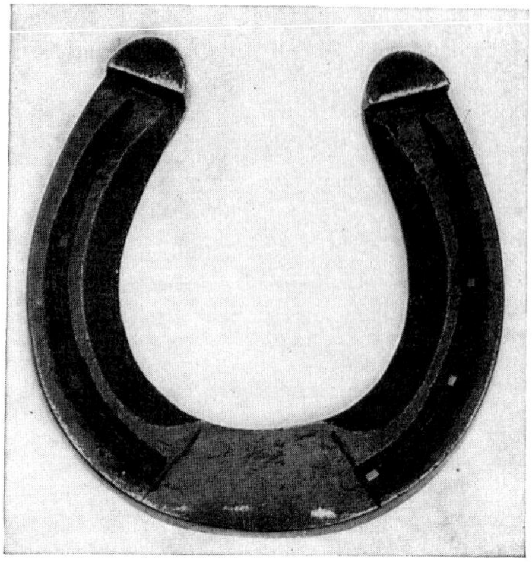

46

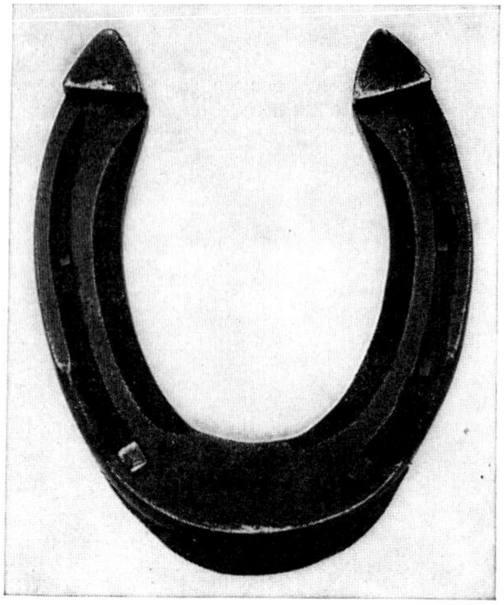

47

Fig. 2.1.20. — 46. Corrective front shoe for overreaching. Note heel blocks and bevel (which should include the toe).

Fig. 2.1.20. — 47. Corrective hind shoe for overreaching, with heel blocks and leather pad nailed to the toe.

signs of injury. This condition can cause stumbling and falling, and so its treatment is a matter of great importance in all ridden horses (three-day-event horses, jumpers, polo horses, show horses, etc.) as well as in Standardbreds. The farrier as well as the attending veterinarian bear the responsibility for the physical safety of man and horse! Shoe pulling is a very common result of overreaching, and spectators at show-jumping contests are especially likely to be injured by a thrown shoe.

With repeated shoe pulling, it may become difficult to nail the shoe securely to the hoof.

Occurrence. Overreaching can occur in all horses, especially three day event horses, jumpers and Standardbreds. Any horse can overreach as a result of fatigue or over-exertion.

Etiology. The major causes lie in the animal's overall conformation as well as limb conformation, methods of trimming, and methods of shoeing the foot. Short, long-legged horses that stand under in front, stand under behind or have sickle hocks, as well as horses with long, sloping forefeet and hind feet shod with shoes that are too heavy, tend to overreach. Horses having a croup higher than the withers and young, inexperienced horses are also predisposed especially following heavy exertion and in the presence of (painful) diseases of the locomotor system. Improper *trimming* is a frequent cause. If the toe (dorsal wall) is left too long on the front and hind feet, the heels are trimmed too low, or if there is excessive growth of the horny wall in general, breakover becomes more difficult. As a result, the front foot is too slow in leaving the ground to avoid the advancing hind foot. Overreaching can also result from front shoes that are too heavy or too long, have a poor breakover, or are calked too high; and from hind shoes that are too heavy, have large, thick toe clips, or have forward-pointing grabs.

The use of grabs should be limited to heavy draft horses! In all other horses, especially racing horses, the use of grabs is dangerous and contraindicated due to the danger of falling.

Diagnosis. Audible in 'forging', otherwise visible from the described injuries or changes in the horny capsule and shoe.

Prognosis. Favorable if the causes can be removed: young horses, improper trimming and/or shoeing.

Treatment. Adequate trimming and corrective shoeing. With all athletic horses, prevention should be practiced to eliminate possible causes (fatigue). *Shoeing:* front shoe with roller or rocker motion, short branches that end at the heels of the foot, full bevel; slipper shoe with beveled and rounded heels, possibly combined with low screw calks or heel blocks (fig. 2.1.20. — 46).

A wider toe (toe-weight shoe) may be used in suitable cases. The hind shoes have a straighter toe that is set back from the edge of the anterior hoof wall by about half the wall width; the front edge is forged and rounded for base-narrow correction (fig. 2.1.20. — 47). Quarter clips are used in preference to toe clips. Rocker- or square-toe shoes and shoes with a heavy outside branch (side-weight shoes) may also be tried.

Prophylaxis. Horses at risk for overreaching should wear protective leg gear.

2.1.20.2.19. Shuffling, Foot Dragging

Definition. A shuffling gait is characterized by a poor breakover of the bearing surface of the anterior wall, usually of the hind foot, after weight-bearing. As a result, the toe is dragged a short distance on the ground as it is advanced. At this time the bearing surface of the heel is raised from the ground and forms an angle with the ground of up to 90°.

Occurrence. The hind feet are more commonly affected.

Symptoms and Diagnosis. There is characteristic wear to the toe of the shoe that may also involve the anterior hoof wall, depending on the angle at which the foot is dragged. Normally the front shoe edge is rounded and blends smoothly with the ground surface of the toe. But with a shuffling gait, the front edge of the shoe appears flat, and the upper edge may be frayed and driven into the worn anterior hoof wall.

Sometimes foot dragging is directly observable at the trot.

Etiology. Besides fatigue, immaturity and overexertion, a variety of pathologic conditions can cause foot dragging by interfering with normal breakover. A shuffling gait is frequently associated with swinging-leg lameness, for example. In the forefoot, shuffling is often combined with bucked knees.

Treatment. Causes originating in the proximal locomotor system are corrected. The foot is shod with a rolled toe to assist breakover, or higher clips are applied over leather pads.

2.1.20.2.20. Pivoting of the Hind Foot

Definition and Symptoms. This is a rotary movement of the hind leg and foot that occurs immediately before breakover, the heels being turned outward and the dorsum inward. This can cause contact with the adjacent hind limb in a manner similar to interfering. The area of the fetlock joint is most commonly injured.

Etiology. Cow hocks, bow legs and a camped-behind configuration predispose to pivoting. Shoeing with calks and grabs exacerbates the fault.

Treatment. Defects of limb and foot conformation are improved, broken digital axes are corrected in young horses, and adult horses are put in flat shoes. Protective leg gear is worn for interfering.

References

ADAMS, O. R.: Chip fractures of the first phalanx in the metacarpophalangeal (Fetlock) joint. J. Amer. vet. med. Assoc. *148:* 360 (1966).

ADAMS, O. R.: Lameness in horses; 2nd ed. (Lea & Febiger, Philadelphia 1966).

ADAMS, O. R.: Constriction of the palmar (volar) or plantar annular ligament in horses. Vet. Med. and Small Animal Clinician *69:* 327 (1974).

BÉRUBÉ, R.: Les fractures de la première phalange chez le cheval. Canad. J. comparat. Med. vet. Sci. *26:* 167 (1963).

BESSIGNANA, G.: Neurotomy in fractures of sesamoid bones. Veterinaria, Milano *16:* 126 (1967).

BOYES, J. H.: Bunnell's surgery of the hand; 4th. ed. (Lippincott, Philadelphia).

BREUER, D.: Fesselbeinfraktur beim Pferd. Sonderdruck, anonym.

CHURCHILL, E. A.: Surgical removal of fractured fragments of the proximal sesamoid bone. J. Amer. vet. med. Assoc. *128:* 58 (1956).

CLAPP, N. K.; CARLSON, W. D.; MORGAN, J. P.: Radiation therapy for lameness in horses. J. Amer. vet. med. Assoc. *143:* 277 (1963).

COLLES, C. M.: Pathogenese der Podotrochlose und ihre Therapie mit Cumarinderivaten. Sonderh. III. Tagung über Pferdekrankheiten, Equitana, Essen 1979.

DALIN, G.; DREVEMO, S.; FREDRICSON, J.; JONSON, K.; NILSSON, G.: Ergonomic aspects of locomotor asymmetry in standardbred horses tracting through turns. An investigation with special reference of the fetlock joint, using high-speed-cinematography and thermography. Acta vet. scand. *44:* suppl. 111 (1973).

DANIELS, H.: Grundlagen der AO-Osteo-Synthese bei Gross- und Kleintieren. Prakt. Tierarzt *53:* 473 (1972).

DIETZ, O.; GÄNGEL, H.; RICHTER, W.; SCHWAN, G.: Behandlungsergebnisse und Prognose der Fesselbeinfraktur des Sportpferdes. Mh. Vet.-Med. *29:* 181 (1973).

DIETZ, O.; MILL, J.; RICHTER, W.: Klinik und Therapie der Gleichbeinfraktur. IV. Tagung über Pferdekrankheiten, Equitana, Essen 1981.

DIETZ, O.; NAGEL, E.; RECHENBERG, R.: Beitrag zur Gliedmassenchirurgie bei Vollblutgalopp- und Vollbluttraberpferden. Mh. Vet.-Med. *18:* Sonderheft 1, 5 (1963).

DIXON, R. T.: Radiation therapy in horses. Austral. vet. J. *43:* 508 (1967).

DUBS, B.; NEMETH, F.: Therapie und Prognose der Fesselbeinfrakturen. Schweiz. Arch. Tierheilk. *117:* 299 (1975).

EISENMENGER, E.: Experimenteller Beitrag zur intraartikulären Injektion von Mukopolysaccharid-polyschwefelsäureester (Eleparon). Berliner Münchener tierärztl. Wschr. *81:* 382 (1968).

EISENMENGER, E.: Gelenkpunktion für Diagnostik und Therapie. Nutzen und Risiko. tierärztl. praxis *2:* 401 (1974).

FACKELMANN, G. E.: Sagittal fractures of the first phalanx (pl) in the horse: fixation by the lag screw principle. Vet. Med. and Small Animal Clinician *68:* 622 (1973).

FACKELMANN, G. E.; CLODIUS, L.: Surgical correction of the digital hyperextension deformity in foals. Vet. Med. and Small Animal Clinician *67:* 1116 (1972).

HAAKENSTAD, L. H.: Chronic bone and joint diseases in relation to conformation in the horse. Equine vet. J. *1:* 248 (1969).

HEINZE, C. D.: Equine orthopedic surgery. Mod. vet. Pract. *47:* 63 (1966).

HOUDESHELL, J. W.; BLOOMFIELD, N. J.: Field trials of a new longacting corticosteroid in the treatment of equine arthropathies. Vet. Med. and Small Animal Clinician *64:* 782 (1969).

HUSKAMP, B.: Möglichkeiten und Grenzen der operativen Knochenbruchbehandlung beim Pferd. Prakt. Tierarzt *53:* 469 (1972).

KUBITZA, G.: Zur Therapie degenerativer Gelenkerkrankungen bei Pferden und Hunden. Tierärztl. Umschau *21:* 402 (1966).

LEWANDOWSKI, M.: Próby operacyjnego leczenia szczudlowatości pochodzenia ściegnowego przeciecie ściegnistej (Caput tendineum). Med. weteryn. *23:* 321 (1967).

LYSHOLT, B.; SOENNICHSEN, H. V.: Senestyltefod hos fol og plage. Nord. Vet.-Med. *21:* 601 (1969).

MAROLT, J.; ZUKOVIL, N.; MOLAN, M.: Die Onchocercosis beim Pferd. Beitrag zur Ätiologie der Lahmheiten, Haut- und Augenkrankheiten. Dtsch. tierärztl. Wschr. *73:* 130 (1966).

MILNE, F. J.: Clinical examination and diagnosis of the diseased equine foot. J. Amer. vet. med. Assoc. *151:* 1599 (1967).

Myers, V. S.; Lundvall, R.: Corrective trimming for weak flexor tendons in a colt. J. Amer. vet. med. Assoc. *148:* 1523 (1966).
Nemeth, F.: Sesamoiditis in the horse. Tijdschr. Diergeneesk. *98:* 15 (1973).
Nemeth, F.: Prognose, Therapie und Pathogenese der Gleichbeinlahmheit. tierärztl. praxis *3:* 287 (1974).
Nilsson, G.; Olsson, S. E.: Radiologic and patho-anatomic changes in the distal joints and the phalanges of the standardbred horse. Acta vet. scand. *44:* 1 (1973).
Numans, S. R.; Wintzer, H. J.: Zur Knochen- und Gelenkchirurgie beim Pferd. Wiener tierärztl. Mschr. *51:* 217 (1964).
Pettersson, H.: Osteosynthese der Gleichbeinfraktur. IV. Tagung über Pferdekrankheiten. Equitana, Essen 1981.
Richter, W.; Weser, H.: Dislokation (Luxation) der Gleichbeine nach Ruptur der distalen Gleichbeinbänder. Mh. Vet.-Med. *19:* 224 (1964).
Rooney, J. R.: Distal condylar fractures of the cannon bone in the horse. Mod. vet. Pract. *55:* 113 (1974).
Rydell, N. W.; Butler, J.; Balazs, E.: Hyaluromic acid in synovial fluid. VI. Effect of intraarticular injection of hyaluronic acid on the clinical symptoms of arthritis in track horses. Acta vet. scand *11:* 139 (1970).
Salis, B. von: Osteosynthese beim Pferd, neueste Fortschritte und Anwendungsmöglichkeiten in der Privatpraxis. Proc. 18th Ann. Conv. Equine Pract. 193, ref. in Schweiz. Arch. Tierheilk. *116:* 38 (1972).
Sevelius, F.; Tufvesson, G.: Treatment for fractures of the sesamoid bones in horses. J. Amer. vet. med. Assoc. *142:* 981 (1963).
Schneider, W.: Weitere Untersuchungen über die Wirksamkeit von Arumalon ad us. vet. bei degenerativen Gelenkerkrankungen der Pferde. Tierärztl. Umschau *27:* 132 (1972).
Soennichsen, H. V.: Fractures of phalanges. Nord. Vet.-Med. *15:* 251 (1964).
Stihl, H. G.: Frakturen als orthopädisches Problem beim Sportpferd. Schweiz. Arch. Tierheilk. *110:* 309 (1968).
Tronicke, T.: Zur Tomanol-Therapie bei Bewegungsstörungen des Pferdes. Tierärztl. Umschau *24:* 188 (1969).
Wheat, J. D.; Rhode, E. A.: The surgical treatment of fractures of the proximal sesamoid bones in the horse. J. Amer. vet. med. Assoc. *132:* 378 (1958).
Wirstad, H. F.: Fractures of the proximal phalangeal sesamoid bones. Vet. Rec. *75:* 509 (1963).

2.1.20.3. Diseases of the Coronet, Pastern Joint and Middle Phalanx (P2)

2.1.20.3.1. Injuries of the Coronet

Definition and Occurrence. Injuries of the coronet are relatively common in the horse (fig. 2.1.20. — 48). They may be superficial or deep and often due to contact with an adjacent leg: *coronet striking* (cf. Overreaching).

Symptoms. The manifestations are variable and range from excoriations with slight contusion — *superficial coronet strike* — to more severe contusions and lacerations of the skin, perioplic and coronary matrix with associated destruction of the perioplic band and horny wall (tubular and laminar layer) — *deep coronet strike* — to injury of the extensor tendon, lateral cartilage, extensor process of the distal phalanx, or even the joint capsule (contusion with secondary necrosis or primary opening) — *perforating coronet strike.* Given the extensive vascular plexuses of the coronary tissues, injuries usually cause profuse hemorrhage in the acute stage; immediate lameness is less frequently observed. Lameness is most common with injuries to the heel bulbs, which appear to be more painful than lesions elsewhere on the coronet. With a deep or perforating coronet strike, lameness develops imme-

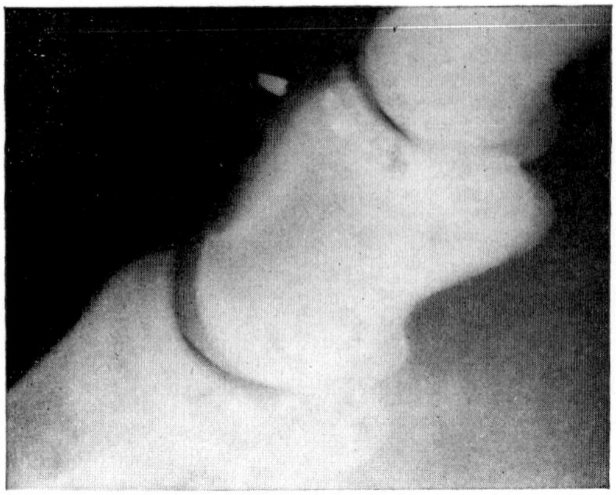

Fig. 2.1.20. — 48. Foreign-body injury above the coronet.

diately if the extensor process is avulsed. By contrast, injuries that open the coffin joint may cause no noticeable lameness in the acute stage. As inflammation progresses, however, a pronounced supporting-leg lameness develops following all coronet injuries. The lameness has typical features, depending on whether the injury involves the coronet of the dorsum, quarters or heel. For example, following a strike to the dorsal coronet of the hind foot, a rapid plantar flexion is seen in the phalangeal joints at the moment of breakover, coupled with a stringhalt-like gait. A deep coronet strike injuring the keratin-producing structures causes an interruption of horn production, which, after infection has subsided, results in the formation of a wide crack or defect in the horny wall.

It is important to understand that the horn of the hoof is produced not by the corium, but by the epidermis! Accordingly, we may divide the horn-producing epidermis of the foot into six parts: the *perioplic*, *coronary*, *laminar*, *sole*, *frog* and *heel-bulb epidermis*. The term 'matrix' may also be used to designate these horn-producing tissues. An example is the perioplic matrix, which secretes the soft horn of the perioplic band (junction between outer skin and horny capsule). This soft horn forms a glaze-like layer which covers the horny wall.

Even superficial excoriations of the skin can become complicated by infection. The conditions in contused coronet tissues are especially conducive to the establishment of tetanus. Various other bacteria can cause inflammation that frequently leads to cellulitis *(coronary or subcoronary cellulitis)*, *abscessation* or *lymphangitis*. After necrotic tissues are sloughed, granulation tissue forms which is gradually replaced with scar tissue. Even large tissue losses can heal completely in this fashion. If the process spreads to deeper levels or originates there in connection with a deep primary injury, the extensor tendon, lateral cartilage or coffin bone and coffin joint may become involved. Damage to the horn-producing structures gives rise to repair processes in these tissues that are eventually manifested by a resumption of new horn growth. A prerequisite for this is the restoration of the matrix. Only then can '*cicatrical horn*' be expected to appear. This horn is distinguished by its fissured, wavy surface and in some cases by its lack of pigmentation. Often this replacement matrix becomes displaced, resulting in *cicatricial* granulation tissue that projects past the coronet, as well as *horny excrescences* that grow outward from the horny wall and bizarre forms of 'cutaneous horns'. Other horny thickenings, called *horn calluses* (q.v.), grow inward from the wall. Coronary abscesses may erupt either outward or inward (e.g., into the coffin joint).

Perforating coronet strikes may open the coffin joint where it is subcutaneous between the extensor process of the distal phalanx and anterior upper angle of the lateral cartilage, or may cause a secondary infectious arthritis as a result of primary tissue damage. The discharge of synovial fluid, swelling of the coronet, the degree of lameness (if present), and possible systemic signs confirm the diagnosis of *infectious podarthritis*.

The probing of such injuries is contraindicated due to the danger of perforating the joint capsule. Repeated contusions can cause periarticular lesions.

The coronet is also susceptible to *thermal and chemical burns*. Finally, numerous lesions of the volar fetlock, eczemas, dermatitides, etc. can spread to the coronet, causing characteristic symptoms.

Etiology. Injuries of the coronet and especially coronet strikes may be self-inflicted (interfering, overreaching, foot dragging, resting one foot on the other). They may also result from slipping, sharp turns, side-stepping, side gaits in inexperienced or fatigued horses, the sudden release of a raised foot, kicks from other horses, and other injuries at the coronet.

Predisposing factors are defects of limb and digital conformation and breaks in the digital axes, which lead to faults of gait and possibly to coronet injuries. Neglected or improper trimming and a number of shoeing errors can also be significant: excessive shoe width, crooked calks, projecting inside quarter clips, projecting nails, etc. Coronet strikes are very often seen in horses affected with central nervous pathology (dummy syndrome).

Pruritus of the limbs associated with filthy bedding, eczema, grease heel or foot mange causes continuous scratching with possible injury and infection.

Thermal burns of the coronet can occur during stable fires, and chemical burns can be caused by various chemical agents (quicklime, mineral fertilizers, herbicides, etc.).

Jumping horses can sustain injuries to the coronet while going over hurdles. Also, unscrupulous owners or attendants have been known to injure the limbs of performance horses intentionally in order to achieve a short-term performance enhancement.

Finally, coronet injuries can have *iatrogenic causes:* injuries that are self-inflicted following firing or blistering as a result of improper aftercare and restraint.

Differential diagnosis must be made from 'separation of the *perioplic band'* following superficial purulent pododermatitis, and *discharge at the coronary band* following deep purulent pododermatitis, due for example to a puncture in shoeing. Fistulae of the collateral cartilage can have causes other than coronet strikes. Swellings and injuries of the coronet region can also occur in connection with *chronic inflammation of the perioplic and coronary epidermis*.

The *diagnosis* is readily made from clinical signs.

Prognosis. Coronet injuries and coronet strikes must be considered serious foot disorders, especially from the standpoint of potential sequelae. The prognosis depends mainly on the location, extent and age of the injury, the degree of swelling, and the severity of the lameness.

Superficial injuries usually have a favorable prognosis. The prognosis is guarded to unfavorable if the injury involves the coffin joint, and in the case of older, more extensive lesions of the extensor process and hoof cartilage. Hoof cartilage injuries can lead to the formation of fistulous tracts. Injuries of the extensor tendon are often very slow to heal, and if they are complicated by an avulsion of the extensor process, an unfavorable prognosis is indicated. With extensive infectious processes of the matrix and cellulitis, loss of the hoof wall is also a danger.

Possible complications are tetanus, periarticular processes, decubitus, hoof deformities and septicemia.

Cicatricial horn formation can *lessen the value of the horse* and even lead to permanent lameness.

Treatment. With even the smallest of injuries, immediate treatment is imperative. This includes proper foot care, preferably on a daily basis. Tetanus prophylaxis is best achieved by immunizing the young horse. Contusions are treated with cold irrigation and cold, moist compresses. These are replaced with warm compresses after about 24 hours. The wound area is cleansed, the hair is clipped, and the wound is closely inspected to ascertain its depth and extent. If the horny wall is included in the injury, or if it appears that purulent material may form behind the horny wall, a sufficiently large piece of wall horn should be removed without delay. This piece is usually crescent-shaped, and its edges should be beveled to inhibit crack formation. Necrotic tissue is removed, and antiseptic treatment is administered including sulfonamide or antibiotic powder, gauze sponge and a pressure bandage. With impending septicemia, long-term parenteral antibiotic therapy is initiated. In many critical cases (cellulitis, podarthritis, lymphangitis), the additional i.v. administration of suitable antibiotics in very large doses (e.g., penicillin 2—3 daily doses of 15 million units) has proved beneficial.

In all operative procedures on the horny capsule, the need for adequate horn resection must be weighed against the consideration that horn replacement is a very slow process. Horn replacement can be hastened by walking the horse frequently or permitting light exercise under a rider. Often this exercise cannot be performed unless the horse is shod. Consequently an effort should be made to spare the wall and sufficiently large portions of the bearing surface if possible so that a shoe can be applied.

Postoperative recovery is aided by giving warm foot baths containing mild disinfectants. Early exercise, even if the horse is still lame, is favorable from the standpoint of preserving foot shape (contraction can occur with prolonged standing) and improving general condition. Moist foot packs (coronet packs) are also recommended, and this should be combined with intensive foot care: daily massage of the coronet with agents such as laurel oil, as well as cleansing and trimming (to stimulate growth).

Prophylaxis centers on regular trimming, proper shoeing and adequate exercise. Good results cannot be achieved overnight; therefore changes must be made gradually. Development of the locomotor system and conditioning of the performance horse require time and patience.

2.1.20.3.2. Diseases of the Pastern Joint

Sprain

Definition. This is a ligamentous injury of the proximal interphalangeal joint.

Occurrence. Pastern joint sprains are a frequent injury, especially in athletic horses, and are usually combined with a sprain of the coffin or fetlock joint.

Symptoms and Diagnosis. There is a sudden, usually severe supporting-leg lameness with marked evidence of pain on passive movement, especially rotation. Inflammatory swelling and joint distension (fluctuation of joint pouches) may appear soon after the injury. The joint and surrounding tissues feel warm to the touch.

Etiology. Sprains result from excessive load, missteps, stumbles, slips, falls, leg entanglements, etc. Weak joints, faults of limb and digital conformation, and improper trimming and shoeing are predisposing factors. Sprains are most common in poorly-conditioned, fatigued horses.

Differential Diagnosis. Complete and incomplete fractures and joint mice should be considered. Radiographs should be taken as soon as possible to exclude lesions of the distal phalanx.

Prognosis. The course is variable. The animal may recover within a few days. Often, however, a painful lameness persists for some time, and the acute inflammation progresses to a chronic arthritis and periarthritis of the pastern joint with ligamentous involvement (articular and periarticular ringbone or chronic ossifying periostitis on the palmar or plantar surface).

Treatment. Acute inflammation is treated with cold applications: Burow's mixture, irrigations, cold baths. Physical therapy in the form of prolonged pasturing or even swimming is indicated.

Prophylaxis. Sound, regular trimming and proper shoeing are the best preventive measures. Shoes with 'grabs' can halt foot motion too abruptly, requiring the phalangeal joints to absorb large amounts of energy; sprains are a frequent result (cf. 'tartan syndrome').

Aseptic Arthritis

Definition and Occurrence. Aseptic inflammation of the pastern joint mainly occurs as a serous arthritis of the forelimb.

Symptoms and Diagnosis. With acute serous arthritis of the pastern joint, the horse exhibits a moderate to severe supporting-leg lameness. The joint is distended with fluid, and fluctuation can be elicited in the joint pouches. Heat is palpable in the joint and surrounding area, and increased pulsation is felt in the palmar artery. Passive movements of the joint — flexion, extension and rotation — are painful. Local anesthesia at the level of the fetlock joint is positive. Intra-articular injections are not recommended for either diagnosis or therapy.

Etiology. The etiology is trauma associated with jumps, cross-country rides, slipping, entanglement, etc.

Differential Diagnosis. Sprains of the pastern joint are difficult to differentiate and often progress quickly to an acute aseptic arthritis. Acute trauma to the foot and pastern should also be considered, however. Doubts can be resolved by obtaining radiographs, but these should be taken only after the seat of the lameness has been localized.

Treatment. The cause is removed, and anti-inflammatory treatment is administered. The horse is confined to a box stall or paddock; cold is applied initially and later replaced with heat to promote absorption of effusion. Glucocorticoids are best administered in ointment form, rather than by injection.

Infectious Arthritis

Definition, Occurrence, Etiology. The pastern joint can become infected secondary to a traumatic opening of the joint cavity (coronet strike, pitchfork wound, overreach injury of the hindfoot, compound fracture), the extension of suppurative processes from adjacent tissues, or, not infrequently, iatrogenic causes. Careless intra-articular injections, especially of glucocorticoids, also frequently lead to pyogenic arthritis (add antibiotics to the injection solution!).

Symptoms. Typical symptoms are a severe supporting-leg lameness, increased warmth of the pastern joint and surrounding area, increased pulsation in the palmar

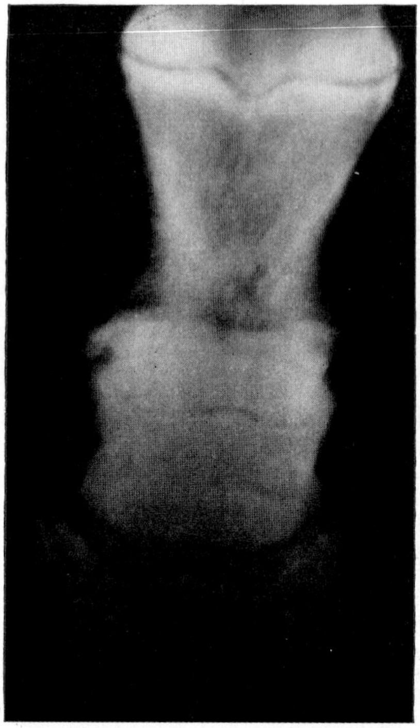

49

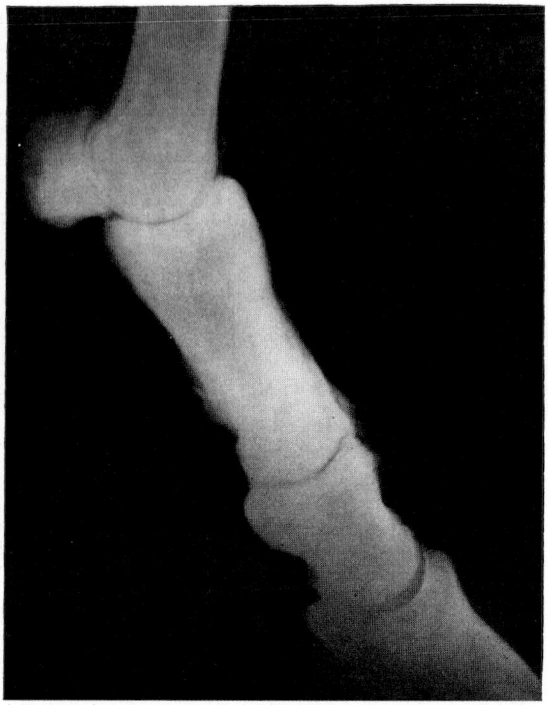

50

Fig. 2.1.20. — 49. Periarticular ringbone of the pastern joint (dorso-palmar projection).
Fig. 2.1.20. — 50. Periarticular ringbone of the pastern joint (latero-medial projection).

artery, and often extensive swelling of the entire digit. Spontaneous eruption may occur, characterized by the discharge of a foul-smelling, discolored, purulent exudate. Cellulitis is also possible. Systemic signs are present in advanced cases.

The *diagnosis* is readily made from the symptoms described.

Prognosis. If important structures are destroyed (joint cartilage, bone, etc.), the prognosis is guarded to unfavorable in terms of functional recovery, but is usually favorable in terms of survival, provided septicemia does not supervene. When arthrodesis of the pastern joint is carried out, the horse may again be fit for work under saddle; this procedure is deferred until ringbone of the pastern joint has developed.

Treatment. Immediate arthrocentesis or puncture of the joint and irrigation with physiologic saline or mild antiseptics. After the organisms have been identified and their sensitivity determined, specific local and parenteral antibiotic therapy is administered.

Chronic Degenerative Arthritis and Periarthritis (Ringbone of the Pastern Joint)

Definition and Occurrence. Ringbone of the pastern joint refers to any chronic inflammation of the proximal interphalangeal joint that is accompanied by new bone growth (osteophytes, exostosis). The two basic forms are articular and periarticular (non-articular) ringbone. Articular ringbone may be further classified as marginal or central, and periarticular ringbone as complete or partial (lateral, medial, bilateral, dorsal, palmar, plantar) (figs. 2.1.20. — 49 through — 52). The front foot is more commonly affected.

51 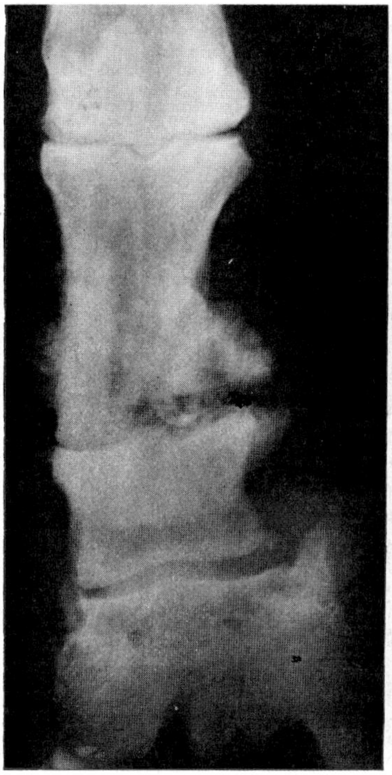

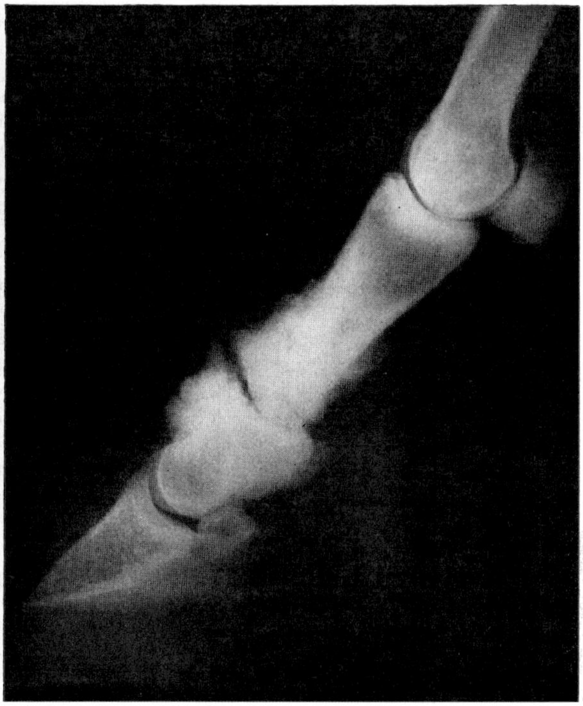 52

Fig. 2.1.20. — 51. Periarticular and articular ringbone of the pastern joint (dorso-palmar projection).

Fig. 2.1.20. — 52. Periarticular and articular ringbone of the pastern joint (latero-medial projection).

Etiology. Causes may be *endogenous* or *exogenous:*

a) *Endogenous* or *predisposing causes* are irregularities of limb and digital conformation (base-narrow, base-wide, bow legs, knock knees, toe-in, toe-out) and breaks in the digital axes producing unequal loads on different parts of the joint (e.g., unilateral overload, contusion, erosion, ligamentous lesions). Such causes include an excessively upright or sloping pastern, narrow, weakly-developed joints, weak tendons and ligaments, and trimming errors, such as trimming the wall uneven on one side, trimming the heels too low and leaving the toe too long (broken foot and pastern axis), or improper shoeing.

b) *Exogenous causes* are overexertion, premature use of racing and riding horses, sprains and contusions. In the less-frequent articular ringbone, increased contact pressure leads to severe abrasion of the articular cartilage and to gradual fusion (ankylosis) of the proximal and middle phalanges. This condition has been described as an 'arthrosis'. Other possible causes are articular fractures of P2 and 'traumatic ringbone' due, for example, to coronet striking.

Ringbone in yearlings is a special form of the disease and is seen with epiphysitis.

Symptoms. Lameness is usually gradual and of the supporting-leg type. With sprains or other trauma, however, the loss of function is immediate. Most horses exhibit a 'cold' lameness that improves after the start of exercise. In the standing position, the affected limb is carried cranially. If there is disability of long standing,

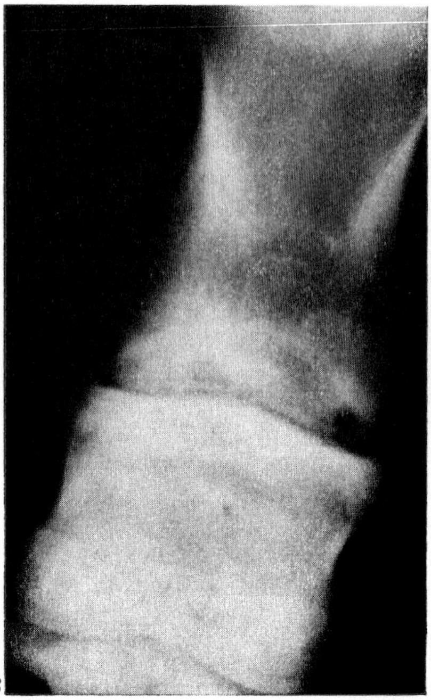
53

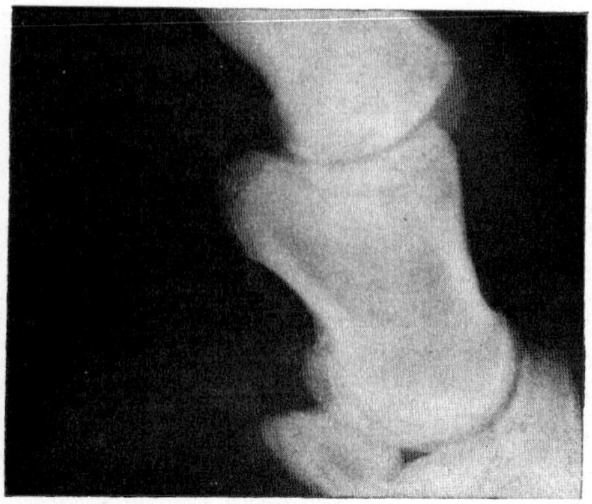
54

Fig. 2.1.20. — 53. Subchondral cyst of the pastern joint.
Fig. 2.1.20. — 54. Subluxation of the pastern joint of the left forelimb due to tendon damage.

atrophy will be evident in the muscles of the shoulder or croup. Inspection will reveal marked swelling in various parts of the pastern joint, especially in unilateral cases. Findings should be compared with the contralateral digit. Pain is usually produced by passive manipulation of the pastern joint, especially rotation. In many cases the periarticular changes are palpable as hard, usually painless enlargements in the vicinity of the pastern joint.

An internal (articular, occult) or external (periarticular) ankylosis of the joint gradually develops over a period of months or even years, accompanied by persistent lameness.

Radiographs are of value, especially in cases of articular ringbone. This examination should be done only after the seat of the lameness has been localized by a palmar (or plantar) nerve block at the fetlock joint.

Lesions. The enlargements consist initially of soft, highly-vascularized fibrous tissue that gradually ossifies. The ends of the proximal and middle phalanges acquire a knobby, grooved appearance, exhibit numerous exostoses and osteophytes, and gradually fuse together: i.e., ankylosis. Bone-destroying processes coexist with bone-forming processes. The articular cartilage shows a loss of normal luster, increasing yellow-brown discoloration, abrasion and destruction; wear lines and spots of varying shape are visible on the cartilage surface. Eventually the cartilage-denuded bony ends undergo fusion, or 'internal ankylosis'. Ligamentous changes are also usually present and consist of firm thickenings and bony inclusions, mainly at the ligamentous attachments (traction osteophytes). Nearby tendinous and capsular tissues may also undergo gradual ossification.

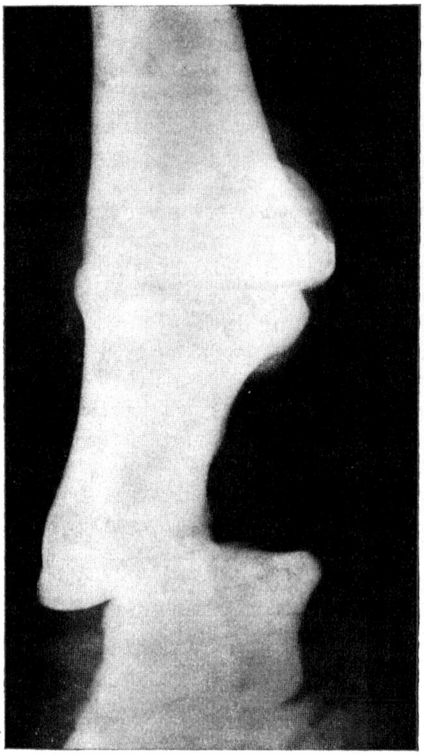

55

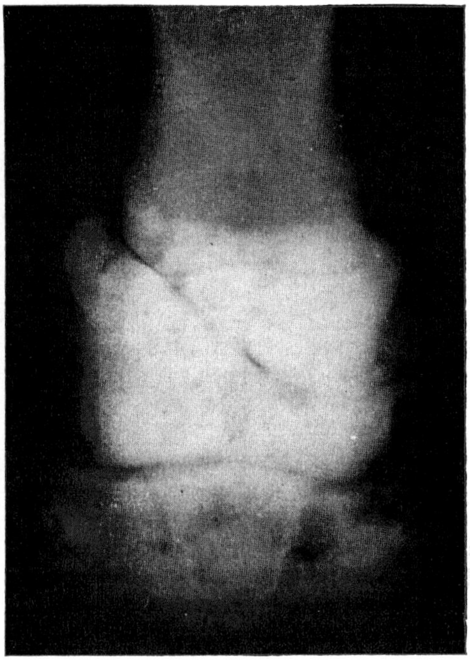

56

Fig. 2.1.20. — 55. Pastern joint luxation in an 8-year-old jumper.
Fig. 2.1.20. — 56. Fracture of the middle phalanx.

Diagnosis is not difficult in advanced cases. In the early stage, radiographs are necessary to verify the diagnosis.

Prognosis and Treatment. Once begun, the process of ringbone formation can seldom be arrested. Treatment is directed toward the cause, eliminating it if possible: trimming and shoeing are directed mainly toward achieving a level foot landing. In the past the treatment of early ringbone has varied from the use of topical rubefacients to firing (superficial or perforating). Good results are achieved in some cases with arthrodesis (artificial ankylosis).

Luxation and Subluxation of the Pastern Joint (Luxation of the Second Phalanx)

Dislocations of the pastern joint are relatively uncommon. Subluxations (fig. 2.1.20. — 54), usually in an anterior direction, can result from ligamentous laxity. They are more frequent than luxations (fig. 2.1.20. — 55), which are trauma-related (jumping, traffic injuries, leg entanglement). Often such luxations are accompanied by comminuted fractures of the middle phalanx (P2). Some of these fractures are open, resulting in a guarded prognosis at best.

Fracture of the Second Phalanx

Occurrence and Classification. Fractures of P2 are less common than those of the P1 and P3. According to the statistics of PEITL [1971], the P2 shows a fracture rate of 3.17 % as opposed to 4.52 % for the coffin bone and 26.63 % for P1 (highest for all bones!) P2 may sustain a comminuted fracture, a ligamentous sprain-fracture, or, less frequently, an avulsion of the flexor tendon attachment. Comminuted fractures may be simple or open. In open fractures the soft-tissue envelope may be damaged either from the inside by bony spicules, or from the outside by trauma (coronet strike, kick, etc.) (fig. 2.1.20. — 56).

Symptoms. A severe supporting-leg lameness develops immediately. Initially there is slight swelling, tenderness to palpation, crepitation (with a comminution) and an abnormal (lateral) mobility of the hoof. Soon after a comminuted fracture occurs, a painful swelling develops around the coronet and makes accurate palpation difficult.

Etiology. The causes are external trauma: excessive loading during jumps, missteps, coronet strikes, kicks, traffic accidents, slipping, tripping over roots, catching the foot in grates or frozen wheel ruts, etc. Endogenous factors such as osteitis, osteoporosis and post-neurectomy disturbances are predisposing. *Note:* Diagnostic anesthesia of the digital nerves can convert a fissure fracture of P2 to a complete fracture!

Differential Diagnosis. Fracture of P1, P3 or tendon rupture.

Diagnosis. No changes are apparent in other portions of the limb and digit. The onset of lameness is sudden. The diagnosis is confirmed by radiographs, which also have prognostic value. Diagnostic anesthesia is contraindicated if a fracture is suspected.

Prognosis. The prognosis is guarded to unfavorable, especially with open fractures. Involvement of the pastern and coffin joints is present in most comminuted fractures. A chronic supporting-leg lameness usually persists.

Treatment. With fresh *chip fractures*, the fragments are extirpated or, in suitable cases, are reattached to the bone with Kirschner wires or screws.

With comminuted fractures and open fractures of P2, the animal should be moved to a well-equiped hospital and an attempt made to immobilize the fragments in situ by means of screws. In some cases an arthrodesis of the pastern joint should also be performed at the same operation, taking special care to preserve function in the coffin joint. We have repeatedly seen very good functional recoveries in riding horses that have had an arthrodesis of the pastern joint.

Comments. Euthanasia can always be considered if treatment is unsuccessful.

2.1.20.4. Diseases of the Hoof

Definition. The term 'hoof' denotes the horny capsule and enclosed structures; Zietzschmann uses the term *digital end-organ*. Every lameness examination starts with the hoof, because a great many lameness causes have their seat in or on the hoof.

2.1.20.4.1. Pododermatitis (Inflammation of the Epidermis of the Hoof)

Classification. Inflammatory lesions of the hoof matrix closely resemble inflammation of the skin. The differences in terms of pathogenesis, form, course and evaluation are based upon the anatomic structure of the hoof, the firm horny capsule, the powerful development of the stratum papillare, the stratum germinativum, and the near absence of subcutaneous tissue in the horny capsule. The shape changes that the hoof undergoes within the framework of hoof mechanics as weight is alternately placed upon and taken off the foot are expressed both in the course of the inflammation and the manner in which it spreads.

The classification of pododermatitides has undergone many changes over the years and is based upon various criteria:

1. Extent: superficial pododermatitis, deep p., cirumscribed p., diffuse p.
2. Duration: acute p., chronic p.
3. Etiology: aseptic p., infectious p.
4. Character: serous p., hemorrhagic p., suppurative p., gangrenous p., hyperplastic p.

Symptoms. As in any inflammation, the cardinal symptoms are redness, heat, swelling, pain, and loss of function.

Redness and *swelling* are evident only at the coronet and heel bulbs. *Heat* can be detected by palpation and comparative examination of the opposite hoof. *Pain* is among the most important symptoms of pododermatitis and is especially marked when the inflammation is deep-seated, for the major portion of the affected layers are tightly confined in the space between the coffin bone and inelastic horny capsule. The pain is manifested by varying degrees of supporting-leg lameness during progression and by characteristic favoring of the digit while standing. Pain is detected and elicited by the use of palpation, percussion (hammer) and compression (hoof tester) during the course of the examination. Especially in acute cases, increased pulsation is felt in the palmar artery and/or the palmar digital arteries, and swelling is observable over the coronet and proximal to it.

Etiology. Pododermatitis is caused mainly by external influences. Blunt *mechanical trauma* leads to contusions (corns) and strains, while sharp trauma leads to tissue disruption (laceration or puncture wound of the sole, coronet strike, shoenail injuries, etc.). Other external causes are strenuous work on hard ground with improperly trimmed and shod hooves. *Thermal injuries* can result from the prolonged application of a shoe during hot-fitting, or may occur in connection with stable fires, which can cause burns of the coronet and heel bulbs. These tissues can also become frostbitten on prolonged exposure to extreme cold. *Chemical injuries* from acids and caustic substances also occur but are of minor importance.

Most cases of pododermatitis are caused by infections with various organisms, whose virulence determines the duration of the disease and its outcome.

Prognosis. The prognosis depends on the character, location, extent and duration of the disease. It is guarded to unfavorable in cases of deep suppurative and deep gangrenous pododermatitis, because complications may arise such as subcoronary cellulitis, hoof cartilage fistulae (quittor), cellulitis of the frog, necrosis of the deep flexor tendon, disease of the coffin joint and septicemia.

Treatment is aimed at removing the cause: removal of foreign bodies (e.g., shoenail or foreign nail), proper trimming and shoeing. Aseptic inflammation often responds well to 1—2 days' rest and cold application: cold water compresses, ice, Burow's mixture, poultices, flowing water or continuous irrigation, antiseptic poultices (cataplasms).

Whenever a *suppurative process* of the matrix is presumed (increased pulsation, hoof tester), an effort should be made to establish prompt drainage by making an opening on the white line. If purulent exudate has already appeared following separation of the perioplic band, a counteropening should still be made on the white line at the site where the horn tubes running downward from the area of separation meet the bearing surface. The hoof should be cleansed thoroughly before this opening is made. The area is covered with sulfonamide powder, gauze, cotton, and a bandage that exerts enough pressure to prevent prolapse of the matrix. In some cases the bandage can be secured in the area of the bearing surface by the horseshoe, and to the sole and frog with a splint bandage or covered shoe. In *deep suppurative pododermatitis*, the focus should be exposed over a broader area (horn aperture of at least 15 mm), well disinfected and protected with a pressure bandage as a safeguard against pus retention, further infection and prolapse of the matrix. If drainage is inadequate, there will be spontaneous *drainage at the coronary band.*

Swimming-pool exercise has proved very useful as a means of offsetting the training loss in racing and show horses. This may be prescribed for practically all horses with hoof diseases almost immediately after surgery, whereas ordinary track excercise must be deferred for days or weeks.

Below we shall discuss some acute and chronic inflammatory conditions of the hoof epidermis, which are presented in order of frequency:

Acute Inflammation

Shoenail Injuries

Definition. These are injuries of the hoof matrix (wall and sole epidermis) that occur when nails are driven into the foot for shoeing.

Shoenail injuries may be *direct* or *indirect*. Indirect injuries are caused by compression, while direct injuries are the result of puncture wounds. In *shoenail compression*, the nail enters the innermost tubular layer of the hoof and causes the lamellar horn to bow inward against the wall epidermis, resulting in inflammation. A *prick in shoeing* occurs when the nail is driven partially into the hoof epidermis and then immediately drawn. A *true shoenail puncture* is present when the nail injuring the hoof epidermis, lateral cartilage or even the coffin bone is left in place for some time.

Occurrence. Shoenail injuries are more common in the forefoot than in the hind foot. When the shoe is applied by a well-trained farrier, this type of injury is a rarity. But by the same token, the farrier is often held responsible by the owner or attendant when such an injury is incurred.

Symptoms. In cases of *shoenail compression*, the horse manifests unrest during shoeing and especially during clinching; in many cases the aforementioned bowing of the lamellar horn is produced by the nail curvature, which is in the direction of the hoof matrix. Immediately after shoeing the horse exhibits a stilted gait and in rare cases a supporting-leg lameness, though this usually first appears after 3—4 days or even 2—3 weeks together with the symptoms of superficial suppurative pododermatitis.

If the horse flinches noticeably during the driving of a nail, a *prick in shoeing* is indicated, and the offending nail should be pulled and redriven.

A nail prick can be difficult to diagnose in horses that show sensitivity to each blow of the shoeing hammer (young horses, thin walls). If the nail is drawn immediately, blood will be found on the tip and possibly on the shank, and small drops of blood will usually ooze from the nail track.

A *true shoenail puncture* is recognized by the discharge of blood from the exit hole on the horny wall and/or between the bearing surface and shoe. Horses with this injury will place weight only on the toe of the affected foot, will avoid dorsiflexion of the fetlock joint, and will resist attempts to lift the sound opposite foot. In nearly all cases the animal will be lame when first walked after shoeing.

The suspicion of a shoenail injury is well-founded if a freshly-shod horse goes lame, if the hoof wall appears to be lowered excessively, if the wall has been over-rapsed, and if the nails emerge too high. If pain has been elicited by percussion or hoof tester in the region of the nails, then the shoe should be carefully removed. At this time each nail should be pulled *individually*, and a check made for the presence of blood or pus. An evaluation of the entry and exit holes and careful probing of the nail tracks will enable a diagnosis to be made. One should also note the location of the entry hole, which should be at the *outer aspect of the white line*.

Etiology. Shoenail injuries can result from excessive lowering of the horny wall; a weakening of the wall by improper rasping; the use of shoes that are improperly and too deeply creased, have incorrect hole placements, or are poorly-fitted; the use of faulty (incomplete) nails; or driving the nail in too deeply or with the bevel toward the outside. In addition, there may be factors such as a thin, cracked, macerated or brittle horny wall, nail remnants, or viciousness on the part of the horse for which the farrier cannot be held responsible. Nevertheless, the farrier's profession calls for patience and an adequate knowledge of equine behavior; this is especially true in the shoeing of young and highly temperamental horses. If an occasional horse proves too vicious or unmanageable for shoeing to be attempted, then the veterinarian should intervene with sedative measures. The beating or mistreating of a fractious horse is never justifiable.

The shortage of competent farriers is leading to an increasing reliance on prefabricated shoes, which frequently are set by laymen. All too often in such cases the foot is fitted to the shoe! Horseowners should again recognize the tremendous value of an expertly hand-forged and fitted shoe, which can be adapted to the many variations of the equine foot that occur normally as well as in disease. Where the hoof is concerned, there is no substitute for individualized care.

The work of the modern farrier takes him to riding stables, show rings and racetracks, where he must work on well bred, valuable and often excitable horses, always under the scrutiny of a knowledgable owner or attendant. This job is not an easy one and merits the full support of the veterinarian! Conversely, every equine practitioner will benefit from having at least one competent farrier in his district. Cooperation between the two professions is valuable and is a goal worth pursuing.

Prognosis. The earlier a shoenail injury is detected and its full extent appreciated, the more favorable the prognosis. If there is extensive suppuration with necrosis of the distal phalanx or lateral cartilage, a protracted convalescence may be expected. Tetanus is best controlled by vaccinating the animal at an early age and following this with booster injections annually.

Treatment. Whenever a shoenail injury is detected, the shoe should be removed at once. For a fresh *injury of this nature*, tincture of iodine should be dribbled into the nail opening, and some cotton packed into the nail track, which is then sealed with *adhesive hoof wax*. In favorable circumstances the shoe (full bar with leather pad) may be reset right away, taking care not to drive a nail into the injured spot. When a direct or indirect shoenail injury is discovered several days after shoeing, an opening is cut in the horny wall. The size of this opening depends on the type of lesion that is present. The matrix is flushed and irrigated with mild antiseptics, and sulfonamide or antibiotic powder is applied, followed by pressure bandaging. In cases of extensive suppurative pododermatitis, parenteral antibiotics are administered. In all cases it is important to establish drainage through an opening in the horn; otherwise liquefaction, possibly involving the distal phalanx, will occur despite costly antibiotics (cf. Puncture Wounds of the Foot).

With any wound of the foot, it is essential that tetanus antitoxin or toxoid booster be administered. Neglect on this score is tantamount to malpractice.

Comments. Nowadays shoenail injuries are often caused by the owner, attendant, etc., and the veterinarian should bear this fact in mind during his evaluation. Prompt veterinary care has a critical bearing on the prognosis.

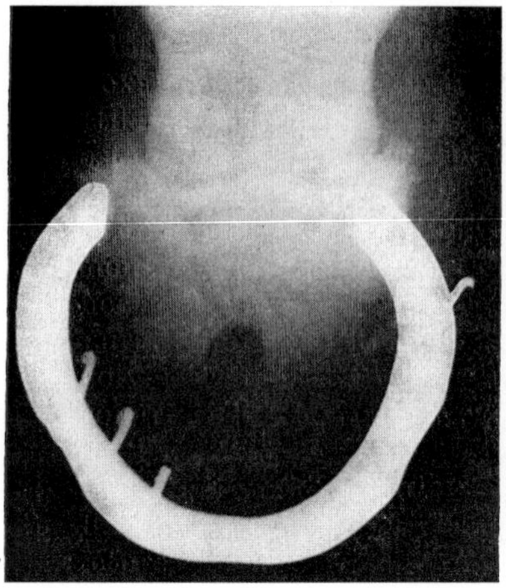
57

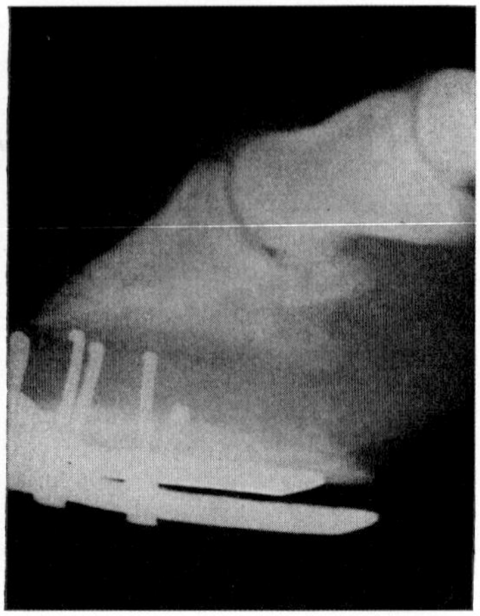
58

Fig. 2.1.20. — 57. Subsolar abscess in a Thoroughbred racehorse (dorso-palmar projection).
Fig. 2.1.20. — 58. Subsolar abscess in a Thoroughbred racehorse (latero-medial projection).

Puncture Wounds of the Foot

Definition. Puncture wounds of the foot are injuries of the ground surface of the hoof inflicted by sharp or pointed foreign objects.

Occurrence. The hind feet are most commonly affected. Sites of predilection are the sulci of the frog.

Symptoms. Most puncture wounds cause a supporting-leg lameness of sudden onset. Often a thorough examination will reveal the foreign body still embedded in the horn tissue of the frog. Remember that the embedded portion may be bent or curved, and so the object should be removed with caution to avoid further tissue injury.

The owner or attendant should call the veterinarian when the injury is first noticed and point out the location of the wound when the veterinarian arrives. By noting the *direction* and *depth of penetration* of the foreign body, the veterinarian should be able to determine which structures have been injured, plan his treatment accordingly, and make a prognosis.

The peculiar anatomic structure of the hoof tends to prevent the drainage of pus. Unless a drainage hole is made in the horn, the pus will spread extensively within the hoof causing the liquefaction of further tissues, even the bone (figs. 2.1.20. — 57 and — 58).

Hoof mechanics plays an important role in puncture wounds of the foot. What can be injured?

1. The *hoof epidermis* (matrix). A purulent pododermatitis develops that may be circumscribed or diffuse, deep or superficial, depending on the structures involved in the injury and the type of treatment given. Unless drainage is established, the purulent exudate, driven by hoof mechanics, will spread along the inner surface of the hoof wall. Large portions of the horny frog and horny sole can become undermined in this way until finally the perioplic band separates from the epidermis, usually at the heel bulb.

2. The *plantar cushion.* Puncture wounds of the plantar cushion, which is composed of connective and fatty tissue, lead to purulent tissue liquefaction around the puncture track, and possibly to the development of cellulitis in the connective tissue. In

most cases, however, healing is relatively rapid, even in cases where, for example, the foreign object has migrated from the frog to the heel-bulb fossa, where it is found on examination. It is possible for the suppurative process to spread to the lateral cartilages or tendon sheath. When there is pain in the heel area, the horse will place most of its weight on the toe and will try to avoid dorsiflexion of the fetlock.

3. The *deep flexor tendon* and *navicular bursa*. Injuries of these structures can lead to tendon necrosis and infectious bursitis. In both cases a severe supporting-leg lameness develops soon after the injury and is usually accompanied by fever and other systemic signs. A normal or turbid synovial fluid may drain from the wound. If surgical intervention is delayed, the tendon sheath and/or coffin joint may become involved, cellulitis may develop in the frog and heel bulbs, and a coronary or sub-coronary cellulitis may develop with considerable risk of loss of the hoof wall.

4. The *navicular bone*. There may be damage to the bone itself (including fractures) or to its articular surface.

5. The *distal phalanx*. The central parts of the bone are usually affected. Chip fractures, fissure fractures and complete fractures can occur. Osteomyelitis and abscessation are possible in long-standing cases.

6. The *coffin joint*. Coffin joint injuries are perhaps the most serious complication of puncture wounds of the foot. They occur when the foreign body perforates the deep flexor tendon and opens the navicular bursa (see above). The synovial fluid discharged from the puncture track may originate from the bursa or from the coffin joint itself. This question can often be resolved by the diagnostic injection of a sterile liquid into the joint. If the joint has been opened, the liquid will flow from the puncture track, provided the latter has not been occluded by adhesions. A definitive diagnosis usually can be made only after the deep flexor tendon has been partially resected and the ligament exposed. When the foot is passively moved, a turbid or purulent synovial fluid will drain from the opening in the joint capsule (purulent podarthritis).

Infections of the coffin joint can also occur secondarily. In such cases existing lameness worsens, fever develops, and swelling may appear around the coronet (coronary or subcoronary cellulitis; see above).

Etiology. Puncture wounds of the foot can be caused by a variety of objects: nails, pins, wood splinters, wires, rocks, broken glass, loose shoe clips, and even pieces of ice. Puncture wounds can also occur during the shoeing of excitable horses that pull the foot away before shoeing is completed, then step down onto a nail or clip.

The most common puncture sites are the lateral sulci and midportion of the frog, about 30—40 mm behind the apex. Objects entering these areas at or near a 90° angle must traverse only a short distance to reach the coffin joint. The wound becomes infected with pathogenic organisms introduced by the foreign body, and there is a danger of tetanus.

Diagnosis. If the foreign body is still in the wound at examination, the extent of the injury can be estimated from the location, direction and length of the embedded portion. The immediate history can provide helpful clues. Even if no foreign body is found, the involvement of specific tissues can still be deduced from the severity of the lameness (if present), the nature and volume of the discharge, the presence of phlegmonous swelling, and systemic manifestations.

Fresh puncture wounds of the foot should not be probed! Probing can distribute pathogenic organisms to deeper tissues or pave the way for secondary infection. Radiographic contrast studies are contraindicated on similar grounds.

Prognosis. Fresh puncture wounds naturally have a better prognosis than old wounds. If the deep flexor tendon has been perforated, or if the navicular bursa or coffin joint has been opened, the prognosis is generally poor, although treatment should be attempted in valuable animals.

Treatment. With every puncture wound of the foot, tetanus prophylaxis should be administered to horses that are not already on an immunization program. We have found that both antitoxin and toxoid vaccine can be administered at the same time as long as they are injected separately to avoid anaphylactic reactions. Neglect of tetanus prophylaxis constitutes malpractice.

Following tetanus prophylaxis, the sole and horny frog are trimmed to remove contaminants. Subsequent treatment depends on the structures involved in the injury. In most cases, however, these are not known with certainty, and so surgery must be limited to paring away the puncture track down to the flexor tendon, plantar cushion or coffin bone, as the case may be. The usual drainage hole is made in the horn, the wound is treated with antibiotic or sulfonamide powder, and a pressure bandage is applied to prevent prolapse of matrix tissues. This treatment is sufficient to prevent the retention of exudate by the hoof wall. With superficial injuries of the matrix, a covered shoe (with removable plate) may be applied. This will aid healing by enabling the horse to exercise at pasture.

Often the process will spread despite this primary care, especially if the full extent of the injury was not appreciated on initial examination. In such cases the horse should be given a general anesthetic, and the wound thoroughly explored by careful probing. Radiographs will disclose any bony lesions of the P3 or navicular bone, as well as any radiopaque foreign-body fragments that may have been left behind.

In the presence of tendon injuries, an attempt should be made to get by with a *partial* resection of the deep flexor tendon in order to minimize function losses (street nail operation). The horny frog and plantar cushion are resected in their anterior portions together with an approximately 3-mm-wide adjacent portion of the bars so that the lateral extent of the process can be seen. Sparing resection of the frog can lead to troublesome recurrences.

Surgical treatment is supported with local and parenteral sulfonamides and/or antibiotics. This therapy does not obviate the need to create a drainage opening in the horn, however.

In cases of septic podarthritis, irrigation of the joint from its dorsal pouch (e.g., with physiologic saline) while maintaining a patent distal primary opening has proved beneficial. Specific chemotherapy is also recommended.

Comments. Puncture wounds of the foot can be prevented or quickly recognized through observance of general safety measures, such as ground cleanup at construction sites, picking up nails after shoeing, and frequent attention to the hoof as part of a program of foot care.

2.1.20.4.2. Evaluation of the Locomotor System

The scheme used by the Viennese School for classifying the healthy and diseased foot is shown in Table 2.1.20. — 1 (p. 177). The foot diseases are classified into three groups. Note that while laminitis belongs to the 3rd group, its product, the 'foundered foot', is assigned to the 1st group.

Horses with wide feet are predisposed to the development of flat feet or dropped sole, while base-wide and base-narrow horses are susceptible to contracted foot, crooked foot or ossification of the lateral cartilages. Thrush frequently develops in the contracted foot, hoof cracks in the 'peg foot' and contracted foot, and chronic corns in the contracted foot or foot with ossified cartilages.

Relation of the Foot to the Limb

The foot can be thought of as a pedestal that supports the 'column' of the limb. Forces associated with body weight and ground pressure act upon it. The arrangement of the limbs on the body and the proportions of their parts, as well as the limb 'conformation', have a significant effect on weight-bearing and locomotion, and thus on the animal's ability to perform work. The show horse is an excellent example of the integral relationship between conformation and performance.

Evaluation of the equine locomotor system encompasses a number of external criteria: axial skeleton, spinal segments, carriage of head and neck, tail, limb conformation, digital conformation, angulation of the digital axes, and foot shape. Included in this evaluation are the animal's development (constitution, condition), musculature, skin and haircoat, as well as its character and temperament. The expert can form many conclusions simply by observing the horse at rest and for a brief time during progression. Of course, few if any horses can be said to have a perfect conformation, character and temperament. Nevertheless, time-tested rules of horse breeding and care, as well as current knowledge concerning the physical development and conditioning of the modern performance horse, can contribute much to the elimination of faults that hamper a horse's performance and predispose it to disease.

The components of the locomotor system should always be evaluated in terms of the use to which the animal is put. The examination made for the purchase of a horse is an important area of veterinary responsibility. The characteristics of the animal will be summarized in an overall evaluation that will determine the price paid.

Conformation of the Limbs

The conformation of the limbs refers to their arrangement on the body and the position of their axes in relation to the ground. It is important to understand that the limb conformation, digital conformation, position of the digital axes and foot shape can all be influenced by trimming, shoeing and use (and, of course, by operative means). This influence can be positive or negative. A decidedly positive effect can be achieved in young, growing horses up to about the age of five, before full maturity is reached. This is usually accomplished through measures that, while relatively simple, must be applied on a continuing basis: corrective trimming, corrective shoeing, adequate exercise, proper care and nutrition. Unfortunately, much harm is done by neglect of these measures and by placing unreasonable physical demands on immature, improperly nourished horses.

A limb conformation that is normal, or regular, when viewed from all sides leads to a uniform distribution of body weight, equal pressures on the bones, and balanced tension in the collateral ligaments.

Conformation of the Forelimbs

The forelimbs bear some 60—65 % of the weight of the horse. The conformation of the forelimbs is evaluated on a level surface, the horse standing with the weight evenly distributed among all four limbs and feet. If this is not possible, then the animal must have a significant deviation or a lesion that is causing lameness: a limb that is painful or otherwise damaged cannot bear weight normally. Conformation is evaluated by examining the horse from the front and from both sides.

Normal conformation from the anterior view: the forelimbs are straight and perpendicular to the body. A line dropped from the middle of the shoulder joint divides the leg into approximately equal halves, passes through the middle of the carpal and

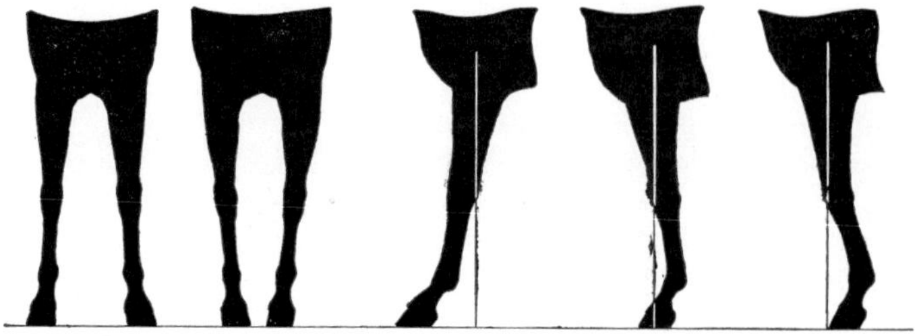

Fig. 2.1.20. — 59. Faults of conformation in the forelimbs.
a = base-wide; b = base-narrow; c = camped in front; d = standing under in front; e = standing under, with cranial deviation of the carpus.

fetlock joint and bisects the anterior hoof wall. The distance between the two front feet may correspond to the greatest width of a (healthy) foot. In a 'wide' conformation the feet are farther apart, but the limbs are still perpendicular to the ground (e.g., in a broad-chested horse); in a 'narrow' conformation they are closer together (narrow chest).

Faults of conformation: In the *base-wide* conformation (fig. 2.1.20. — 59a), the limbs diverge from the chest downward, throwing more weight on the inside of the hoof. In the absence of other deviations of limb conformation from the lateral view or faults of digital conformation or angulation, the foot may acquire a characteristic base-wide shape.

In the *base-narrow* conformation (fig. 2.1.20. — 59b), the limbs converge from the shoulder down, and the fetlock joints may touch in severe cases.

In the *knock-knee* conformation the limbs converge or are straight from the shoulder to the carpus, then diverge from the carpus downward. The opposite of this is the *bow-leg* conformation, in which the limbs are farther apart at the carpal joints than at the shoulder and fetlock.

Normal conformation from the lateral view: a line dropped from the middle of the elbow joint bisects the limb as far as the fetlock. The pivot of the scapula and coronet of the heel are not useful for evaluation due to the varying slope and position of the scapular pivot and variations in pastern length. Normally there is an angle of about 55—78° between the scapula and the body, 85—100° between the scapula and humerus, 120—138° between the humerus and radius, and 125—135° between the 3rd metacarpal bone and proximal phalanx.

Faults of conformation from the lateral view are:
— camped in front (fig. 2.1.20. — 59c),
— standing under in front (fig. 2.1.20. — 59d, e).

Anterior deviation of the limb is usually congenital, while *over in the knees* is an acquired fault in which constant attempts are made to extend the carpus. *Posterior deviation* can also occur.

Conformation of the Hind Limbs

For practical reasons the hind limbs are usually viewed initially from the side. With *well conformed* limbs, a line dropped from the tuber ischii will hit the point of the hock, while a line from the middle of the hip joint (greater trochanter) will hit the hoof wall at the quarters. *Faults of conformation* are:

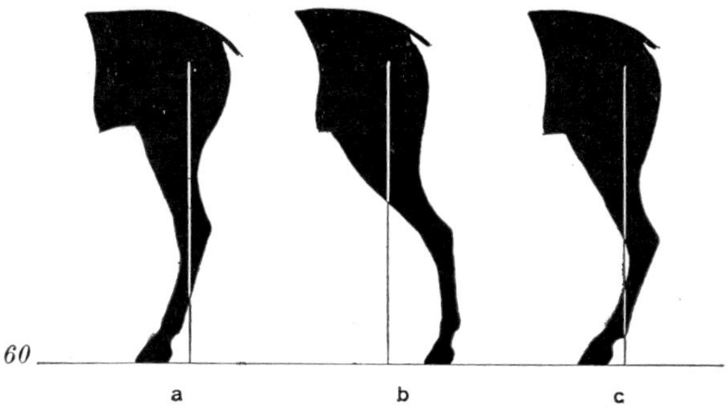

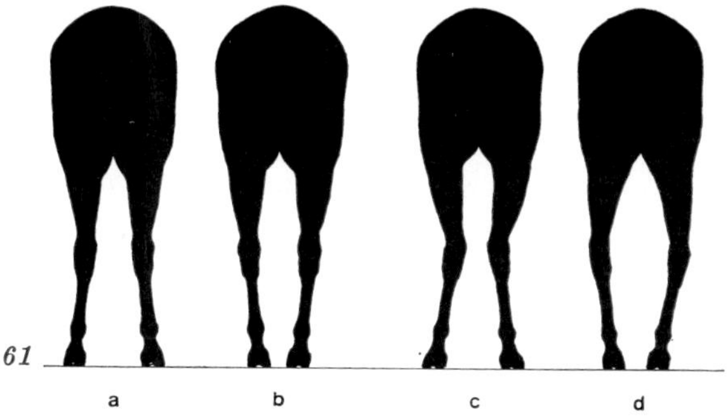

Fig. 2.1.20. — 60. Faults of conformation in the hind limbs (lateral view).
a = standing under behind; b = camped behind; c = sickle hock.

Fig. 2.1.20. — 61. Faults of conformation in the hind limbs (caudal view).
a = base-wide; b = base-narrow; c = cow hocks; d = bow legs.

— standing under behind (fig. 2.1.20. — 60 a),
— camped behind (fig. 2.1.20. — 60 b),
— sickle hocks (fig. 2.1.20. — 60 c) with excessive angulation of the hock joint.

Straight hock is a conformation in which there is too little angulation of the hock joint. A combination of straight hock with a straight stifle joint ('too straight behind') predisposes to such conditions as spavin and upward fixation of the patella.

Evaluating the hind limbs from the side may prove difficult due to individual variations of conformation.

Viewed from behind, the hind limbs have a *normal conformation* if a line dropped from the middle of the tuber ischii bisects the limb and passes through the middle of the hock joint (tuber calcis) and fetlock joint.

Faults of conformation in the hind limb viewed from behind are:
— base-wide (fig. 2.1.20. — 61 a),
— base-narrow (fig. 2.1.20. — 61 b),
— cow hocks (fig. 2.1.20. — 61 c),
— bow legs (fig. 2.1.20. — 61 d).

Conformation of the Digit

The digit is the portion of the limb distal to the fetlock joint. Its conformation is evaluated separate from and following the evaluation of limb conformation. *Normal conformation:* the digital axis is parallel to the median plane of the body when viewed from the front or from behind. *Faults of digital conformation* are the *toe-out* and *toe-in* conformation. The rotation responsible for the fault may have its seat in the fetlock joint or farther up the limb. It is useful to specify the degree of a given fault, using the foot width as a reference: slight (up to $^1/_2$ foot width), moderate (up to 1 foot width), and pronounced (greater than 1 foot width).

Viewed from the side, digital conformation is *normal* if the angle between the ground surface and the digital axis (an imaginary line passing through the center of the phalanges) is between 45 and 47° in front and between 50 and 55° behind. Accordingly, *faults of digital conformation* are present when the digital axis is less than 45 or 50° (foot axis *too sloping*), or greater than 50 or 55° (foot axis *too steep*).

Relation of Foot to Pastern Axis

The foot axis should be continuous with the pastern axis when viewed from the side and from behind. In other words, no break should be evident in the digital axis.

Breaks in the digital axis may be *lateral* or *medial* when viewed from the front, or *anterior* or *posterior* when viewed from the side.

Guides for Corrective Trimming and Shoeing

We shall again summarize the views of the Viennese School with regard to trimming and shoeing: In the immature horse (up to age 5), gradual and sustained efforts are made to straighten the digital axis and if possible achieve a normal digital and limb conformation at the expense of an 'even foot landing'. In the fully mature horse, and with incurable diseases of the foot, an even foot landing is the primary goal.

Evaluation of Foot Shape

The shape of the foot is evaluated by viewing it from the front, from the side, from behind, and from the ground surface. A number of instruments can be used for this purpose (protractors, rulers, calipers, drawing instruments).

The foot is an elastic structure that possesses a specific, highly purposeful shape. More than 60 measurements are needed to accurately reconstruct the equine foot geometrically [Meier, 1917]. Even the slightest shift of body weight in the standing position alters the shape of the hoof wall. When evaluating the foot, a good visual estimate is usually sufficient for practical purposes.

In the *normal and regular* foot, the quarters have a slope of 80° with respect to the ground surface. The foot is said to be *wide and regular* if this slope is less than 80°, and *narrow and regular* if greater than 80°.

Irregularities of foot shape (Table 2.1.20. — 1) include the *base-wide* foot, *base-narrow* foot, *diagonal* foot, a *too steep* or *too sloping foot axis*, and the *coon foot*.

Additional details can be found in the specialized literature. During practical evaluations, the conformations and foot shapes described sequentially here will be determined contextually. A sample evaluation might be stated as follows: Forelimb from the front: slight base-wide, moderate toe-out limb conformation, medial break in both digital axes, diagonal foot shape.

Behavior of the Foot during Progression

A horse with normal conformation has a straight foot path. When conformation is faulty, the foot is advanced in an arc.

Interfering (see Sec. 2.1.20.2.17.),
Pivoting behind (see Sec. 2.1.20.2.20.),
Overreaching (see Sec. 2.1.20.2.18.),
Foot dragging (see Sec. 2.1.20.2.19.).

Table 2.1.20. — 1. Classification of the healthy and diseased foot

Healthy Foot

Regular foot:	Irregular foot:
normal & regular foot	base-wide foot
narrow & regular foot	base-narrow foot
wide & regular foot	diagonal foot
	foot axis too sloping
	foot axis too steep
	coon foot

Diseased Foot

Pathologic changes in foot shape:	Pathologic changes in horn properties:	Inflammatory processes affecting internal foot structures:
1. Flat foot	1. Wall cracks	1. Shoenail lesions
2. Dropped sole	2. Transverse cracks	2. Injuries of solar epidermis
3. Club foot (acq. upright foot)	3. Loose wall	3. Puncture wound of the foot
4. Peg foot	4. Hollow wall	4. Coronet strike
5. Contracted foot	5. Brittle foot, soft foot	5. Corns
Contracted heel	6. Thrush	6. Inflammation of heel-bulb matrix
Coronary contr.		7. Chronic inflammation of perioplic and coronary epidermis
Solar contr.		8. Lat. cartilage fistula
B.-surf. contr.		9. Canker
6. Crooked foot		10. Keratoma
7. Sidebones		11. Loss of hoof wall
8. Foundered foot (curled foot)		

2.1.20.4.3. Diseases Involving Changes in Foot Shape

Flat Feet

Definition. A flat foot is one in which the weak (thin) horny sole is level with the bearing surface of the wall.

Occurrence. Mainly in the forefeet of heavy breeds, though light horses are also affected.

Symptoms and Diagnosis. Flat feet are usually wide feet with a highly sloping foot axis. Usually there is heavy ring formation in the hoof wall parallel to the coronary band. In some cases only half of the weak horny sole is level with the bearing surface: partial, base-wide or base-narrow flat foot. Separation is often evident between the horn of the wall and sole in the area of the white line at the quarters: loose wall. The wall is low at the heels and may be turned under. The horny frog *appears* to be well developed because it is displaced downward; its clefts are wide and shallow. In the interior of the horny capsule a depression corresponding to the navicular bone is present over the crura of the frog ('navicular depression'). Changes also develop in the distal phalanx: its solar surface becomes flattened, and its dorsal surface

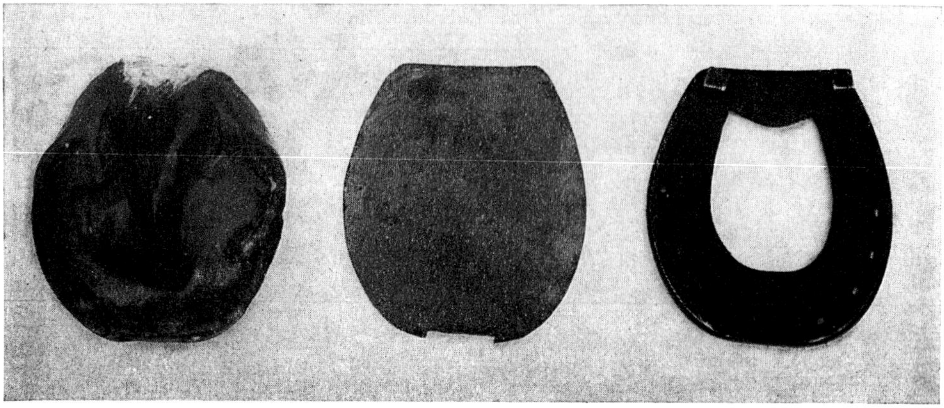

Fig. 2.1.20. — 62. Full-bar shoe with screw calks and full leather foot pad.

shows osteophyte formation with a proliferation and enlargement of the vascular foramina.

Etiology. Causes may be intrinsic or extrinsic. The major intrinsic cause is inherited disposition. The main extrinsic cause is prolonged pasturing on damp ground, which sometimes leads to flat feet through errors of trimming — weakening of the union between sole and wall and undue reduction of the area of shoe contact with the bearing surface, thus giving little or no support to the sole. The use of narrow shoes or shoes with an arched hoof surface can also lead to flat feet.

Differential Diagnosis. Dropped sole, wide foot.

Prognosis. The condition is incurable. The suitability of the horse for work depends upon the competence of the farrier, who trims the foot and applies a hand-forged corrective shoe, generally a full-bar shoe with or without a pad.

Treatment. Treatment consists of corrective trimming and shoeing, whose purpose is to prevent the condition from progressing to a dropped sole.

The horny sole is not trimmed, the circumference of the bearing surface is pared down, any involuted edges are removed, and the horny frog is carefully trimmed. The foot is shod with a thick-branched flat shoe, a calked shoe, or a full-bar shoe with leather pad (fig. 2.1.20. — 62) or perforated Norberg cushion.

Dropped Sole

Definition. In this condition the weak horny sole has dropped below the level of the bearing surface of the wall in the region of the crura of the sole. Dropped sole may be *partial* — base-wide or base-narrow in connection with limb conformation — or *complete*, in which case the entire horny sole is dropped.

Occurrence. The condition affects the front feet and is most common in heavy breeds.

Symptoms. Dropped sole is a more severe form of flat foot; hence its symptoms are similar but more pronounced. The foot is wide and has a highly sloping anterior wall (26—44°). The horny wall shows heavy ring formation parallel to the coronary band. A sign that is pathognomonic for dropped sole is a wedge-shaped or pitlike depression in the wall at the junction of the medial quarter and heel, which, at least in some cases, is genetically linked [Habacher, 1928]. The most pronounced changes are evident on the ground surface of the foot. Besides the dropped, weak horny sole, there are extensive areas of loose wall, low heels that are often turned under at the bearing surface, outward displacement of the bars, a large, low-set frog with shallow sulci, and low-set heel bulbs. The matrix and distal phalanx also show characteristic changes. Alterations in the shape of the lamellae of the wall corium with signs of chronic inflammation indicate strain on the suspensory apparatus of the P3. The shape of the P3 corresponds to that of the horny capsule. It is low, the solar surface is more or less concave, the parietal surface is studded with exostoses, and the wings show signs of rarefying osteitis. In the interior of the hoof wall, the 'navicular depression' previously described for the flat foot is apparent, in addition to changes in the horny lamellae.

Etiology. As in all feet that have undergone a pathologic shape change, *hoof mechanics* are a major cause. The wide shape of the foot apparently predisposes it to dropping of the sole, as does the excessive slope of the anterior wall and in some cases a 'camped in front' conformation (probably symptomatic) that throws more weight on the heels. The increased stress on the deep flexor tendon, which increases further at breakover putting undue stress on the entire suspensory apparatus of the P3, leads to straining of the lamellae, periostitis, and chronic pododermatitis.

All factors that act to weaken the sole promote the development of dropped sole: wet pasture, heavy trimming, especially at the union between wall and sole (white line), weakening of the bars, and the use of open-heeled shoes that are too narrow (!), have a concave or arched hoof surface, or have grabs or calks that remove pressure from the frog. Failure to reset the shoes at regular intervals can lead to anterior elongation of the horny wall and an anterior shift of the bearing surface, which again places increased loads on the caudal half of the foot with increased stress on the deep flexor tendon.

The symptoms listed above are frequently accompanied by a deterioration in the quality of the horn ('pumiced foot'). Matrix lesions are the cause.

As in flat feet, an inherited disposition is presumed.

Differential Diagnosis. In the *flat foot*, the sole is level with the bearing surface. In the *foundered foot*, only the portion of the sole cranial to the apex of the frog is dropped. *Hollow wall* is also associated with a flattening or dropping of the sole in this area.

Diagnosis. The diagnosis is easily made from clinical signs and may be obvious by the manner of weight-bearing. Supplementary radiographs are also helpful and can assist in corrective trimming and shoeing.

Prognosis. No cure is known. The condition can greatly lessen the animal's value, depending on the type of work it performs. Horses with dropped sole require meticulous foot care and special shoeing. Coexisting diseases worsen the prognosis (ossification of the lateral cartilages).

Treatment. The sole is spared during trimming. Only horn that is in the process of being sloughed should be removed. The circumference of the bearing surface should be reduced, the involuted margin of the bearing surface of the heel is pared away, and the horny frog is carefully trimmed (it is dropped and therefore appears thicker than it is). Often it is necessary to create an artificial seating for the shoe by the use of plastic, felt or leather strips. The 'seating' of a horseshoe refers to those parts of the horn that are in contact with the shoe. In the normal foot these are the bearing surface of the wall, the white line, and an equally-wide strip of horny sole. When dropped sole is present, a wider portion of the sole (several times the thickness of the wall) must assist in weight-bearing, depending on the severity of the condition. It should be noted that the weak horny sole drops as a consequence of hoof mechanics, and wide shoe contact is indicated only in cases where the sole

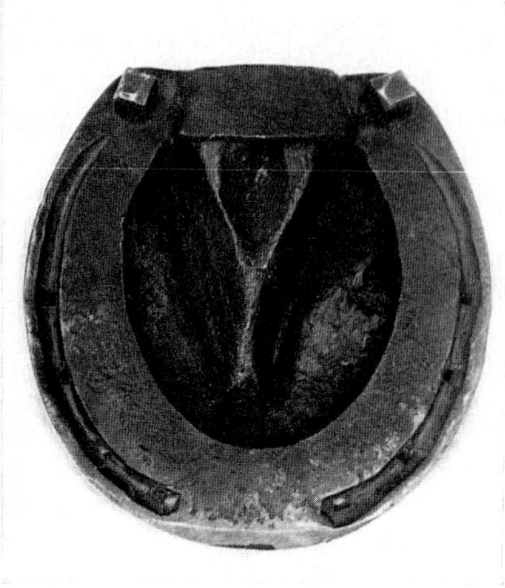

63

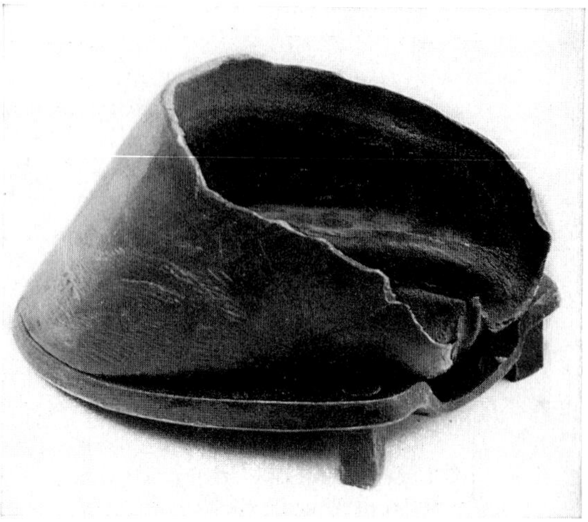

64

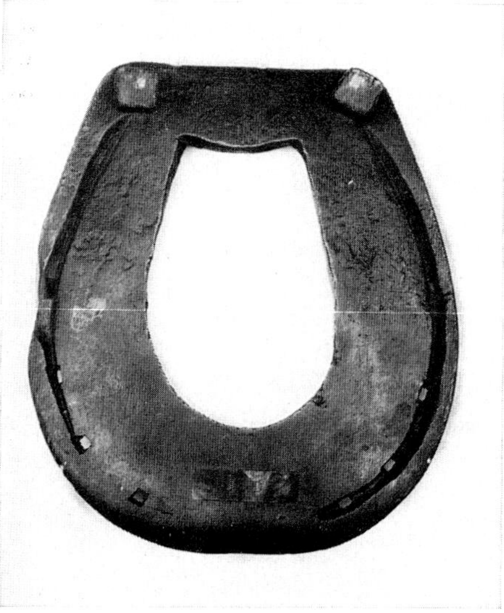

65

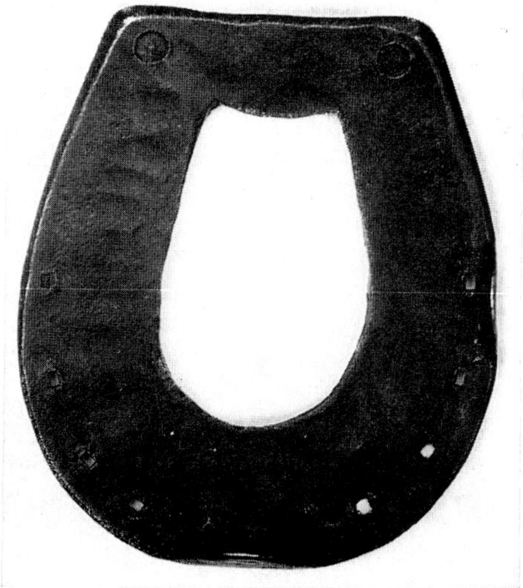

66

Fig. 2.1.20. — 63. Full-bar shoe with heel calks.

Fig. 2.1.20. — 64. Full-bar calked shoe nailed to foot, side view.

Fig. 2.1.20. — 65. Used full-bar shoe with heel calks for dropped sole in a draft horse, ground-surface view.

Fig. 2.1.20. — 66. Used full-bar shoe with heel calks for dropped sole in a draft horse, foot-surface view.

is markedly convex; otherwise matrix contusions and lameness can result. The foot may be shod with a wide-webbed flat shoe or with a full-bar calked shoe (figs. 2.1.20. — 63 through — 66). A skilled farrier is needed to prepare the hoof surface of the shoe. These special shoes cannot be made from factory iron or preformed steel, but must be individually hand-forged from rod stock. Foot pads made from leather or other materials have proved beneficial.

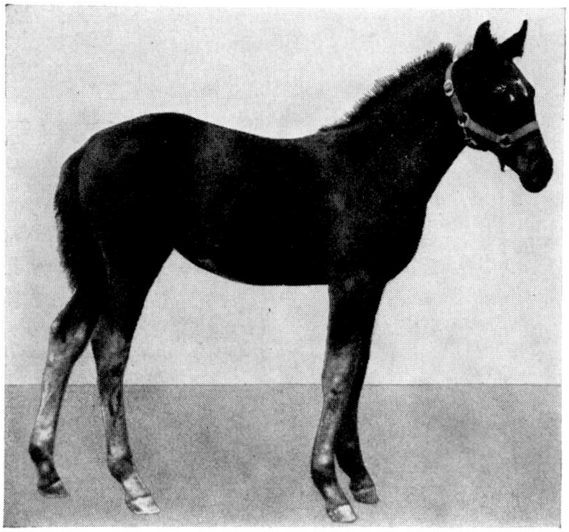
67

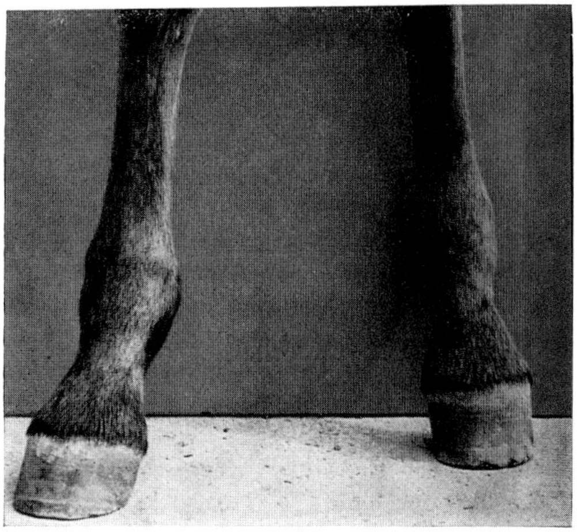
68

Fig. 2.1.20. — 67. Foal with acquired upright front feet.
Fig. 2.1.20. — 68. Foal with acquired upright front feet, cranial view.

Comments. Because many farriers know little about the etiology of dropped sole, cooperation between the veterinarian and farrier is especially important in this condition.

Sometimes a dropped sole is found in very valuable horses, whose further use relies upon proper corrective shoeing.

Club Foot and Acquired Upright Foot

Like flat feet and dropped sole, *club foot, acquired upright foot* and *'peg foot'* are interrelated in the sense that club foot can progress to acquired upright foot and peg foot.

Definition. A *club foot* is one whose anterior wall is abnormally upright but straight (foot axis 60° or more), and in which the heels are too high in relation to the toe.

In *acquired upright foot,* the anterior hoof wall is concave in addition to being abnormally erect (figs. 2.1.20. — 67 through — 69).

Occurrence. Both forefeet are usually affected in young horses, while a single front or hind foot tends to be affected in older animals.

Symptoms. Besides the unphysiologic dorsal angulation of the foot and disproportion between heel and toe, heavy ring formation is visible on the horny walls; these rings diverge at the heel. The horny sole is heavily dished, the frog is deep-set between the bars, and the sulci of the frog are narrow but deep. Weight is borne on the toe at rest and during progression, and the heels bear no weight or do so only momentarily. This faulty weight-bearing can result in crack formation at the toe. The distal phalanx usually shows signs of rarefying osteitis in its dorsal portions.

Etiology. All diseases that interfere with normal dorsiflexion of the fetlock joint can be the cause. These causes may be short- or long-acting: diseases of the tendons, tendon sheath and joints (spavin), bucked knees. Mild forms can result from repeated improper trimming that neglects the principles of the foot and pastern axes. Congenital cases of club foot have also been reported. There is little doubt that modern methods of horse care and nutrition have a significant impact on the development of the extremities, especially the joints, ligaments and tendons.

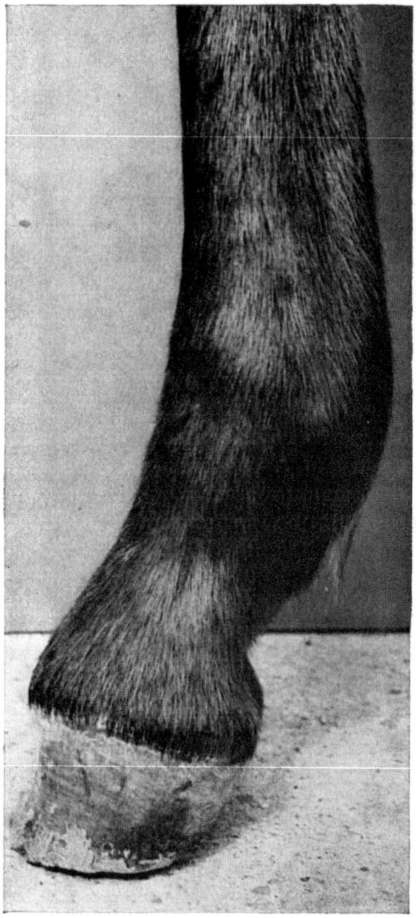

69

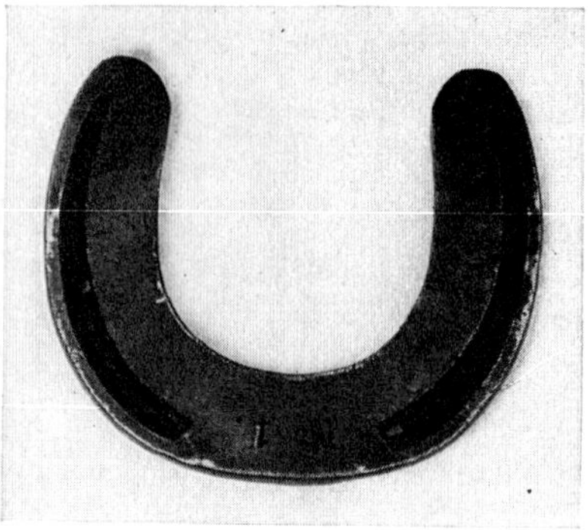

70

Fig. 2.1.20. — 69. Foal with acquired upright front feet, side view of left forefoot. Note concave dorsal wall.

Fig. 2.1.20. — 70. Tip shoe.

Unilateral cases are usually the result of an injury that hampers normal use of the limb. In bilateral cases, inheritance or nutritional deficiencies may be a cause.

Differential Diagnosis. A *steep foot axis* is distinguished by a dorsal angle less than 60°. *Injuries to the caudal part of the foot* (puncture wounds) can produce similar alterations of gait.

The *diagnosis* is readily made from the symptoms described. In young horses the family history and conditions of raising and care should always be investigated. Laboratory tests such as serum calcium, phosphorus, magnesium, alkaline phosphatase, can be performed, but are frequently normal.

The *prognosis* is favorable if the cause can be removed. Possible hereditary defects and/or predispositions should be identified and eliminated.

Treatment. The cause (e.g., tendon or joint disease) is treated. This is supported by corrective trimming and shoeing, as well as proper care and nutrition. With excessive toe wear, a *tip shoe* is applied (fig. 2.1.20. — 70) and may be extended somewhat cranially if necessary to encourage dorsiflexion. Larger (older) horses are shod with thick-branched flat shoes, if necessary with a steel plate welded to the toe in place of a toe clip to reduce wear. Also recommended are shoes with fixed calks whose wear indicates the desired weight shift to the heels, or screw calks that are periodically replaced. Flat shoes with an attached wooden wedge are indicated in more severe cases.

Peg Foot

Definition. 'Peg foot' is the more severe form of club foot or acquired upright foot.

Occurrence. A peg-shaped foot is seen in most cases of knuckling, the conformation fault in which the pastern is upright or deviated forward. Initially weight is borne only on the toe; later the fetlock knuckles over.

Symptoms. The anterior wall angle may be 90° or more. The weak dorsal wall is frequently concave. In many cases the horn acquires a bark-like quality, and rings form that diverge toward the heels as a result of compression in the dorsal wall region. Within the horny capsule, the coronary groove is often twice as wide but much shallower than in the normal foot. This indicates a thin horny wall, a circumstance that must be considered, for example, when repairing wall cracks by clinching. The wall is often considerably higher at the heels than at the toe. The dorsal portion of the horny sole is flattened, and the frog is low. Pressure lesions are evident on the dorsal solar border of P3. In long-standing cases the pathologic loads also result in damage to the articular cartilage of the phalangeal joints and structural changes in the bone.

Etiology. Peg foot is a consequence of knuckling, whose cause may be *arthrogenic*, *tendogenic* or *osteogenic* [Bretschneider, 1909], as described earlier (cf. Sec. 2.1.20.2.12.). A distinction is made between *congenital knuckling*, *acquired knuckling in the foal*, and *knuckling in the mature horse*.

Differential Diagnosis. Knuckling may be confused with puncture wounds of the foot, and in some cases with radial or tibial nerve paralysis.

Diagnosis. Usually a diagnosis is suggested by the history and clinical signs. The clinical diagnosis should be supported with laboratory tests if possible, so that specific treatment can be given.

Prognosis. Favorable to unfavorable, depending on the cause and the age of the horse.

Treatment. See under corresponding tendon and joint diseases. Extended-toe shoe of Neuschild, flat shoe with wooden shim, fiberglass (Lightcast®) casts (strong and lightweight), plastic shims, etc.

Comments. As in other orthopedic conditions of the foot, cooperation between the veterinarian and a skilled farrier is the key to success.

Contracted Foot

Definition. The contracted foot is one whose horny capsule is narrowed in specific areas, leading to reduced space and increased pressure within the hoof. The contraction may affect the heel, coronet, sole, or bearing surface of the wall.

Occurrence. Contractions occur mainly in the front feet of lighter horses, are often bilateral, and sometimes occur as a secondary condition (e.g., to navicular disease) but may also result from lack of exercise.

Contracted Heel

Symptoms. One or both heels are indrawn toward the median plane of the foot. One may speak of 'base-wide' or 'base-narrow' contracted heel, depending on whether the medial or lateral wall is displaced. Often this is associated with an upward displacement of the heel bulb, which is higher than on the unaffected side of the foot. The size of the frog space is correspondingly reduced, and the bar(s) run in arc-shaped fashion to the apex of the frog. The frog is atrophied and is frequently affected with thrush. Sole bruises and 'corns' are also present. Wall cracks are not unusual. In long-standing cases the distal phalanx may become deformed as a result of rarefying or sclerosing osteitis. The pressure increase within the horny capsule predisposes to sidebone.

The horse usually stands with the foot set forward. During progression the animal is inclined to walk on the toe in bilateral cases, manifests a stiff gait, stumbles or goes lame. Compression or percussion of the heel area elicits pain. Palpation usually reveals heat and an increased digital pulse.

The main sequelae are wall cracks, 'corns' and sidebones.

Etiology. Contracted foot results from *intrinsic*, predisposing and *extrinsic* causes. The base-wide foot, base-narrow foot, and foot with a highly sloping axis are all predisposed to contraction of the heel. Moreover, contraction of both heels can occur secondarily to navicular disease or deep thrush. All processes that impair normal dorsiflexion of the fetlock contribute to contracted heel. The condition may also result from inadequate exercise and from a number of trimming and shoeing errors: excessive shortening of the heel, weakening of the bars and frog, or the use of shoes that are too wide, do not support the buttresses, or have a foot surface that is beveled inward.

Differential Diagnosis. The gait is stiff with unilateral involvement of a front foot, and lameness often develops when pain predominates in one limb. When *both* front feet are affected, the gait is stiff and stilted, especially under a rider, and may create the false impression that the seat of the lameness is in the proximal part of the limb, or even in the shoulder joint. Errors of this kind are prevented by conducting a systematic, distal-to-proximal examination of the limb. The experienced examiner knows also that whenever a lameness or locomotor disturbance is present, it is necessary to examine the entire locomotor system, and even the entire animal, during which time a *number of causes* are likely to be discovered. In the foot itself, the changes are highly characteristic, and it is unlikely that contracted heels will be confused with any other disease. Occasionally a mild contraction affecting only one heel may be confused with a base-wide or base-narrow foot.

Diagnosis. The diagnosis is easily made from clinical signs: stiff, stilted gait or lameness, pain at the indrawn heel wall produced by compression and percussion, atrophy of the frog, arc-shaped bars, possible 'corns' at the angle of the sole or wall, and in some cases an increased digital pulse. Diagnostic palmar or plantar nerve block at the fetlock is positive.

Prognosis. The prognosis is favorable if the cause(s) can be removed and normal hoof mechanics can be restored. Other considerations are the age of the horse, its limb and digital conformation, foot shape, the severity of the contraction, the presence or absence of complications, and the use of the animal.

Treatment. When contracted foot is secondary to other disorders, the primary cause must be treated (severe thrush, navicular disease). Thus, expansion of the heels is usually observed following a neurectomy to aid navicular disease. Emphasis is also placed upon sound care and adequate exercise, which is essential for the proper functioning of many systems in the horse.

Many methods are available for expanding the contracted foot, and these are adapted as needed to the individual patient. After first softening the horn, e.g. with moist compresses, baths, or exercise on moist pasture, the condition often can be cured simply by letting the horse go barefoot. Alternatively, corrective shoeing offers many possibilities for foot expansion, and a number of surgical procedures can be performed on the heels.

Corrective trimming: The frog and bars are left untouched; they should continue to exercise their natural function of maintaining (or restoring) normal posterior foot width. The shape of the frog space will indicate whether or not the condition has been corrected. Lines connecting the angles of the wall with each other and with the apex of the frog should form an equilateral triangle, and the bars should be *straight*, not arched. The toe of the foot should be shortened if possible to improve or correct the posterior break in the pastern axis that usually accompanies contracted heel. Much depends upon new horn growth (approx. 8 mm/month), and regular foot care is important from this standpoint.

Corrective shoeing: A thick-branched flat shoe may be used and is applied in such a way that the frog receives ground pressure and thus can exert an expanding action on the foot. The wedge-shaped shoe and tip shoe are also used (figs. 2.1.20. — 71 through — 73), as is the full-bar shoe, usually with a foot pad. At the Viennese Clinic, shoes with an oakum-filled leather pad have been used on many thousands of horses, usually after first making cuts in the hoof wall by the method of Collin [1878] as modified by Habacher [1920]. The actual degree of expansion achieved has been measured in many feet, and the alteration of hoof mechanics has been recorded telemetrically by the use of strain gauges [Knezevic, 1962]. The cushion recommended by Norberg [1968] (fig. 2.1.20. — 74) is also highly beneficial. It is cast to individual shape and hardens through polymerization to form a firm yet soft, permanent mass. The underlying pad of polyurethane or similar material and the cushion itself are *perforated* over the frog as a precaution against thrush. The pressure exerted by this cushion on the sole, frog and bars is excellent for promoting foot expansion, or at least preventing further contraction (fig. 2.1.20. — 75).

An expanding effect is also exerted by shoes in which the web in contact with the wall at the quarter and heel is tapered outward ('slippered') to allow foot expansion.

Surgery of the Heel Wall. In some cases the heel can be thinned with a rasp to quickly reduce pressure within the hoof. This must be done with caution, however, due to the consequent loss of heel stability. A more popular method, therefore, is to place various cuts in the horny wall with the object of weakening the wall in specific areas. Most common are the Collin's cuts as modified by Habacher [1920], and the grooves of Messler, also in a modification that permits favorable attachment of the shoe. The grooving methods of Lungwitz [1910], Smith, Bauer and others are less commonly used. All these cuts and grooves create unsightly blemishes that persist for several months, and the owner should be advised of this before such methods are used.

Wall grooves can be masked if necessary with small cotton rolls and adhesive wax (not, of course, for deceptive purposes).

Coronary Contraction of the Foot

Definition. Coronary contraction of the foot is a contraction at the heels confined to the horn just below the coronet.

Occurrence. Not so common as contracted heels, coronary contraction mainly affects horses that are accustomed to soft going and are made to do work on hard ground (country → city: draft horses). It can also result from other factors that produce a change in hoof mechanics. The front feet are generally affected.

Symptoms. Like contraction of the heels, a coronary contraction may involve the medial or lateral side of the foot, or both. 'Complete' coronary contraction is characterized by hourglass-like constrictions in the area of the heel wall. Affected horses

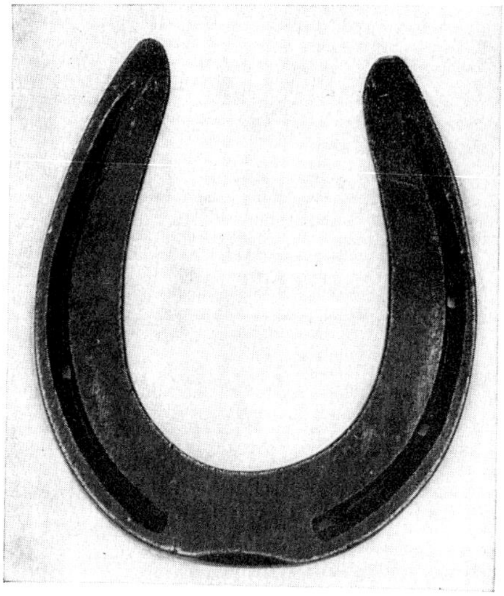

71

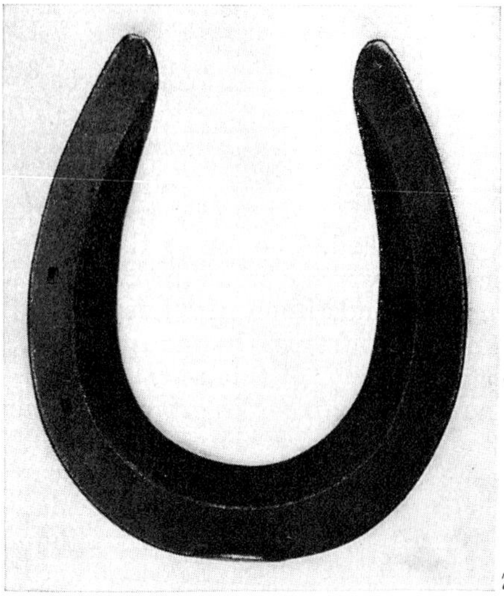

72

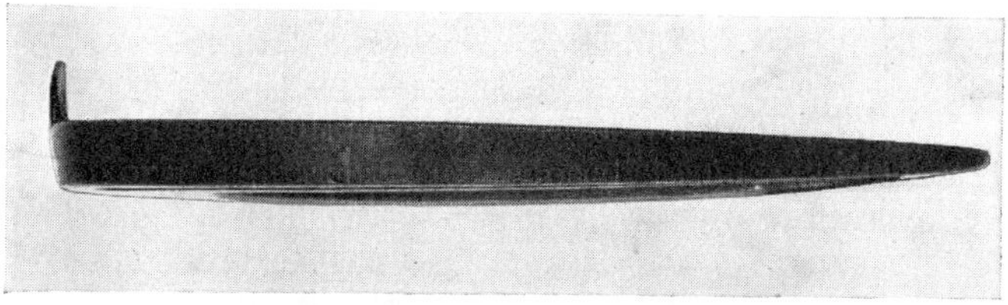

73

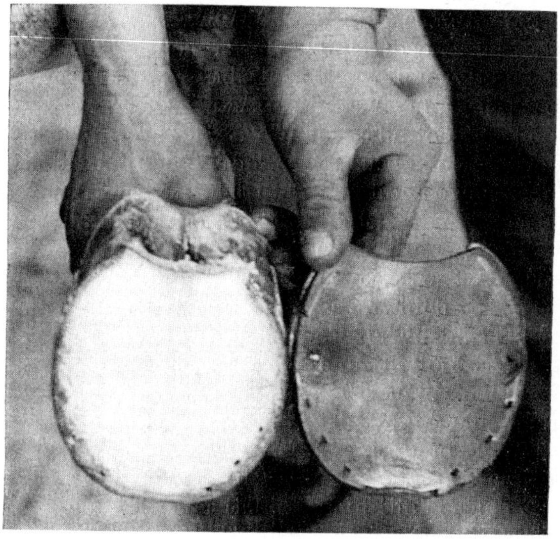

74

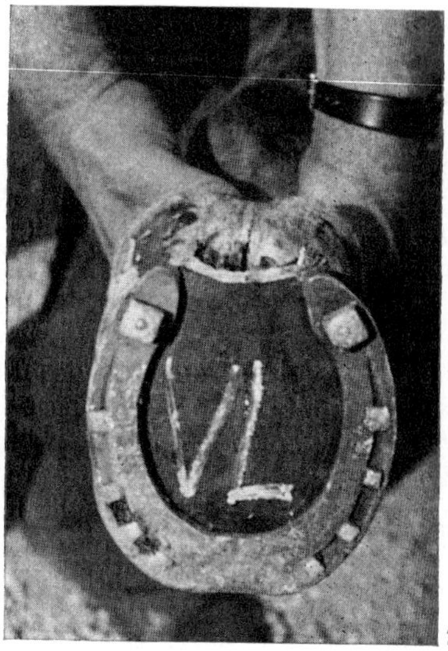

75

Fig. 2.1.20. — 71. Wedge-shaped flat shoe, ground-surface view.
Fig. 2.1.20. — 72. Wedge-shaped flat shoe, foot-surface view.
Fig. 2.1.20. — 73. Wedge-shaped flat shoe, side view.
Fig. 2.1.20. — 74. The Norberg cushion.
Fig. 2.1.20. — 75. The Norberg cushion inserted between foot and shoe (left front).

show a stiff gait or go lame. Pain is produced at the site of the constriction by percussion or by compression with a hoof tester. With a 'partial' coronary constriction, the heel wall is concave on the affected side of the foot.

Etiology. Besides a change in ground pressure, the disease may be caused by excessive wall growth, shoeing with open-heeled calked shoes, or neglect of foot care. As in contracted heels, a pathologic change in hoof mechanics is the precipitating factor.

Diagnosis. The hourglass-like constriction in complete coronary contraction and the unilateral concavity of the heel in partial coronary contraction, with associated tenderness to compression and percussion, are easily recognized and are unlikely to be confused with other disorders.

Prognosis. The prognosis is generally favorable in young horses, and in cases where a skilled farrier is available.

Treatment. Severe cases are treated by grooving the wall over the heel (MESSLER'S method) and applying moist compresses. A full-bar shoe is accurately fitted to the hoof. If pain is severe, the bearing surface at the heel does not touch the shoe, but the angle of the wall is carefully supported. A full-bar shoe with leather foot pad offers the best protection against coronary contraction in many heavy draft horses as well as in light horses that do work on paved surfaces.

Solar Contraction of the Foot

This condition is very rare. The concavity of the sole is increased ('dished sole'), exerting pressure on enclosed structures. The longitudinal diameter of the hoof is greatly reduced. The anterior hoof wall is convex, as in coon-footed horses. The heels are turned under.

Etiology. Thick hoof wall, neglect of foot care, short shoe.

Differential Diagnosis. In coon-footed horses the foot has the same appearance, but the sole is not tender to pressure. If lameness is present, navicular disease and pododermatitides of other etiology must be excluded.

Prognosis and Treatment. The increased concavity of the sole may be difficult or impossible to correct. The foot is shod with a tip shoe or H-shaped flat shoe so that natural ground pressure is placed on the toe and heels.

Comments. Farriers and horseowners should be informed about the harmful effects of shoes that are too short.

Bearing-Surface Contraction of the Foot

This is a rare disorder in which the circumference of the bearing surface is reduced, causing pressure to be exerted on enclosed structures. Viewed from the front, the coronary circumference of the foot appears larger than the bearing surface.

Etiology. RUTHE [1950] suggests that the contracted bearing surface represents the persistence of a normal ontogenic form of the hoof.

Differential Diagnosis. At about the age of 9 months, the foot of light horses possesses this inverted conical shape. Later the circumference of the bearing surface becomes greater than that of the coronary band.

Treatment. The horse is left unshod or is shod with a full-bar shoe and Norberg cushion.

Crooked Foot

Definition. A 'crooked foot' is one in which the quarter and heel are concave on one side and convex on the other. Usually the longer half of the wall is convex, and the shorter concave.

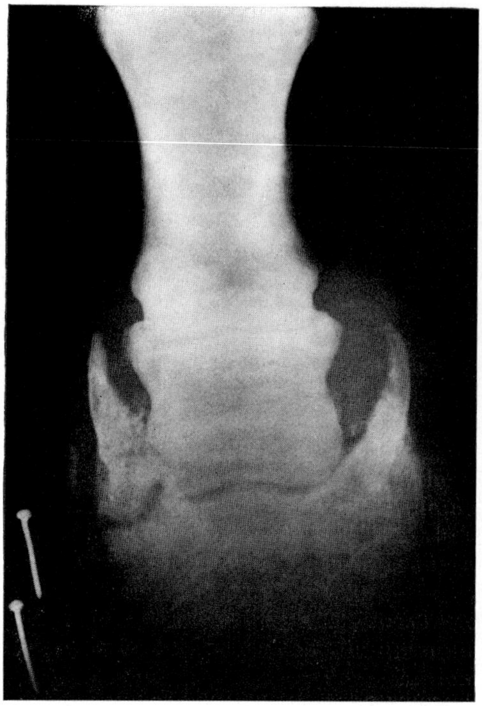

76

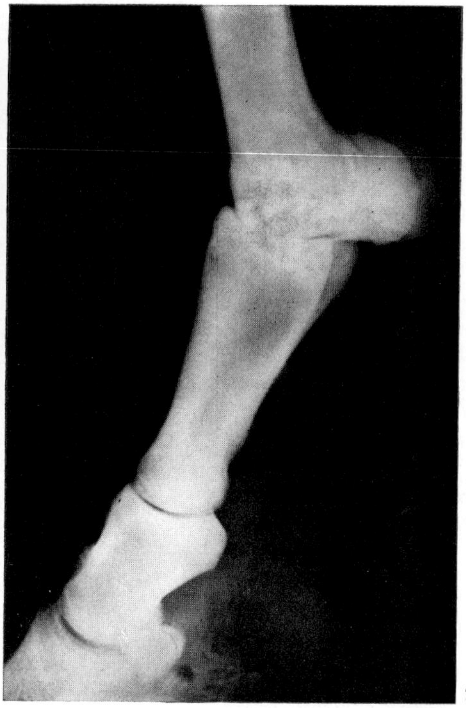

77

Fig. 2.1.20. — 76. Partial ossification of both lateral cartilages (right front, dorso-palmar projection).

Fig. 2.1.20. — 77. Partial ossification of both lateral cartilages (latero-medial projection).

Occurrence. The hind feet are most commonly affected.

Symptoms. In the shod horse, the front feet tend to be concave on the *medial* side, and the hind feet on the *lateral* side. The deformity may be so severe that the convex wall becomes the bearing surface. Often a lateral break is present in the digital axis. The heel bulb tends to be higher on the convex side. The portion of the sole bordering on the concave quarter is flattened, and the horny frog and bars are displaced. Wall cracks and loose walls are often encountered. Ligamentous and tendinous changes have also been described. The transverse axes of the joints may be sloping. The phalanges become deformed and are rotated about their long axis. Osteitis and osteophyte formation at ligament insertions are common. The foot axis is out of alignment with the pastern.

Etiology. Crooked foot is caused by uneven foot wear associated with load disparities and neglected foot care, especially in animals at pasture. It can also result from faulty trimming and shoeing. A wall that is repeatedly left too long at shoeing and is supported by a branch that turns in too much at the quarter and heel causes unequal loads to be placed on the foot, resulting in hoof deformity. In particular, the *lateral shear force* that is often associated with faults of limb and digital conformation leads to the development of crooked foot.

Differential diagnosis. Crooked foot may be confused with the base-wide or base-narrow foot or with partial contraction of the foot on superficial examination.

Diagnosis. Generally the characteristic hoof deformity is readily apparent even when the horse is viewed from the front.

Prognosis. The prognosis depends on the degree of pathologic changes that have developed, coexisting faults of digital and limb conformation, and the gait and age of the horse. Severe articular changes (radiography) indicate a poor prognosis.

Treatment. Primary treatment is directed toward the causes of faulty conformation and gait. Excellent results, even cures, can be achieved by taking a vigorous, consistent approach to the treatment of foals and young horses. One should not hesitate to employ operative means if necessary (transphyseal bridging (stapling), wedge osteotomies, etc.) as well as corrective wraps and bandages combined with an individualized program of exercise therapy. Development of techniques in this area of equine orthopedics correspond closely to those in human orthopedics.

Corrective trimming and shoeing also form an essential part of the treatment regimen. The high convex portions of the wall are lowered, and the bearing surface on the concave parts of the wall is reduced by vertical rasping. The special hand-forged shoe is set wider (creased more deeply) on the convex side of the hoof. If this branch is on the lateral side, there will be no danger of interfering, and one can go farther out and even have a *base-wide* correction on the outside edge of the shoe. The branch for the concave side of the hoof has a shallower crease — the crease must always face the outer edge of the white line — and has base-narrow correction (inside branch) if interfering is a danger.

The condition is considered to be cured when the foot has a normal or nearly-normal shape, shows acceptable deviation in ground contact, and is in satisfactory alignment with the pastern and remainder of the limb.

Comments. The trimming and shoeing of a crooked foot require orthopedic knowledge on the part of the farrier. Consistency is also called for as gradual progress is made. A competent, reliable farrier working hand in hand with the veterinarian is of great value in the treatment of this condition.

2.1.20.4.4. Ossification of the Lateral Cartilages

Definition. Ossification of the lateral cartilages, also called 'sidebones', is a disease in which the elastic hoof cartilage becomes transformed into bony tissue (figs. 2.1.20. — 76 and — 77).

Occurrence. Sidebones affect mainly the front feet of heavy breeds. Lateral sidebone is more common than medial sidebone. Sidebones are occasionally seen in the athletic horse but are rare in the Thoroughbred. The disease has also been reported in young horses.

Symptoms. Sidebones cause a supporting-leg lameness in unilateral cases, or produce a stiff, choppy, stilted gait when *both* front feet are affected. The cause of the gait disturbance is pain stemming mainly from contusions ('corns') of the wall and sole matrix.

Ossification confined to the distal parts of the cartilages cannot be palpated directly but an experienced examiner can make a presumptive diagnosis from the unusual rigidity of the non-ossified portion. The diagnosis is established by radiography. The coronary band of the affected foot is widened. The ossified hoof cartilage presents an often knobby, sievelike surface with numerous osteophytes. The proximal border of the affected cartilage is thickened and uneven compared to the narrow, smooth border of the healthy cartilage. The wings of the P3 usually show changes characteristic of rarefying osteitis. Often what appears to be a fracture occurs in the ossified cartilage. However, this presumed fracture could be interpreted as a 'hinge' that develops as a consequence of hoof mechanics (cartilage mechanics). Sometimes the ossification spreads to involve the ligaments that connect the lateral cartilages with the P1, P2 and navicular bone, as well as the plantar cushion and coffin joint ('ringbone of the coffin joint').

Etiology. Causes may be predisposing or precipitating (immediate). Some authors suggest that the disease is inherited. *Predisposing causes* include body weight, use (types of gait), ground characteristics, limb and digital conformation, and certain foot diseases and conformation faults: base-wide, base-narrow, dropped sole, and especially contracted foot (contracted heels). Precipitating causes are repeated, severe concussions, especially in feet with poor support (improper trimming and shoeing). Other causes are calked shoes, disparaties of wall height, and uneven foot landing with tipping of the foot (thrown calks, uneven terrain) causing constant strain on the hoof cartilage and its ligaments, especially at the wings of P3 where the lateral cartilages are attached. Except in cases of 'insular' sidebone, this is the area where the ossification process begins. Constant strains at the junction of P3 and lateral cartilage lead to tissue irritation and chronic inflammation, and the inflamed wing resumes its earlier growth. According to WESTHUES and MUSZAR, this growth of the wing into the lateral cartilage proceeds from the upper (proximal) process of the wing. In some cases the lower (distal) process of the wing may also show growth resumption, but this process tends to elongate horizontally in the direction of the solar border of P3. The ossified portions of the cartilage lead to contusions of the wall and sole matrix ('corns').

Differential Diagnosis. Low ringbone periostitis, periarthrosis. The diagnosis is confirmed by radiography: two standard views supplemented with oblique and tangential views of the wings of the distal phalanx.

Diagnosis. Inspection, palpation, and finally radiography enable a definitive diagnosis to be made.

Prognosis. The prognosis depends on the degree of ossification, the age of the horse, its use, and the presence or absence of complications (dropped sole, contracted foot, ringbone, brittle foot).

Treatment. The goal of treatment is to relieve lameness. In early cases this can often be done by the use of cuts or grooves to expand the wall (modified from COLLIN or MESSLER and LUNGWITZ) in connection with corrective trimming and the application of a fitted, full-bar shoe with leather pad.

We have had success with partial extirpation of the ossified cartilage by the method of RIEHLEIN-MEIER, in which the cartilage is approached through a proximal skin incision.

Corrective trimming, shoeing, and the early placement of expansion cuts in the wall are the best preventive measures.

2.1.20.4.5. Laminitis

Definition. Laminitis, or founder, is a multifactorial disease, of which diffuse septic pododermatitis is only one aspect.

Occurrence. One, two, or all four feet may be affected, depending on the cause, but in most cases only the front feet are involved.

Symptoms. The symptoms of laminitis from all causes are similar. A distinction is made between the acute and chronic form.

Acute laminitis has a sudden onset and is accompanied by systemic and local manifestations. Systemic signs include an elevation of temperature (39—41 °C), increased pulse and respiratory rate, sweating and muscular tremors. Often the appetite is unaffected. Other signs are pain in the toe and sole area, leading to the characteristic stance in which the feet are placed forward of their normal position. The gait is stiff and halting with a *two-beat foot landing:* first on the heel, then on the toe. Progression, especially turning, causes obvious pain, and this is reflected in the animal's behavior. This mode of behavior is explained by the localization of the painful lesions in the cranial half of the foot. Tenderness to pressure (hoof tester) and percussion is evident in the cranial part of the sole and in the area of the dorsal wall. If all four feet are involved, it is difficult even to lift the legs for examination. Heat is palpable in these parts of the foot and in the dorsal coronet, and increased pulsation is felt in the palmar digital arteries and palmar artery or in the plantar arteries. Colicky symptoms may also appear in some cases.

Rotation of the P3 is a rightly feared and irreversible complication of laminitis. It may occur within 3 days after symptoms first appear. Rotation of the P3 may be inferred from a palpable indrawing of the coronet or can be demonstrated with radiographs. The course is variable. Either spontaneous healing occurs within 8—14 days, or the condition becomes chronic, resulting in the typical 'foundered foot'. Pressure from the displaced bone can cause pressure necrosis of the solar matrix and later a perforation of the sole. Other possible complications are loss of the hoof wall, metastatic pneumonia, and septicemia.

Chronic laminitis is seldom primary and usually develops from the acute form. Chronic laminitis with acute flareups is not uncommon. The *foundered foot* or *curled foot* is a common feature of chronic laminitis and develops subsequent to rotation of P3. In other cases the 3rd phalanx may simply recede from the anterior wall without rotating (radiography). Rotation of the phalanx is accompanied by an indrawing of the dorsal coronet. The horny walls of the foundered foot show a characteristic pattern of ring formation: rings close together at the dorsal wall (or dorsal coronet) and farther apart at the heels. Particular attention should be given to this symptom when examining a horse for purchase. The rings can also be used forensically to estimate the age of the condition. A curl composed of laminar horn develops in the distal part of the anterior wall (fig. 2.1.20. — 78), and this also results in a widening of the white line. The walls are high at the heel, and the bottom of the foot acquires a convex shape. The distal phalanx may even protrude through the horny sole. In most cases a 'hollow wall' is present at the toe. The horn is friable and is often broken away at the ground border. The distal phalanx may show signs of rarefying osteitis, a hat-brim-like curl of its dorsal solar border, and eventual atrophy (radiographs).

Etiology. Recent studies point to certain correlations, or risk factors, in the etiology of laminitis. These include age, sex, season and breed. Risks are equally high for males and females, although castration in the male apparently reduces the risk nearly by half. Ponies are at significantly greater risk than large horses. Mares are most comonly affected between the ages of 4 and 7 years, and stallions between the ages of 7 and 10.

Experiments conducted in recent years with acute 'grain founder' have repeatedly demonstrated the presence of circulatory and hematologic changes (heart rate, arterial and venous blood pressure, hematocrit, leukocytes, total protein) in addition to fluctuations of rectal temperature. All horses manifested these blood changes prior to the appearance of lameness or locomotor disturbances. Histopathologic changes are thought to be related to *decreased* perfusion of the matrix. Besides the known

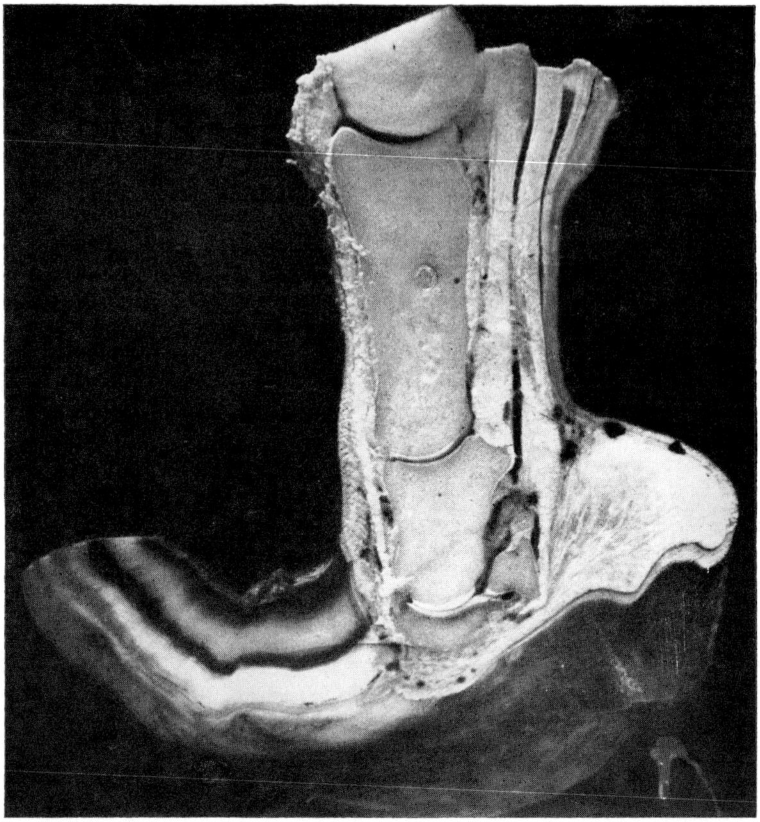

Fig. 2.1.20. — 78. Curled foot in chronic laminitis (longitudinal section).

symptoms and those just described, an elevation of blood pressure has also been observed in both acute and chronic laminitis.

Fast work on hard ground, long-distance rides, riding and driving at fast gaits, and even prolonged standing in transportation vehicles or on hard ground with the foot improperly trimmed and shod can lead to *traumatic laminitis* ('road founder'). Included in this category is the increased stress placed on the sound foot as a result of disease in the adjacent limb: *stress laminitis*.

Toxic laminitis is observed following the ingestion of fresh grain feeds such as corn, barley, wheat, oats, bran and rye, as well as molasses, legumes or fresh hay: *grain founder*. The toxin histidine, which is formed during the digestion of grains, is decarboxylated to histamine, and this causes the laminitis, as experiments have confirmed [ÅKERBLOM, 1934]. Cooking, steaming or soaking the grain inhibits the histamine effect. Laminitis can also be caused by pharmaceutical products such as aloe and tartar emetic, by the topical use of petroleum, crude oil, etc., by the ingestion of locust tree bark, cuckoo-flower *(Cardamine pratensis)* and castor seeds, as well as by herbicides and, in recent years, by the administration of corticoids and phenylbutazone. The form known as *postparturient laminitis* should probably be included in the 'toxic' category.

Metastatic laminitis can develop as a sequel to severe infectious diseases (contagious pleuropneumonia, influenza). An endarteritis can follow viral respiratory diseases in the horse.

Pathogenesis. As mentioned earlier, laminitis is a systemic illness in which pathologic processes in the foot produce a highly characteristic set of symptoms.

The early stage of acute laminitis is marked by hyperemia, serous suffusion and cellular infiltration of the anterior-wall matrix. This may spread to involve matrix tissues of the quarters and adjoining sole. This serous, serofibrinous and/or hemorrhagic exudation eventually leads to separation between the matrix and anterior horny wall, and apparently affects the entire suspensory apparatus of the P3 in such a way that this bone is allowed to rotate and descend. It is thought that the forward placement of the limbs in the 'founder stance' promotes this rotation by placing increased tension on the deep flexor tendon and other structures. The rotation is accompanied by a sagging of the dorsal coronet and kinking of the horn tubules, causing annular grooves to form in the hoof wall.

Differential Diagnosis. Laminitis must be differentiated from acute pododermatitides of other etiology, contusions, and purulent pododermatitis.

Diagnosis. Most cases of laminitis are easily diagnosed from observable signs. The history alone provides important clues.

Prognosis. Generally a guarded prognosis is indicated. The outcome depends upon the cause, the number of feet involved, the shape of the feet, the quality of foot care, the body weight of the horse, etc. Horses with P3 rotation are suited only for very limited work (breeding) on account of their shuffling, stumbling gait.

Treatment. Treatments vary widely depending on the cause. However, the time elapsed between the onset of the symptoms and initiation of treatment is a crucial factor in all cases. Thus, laminitis, like colic or fractures, must always be dealt with as an emergency.

General Therapy. The cause or causes are removed. Grain and hay feeding are suspended. The shoes are pulled, and the horse is confined to a roomy box stall with adequate bedding. Treatment has included the i.v. administration of 8% sodium bicarbonate (4—8 liters, depending on size and circulatory status), antihistamines, circulatory agents, dextrose and electrolytes as needed (especially with diarrhea), spasmolytics (metapyrine = noramidopyrine methane sulfonate sodium). Gentle exercise is also beneficial if the animal is able to walk. In the past, other nonspecific treatments have included heavy bloodletting.

Treatment of the Foot with Acute Laminitis. Generally it is best to remove the shoes. The anterior walls are thinned with a rasp. In some cases good results have been achieved (prevention of P3 rotation) by filling in the sole with plaster under a covered shoe or by applying an acrylic (Technovit) with a hardwood sole combined with exercise.

Treatment of the Foundered Foot (Curled Foot). The curled toe is removed by sawing or rasping, and the heels are lowered to reestablish a normal relation between the distal phalanx, hoof wall and ground. The sole is not trimmed due to the danger of perforation.

Corrective Shoeing. The toe of the shoe is wide and extends back to the apex of the frog. The foot surface of the shoe is beveled so that the hoof mechanics of the convex anterior sole is not disturbed; the ground surface is flat. Either a thick-branched flat shoe or full-bar shoe with leather pad or Norberg cushion may be used. The shoe must be comfortably seated on the foot. The nail holes should be located at the quarters and heels. If the ground border of the toe is broken away, it is replaced with a suitably shaped leather strip. The shoe must fit but should not be too heavy.

This is where the farrier's skills come into play. A competent blacksmith can restore this seriously diseased foot to serviceable condition. The founder shoe of Bolz [1939] has also been successfully used in some cases.

We have not found that grooving of the hoof wall [Gross; Bayer, 1890; Hanslian] significantly improves results.

Comments. It is important that owners, riders and attendants be well informed as to the signs and dangers of laminitis, inasmuch as hoof deformity can be prevented by early treatment. If the laminitis becomes chronic, all efforts are directed toward the prevention of acute flareups. Trimming and special shoeing are the job of the farrier. A program of meticulous foot care is also indicated.

2.1.20.4.6. Conditions Involving Changes in the Horn

Wall Cracks

Definition. These are disruptions in the continuity of the hoof wall that run in the direction of the horn tubules. The crack may originate at the bearing surface and extend up the hoof wall, or may originate at the coronary band and extend downward. Cracks are identified with the part of the hoof affected: toe, quarter, heel, sole, bar or frog. They may also be characterized as superficial or deep, or as 'complete' if they involve both the the coronary band and the bearing surface. Wall cracks may become complicated by infection or suppuration.

Cracks Involving the Coronary Band. These may occur at the toe, quarter or heel. They are most common in abnormally-shaped or diseased front feet and usually affect the medial side. A steep or vertical foot axis also predisposes to cracking at the toe.

Symptoms. Fresh wall cracks usually present as fine fissures about 2—3 cm long with smooth edges that are soiled with fresh or dried blood. Most cracks cause some degree of lameness, which prompts the owner to seek veterinary help. Often the crack goes unnoticed in its early stage, especially if it causes no lameness or locomotor disturbance. Later, however, the crack will become obvious as it grows longer and wider, presenting edges that are smooth, zigzagged or overlapping. If the hoof is examined closely as pressure on it is alternately exerted and released during walking or standing, an alternating expansion and contraction of the crack will be evident as a consequence of hoof mechanics. Toe cracks close when weight is placed on the foot and open when the foot is raised; heel and quarter cracks work in the opposite way. Deep cracks involving the sensitive laminae can become infected, leading to a suppurative pododermatitis that may progress to a subcoronary cellulitis or even to a lateral cartilage fistula (quittor). With prolonged inflammation of the hoof matrix, keratoma formation is not uncommon. Prolapse of the matrix can result from improper treatment that causes expansion of the crack or creates a space between the horseshoe and angle of the wall. Generally a wall crack is not difficult to detect, although it may be accidentally or purposely hidden from view by mud, tar, wax, long hairs, etc. This should be considered during pre-purchase examination. Once detected, a wall crack should be identified as being deep or superficial; usually this presents no difficulties.

Etiology. Causes may be predisposing or extrinsic.

Predisposing causes: Horses with faults of limb and digital conformation are predisposed due to the unequal loads on the feet that place undue strain on the coronary band and other structures. Feet with weak, thin horny walls are commonly affected with cracks. The deficient production of keratin contributes much to the development of wall cracks. The significance of hereditary factors in this deficiency remains unclear. Additional predisposing causes are partial contraction of the foot with displacement of the heel, the 'peg foot' with its thin, weak anterior wall, and feet with chronic inflammation of the perioplic and coronary epidermis. In feet with an abnormally steep axis (acquired upright foot, club foot, peg foot), the upright position of the pastern causes excessive strain to be placed on the dorsal coronet as the foot is pushing off, causing the thin anterior wall to split at the upper part of the coronary band. Season also appears to be a factor, wall cracks being most prevalent during the spring and fall.

Extrinsic causes: These causes are mainly responsible for the increased incidence of wall cracks and are based largely on neglect of foot care, errors of trimming and shoeing, and work on hard ground. Improper foot care leads to excessive drying of the horn, with a consequent weakening of the wall. Rancid, acid-containing hoof ointments have a similar effect. Improper trimming of the foot can have lasting adverse effects. Walls of unequal height that do not correspond to the limb conformation cause greater pressure and counterpressure to be exerted on one half of the foot, causing an abnormal expansion of the coronary band. Short shoes with close-set heels have a similar effect. A frequent cause is an absence of contact between the shoe and angle of the wall. Lowering of the heels for severe dropping of the fetlock places increased tension on an area of the coronet that is unable to resist the internal hoof pressure and pull of the unsupported heel, causing a crack to form in that area. If a line is drawn perpendicular to the plane of the bearing surface at the site where shoe support is absent, this line will intersect the coronet at a point where initial crack formation is most likely to occur. This is especially true in the case of heel cracks. In addition, wall cracks often develop following coronet strikes due to partial destruction of the papillary body of the perioplic and coronary epidermis. Not infrequently, hoof cracks are observed following removal of the heel wall subsequent to purulent or gangrenous pododermatitis. Fast work on hard ground can also contribute to the occurrence of the disease. This is frequently observed in riding horses and especially in Standardbreds, which race at a forced gait, often have thin hoof walls, and commonly suffer from contraction of the foot.

Prognosis. When cracks form in the otherwise healthy foot, a favorable prognosis is usually indicated. In some cases an *inherited defect* is the cause. Bilateral involvement can cause a lameness or locomotor disturbance that renders the horse unsound for work. Some wall cracks cause purulent inflammation that may lead to serious sequelae such as subcoronary cellulitis, lateral cartilage fistula (quittor), cellulitis of the plantar cushion, necrosis of the deep flexor tendon, septic arthritis, and even loss of the hoof wall. This condition is difficult to control in *deformed hoofs*, e.g., in cases of toe crack or ringbone of the dorsal coffin or pastern joint, and in feet that are subject to faults of limb conformation. The use of the animal should be considered during the evaluation. The presence of wall cracks necessarily lessens the value of the horse and will affect its selling price. Cracks heal by 'growing out', i.e., by the growth of new, undisrupted horn from the perioplic, coronary and wall matrix.

Treatment. The goal of treatment is to close the wall crack and secure the closure until new horn growth repairs the defect. A split in the horny wall can never be made to 'grow back together'. Nevertheless, it is important that the edges of the crack be immobilized in close approximation, for otherwise hoof mechanics will compel relative movement of the edges, causing irritation of the matrix with undesired 'healing' by excessive keratin production (keratoma). Secure fixation will also prevent extension of the lesion. As in other diseases, moreover, therapy directed at the cause is emphasized: the cause of the wall crack is identified and removed if possible. Healing usually occurs if prompt, suitable treatment is given. Control of weight bearing generally is crucial to successful healing. Therefore, much emphasis is placed upon correct trimming and proper seating of the shoe. As mentioned, immobilization of the crack edges is an important adjunct to therapy. This can be accomplished by the use of fixed dressing (see below), clips, pins, metal plates, or PVC films. In addition, the modified operation of Collin or other stress-relieving measures are often very useful, especially in the contracted foot. The operative treatment of suppurating wall cracks requires special care due to the danger of complications. In the early stage of inflammation, cooling antiseptic poultices and several days' rest are indicated.

The goal of trimming is a level foot landing, and especially the relief of stress on the affected parts of the wall, which often are too high. By trimming the foot in this fashion and then allowing the horse to go barefoot, many wall cracks will heal spontaneously. Unfortunately this method is suitable in only a select patient group. The modern 'plastic shoes' (usually polyurethane), which sometimes are used in Standardbreds owing to their light weight, are soft and do not give the foot adequate protection. Defects and cracks in the bearing surface are the result. The foot may be shod with a full-bar shoe with leather pad or Norberg cushion, a thick-branch flat shoe or an ordinary flat shoe. Care must be taken that the angle of the wall is well supported when fitting the shoe. Before the shoe is attached, the bearing surface of the wall should be lowered by about 2 mm between two points defined as follows: (1) the point where a line dropped from the start of the crack at the coronet intersects the ground border, and (2) the point on the ground border intersected by a linear extension of the crack line. This procedure is called 'lowering the wall from the shoe'.

Sometimes it is advisable to attach a small leather strip to the shoe branch to protect the delicate angle of the wall. This will absorb shocks, yet still provide support for the wall angle. This simple measure has proved to be of very great value in feet with corns.

Various methods are available for immobilizing the crack edges to promote healing and prevent extension:

1. A *fixed dressing* consisting of a 2-cm-wide twill tape can be applied to hoofs with an extremely thin wall. This tape acts to limit the mobility of the crack edges and lower the risk of infection. A twill tape of suitable length, usually 2—3 meters, is coated on one or both sides with adhesive hoof wax, rolled, and then applied to the degreased hoof. The hairs at the coronet should be clipped beforehand so that they will not be incorporated into the dressing, as this may cause pain with associated disturbances of gait.

2. *Clasps* are wire clamps about 2 mm thick whose tips are bent and sharpened. They are driven staple-fashion into the horny wall and are an effective means of holding the borders of a crack together. The instruments needed to apply the clasp are a firing iron and a forceps for closing the clasp into place (clamping iron). With the red-hot firing iron, two notches are burned into the wall, one on each side of the crack and about a finger's width from it, at the distal border of the coronary groove and parallel to the coronet. The tips of the clasp are driven into these notches with the clamping iron; usually half the thickness of the seated clasp projects above the level of the wall. Before the clasp is applied, it is important to confirm that the width of the firing iron coincides with the width of the clamping iron, lest difficulties arise. To ensure that the sharp tips of the clasp close equally and that one tip does not penetrate too deeply (possibly pricking the matrix and leading to a suppurative inflammation), the clamping iron should be closed by only about half when first securing the clasp, and then turned over before closing the rest of the way. Clasps

are excellent for repairing quarter and heel cracks. If the crack shows considerable gaping, the space should be filled with a leather strip or with soft plastic, and the clamps should not be closed too tightly. Wound care also is administered.

3. *Clinches.* Clinching, or cross-pinning, is an effective means of immobilizing toe cracks. For this purpose a small notch is again cut or burned into the wall about 2 cm from the crack on each side at the lower edge of the coronary band. From each notch a drill hole is made through the horn to the middle of the crack, extending in depth to about half the wall thickness. The appearance of horn shavings in the fissure indicates that the crack has been reached. Each pair of drill holes should lie on a straight line that is parallel to the coronary band. The diameter of the hole must correspond to that of the clinch, which consists of a pin of tough iron or a large horse-shoe nail (2 or 2.2 mm size). The pin or nail is driven into the predrilled channel and its ends bent over. Then the edge of a rasp is placed against one end of the pin and a clinching tool against the other, and the pin is clinched with a few hammer taps. Finally the ends of the clinch are cut and filed smooth, in the same way that nails are rasped after shoeing. The clinching of toe cracks in the peg foot requires special caution due to the wide coronary band and thin anterior wall. Usually 2—3 clinches spaced 10—15 mm apart are sufficient.

4. *Metal plates.* A small metal plate about 2 mm thick, 12—14 mm wide and 35—40 mm long is provided with 6 holes, heated, and then pressed transversely over the wall crack near the coronary border to make a slight depression in the horn for better seating of the plate. After cooling, the plate is fitted into the prepared seat and attached with small wood screws (flat-head wood screws) whose length corresponds to the wall thickness. This technique has proved particularly useful for closing cracks with *overlapping edges.*

For heel cracks in contracted feet, the Habacher modification of Collin's operation is carried out, and the crack edges are immobilized with a fixed dressing or clasp.

The efficacy of all the foregoing methods is enhanced by sound concurrent foot care.

5. *PVC films.* Noninfected wall cracks and especially heel cracks involving the coronet can be securely immobilized by attaching PVC (polyvinylchloride) films to the hoof with a two-component fast-setting adhesive. The technique is relatively simple and inexpensive and has numerous advantages over traditional methods.

Following corrective trimming and lowering of the bearing surface from the shoe (see above), a full-bar shoe is applied to the foot. Then the area surrounding the wall crack is smoothed with a rasp and finally with sandpaper. The hoof is then carefully degreased by repeated cleaning with grease solvents (trichloroethylene). The PVC film, about 0.3 mm thick, is cut to proper size. After the crack has been treated with sulfonamide or antibiotic powder, the film is coated with adhesive, applied over the crack, and pressed out carefully to eliminate air bubbles. This is most easily done with a piece of cellophane laid over the PVC film. After about 4 minutes when the adhesive is dry, the cellophane is removed together with any excess glue.

Normally the film will last for at least one shoeing period and will grow down toward the bearing surface along with the crack. Both the film and adhesive can be trimmed and rasped with the horn.

Transverse Cracks

Definition. A transverse crack is a disruption of the horny wall that runs perpendicular to the direction of the horn tubules.

Occurrence. Most transverse cracks occur at the toe and quarters of both the front and hind feet.

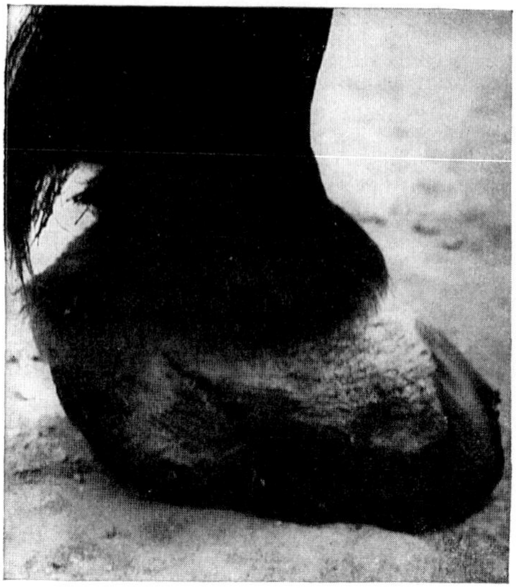

79

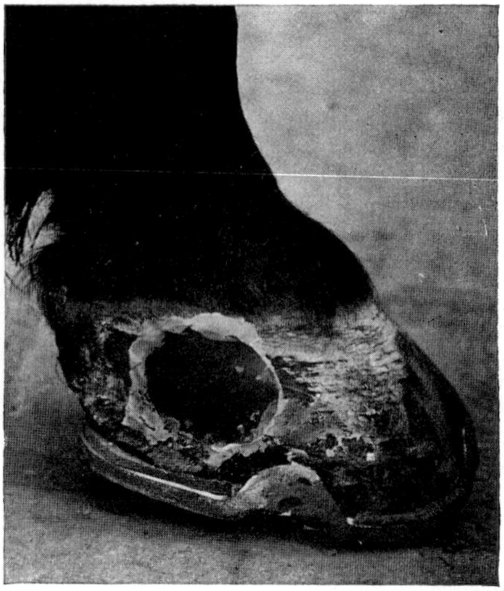

80

Fig. 2.1.20. — 79. Complete heel crack.
Fig. 2.1.20. — 80. Complete heel crack repaired with PVC film and adhesive.

Symptoms and Etiology. Disruptions of continuity resulting from coronet strikes or other injuries, separation of the perioplic band associated with superficial purulent pododermatitis, mechanical avulsion, overreaching, or resting one foot upon the other can cause transverse cracks to form. Injuries of the matrix lead to an interruption of horn secretion, and usually this is associated with an infection of the matrix that extends and perpetuates the inflammatory process, thereby enlarging the transverse crack.

Diagnosis. Easily made from symptoms.

Prognosis. Favorable. Overreaching and foot-resting should be considered during pre-purchase examination.

Treatment. Exposed matrix should be attended to, and infections treated. If the crack extends into the area of the shoenails or bearing surface of the wall, the nails should be redistributed or the absent horn replaced.

Loose Wall

Definition. 'Loose wall' is defined as a disruption in the continuity of the horny wall and horny sole in the area of the white line.

Occurrence. Loose wall is very common in the front feet, especially if the feet are wide, and is less common in the hind feet. It is the most common hoof disease.

Symptoms and Diagnosis. The unpigmented horn of the white line is absent in circumscribed areas of the bearing surface or is absent in all areas, including the bars; this is almost the rule in flat foot and dropped sole.

Etiology. Causes are foot shape, improper shoeing, and neglect of foot care. Wide feet are frequently difficult to trim and shoe properly. If the bearing circumference is reduced too much by vertical rasping, then the weak horny wall will give inadequate support, and 'loose wall' will result. The opposite situation, i.e., inadequate support by the horny sole (e.g., due to wide-set shoes or poor-fitting factory shoes), is frequently seen. Narrow shoes with uneven foot contact can also cause loose wall. The

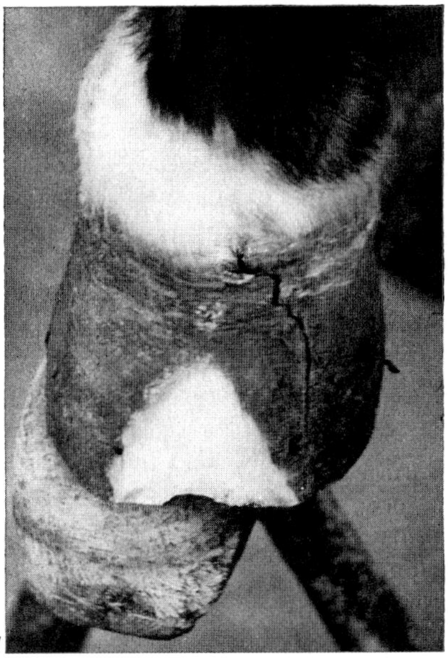
81

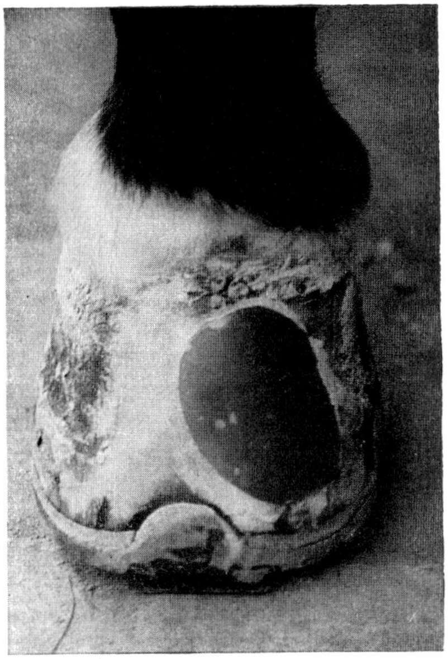
82

Fig. 2.1.20. — 81. Zigzag toe crack.
Fig. 2.1.20. — 82. Zigzag toe crack repaired with PVC film and adhesive.

hot-fitting of shoes can have adverse effects, especially on the horn and white line. The same applies to unhygienic stabling, which can lead to putrefactive processes (as in thrush) that destroy the soft horn of the white line. Finally, work on hard, dry ground and excessive drying of the horn can be a cause. In the contracted foot, it is thought that the change in foot shape may result in a deterioration of horn quality.

Prognosis. Tends to be favorable, except in wide feet.

Treatment. The cause is removed, and new horn growth is promoted. Emphasis is placed upon proper corrective trimming and shoeing, correct shoe contact with the foot, and proper shoe width. Defects are packed with oakum and pine-tar, and *not with hard materials* such as leather cement, Technovit, etc. Regular foot care and hygienic stabling are an important adjunct.

Hollow Wall

Definition. 'Hollow wall' refers to a separation between the lamellar and tubular layer of the horny wall that may extend from the ground surface up to the coronary band.

Occurrence. Uncommon; usually affects toe and quarters of front or hind foot (figs. 2.1.20. — 79 through — 82).

Symptoms and Diagnosis. A bulge may be evident in the wall that gives a hollow sound on percussion. Supporting-leg lameness is present if separation is extensive. Often there is only a very narrow cavity that is difficult to probe. Hollow wall is very common on the anterior wall of the foundered foot.

Etiology. Hollow wall is usually secondary to inflammation of the wall matrix (laminitis, shoenail injury, coronet strike). It often represents an extension of loose wall and may also result from repeated hurdle contact in jumpers.

The *prognosis* is guarded, especially if the defect is extensive and horn quality is poor.

Treatment. The cause is removed. The separated horn must grow down and be replaced with healthy horn. Larger defects are loosely packed with gauze. No hard materials are introduced; they act like a wedge and exacerbate the condition. In many cases a transverse cut is effective in the early stage. It extends into the hollow space and is intended to keep the defect from extending toward the coronet.

In jumpers, a very large clip of sheet metal can be applied to cover the defect and exert pressure upon it. The clip must be welded or soldered to the shoe. Removal of the hollow wall horn is not recommended.

Forensic Aspects. Hollow wall of minimal extent that is unaccompanied by lameness is usually not an inherited defect.

If the hollow wall accompanies laminitis, dropped sole or other diseases that alter foot shape, and horn quality is poor, then a serious defect is considered to be present. The same applies to cases in which lameness coexists. It should also be considered that such feet are difficult to shoe, and the shoe will not remain in place for long, which greatly compromises the usefulness of the horse.

Because hollow wall is not visible until the shoe is removed, it must be considered an 'occult' disease.

Brittle Foot, Soft Foot

Definition. In these conditions the foot exhibits a change in physical properties, in the one case being extremely hard or brittle, and in the other abnormally soft.

Occurrence. Generally the brittle foot is more common than the soft foot. All four feet are susceptible.

Symptoms and Diagnosis. (a) In brittle foot, a chipping and fraying of the horn is evident at the bearing surface and around shoe nails. (b) In soft foot the horn and especially the periople are less compact than normal, making it difficult or impossible to drive and clinch shoe nails securely. The shoe soon loosens and is thrown.

Etiology. (a) In brittle foot, according to LUNGWITZ and TSCHERNE [1910], the horn has an unphysiologic structure that is based in part on genetic factors. But extrinsic factors can also play a role: improper foot care; dry, hard ground (sawdust, peat); destruction of the periople by rasping the horny wall; prolonged hot-fitting of shoes; oversized shoe nails, etc. (b) As in brittle foot, poor horn quality, excessive moisture (pasture), poor foot care and unhygienic stabling, especially in horses with wide feet, are of causal importance.

Prognosis is favorable if exogenous factors can be controlled. Endogenous factors such as structure and horn characteristics (keratin production) are extremely difficult to influence.

Treatment consists of meticulous foot care, combined with measures to keep the hoof wet or dry, as needed. The foot is carefully trimmed and shod with hand-forged, light-weight, well-fitting shoes, which are nailed higher than usual; nailing should include the heel area. Larger quarter clips are used, and more than one clip per side may be indicated. A skilled farrier can be of great benefit in protecting and strengthening the brittle or soft foot.

Thrush

Definition. Thrush is a destruction of the horny frog due to putrefaction.

Occurrence. Thrush is common in the hind feet.

Symptoms and Diagnosis. The extrinsic destructive process usually begins in the central sulcus and then spreads to involve adjacent tissues. The horn tissue of the frog shows fissures, and a grayish-black, foul-smelling discharge is found within the fissures and sulci. If treatment is delayed, the process will spread toward the horn of the heel bulbs and the coronary band. If the frog is destroyed, the crura of the frog will migrate toward the midline of the foot, narrow the frog space, and result in a contracted foot. Lameness can develop if the matrix is exposed. The characteristic 'thrush rings' will form if the perioplic matrix becomes involved.

Etiology. Improper cleaning of the feet, inadequate exercise, and unhygienic stabling are the principal causes. Excessive trimming of the horny frog and shoeing with open-heeled, calked shoes predispose the foot to thrush by removing frog pressure. It is thought that ischemia of the frog matrix leads to a decrease in horn production. In this situation prolonged stabling can easily cause disruptions to develop in the horn tissue of the frog. Thrush is often seen in contracted foot and other diseases that alter foot shape.

Differential Diagnosis. Canker is the only condition to be differentiated from thrush. It is characterized by vegetative growth of the matrix with an offensive odor and destruction of the horn tissues from within.

Prognosis is generally favorable. Many authors believe that thrush predisposes the foot to canker.

Treatment. Ample exercise, good foot care, dry bedding. The hoof is cleaned, all degenerated horn is removed, and drying agents are applied (especially pine tar or liquid pitch). A bandage or covered shoe should be applied if the frog matrix is exposed.

Some authors describe 'wall rot', a less common condition that in essence corresponds to thrush.

2.1.20.4.7. Inflammatory Processes Involving Internal Foot Structures

Besides diseases of the coffin joint and associated bones, the main conditions to be discussed are:

1. Shoenail injuries
2. Injuries of the solar epidermis
3. Puncture wounds of the foot
4. Coronet strike
5. Corns
6. Inflammation of the heel-bulb matrix
7. Chronic inflammation of the perioplic and coronary epidermis
8. Lateral cartilage fistula (quittor)
9. Canker
10. Keratoma
11. Loss of the hoof wall.

Shoenail Injuries (see Sec. 2.1.20.4.1.)

Injuries of the Solar Epidermis

Definition. These injuries are divided into three categories:

a) Road injuries
b) Trimming injuries
c) Firing injuries.

Occurrence. Road injuries of the solar epidermis occur mainly at the toe, while trimming injuries are observed in the frog area or at the quarters. Firing injuries are most commonly seen in the heel area.

Symptoms and Etiology. (a) In horses that work barefoot on hard ground or throw a shoe that is not replaced (with a boot, etc.) during long-distance rides, the horny sole will soon be worn thin. The thin sole will yield to digital pressure, and tenderness may be evident. The solar matrix becomes contused, and an acute aseptic pododermatitis develops that can progress very quickly to a purulent pododermatitis if infectious organisms gain entry through perforations caused by pebbles, sand or other objects.

If the resulting lameness or alteration of gait is neglected, a complete penetration of the sole can occur. This usually happens as a result of friction at the toe, causing a sickle-shaped area of the solar matrix — the solar epidermis — to be exposed. It is usually contaminated with dirt and bleeds in the acute stage. Later a purulent pododermatitis develops.

The edge of the bearing surface is rounded as a result of friction, and the foot appears unusually small. Parts of the horny wall may be chipped away. (b) The cause of trimming injuries often lies in a deficient knowledge of anatomy, or in excessive trimming of the hoof at the request of the owner or rider in order to obtain a 'petite' foot. (c) The causes of firing injuries also lie in an ignorance of anatomy, as well as the fact that it is much easier to lower the wall by firing than by orthopedic trimming. The shortage of competent farriers has made this a common injury.

Prognosis. It is favorable provided the hoof matrix is not seriously injured. Once the coffin bone has been exposed, the prognosis is guarded at best.

Treatment. Following general wound care, a full-bar shoe with leather pad is applied or the foot is bandaged, depending on the condition of the matrix and the depth and extent of the lesion. The treatment of suppurative and gangrenous pododermatitis follows general rules: antibiotics are administered locally as well as parenterally if fever is present. Tetanus antitoxin or toxoid booster is also administered.

Puncture Wounds of the Foot (see Sec. 2.1.20.4.1.)

Coronet Strike (see Sec. 2.1.20.3.1.)

Corns

Definition. Corns are contusions of the hoof matrix that can lead to aseptic and purulent inflammation. The hoof wall is not disrupted.

Occurrence. Corns occur most frequently on the medial half of the shod front foot in the wall matrix of the heel, the solar matrix at the angle of the sole, and in the bar matrix. Conditions that alter foot shape predispose to the development of corns.

Symptoms. Three forms are recognized:

a) Dry corn, or hemorrhagic pododermatitis
b) Moist corn, or chronic serous pododermatitis
c) Suppurating corn, or purulent pododermatitis.

At least initially, all three forms involve a circumscribed lesion of the matrix that is confined to a typical area.

Dry corn presents as a discoloration of the horn occurring at the typical sites listed above or in the area of the white line. It represents a hematoma of the horn in which an initially bluish-black, then red and finally yellow-green stain appears due to the gradual breakdown of hemoglobin — analogous to a 'black eye' in humans. The horn at that site often has a yellowish, waxy appearance and tends to flake easily. If the contusion is mild, and especially if stains are not yet visible on the horn (they must grow out gradually with the horn), a contusion of the matrix may be presumed from tenderness to compression with a hoof tester. Dry corns may produce a mild to moderate supporting-leg lameness or a stiffness of the gait if both front feet are involved.

Moist corn (chronic corn, habitual corn) is a discoloration due to the prolonged action of factors that are often difficult to control (abnormal foot shape, sidebones, periosteal new bone growth). There is frequent flaking of the horn, which sometimes contains blood- or serum-filled cavities. A constant, mild to moderate lameness is present.

Suppurating corn occurs when the contused matrix becomes infected, leading to a superficial or deep suppurative pododermatitis with all the typical signs of inflammation and severe lameness.

Etiology and Diagnosis. Any contusing force exerted on the caudal half of the foot will result in the tearing of small blood vessels in the matrix. Predisposing factors include faults of limb and digit conformation, foot disease or abnormalities of foot shape, improper trimming and shoeing, overexertion of poorly-conditioned horses, and neglect of the feet. The practice of 'cutting out' corns sometimes employed by laymen and farriers is highly detrimental.

Prognosis. Generally favorable if the cause can be removed. The presence of deep suppurating inflammation, necrosis of the hoof matrix, subcoronary cellulitis, lateral cartilage fistula, etc. indicates a guarded or unfavorable prognosis.

Treatment. Often *dry corns* can be cured simply by removing shoe contact at the contused site. Cold compresses are applied, and the cause is removed if possible. Full-bar shoes with leather pads are beneficial.

With a *suppurating corn*, it is necessary to establish immediate drainage of the pus. Further treatment is like that for suppurative pododermatitis.

Moist corns, which occur mainly in feet with pathologic shape changes, require careful trimming, well-fitting shoes and meticulous foot care. These measures are also effective in preventing this common foot disorder.

Inflammation of the Heel-Bulb Matrix

Occurrence. This disease is observed in both the shod and unshod foot. The front feet are most commonly affected.

Symptoms and Diagnosis. The horse will be lame or will manifest a stiff gait if more than one foot is involved, especially on hard ground or hilly terrain. There is increased dorsiflexion of the fetlock, swelling, heat, redness, hemorrhage, tissue destruction, and suppuration at the heel bulb with marked tenderness to pressure. Separation of the damaged horn tissue of the heel bulb is common.

Etiology. The causes are contusions and wounds of the heel bulb, due especially to work on uneven, stony ground, frozen roads or fields with coarse stubble; severe overreaching or being struck from behind in a race; frostbite and burns (stable fires); or pressure from a poorly-fitted covered shoe.

The *prognosis* is generally favorable.

Treatment consists in removing the cause and treating the injuries. Protective foot gear may be worn to shield the heel bulbs from injury.

Chronic Inflammation of the Perioplic and Coronary Epidermis

Definition. Chronic inflammation of the perioplic and coronary epidermis interferes with horn production as a result of a sustained hyperplastic inflammatory process. This causes the horny wall to acquire a fissured, bark-like appearance.

Occurrence. The disease most commonly affects both the front feet, especially the toe and heel areas. Involvement of all four feet is rare. The disease is particularly common in Standardbreds with steep foot axes as well as in donkeys and mules.

Symptoms. The cardinal symptoms of inflammation — redness, heat, swelling and pain — may be present in the early stage. Rarely is lameness or altered gait apparent at this time. Gradually, changes appear in the hairs at the coronet, in the perioplic band and in the periople. With inflammation of the coronary epidermis, deep fissures or even cracks develop in the tubular horn. The gait becomes stiff and stilted, or a mild to moderate supporting-leg lameness appears.

Etiology. The major cause is chemical irritants (acid-containing hoof ointments, sprays, etc.). Mechanical causes such as interfering, overreaching and coronet striking are less frequent. The high incidence in Standardbreds may be due to the increased wall compression that occurs when the upright forefoot comes down on a hard track surface.

Differential Diagnosis. Skin and horn changes asscociated with ringbone of the coffin joint, lateral cartilage fistula, canker, grease heel, etc. must be differentiated.

Diagnosis. The diagnosis is easily made from the fissured, bark-like appearance of the hoof wall in advanced cases.

Prognosis. Favorable to guarded, especially if extensive matrix lesions are present.

Treatment. The cause, if known, is removed. The horn is cleaned, crusts are rasped away, antiseptic bandages are applied. Horn growth is stimulated by exercise on grass pasture. Hoof ointments and sprays with vitamin A may be applied; the coronet should be massaged with ointment daily.

Chronic inflammation of the wall epidermis is also occasionally observed. The literature contains references to 'chronic hoof ulcer' [Schleg, 1886] and 'internal or ulcerous hollow wall' [Pillwax, 1892; Bayer et al., 1890]. The condition is undoubtedly rare and affects the distal portions of the cranial hoof wall. Injuries of the wall matrix, loose wall and hollow wall are believed to be causes. Treatment corresponds to that for matrix injuries.

Lateral Cartilage Fistula ('Quittor')

Definition. Lateral cartilage fistula or quittor is a suppurating fistula that is sustained by necrosis of the collateral cartilage. It is most common in the area of the posterior coronet, but can also occur at the angle of the sole or on the horny wall.

Occurrence. Most lateral cartilage fistulae are observed on the medial side of the front foot. Their prevalence has decreased significantly in recent years, and they are classified among the rare equine foot disorders.

Symptoms. Many horses with lateral cartilage fistulae show little or no lameness, and this often causes the disease to be underestimated in its severity and extent.

The early stage is marked by a painful swelling of the coronet in the area of the lateral cartilage. One or more fistulous openings appear in this area, and usually these discharge a viscous, yellow-white pus that sometimes contains necrotic pieces of lateral cartilage showing a greenish discoloration. The fistulous openings may close for a time, only to reopen later on.

A supporting-leg lameness will develop if drainage of exudations is blocked, as well as during flareups associated with cellulitis of surrounding tissues. The horny wall is soiled by the exudate, and the hairs around the fistulous opening are matted. Generally an increased digital pulse is palpated, and pain is produced by hoof-tester compression or percussion of the corresponding portion of the wall. This acute stage lasts only a few days and is followed by a chronic stage with less pronounced symptoms. In long-standing cases, and if matrix tissues that produce the wall horn become involved, ring formation may be evident on the hoof wall.

Etiology. Direct causes of lateral cartilage fistulae include interfering, overreaching, coronet striking, pitchfork injuries, and similar trauma. Fistulae can also result from the spread of suppurative processes following puncture wounds of the foot, cellulitis of the plantar cushion, necrosis of the deep flexor tendon, purulent inflammation of the navicular bursa, shoenail injuries, suppurating corns, infected wall cracks, etc. These can cause the parachondrium and even the perichondrium and lateral cartilage itself to undergo liquefaction and necrosis. Due to the tendency of pus to form, and to the constant upward and downward movement of exudate that occurs as a consequence of hoof mechanics, spontaneous recoveries are uncommon.

Differential Diagnosis and Diagnosis. In *coronary* and *subcoronary cellulitis*, the entire coronet is involved and swollen, and this swelling may extend up to and above the fetlock joint. With quittor on the other hand, swelling is confined to the fistulous area. The probing of lateral cartilage fistulae should be done with extreme caution, especially in proximity to the joint (local anesthesia). In many cases the fistulous tracts will take a tortuous course and have an extremely small caliber, making them difficult to demonstrate even with contrast radiographs.

Prognosis. The prognosis is favorable if the necrotic focus or foci in the lateral cartilage can be surgically removed together with the fistulous tracts. The many traditional, conservative treatments using various pharmaceutical agents are obsolete. The prognosis is guarded to unfavorable if the coffin joint is involved and tissue destruction is extensive, making it likely that ankylosis will develop.

Treatment. At one time, three treatment methods were recognized: conservative, radical and mixed. Today, serious attention is given only to surgical removal of the entire lateral cartilage or large portions of it, together with the fistulous tract. In this way healing time is substantially reduced.

Of the many operative methods available, the Viennese School mainly practices three: the Bayer-Schmidt operation, the Möller-Imminger operation, and the Riehlein-Mayer operation.

The last of these methods is the least traumatic, for it injures neither the hoof wall nor the matrix. Hence, it is preferred over other methods. Its great disadvantage is that the lateral cartilage must be removed without benefit of visual control. This may cause necrotic tissues to be left in the foot, leading to a recurrence.

In the lateral cartilage resections of Bayer-Schmidt, Möller-Imminger and others, large pieces of the horny wall are removed; the coronary, perioplic and wall matrices are sectioned at least once; and suitable skin flaps must be developed so that the lateral cartilage can be visualized almost in its entirety. It is unlikely that necrotic tissues or fistulous tracts will be overlooked with this technique. On the other hand, this method entails the destruction of keratogenous tissues with their extensive, complex vascular supply (necrosis of matrix flaps), thereby prolonging healing time and leading to hoof deformity.

In Riehlein-Mayer operation, the horse is placed under general anesthesia with the affected side uppermost. Beforehand, several radiographs are taken to decide if, and to what extent, the affected lateral cartilage has become ossified. Then a skin incision is made at the proximal border of the cartilage, and through this incision the entire cartilage is removed with an oval hoof knife or, if the cartilage is ossified, with curved gouges of suitable size. Particular attention is given to the wing of the distal phalanx, for that is where many fistulae originate. Positioning the digit in extension will protect the coffin joint from injury. A snug-fitting pressure bandage is applied postoperatively. If hoof wall properties are favorable and the horse has a quiet temperament, it is usually confined barefoot to a box stall. Shoes may be applied after 3—4 weeks when the animal is at pasture.

Comments. The atraumatic partial resection of RIEHLEIN-MEYER is highly recommended. Especially in athletic horses, results are good, and rehabilitation time is shortened. It is important that the surgery be followed by corrective trimming and suitable shoeing.

Canker (Pododermatitis chronica verrucosa migrans)

Definition. Canker may be defined as a chronic inflammation of the hoof matrix that is associated with vegetative growth of the papillary body and an interruption and alteration of hoof secretion (parakeratosis).

Occurrence. Canker is seen most frequently in draft breeds and may involve any of the feet, though it is most common in the hind feet. It is rare for all four feet to be affected. Changes may involve the frog, bars, sole, wall or periople.

Symptoms. In the initial stage the horny frog, and especially the lateral sulci, show areas where the horn is friable, soft, greasy, and loosens easily. The somewhat pale epidermis often shows enlarged, club-shaped villi even in the early stage. Later these changes become more pronounced, and blood-engorged groups of papillae appear that have a columnar, ridge-shaped, cauliflowerlike or feathery appearance. A grayish-white, greasy material with an offensive odor is found in the spaces between the papillary groups. The frog is often greatly enlarged and has a spongy appearance. From the frog, the disease spreads to involve other tissues, especially the matrix of the sole and wall. The hypertrophy of the lamellae of the wall matrix and disturbed keratinization gradually lead to a localized separation of the hoof wall with its mechanical consequences (local bowing and expansion of the wall), and to a dropping of P3 in the area of the sole.

'Canker of the bars' produces characteristic changes. The destruction of the bars in this condition serves to demonstrate their important role in maintaining a normal heel width. The bars extend from the angles of the wall to the apex of the frog, and join anterior to the apex to form an arch. The caudal part of the bars is composed of both tubular and lamellar horn, like the rest of the horny wall. But the anterior part including the arch consists of tubular horn only. The bars are not covered by periople. Owing to their structure and their arrangement in the hoof wall, the intact, unweakened bars behave as an elastic spring. They control hoof mechanics in the caudal part of the foot and prevent undue expansion and contraction of the hoof wall. If horn production is disturbed by canker of the bars, the weight of the body will produce an abnormal expansion of the foot at the heels. The solar surface of the foot will acquire a heart shape that is a characteristic feature of this disease.

Lameness does not appear until the late stage. Systemic manifestations are observed only in severe cases where several feet are involved.

Many authors make a distinction between the *benign* and *malignant* form of canker, the latter showing particularly severe pathologic changes and a more rapid spread.

BÜRGI [1910] performed histologic studies of canker and chronic verrucous dermatitis and concluded that both diseases are identical. We, too, have found that the two conditions very often coexist in the same foot.

Etiology. The etiology of canker remains unclear. It is definitely not a neoplastic disease; metastases have never been observed. A bacterial etiology is unlikely. HABACHER [1931] was unsuccessful in his attempts to produce the disease experimentally. Parakeratosis is a symptom, rather than a cause, of this disease. However it appears likely that biochemical and histologic investigations of keratin and especially of keratinization could help to clarify unanswered questions concerning the etiology of canker. To date no protein analysis of keratin has been performed.

Differential Diagnosis and Diagnosis. The signs of canker are unmistakable to anyone who has ever seen and smelled the affected foot. Thrush is the only condition to be differentiated, but response to treatment should resolve all doubts in this regard. Disturbances of horn production associated with vegetative growth of the matrix are necessary for a diagnosis of canker to be made.

Prognosis. The prognosis depends on the extent of the disease. If several feet are affected, the disease is far advanced, and the horse is restless and difficult to approach (typical of animals previously treated by laymen), a guarded prognosis is indicated. Otherwise, recovery almost invariably occurs when vigorous treatment is rendered by someone with patience.

Treatment. Innumerable medicaments, caustics and astringents have been used in the treatment of canker. Three types of therapy are recognized:

Drug therapy
Radical surgical therapy
Mixed therapy.

The latter is most commonly employed. With the horse recumbent and anesthetized, all diseased matrix tissues are removed until healthy matrix is reached. A broad excision of healthy hoof wall is necessary in this procedure, for the horn often conceals matrix vegetations. The surgery is done under tourniquet control to obtain a bloodless, unobstructed field. Following the removal of diseased tissues, it is sufficient to overlay the matrix with a gauze pad, covering this with a Hilbert plaster bandage that encloses the entire hoof wall. This bandage should exert pressure on the operative area and must be 2—3 cm thick so that it can be worn for about 10—12 days. It is also recommended that Lightcast® fiberglass tape be wrapped around the periphery of the plaster cast. This enables a thinner plaster cast to be used, and the entire bandage is very firm and resistant to breakage.

No matter how thorough and careful the operation, there will often be areas, usually at the periphery of the field, in which the process is still active and matrix vegetations are still present. These areas should be carefully resected under anesthesia, and the foot protected with a covered shoe or, if a shoe cannot be applied, with a compression bandage. Anesthesia is important both from a humane standpoint and to facilitate raising of the foot for surgery.

Erkurt [1955] claims to have cured canker with large doses of parenteral penicillin.

Keratoma

Definition. Keratoma, or keraphyllocele, is a columnar or conical thickening on the inner aspect of the horny wall. If the thickening has a broad, flat appearance, it is called a 'horny callus'. Either the wall or the coronet may be involved. Some types of keratoma, called 'horn pearls', are spheroidal or bean-shaped structures of varying size that rarely involve the matrix but may be found embedded in the distal phalanx [Knezevic, 1962].

Occurrence. Keratomas occur most frequently at the toe and quarters of the front and hind feet.

Symptoms. Changes may be evident on the outer surface of the horny wall: groove-like depressions, scar contractions at the coronet, wall cracks or ridges. Intermittent lameness may also be present. Finally, removal of the horseshoe may reveal a mass at the white line pointing toward the center of the foot if the keratoma or horn callus has already reached the bearing surface as a result of downgrowth of horn. The horn of the keratoma is usually yellow in color and is sharply delineated from surrounding tissues. Often a funnel-shaped depression or crack is visible, whose dark border contrasts sharply with adjacent horn. Frequently this area is coated with grayish-black pus, as is the corresponding site on the shoe ('suppurating keratoma'). The source of the pus is a superficial purulent pododermatitis. Lameness is invariably present in such cases.

Often the foregoing symptoms are absent, and the disease must be diagnosed by exclusion. In these cases percussion of the horny wall revealing variations of sound quality can provide valuable clues to the presence of a keratoma or horn callus. If the lesion is large enough to cause involvement of P3 (pressure atrophy, erosion of the solar border), radiographs will be rewarding. Some authors recommend that drill holes be made to evaluate the thickness of the horny wall.

Necropsy reveals changes in the matrix, horny capsule and distal phalanx. The matrix shows signs of hyperplastic or suppurative pododermatitis, depending on whether the keratoma has developed from an aseptic or suppurative inflammation. The lesion consists either of cicatricial lamellar horn or of horn tubules only. It presents a smooth or fissured surface and often contains cavities. The constant pressure from the keratoma leads to atrophy of the wall matrix and P3, manifested by a pitlike depression (wear spot) in the bone whose shape and size correspond to the horny wall thickening.

In all horses, the midportion of the solar border of P3 presents a round, more or less hemispherical depression up to 8 mm deep. This is made by a corresponding thickening of the lamellar horn in the opposing area of the wall (ground-border notch and spurlike rib in the epidermal horn) [Bittner, 1927], and is especially pronounced in the presence of flat foot or dropped sole.

Etiology. Keratomas develop as a sequel to chronic, hyperplastic, aseptic or suppurative pododermatitides resulting from wall cracks, coronet strikes, shoenail injuries, corns, etc.

Keratomas are distinguished from *horny excrescences*, or thickenings of the horny wall on its outer aspect. These result from the traumatic displacement of matrix tissues.

Differential Diagnosis. Diagnosis may prove difficult if the aforementioned changes in the coronet, wall and white line are absent, and it may prove necessary to diagnose the condition by exclusion from contusions of the coronary and wall matrix, and from complete or incomplete fractures of the P3.

Good radiographic views of the distal phalanx and its solar border, as well as conduction anesthesia, can assist greatly in establishing a diagnosis.

Diagnosis. Diagnosis is simple if typical symptoms are present; otherwise diagnosis by exclusion is necessary. Sometimes it is difficult to prove that an existing lameness is caused by a keratoma. If a purulent or suppurative pododermatitis is present, there will be lameness, pain on palpation and percussion, and a increased digital pulse. Valuable information is also provided by palmar or plantar nerve blocks followed by radiography.

Prognosis and Treatment. The prognosis is guarded, because keratomas may regrow after being surgically removed.

If a keratoma is detected incidentally in a horse that is not lame, the lesion is usually an aseptic one. In this case conservative therapy is recommended, i.e., lowering the bearing surface from the shoe, thinning the affected wall, moving the shoe clips, and applying warm, moist foot compresses.

In draft horses with suppurating keratoma, a functional recovery is often achieved by creating a drainage opening in the horn at the bearing surface. In all other cases of suppurating keratoma, surgical excision of the affected horny wall is the only recourse. No more horn should be removed than is absolutely necessary, of course, due to the slow rate of new horn growth (see surgical text for details).

Comments. Often one or even two keratomas are found incidentally while the foot is being trimmed, having caused no previous symptoms. Many spontaneous recoveries over a period of several years have been reported.

Loss of the Hoof Wall (Exungulation)

Definition. This is a condition in which cleavage develops between the hoof wall and the hoof matrix (hoof epidermis). The loss may be *partial* or *complete, primary* or *secondary*.

Occurrence. Any of the feet may be affected. The concurrent involvement of all four feet is very rare.

Symptoms and Etiology. A primary, complete loss of the hoof wall can occur traumatically (hoof avulsion) when the foot or shoe becomes caught on roots, hurdles, rails, sewage grates, or similar objects. The avulsion causes matrix damage, hemorrhage, and in most cases a very severe lameness, which may first appear some time after the accident (after the fright reaction has subsided). A primary or secondary, partial or complete hoof loss can also occur when the foot is run over by a wheeled vehicle. Often the horny capsule is primarily separated from the matrix by the trauma, frequently accompanied by P3 fractures (chip fractures or, if the foot is crushed, comminuted fractures).

Secondary loss of the hoof wall is usually manifested by a separation of the perioplic band and the discharge of exudate. This is preceded by a painful swelling of the coronet, often with fever and pronounced lameness. The hoof loss often occurs suddenly when the horse rises to its feet, accompanied by minor bleeding. Hoof losses of this type are observed following retention of pus in the hoof wall, when the exudate has undermined large portions of the horn (shoenail injury, puncture wound, keratoma, cellulitis), as well as after severe burns, frostbite, chemical burns, faulty blistering, laminitis, canker, and trophic disturbances secondary to surgical division of both palmar or plantar nerves at the fetlock. It should be noted that a correctly-performed neurectomy of the palmar or plantar rami on the *flexor surface* of the fetlock joint (e.g., to aid navicular disease) never leads to loss of the hoof wall.

Differential Diagnosis. Separation of the perioplic band associated with localized, superficial suppurative pododermatitis.

Diagnosis. A diagnosis is easily reached by conducting a careful examination and taking into account all symptoms.

Prognosis. The prognosis is favorable if the loss is partial and there is no serious injury to enclosed structures, especially the distal phalanx. A guarded or unfavorable prognosis is indicated if there is complete loss of the hoof wall and the aforementioned complications arise. The prolonged healing time and danger of gangrene with septicemia make humane euthanasia the recommended course of action in such cases.

Treatment. For partial hoof loss with purulent exudation, openings should be made in the horn to permit drainage. It is better to make several drainage holes than remove parts of the hoof wall. Cavities in the horny sole should be flushed with 3% H_2O_2 and mild antiseptic solutions, and then treated with antibiotics.

Prophylaxis. The danger of foot entanglement can be reduced by using shoes with short heels and small calks; *grabs should never be used in riding horses.*

2.1.20.4.8. Diseases of the Coffin Joint

In diseases of the coffin joint as in all articular diseases, a basic distinction is made between arthritis and arthrosis.

The following conditions may affect the coffin joint, listed in order of clinical frequency:

a) podarthrosis,
b) aseptic podarthritis,
c) infectious podarthritis.

Podarthrosis

Definition: Arthrosis (arthropathy, degenerative joint disease) is the term applied to joint disease caused by erosive processes due to conformation faults, disparities of load distribution, excessive loads, disproportion between load and load-bearing

Table 2.1.29. — 2. Differentation between arthritis and arthrosis (general)

	Arthritis	Arthrosis	Healthy joint
1. Inflammation	+ to +++	— to (+) (flareups)	—
2. Pain	+ to +++	+ to ++ typ. 'cold lameness'	—
3. Loss of function	+ to +++	+ to ++	—
4. Synovial fluid increase	— to +++	— to +	—
5. Cell content of synovial fluid	increased	normal or reduced	normal $< 200/mm^3$
6. Arthroscopic appearance of cartilage	surface: dull luster color: bluish	surface: dull and velvety with erosive lesions color: gray to brown	young animals: bluish-white old animals: yellow-brown
7. Arthroscopic appearance of synovial membrane	surface: glistening color: reddish, yellow, vascular congestion frequent	surface: duller than normal; color: brown to grayish-brown, vascular congestion rare	glistening, light gray or white
8. Course	acute to chronic with acute flareups	generally chronic	—
9. Lipping	—	++	—
10. Outcome	Recovery or?	Joint destruction, ankylosis	—
11. Joint mice	—	++	—
12. Occurrence, onset	in many joints, in small joints	usually in one joint, in large joints?	—
13. Cause(s)	Fault of weight bearing Infections	Conformation fault Fault of weight bearing Excessive loading Metabolic disorders	—
14. Joint capsule	usually distended, thin	shrunken, usually thickened	—
15. Treatment	anti-inflammatory, rest	cartilage extracts, adequate exercise	—

capacity, metabolic disorders, etc. (table 2.1.20. — 2). Inflammation is present but is not the dominant feature of the disease.

In the diagnosis of arthrosis in veterinary medicine, *arthroscopy* has proved a particularly valuable tool. Arthroscopy, especially of the large proximal joints (stifle joint, shoulder joint, talocrural joint), furnishes information that cannot be obtained with any other diagnostic method.

Occurrence. Podarthrosis is frequently found in the coffin joint of the forelimbs and is common even in very young horses.

Symptoms. Achronic supporting-leg lameness of moderate degree is apparent. In many cases both front coffin joints are affected concurrently but in varying degrees. This results in a *locomotor disturbance* with a stiff, constrained gait. Often marked pain is evident on turning. Diagnostic anesthesia of the coffin joint usually improves the gait but does not correct it completely. This is firstly because the disturbance is partly *mechanical* due to extensive cartilage damage, and secondly because the fetlock and pastern joints also may show arthritic change. Pain may be produced by passive rotation of the digital joints.

Radiographs show distinct lipping, especially at the dorsal articular margin of the middle phalanx (P2). A widening of the coffin joint space is usually apparent.

Etiology. Arthrosis of the coffin joint develops as a result of breaks in the digital axes, especially in a medial or lateral direction; faults of digital conformation (toe-out or toe-in, too sloping or too steep) and/or limb conformation (base-wide, base-narrow, knock knees, bow legs, kneesprung, anterior or posterior deviation, cow hocks, sickle hocks, straight hocks).

These faults lead to microtrauma and excessive straining of certain joint areas on hard ground, uneven terrain and during jumping. *Cartilage damage* occurs and leads gradually to a 'denuding' of the bone (exposure of subchondral bone), which in time causes an internal ankylosis of the joint.

This *arthrotic ringbone of the coffin joint* can progress to a periarthritic ringbone, or the latter may develop as a primary condition.

Lack of exercise (e.g., prolonged confinement to a small box stall) as well as overexertion of the poorly-conditioned horse will cause rapid exacerbation of the arthrosis. Horses are running animals, and arthritic horses in particular require adequate exercise if ankylosis is to be avoided.

Differential Diagnosis. Often it is difficult to distinguish an arthritis from an arthrosis. The criteria in table 2.1.20. — 2 are helpful in making a differentiation.

Diagnosis. The diagnosis is based on all findings: history, clinical symptoms, anesthesia, radiography, and if possible arthroscopy (figs. 2.1.20. — 83 and — 84).

Prognosis. The prognosis of arthrosis is generally guarded to unfavorable. The task of the veterinarian is to slow the advance of the disease process.

Treatment. The cause or causes of the podarthrosis are removed if possible: corrective trimming and shoeing, Norberg [1968] cushion, leather foot pad, appropriate exercise (exercise program!), hyperemic therapy. In Europe point cautery and blistering of the coronet has been used. Perforating cautery may be tried in near-hopeless cases. We have seen no improvement following the administration of cartilage and bone-marrow extracts alone. Glucocorticoids should be used with caution!

Comments. With the increase in equestrian events, the arthritic diseases are assuming greater importance and now rank first among the lesions that cause lamenesses and locomotor disturbances. Hence, the veterinarian must make a constant effort to ensure that adequate exercise programs are formulated and adhered to. The popular practice of taking horses on weekend rides while keeping them idle for the rest of the week is not recommended for an animal that is, by nature, highly active.

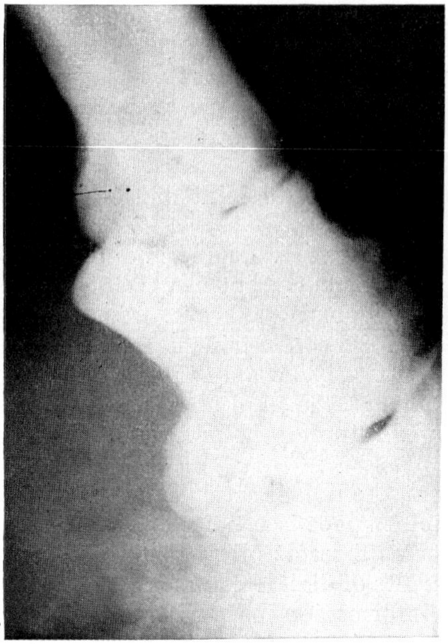
83

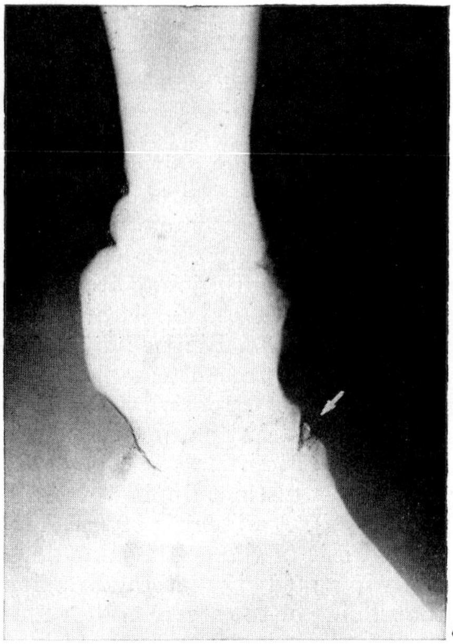
84

Fig. 2.1.20. — 83. Podarthrosis and periarthritis.
Fig. 2.1.20. — 84. Loose body in the coffin joint (podarthrosis).

Aseptic Podarthritis

Definition. Aseptic podarthritis is an aseptic, usually serous inflammation of the coffin joint.

Occurrence. Aseptic podarthritis mainly affects the front feet and is often bilateral.

Symptoms and Etiology. Symptoms vary depending on the cause (misstep, sprain, entanglement, slipping, contusion, concussion on hard ground). Acute inflammation is characterized by heat in the joint region, distension and fluctuation of the joint cavity, and pain on passive extension, flexion or rotation of the coffin joint.

The horse will show a mild to moderate supporting-leg lameness on hard ground. It stands with the affected foot set forward somewhat, with weight borne only on the toe.

Differential diagnosis is made from hemarthrosis and infectious arthritis.

Diagnosis. Joint distension associated with mild la menessforms the basis for diagnosis. Joint anesthesia should be used with restraint, even when antibiotics are added. Diagnostic nerve blocks are followed by radiographs taken in specific views.

Prognosis. Generally favorable.

Treatment. Mild inflammations often regress spontaneously within a few days. Cold may be applied by means of a cold water stream or cold baths. A soft ground surface is provided. Mild hyperemia is stimulated to promote the absorption of effusions (rubbing the coronet with ointment or liniment). In many cases the effusion is stubborn, and a mild supporting-leg lameness may even persist. After it has been determined whether any other causes are responsible for the lameness, the foregoing measures are applied more vigorously. Arthrocentesis and steroids are contraindicated. Their value is limited, and they will probably lead to an exacerbation or even to the loss of the animal.

Healing is supported by corrective trimming and shoeing. We recommend using flat shoes without calks, or letting the horse go barefoot in a paddock. Cushions [Norberg, 1968] and leather pads can be used with a full-bar shoe to absorb shocks.

Infectious Podarthritis

Definition. Septic inflammation of the coffin joint.

Occurrence. All four feet are susceptible.

Symptoms and Etiology. Purulent inflammation of the coffin joint results either from a perforating wound (puncture wound, coronet strike) or from the extension of septic processes from surrounding tissues. Coronet strikes on the side of the foot between the extensor tendon and lateral cartilage may open the coffin joint primarily or damage the tissue so severely that a joint infection soon follows.

Foreign bodies entering the foot vertically through the central or lateral sulci of the frog need not penetrate too deeply in order to perforate the deep flexor tendon and open the coffin joint between the navicular bone and distal phalanx. The resulting septic arthritis does not always take as dramatic a course as many laymen believe. This may cause it to be overlooked in the early stage. A purulent discharge from the joint is rarely observed following puncture wounds of the foot. Usually the only observable discharge is that from a coexisting purulent pododermatitis.

If synovial fluid appears, it may originate either from the navicular bursa or from the joint.

Besides the symptoms of puncture wounds or coronet strike, additional signs of infectious podarthritis are: joint distension, markedly increased pulse in the metacarpal and digital arteries, pain on passive flexion, extension or rotation, and a moderate to very severe supporting-leg lameness. Often the body temperature becomes elevated within a day or so after symptoms first appear. The puncture track should not be probed due to the danger of introducing or distributing infection.

Differential Diagnosis. Coronet strike, puncture wound with infection of the navicular bursa.

Diagnosis. Diagnosis may prove difficult in some cases, but is readily established by radiographic examination after several days have passed. Often many conclusions can be drawn from the clinical course.

Prognosis. Severe damage to joint tissues (cartilage, synovial membrane, bony joint members) is followed by ankylosis and chronic lameness. Septicemia is another danger. Thus, purulent coffin joint inflammation usually carries a guarded to unfavorable prognosis.

Treatment. In acute cases the animal is confined to a box stall (enforced rest), the joint is irrigated with warm isotonic saline, and antibiotics are administered intra-articularly *and* parenterally. Preferably this is done after the sensitivities of the organisms have been ascertained. Intravenous therapy is administered to improve circulatory status. If the cause is a puncture wound, drainage is established by partial resection of the deep flexor tendon.

With a coronet strike, a crescent-shaped piece of horn is excised, and a partial resection of the lateral cartilage is carried out. Joint irrigation should be repeated daily if possible.

The horse will be recumbent much of the time, and so soft bedding is provided to prevent decubitus. Measures are also taken to prevent laminitis. All shoes are removed. Tetanus antitoxin or toxoid booster is administered. The healing of a purulent podarthritis is often followed by ankylosis. If this occurs, an arthrodesis can be performed to preserve the breeding soundness of the animal.

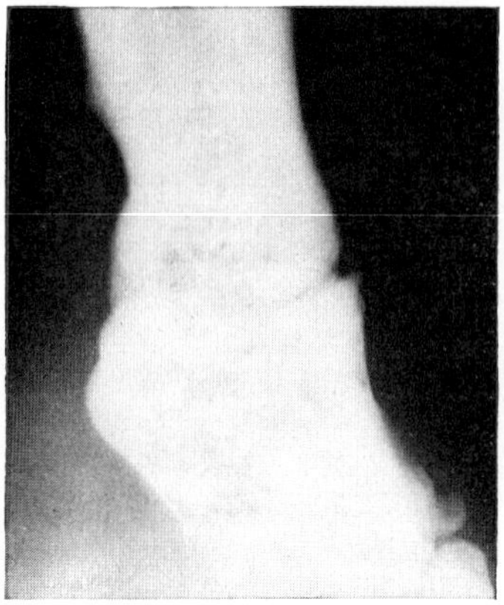
85

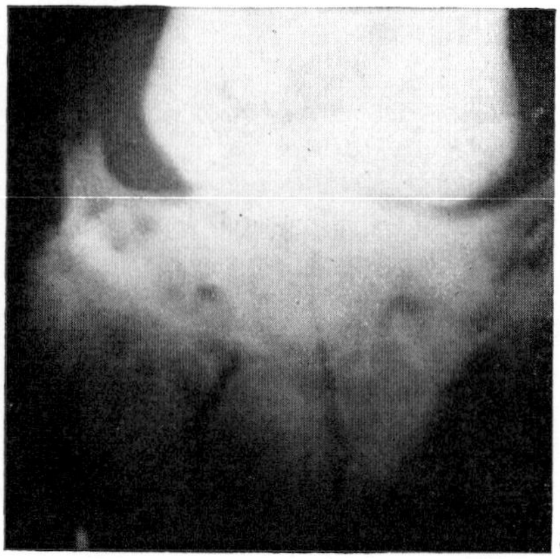
86

Fig. 2.1.20. — 85. Articular chip fracture of P3.
Fig. 2.1.20. — 86. Central fracture of P3.

2.1.20.4.9. Luxation of the Distal Phalanx (P3)

Luxations of the P3 are rare. Most occur in a dorsal direction; medial, lateral and palmar (or plantar) luxations are less common. Avulsions of the deep flexor tendon and navicular bone from the P3 have been described following incorrectly-performed neurectomies for navicular disease; these were accompanied by a *dorsal* subluxation of the P3. For this to occur, there must be severe damage to the ligaments of the coffin joint. The prognosis is guarded to unfavorable. An arthrodesis of the coffin joint should be attempted in suitable candidates.

2.1.20.4.10. Fracture of the Distal Phalanx (P3)

Classification. Fractures of the P3 are classified as follows, in order of frequency: chip fractures of the solar border, fractures of the extensor process, wing fractures, and fractures through the center of the bone (the latter with articular involvement). In many cases a true fracture is preceded by an incomplete fracture. Distal phalangeal fractures may be closed or open.

Occurrence. Uncommon; mainly occur in the front feet.

Symptoms. The supporting-leg lameness associated with incomplete P3 fractures is mild and therefore easily overlooked. With articular fractures, a severe to very severe supporting-leg lameness is usually present. The horse tends to stand on 3 legs, either bearing no weight on the affected foot or doing so very gingerly and on the toe only. There is distension of the coffin joint and fluctuation of the dorsal pouch (front of coronet medial and lateral to common extensor tendon). Percussion of certain parts of the wall produces pain, as does compression of the heels with a hoof tester. Pain is also produced by passive extension, flexion and rotation of the foot.

Etiology. Chip fractures of the solar border of P3 can result from shoenail injuries, and the curled solar border in the foundered foot may break away from the rest of the bone.

Fractures of the extensor process (fig. 2.1.20. — 85) are caused by coronet strikes, crushing of the foot by a wheeled vehicle, and by abruptly dropping the raised foot, allowing the toe to strike the ground with force.

Wing fractures and sagittal fractures (fig. 2.1.20. — 86) through the center of P3 can result from jumps, crushing by a wheeled vehicle, catching the foot on roots, etc.

Rarefying osteitis of P3 (e.g., following laminitis) as well as erosive lesions caused by keratomas predispose to fractures.

Differential diagnosis is made from all foot and limb diseases that cause sudden lameness, puncture wounds of the foot, shoenail injuries, sprains, contusions, etc.

Diagnosis. The diagnosis is established by radiography. It is important that the horn be trimmed and the clefts of the frog packed with a homogenous material (e.g., soft soap). A fracture line will be demonstrated only if it is struck straight-on by the central beam. As a rule, several views must be obtained in the dorso-palmar (or plantar) and latero-medial projection.

Diagnostic anesthesia is contraindicated whenever a complete or incomplete fracture is suspected!

Prognosis. Closed fractures generally have a favorable prognosis. With intra-articular fractures, it is necessary to restore the articular surface, which can be accomplished with two screws [Dubbs and Nemeth, 1972].

Treatment. All P3 fractures benefit from proper shoeing. With concurrent box stall confinement, many fractures will heal in 2—3 months. If conventional shoeing is not possible, a wire-reinforced Technovit shoe has proved beneficial in suitable cases. Stall confinement is maintained for 2—3 months.

For fractures involving the coffin joint, screw fixation of the fragments is desirable in order to prevent *post-traumatic arthrosis*. Dubs and Nemeth [1972] have described a drill guide for that purpose.

Petterson [1976] reviewed a series of 79 fractures of P3 in various classes of horses. Forty-five horses with wing fractures were treated conservatively, and 11 by immobilization of the fragment with a compression screw. With extra-articular fractures, conservative therapy was usually successful. Intra-articular fractures managed conservatively had a good prognosis in horses less than 3 years old. In older horses, operative treatment is the method of choice. Only 1 out of 23 fractures of the extensor process was treated operatively. The prognosis was not always good, because a secondary osteoarthritis of the coffin joint occasionally developed.

2.1.20.4.11. Fracture of the Navicular Bone

Occurrence. Fractures of the navicular bone are rare and occur mainly in the front feet of riding, jumping and racing horses.

Symptoms. Generally a moderate to severe supporting-leg lameness appears immediately after the fracture occurs. Pain is sometimes produced by hard percussion of the middle third of the frog, and occasionally by compression of that area with a hoof tester. An increased pulse is usually felt in the palmar digital and palmar arteries.

Etiology. Navicular fractures may be primary or secondary. Primary fractures have a traumatic origin and may result from severe stresses that arise in connection with joint mechanics, or from direct injury by a penetrating foreign body (harrow spike, etc.). Secondary fractures mainly result from osteoporosis of the navicular bone due to severe navicular disease (fig. 2.1.20. — 87). They may also be secondary to a suppurative navicular bursitis or puncture wound of the foot.

Diagnosis. Diagnosis is made by radiography using the technique of Oxspring [1935], in which the navicular bone is projected through the middle phalanx. A latero-medial view is also obtained (standard views). Sometimes a navicular fracture is detected during a resection of the deep flexor tendon.

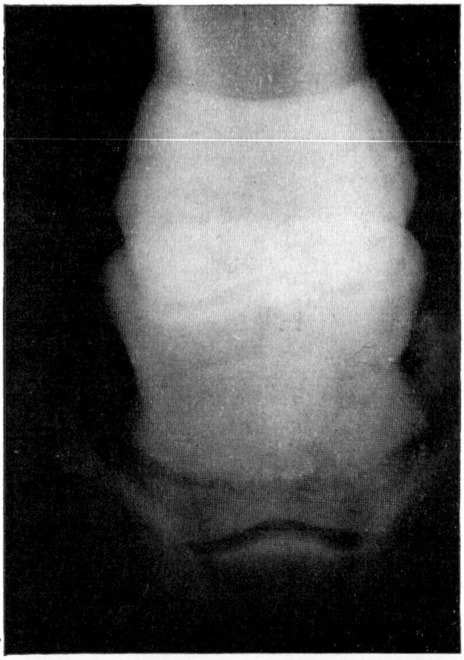

87

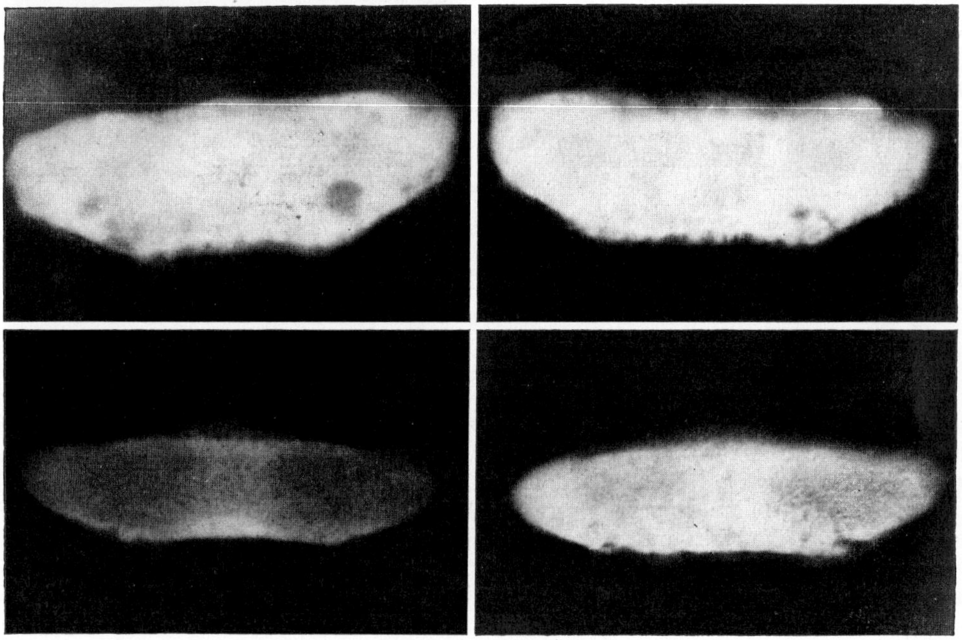

88

Fig. 2.1.20. — 87. Pathologic fracture of the navicular bone.
Fig. 2.1.20. — 88. Isolated navicular bones in navicular disease.

Prognosis and Treatment. Treatment of an infected navicular fracture is useless in most cases. A complete or partial resection of the navicular bone combined with arthrodesis of the coffin joint may be attempted in valuable horses. Simple fractures usually heal well with stall rest and suitable shoeing: elevated heel, roller-motion toe, full bar with leather pad; *the bar should not come in direct contact with the foot!*

2.1.20.4.12. Diseases of the Podotrochlea

Definition. The podotrochlea is formed by the navicular bone, the navicular bursa and the overlying portion of the deep flexor tendon. The joint between the navicular bone and the distal phalanx (part of the distal interphalangeal articulation) plays an important role in the joint mechanics of the foot. The capsule of the coffin joint is reinforced in this area by the distal ligament of the navicular bone (sesamoid impar ligament).

Function. The navicular bone and navicular bursa act as a fulcrum for the deep flexor tendon while also serving to enlarge the articular surface of P3 for receiving the head of the middle phalanx.

Classification. Two main forms of podotrochlear disease are recognized clinically:

a) navicular disease (podotrochleosis),

b) podotrochleitis (infectious p.).

Navicular Disease (Podotrochleosis)

Definition. Navicular disease is a typical *arthrosis,* or *erosive lesion,* affecting the navicular bone, navicular bursa and adjacent deep flexor tendon. Inflammatory symptoms are not predominant.

Occurrence. Navicular disease affects horses almost exclusively. It is most often seen in riding horses and is less common in draft horses. Navicular disease generally affects *both front feet* in varying degrees; the hind feet are rarely if ever affected. Even horses that have never been shod or ridden are susceptible.

Symptoms. The disease develops gradually and often goes unnoticed in its early stages. When *both* forefeet are affected more or less simultaneously, a *locomotor disturbance* develops, rather than lameness. The action of the forelimbs is reduced, the stride becomes shorter, and the foot tends to land on the toe.

Mild locomotor disturbances are apparent only when the horse is exercised on hard, flat ground (concrete, asphalt).

The gait changes are nonspecific. Sometimes the animal will show obvious *pain on turning,* especially at the start of exercise. Under a rider the locomotor disturbance will initially worsen when the animal is ridden cold but will disappear as exercise is continued; after a while it does not. Often a general decline of performance is noted.

When standing, the horse takes weight off the front feet by pointing alternately with one foot and then with the other, or by standing with both feet set forward. Gradually contraction of the heels may develop due to a lack of pressure on the caudal part of the foot (incomplete dorsiflexion). For the same reason an increasing erectness of the digital axis and foot may be observed. If one foot is mainly affected, muscular atrophy may be evident in the more severely affected limb; atrophy of the foot has also been described.

Examination of the foot with a hoof tester will sometimes elicit pain when pressure is applied to the middle third of the frog. Compression of the walls at the heel will also be painful if contraction has developed. Hard percussion of the center third of

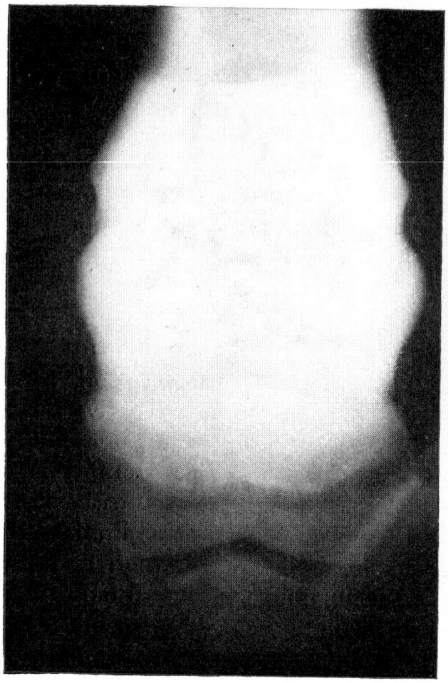

89

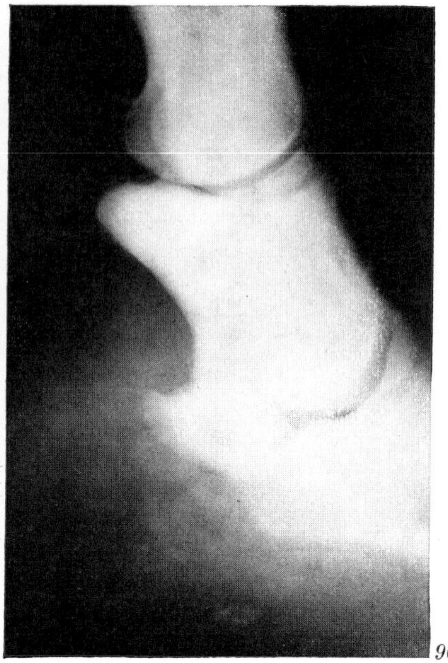

90

Fig. 2.1.20. — 89. Second-degree navicular disease.
Fig. 2.1.20. — 90. Navicular disease (latero-medial projection)

the frog (e.g., with a closed hoof tester) will also produce pain in some cases. Not infrequently, faulty shoeing with a full-bar shoe will provoke a locomotor disturbance or navicular lameness due to contact between the bar and frog. This method has been utilized diagnostically in circumstances where an x-ray machine was unavailable.

The gait exhibited in navicular disease may erroneously suggest a diagnosis of 'shoulder lameness' unless a careful, systemic examination of both forelimbs is carried out, proceeding from the foot upward.

Etiology. The disease is precipitated by a number of factors that are not yet fully understood. It is known, however, that the specific stresses placed on the podotrochlea in riding horses are probably aided by other factors. These factors include foot shape, faulty trimming and shoeing, limb and digital conformation. Errors of rearing, stabling, conditioning and nutrition lead to the rapid development of erosive lesions in the navicular bone, navicular bursa and adjacent deep flexor tendon. This is especially common in young performance horses that are not given adequate conditioning. The influence of genetic factors is, we believe, more indirect than direct.

In general, it may be said that all riding horses contract navicular disease sooner or later, and that the challenge is to forestall its occurrence, if possible, until old age.

Pathogenesis. WINTZER and DÄMMRICH [1971] state that changes develop in the distal ligament of the navicular bone and its insertions as a consequence of the functional stresses placed on the navicular bone and its ligaments during locomotion, and that the pain of navicular disease is due to these changes. Their studies revealed a distalward, roof-like expansion of the navicular bone on its tendinous surface, a fibrous thickening and shortening of the distal ligament of the navicular bone, an alteration in the shape of the articular surface, and exostosis formation at the insertions of the distal ligament and deep flexor tendon on the flexor surface of P3. Lipping was also demonstrated at the articular margin of P3, as well as chip fractures on the flexor surface of the navicular bone.

Pathologic Anatomy. Pathologic changes are found in the ligaments of the navicular bone (especially the distal ligament), the navicular bone (fig. 2.1.20. — 88), P3, the navicular bursa, and the deep flexor tendon. The changes in the navicular bone, which can be demonstrated *radiographically*, are of particular clinical and diagnostic importance (figs. 2.1.20. — 89 and — 90). Both the structure and the contour of the bone may be affected. Hertsch and Zeller [1976] classify the changes into two groups: 'suspicious' and 'pathologic'. *Age-dependent changes* in the navicular bone are also recognized. Thus, changes that are acceptable in a 7-year-old horse, for example, would be considered pathologic in a 3-year-old.

The bony end-plate of the tendinous surface of the navicular bone is composed of two layers corresponding to stresses imposed by compressive and tensile forces. The vascular channels of the outer layer run parallel to the longitudinal axis of the navicular bone, while those of the inner layer run mainly at right angles to it. The constant action of these forces also produces a gradual change in the shape of the navicular bone, which likewise is age-dependent. The navicular bone of the foal has a nearly square shape in the median longitudinal section. As age increases, the longitudinal cut surface acquires a rectangular or wedge shape.

The apposition of bony tissue causes the flexor surface of the navicular bone to elongate in the direction of P3. Osteoclastic processes lead to a sinuous, lacuna-like expansion of the vascular channels. Splits and circumscribed defects develop in the overlying cartilage. These cause lesions of the flexor tendon and appear as club-shaped lucent areas in the radiograph.

The changes in P3 affect its surface of articulation with the navicular bone. This surface becomes involved in the same type of structural changes that affect the navicular bone itself (fig. 2.1.20. — 88).

The fluid content of the navicular bursa becomes progressively reduced in volume, the wall of the bursa becomes thickened, and adhesions develop.

The gliding surface of the deep flexor tendon shows various changes (tearing and fraying of the fibrils) caused by dry friction, finally resulting in adhesions of the tendon to the navicular bursa and tendinous surface of the navicular bone.

Differential Diagnosis. Early navicular disease may be difficult to differentiate from podarthrosis in the absence of specific radiographic signs. Intra-articular anesthesia is also of little help in such cases (besides being little practiced under ordinary conditions).

Ringbone of the coffin joint (severe podarthrosis) can be verified radiographically. This disease also leads to a mechanical impairment of joint motion and thus to a mechanical lameness (cf. pain lameness).

Ossification of the lateral cartilages is palpable and is demonstrable radiographically, while *fissure fractures of the navicular bone* (q.v.) often cannot be detected radiographically unless struck at the precise angle by the central beam. The same applies to *complete navicular fractures* with an indistinct fracture line.

Osteitis of the wings of the distal phalanx can be demonstrated with radiographs if sufficient demineralization has occurred.

Aseptic pododermatitis is confirmed or excluded by employing a systematic examination routine (hoof testers, percussion of horny capsule).

In doubtful cases a thorough reexamination of the horse under various conditions is helpful: hard ground/soft ground, uphill/downhill, with/without a rider, in harness, over jumps, in terrain, following prolonged exercise, etc.

Diagnosis. The diagnosis of navicular disease relies upon the history, *clinical findings* in the foot and rest of the limb, the disappearance or shifting of lameness in response to a *palmar digital nerve block*, and *radiographic findings*.

The palmar digital nerves are blocked by injecting no more than 2—3 ml of anesthetic on each side of the deep flexor tendon on the back of the pastern, about halfway between the fetlock and the coronary band. More than 2—3 ml might also block the anterior branches, making diagnosis difficult. If the injection is correctly done, there will be no cutaneous field for verifying the correct location of the block, as there is when a nerve block is done, say, at the level of the fetlock joint. An improvement of gait or the disappearance or shifting of lameness is the only indication of a successful block. The nerve block should precede radiographic examination.

Radiographic evidence must be present before a definitive diagnosis of navicular disease can be made. However, it is important to note that the disease cannot be diagnosed on the basis of radiographic findings alone!

Many shoulder joints have been unnecessarily treated because of navicular disease located a meter or more away from the presumed seat of the disorder.

A 'shifting' of the lameness indicates that a painful condition is present in the adjacent limb. In such cases that limb, too, must be carefully examined, working from the foot upward. A thorough examination should encompass the entire locomotor system, including the spine, muscles, nerve roots, blood vessels and other structures.

Before radiographs are taken the horseshoe should be removed and the foot thoroughly cleaned. Excess horn is trimmed, and the hollow of the sole and the sulci of the frog are packed with a homogenous material (soft soap, fine horn cuttings with putty) to eliminate the possibility of a misdiagnosis (navicular fractures!).

Radiographic Examination of the Navicular Bone. We use the Oxspring technique, a dorso-palmar projection in which the navicular bone is projected through the middle phalanx, producing a summation of shadows. One should avoid projecting the articular border of the navicular bone onto the line of the coffin joint, as this would hamper evaluation of these important areas. Once the examiner has become familiar with the topography of the navicular bone at varying angles of the dorsal hoof wall, little can happen that will seriously interfere with the radiographic interpretation. The AP view is obtained by using a specially constructed wooden stand that holds the dorsal wall upright; the film cassette is placed vertically behind the foot. Many colleagues radiograph the digit with the foot hanging free, even though this method entails a slight radiation hazard. Hertsch and Zeller [1976] have compiled a list of guidelines for radiographic examination of the navicular bone. Morgan [1972] also describes a dorso-ventral technique for demonstrating the contour of the flexor surface of the navicular bone. In all cases a lateral view should also be obtained to demonstrate the profile of the bone. This view, together with the AP, are the two standard views for navicular bone radiography. The age-related changes in the navicular bone were described previously. In the AP view we give particular attention to the articular border of the bone, watching for such changes as toothlike exostoses, lucent areas, enlarged vascular channels, and the presence of lacunae in the body of the bone (lucent areas, usually club-shaped and sometimes occurring in succession, osteoporosis, sclerosis). Hook-shaped exostoses of variable size are sometimes visible at the extremities of the navicular bone, and osteophytes of varying shape may be present on its free border.

The lateral (latero-medial) view demonstrates the profile of the bone and may reveal spurlike exostoses and other changes. The lateral view is usually less rewarding than the AP view.

The absence of radiographic changes does not prove that navicular disease is not present. Conversely, positive radiographic findings must be evaluated in terms of the the age of the horse and the type of work it has performed.

In many horses of all breeds, radiography sometimes shows marked changes in the navicular bone, even though no lameness or locomotor disturbance is apparent. The previous diagnostic nerve block, correctly performed, is also negative in the absence of navicular disease.

Generally, radiographic changes are not evident at the onset of navicular disease. In advanced cases, on the other hand, the radiographic changes seem to follow the development of locomotor signs.

At the Orthopedic Clinic of the University of Veterinary Medicine in Vienna, a radiographic examination of the navicular bones of both forefeet and the hock joints of both hind limbs is mandatory for every new horse that is acquired. Examinations of this type can even have prognostic value in experienced hands.

The value of radiographic examinations in young horses is undisputed, especially for the early diagnosis of disease as part of a preventive health-care program.

Prognosis. The prognosis in terms of functional recovery is guarded to unfavorable. The main task of the veterinarian, working in cooperation with the farrier, is to slow the progress of the disease. Proper loading of the navicular area within the framework of a sound exercise program will prolong the horse's usefulness. Several months of exercise at pasture almost always leads to transitory improvement.

In more severe cases, neurectomy of the palmar digital nerves is recommended.

Treatment. The walls at the heel are left long in order to obtain a more upright foot axis. Leather or plastic shims will also fulfill this requirement, as will shoeing with thick-branched flat shoes, though this results in a greater shoe weight. The toe is rolled to facilitate breakover and extend the life of the shoe.

Point firing followed by blistering is a treatment regimen of the past and is seldom beneficial. The injection of various drugs into the navicular bursa (glucocorticoids, anesthetics, cartilage extracts, etc.) will do more harm than good!

Bilateral palmar digital neurectomy performed for more severe cases of navicular disease will relieve lameness symptoms for 2—3 years on the average and is a suitable treatment method for all classes of performance horses. Regulations in some states may prohibit its use in racehorses. Because it relieves the pain of navicular disease, this operation is also favorable from a humane standpoint. It is a palliative treatment only, however, and does not alter the disease process. We do not advocate a palmar digital neurectomy for horses that are ridden or driven recklessly. Treatment with coumarin derivatives recommended by Colles [1979] requires further testing.

Comments. Next to spavin, navicular disease is one of the major causes of locomotor disability in horses. Whenever a horse with a lameness or locomotor disturbance is to be purchased, the podotrochlea should be checked for disease by administering a palmar digital nerve block *and* by taking radiographs. If navicular disease is present, it may be possible to estimate the age of the disease from the degree of muscular and/or foot atrophy that has occurred, eyewitness accounts, and neurectomy scars.

Infectious Podotrochleitis

Occurrence. This disease occurs mainly in the hind feet following injuries to the navicular bursa or navicular bone due to puncture wounds of the foot. Infectious podotrochleitis may also develop secondarily due to the extension of suppurative processes from adjacent tissues.

Symptoms. Systemic manifestations may be severe. The pulse is increased in the plantar arteries. The horse exhibits a severe supporting-leg lameness and bears weight gingerly on the toe of the foot. A puncture wound may or may not be visible in the lateral or central sulci of the frog (the soft horn of the frog tends to close over wounds made by thin foreign bodies). Usually a bloody, purulent (grayish-black) exudate drains from the wound, indicating the presence of a suppurative pododermatitis. In rare cases, synovial fluid is discharged from the navicular bursa and has a scrambled-egg-like appearance when coagulated. It is advisable to pare down the horn tissue of the frog somewhat, as the foreign body or pieces of it can sometimes be located in this way.

The fossa of the heel may be effaced, and corresponding inflammatory symptoms will be evident if abscessation is present. Cellulitic processes are manifested by a firm, hot, painful swelling at the coronary band that extends upward to the fetlock joint. The swelling may extend to the tarsal or carpal joint, or even to the elbow or stifle.

Etiology, Differential Diagnosis and Diagnosis. See Puncture Wounds of the Foot.

Prognosis. Recovery depends to a large extent on a prompt diagnosis. Often damage to the bursa is not apparent until some days after the injury. Navicular fractures may also be present. Even with operative wound care, such complications as purulent tendovaginitis, infectious podarthritis, and adhesions of the deep flexor tendon to the navicular bone cannot always be avoided. The prognosis in terms of functional recovery is guarded, therefore.

Treatment. The wound edges are excised, and if necessary a partial resection of the deep flexor tendon is carried out so that the navicular bursa can be opened and treated with antibiotics. Parenteral antibiotics are also given. Tetanus antitoxin or booster is administered, a pressure dressing is applied, and the horse is confined to a box stall.

2.1.20.5. Fundamentals of Foot Care and Shoeing

Foot care refers to all measures that serve to maintain the health and functional integrity of the equine foot. The importance of the foot to the overall soundness of the horse is reflected in such aphorisms as 'no foot, no horse' and 'the horse has but one foot'.

The broad area of foot care can be divided into two main categories: *care of the unshod foot* (especially, foot care in foals) and *care of the shod foot*.

2.1.20.5.1. Care of the Unshod Foot

Foot Care in Foals

The first concern is the correct sloughing or wear of the soft horny pad that covers the hoof and protects the uterus from injury before and during parturition. It is very important to start handling the foal's feet soon after birth so that it will become accustomed to it and will not be frightened when trimmed and shod later on. Of course the attendant, rider, farrier, veterinarian, and others must be aware of proper handling methods and recognize the importance of *time and patience* in the handling of animals. Especially in performance horses, the goal is to establish a sense of complete trust between man and horse so that contact with the animal will be safe at all times. Thus, it should be possible to carry out mildly painful procedures, like giving an injection, without resorting to forcible measures and with no more preparation than a reassuring pat on the neck. More involved procedures are performed under general anesthesia.

The first contact with the horse is vocal; the horse is called by name and spoken to gently. The next contact is tactile and consists of patting the horse on the neck, stroking the limbs, palpating areas of suspected disease, etc., avoiding any manipulations that might cause pain. These are carried out gradually at the end of the examination and should employ the minimum force necessary to confirm or exclude the presence of pain (e.g., 'tenderness to pressure over the lateral splint bone').

Through expert foot care in the foal, as well as through proper corrective trimming and good general care, it is possible to improve or eliminate faults of limb and foot conformation and thus significantly improve performance when maturity is reached. It need hardly be stated that the well-conformed horse is better able to run in a balanced fashion and stride out properly than the poorly-conformed horse.

At one time these elementary rules of horse care were much better known than today owing to the reliance on horses for agricultural, military and other uses, and the greater density of horse populations.

An important element of early foot care is *exercise*, which can contribute greatly to the development of a well-shaped foot and to the horse's working capacity in general. Foals should be exercised on dry, moderately soft ground; a good pasture is best. Ground that is constantly damp or rocky is less favorable for foot development. The foal's hoof initially has a larger circumference at the coronet than at the bearing surface (inverted conical shape) until about the age of 8—10 months, when the hoof is more or less cylindrical. Later the ground circumference becomes larger than the coronary circumference. (We are speaking of the widest part of the coronet and bearing surface as viewed from the front.) These processes are the result of 'hoof mechanics'. Early exercise of the 8- to 10-day-old foal sets these processes in motion, besides promoting blood circulation through the foot, *keratinization* and the growth of new horn. It would be a mistake, however, to allow hoof development to proceed without interference, since faults of development can occur despite pasturing. Particular attention should be given to the limb and digital conformation, for faults in these areas are generally amenable to correction before about the 5th year of life when growth is completed and skeletal maturity is reached.

Faults of limb and digital conformation place uneven loads on the foot and predispose to 'crooked foot' and other hoof deformities. Base-wide and base-narrow feet with their associated conformation faults are also damaging to the performance horse. Eventually the load disparities will lead to disease of the joints, ligaments, tendons and muscles, as well as permanent foot deformity. It is mandatory, therefore, that the feet be *inspected and trimmed* by a competent farrier every 4—6 weeks, or more frequently if indicated. Uneven horn wear is prevented if necessary by corrective shoeing, which will also improve conformation faults. Lightweight, hand-forged, individually-fitted flat shoes or *three-quarter shoes* are suitable for this purpose. If toe wear is excessive or club foot is present, tip shoes are indicated; these may extend beyond the toe in severe cases. Once the foot has shown satisfactory improvement following these corrective measures, it may again be left unshod. As a general rule, *shoeing should be deferred until absolutely necessary* This will also prevent premature use of the horse, which is a major cause of early retirement.

Because horn growth in the foal and young horse proceeds at a much faster rate (up to 14 mm per month) than in the mature horse (8 mm per month on the average), the foot should be trimmed at more frequent intervals — every 4—5 weeks or so. This will also serve to stimulate horn growth.

It is good practice to lift the foal's hoof and tap it to simulate shoeing, so that the animal will not become frightened later when the feet are picked up and shod. Adult horses that *resist shoeing* have no value as working animals.

Foals that are stabled during the winter require a particularly careful and intensive foot care. The *self-cleaning mechanism* of the normal foot cannot function well under such conditions and must be replaced or supplemented by human intervention: The ground surface is cleaned, debris is removed with a hoof-pick, the horny walls are washed with water and a brush, the sensitive skin on the back of the pastern is dried, the fissured horn tissue of the frog is trimmed with a hoof knife, and the edges of the bearing surface of the wall are smoothed with a hoof rasp. Thrush can be remedied by paring away the macerated horn of the frog and then applying oak-bark powder, pine tar, etc. Good, clean straw bedding is provided. Foals are kept with their dam in a large box stall.

Knuckling, resulting in an upright foot and pastern axis, is treated by correcting any calcium-phosphorus imbalance providing a sufficient vitamin D intake, adequate exercise, and by specific measures such as extension casts (e.g., Lightcast®). We have obtained very good results with these techniques in a number of cases. In severe cases acrylics can be applied to the foal's hoof to take the place of corrective shoeing (cf. corrective shoeing for peg foot).

Care of the Unshod Foot in Older Horses

In older horses that go barefoot (dams), the feet should be trimmed every 4—6 weeks according to the guideline outlined above, and the edge of the bearing surface should be rounded to reduce the risk of horn damage. Similar considerations apply to Thoroughbred racehorses, circus horses, show horses, ponies, and other horses that usually wear shoes only on the forefeet or go unshod.

2.1.20.5.2. Care of the Shod Foot

In the shod foot, emphasis is placed upon regular resetting of the shoe, cleaning, exercise and stable hygiene. Shoeing, even in the most skillful hands, represents a 'necessary evil' that entails certain disadvantages. Shoes invariably remove some ground pressure from the foot and effect a fundamental change in hoof mechanics. Ground moisture has little or no access to the horny tissues, which reduces the elasticity of the hoof. When shoeing is not done properly, its harmful effect on the foot, the conformation of the digits and limbs, and the gait can be observed daily. The foot should be trimmed and the shoe reset every 4—6 weeks. Even if shoe wear is minimal, the horn continues to grow and requires periodic trimming. Neglect in this area is an invitation to locomotor impairment or lameness.

The modern farrier must travel to farms, riding stables, show arenas and racetracks to practice his trade and usually must rely on untrained persons for assistance. We can help to improve this situation by rendering support where needed, and by watching for competent young riders and drivers that would make good candidates for training as farriers. The high-performance athletic and show horses of today place considerably greater demands on the farrier than did the agricultural horses of yesterday. He must cope with such problems as thin horny walls, unfavorable horn properties (brittle or soft), and hoofs that are irregular or even diseased, even in many top-performance animals. The modern farrier must know something about riding, racing and driving, and should himself be a rider or driver if possible.

The feet should be inspected daily so that such problems as loose-fitting shoes, lost calks, projecting nails, etc. can be quickly recognized. The rider and driver are generally well-informed about such matters, and this knowledge is required in order to pass the tests for rider or driver certification. The feet should be cleaned routinely after workouts: the sole and sulci of the frog are cleaned with a hoof pick, the foot is scribbed with water and a brush, the skin on the back of the pastern is dried, and suitable hoof ointments or sprays are applied. These products should be acid-free and should not blacken the horn. Ointments that contain vitamin A can be rubbed daily into the skin of the coronet to promote horn growth and improve horn quality.

Moisture that enters the horn from the blood via the matrix is kept from evaporating by the intact perioplic layer. When work is done on rocky or sandy ground, the distal portions of this layer become disrupted and should be replaced with suitable hoof ointments. When applied in an extremely thin layer, these ointments effectively prevent the rapid evaporation of exogenous and endogenous hoof moisture.

The horn tissue of the hoof possesses a functional, somewhat complex structure that is elegantly reflected in the various processes that enter into 'hoof mechanics'.

Opinion is divided concerning the importance of the pigment with respect to horn quality. However, it may be safely assumed that its influence is a favorable one.

Rancid fats, motor oil, petroleum jelly, blackened hoof ointments, shoe greases, etc. are harmful. They cause crusts to form, below which the horn is soft and friable. Often they cause chronic inflammations of the perioplic and coronary epidermis, causing the horn to acquire a bark-like appearance. In the properly-cleaned hoof, the natural color of the horn will shine through. Excessive drying of the horn is prevented with baths or poultices made with loam, linseed meal, bran or sawdust. In Europe hard, brittle horn responds well to sauerkraut poultices, in which case lactic acid serves as the moisturizing agent! One can also use rubber or leather shoes with sponge inserts. The use of cow manure is not advised.

The beneficial effect of adequate exercise on horn quality is reemphasized.

Finally, it is important that good, dry bedding be provided. Of the various bedding materials available (straw, sawdust, peat, tannin bark), straw has proved the most suitable. Peat is a good bedding material for sensitive feet (laminitis) and may be covered with a layer of straw if desired.

Various means are available for *accelerating horn growth:* the vitamin-A ointment mentioned above, adequate exercise, regular trimming and proper nutrition: whole oats and good pasture hay.

2.1.20.5.3. Fundamentals of Shoeing

'Shoeing' refers basically to the protection of the horn from excessive wear by suitable implements made of metal (steel, aluminium, silver, gold) or other materials (plastic, polyethylene, PVC, polyurethane, rubber, etc.). But beyond its purely protective function, the shoe is fashioned in such a way that it aids the horse in the performance of its assigned tasks, or provides needed correction in the presence of conformation faults or disease. Shoeing can also contribute to the prevention of many foot diseases.

Shoeing should always be preceded by orthopedic trimming of the foot. Then the shoe is selected according to the principles discussed above. In the great majority of cases, the hand-forged, individually-fitted shoe will be far superior to any semi-finished or ready-made product ('factory shoe') that may be available. Only the hand-made shoe has the exact size, shape, width, thickness, length and crease size that is optimum for a given foot. If this is true for the healthy but irregular foot, it is especially true in the case of the diseased foot, such as the flat foot or foundered foot, whose many variables demand treatment with special corrective shoes that are hand-forged to individual specifications.

The full-bar shoe with leather pad has proved useful in the treatment of diseased feet, as well as in preventing such diseases as contracted foot.

The Norberg cushion has proved effective in the treatment of contracted foot and in preserving the concavity of the sole, thereby aiding in the prevention of flat foot and dropped sole. The much-publicized 'plastic shoes' are in many cases attached with conventional horseshoe nails and are occasionally used in Standardbreds mainly owing to their light weight. These shoes last only a very short time, however.

Another type of plastic shoe has a steel insert and is applied to the foot with adhesive. It can be adapted somewhat to the shape of the foot. Stable attachment is ensured by a rim about 3 cm high which encloses the distal portions of the horny wall. Experience with this shoe is not yet adequate for an evaluation to be made.

For details on shoeing, the reader is referred to the large specialized literature. Corrective principles have already been discussed under Faults of Gait.

Every veterinarian who specializes in equine diseases should have a thorough knowledge of corrective shoeing as well as the shoeing of the normal foot.

References

Ackermann, N.; Garner, H. E.; Coffmann, J. R.; Clement, J.: Angiographic appearance of the normal equine foot and alterations in chronic laminitis. J. Amer. vet. med. Assoc. *166:* 58 (1975).

Adams, O. R.: Vascular changes in experimental laminitis. Proc. 18th Ann. Conv., Amer. Assoc. Equine Pract., p. 359 (1972).

Åkerblom, E.: Über die Ätiologie und Pathogenese der Futterrehe beim Pferd. Skand. Arch. Physiol. *58:* 1 (1934).

Bayer, J.: Lehrbuch der Veterinär-Chirurgie (Wilhelm Braumüller, Wien und Leipzig 1890).

Bittner, H.: Hufbein der Pferde. Arch. Tierheilk. *56:* 84 (1927).

Bolz, W.: Behandlung der chronischen Hufrehe. Tierärztl. Rdsch. *45:* 651 (1939).

Bretschneider: Die Veränderungen des Hufes beim Stelzfuss des Pferdes. Der Hufschmied *27:* 93, 107 (1909).

Bürgi, O.: Untersuchungen über den sog. Hufkrebs und Straubfuss des Pferdes. Schweiz. Arch. Tierheilk. *52:* H. 3, 4, 5 (1910).

Coffmann, J. R.; Johnson, J. H.; Guffy, M. M.; Finocchio, E. J.: Hoof circulation in equine laminitis. J. Amer. vet. med. Assoc. *156:* 76 (1970).

Colles, M.: Pathogenese der Podotrochlose und ihre Therapie mit Cumarinderivaten. III. Tagung über Pferdekrankheiten, Equitana, Essen 1979.

Dubs, B.; Nemeth, F.: Therapie und Prognose der Hufbeinfrakturen. Schweiz. Arch. Tierheilk. *114:* 423 (1972).

Erkurt, O.: Erfahrungen über die Behandlung des Hufkrebses bei Pferden mit Penicillin. Tierärztl. Umschau *10:* 164 (1955).

Garner, H. E.; Coffman, J. R.; Hahn, A. W.; Ackermann, N.; Johnson, J. H.: Equine laminitis and associated hypertension. J. Amer. vet. med. Assoc. *166:* 56 (1975).

Habacher, F.: cited after Haun, R.: Vet.-med. Diss., Wien (1921).

Habacher, F.: Der Vollhuf; in: Stang; Wirth, Tierheilkunde und Tierzucht. Enzyklopädie (Urban & Schwarzenberg, Berlin 1928), p. 449.

Habacher, F.: Beiträge zum sog. Hufkrebs. Wiener tierärztl. Mschr. *18:* 417 (1931).

Hertsch, B.; Zeller, R.: Röntgenologische Veränderungen am Strahlbein und ihre Beurteilung. Collegium vet., p. 14 (1976).

Hilbert, W.: Erfahrungen über operative Hufkrebsbehandlung mit Gipsgußverband. Z. Veterinärk. *55:* 152 (1943).

Knezevic, P.: Untersuchungen über die beschleunigende Wirkung verschiedener Salben auf das Wachstums des Huf- und Klauenhornes. Wiener tierärztl. Mschr. *46:* 70 (1959).

Knezevic, P.: Hornperle in der Huflederhaut. Berliner Münchener tierärztl. Wschr. *75:* 141 (1962).

KNEZEVIC, P.: Klinik des Trachtenzwanghufes und Grundlagen der Ungulographie mit Dehnungsmeßstreifen beim Pferd. Wiener tierärztl. Mschr. *49:* 777, 869, 944 (1962).
KNEZEVIC, P.: Therapy of hoof cracks by application of adhesive sheets. Proc. VIIIth Congr. Europ. S. Vet. Surg., Bologna 1968.
KNEZEVIC, P.: Spezielle Untersuchung des Hufes. tierärztl. praxis *3:* 45 (1975).
KNEZEVIC, P.: Hufabszess, Steingallen — Therapie und Prognose. tierärztl. praxis *3:* 205 (1975).
LUNGWITZ, M.; TSCHERNE, L.: Untersuchungen über die Qualität des Wandhorns beim Pferdehufe. Vet.-med. Diss., Leipzig (1910).
MORGAN, J. P.: Radiology in veterinary orthopedics (Lea & Febiger, Philadelphia 1972).
MUSZAR: Beitrag zur Anatomie und Pathologie des Hufbeins. Vet.-med. Diss., München (1930).
NORBERG, Å.: Silicone rubber hoof pad. Proc. AAEP (1968), p. 336.
OXSPRING, G. E.: The radiology of navicular disease, with observations on its pathology. Vet. Rec. *15:* 1433 (1935).
PETTERSON, H.: Fractures of the pedal bone in the horse. Equine Vet. J. *8:* 104 (1976).
PILLWAX, J.: Lehrbuch des Huf- und Klauenbeschlages; 5. Aufl. (Wilhelm Braumüller, Wien und Leipzig 1892).
RUTHE, H.: Eine neue Zwangshufform. Mh. Vet.-Med. *5:* 330 (1950).
SCHEBITZ, H.: Zur Podotrochlose. Spätergebnis nach Neurektomie der Rami volares. Berliner Münchener Tierärztl. Wschr. *78:* 21 (1965).
SCHEBITZ, H.; WILKENS, H.: Atlas der Röntgenanatomie des Pferdes; 3. Aufl. (Parey, Hamburg 1978).
SCHLEG: Chronisches Hufgeschwür (Fleischwandgeschwür) der Pferde. Der Hufschmied *6:* 85 (1886).
WINTZER, H.-J.; DÄMMRICH, K.: Untersuchungen zur Pathogenese der sog. Strahlbeinlahmheit des Pferdes. Berliner und Münchener tierärztl. Wschr. *84:* 221 (1971).

2.2. Bacterial, Mycotic and Viral Infections

2.2.1. Infectious Diseases of the Skin

2.2.1.1. Malignant Edema

Definition. Malignant edema is an acute to hyperacute wound infection caused by *Clostridium septicum.* It is marked clinically by a rapidly-spreading, inflammatory, emphysematous edema that progresses to a necrotizing cellulitis. Death may occur in 4—5 days.

Symptoms. Grossly contaminated wounds of the skin, subcutaneous tissue, fascia and muscle will be present. The vulva and vaginal mucosa may become injured, contused and torn at parturition. These wounds, which contain little or no viable tissue, are an ideal site for invasion by clostridia. Within hours, or within 2—3 days at the latest, rapidly-spreading, gassy, cellulitic swellings develop at the site of the infection. All gas-permeated tissues succumb to necrosis within 24—48 hours. The area surrounding the gaseous cellulitis is very painful and initially shows a rubbery swelling. A crepitant sound is noted on palpation of the tissue. The puffy tissues appear balloon-like when percussed, and a tympanitic sound is produced. Air bubbles and foam sometimes exude from the wounds. During the first few hours the wounds give off an odor reminiscent of malic acid; later this odor turns foul and putrid.

Within hours the gaseous cellulitis spreads from the wound area to involve the entire limb, head, neck and back. Swelling also becomes evident in the anal and pubic region.

The discharge from the wound is initially watery and contains decomposed blood. The necrotic muscle is blue in color and can be easily picked apart, as if boiled. In extreme cases a pulpy degeneration of the muscles is evident. If the infectious process is arrested, the necrotic skin, fascial and muscle tissues will become completely demarcated within 2—3 weeks.

Within hours after the onset of a gas gangrene infection, severe systemic manifestations appear as a result of toxins produced by the causal organism and by endogenous tissue degeneration. Pronounced circulatory and respiratory changes appear, and the body temperature rises to 40.0—42.0 °C.

If the gas gangrene infection is stopped, it will take some time for systemic signs to disappear.

Etiology. Besides *Clostridium septicum,* other possible organisms of malignant edema are *Cl. histolyticum, Cl. perfringens* and *Cl. chauvoei.* A grossly contaminated and heavily traumatized wound always serves as the portal of infection. In the horse, injuries with rusty metals, rotten wood or other heavily contaminated objects are the most common mechanisms whereby clostridia gain entry to soft-tissue wounds.

Differential Diagnosis. Subcutaneous edema is unaccompanied by systemic signs. It is usually associated with the presence of small puncture wounds or incised wounds in areas that are subject to much movement (stifle, submaxillary region, olecranon).

Putrid wound infections spread only along the connective tissues, whereas gaseous cellulitis always spreads to involve the muscle.

Diagnosis. Infections with *Cl. perfringens* do not spread as rapidly as infections with *Cl. septicum*, *Cl. novyi* or *Cl. histolyticum*, which are rapidly progressive and fatal.

A bacteriologic diagnosis is usually too late to be of therapeutic value.

Prognosis. The prognosis is always unfavorable. Even if infection is controlled, weeks of convalescence will be needed. A return to athletic soundness is doubtful.

Treatment. Prompt, vigorous surgical treatment is indicated. Exposure to any amount of oxygen is harmful to the offending anaerobes. Thus, deep incisions and counterincisions are made in the healthy tissue. The wounds are irrigated, if necessary at 2-hour intervals, with 5% hydrogen peroxide solution or potassium permanganate solution. One may also try introducing oxygen directly into the tissue. It is useless to irrigate the wounds with ordinary antiseptic solutions. Once demarcation has occurred, conventional treatment may be given like that for a granulating wound. Suitable antibiotics are the tetracyclines and chloramphenicol.

Large doses of a polyvalent clostridial anti-serum (100—500 ml) can be administered i.v. to treat the systemic disease.

At the same time, tetracycline or chloramphenicol is administered i.v. together with glucose, electrolyte solutions, dextran or whole blood by continuous intravenous drip.

Prophylaxis. Whenever any grossly contaminated, contused wound of the subcutaneous and muscle tissues is present, 20—40 ml of a polyvalent gas edema serum should be administered as a precaution.

2.2.1.2. Vesicular Stomatitis

Definition. Vesicular stomatitis is a disease caused by an epitheliotropic virus of the rhabdovirus group that is associated with the formation of vesicles, erosions and small macules. As in foot-and-mouth disease, the vesicles and erosions may appear in the mucous membranes of the mouth or on the coronary band, udder, scrotum or prepuce.

Symptoms. Natural or experimental infection is followed by an estimated incubation period of 1—3 days. The initial symptom in the horse is excessive salivation, which increases further during eating. Initially food ingestion is not impaired. A large amount of frothy and liquid saliva is found in the feed trough. At this stage the temperature may rise to 40 °C. The fever usually persists for 3—5 days and shows little or no response to antibiotics and sulfonamides. By the 3rd or 4th day the horse drinks water copiously, but feed is consumed slowly, carefully and in smaller amounts. On the 1st or 2nd day vesicles are already evident on the lips, later appearing on the ventral and lateral surfaces of the tongue and then on its dorsal surface. The vesicles rupture within 48 hours leaving raw, bleeding erosions surrounded by necrotic mucosa at the margin. Often several vesicles coalesce before rupturing, creating a larger erosion that may cover half the lingual surface. The more extensive the erosions, the more copious the salivation.

On the foot, changes appear in the area of the coronet.

The corium of the foot may become involved, and this may lead to the development of an aseptic pododermatitis. If the affected horse is forced to move, its gait is similar to that seen in laminitis. Loss of the hoof is possible but is very rare [Heiny, 1945].

Even rarer is the appearance of vesicles on the udder, prepuce and scrotum.

Etiology and Pathogenesis. Two serologically distinct types of stomatitis virus are known [Hanson, 1972], and the diseases they produce are clinically indistinguishable. Vesicular stomatitis was first observed by Theiler in South Africa in 1901, who described it as 'contagious stomatitis'. During World War I the disease was first diagnosed in North America [Teidebold et al., 1916; Gregg et al., 1917]. The stomatitis viruses are named after the American states in which they were first isolated, New Jersey and Indiana. The Indiana virus has 3 serotypes [Federer et al., 1967]. The size of the stomatitis virus is 70 to 100 nm. At a temperature of 56 °C it retains its activity for 10—20 minutes, and at 37 °C for 3—4 days. At —20 °C it may remain viable for more than a year. It is relatively stable in a basic milieu.

The virus is readily cultivated in guinea pigs, mice, chicken embryos and tissue cultures [Wagener, 1932; Cox and Olitsky, 1933; Canha et al., 1955]. Cell cultures are best suited for the production of antigens.

All horses that do not have antibodies to vesicular stomatitis are susceptible to infection with the VS virus. According to Gregg et al. [1917] and Heiny [1945], from 30 to 95 % of exposed horses become infected. Mules do not appear to be as susceptible as horses.

The VS infection is transmissible to other mammals, including man. Its course is similar to that of influenza.

Epizootiology. At present the disease exists only in the Americas. According to Hanson et al. [1968], the New Jersey virus has been isolated from Canada to Peru. The Indiana virus type I is reported to occur in the southwestern United States, Mexico, Panama, Colombia, Venezuela and Ecuador. Type II Indiana virus has been isolated in Venezuela and Argentina. Type III Indiana virus has been found in Brazil.

The disease has always spread along waterways and arteries of traffic. It may persist on wooded pastures for very long periods. Some 90 % of cases occur in August and September. Camargo [1954] reports that the disease occurs almost entirely during the rainy season.

Vesicular stomatitis appears to have a reservoir in the frost-free areas of America. The spread of the disease along waterways and roadways, as well as its seasonal prevalence, would suggest that a carrier, or vector, is involved. Evidence points to biting Diptera as the most probable vector, especially stable flies, mosquitoes and horseflies. Indiana-type virus has been isolated from mites [Jonkers, 1967], tropical sand flies [Shalokov and Peralta, 1967] and from mosquitoes [Sudia et al., 1967]. The vector population can vary from year to year, and from one area to the next.

Diagnosis. A presumptive diagnosis of vesicular stomatitis is readily made from clinical symptoms, course, and the enzootic character of the disease. A definitive diagnosis is made by isolating the virus or by demonstrating a rise of antibody titers.

A sample of saliva, epithelium or vesicular fluid from an infected horse is used. The presence of virus can usually be demonstrated within 48—72 hours using virologic methods. Antibodies can be detected by the neutralization test or complement-fixation test.

Differential Diagnosis. There is no other viral or bacterial infection in the horse that is apt to be mistaken for vesicular stomatitis. Cattle and swine are susceptible to equine VS as well as to foot-and-mouth disease, and pigs are additionally susceptible to vesicular exanthema of swine. However, foot-and-mouth disease and swine vesicular exanthema do not occur in horses.

Contact with caustic agents or photosensitizing substances may produce lesions that resemble VS, but cases of this type will lack the enzootic character that distinguishes the VS infection.

Prognosis. The prognosis is very favorable. The disease is self-limiting, and recovery is complete within 8—14 days.

Treatment. Treatment is symptomatic. The oral cavity is rinsed 2 or 3 times daily with weak solutions of $KMNO_4$. Ample water and soft feed are provided. Potassium permanganate solutions are also placed in separate containers or poured into the feed trough so that the horse can rinse its own mouth. During the viremic phase, fever-reducing drugs or sulfonamides and antibiotics are given to prevent secondary infection. Vitamin A and calcium gluconate solutions may also be administered to promote epithelialization and reduce vascular permeability. Stall confinement is indicated. Affected horses generally may resume work or training 2 to 3 weeks after the onset of the disease.

Comments. The antibody titer remains at a high level for months and protects the animal from reinfection. Neither killed- nor live-virus vaccines have yet been used to immunize horses. A horse that is kept stabled and protected from insects is reasonably safe from infection even in enzootic areas. The risk of infection is also low on pastures located in upland areas.

References

Camargo, N. C.: A contribution to the study of vesicular stomatitis in Mexico. Proc. US Livestock Sanit. Assoc. *58:* 379 (1954).

Canha, R. G.; Eichhorn, E. A.; Mata, F. O.: Differentiation between foot-and-mouth disease and vesicular stomatitis viruses by means of mouse inoculation. Amer. J. vet. Res. *16:* 472 (1955).

Cox, H. R.; Olitsky, P. K.: Neurotropism of vesicular stomatitis virus. Proc. Soc. Exp. Biol. Med. *30:* 653 (1933).

Federer, K. E.; Burrows, R.; Brooksly, J. B.: Vesicular stomatitis virus — the relationship between some strains of the Indiana serotype. Res. Vet. Sci. *6:* 103 (1967).

Gregg, J.; McGuire, F. X.; Glover, G. J.; Gillespie, A.; Gregory, G.: Vesicular stomatitis contagiosa. Amer. J. Vet. Med. *12:* 221 (1917).

Hanson, R. P.; Eustupinan, J.; Castaneda, G. J.: Vesicular stomatitis in the Americas. Proc. PAHO conf. on vesicular diseases and zoonosis, Washington, DC, March 1968.

Hanson, R. P.: in Catgott; Smithcors, Equine medicine and surgery, 2nd ed. (Amer. Vet. Public. Inc., Wheaton/Ill. 1972).

Heiny, F.: Vesicular stomatitis in cattle and horses in Colorado. North Amer. Vet. *26:* 726 (1945).

Jonkers, A. H.: The epizootiology of the vesicular stomatitis viruses: a reappraisal. Amer. J. Epidemiol. *86:* 286 (1967).

Shalokow, A.; Peralta, P. H.: Vesicular stomatitis virus, Indiana type: an arbor-virus infection of tropical sandflies and humans? Amer. J. Epidemiol. *86:* 149 (1967).

Sudia, W. D.; Fields, N. B.; Calisher, C. H.: The isolation of vesicular stomatitis virus (Indiana strain) and other viruses from mosquitoes in New Mexico. Amer. J. Epidemiol. *86:* 598 (1967).

Teidebold, T. C.; Mather, C. S.; Marrilat, L. A.: Gangrenous glossitis of horses. Proc. US Livestock Sanit. Assoc. *20:* 29 (1916).

Theiler, S.: Eine contagiöse Stomatitis des Pferdes in Süd-Afrika. Dtsch. Tierärztl. Wschr. *9:* 131 (1901).

Wagener, K.: Foot-and-mouth disease and vesicular stomatitis. J. Amer. vet. med. Assoc. *80:* 39 (1932).

2.2.1.3. Papillomatosis

Definition. Cutaneous papillomatosis is a localized, epitheliotropic viral disease of young horses up to 3 years of age, characterized by the formation of multiple small warts on the skin.

Symptoms. The disease may affect foals only a few months old or young horses up to about 3 years of age. The papillomas (warts) most commonly appear on the muzzle between the nostrils, at the junction of the nostrils and upper lip, and around the corners of the mouth, sometimes spreading to involve the lower lip. The warts range in number from a few to a hundred or more. They project several millimeters above the skin surface and measure up to 10 mm in diameter. They are small, fleshy, circumscribed, and are covered by keratin-containing masses. In young horses having only a few warts, the lesions may grow to a larger size. The warts appear within a few days without apparent cause. Generally they will disappear spontaneously in 3–4 months. The warts are bothersome to the horse. Sometimes they cause an obvious pruritus, for the animal rubs the affected area, causing some of the warts to bleed. Over a period of 3—4 months the warts shrink and fall off without leaving scars. Surgical removal leaves depigmented areas on the muzzle.

Etiology. As CADAEC showed experimentally in 1901, and COOK and OLSON in 1951, cutaneous papillomatosis in the horse is caused by a filtrable virus that is infectious only for equids. The infection can be transmitted by intradermal injection or by inoculating the scarified skin. The incubation period is 2—3 months. The natural route of infection is by way of small wounds, lesions and bites from blood-sucking insects. It is assumed that the habit of foals and colts to 'nuzzle' various objects results in skin breaks about the nose and muzzle that permit entry of the virus. Contaminated curry combs and similar tools can also spread the disease. The virus is relatively resistant and may exist on stable walls, fences and railings. How long it can remain infectious is not known.

Diagnosis. The diagnosis is based upon the age of the horse and localization of the lesions about the nose and lips.

Differential Diagnosis. Fibromas in this age group do not occur as multiple neoplasms in the muzzle area.

Treatment and Prognosis. The prognosis is always favorable. The owner should be informed that the disease is self-limiting, and that the warts will heal spontaneously in 3—4 months. Recovery confers a long-lasting immunity.

Surgical removal of the warts leaves small scars and depigmented areas. This should be explained to the owner if he insists on treatment. Treatment with bovine papillomatosis-formol vaccine is useless, because the equine papillomatosis virus is species-specific, and so immunization is not achieved with bovine vaccine.

If the disease is a problem among 1- to 3-year-olds on breeding farms, the stables and perhaps also the paddock fences should be disinfected with formalin.

References

CADEAC: Sur la transmission experimentele des papillomes des diverses especes. Bull. Soc. Sci. Vet. *4:* 280 (1901).

COOK, RH.; OLSON, C.: Experimental transmission of cutaneous papilloma of the horse. Amer. J. Pathol. *27:* 1087 (1951).

2.2.1.4. Sarcoid

Definition. Sarcoids are nodular, sarcomalike tumors of the skin that can occur in various parts of the body. Horses in all age groups are susceptible. The neoplasm is transmissible, fibroblastic, and is characterized by epithelial destruction and ulcerous degeneration of its surface.

1
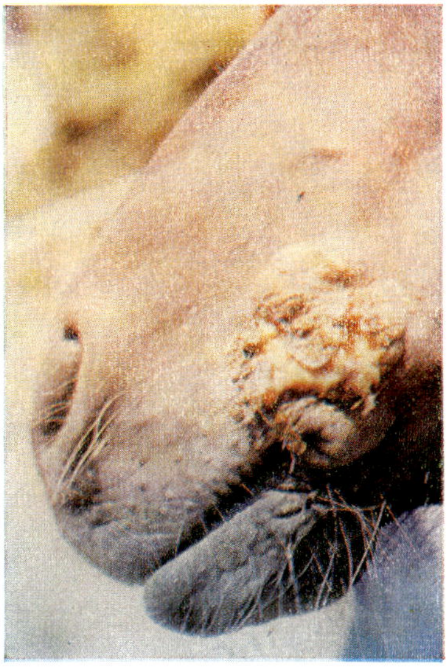

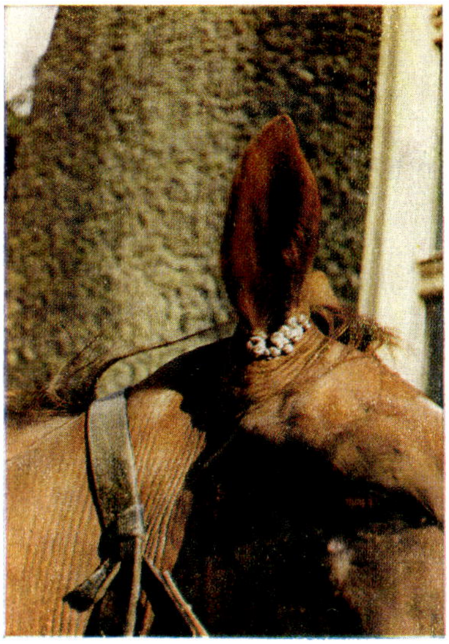
2

3
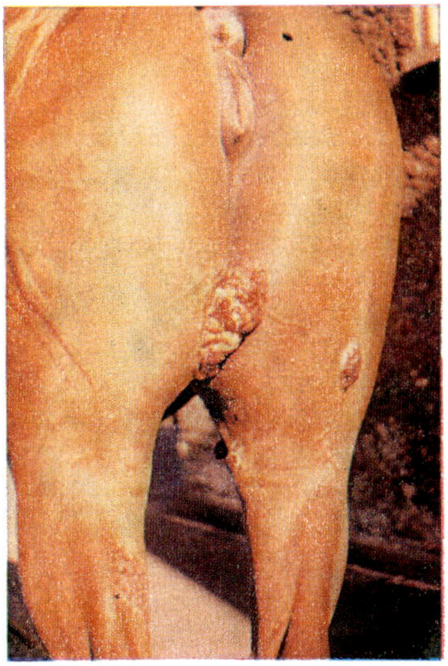

Fig. 2.2. — 1. Sarcoid at the angle of the mouth.
Fig. 2.2. — 2. Sarcoid at the base of the ear.
Fig. 2.2. — 3. Sarcoid in the perineal region.

Symptoms. Sarcoids occur on the head, neck, ear, shoulder, limbs, flanks and ventral abdomen (figs. 2.2. — 1 through — 3). The initial lesion resembles a papilloma, but later the epithelium degenerates and an ulcer may form. Even in the initial stage, however, palpation will reveal a broadly sessile mass that has firm attachment with the subcutaneous connective tissue. As the tumor increases in size and the epithelium degenerates, a superficial bacterial infection will occur. The surface of the tumor appears knobby at this stage, and the tumor is covered with purulent and sanguinous crusts that flake easily. The area surrounding the tumor shows chronic inflammatory changes with induration of the skin and subcutaneous tissue. The tumor itself appears firm.

Equine sarcoid is relatively rare in the Central European countries and is more common in England and America. At our clinic in the GDR we have seen only a few cases over a period of several years. The first case had two sarcoids, one located on the ventral abdomen and the other on the inside of the gaskin. Five years later the same patient presented with recurrences on the ventral abdomen, gaskin and inguinal region; this time the lesions were multiple. Radical surgery was again performed, and an uneventful recovery followed. Like OLSON [1948], we found the recurrences on the same side of the body as the initial lesions. RAGLAND et al. [1966] described an outbreak in 5 horses in a band of about 45.

OLSON [1948] states that equine sarcoid can occur in horses, mules or donkeys of any age.

No systemic signs occur. The tumors may grow to fist-size or even twice that size in some cases. Their removal is recommended on hygienic grounds alone. Equine sarcoid is most commonly observed in North America and England.

Olson described one case of sarcoid in a mule. This animal suffered a lengthy series of recurrences in various body areas, separated by intervals of about 6 months.

Etiology. According to OLSON [1948], sarcoids can be transmitted to other body areas of a horse that is already affected, as well as to unaffected horses. Small skin wounds or scarified areas are necessary in order for transmission to occur. Under such conditions, according to VOSS [1969], sarcoid lesions develop within 49 to 164 days. A virus is the presumed causative agent.

Diagnosis. A presumptive diagnosis can be made on clinical evidence and is confirmed histologically. Typical sarcoids closely resemble Schwann-cell tumors or fibrosarcomas in histologic section.

Differential Diagnosis. According to studies by OLSON and COOK [1951] and RAGLAND and SPENCER [1969], horse skin reacts to bovine papilloma virus by developing sarcomalike growths with little or no epithelial reaction. In these experimental infections, tumors usually develop 3—4 weeks after intradermal inoculation. Histologically, the tumors produced by bovine papilloma virus closely resemble naturally occurring equine sarcoids.

Prognosis and Treatment. The prognosis is good in terms of survival. It is difficult to predict the timing of recurrences. Sarcoid tumors have never been known to metastasize to internal organs. Our own experience indicates that surgical removal is successful if the individual tumors can be extirpated well into healthy skin and if the local lymph nodes are also removed. Lymphadenectomy appears to be crucial for the prevention of recurrences.

A final judgement cannot yet be made concerning the therapeutic value of autogenous vaccines [WHEAT, 1964; PAGE et al., 1967].

References

KÖRNER, H.: Das equine Sarcoid und eine Möglichkeit der Behandlung. Tierärztl. Umschau *31:* 436 (1976).

OLSON, C.: Equine sarcoid, a cutaneous neoplasm. Amer. J. Vet. Res. *9:* 333 (1948).

OLSON, C.: in CATGOTT; SMITHCORS; Equine medicine and surgery; 2nd ed. (Amer. Vet. Med. Public. Inc., Wheaton/Ill. 1972).

OLSON, C.; COOK, R. H.: Cutaneous sarcoma-like lesions of the horse caused by the agent of bovine papilloma. Proc. Soc. Exp. Biol. and Med. *77:* 281 (1951).

PAGE, E. H.; TIFFANY, L. W.; RUSSELL, H. T.: Use of an autogenous equine fibrosarcoma vaccine. J. Amer. vet. med. Assoc. *150:* 177 (1967).

RAGLAND, W. L.; KEOWN, G. H.; GORHAM, J. R.: An epizootic of equine sarcoid. Nature *210:* 1399 (1966).
RAGLAND, W. L.; SPENCER, G. R.: Attempts to relate bovine papilloma virus to the cause of equine sarcoid. Equidae inoculated intradermally with bovine papilloma virus. Amer. J. Vet. Res. *30:* 743 (1969).
VOSS, J. L.: Transmission of equine sarcoid. Amer. J. Vet. Res. *30:* 183 (1969).
WHEAT, J. D.: Therapy of equine sarcoids. Modern Vet. Pract. *45:* 62 (1964).

2.2.1.5. Botryomycosis

Definition. Botryomycosis is an old term for a staphylococcal infection that may spread to the skin, muscles, spermatic cord, udder, and in rare cases to internal organs such as the lung and diaphragm. Typical cases are marked by the development of local or diffuse, nonpainful connective tissue proliferations and suppurations during the course of a chronic inflammation secondary to a skin infection.

Symptoms. The disease begins with a cellulitic swelling in an infected skin area. This swelling rarely leads to abscessation; instead, a thickening of the skin gradually develops. Proliferation of subcutaneous connective tissue is usually present as a result of chronic inflammation. The first clinical signs, which may take days or weeks to develop, are fibromalike lesions that may present a knobby, tumorlike surface. These lesions may grow to the size of a soccer ball or breadloaf over a period of months. Sometimes nodular thickenings may persist on the skin for years before suddenly enlarging. In other cases the skin swellings are flatter or more diffuse in nature and present small surface protuberances; this tends to be true of lesions occurring on the limbs, withers or neck-and-shoulder area. The lesions feel hard on palpation and show little or no tenderness to pressure. Pea-size nodules (botryomycomas) are found in the tissue, and when incised, these are found to be filled with a mucoid fluid. The connective tissue, on the other hand, is hard, lardaceous and grayish-white in color. It often contains a great number of botryomycotic foci which crackle under the knife or, if they have opened spontaneously, are found to consist of loose, degenerating granulation tissue. Smaller foci or nodules with their connective tissue sheaths may coalesce. These lesions contain a thick, yellow, creamy pus and are prone to abscessation. One then finds mainly cherry-size abscess cavities with a loose granulation tissue that bleeds easily. The mucoid clumps from small botryomycomas look like sago grains on a microscope slide.

Under the microscope these granules appear as grapelike clusters of staphylococci, which are always enclosed in a mucous film. These small clumps can be crushed completely between the fingers, leaving no residue. Smaller botryomycotic abscesses that have drained do not heal spontaneously, but produce fistulae. These fistulae remain patent for some time, perhaps for many months. New eruptions also occur in adjacent tissues. Surrounding tissues may also undergo cellulitic changes, resulting in renewed abscessation with secondary infection.

'Cutaneous botryomycosis' in the horse may occur under the harness, on the head, the anterior and lateral thorax, the withers, and the outside of the gaskin. In rare cases they are seen on the coronet or fetlock, and in areas that are exposed to rubbing or abrasion, such as the base of the tail or submaxillary region. Secondary involvement of the local lymph nodes is the rule. In such cases daughter nodes arise which slowly enlarge until finally, after some months, extensive, painless thickenings develop. These masses are firm and tumorlike and have a knobby surface. Cutaneous botryomycoses are easily moved relative to underlying tissues. The hair over such lesions is always shed. Abscessation occurs, leaving behind fistulous tracts. These fistulae may close spontaneously leaving indrawn scars. Ulcerous changes are sometimes evident in the skin surface.

Muscular botryomycosis in the horse arising from a skin abrasion presents as a swelling in the region of the brachiocephalic muscle anterior to the shoulder joint, in the area below the harness. A spindle-shaped swelling gradually appears in the muscle and later may become fist-size or even larger.

In the process, the muscle undergoes a fibrous-tissue degeneration, and numerous botryomycotic foci appear at its center. These may take the form of small abscesses that later coalesce to form larger abscesses. They are always surrounded by a thick fibrous-tissue capsule. The superficial cervical lymph nodes are generally involved. The swelling in the muscle may grow so large that the hand can no longer be placed around the muscle during palpation.

Botryomycosis of the spermatic cord ('funicular botryomycosis') is not uncommon following castrations performed by antiquated methods. However, it does not develop until several months postoperatively. Fistulous openings appear in the area of the old castration wound. From there the spermatic cord stump thickens proximally in bottle fashion. A probe inserted through the fistulous opening will usually pass to the center of the cord stump. Sometimes numerous fistulous openings are found in the scrotal skin. In rare cases the botryomycotic changes spread dorsad along the spermatic cord to the inguinal region. Rectal examination in such cases will disclose nodular thickenings in the inguinal ring. The inguinal lymph nodes are always involved.

Mares are susceptible to botryomycosis of the udder. Hard, diffuse or nodular thickenings are found in one or both halves of the udder. The skin is immobile and also thickened. Sometimes numerous fistulous openings are present and exude a grayish-brown pus that is permeated with granules. The process may spread to the abdominal wall or inside of the thigh.

Botryomycosis of the internal organs has been observed in the lungs, peritoneum, uterus, spleen, endocardium, kidneys and liver. In such cases the staphylococci gain access to the organs from the lung or intestinal tract. Metastatic spread is usually involved.

Etiology. The causative agent of botryomycosis, which formerly was indentified with such organisms as *Staphylococcus ascoformans* or *Botryomyces equi*, is identical to *Staphylococcus aureus*. The cocci are encapsulated to form granules ranging from 5 to 10 μm in size. Several such granules combine in turn to form a gelatinous, grape-like or blackberrylike cluster ranging in size from a pinhead to a millet seed (up to a millimeter in diameter). A skin wound is the usual portal of infection.

Diagnosis. The microbiologic diagnosis is established by the demonstration of staphylococci in the pus or granulation tissue.

Differential diagnosis must be made from epizootic lymphangitis and nocardiosis. A microbiologic examination is necessary to make this differentiation.

Treatment. The results of chemotherapy are uncertain. Such therapy, if used, should be preceded by a determination of drug resistance. Local or systemic iodine therapy is beneficial in only a small number of cases.

Best results are obtained by radical surgical removal of the affected tissue, combined if possible with a regional lymphadenectomy. The resection must be carried into healthy tissue; if remnants of botryomycotic tissue are left behind, a recurrence is inevitable.

Hard, thickened skin areas that are adherent to underlying tissues are resected into healthy tissue, whereupon a skin graft is applied if necessary. For muscular botryomycosis, the thick connective-tissue capsules are included in the exstirpation. Spermatic cord affected with botryomycosis is amputated well into healthy tissue.

In udder botryomycosis, a unilateral or bilateral amputation of the udder must be carried out. In pregnant mares with unilateral disease, it is possible to do a unilateral extirpation of the udder without inducing abortion. Half an udder is sufficient for nursing.

For botryomycoses of the internal organs, systemic antibiotic therapy may be tried after drug resistance has been determined.

Prognosis. The prognosis depends upon the nature of the affected tissue. It is favorable if the disease is confined to the skin or brachiocephalic muscle. In funicular botryomycosis, the prognosis is favorable if the cord or cords can be amputated into healthy tissue, and there is no involvement of the abdominal wall. With unilateral botryomycosis of the udder, a favorable prognosis is always indicated.

2.2.1.6. Nocardiosis

Definition. Nocardiosis is characterized by skin changes very similar to those of botryomycosis — nodule formation, abscessation and ulceration. The causative organisms are of the genus *Nocardia*; the species *N. asteroides* and *N. farcinica* are considered pathogenic to animals. These organisms occur widely in nature, are especially abundant in soil, and gain entry to the skin and subcutaneous tissue via small wounds. The disease was formerly called streptotrichosis.

Symptoms. Small puncture wounds or abrasions of the skin are followed by the development of diffuse cellulitic changes or circumscribed nodular thickenings. The areas most commonly affected are the angle of the jaw, the withers, the intermandibular area, the buccal region, the croup, and the region of the costal cartilage. Later the individual nodes may undergo abscessation, leaving ulcers or fistulous openings. Involvement of the regional lymph nodes is generally present. They are enlarged and tender to pressure, and their lobulation is no longer palpable. Cutaneous or subcutaneous abscesses form in the skin itself. The pus has a watery consistency, is reddish-brown in color, and is permeated with small yellow granules. As in bovine actinomycosis or equine botryomycosis, these granules crackle under the knife and are visible with the naked eye. In other cases the skin may show a patchy thickening that persists for some time. These skin tickenings are not especially painful and are bordered by reddish zones. Spontaneous abscessation at such sites may take weeks or even months to occur. At that time loose, violet-red granulations that bleed easily are found in the depths of the abscess cavities. The course is always chronic.

Etiology. The infection gains entry by way of contaminated skin wounds. The causal organisms mentioned above, *Nocardia asteroides* and *Nocardia farcinica*, may be transmitted by grooming tools or stable equipment. Lymphatic vessels appear unusually prominent in the area surrounding the affected skin. In the horse it is very rare for the infection to metastasize to internal organs. The causal organisms, especially *N. asteroides*, are present ubiquitously in the soil.

Diagnosis. The *Nocardia* organisms are gram-positive, weakly acid-fast rods. Some are coccoid in form, while others occur in filament-like and branched chains. The organisms can be demonstrated both directly in clinical specimens and in culture.

Differential Diagnosis. Cutaneous botryomycosis and epizootic lymphangitis must be considered. Differentiation is possible only by bacteriologic or mycologic examination.

Prognosis. The prognosis in the horse is more favorable than in the dog.

Treatment. Large doses of chloramphenicol or streptomycin are administered systemically for 8—10 days. If affected skin areas are small, radical surgery should be done without delay (immediately after systemic therapy at the latest). Altered skin is excised into healthy tissue if possible. In certain areas (withers, submaxillary region) this may create defects that necessitate plastic repair. Abscesses and fistulous tracts are incised, followed by the application of chloramphenicol ointments or furacin gel. Tincture of iodine may also be locally applied. The intravenous use of potassium iodine and sodium iodine has not proved effective in the treatment of equine nocardiosis.

Comments. The thorough disinfection of stable equipment and grooming tools is an important prophylactic measure.

2.2.1.7. Dermatomycoses

Definition. Fungi which are pathogenic to the skin cause a superficial dermatosis, or 'dermatophytosis'. The fungi characteristically affect the superficial, keratinized layers of the body surface: the skin, hair, and even the horny capsule of the hoof. In the horse, dermatomycoses are caused by various species of dermatophytes, especially those of the genus *Microsporum* and *Trichphyton.* The terms 'ringworm' and 'favus' are commonly used in reference to the horse and serve to characterize the clinical appearance of the corresponding dermatomycosis. Either a microsporosis or trichophytosis is present.

Ringworm, caused by *Microsporum canis* (or *M. equinum*), produces rounded skin lesions about 3 cm in diameter that are hairless and covered with small crusts. This infection is particularly common in cases where leather tack items come in contact with the skin.

Infection with *Microsporum canis* can be transmitted to man, other horses and other domestic animals. Similarly, retransmission from other domestic animals and from man to the horse is possible. Crust formation tends to be heavier in infections with *M. gypseum* than with *M. canis. M. gypseum* is a ubiquitous dirt- and soil-dwelling fungus and also causes ringworm in horses, donkeys and mules. The lesions occur around the eyes, around the nostrils, on the neck, chest, flanks and back. Again, abrasions from tack items are an important predisposing factor. The lesions appear as multiple circular areas. The affected skin is either completely hairless, or some hairs remain and protrude through the thick crusts covering the lesions. These crusts are rather firmly adherent to the base of the lesion. In both the *M. canis* and *M. gypseum* infection, the round spots may gradually become larger. An infection with either Microsporum species is manifested initially by only a slightly swollen, circular skin area that within days becomes covered with scales, small vesicles or papules. A slight redness may also become apparent in unpigmented skin areas. The vesicles quickly rupture and form additional crusts. Later these may leave dry, hairless, scaly areas that have a moth-eaten appearance. These spots may enlarge and coalesce over a period of weeks or months. A new crop of lesions may appear in other areas of the body. In rare cases, hairless areas are distributed over the entire body surface. When very thick crusts are forcibly removed, a moist, deep-red area is uncovered. The lesions caused by *M. gypseum* are usually larger and show a greater degree of perifocal inflammation. All fungal infections of the skin may give rise to severe, purulent dermatitides. This is especially likely if pruritus is severe and there is constant rubbing of affected areas.

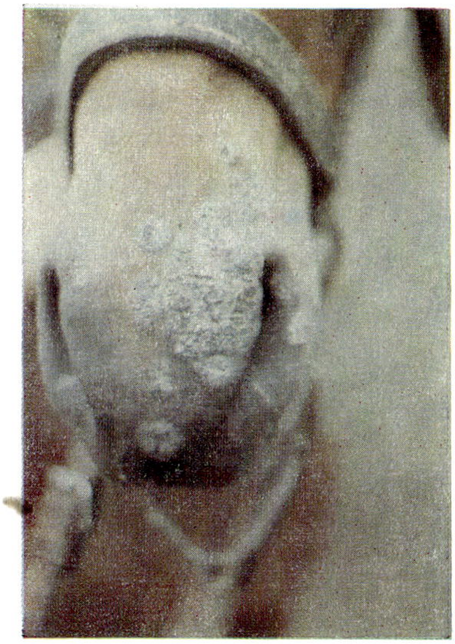

Fig. 2.2. — 4. Ringworm caused by *Trichophyton mentagrophytes.*

Dermatomycoses in the horse are also caused by *Trichophyton mentagrophytes*, *T. equinum*, *T. verrucosum* and *T. schoenleini*. *Trichophyton mentagrophytes* can infect the horse as well as other domestic animals. It is believed that rodents play an important role in the transmission of this infection. The skin lesions caused by this fungus vary in size and are highly irregular in shape. They can occur on the head, neck, base of the tail, and limbs. In extreme cases the entire body surface may be covered with irregularly-shaped spots. These spots are always hairless and covered with thick, gray crusts, which may contain short stumps of hair. This disease, too, begins with very small, hairless lesions which enlarge to form round spots that later fuse into irregularly-shaped areas (fig. 2.2. — 4). Pustules and vesicles may also be present initially; these usually occur at the periphery of hairless areas. If the heavy crusts are removed, a suppurative dermatitis is always discovered beneath. Healing, if it occurs, starts at the center of the lesions. Pruritus is not so severe as in the *Microsporum* infections.

Trichophyton equinum also causes a ringworm-like skin infection. Young horses are especially susceptible to this infection, and its spread in foal nurseries is very rapid. *T. equinum* is highly resistant and can remain infectious for years on contaminated grooming tools, saddles, blankets and stable walls.

The skin lesions caused by *T. equinum* appear as very small, round spots varying in diameter from a few millimeters to a maximum of $1^1/_2$ to 2 cm. These spots are hairless and are covered with tiny, thin scales. When these spots enlarge, small vesicles may be felt on their surface. These vesicles may rupture to form crusts. As in the previous infection, healing always starts at the center.

The *T. equinum* infection causes very severe pruritus. It is transmissible to man.

Trichophyton verrucosum infection occurs in large and small ruminants, and these animals may infect a horse that grazes the same pasture.

Trichophyton schoenleini produces irregularly-shaped, hairless skin lesions that are covered with crusts and may occur on various parts of the body surface. Infected skin areas give off a characteristic acrid odor.

A dermatomycosis caused by *Trichophyton ajelloi* has been described in the United States by PIER et al. [1961]. To date the disease has not yet been described in the German literature.

Etiology. Most dermatomycoses, as stated earlier, are caused by *Microsporum* species. In the horse these are *Microsporum canis (M. equinum)* and *Microsporum gypseum*. The major *Trichophyton* species are, as mentioned. *T. mentagrophytes*, *T. equinum*, and, to a lesser extent, *T. verrucosum* and *T. schoenleini*. Dermatophytes grow especially well on horse hair. Penetration of the skin starts with the affinity of the fungus for the stratum corneum, leading to the formation of threadlike hyphae. When these hyphae reach the hair follicle, they grow down between it and the follicle wall, at which time some branches of the mycelium invade the hair itself and continue to grow there. In the extrapapillary mycelium the hyphae break up into numerous small spores. The fungal growth within the hair weakens it and causes it to split or break off. Because the hyphae stop short of the hair root or bulb, the hair continues to grow. In this way the spore layer can become pressed out of the follicle and thus reach a considerable length, assuming the hair does not break. The clinically observable skin changes are dependent on the toxicity of the fungi, the amount of hair present in the infected area, and on whether secondary infection by pathogenic organisms complicates the dermatomycosis. Given the mechanism of skin infection by dermatophytes, inflammatory symptoms tend to be mild and accompanied by minimal crust formation in areas where hair is sparse. On the other hand, fungal infections of thick skin with a heavy haircoat lead to more extensive changes with clinical symptoms of folliculitis and perifolliculitis, and a severe dermatitis with edematous swelling of the surrounding skin.

Horses that are debilitated or malnourished are particularly susceptible to the dermatomycoses. The diseases are observed more frequently during the winter months in cold, wet stables than during the summer months and when hygienic stabling conditions are maintained. Transmission is usually by direct contact with affected animals or by indirect infection from contaminated brushes, combs, blankets, harnesses or other tack.

Dermatophytes can remain viable for more than a year in a dried state. When placed in water, they lose their ability to reproduce within about a week; this takes several hours in 1% sodium hydroxide solution, and about an hour in 1% acetic acid.

A fungal infection can become established only in the presence of macerated skin or small wounds. The incubation period of the dermatomycoses ranges from one week to one month. Infection can be artificially transmitted through scarified skin in 8 to 14 days.

Diagnosis. Affected hairs and a skin scraping must be examined microscopically. The skin scraping should be taken from the periphery of the affected area with a curette or scalpel. A *Microsporum* infection is best identified by gross examination under a Wood's light. Hairs infected with *Microsporum canis* will show a distinct greenish fluorescence under the filtered ultraviolet light in a darkened room. *M. gypseum* and the *Trichophyton* fungi show little or no fluorescence under Wood's light. For microscopic examination, the material is placed on a sterile glass slide and treated with a few drops of a 10—15% sodium hydroxide solution and a drop of glycerin. It is examined under low- and high-power dry objectives using a suitable diaphragm for light reduction. In *Microsporum* infections the small spores are irregularly arranged in a sheath surrounding the affected hair. In *Trichophyton* infections the spores tend to be arranged in regular chains of varying length on the surface of the hair or within its substance. In both types of infection the mycelium may be inside or outside the hair shaft, and the branching, refractive hyphae can be seen in skin scrapings. The two genuses cannot be differentiated on the basis of mycelial appearance. Instead of sodium hydroxide, potassium hydroxide or a solution of lactophenol cotton blue may be used. This stains the fungal elements a deep blue, while tissue elements are stained a light blue.

The differentiation of fungal species can be made only by the culturing of clinical material. This procedure is reserved for specially-equipped laboratories. Culturing normally takes 2—4 weeks. The fungi are then differentiated according to their shape and color and on the basis of various microscopic characteristics.

Differential Diagnosis. Other eczemas of endogenous cause, including allergic skin reactions, must be considered. Differentiation is difficult if severe suppurative skin changes coexist with the fungal infection.

Treatment and Prognosis. Most dermatomycoses have a good prognosis. If hygienic stabling and environmental conditions are provided, including good climate control, many fungal infections will heal spontaneously within 8—10 weeks, assuming that reinfection is avoided and grooming tools, tack items, buildings, etc. are adequately disinfected.

Many dermatomycoses in young horses will regress very quickly when the animal is put on pasture. After the lesions heal, hairless areas will acquire a new haircoat unless secondary pyogenic dermatitides have complicated the infection.

The hairs surrounding affected skin areas are clipped short or carefully shaved. Thick crusts or heavy scales are softened with the aid of soap baths or oils. Most older fungicides are less effective in killing the fungi and spores than in promoting the healing of local lesions. Thus, topical treatment with salicylic acid, benzoic acid, iodine and sulfurous compounds, as well as ichthammol, petroleum and creolin, can be recommended with some reservations.

Mercury compounds, especially mercury ointments, can also be used in the horse to effect a rapid improvement. In recent years caprylic acid and propionic acid have also proved to be highly effective. Griseofulvin is a well-known antibiotic with fungicidal properties. It may be administered in ointment form or orally, though oral griseofulvin must be maintained for some weeks. The medicated feed given to young cattle has proved effective in young horses with dermatomycoses.

Contaminated stable equipment and tack items are disinfected with Lysol or formalin solution. Stable walls also should be disinfected with 5% formalin. Clipped hairs should be disposed of by burning.

Comments. A major concern in dermatomycoses is to prevent further transmission. Environmental hygiene is therefore of critical importance.

References

Georg, L.; Kaplan, W.; Cam, L. B.: Equine ringworm with special reference to Trichophyton equinum. Amer. J. Vet. Res. *18:* 798 (1957).

Gierløff, B.: Dermatophytosis: Glatzflechte und Erbgrind. In: Handlexikon der tierärztlichen Praxis, Medical Book Company, Kopenhagen 1958.

Hiddleston, W. A.: Antifungal activity of Penicillium griseofulvin mycelium. Vet. Rec. *86:* 75 (1970).

Hoerlein, A. B.: Studies of animal dermatomycosis. Cornell Vet. *35:* 299 (1945).

Hofmann, W.; Nieper, L.: Zur Behandlung von Pilzerkrankungen bei Pferden und Rindern mit Griseofulvin-Supplement. Tierärztl. Umschau *27:* 348 (1972).

Jung, H. D.: Die Dermatomykosen und ihre aktuelle Problematik für Human- und Veterinärmedizin. Mh. Vet.-Med. *16:* 329 (1961).
Kaplan, W.; Georg, L.; Fosnaugh, C. J.: Isolation of the dermatophyte Microsporum gypseum from a horse with ringworm. J. Amer. vet. med. Assoc. *129:* 381 (1956).
Pier, A. C.: Isolation of Keratomyces ajelloi from the skin lesions of a horse. J. Amer. vet. med. Assoc. *138:* 484 (1961).

2.2.1.8. Horsepox (Variola)

Definition. Horsepox is a benign disease characterized by a local, papulovesicular eruption of the skin or mucous membranes.

Symptoms. If the disease occurs on the back of the pastern (the 'leg form'), a weeping grease heel develops. Here as elsewhere, the disease goes through several stages, though these may not always be visible if much hair is present. The three characteristic stages are the papular stage, vesicular stage and pustular stage. The pustules rupture quickly, resulting in a serocrustal or eczematous grease heel. Also, inflammation of the skin gives rise to a mild supporting-leg lameness in the 2nd phase. Lesions may become secondarily infected with pyogenic bacteria, causing the formation of a greasy coating and marked swelling of the skin.

Less frequently the horsepox infection is localized in the mouth ('buccal form'), with lesions occurring on the lips, buccal mucosa, lateral and ventral surface of the tongue, and the hard palate. These take the form of small vesicles and pustules that rupture leaving circular epithelial defects. Spreading of these lesions is rare. Affected animals salivate excessively and have difficulty eating.

Sometimes lesions on the lips spread to involve the nasal mucosa. A slight rise of body temperature is noted on the 2nd and 3rd day of the disease. Fever tends to be more prolonged in affected foals.

Etiology. Horsepox is caused by an epitheliotropic virus that can multiply in the skin and mucous membranes. It is a large virus, having a size of 150—180 μm. Variola viruses are highly resistant to drying. Infection occurs by transmission from animal to animal or by attendants. The initial lesions are small, red stipples that subsequently change into nodules, vesicles or pustules. Crusts form in the final stage. The virus can be demonstrated microscopically by staining, in which case it is termed an elementary body or Paschen's body. Within the cell, 'inclusion bodies' or 'Guarnier's bodies' form in response to the invading virus. Sometimes the virus can be isolated in pure culture in material from the vesicles and pustules. During the brief febrile period, the virus can also be isolated from the blood (viremic phase). The horsepox infection leaves a long-lasting immunity.

Treatment and Prognosis. The prognosis is always good in mature animals. In foals that have prolonged fever or in which the disease has become generalized, the prognosis is unfavorable. Pox lesions on the back of the pastern are treated with dessicating and disinfecting ointments, such as 10 % tannin ointment, or with antibiotic or sulfonamide powder. In the buccal form the oral cavity is rinsed with 0.1 % permanganate solution or 1 % hydrogen peroxide solution, or tincture of myrrh is applied topically to affected areas. The horse should be given access to potassium permanganate solution so that it can rinse its own mouth. Soft feed or fresh green feed is provided during the disease.

2.2.2. Infectious Diseases of the Lymphatic System

2.2.2.1. Epizootic Lymphangitis (Pseudoglanders)

Definition. Epizootic lymphangitis is a chronic, contagious, suppurative inflammation of the subcutaneous lymphatic vessels and regional lymph nodes caused by the fungus *Histoplasma farciminosum.*

Symptoms. The disease usually affects several horses in a given population. Pale-red granulations that bleed easily and have fine fistulous openings appear on the limbs, neck, head, withers, or in the saddle area. These initial lesions are followed by swelling of the lymphatic vessels, with 'string-of-beads' nodules developing on the head and neck along the course of the lymphatics. These nodules rupture discharging a creamy pus. The affected lymph vessels appear as firm, finger-thick, often painless cords that are adherent to the skin. The regional lymph nodes usually enlarge to form fist-size, painless masses that occasionally rupture and may discharge pus. As the disease progresses, millet-seed-size nodules and ulcers with raised borders appear on the nasal mucosa near the opening of the nostril (pseudoglanders [Hutyra et al., 1954]).

Systemic signs are mild or absent. The temperature becomes elevated only in the presence of pyogenic mixed infections. Symptoms may regress completely within 4—6 weeks, or the disease may persist for months.

Diagnosis. The gradual development of nodules and ulcers, and the 'cording' of the lymphatic vessels and suppuration of local lymph nodes provide a basis for diagnosis.

Differential diagnosis is made from glanders, sporotrichosis and streptococcal infection by microscopic demonstration of *Histoplasma farciminosum* in the pus.

Prognosis. The prognosis is favorable if the disease is confined to the torso, neck or head, although recurrences are possible. With involvement of the respiratory tract, the prognosis is usually poor.

Treatment. There is no economical treatment for epizootic lymphangitis at the present time. Besides exposure to light and sun, good nutrition and complete rest are recommended. If chemotherapy is desired, procaine penicillin is administered in large doses (see Ulcerative Lymphangitis), possibly combined with the i.v. administration of sulfonamide-trimethroprim preparations. Potassium iodide given orally in increasing doses of 15—20 g daily can be a useful adjunct. Surgical measures and meticulous wound care are beneficial for healing.

2.2.2.2. Sporotrichosis

Definition. Sporotrichosis is a chronic disease caused by the infection of wounds with *Sporotrichum* fungi. Its symptoms are similar to those of ulcerative lymphangitis. It is rare in Europe but is seen in North America.

Symptoms. Systemic signs are absent. Firm nodules appear along the course of the lymphatic vessels, mainly on the limbs, and later rupture. The lymph nodes themselves are unaffected. Metastasis does not occur. A thin, sanguinous pus exudes from the ruptured nodules, and ulcerative skin defects may form. Infection results from inoculation of the fungus into small skin wounds.

The *diagnosis* is made by demonstrating *Sporotrichum schenkii* or other *Sporotrichum* species in the pus.

Epizootic lymphangitis must be differentiated.

Treatment. Surgical treatment with vigorous wound care and frequent medication changes is recommended. Potassium iodide should be given orally in increasing daily doses of 5—10 g until iodism appears.

2.2.2.3. Ulcerative Lymphangitis

Definition. Ulcerative lymphangitis is a chronic disease caused by wound infection. It is characterized by an inflammation of the subcutaneous lymphatic vessels with a tendency toward nodule formation and ulceration. The regional lymph nodes are not involved.

Symptoms. The disease usually affects the hind limbs, appearing initially as diffuse, mildly painful swellings from the coronet to the hock joint. Later the lymphatic vessels enlarge to finger-size, and nodules develop along their course in string-of-beads fashion. The nodules begin to fluctuate and rupture to the outside, discharging a purulent exudate with varying properties (thin or viscous, purulent, sanguinous). The resulting ulcers vary in size and have a yellowish-gray base, and poor granulation tissue is formed. The associated lymph nodes rarely show marked enlargement or tenderness. The disease may take a course of weeks or months, and apparent cicatricial healing is followed repeatedly by renewed nodulation and ulceration. Occasionally the disease spreads to the head, neck and torso, and dissemination to internal organs is possible [Wirth et al., 1950]. Systemic signs are of no consequence, and only mild temperature elevations occur. A marked improvement of the animal's condition is noted during the summer months.

Etiology. Ulcerative lymphangitis is a separate entity in clinical terms, but not etiologically.

Besides the primary causal organism *Corynebacterium pseudotuberculosis*, micrococci, staphylococci and streptococci may play a role in spreading and perpetuating the disease [Bridges, 1972].

Natural infection occurs through skin lesions in the area of the coronet and fetlock on the hind limbs, as these areas are most heavily exposed to feces and urine.

Diagnosis. The clinical picture is obvious. Glanders is excluded on the basis of negative mallein and serum tests. Epizootic lymphangitis takes a more malignant course than the ulcerative form. It is also distinguished by local lymph node involvement and the development of exuberant, fungiform granulations within the ulcers. In addition, specific causal organisms *(Histoplasma farciminosum)* can be demonstrated in the epizootic form.

Prognosis. The disease may persist for weeks despite intensive therapy and in many cases heals with unsightly scarring. Death may occur if the disease metastasizes to internal organs. When treatment is initiated, it must be understood that the horse will be incapable of working for some time, and that its working capacity may be impaired.

Treatment. Early cases are treated with procaine penicillin given in very large doses (20 million I.U./day) for at least 6—8 days, or with oxytetracycline administered i.v. in a dose of 40—50 ml for 5 days [Bridges, 1972].

In advanced cases, vigorous daily wound care and general nursing measures are of critical importance. Wound care involves the incision of abscesses and daily irrigation with chlorine preparations, acridine dye solutions and potassium permanganate used in an alternating regimen. Nonspecific irrigation therapy can be useful in promoting healing.

References

BRIDGES, C. H.: in CATGOTT; SMITHCORS, Equine medicine and surgery, 2nd ed. (Amer. Vet. Public. Inc., Wheaton/Ill. 1972).

HUTYRA, F. v.; MAREK, J.; MANNINGER, P.; MÓCSY, J.: Spezielle Pathologie und Therapie der Haustiere; 10. Aufl. (VEB Gustav Fischer Verlag, Jena 1954).

SCHULZ, W.: in BEER, Infektionskrankheiten der Haustiere; 2. Aufl. (VEB Gustav Fischer Verlag, Jena 1980).

WIRTH, D.; DIERNHOFER, K.-L.: Lehrbuch der inneren Krankheiten der Haustiere (Enke, Stuttgart 1950).

2.2.3. Infectious Diseases of the Respiratory System

2.2.3.1. Equine Influenza (Hoppgarten Cough, Newmarket Cough, Infectious Catarrh of the Upper Respiratory Tract, Infectious Equine Bronchitis)

Definition. This highly contagious, epizootic disease affects equidae in all age groups and is caused by influenza viruses A-equi-1 and A-equi-2.

Symptoms. An incubation period of 2—3 days is followed by depression and a high fever of 39—41 °C, which generally returns to normal in 1—3 days. Some animals develop symptoms such as severe muscular weakness and an unsteady gait. There is marked redness of the visible mucous membranes, and a slightly serous nasal discharge may be present. The pulse rate may rise to more than 60/min in both young and old animals. The mandibular lymph nodes are slightly swollen and tender to pressure. A dry, hacking cough develops after a few hours and rarely more than 2 days after the onset of the disease. The disease is easily recognized in large bands of horses, for the majority of animals tend to develop the same symptoms within a period of 2—3 days. Coughing is easily produced by pressure on the larynx and upper tracheal rings. Respiration is shallow, and the respiratory rate is markedly increased depending on the severity of the disease. Auscultatory findings are characteristic of the causative viral type. With the A-equi-1 type, auscultation of the lungs is negative aside from a coarse vesicular respiration, while in A-equi-2 infections, fine moist rales or crepitation can often be detected over the apical lobes. In rare cases these sounds are also detectable over the diaphragmatic lobes. If complete rest is enforced, the disease usually runs an uneventful course, although a cough may persist for 2—3 weeks. Laryngoscopy in such cases reveals a mild laryngitis. Occasionally the disease is confined to the larynx. If the horse is returned to work despite the cough, complications may arise. The greatest danger is that the disease will progress to a chronic bronchitis and thence to an alveolar emphysema, or that a secondary infection will supervene leading to a purulent bronchitis and bronchopneumonia. Exacerbation is characterized by a recurrence of fever and the development of a mucopurulent to purulent nasal discharge. Auscultation of the lungs in such cases reveals moist and dry rales and possibly bronchial respiration. Additional complications such as sinusitis and guttural pouch diseases are not uncommon. The causal relationship between influenza and laryngeal hemiplegia remains unclear [GERBER, 1970].

Etiology. The equine influenza virus is an RNA virus belonging to the group of myxoviruses. It has the same ribonucleoprotein as influenza viruses of other species and is assigned to type A. The ribonucleoprotein of the influenza virus produces complement-fixing antibodies and makes it possible to differentiate the three types A, B and C. Only the type-A viruses are important in the horse; these viruses are also found in human influenza. The RNA core of the virus is surrounded by a lipoprotein envelope that possesses two functionally distinguishable components, and this enables further subtypes to be differentiated. One component is a hemagglutinin that is responsible for attachment of the virus to the host cell; the other is an enzyme, neuraminidase, that permits the liberation of the virus from the cell [Fenner; Catcott; Mayr].

The characteristics of the hemagglutinin and neuraminidase form the basis for identifying the two subtypes of equine influenza virus, A-equi-1 and A-equi-2. The A-equi-1 virus generally causes milder disease than A-equi-2. The causal virus is readily cultivated in the amniotic sac of chicken eggs incubated for 9—11 days. Embryonic kidney-cell cultures from cattle, man, monkey and chicken are also suitable. Because the viruses have no cytopathogenic action, however, growth must be demonstrated indirectly by the hemadsorption test.

The influenza virus also shows some antigenic similarity to the causative virus of fowl plague and to human type-A2 Hong Kong 1/68. It has been suggested, therefore, that a reciprocal adaptation may be possible [Paccaud, 1970; Cateigne, 1970; Blaskovic, 1970]. The virus shows little resistance to the antiseptics and disinfectants customarily used for viral infections [Mayr].

Pathogenesis. Infection is contracted by droplet inhalation. The virus becomes trapped by the nasal mucosa, and it selectively attacks and destroys ciliated respiratory epithelium. As the disease progresses, there is damage to the tracheal and bronchial mucosa resulting in a tracheitis and bronchitis. Because the bronchi are always involved, the term 'catarrh of the upper respiratory tract' does not accurately describe the disease. Besides bronchitis, a circumscribed bronchopneumonia can also occur [Gerber, 1970]. In many cases a peribronchitis also develops that appears to perpetuate the cough and may cause chronic disease. Infections with A-equi-1 tend to be relatively mild, while A-equi-2 can cause severe damage, perhaps even to the myocardium and brain. The pneumonia, peribronchitis and myocardial damage suggest that invasion is not exclusively by the air-borne route, and that at least a transitory viremic phase is present. Lesions that are purely viral in origin may heal completely in abour 3 weeks [Bryans, 1966].

Secondary infections can easily develop in unfavorable circumstances and can cause an initially benign bronchitis and pneumonia to progress to a suppurative bronchopneumonia with grave prognosis. Affected foals can also develop serious myocardial damage that leads to death within a short time. Generally virus cannot be demonstrated in nasal swabs until 3—4 days (8 days at most) after the onset of the disease.

Epizootiology. The virus appears to have a worldwide distribution. It is introduced into a given population either by the acquisition of animals during the incubation period or by the congregation of horses in large numbers (riding establishments, racetracks, sales barns). When introduced to a population lacking immunity, equine influenza spreads in an explosive manner and affects all horses within a few days. Most of the animals are already infected following the 1- to 3-day incubation period. The rapid propagation of the disease is promoted by the explosive cough, which spreads the virus over a range of up to 35 meters [Bryans, 1966]. It cannot be said for certain whether there are carriers that still shed virus after a period of weeks [Gerber, 1970]. Neither is it known whether virus can be spread indirectly by the rider or attendants.

Because only one of the viral types, A-equi-1 or A-equi-2, is generally found in influenza epizootics, it appears that immunity is developed only to that particular type. If the other type appears later, the animals may contract influenza twice in one year. Additional studies point to a possible antigenic variability, especially in the A-equi-2 virus, that is similar to that observed in the human virus. While this has not been definitely proven for A-equi-2, it is nevertheless possible that a new antigenic variant of this virus may appear suddenly and lead to major outbreaks.

It is not known with certainty how long immunity to a given viral type persists following a natural infection with that type.

The greatest danger at racetracks is to 2-year-olds that are just starting training. Among jumpers, 4-year-olds are considered to be at greatest risk for contracting influenza [Mayr].

Diagnosis. The diagnosis is based mainly on the clinical course. A presumptive diagnosis of influenza may be made if a number of horses (especially younger animals) become ill within an period of 3—5 days, but a definitive diagnosis requires isolation of the causative agent or proof of a rise in specific antibody titers. A 4-fold increase in titers over a 2-week period is considered proof of infection. When antibodies are demonstrated with the hemagglutination inhibition test, it is possible to identify the specific viral subtype (A-equi-1 or -2) that is causing the disease. Because isolation of the causative agent is a very laborious process, antibody determinations are usually sufficient for routine purposes.

The erythrocyte count is usually in the low-normal range, although a more marked anemia may be present. Leukocyte counts are reduced at the onset of the disease as a result of lymphopenia. The serum bilirubin is slightly elevated. If marked systemic signs are present, there will be an elevation of the specific liver enzyme lactate dehydrogenase as an indication of damage to that organ. Creatine phosphokinase (CPK) may also be elevated, especially in patients with a rapid, weak pulse.

Recovery from the disease confers immunity for about one year toward the corresponding viral type. However, animals may contract influenza twice in one year if exposed to a different type.

Differential Diagnosis. The clinical course of rhinopneumonitis, which is caused by a herpes virus, is similar to that of influenza. However, rhinopneumonitis is not as contagious as influenza, and it causes abortion in pregnant mares.

In viral arteritis, respiratory tract disease is not the predominant feature. The body temperature remains elevated for more than 7—10 days. Infections with adeno-rhinovirus and reovirus also must be considered [Mayr; Hofer et al., 1973]. They are not as contagious as influenza, but serologic tests are necessary for a reliable differentiation.

Treatment. Immediate rest is indicated. At least a 5-day course of antibiotics or sulfonamides should be given as a precaution against secondary infection (penicillin 5—10 million units, sulfonamides). Enforced rest should be maintained for about 3 weeks after fever has subsided. This will offer reasonable protection against a chronic bronchitis and bronchiolitis and will give the respiratory epithelium time to heal completely.

Prognosis. A pure viral infection has a favorable prognosis. Foals with influenza are at some risk for developing a fatal bronchopneumonia, especially in infections with A-equi-2.

The prognosis is much less favorable if secondary infection has developed *(Streptococcus zooepidemicus, S. equi)* leading to purulent bronchopneumonia (evidenced by renewed fever and purulent nasal discharge). The development of an exudative pleuritis also indicates an unfavorable prognosis.

Prophylaxis. When an outbreak is in progress, the isolation of introduced animals for at least 10 days and the avoidance of large concentrations of horses are important precautions.

Prophylactic vaccination is advised. It is done with a chick-embryo vaccine in which the viruses have been killed with formalin or propiolactone, adsorbed on aluminium hydroxide ('full vaccine'), or split with polysorbate 80 and ether ('split vaccine' or 'subunit vaccine' [MAYR; PETERMANN et al., 1970]). The vaccine should contain both A-equi-1 and A-equi-2. The initial vaccination is given in two intramuscular injections 6—12 weeks apart. This is followed by yearly booster injections to give permanent immunity. Generally the vaccine is well tolerated. A local, painful swelling may develop at the injection site, depending on the method of preparation and the presence or absence of adjuvants; this disappears completely in 1—2 weeks. Even if the vaccination does not provide absolute protection (the titer can fall considerably toward the end of the year), infections in vaccinated horses take a much milder course than in unvaccinated animals.

References

BLAŠKOVIČ, D.: Experimental infection of horses with equine influenza viruses. Proc. 2nd Int. Conf. Equine Infect. Diseases. Paris 1969 (Karger, Basel 1970).

BLOOD-HENDERSON: Veterinary Medicine; 5th ed. (Baillière-Tindall, London 1979).

BRYANS, J. T.; DOLL, E. R.; JAMES, C.; WILSON, M. S.; MCCOLLUM, W. H.: Immunization for equine influenza. J. Amer. Vet. med. Assoc. *148:* 413 (1966).

BRYANS, J. T.; GERBER, H.: in CATCOTT; SMITHCORS, Equine influenza. In: Equine medicine and surgery; 2nd ed. (Amer. Vet. Public. Inc., Wheaton/Ill. 1972).

CATEIGNE, G.: A parallel study of the antigens of equine and human strains of Myxovirus influenzae. Proc. 2nd Int. Conf. Equine Infect. Diseases. Paris 1969, p. 94 (Karger, Basel 1970).

GERBER, H.: Clinical features, Sequelae and epidemiology of Equine Influenza. Proc. 2nd Int. Conf. Equine Infect. Diseases. Paris 1969, p. 63 (Karger, Basel 1970).

HOFER, B.; STECK, F.; FERBER, H.; LÖHRER, J.; NILOLET, J.; PACLAUD, M. F.: An investigation of the etiology of viral respiratory disease in a remont depot. Proc. 3rd Int. Conf. Equine Infect. Diseases, Paris 1972, p. 527 (Karger, Basel 1973).

PACCAUD, M. F.: The virology of Equine influenza. Proc. 2nd Int. Conf. Equine Infect. Diseases. Paris 1969, p. 81 (Karger, Basel 1970).

PETERMANN, H. G.; FAYET, M. T.; FONTAINE, M.; FONTAINE, M. P.: Vaccination against Equine influenza. Proc. 2nd Int. Conf. Equine Infect. Diseases. Paris, 1969, p. 105 (Karger, Basel 1970).

ROLLE, M.; MAYR, A.: Mikrobiologie, Infektions- und Seuchenlehre; 4. Aufl. (Enke, Stuttgart 1978).

2.2.3.2. Viral Arteritis (Pinkeye, Epizootic Cellulitis)

Definition. This febrile disease is caused by a specific virus and is highly contagious. Conjunctivitis and edema of the limbs and ventral abdomen are the predominant features in typical cases.

Symptoms. In individual cases the clinical picture may be uncharacteristic, except for 2—3 days of fever (abortive form). If the disease becomes epizootic, however, the features are unmistakable. Transmission occurs by direct contact. A fever of 39.5—41.0 °C develops after an incubation period of $1^1/_2$ to 10 days. Marked depression is evident. Frequent signs are marked palpebral edema, photophobia, and a serous to seropurulent ocular and nasal discharge. Edema of the limbs and ventral abdomen may also appear. The pulse and respiratory rates are always increased during the febrile period. Anorexia is pronounced, and diarrhea is present in severe cases. From 50 to 80 % of pregnant mares abort within 7—14 days after an outbreak. Severely affected animals stamp about restlessly, apparently as a result of muscular pain.

Course. The course depends largely on the resistance of the patient. Foals and aged horses tend to be more severely affected. The disease usually takes a more severe course in horses with preexisting disease (endoparasitisms, malnutrition) and in pregnant mares. On the other hand, it is difficult to predict the pattern of clinical symptoms that will occur. Fever may in some cases be associated only with slight palpebral edema and photophobia, or the patient may show mild colic and diarrhea. In other cases the animal's condition deteriorates daily, accompanied by a steady rise in the pulse and respiratory rates. Death from massive septicemia can occur in 4—7 days. A marked leukopenia is present early in the disease, and a neutrophilia develops as the disease progresses. The lymphocytes are always depressed, however [Doll, 1972].

Other changes during the acute phase are a reduction of platelet counts, a prolonged coagulation time, and delayed clot retraction [Crawford and Henson, 1973]. A marked proteinuria is usually detected, and hemoglobinuria may also be present. The pulse rate remains elevated for some time after fever has abated.

Etiology. The causative agent is an RNA virus that belongs to the family of the togaviruses. Because the virus is not transmitted by arthropods, it is assigned to the genus Pestivirus along with the viruses that cause swine plague and bovine virus diarrhea. The arteritis virus has a diameter of 40—60 nm and shows sensitivity to chloroform, ether and heat. The virus shows a uniform serology, propagates in cytoplasm and is best grown in horse kidney-cell cultures.

Serial passage in horse kidney-cell cultures reduces infectivity but is suitable for vaccine production. The virus is pathogenic only for horses [Rolle and Mayr, 1978].

Pathogenesis. Virus is shed in nasal secretions, saliva, ocular discharges, feces and urine during the febrile period. Aborted fetuses harbor large numbers of virus [Rolle and Mayr, 1978].

Twenty-four hours after entering the respiratory tract, arteritis virus is found in the macrophages of the bronchioles. From there it spreads to the sinusoids of the bronchial lymph nodes, and by the 3rd day after infection it is found in the endothelial cells of the veins and arteries. By day 5 of the infection all three zones of the adrenal cortex show massive invasion by the virus. In very severe cases the virus also propagates in the hepatocytes. From day 6 to 8 the virus is found in the capillary endothelium of all organs and even in the macrophages of the renal interstitial tissue. Propagation of the virus leads to inflammation of the vascular endothelium, damage to the intima, and edema. Although necrosis usually occurs in the capillaries, thrombosis is not observed. Most vascular lesions disappear within 10 days, but focal necroses can still be demonstrated in the muscular layer of the arteries for up to 2 months. The outcome of the disease depends largely on the severity of capillary damage. When the disease becomes generalized, the fluid loss to the interstitium is so great that death occurs from circulatory collapse [McCollum and Bryans, 1973; Crawford and Henson, 1973; Prickett et al., 1973]. Neutralizing antibodies can be detected from the 3rd to 4th day after infection and persist for some months [Crawford and Henson, 1973].

Epizootiology. The disease is transmitted directly from animal to animal. Transmission by biting or sucking insects appears unlikely. The question of whether stallions still shed virus in the semen months after an infection has yet to be resolved [Bryans, 1970]. In earlier years, a major outbreak of equine viral arteritis occurred every 12 years or so, with a large number of animals contracting the disease within a short period [Hutyra]. In recent years the disease has tended to be limited to circumscribed regions. Because the mortality rate is low in natural outbreaks while spread is rapid, epizootics tend to have little economic impact given the general reduction in horse populations. The situation is different on breeding farms, however. Because pregnant mares tend to be affected more severely than barren mares, and the abortion rate commonly exceeds 50 %, the economic loss can be substantial. Horses that have recovered from the disease generally are immune to reinfection for some years.

Differential Diagnosis. When fever, edema of the eyelids and limbs, and a marked leukopenia with absolute lymphopenia are exhibited by several horses at one time, then a presumptive diagnosis of viral arteritis can be made with reasonable confidence. A definitive diagnosis requires isolation of the causative virus. Virus is recoverable from blood or from nasal and guttural pouch swabs during the febrile period.

Serologic tests for antibodies are useful only if 2 blood samples are tested 1—2 months apart. A 4-fold rise in antibody titers between the 1st and 2nd samples is considered diagnostic of an infection [Rolle and Mayr, 1978]. Another disease to be considered is rhinopneumonitis, a viral infection that likewise causes abortion in pregnant mares. The diagnosis is made by examining the aborted fetus for the corresponding virus.

Finally, African horsesickness should be considered in areas where this disease is enzootic. The greater mortality of this infection distinguishes it from viral arteritis.

Lesions. The most obvious gross lesions are the subcutaneous edemas and hemorrhages on the limbs as well as in the omentum, pleura, colon and cecum. Edema and hyaline necrosis of the arterial media are a characteristic histologic feature. Inclusion bodies are absent.

Prognosis. The prognosis is generally favorable. Cases marked by a progressive rise in the pulse and respiratory rates have a guarded to unfavorable prognosis.

Treatment. No specific therapy is available. Systemic antibiotics may be administered to prevent secondary infection. Cardiac glycosides are indicated if a sustained rapid pulse is present.

Prophylaxis. Affected animals are isolated, and isolation is maintained for at least 4—6 weeks after fever has subsided. Stables should be thoroughly cleaned and disinfected. Healthy animals are protected with live-virus vaccine; a single vaccination will provide complete protection for at least 3 years.

References

Bryans, J. T.: Equine viral arteritis. Proc. 2nd Int. Conf. Equine Infect. Diseases, Paris 1969 (Karger, Basel 1970).

Crawford, T. B.; Henson, J. B.: Immunfluorescent, light-microscopic and immunologic studies of equine viral arteritis. Proc. 3rd Int. Conf. Equine Infect. Diseases, Paris 1972 (Karger, Basel 1973).

Doll, E. R.: Viral Arteritis; in Equine medicine and surgery (Amer. Vet. Public. Inc., Wheaton/Ill. 1972).

McCollum, W. H.; Bryans, J. T.: Serological identification of infection by equine arteritis virus in horses of several countries. Proc. 3rd Int. Conf. Equine Infect. Diseases, Paris 1972 (Karger, Basel 1973).

Prickett, M. E.; McCollum, W. H.; Bryans, J. T.: The gross and microscopic pathology observed in horses experimentally infected with the equine arteritis virus. Proc. 3rd Int. Conf. Equine Infectious Diseases, Paris 1972 (Karger, Basel 1973).

Rolle, M.; Mayr, A.: Mikrobiologie, Infektions- und Seuchenlehre, 4. Aufl. (Enke, Stuttgart 1978).

2.2.3.3. Rhinopneumonitis (Equine Viral Rhinopneumonitis, Equine Viral Abortion, Catarrhal Influenza)

Definition. Rhinopneumonitis was often confused with influenza before means were available for identifying the causative virus [Hutyra]. Now that the EVR virus has been accurately characterized, differentiation from influenza is necessary.

Symptoms. Rhinopneumonitis occurs in two principal forms: abortion and respiratory disease. Abortion in pregnant mares can occur from 3 weeks to 4 months following a mild, febrile respiratory infection [Doll, 1972]. However, some abortions follow a silent infection in which no respiratory signs are observed. Abortions may occur at any time from the 7th month of gestation to full term [Prickett, 1970]. Most occur spontaneously without impending signs, and the membranes are usually expelled with the fetus. Complications related to uterine disease are rare, and affected mares can be rebred during the next estrus.

In nonpregnant mares, foals and older horses that are fully susceptible to infection, the temperature may reach 41 °C, and fever persists for 1—7 days. Systemic manifestations vary in severity depending on the degree of fever that is present. Affected horses develop a dry, painful cough, and there is a marked reddening of the palpebral conjunctivae. Initially there is a serous ocular and nasal discharge that may become mucoid or purulent after 1—2 days.

Regurgitation is not uncommon and is the result of pharyngitis. The mandibular lymph nodes are slightly swollen to markedly edematous. In severe cases moist and dry rales are auscultated over the lung, and bronchial respiration is occasionally detected in young animals. Secondary streptococcal infection is quite common in horses that are debilitated due to other causes, exposed to unhygienic conditions, or returned to work before fully recovered. If an outbreak occurs during a strangles epizootic, serious pulmonary complications are likely to ensue. Foals that become infected *in utero* and are born alive are usually weak and exhibit severe respiratory distress. Most do not survive for more than a few days after birth.

Course. In uncomplicated cases the cough very often persists for several weeks. Examination with the rhinolaryngoscope reveals a pronounced folliculitis of the pharynx and larynx. Secondary infection, especially in foals, often leads to the development of a severe purulent bronchopneumonia that may occasionally become necrotic. Complications should be suspected if the temperature remains elevated for a week, mucopurulent nasal discharge persists, and breathing remains labored. An exudative pleuritis should also be considered if the respiratory rate continues to increase. Other possible sequelae are facial nerve paralysis, mild ataxia and transitory pareses [Saxegaard, 1966].

Laboratory Findings. In pure viral infections a leukopenia with lymphopenia is present during the febrile period. With development of secondary bacterial infection, a leukocytosis with neutrophilia and a distinct left shift becomes evident. Other laboratory findings are of little value.

Etiology. The infection is caused by a DNA virus, equine herpesvirus 1 (EHV 1). The virus has an average size of 170 nm, is highly resistant to drying, and retains its virulence for up to 14 days on fomites such as wood, and for up to 42 days on horse hairs [Rolle and Mayr, 1978]. Different strains show slight variations in terms of antigenic makeup and virulence. The virus has antigens in common with human herpes simplex virus, BR/PV and pseudorabies virus. It also shares complement-fixing antigens with equine herpesvirus 2 (cytomegalovirus) and equine herpesvirus 3 (coital exanthema). EHV 1 agglutinizes horse erythrocytes and forms compliment-fixing antibodies. It can be grown in horse, lamb, hamster, swine and rabbit kidney-cell culture and exerts a cytopathogenic effect [Hagan, 1971]. Nuclear inclusion bodies are also observed [Rolle and Mayr, 1978].

Pathogenesis. The initial phase is one of rapid propagation of the virus in the nasal mucosa. From there the virus is carried to all the internal organs (swelling of mandibular lymph nodes and lymph follicles in the pharynx). The virus readily invades the fetus in pregnant mares, causing focal necrosis in the liver and lungs. Experimental studies show multiple foci in the lungs during the febrile period and, 10 days after infection, signs of a reparative bronchopneumonia (especially in the apical lobes) with hyperplasia of the respiratory epithelium. The lymph follicles are hyperplastic and show foci of necrosis [Prickett, 1970].

Epizootiology. Dimock and Edwards [1932] were the first to recognize a virus abortion in horses. Manninger and Csontos first suggested that influenza virus was responsible for epizootics of viral abortion. Bürki [1965] succeeded in isolating the EVH-1 virus in Switzerland in 1965. Today the disease is known worldwide.

The disease is transmitted directly by droplet inhalation or indirectly by ingestion of material contaminated by respiratory discharges or abortion products. Because the virus is highly resistant in the environment, it can also be spread by attendants [Rolle and Mayr, 1978]. The disease is usually introduced to a given population by the acquisition of animals that are in the incubation period or have a clinically silent infection. In fresh outbreaks, all horses in the population become infected within a short period of time. In enzootic populations, young horses are mainly affected. Infected animals develop high titers of neutralizing and complement-fixing antibodies, which decline sharply after about 5 months. The nasal mucosa acquires no lasting immunity, and the animal can become reinfected within a year. Because the disease is often overlooked in horses with partial immunity, these animals play a major role in the reinfection of susceptible horses.

Lesions. Fetuses that are aborted before the 7th month of gestation are usually autolytic, and lesions can be demonstrated only by histologic examination. Fetuses aborted after the 6th month show icterus, petechial hemorrhages on all mucous membranes, subcutaneous edema, excessive fluid in the pleural cavity, pulmonary edema, and small, white necrotic foci in the liver and spleen.

Histologic examination reveals bronchiolitis with some focal necrosis of the bronchioles, pneumonia, and focal hepatic and splenic necroses. Intranuclear inclusion bodies characteristic of herpes infections are found in altered tissues [Prickett, 1970].

Diagnosis. The diagnosis is based on the clinical picture, which may closely resemble influenza, and on isolation of the causative virus. The virus can be isolated from nasal swabs or washings or from suspensions of liver and lung from aborted fetuses and identified in renal cell culture.

Differential Diagnosis. Influenza is less apt to cause abortion but can be reliably distinguished from rhinopneumonitis only by serologic tests or by virus isolation. Infections with *Salmonella abortus equi* lead to abortion between the 4th and 8th months of gestation. The affected mares are generally sick for a longer time, have recurrent fever, and frequently suffer colic or enteritis. The causative organism is easily isolated from fetal tissues. Other causes of abortion include fungi, *E. coli*, *Proteus* species and other pathogenic organisms.

Infections with reoviruses and rhinoviruses can cause respiratory symptoms similar to those of rhinopneumonitis. Differentiation is made by isolation of the causative agent. In Europe, Borna disease should be considered if paralytic symptoms are present. However, this disease generally affects only individual animals, does not cause coughing, and produces a fever of longer duration. Again, doubts are resolved by serologic testing and virus isolation. Rabies is characterized by a rapidly progressive paralysis and death within a few days after symptoms first appear. Fluorescent microscopy may also be used to examine brain tissue for antigen.

Prognosis. When virus abortion occurs on a breeding farm, further abortions may be expected in fresh outbreaks. Respiratory tract disease has a favorable prognosis provided rest is maintained until coughing subsides. If severe pneumonia develops, the prognosis is guarded. With pleuritis, the prognosis is poor. Animals that are worked while pulmonary lesions are still present are at risk for developing a chronic bronchitis with emphysema.

Treatment. No specific treatment is available. Immediate rest should be enforced and maintained for at least a week after fever has passed. Acute cases are treated with antibiotics or sulfonamides for at least 3 days after the febrile period, and antitussives may be given if coughing persists.

Prophylaxis. Without vaccination, prophylaxis is limited to purely hygienic measures. The dried virus can be destroyed by the thorough cleaning and disinfection of stall surfaces. Newly arrived horses should be kept isolated for at least 3 weeks. A modified live-virus vaccine is available [ROLLE and MAYR, 1978] and requires yearly booster injections. See ROLLE and MAYR [1978] for prophylactic and emergency vaccinations on breeding farms.

References

BÜRKI, F.; BÄRISWYL, K.; LINDT, S.: Nachweis des Virus der Equinen Rhinopneumonitis als Ursache von Stutenaborten. Schweiz. Arch. Tierheilk. *107:* 386 (1965).

DIMOCK, W. W.; EDWARDS, P. R.: Infections of fetuses and foals. Bull. 333, Ky Agric. Exper. Station (1932).

DOLL, E. R.: Viral rhinopneumonitis. In: Equine medicine and surgery, 2nd ed. (Amer. Vet. Public. Inc., Wheaton/Ill. 1972).

HAGAN, W. A.: The herpesviruses; in HAGAN's Infectious diseases of domestic animals; 6th ed. (Cornell Univ Press, Ithaca and London 1971).

JACK, J.: Persistent infections with herpesvirus. Progr. Med. Virol. *18:* 160 (1974).

JACKSON, G. G.: Viruses causing common respiratory infections in man. J. Infect. Dis. *127:* 328 (1973).

PRICKETT, M. E.: The pathology of diseases caused by equine herpesvirus I. Proc. 2nd Int. Equine Infect. Diseases, Paris 1969 (Karger, Basel 1970).

ROLLE, M.; MAYR, A.: Mikrobiologie, Infektions- und Seuchenlehre; 4. Aufl. (Enke, Stuttgart 1978).

SAXEGAARD, F.: Isolation and identification of equine rhinopneumonitis virus from cases of abortion and paralyses. Nord. Vet.-Med. *18:* 504 (1966).

2.2.4. Infectious Diseases of the Digestive System

Salmonellosis (Paratyphoid)

Definition. Salmonellosis is an infection with *Salmonella* species characterized by abortion and genital disease as well as by septicemia, enteritis and chronic abscess-forming processes.

Occurrence and Epizootiology. Salmonellosis has a worldwide distribution. A basic distinction is made epizootiologically between the specific salmonella abortion and the other diseases caused by the various salmonella species.

In Europe salmonella abortion is one of the most common causes of abortion in broodmares and can pose a significant threat to the success of breeding operations. It is introduced to breeding farms by infected horses which shed the bacteria through the genital and digestive tract. Within a given population, the infection is disseminated by breeding and by direct or indirect contact with abortion products, which contain the organisms in large numbers. Generally a high incidence of abortion occurs only during the 1st foaling period after the infection is introduced, owing to the immunity that develops in areas where outbreaks have already occurred. In the years that follow, abortion usually is restricted to new arrivals. It is thought that permanent carriers are relatively rare. The infection can also be transmitted pre- or perinatally to the foal. If infection occurs during late pregnancy, the foal is born weak and will probably die within a few days. Effective control measures have greatly lessened the importance of salmonella abortion on modern breeding farms.

In the remaining salmonella infections, the potential sources of infection are extremely varied. The most important of these are contaminated feedstuffs, drinking water, pastures, various contaminated objects, rodents, other domestic animals and infected horses. The route of infection is principally through fecal-oral cycling, and the occurrence and severity of infection are significantly influenced by prevailing hygienic conditions.

Foals and aged horses are particularly susceptible. Infections are most prevalent during the warm, moist months (May to mid-September). Carriers are relatively common and often become clinical cases under stress (e.g., following the use of anti-helminthic or laxative drugs, transportation, stable changes, crowded stabling and pasturing, hard training, pregnancy, hunger, thirst, major surgery, other diseases). Major epizootics can occur in this way, like the outbreak in England in which more than 100 horses died *(S. newport)*. Infected horses can shed *S. typhimurium* for at least 107 days. Horses have been known to carry *S. enteritidis* infection for more than 14 months. The number of organisms shed per gram of feces can be considerable (3×10^5/g has been reported). Horses can provide an important reservoir for the organisms and can be a source of infection for other animal species and for man.

Symptoms. Salmonella abortion is characterized by an incubation period of 2—4 weeks, fever, vaginal discharge, swelling of the vulva, colic and occasional mastitis. Premonitory symptoms may be absent, however. The fetus is expelled suddenly along with the fetal membranes. Areas of maceration are evident on the expelled placenta. In other cases the placenta may be retained due to hydrops of the fetal membranes. Most mares that abort recover completely with no impairment of reproductive function, though complications such as metritis and sterility are possible.

Frequently the infection will metastasize, causing tendovaginitis, arthritis, pneumonia, abscessation or laminitis. If infection is contracted during late pregnancy, the mare will give birth to a weak foal with septicemia, arthritis, hemorrhagic diarrhea and respiratory distress. Orchitis and epididymitis develop in stallions and male foals.

The remaining manifestations of salmonella infections represent systemic diseases with highly variable clinical course. Fever, depression, reduced working capacity, incoordination and diarrhea are the initial signs. The peracute form is frequently observed in foals. The onset is sudden and marked by the development of septicemia and toxemia with high fever, profuse diarrhea, depression and anorexia. Death usually occurs within 24—72 hours. Acute cases are characterized by the intermittent passage of watery feces containing blood and mucus. The consequent heavy fluid loss leads to dehydration and a disturbance of the electrolyte balance.

The chronic form runs a course from 3 weeks to several months in duration. The stool has a cow-dung-like appearance. Severe emaciation and dehydration are characteristic. Food is alternately accepted and refused. The body temperature is generally normal, though it may be elevated or even subnormal for several days. Cachexia and recumbency develop, followed by death in 5—8 days or by a convalescence of several weeks.

Hansen et al. [1971] described an intestinal septicemic form of equine salmonellosis, a pyemic form, a moderate form, and a carrier form in which bacteria are shed but symptoms are absent.

Etiology and Pathogenesis. The causative organism of the specific abortion and genital infection is *Salmonella abortus equi*, a salmonella species that shows a high degree of host adaptation. Abortion due to this organism in North America is virtually unknown nowdays.

The remaining manifestations can be caused by a great variety of salmonella species, the foremost of which are *S. typhimurium*, *S. heidelberg*, *S. newport* and *S. anatum* [Morse et al., 1975]. *S. dublin* is also important and has been demonstrated in the German Democratic Republic. Concurrent infections with two or even three salmonella species have been described [Quevedo et al., 1973]. The organisms are relatively easy to isolate and identify in the laboratory. The incidence of infection with a particular species depends upon the territorial prevalence of that species and upon the potential sources of infection for the horse. The ubiquitous nature of salmonellae, their high resistance to environmental influences, their ability to reproduce outside the body, and their ability to acquire virulent characteristics rapidly (virulent plasmids) make these organisms, and especially *S. typhimurium*, a great threat to horse populations. Records indicate that the number of salmonella infections is on the increase. The bacteria usually gain access to the body by ingestion. Small amounts are killed by gastric juices. However, the organisms that reach the intestine propagate there and invade the intestinal mucosa. The endotoxins that are liberated from the intestine, as well as the bacteria themselves, damage the bowel wall and make it permeable to the salmonellae. Following a bacteremic phase, various types of organ damage can occur or a septicemia may develop. Infection via the pharyngeal lymph nodes has also been demonstrated.

Diagnosis and Differential Diagnosis. The presumptive clinical diagnosis must be confirmed by demonstrating the causative organism, which is readily isolated from the fetus or fetal membranes, genitalia, feces, pus from abscesses, and postmortem from the parenchymatous organs. The specific causative species of salmonella can generally be identified within 48 hours with available laboratory methods.

In infections with *S. abortus equi*, the detection of antibodies by the agglutination test has proved a valuable method for assessing the degree of infection present within a given population. Titers of 800 indicate a definite infection, while titers of 400 are considered suspicious. Antibody levels are highest 8 to 14 days after abortion occurs. The titers may persist for years and are subject to large individual variations as well as variations within the individual. Thus, repeated blood tests performed at intervals of about 2 weeks are indicated to ascertain the time of infection. Active immunization produces titers of an approximately equal level that gradually decline over a period of a year.

Serologic diagnosis of the remaining salmonella diseases is a difficult matter. Its usefulness is limited due to the constant possibility of contact with the organism. For differential diagnosis in cases of genital infection and abortion, it is necessary to exclude infections of other origin as well as noninfectious abortions. The serum neutralization test in tissue culture provides the best evidence for a virus abortion. In septicemic forms, other infections that are associated with septicemia, most notably anthrax, must be considered.

In cases with abscess formation and articular disease, Brucella spp. and wound-infecting bacteria should also be considered.

Lesions. Septicemic forms are marked by the changes typically seen in septicemia with hemorrhagic diathesis, parenchymal degeneration and congestion, and hyperemic enlargement of the spleen.

A gastroenteritis may be catarrhal, hemorrhagic or even necrotic in nature. Pronounced swelling of the lymph nodes is apparent.

In chronic forms, necrotic foci and granulomas may be found in the liver, kidneys, spleen or lungs, depending on the nature and extent of organ involvement. The liver also manifests a fatty degeneration and may even show cirrhotic lesions. Examination of the intestine, especially the ileum and large bowel, reveals a diphtheroid-necrotizing inflammation with swelling and dark-red marbleization of the mesenteric lymph nodes. In addition, these granulomas may contain areas of central caseation. Edema in the lungs is frequently accompanied by a purulent catarrhal bronchopneumonia with abscessation. Fibrinous pneumonias with a lobar or lobular character are also observed. Pericarditis and myocarditis are frequently present.

Fibrinous exudations with organ adhesions are found in the thoracic and abdominal cavity. The tendon sheaths and joints contain excessive fluid. The joint capsules are thickened.

Prognosis. The prognosis of genital infections is favorable. As a rule, affected mares will only abort once. Septicemia is rapidly fatal, and treatment is useless.

The various forms of organ damage can be influenced therapeutically to some degree. Advanced intestinal changes usually lead to a fatal outcome. Double infections with *S. anatum* and *S. typhimurium* warrant a guarded prognosis.

Treatment. Affected animals should be isolated at once. The prompt initiation of treatment is crucial to success.

With a genital infection, surveillance of the puerperium is indicated, combined if necessary with antibiotic and sulfonamide therapy. In peracute and acute salmonellosis, intravenous or oral electrolyte therapy is indicated to restore the electrolyte balance and prevent dehydration. Drugs to control diarrhea and stimulate the appetite, as well as dietary measures, are also recommended.

In the experience of some authors [Morse et al., 1976], a specific antimicrobial therapy is questionable. When high bacterial counts are present, treatment with antibiotics can cause a rapid bacterial decomposition accompanied by a massive release of endotoxins. This may cause complications to arise where none existed previously. We recommend chloramphenicol, neomycin, streptomycin, polymyxin B, potentiated sulfonamides and nitrofuran derivatives, given in conjunction with symptomatic therapy and dietary measures. Little can be done to prevent the development of a carrier state, however.

Prevention and Control. Specific and general hygienic precautions for preventing infection and limiting its spread are of primary importance.

With regard to *S. abortus equi* infections, it is important to ascertain that mares are entirely free of such infection before they are bred or transported. Transportation between farms should be kept to an absolute minimum. Stallions should undergo routine examinations as part of a regular hygienic breeding program. In high-risk populations, prophylactic vaccination with commercial or stable-specific vaccines is recommended. Even in the face of an outbreak, active immunization can be used as a means of protecting animals in the band that have not yet been infected. However, the antibody titers associated with the vaccination will invalidate serologic tests as a means of supervising eradication. For mares that have aborted, an interval of at least 3 months should elapse before breeding is resumed.

It is important that all mares showing signs of aborting be isolated from the rest of the band without delay. After abortion occurs, proper sanitary procedures should be followed: disposal of septic materials, thorough cleaning and disinfection with commercial products used in recommended strengths, regular disinfections throughout the foaling period.

The remaining salmonella infections are best controlled by scrupulous cleanliness, regular disinfection and tidiness in stable areas, and precautions to prevent salmonella contamination of feed and drinking water. In horses that are at pasture, meticulous pasture care is of great preventive importance. In bands in which an outbreak has occurred and then been eradicated, every means should be utilized to identify and eliminate permanent carriers.

References

BAKULOV, I. A.: Salmonelloznyj abort kobyl. In: Infekcionnye i unvasionnye bolezni nošadej (Kolos, Moskva 1976).

GIBBONS, D. F.: Equine salmonellosis. A. Review. Vet. Rec. *106:* 356 (1980).

HANSEN, M. A.; FOSSUM, K.; TEIGE, J.: Infeksjon med Salmonella typhimurium hos hest. Nord. Vet.-Med. *23:* 475 (1971).

MORSE, E. V.; DUNCAN, M. A.; PAGE, E. A.; FESSLER, J. F.: Salmonellosis in equidae: A study of 23 cases. Cornell Vet. *66:* 198 (1976).

QUEVEDO, F. D.; DOBOSCH, D.; GONZALES, L. E.: Contamination of horse meat with Salmonella. An ecological study. I. Carrier horses. Gaceta Vet. *35:* 119 (1973).

NN: Salmonellosis in horses. Vet. Rec. *99:* (2), 19 (1976).

2.2.5. Infectious Diseases of the Urogenital System

2.2.5.1. Rhinopneumonitis

(see Sec. 2.1.11.7.)

2.2.5.2. Coital Exanthema

(see Sec. 2.1.10.4.2. and 2.1.11.3.5.)

2.2.5.3. Salmonella Abortion

(see Sec. 2.1.11.7. and 2.2.4.)

2.2.5.4. Contagious Equine Metritis

(see Sec. 2.1.11.5.)

2.2.6. Infectious Diseases of the Nervous System

2.2.6.1. Borna Disease

Definition. Borna disease is a viral infection of equidae and sheep that is characterized by a nonpurulent encephalomyelitis.

Symptoms. The disease can be produced in 4—6 weeks by injecting infected brain pulp into the cerebrum of experimental animals. Observations indicate that natural infections have a considerably longer incubation period. Initial symptoms are nonspecific and include anorexia, a fever that may reach 40.5 °C, and drowsiness. Diarrhea, mild colic and coughing may also be present. The palpebral conjunctivae are usually mildly icteric. As the disease progresses, central nervous signs become increasingly predominant. Patients show an incoordination of gait, ataxia, nystagmus, pareses of the limbs, and disturbances of equilibrium. The latter are especially marked when the animal is blindfolded. A stage follows in which the animal adopts unphysiologic postures and performs compulsive movements. Initially there is hypersensitivity to pain in the head and neck area, but later a pronounced hypoesthesia is the rule. Usually the course is progressive, so that the animal becomes recumbent after 1—2 weeks and has to be destroyed. The disease may take a gradual course in which there are days or even weeks of transitory improvement. These are usually followed by recurrence with fever and an exacerbation of nervous signs. The mortality in such cases is 90 %. Even if the animal survives, it is likely that residual defects such as ataxia, unsteady gait and unphysiologic posturing will remain.

Laboratory Findings. The hematocrit is slightly elevated, and a neutrophilia (no left shift) and lymphopenia are present. The serum bilirubin is moderately elevated (5.1—86 μmol/l). Liver enzymes are within normal limits. The total protein content of the cerebrospinal fluid is always increased (96—176 g/l; normal = 22—27 g/l). An increase in mononuclear cells is possible but may be absent in chronic cases (personal oberservations).

Etiology. The viral etiology of Borna disease was first demonstrated by ZWICK, SEIFRIED and WETTE. The causative virus has not yet been accurately identified, however. According to ELFORD and GALLAWAY, the virus of Borna disease is between 85 and 125 nm in size. It appears to have a complex structure and possesses a complement-fixing, soluble antigen (S antigen). The virus is presumed to be of the RNA type, although its precise structure remains unknown [ROLLE and MAYR, 1978].

The virus is highly resistant to environmental influences. It can remain virulent for up to 30 days at room temperature. It also shows little sensitivity to pH changes in the range from 5 to 12, and thus is resistant to sodium hydroxide. Chloramine and formalin are most effective in killing the virus. The virus has uniform immunologic characteristics, but different strains of the virus show marked differences in terms of virulence and host range. The virus is serologically and immunologically distinct from the viruses that cause other types of encephalitis (eastern equine encephalomyelitis, rabies, pseudorabies, etc.) [MAYR, 1978].

The Borna virus is readily cultivated in chick embryo and various cell cultures [MAYR and DANNER, 1972].

Pathogenesis. Artificial infection is most readily produced by intranasal or intracerebral inoculation with infected brain pulp. The principal means of natural infection is apparently via the nasal mucosa and olfactory nerve following droplet inhalation. The virus appears to have a specific affinity for the ganglion cells, since the characteristic intranuclear inclusions, the Joest-Degen bodies, are found in these cells. Current evidence suggests that the virus primarily attacks the CNS centripetally along the nerves, and then spreads centrifugally to invade the salivary gland, kidneys, mucous membranes and mammary gland. The most pronounced ganglion changes are found in the olfactory bulb, frontal brain and hippocampus. The changes become visibly less pronounced in a caudal direction, and few if any lesions are found in the cerebellum and spinal cord. The nonpurulent inflammation of the ganglion cells also leads to degeneration of the associated nerves, and thus to irreversible paralyis.

Epizootiology. Borna disease was first described as an epizootic in the Borna region near Leipzig in 1894. It remains epizootic in southern areas of the Federal Republic of Germany, in Hessen, in the Saxony regions of the German Democratic Republic, and in Switzerland. As a rule, the morbidity of Borna disease is not high within a given population. There is much seasonal variation in its occurrence. While most cases tend to occur during the spring, infections are observed throughout the year. It is not known whether true reservoirs for the virus exist. Because the disease can affect sheep as well as horses, and positive titers can be found in these species even in the absence of marked clinical symptoms [Metzler, 1977], both species must be considered potential carriers. The positive titers found in cattle and goats, and the spontaneous cases observed in rabbits, suggest that these species, too, may provide a reservoir. When horses become affected in regions previously thought to be free of Borna disease, it is essential that the origin of the infection be pinpointed as to its location. The geographic distribution of the disease suggests that a soil reservoir may be involved, although the soil itself is probably not of direct importance in this respect.

Diagnosis. A definitive diagnosis of Borna disease is not possible on clinical evidence alone. However, the occurrence of central nervous signs in areas known to be endemic for the disease should always arouse suspicion that Borna disease may be present. The diagnosis is based on serologic tests as well as on isolation of the virus from the brain of animals that die or are destroyed. Tests for serum antibodies are useful only if positive; the CF test in particular may be falsely negative in infected animals. Indirect immunofluorescent serology of the cerebrospinal fluid is a better method. The cerebrospinal fluid tends to contain greater amounts of antibodies than the serum, especially if the infection has been present for more than 14 days [Danner, 1976]. Rises in antibody titers are also important, and so samples should be examined when the animal is first seen and 14 days later, survival time permitting. A ratio of more than 1 : 20 is considered positive.

If the animal dies or is destroyed, the brain should be removed and examined for virus (antigen). The virus may be demonstrated in cell culture or by rabbit inoculation. In positive cases the rabbit will contract a lethal meningoencephalitis within 3—6 weeks. A faster method is to demonstrate complement-fixing antigen in the brain using specific rabbit serum as an antibody source. Finally, the diagnosis can be established by the histologic demonstration of inclusion bodies (Joest-Degen bodies) in the ganglion cell nuclei. These bodies are most commonly found in the ganglion cells of the hippocampus of the caudate nucleus and in the olfactory brain [Nicolau et al., 1929].

Differential Diagnosis. In *rabies*, somnolence is absent, but the patient shows marked behavioral disturbances and may become aggressive or violent. Pharyngeal paralysis develops rapidly. In every case the brain should be removed and examined for specific antibodies. *Pseudorabies* (Aujeszky's disease) is characterized by high fever and severe pruritus, as well as by a rapid course. Pseudorabies in the horse is always associated with a previous or concurrent outbreak in pigs. Serologic tests or virus isolation are helpful in diagnosis.

Listeriosis in the horse is rare and is practically always associated with the feeding of spoiled corn silage. Fever and meningitic symptoms (head extension) are the most salient features. Histologic examination of the brain is diagnostic. *Botulism* in the horse is also relatively uncommon. It is associated with the eating of spoiled feeds (eg. dead cat in haystack). The disease is nonfebrile. There is rapid paresis and paralysis of the limbs, the tongue and pharynx become completely paralyzed, and blindness develops. No changes can be demonstrated in the brain or other organs by gross examination or by serologic or histologic methods.

Treatment. No specific treatment exist. Brain edema in acute cases can be reduced at least temporarily by the i.v. administration of mannitol (1 g/kg BW of 10% solution) or urea (60—250 g of 5% solution) to induce diuresis. The same effect can be achieved by cisternal puncture. Adrenocortical hormones may be given to reduce inflammation. All such treatments are of only temporary benefit in most cases, however.

Prognosis. The prognosis is generally unfavorable. Mortality is about 90%. The prognosis is very poor in cases where symptoms worsen within a week. The same is true if recumbency develops. In mild cases 'dummy' symptoms are likely to appear as the disease progresses.

Prophylaxis. Given the limited value of treatment, prophylactic vaccination should be considered in areas where Borna disease is epizootic. The live-virus vaccine of Zwick [Hahn] derived from the brain of infected rabbits is most commonly used at present. Immunity develops within 3 weeks following the subcutaneous injection of a 10-ml dose. Because live virus is used, the vaccine should be given only in epizootic areas. Foals less than 1 year old and mares in late pregnancy should not be vaccinated. Horses between 1 and 2 years old, ponies and donkeys are given a half dose. Additional precautions are recommended: Horses, sheep and goats should be housed separately. Horses from epizootic areas should be quarantined for 2 months and tested serologically for specific antibodies in paired tests conducted 1 month apart. Even if an outbreak is limited to sheep, the prophylactic vaccination of horses on the same farm is considered a wise precaution [Nitzschke, 1957].

References

Danner, K.: Labordiagnose der Bornaschen Krankheit über den Nachweis von Antikörpern im Zentralnervensystem. Zbl. Vet.-Med. R. B. *23:* 865 (1976).

Ernst, W.; Hahn, H.: Bestehen Aussichten gegen die seuchenhafte Gehirn-Rückenmark-Entzündung der Pferde (Bornasche Krankheit) zu immunisieren? Münchener tierärztl. Wschr. *77:* 477 (1926).

Eikmeier, H.: Bornasche Krankheit des Pferdes und Schafes. Handlexikon der tierärztlichen Praxis, p. 120 (Medical Book Company, Kopenhagen 1965).

Joest, E.; Degen, H.: Über eigentümliche Kerneinschlüsse bei der enzootischen Gehirn-Rückenmark-Entzündung der Pferde. Z. infekt. Krankh. d. Haustiere *6:* 348 (1909).

Mayr, A.; Danner, K.: Production of Borna Virus in tissue culture. Proc. Soc. exp. Biol. Med. *140:* 511 (1972).

Mayr, A.: In Rolle; Mayr, Mikrobiologie, Infektions- und Seuchenlehre; 4. Aufl. (Enke, Stuttgart 1978).

Metzler, A.: Die Diagnose der natürlichen Bornavirus-Infektion bei Schafen und Pferden. Ein Vergleich verschiedener Methoden. Vet.-med. Diss., Zürich (1977).

Metzler, A.; Minder, H. P.; Wegmann, Ch.; Zindel, W.: Die Bornasche Krankheit, ein veterinärmedizinisches Problem von regionaler Bedeutung. Schweiz. Arch. Tierheilk. *121:* 207 (1979).

Nicolau, S.; Dimanescu-Nicolau, O.; Galloway, J. A.: Etude sur les septinévrites a ultravirus neurotropes. Ann. Inst. Pasteur *43:* 1 (1929).

Nitzschke, E.: Über den Nachweis eines komplementbindenden Antigens und komplementbindender Antikörper bei weißen Ratten, Meerschweinchen und Pferden, die mit dem Virus der Bornaschen Krankheit infiziert waren. Zbl. Vet.-Med. *4:* 289 (1957).

Infektionsschutz des Tieres. Kompendium für die Veterinärmedizin (Hoffmann, Berlin 1972).

2.2.6.2. Eastern Equine Encephalomyelitis (EEE) (Blind Staggers, Sleeping Sickness)

Definition. EEE is an acute viral disease that occurs in the United States. It has a marked seasonal incidence, and is transmitted to humans and horses (and other equidae) by mosquitoes. In the horse, EEE generally is associated with central nervous signs and a high mortality.

Occurrence. The disease derives its name from its principal occurrence along the Atlantic Coast of the American continent in all areas that have direct access to the Atlantic Ocean or that border on the Gulf of Mexico or lie within its waters. It is not restricted to coastal areas, but extends relatively far inland. For example, cases have been reported in Texas as far as 100° west longitude. Every few years epizootics of EEE occur during the months from August to October. Descriptions of the disease from the previous century (1831 in Massachusetts) prove that viral encephalomyelitis in equidae always had its natural origin in America and was not introduced by the horses of immigrants. The percentage of earlier deaths in horses referable exclusively to EEE remains unclear. It was not until 1933 that the virus was first isolated and EEE recognized as being a separate entity from the clinically indistinguishable western equine encephalomyelitis (WEE).

Outside of America, cases of EEE have been reported in Egypt, Syria, Italy and the Philippines. The ecological factors that maintain a reservoir of infection and lead to epizootics have not yet been fully researched. Two host-virus cycles exist, one enzootic (silvatic) and the other epizoodemic (fig. 2.2. — 5).

The enzootic cycle of infection is maintained by various swamp-dwelling birds along the Atlantic Coast and Gulf of Mexico and possibly by cold-blooded vertebrates. These animals serve as the primary reservoir. The swamp mosquito *Culiseta melanura* is the primary vector. Ticks and mites may also play a role. This cycle can keep the EEE virus alive for years without involving the horse or man. Apparently the

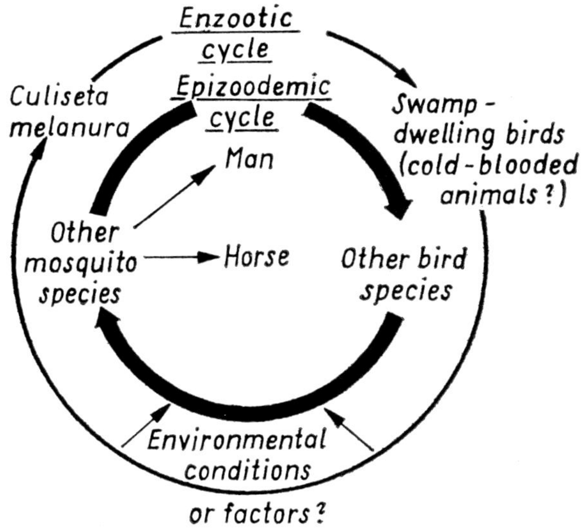

Fig. 2.2. — 5. Cycles of infection with EEE virus.

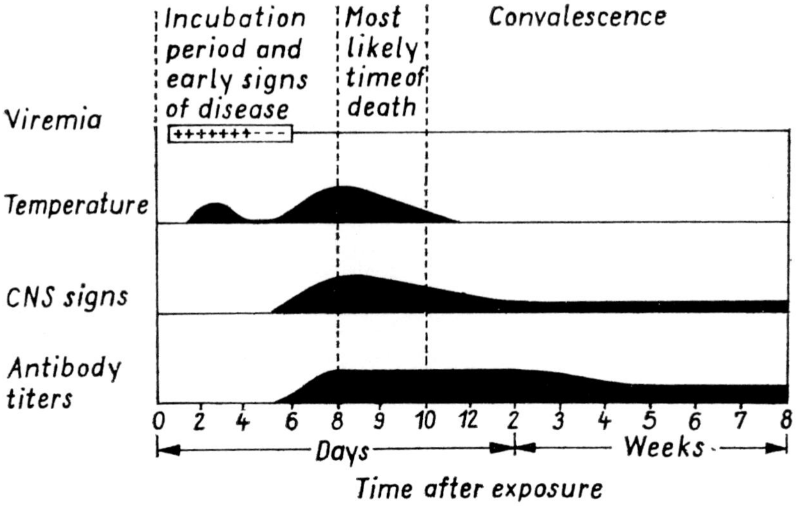

Fig. 2.2. — 6. Response of horses to EEE virus (after BYRNE [1969]).

infection spreads from the enzootic cycle to involve other bird species as a result of environmental factors that are not yet known. The infection is then spread from these birds by other mosquitoes and biting insects which attack horses and man, initiating the epizoodemic cycle of infection.

Although it is theoretically possible for the virus to be transmitted by vectors from infected horses to healthy ones, EEE differs from Venezuelan equine encephalomyelitis (VEE) in that affected horses do not significantly amplify the epizootic infection.

Symptoms. An incubation period of 24—48 hours is followed by a transitory febrile period that coincides with the viremic phase. Afterwards the body temperature returns almost to normal for 1—2 days, then rises again to reach peak levels within 24—48 hours. This biphasic fever pattern is a characteristic feature of EEE (and WEE). The horse responds to the 2nd febrile period with marked depression and anorexia. Within hours, cerebral manifestations appear in the form of somnolence, teeth grinding, diminished cutaneous reflexes, drooping of the lower lip, and nystagmus. Visual disturbances and dysphagia may also be present. The horse shows a distinct reluctance to move and will resist attempts by handlers to turn it in the stable. The final stages are marked by bizarre excitation states in which the horse may batter down walls or attempt to climb obstacles. Disturbances of coordination increase until the horse is no longer able to stand, collapses suddenly and is unable to rise. The animal lies on its side and makes continuous running movements with the forelimbs. The cerebrospinal fluid is increased in volume and contains up to 30 lymphocytes or leukocytes per ml. Death frequenly occurs within 2—3 days after symptoms first appear (fig. 2.2. — 6).

The chance of survival is poor if cerebral manifestations develop. In the few animals that survive the disease, the body temperature first returns to normal before CNS signs gradually regress. All horses do not recover completely, and some are left with permanent motor (or sensory) impairment.

Some horses with EEE do not develop central nervous signs; most of these animals recover completely and experience no sequelae.

Table 2.2. — 1. Important representative members of group A and B arboviruses

Arbovirus group	Major Representatives
A (alpha)	Sindbis Eastern equine encephalomyelitis (EEE) Western equine encephalomyelitis (WEE) Venezuelan equine encephalomyelitis (VEE)
B (flavo)	Yellow fever Dengue type 1—4 Japanese B encephalitis (JBE) Kyasanur forest disease Louping ill Omsk hemorrhagic fever St. Louis encephalitis (SLE) Tick encephalitis (Central European and Far Eastern) Murray valley encephalitis West Nile fever

Etiology. The causative agent of EEE is an RNA virus with a diameter of 45—58 nm. It is assigned to the A group of arboviruses (table 2.2. — 1) and shows some similarities to the WEE and VEE viruses in the hemagglutination reaction. Viruses isolated in various parts of North America show uniform serologic characteristics, but their antigenic makeup and pathogenicity differ somewhat from EEE viruses isolated in South American countries.

The EEE virus is highly pathogenic for guinea pigs, mice, rabbits and chicks and can be cultivated in chick embryos and tissue culture. Calves, pigs, sheep, goats, dogs, pigeons, ducks, and several species of wild bird are also susceptible to the virus.

Pathogenesis. The virus is transmitted to horses by biting and blood-sucking arthropods. After only 24 hours there is extensive proliferation of virus in the blood. The viremia persists for several days, usually until death occurs. The markedly neurotropic virus passes to the central nervous system in the blood stream, where it produces symptoms by damaging neuronal cells. The viremic phase is followed by the appearance of hemagglutination-inhibiting, complement-fixing and virus-neutralizing antibodies in the serum, which reach maximum titers 2—3 days later (fig. 2.2. — 6). The duration and intensity of the viremic phase are thought to have a critical bearing not only on the level of antibody titers, but also on the development and severity of CNS signs.

Differential Diagnosis. Sporadic cases occurring in regions where several types of viral equine encephalomyelitides coexist can present a challenge to differential diagnosis. EEE is clinically indistinguishable from WEE and VEE. Only laboratory studies (virus isolation, serology) will enable a differentiation to be made.

Other diseases to be considered are rabies, tetanus, and botulism. Rabies is distinguished by pruritus, bite wounds on the extremities, and dysphagia in typical cases. The prevalence of rabies in the area is also a useful guide. Tetanus (neck rigidity, 'sawhorse' stance) and botulism (normal temperature and appetite, dyspnea, tachycardia, paralytic symptoms) lack the signs of CNS excitation that characterize EEE. Encephalitides with dummy-like behavior, space-occupying intracranial lesions (tumors, parasites) and hydrocephalus are characterized by a subacute or chronic course. Intoxications generally take an afebrile course.

Diagnosis. Besides clinical findings, the diagnosis is based on the location of the affected animals (high-risk area) and the season (summer, fall). Clinical signs of EEE are a high, biphasic fever, the presence of CNS signs, and a fulminating course that is rapidly fatal in most cases. The clinical diagnosis is confirmed in surviving animals by means of laboratory studies (serology). A 4-fold rise of antibody titer in paired serum samples taken when the animal is first seen and a week or so later confirms the diagnosis. An absence of antibodies excludes the disease. In animals that die or must be destroyed, an effort should be made to demonstrate EEE virus in the brain. The virus is extremely dangerous in the laboratory, and extreme precautions should be taken during removal of the brain (rubber gloves!).

Lesions. Characteristic cerebral lesions are found at necropsy. These consist of an acute, primary degeneration and necrosis of nerve cells, neuronophagia, and massive infiltration with varying proportions of polymorphonuclear leukocytes and lymphocytes, occurring both diffusely in the cerebral parenchyma and in direct proximity to the cerebral vessels. Inflammatory changes are usually more pronounced in the gray matter and mainly affect the cerebral cortex, thalamus and hypothalamus; the striate body, brain stem and spinal cord are affected to a lesser degree. Secondary extension of the inflammatory process to the meninges is evident. Oxyphilic nuclear inclusions are occasionally found in ganglion cells, but these inclusions are not considered pathognomonic for EEE.

Prognosis. The prognosis is extremely grave. The mortality is as high as 90%, with most deaths occurring from myocardial asthenia, general debility, aspiration pneumonia, or septicemia resulting from decubital lesions. Horses that survive recover very slowly and often are left with permanent brain damage.

Treatment and Prophylaxis. Treatment is of little avail, although supportive measures are beneficial. Intravenous therapy is given to support the circulation and prevent dehydration (glucose), and laxatives are given for constipation. Sulfonamides may be indicated to control or prevent bacterial infection. The animal should be protected from injury, and slinging may be advised. Immune sera are useless in animals with clinically overt infection, but hyperimmune serum can give passive protection to animals being exposed.

Bivalent live-virus vaccines derived from cell culture have proved effective for active immunization. When injected intradermally, these vaccines induce at least a 4-fold rise in serum antibody titers in more than 80% of vaccinated animals, giving simultaneous protection against both EEE and WEE. Several weeks are required for complete immunity to develop. VEE vaccine also affords immunity to EEE.

Comments. EEE is one of the most dreaded viral equine encephalomyelitides on the American continent. Its high virulence and epizootic character make it a potential killer of great magnitude. The spread of infection can be contained only by prompt, active vaccination of endangered horse populations, and through vigorous insect control. These measures are also important from a public health standpoint, although clinically frank EEE infections in man are less common than other arbovirus infections (WEE, VEE).

References

Byrne, R. J.: Immunity against Eastern und Western Equine Encephalomyelitis viruses. J. Amer. vet. med. Assoc. *155:* 365 (1969).

Byrne, R. J.: Neurotropic viral diseases. In: Equine medicine and surgery; 2nd ed. (Amer. Veterin. Public. Inc., Wheaton/Ill. 1972).

Byrne, R. J.: The control of arboviral encephalomyelitis of horses. Proc. 3rd Int. Conf. Equine Infectious Diseases, p. 115 (Karger, Basel 1973).

Hanson, R. P.: Virology and epidemiology of Eastern an Western arboviral encephalomyelitis of horses. Proc. 3rd Int. Conf. Equine Infectious Diseases, p. 106 (Karger, Basel 1973).

Jochim, M. M.; Barber, T. L.: Immune response of horses after simultaneous or sequential vaccination against Eastern, Western, and Venezuelan Equine Encephalomyelitis. J. Amer. Vet. Med. Assoc. *165:* 621 (1974).

Vasilenko, V. A., et al.: Investigation of the antigenic structure of arboviruses isolated in Cuba during epidemic of Eastern Equine Encephalomyelitis, May 1969. Voprosy Virusologii *16:* 682 (1971).

Williams, J. E., et al.: Relationship of density of Culiseta-Melanura mosquitos to infection of wild birds with Eastern and Western Equine Encephalitis viruses. J. Med. Entom. *11:* 352 (1974).

2.2.6.3. Western Equine Encephalomyelitis (WEE) (Kansas Horse Plague, Western Viral Encephalitis)

Definition. WEE is an acute viral infection affecting horses and humans. The disease is transmitted by mosquitoes and shows a seasonal incidence. Epizoodemic outbreaks are not uncommon.

Occurrence. WEE was first described in 1912. In that year some 25,000 horses in Colorado, Kansas, Missouri, Nebraska and Oklahoma died during an epizootic of WEE. The viral nature of the disease was discovered in 1930 with an outbreak among horses and mules in California. A later epizootic in 1938 claimed nearly 100,000 horses.

WEE occurs primarily in the western and midwestern U.S., extending as far east as Illinois. It also occurs in Texas, Louisiana and Florida, together with EEE. The WEE virus has been recovered from birds and mosquitoes in a few eastern states. Outside the U.S., the WEE virus was isolated in Czechoslovakia in 1957 from ticks and mice within a limited geographic area; one human fatality occurred.

Within the U.S. the greatest number of cases are recorded from July to September. The epizootiology of WEE is similar to that of EEE. Wild birds are considered to be the primary reservoir, at least during epizootic periods. WEE virus has also been found in wild mammals and reptiles. The role of domestic fowl in transmitting the virus is still unknown. The mosquito *Culex tarsalis* is the primary vector of WEE, serving as the connecting link between the enzootic and epizoodemic cycles of infection. It is also a vector of St. Louis encephalitis, which occurs in many of the same areas as WEE. The main breeding areas for this mosquito are located along the western coast.

The horse is considered a dead-end host for the WEE virus, because blood virus levels in infected horses are too low to infect blood-sucking vectors and amplify the epizootic.

Symptoms. The symptoms of WEE are essentially the same as those of EEE. Differences relate to the fact that WEE takes a less fulminating course than EEE, and thus allows cerebral manifestations (which develop in at least 30% of affected horses) to become more apparent. In severe cases, however, death may be fairly rapid, occurring by the 4th day of the disease. Mild cases show marked improvement after 4—8 days. Of the animals that recover, only about 2% have permanent neurologic losses. Hemagglutinizing antibodies are demonstrable within 11 days following recovery from an infection. Complement-fixing and virus-neutralizing antibodies appear several days later.

Etiology. The causative virus was isolated in 1930 and is assigned to the A group of arboviruses based on its antigenic structure (table 2.2. — 1). It is an RNA virus with a diameter of 45—58 nm. The WEE virus is related serologically to the EEE and VEE viruses.

The same animal species are susceptible to the WEE virus as to the EEE virus. Both viruses are highly pathogenic for one-day-old chicks and (on intracerebral inoculation) for mice.

Pathogenesis. The virus has a strong affinity for the central nervous system, which it attacks by the hematogenous route during the brief viremic phase. There it produces central nervous signs by damaging neuronal elements.

Differential Diagnosis, Diagnosis, and Lesions. What has been said on these aspects of EEE, also applies to WEE.

Prognosis. WEE has a more favorable prognosis than EEE, and its mortality rate is about 50 %. Prognosis tends to be poor if the body temperature falls below normal and the animal goes down. Ponies are relatively resistant.

Treatment and Prophylaxis. See corresponding discussions for EEE (p. 264). Live-VEE-virus vaccines give at least partial immunity to WEE.

Comments. WEE is one of the most feared equine viral encephalomyelitides in the U.S. Devastating losses from epizootics can be effectively prevented by prompt vaccination of endangered horse populations.

WEE poses a considerably greater risk to public health than EEE. Outbreaks in man have been more numerous, more severe, and have been associated with a greater mortality. Outbreaks in humans are usually preceded by outbreaks in horses, and so the horse may be considered a sentinel for the disease. Systematic, intensive mosquito control measures, together with vaccination, offer the most effective means for preventing and controlling epizootics.

References

Byrne, R. J.: Neurotropic viral disease. In: Equine medicine and surgery, 2nd ed. (Amer. Vet. Public. Inc., Wheaton/Ill. 1972).

Byrne, R. J.: The control of arboviral encephalomyelitis of horses. Proc. 3rd Int. Conf. Equine Infectious Diseases, p. 115 (Karger, Basel 1973).

Doby, P. B.; Schnurrenberger, P. R.; Russel, J. M.; Hanson, L. E.; Sherrick, G. W.; Schoenholz, W. K.: Western encephalitis in Illinois horses and ponies. J. Amer. vet. med. Assoc. *148:* 422 (1966).

Gutekunst, D. E.: Immunity to bivalent tissue culture origin equine encephalomyelitis vaccine. J. Amer. vet. med. Assoc. *155:* 368 (1969).

Hanson, R. P.: Virology and epidemiology of Eastern and Western arboviral encephalomyelitis of horses. Proc. 3rd Int. Conf. Equine Infectious Diseases, p. 106 (Karger, Basel 1973).

Kirk, L. J., et al.: Rapid identification of WEE virus. Canad. J. Microbiol. *20:* 215 (1974).

2.2.6.4. Venezuelan Equine Encephalomyelitis (VEE) (Pesta Loca)

Definition. Venezuelan equine encephalomyelitis is a viral disease that occurs periodically as an epizootic, and whose cycle of infection involves arthropods, animals and man. Infection is characterized by febrile systemic manifestations that usually are associated with CNS signs.

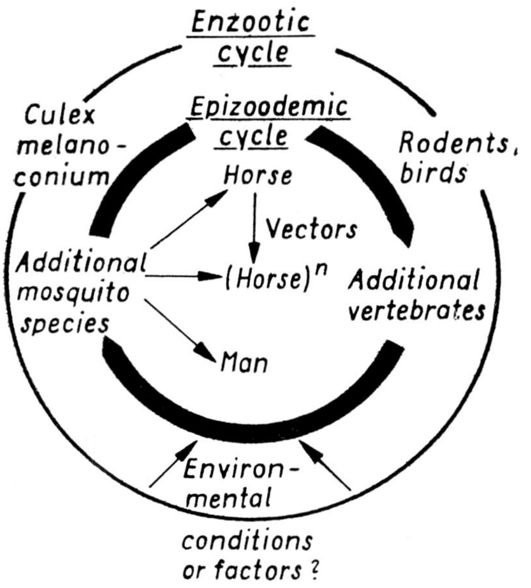

Fig. 2.2. — 7. Cycles of infection with the VEE virus.

Occurrence. VEE occurs in the northern countries of South America (Venezuela, Colombia, Ecuador, Peru), in Central America since 1969 (Costa Rica, Nicaragua, Honduras, El Salvador, Guatemala, Mexico), and in the U.S. since 1971 (Texas). The name 'Venezuelan' derives from the fact that the disease was first reported in Venezuela (Guajira Peninsula) in 1936—1938. VEE caused total damages of \$ 10 million in Colombia in 1967, and \$ 1.2 million in Ecuador in 1969. VEE has its origin in natural enzootic foci located in tropical rain forests and swamps of South and Central America. These areas are seldom more than 1,000 meters across and can be divided into two types:

a) nonpathogenic for equidae and man (e.g., Brazil),

b) nonpathogenic for equidae but sporadically pathogenic for man (Central America).

The principal reservoirs of the virus are small rodents such as the cotton rat *(Sigmodon hispidis)* and cotton mouse *(Peromyscus gossypinus)*, birds, and mosquitoes of the species *Culex melanoconium* that inhabit these biotopes. The Culex mosquito can also serve as a vector. Under the influence of environmental factors that are yet unknown, the cycle of infection is expanded beyond virus-harboring vertebrates and mosquitoes to include other genera and species, particularly species of mosquito that feed avidly on horses. It is these arthropods that then initiate the epizoodemic cycle of infection by transmitting the virulence-enhanced organism to horses and man. Because affected horses temporarily acquire high blood-virus levels, they amplify the transmission of virus to other horses through active and passive vectors (and by contact) (fig. 2.2. — 7).

The natural virus-vector-host relationships are not yet fully understood. Under experimental conditions, numerous mosquito species of the genera *Culex, Aedes,*

Anopheles, *Mansonia* and *Psorophora* have proved capable of transmitting the virus in varying degrees.

Symptoms. VEE appears in equines as a generalized, febrile systemic disease that may or may not be accompanied by CNS signs. Symptoms vary in degree depending on the type and severity of the infection. The morbidity varies between 3 and 90 %.

In the *generalized form* (without CNS involvement), an incubation period of 24 to 78 hours is followed by a (viral strain-dependent) mono- or biphasic temperature elevation up to 41 °C that persists for 2—6 days or up to 9 days in some cases. The horse appears dull, listless, and refuses to eat. Gastrointestinal disturbances with diarrhea or constipation are observed. The pulse is rapid and bounding. The animal becomes visibly weaker, loses body weight rapidly, and lies down frequently. In severe cases it is unable to rise and dies following a 2- to 4-day course of illness. In milder cases the body temperature returns to normal within 2—3 days, and this is followed by a prolonged convalescence.

The prodromal signs of the *cerebral* or *encephalitic form* are those of the generalized form, i.e., high fever, anorexia and depression. This stage is followed by the development of central nervous signs that are either irritative or depressive in character. In the former case, the animal will pull against its lead and display vicious behavior such as kicking and biting. Foam may appear about the lips, and spasms are evident in certain muscle groups. On walking there is obvious incoordination, and circling is common. When signs are depressive, the horse stands in straddle-legged fashion to maintain its balance. It lays its head on available objects or supports it against the wall or against a dark corner of the stall and lapses into a somnolent state. Unnecessary movements are avoided.

The terminal stage, seen in 80—90% of cases, is marked by loss of equilibrium leading to collapse. The animal lies on its side and makes continuous running motions with its forelimbs. When death comes, the animal is in a state of extreme exhaustion and has a subnormal body temperature. The course of the disease rarely exceeds 2—4 days.

In the few horses that survive, recovery is very gradual. The animal eats poorly, remains weak and emaciated for some time, and has difficulty walking. Tufts of hair may be lost in certain body areas (dorsum, tail). Hematologically, both forms of VEE are characterized by leukopenia coinciding with the onset of viremia, and anemia; hemoglobin values fall to 4—5 g/100 ml. Differential blood counts show a decrease in polymorphonuclear leukocytes and lymphocytes.

Etiology. The causal agent of VEE is an RNA virus that was first isolated in 1938 [Beck and Vyckoff] and is assigned to the group-A arboviruses (table 2.2. — 1). In the hemagglutination test the VEE virus shows antigenic similarities to the EEE and WEE viruses. Four major subtypes of the VEE virus are known which vary in serology, epizoodemiology, and geographic distribution. Subtype 1 (varieties A, B and C) is highly virulent for horses and is the cause of epizootics. Unlike the enzootic viral strains, which are distributed primarily in the rain-forest and swamp areas mentioned above, the epizoodemic strains show a high degree of ecologic adaptability, in that they can adapt to a wide range of vectors, reservoirs and hosts. Common laboratory animals (rat, mouse, guinea pig, rabbit, hamster) have proved susceptible to VEE virus.

Pathogenesis. The VEE virus is transmitted from one horse to another by blood-sucking arthropods and by direct contact. Viremia develops within 24—78 hours and persists for 72—146 hours or, in severe cases, until death. High titers of virus are also found in the pancreas, and in the CNS of animals contracting the encephalitic form. Virus is contained in the discharges of affected horses.

In horses surviving the viremic phase, virus-neutralizing, complement-fixing and hemagglutination-inhibiting antibodies appear in the serum 6—12 days after infection. The titers of these antibodies are maximal after an additional 2—3 days.

Differential Diagnosis. In sporadic cases the differential diagnosis of VEE presents problems even to experienced veterinarians. EEE, WEE and VEE are clinically indistinguishable. The monophasic febrile response to VEE is strain-dependent and so does not serve to differentiate the condition from the biphasic fever patterns of WEE and EEE. Laboratory conformation (detection of antibodies, virus isolation) is necessary to identify the specific causative agent.

In addition, the generalized form of VEE may be confused with a great variety of febrile infectious diseases such as leptospirosis, African horsesickness, equine infectious anemia (chronic course!), etc. Again, laboratory confirmation may be needed to make a differentiation.

The cerebral form of VEE has certain features in common with rabies, but pruritus, the presence of bite wounds, and dysphagia serve to distinguish the latter disease. Botulism is distinguished by normal temperature and appetite and a rapidly progressive tachycardia and respiratory distress. Tetanus is characterized by neck rigidity and a saw-horse stance.

Diagnosis. Diagnosis must take into account the overall epizootiology of the affected region, and in individual cases is based upon the following symptoms:

a) high (mono- and biphasic) fever, systemic signs, leukopenia, anemia (= generalized form);

b) coexisting CNS signs that are either irritative (viciousness, motor incoordination) or depressive in nature (somnolence, loss of equilibrium = cerebral form).

In surviving animals the clinical diagnosis can be confirmed retrospectively by the detection of virus-specific antibodies in the serum. In animals that die with VEE, virus can be demonstrated in the brain by immunofluorescence. Isolation of the causative agent is frequently unsuccessful.

Lesions. Necropsy reveals signs of depletion of the hematopoetic tissues, hemorrhages in the mucosae of the gastrointestinal tract, and multiple necrotic foci in the spleen, lymph nodes and pancreas. In the encephalitic form these changes are accompanied by inflammatory lymphocytic infiltration of the cerebral cortex and, to a lesser degree, of the midbrain, cerebellum and medulla oblongata. The perivascular lymphocytic infiltrate may contain a neutrophilic leukocyte component. In addition, foci of glial-cell proliferation are found in the cerebellum and medulla oblongata. Thrombosis and necrosis are frequently observed in the small cerebral arteries and are considered relatively characteristic of VEE.

Prognosis. The prognosis is favorable in the generalized form of VEE and grave in the cerebral form. The mortality is 70—90%. When affected horses go down, there is usually no hope of recovery.

Treatment and Prophylaxis. Treatment is at best supportive: blood volume maintenance, fluid replacement, protection from injury during excitation states. The i.v. administration of pure terpentine (10—20 mg/day) is reported to have a salutory effect!

The administration of immune serum is useless when overt infection is present. Experience is still lacking on the possible efficacy of passive immune prophylaxis.

The active immunization of horses may be done with live and inactivated vaccines. Attenuated vaccines developed in the U.S. (TC 50; TC 83) have proved effective in populations threatened by serious outbreaks. Immunity is usually retained for at least 1 year. The live vaccines also afford complete or partial immunity to EEE and WEE.

Comments and Control of Epizootics. VEE is one of the most destructive viral encephalomyelitides in Latin America. The threat of outbreaks in the U.S. has intensified efforts toward systematic prevention and control. Given the epizootic character of VEE, major losses among equidae can be prevented only if control efforts are directed toward the rapid establishment and maintenance of an adequate level of immunity in endangered horse populations. Due to the danger of contact transmission among horses and the fact that infected horses can transmit the virus to potential vectors, affected animals must be isolated and shielded from mosquitoes.

In man, the disease has a high morbidity and causes influenza-like symptoms that may be associated with cerebral signs (0.5% mortality). From a public health standpoint, therefore, contact with infected horses should be minimized, and much emphasis should be placed upon disinfection and intensive mosquito control measures.

References

Eddy, G. A.; Martin, D. H.; Johnson, K. M.: Epidemiology of the Venezuelan equine encephalomyelitis complex. Proc. 3rd Int. Conf. Equine Infectious Diseases, p. 126 (Karger, Basel 1973).

Erickson, G. A.: Rapid diagnosis of VEE by fluorescence microscopy. Amer. J. Vet. Res. *36:* 167 (1975).

Omohundro, R. E.: VEE emergency operation. J. Amer. Vet. Med. Assoc. *161:* 1516 (1972).

Stellmann, C.; Santucci, J.: Le complexe des Encephalomyelitis équines Vénézuéliennes. Bulletin de l'Office Int. des Epizooties *75:* 1027 (1971).

Sudia, W. D., et al.: Epidemic VEE in North-America. Amer. J. Epidemiol. *101:* 1 (1975).

Zehmer, R. B.: VEE epidemic in Texas. Health Serv. *89:* 278 (1974).

2.2.6.5. Japanese B Encephalitis (JBE) (Japanese Encephalitis, Japanese Equine Encephalitis)

Definition. JBE is an acute, arthropod-borne viral disease that is widespread throughout the Far East. Epizootics occur periodically and cause central nervous symptoms in horses with some mortality. Clinical infections also occur in other domestic species and in man.

Occurrence. Besides Japan, JBE occurs in Korea, Malaya, Singapore, the Pacific islands, and the far eastern part of the Soviet Union. It is most prevalent during the summer and fall (July to October). The major epizootics of 1936/37 and 1947/50 in Japan caused heavy losses among horses. The disease in swine, leading to abortion, stillbirths and high mortality among newborn pigs, is of main economic concern at the present time. Serologic studies in Malaysia showed that 90% of swine, 70% of cattle and 25% of goats and sheep had virus-specific antibodies in the serum, i.e., had been exposed to the virus.

Swamp-dwelling birds are considered the natural reservoir of the virus. While the virus is not pathogenic for these birds, they produce blood-virus levels high enough to infect blood-sucking insects, which in turn transmit the infection to humans and domestic animals. The mosquito *Culex tritaeniorhynchus* is the primary vector in this regard. The heavy enzootic distribution of the virus among pigs also makes this species a significant reservoir. Infected horses are not considered significant amplifiers of epizootics.

Symptoms. Following an incubation period of 2—4 days, infected horses respond with anorexia and a fever of about 39 °C that may rise to 41 °C in subsequent days. Depression, photophobia, tremors, locomotor disturbances, hindquarter ataxia, and hyperasthesia about the head and neck are characteristic features. The animal's weakened condition compels it to lie down. Respiration becomes labored, and condition is rapidly lost. Finally the animal is unable to rise. In other cases the animal may collapse suddenly. Most deaths occur after a 3- to 5-day course of illness.

The majority of infected animals survive, however. Some are only mildly affected and develop no CNS signs, while others acquire only a latent infection. Low-grade fever is the only symptom in many cases and usually goes unnoticed.

Aside from a leukocytosis with an increase of juvenile neutrophils in the early stage, no hematologic changes can be demonstrated.

Etiology and Pathogenesis. JBE is caused by an RNA virus that is assigned to the B group of arboviruses on the basis of its antigenic properties and vector-host relationships (table 2.2. — 1). It differs antigenically from the EEE and WEE arboviruses but shows serologic similarities to the causal viruses of St. Louis encephalitis and the infectious equine encephalomyelitides occurring in the Soviet Union. Animal studies have shown that, unlike the North American encephalomyelitis viruses, the JBE virus is not pathogenic for chicks or any other avian host.

In infected mammals, the virus passes to the brain (among other organs) during the viremic phase. There it proliferates and causes damage to neuronal tissue, with consequent neurologic symptoms.

Differential Diagnosis and Diagnosis. Febrile systemic diseases of other etiology may prove difficult to distinguish from cases of JBE that are unaccompanied by signs of cerebral involvement. If such signs are present, then diseases such as rabies, tetanus, listeriosis and staggers must be excluded; botulism should also be considered. The diagnosis is based on the presence of high fever and CNS signs in horses that are either in, or have been imported from, enzootic areas. Retrospective confirmation is obtained by demonstrating virus-specific antibodies in the serum or by a rise of antibody titers in paired blood samples. At necropsy the virus can be demonstrated in the brain.

Lesions. Gross changes include small hemorrhages on serous surfaces (pericardium, endocardium, pleura, peritoneum). The principal changes, however, are found in the brain. The brain tissue is edematous, the vessels are congested, and petechial hemorrhages are visible on the meninges. The histologic picture is one of panencephalitis with perivascular infiltration of leukocytes and later of lymphocytes. The cerebral cortex, thalamus and quadrigeminal zone are mainly affected, while the pons, medulla oblongata, cerebellar cortex and spinal cord show little or no evidence of inflammation.

Prognosis and Treatment. The prognosis of JBE depends on the course of the disease and on its prevalence in a given area. Sporadic cases in enzootic areas have a favorable prognosis; the mortality is about 5 %. Epizootics are associated with a much higher prevalence of cerebral manifestations, and thus with a significantly higher mortality. All cases with cerebral involvement have an unfavorable prognosis. Treatment is supportive, and large doses of penicillin (8 million I.U./day i.m.) may be given to prevent bacterial complications. Slinging may be indicated for debilitated animals or animals weak in the hindquarters.

Comments. Epizootics pose a serious threat to horse populations, especially in areas where JBE rarely occurs or is newly introduced. In enzootic regions, horses with latent or mild infection acquire a solid immunity.

JBE should be feared when horses from JBE-free regions are transported to enzootic regions or congregate with infected animals (e.g., race tracks). It is thought that the transitory febrile diseases that occasionally affect horses at racing centers, such as Malaya, and disrupt racing schedules may also be caused by the JBE virus.

Reference

KHENG, C. S.: JBE in a horse. Austral. vet. J. *44:* 23 (1968).

2.2.6.6. Saint Louis Encephalitis (SLE)

Definition. SLE is a viral arthropozoonosis that occurs seasonally in the U.S. and produces meningoencephalitic symptoms in humans. Simultaneous infections in horses are observed.

Occurrence, Etiology and Epizootiology. The disease has been known in humans since a 1933 outbreak in St. Louis and Kansas City, Missouri. At present SLE occurs in the central and western states of the U.S. In these areas it occurs endemically or epidemically during the summer months. The detection of virus-specific antibodies in man and animals suggests that the virus also occurs in Central Africa.

Infection in man leads to a febrile systemic disease that may or may not be accompanied by encephalitis. The disease in horses is clinically similar to WEE but takes a milder course and does not assume the same epizoologic or economic importance. The causative viruses of both diseases have roughly the same geographic distribution but show marked antigenic differences.

The SLE virus is a member of the B group of arboviruses (table 2.2. — 1). Serologic cross-reactions are obtained with the JBE virus.

The SLE virus has its natural reservoir in domestic and wild birds, in which the virus causes no morbidity or mortality. The virus is spread among avian hosts by blood-sucking arthropods (mites, mosquitoes). Mosquitoes, particularly those of the genus *Culex (C. tarsalis, C. pipiens)*, transmit it from infected birds to horses and man. Conditions for such transmission are best during dry, hot weather (July—August) in mosquito breeding areas (swamps, ponds, lakes, streams).

The clinical and pathologic aspects of SLE in the horse correspond largely to those of WEE. The frequent detection of virus-specific antibodies in horses suggests that the infection takes a predominantly latent course. Inoculation experiments have also shown that the horse has a relatively low susceptibility to the virus and that the disease is difficult to reproduce experimentally. Thus, horses become infected following intracerebral inoculation with the SLE virus, but not following subcutaneous or intranasal inoculation, although the virus is recoverable from the blood and antibodies may be formed.

Despite serologic relationships that exist between the SLE and JBE viruses, virus-specific (monovalent) vaccines do not afford cross-immunity.

References

LORD, R. D., et al.: Urban St. Louis encephalitis surveillance through wild birds. Amer. J. Epidemiol. *99:* 360 (1974).

MATTHIAS, D.: Die Saint-Louis-Enzephalitis; in RÖHRER, Handbuch der Virusinfektionen bei Tieren *IV*, p. 593 (VEB Gustav Fischer Verlag, Jena 1969).

2.2.6.7. Russian Spring-Summer Encephalitis

Definition. This is a viral infection of horses, apparently of diverse etiology, that occurs in the Soviet Union and has epizootic characteristics. The causative viruses are transmitted by blood-sucking insects and can cause disease in humans.

Epizootiology and Etiology. The disease shows a seasonal prevalence, appearing in the late spring (May) and reaching its peak incidence in the fall (September, October). Nearly 10 % of the horses in a given population or region can become infected within a few months. Birds and rodents are the presumed reservoirs of the virus. It is transmitted to horses (and humans) by mosquitoes, biting flies or ticks (e.g., *Dermacentor marginatus* and *Haemalastor detritus*). The horse is a side-link in the chain of infection and contributes little to the spread of infection. Contact infections are of negligible importance.

The etiology of Russian spring-summer encephalitis has not been adequately researched to permit identification and classification of the causative agents. Regional differences in the course of the disease suggest that at least two different varieties of virus are of causal importance. There are reports relating the disease to louping-ill.

Symptoms. Latent or silent infections appear to be common in horses, judging by serologic findings. Clinically overt infections take an acute to peracute course, and death within 3—5 days is not unusual. States of excitation and depression are observed, with associated disturbances of coordination and equilibrium. The incubation period may range from a few days (3—5) to several weeks (40 days), apparently depending on the specific virus.

Lesions. Hemorrhages are visible on the gastric mucosa, in lymph nodes, below the serosa of the lung, liver, spleen and kidneys, and in the CNS. The gray matter of the cerebrum and cerebellum shows acute edema, hyperemia, hemorrhages, and inflammatory changes. Unlike Borna disease, no inclusions are found in the brain cells.

Prognosis. The prognosis is unfavorable to poor. The mortality rate is on the order of 40—90 %.

The outbreak of hemorrhagic encephalomyelitides among riding horses in Austria in 1974 showed strong similarities to Russian spring-summer encephalitis in terms of clinical and necropsy findings. Apparently the disease, which disappeared within a month, was introduced by horses that had taken part in an international riding and jumping competition held outside the country. The mode of transmission, however, was by contact.

References

BURTSCHER, H.: Hämorrhagische Enzephalomyelitis-Epizootie bei Pferden in Österreich. Wiener tierärztl. Mschr. *61:* 157 (1974).

HEINIG, A.: Die infektiöse Enzaphalomyelitis der Pferde in der UdSSR; in RÖHRER, Handbuch der Virusinfektionen bei Tieren, *IV*, p. 151 (VEB Gustav Fischer Verlag, Jena 1969).

2.2.6.8. Tetanus

Definition. Tetanus is a noncontagious wound infection. The causative organism, *Clostridium tetani*, produces a toxin (tetanospasmin) that leads to a spasmodic, tonic contraction of the skeletal muscles.

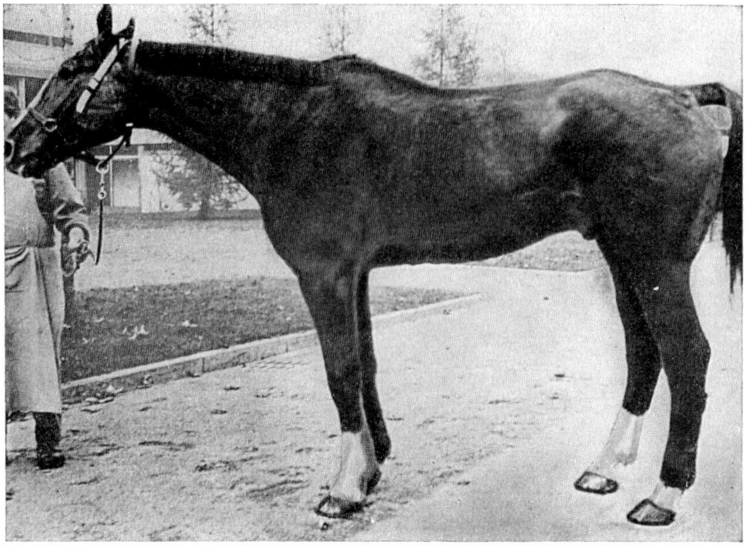

Fig. 2.2. — 8. Typical stance in tetanus.

Symptoms. The incubation period varies from a few days (especially in foals) to several weeks. A reluctance to feed or a stiff gait is usually the earliest sign. Depending on the amount of toxin produced, the clinical symptoms may worsen rapidly within a 24-hour period (acute tetanus), or the muscle spasms may increase gradually over a period of several days (subacute tetanus). The spasms are easily recognized when the patient is observed closely. An obvious and characteristic 'sawhorse' stance is adopted. The head and neck are rigidly extended, and the horse is no longer able to feed off the ground. The ears are held erect, and normal ear movements are reduced or absent. The tail is stiff and raised away from the body (fig. 2.2. — 8). Turning the animal within a narrow stall is extremely difficult. The limbs are not lifted, and the gait is exceedingly stiff and stilted. The limbs can be flexed only to a very small degree; as a result, the animal is inclined to stumble over the smallest obstacles (catching the foot in bedding, etc.). A wide dilatation and fixation of the nostrils is apparent when the animal is viewed from the front. In severe cases the third eyelid is prolapsed; this is most easily appreciated when the muzzle is lifted (fig. 2.2. — 9). In acute cases the pulse rate and temperature may be markedly elevated, while in subacute cases they remain within normal limits.

Respiration, on the other hand, is always rapid and shallow. The animal will have great difficulty eating and drinking or will be unable to do so. The mouth can be actively opened only to a small degree if at all. In severe cases the jaws are clamped tightly shut and cannot be separated by the examiner. Normally trivial stimuli provoke exaggerated responses, and any sudden light or noise will further exacerbate the tetanic spasms.

The course of the disease is mainly a function of toxin production. The more toxin that is formed within a short period, the shorter the incubation period, and the more severe the tetanic states. If the clinical picture is full-blown within 24—48 hours and the trismus so severe that even fluid ingestion becomes impossible, death will

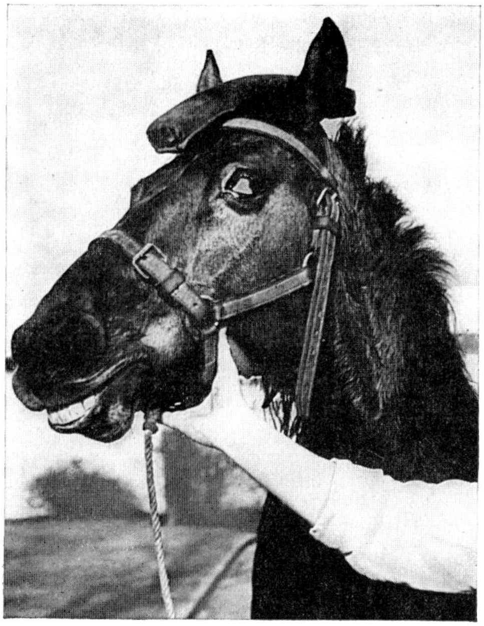

9

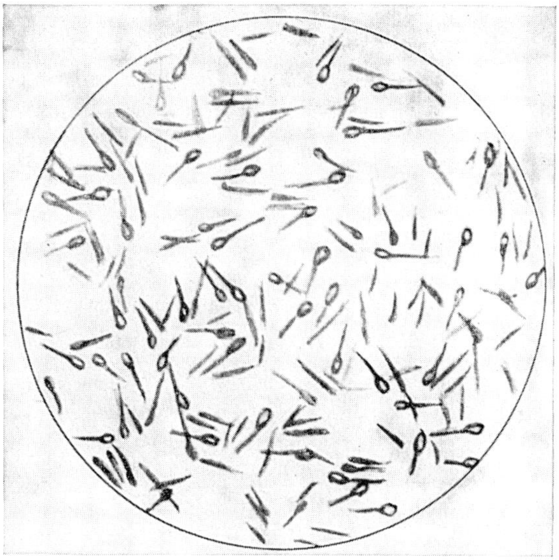

10

Fig. 2.2. — 9. Prolapse of the third eyelid in tetanus.
Fig. 2.2. — 10. Clostridium tetani.

generally follow within 1—4 days. On the other hand ,if the muscle spasms develop slowly and the animal retains its ability to eat and drink, recovery may be anticipated. There is always a danger, however, that dysphagia will lead to an aspiration pneumonia as the disease progresses. This should be suspected if the temperature rises sharply above 39 °C and there is a marked increase in the respiratory rate. Coughing is not always present. However, the pulse rate will rise in aspiration pneumonia, and there will be a noticeable deterioration of condition. After 2—3 days a grayish-red, sweetly malodorous nasal discharge will appear. Death from cardiac failure usually follows within a week.

The massive spasms of the neck and back muscles can cause spontaneous fractures of individual cervical or dorsal vertebrae [Haluzicky, 1961]. A vertebral fracture should be suspected if the horse suddenly goes lame and is unable to remain standing as the spasticity subsides.

Laboratory Findings. Hemoconcentration with a hematocrit in excess of 0.45 (45 vol.%) denotes a significant fluid loss that requires therapy. Severe cases may show a marked neutrophilic leukocytosis with a shift to the left, while mild cases show no change in white cell values. If aspiration pneumonia develops, a leukopenia may be present in the early stage. A pronounced shift to the left with more than 30% nonsegmented neutrophils is not unusual in such cases.

In our experience, determination of the muscle enzyme creatine phosphokinase (CPK) is of prognostic value in horses with tetanus. A 10- to 20-fold increase denotes a significant degree of muscle damage. A further rise of CPK during the course of the disease indicates an unfavorable prognosis. (These findings have also been confirmed in human patients [Banerjee et al., 1975]).

Lesions. In horses that die within 48 hours or show a marked rise of CPK values, examination of the skeletal muscles at necropsy reveals hemorrhages, a loss of cross-striation, and atrophy of the myofibrils.

Etiology. The causative organism, *Clostridium tetani,* is an anaerobic bacillus that develops a terminal spore, which gives it the familiar drumstick appearance (fig. 2.2. — 10). It is a motile rod 2—5 μm long and 0.5 μm wide [Rolle and Mayr, 1978; Hagan, 1973; Gillies, 1977] that is gram-positive in fresh cultures but tends to be gram-negative in older cultures. Nicolaier isolated the organism from a mouse that he had infected with garden soil, and Kitosato was able in 1889 to grow the bacillus in pure culture. *Cl. tetani* is commonly found in the intestine of herbivorous animals and is especially abundant in soil that has been fertilized with manure. The spores can persist in the environment for years, which is why wounds contaminated with manured soil are especially prone to clostridial infection. The tetanus organisms produce a thermolabile H antigen that originates from the flagellae. Ten varieties of *Cl. tetani* are distinguished on the basis of the H antigen. A somatic, thermostable O antigen is also formed; it is common to all varieties and is responsible for the spasms [Schmidt, 1940]. The amount of toxin produced apparently depends on the conditions that the organism encounters in the wound. The better the anaerobic conditions, the more toxin is produced. Proliferation of the organism and the production of toxin are promoted by concurrent infection with *E. coli* and staphylococci, tissue necrosis, and exudation within the wound. The more toxin is released, the shorter the incubation period and the more severe the syndrome [Schmidt, 1940].

Pathogenesis. The bacilli proliferate at their site of introduction. Favorable anaerobic conditions like those associated with deep puncture wounds (e.g., nail punctures of the foot) or tissue necrosis in the presence of pyogenic organisms (castration wounds, blunt injuries, umbilical infections, etc.) create favorable conditions of growth, and thus of toxin production. Although tetanus is generally classified as a wound infection, a portal of entry is found in only about 50% of affected horses. Because the bacillus is a common inhabitant of the intestine of the horse, it is possible for tetanus organisms to invade wounds of the intestinal mucosa inflicted by strongyles, or to reach internal organs from the intestine by the hematogenous route, where, if conditions are favorable (contusions), they will start to multiply and produce toxin [Knight, 1972].

The exact means by which the toxin is disseminated in the body remains unknown. Based on the observation that the disease can spread in an ascending fashion, it appears that the toxin migrates along the axis cylinders of the motor nerves to the anterior horns of the spinal cord or along the perineural lymphatic channels [Meyer and Ransom]. On the other hand, a hematogenous spread of toxin has been demonstrated by Abel et al. in experimental dogs. It appears that the blood-cerebrospinal fluid barrier is also easily crossed [Abel et al.]. The main evidence for this is the fact that a severe generalized tetany can develop within a 24-hour period. This theory is also supported by the results of Muylle [1975], who could stop the progress of the disease by injecting tetanus antitoxin into the suboccipital space. It is known that tetanospasmin is fixed very rapidly to the neuromotor end-plates by the gangliosides of the anterior horns of the spinal cord and of the cranial nerves. Apparently this inhibits the breakdown of acetylcholine by cholinesterase, leading to spasmodic, tonic contractions of the muscles.

Tetanospasmin is an extremely potent bacterial toxin, and the horse is the most susceptible of the domestic species. Thus 1 ml of culture filtrate is sufficient to kill a horse [v. Hutyra and Marek].

The toxin can no longer be demonstrated after binding to the motor end-plate. It is not yet known how the toxin is broken down or how ultimate recovery can occur. It is significant that animals that recover from tetanus frequently have no immunity and thus are susceptible to a recurrence.

Epizootiology. Clostridium tetani has a worldwide distribution and is abundant in manured soil [Nicolaier]. Hence, all puncture wounds or injuries with necrosis and retained secretions that become contaminated with soil or feces are liable to tetanus infection. Though tetanus in the horse has mainly an individual, sporadic occurrence, it is nonetheless feared because of its high mortality (up to 80 %). One survey showed that 1.9 % of equine deaths during the period 1950—1963 were attributable to tetanus [Ammann].

Prognosis. The more rapid the development of generalized spastic symptoms, the poorer the prognosis. If the trismus cannot be relieved by drug therapy to the point where the horse can ingest liquid feeds spontaneously, the prognosis is very poor. Animals that are still able to ingest solid and liquid feeds have a good chance of surviving.

If tetanic symptoms are full-blown within 24 hours, the mortality is 80—100 %. If symptoms progress more gradually over a period of 3—6 days, on the other hand, the mortality decreases to 30—40 % [Bryans; Hengeler; Leemann, 1975].

Differential Diagnosis. It is unlikely that tetanus will be confused with other diseases when all clinical symptoms are taken into account.

Treatment. The patient should be placed in a quiet, darkened stall and moved as little as possible. If transportation becomes necessary, the patient should be sedated beforehand (e.g., with Combelen) and secured so that it cannot fall during transport.

It is important that injuries be tended to. Obvious wounds, even those that have already formed a scab, should be surgically debrided. All necrotic tissues are removed, and drainage is established for secretions. Wounds should be left open. Penicillin may be applied locally to inhibit further proliferation of the bacilli. The wound is cleaned with 1% H_2O_2 solution, and antitoxin serum is injected around the wound [Scherer, 1975; Muylle et al., 1975]. At the same time, 2 ml of a toxoid vaccine are administered i.m. to stimulate antibody production. Larger animals should be placed in a sling to keep them from going down. In Europe, peat is the recommended bedding material.

Horses that are unable to stand are sedated and placed in a sling. Foals should be turned every 4 hours as a precaution against decubitus.

There is diversity of opinion as to the value of antitoxin sera. Löhrer and Radvilla [1965, 1970] recommend giving massive doses of antitoxin, 2—3 liters i.v., spread over a 3-day period, while others question the value of such therapy [van Beukelen, 1975; Muylle et al., 1975]. At best, the serum will only neutralize toxin that is circulating in the blood stream; toxin already fixed to gangliosides must be broken down by the body itself. Moreover, a dose of 50 ml antitoxin is entirely adequate to effect the desired neutralization. In severe cases Muylle et al. [1975] recommend that the antitoxin be administered by cisternal puncture. Following the withdrawal of 50 ml cerebrospinal fluid, 50 ml of antotixon serum (1,000 U/ml), warmed to body temperature, are slowly infused in the adult horse. A 30-ml dose is used in foals.

If the patient is able to eat and drink without much difficulty, additional treatment generally is unnecessary. Attention must be given to nutritional intake, water intake, temperature changes, pulse rate and defecation. On the other hand, if significant trismus is present and the animal is unduly excited, preparations such as Vetranquil, Combelen or Valium should be injected i.m. or i.v. These drugs often afford a muscle relaxation sufficient to permit eating and drinking. The dose is individualized and varies between 50 and 100 mg/500 kg BW. Because injections must be repeated at 6- to 8-hour intervals, an indwelling intravenous catheter is advantageous. If the trismus cannot be relieved with drug therapy, the patient must be fed artificially by nasogastric tube. Because of the excitation caused by passage of the tube, prior sedation is indicated. Suitable feeds include green meal, bran and oatmeal gruel. If a nasogastric tube cannot be passed, Ringer's solution may be administered by intravenous drip. The dose is determined by the hematocrit which should not be allowed to exceed 0.4 (40 vol.%). Feeding with a bran, linseed and green-meal mash may be started if trismus improves. Warm enemas are indicated for relief of constipation. The animal should be kept in a sling until able to stand unassisted.

Penicillin should be given in a dose of 10—15 million I.U./day i.m. to prevent secondary infections and control pneumonia associated with dysphagia. This systemic antibiotic therapy should be continued until the animal is again able to eat without difficulty. As hyperexcitability and limb spasticity subside, mild daily exercise may be started. In uncomplicated cases, a full recovery may be expected in 2—3 weeks.

Prophylaxis. Because recovery from tetanus does not necessarily confer immunity, horses should be actively immunized with a toxoid vaccine. Two doses of an adsorbed toxoid are given 6—8 weeks apart by i.m. injection. Each dose is 1—2 ml, depending on the preparation. A booster injection is given a year after the initial injections and usually will ensure immunity for life. In horses that sustain contaminated wounds 5—6 years after vaccination, one booster injection is usually sufficient to ensure protection.

Horses that have not been actively vaccinated should be passively immunized following wounds, surgery, etc. by administering 10 ml of antitoxin serum. It is advantageous to administer the antitoxin and toxoid at the same time, thus combining active and passive immunization. Failure to give antitoxin to a horse that has not been actively immunized constitutes gross negligence on the part of the veterinarian.

References

Abel, J. J.: cited after Schmidt.

Abel, J. J., et al.: cited after Schmidt.

Ammann, K.: personal commun.

Abmayr, H.; Abmayr, H.: Die Behandlung des Starrkrampfes beim Pferd mit Relaxan. Tierärztl. Umschau *4:* 347 (1949).

Bannerjee, A. P., Gokarni, S.; Kamat, S. R.: Creatine phosphokinase and other enzyme values in diagnosis of tetanus. Cit. Excerpta Medica, Sect. 6, *32:* 608 (1975).

Beukelen, P. van: Experience in the treatment of tetanus. Proc. third meeting Acad. Soc. large animals. Vet.-Med. Zürich 1975.

Eberlin, J. J.; Michael, B.: Zur Therapie des Tetanus mit hohen Antitoxin-Dosen. Arch. Klin. Chirurgie *300:* 287 (1962).

Gillies, R. R.; Dodds, T. C.: Illustrierte Bakteriologie (Huber, Bern 1977).

Hagan, W. S.: Hagan's infectious diseases of domestic animals; 6th ed. (Cornell Univ. Press, Ithaca 1973).

Haluzicky, M.: Vertebral fracture in tetanus. Zbl. Chirurgie *86:* 2195 (1961).

Kitosato, cited after Marek et al.

Knight, H. D.: Equine medicine and surgery; 2nd ed., pp. 94—98 (Amer. Vet. Public. Inc., Wheaton/Ill. 1972).

Leemann, W.: Zur Prognose und Therapie des Tetanus beim Pferd. Proc. third meeting Acad. Soc. large animals. Vet.-Med., Zürich 1975.

Löhrer, J.; Radvilla, P.: Behandlung des Starrkrampfes beim Pferd mit hohen Serumdosen. Schweiz. Arch. Tierheilk. *107:* 305 (1965).

LÖHRER, J.; RADVILLA, P.: Aktive Tetanusprophylaxe beim Pferd und Immunitätsdauer. Schweiz. Arch. Tierheilk. *112:* 307 (1970).
MAREK, J.; MANNINGER, R.; MÓCSY, J.: Spezielle Pathologie und Therapie der Haustiere; 9. Aufl., 1. Band (Gustav Fischer Verlag, Jena 1945).
MEYER; RANSOM, cited after SCHMIDT.
MUYLLE, E.; OYAERT, W., OVNES, L.; DECRAEMERE, H.: Treatment of tetanus in the horse by injections of tetanus antotoxin into the subarachnoid space. J. Amer. vet. med. Assoc. *167:* 47 (1975).
NICOLAIER, cited after MAREK et al.
PAVLOVIC, J.; JORGACEVIC, D.: Therapy of tetanus during 1967—1969. Cit. Exerpt. Med. Sect. 6, *27:* 287 (1972).
PRYS, R. C.; CORBETT, J. L.; KERR, K. H.: Treatment of sympathetic overactivity in tetanus. Lancet *69:* 542 (1969).
ROLLE, M.; MAYR, A.: Mikrobiologie und allgemeine Seuchenlehre; 4. Aufl. (Enke, Stuttgart 1978).
SCHERER, F.: Tetanusproblem nicht unterbewerten. Med. Trib. *7:* 9 (1975).
SCHMIDT, H.: Grundlagen der spezifischen Therapie und Prophylaxe bakterieller Infektionskrankheiten (Schulze, Berlin-Grunewald 1940).

2.2.6.9. Rabies (Lyssa, Hydrophobia)

Definition. Rabies is a viral disease of man and animals that is transmitted chiefly through bite wounds, produces a nonpurulent encephalomyelitis, and is manifested by central nervous symptoms. All mammalian species are susceptible, including man. Carnivores are responsible for maintaining and transmitting the infection, and equidae may be considered a dead-end host for the rabies virus.

Occurrence. The occurrence of rabies in horses is dependent upon a sporadic or enzootic viral infection among carnivores in the affected area. The main source of infection in urban rabies (rabies of domestic animals) is the dog. The main source animals in sylvatic (wildlife) rabies are wild carnivores such as the fox (Central Europe, North America), skunk (North America), wolf (Southeastern and Eastern Europe), jackal (Asia, Africa), etc. The disease is usually transmitted to horses from the bites of rabid carnivores. Thus, stabled horses are at far less risk than pastured animals, which are exposed to attack by infected wildlife or stray dogs. Horses at pasture can account for up to 5% of total rabies cases among domestic animals (e.g., U.S. during the period 1960—1969). In Central Europe, rabies is relatively rare in the horse.

Symptoms. The incubation period varies from 3 weeks to 3 months. This is followed by an initial stage of hyperexcitability and unrest, which become progressively more severe. Restless pawing of the ground and exaggerated tail-swishing are usual at this stage. Pruritus from the bite wound causes the horse to rub or bite the skin incessantly at that site. As the disease progresses, the unrest increases until a 'furious' stage is reached in which markedly aggressive behavior is exhibited. The horse will run into doors and walls and attack inanimate objects, possibly doing itself serious injury. A tied horse will tear violently at its lead shank and make every effort to free itself. At pasture the horse will break suddenly into a gallop for no apparent reason, kick blindly into the air or attack other horses. Symptoms similar to spastic colic may also appear: The animal will roll on the ground, jump to its feet, groan loudly and strain when defecating. Transient periods of sexual excitement may also be observed in both stallions and mares (erection, frequent micturition). Excitation states give way to states of complete exhaustion during which the animal stands motionless, drenched with sweat. Increasingly, tremors or spasms are noticed in specific muscle groups. The animal refuses to eat its feed, shows dysphagia, and may ingest wood or feces. Convulsions at this stage are common. In the terminal, paralytic stage of the disease, hindquarter weakness becomes evident. The pulse and respiratory rates are markedly increased. The animal sways, falls to the ground, and dies within a short time. The course of the disease is from 2 to 4 days.

In the dumb or depressive form of rabies, the symptoms are similar to those of Borna disease.

Etiology. Rabies is caused by an elongated conical rhabdovirus (serologic subgroup B) with a filamentous, RNA-containing nucleoprotein that is arranged in the form of a helical nucleocapsid. Apparently lipids are also a structural constituent of the envelope. Viruses isolated from various geographic areas are uniform in their antigenic features. Rabies vaccine can be prepared with attentuated, 'fixed' virus strains obtained by adapting 'street' virus to specific experimental animals (mouse, rabbit) or biologic substrates (chick embryo, cell culture).

Pathogenesis. Having gained entry to a bite wound in virus-contaminated saliva, it is thought that the virus 'migrates' along nerve pathways via the spinal cord to the brain. Although the virus is capable of propagating in nonneurogenic tissue (e.g., salivary glands, cell cultures), the brain is the main site of proliferation. There the virus attacks ganglion (and glial) cells and in advanced stages produces clinical symptoms by damaging neuronal elements. Symptoms are probably also produced indirectly by the resultant cellular and viral decomposition products. The titers of virus vary from one brain area to the next; virus is found with greatest regularity in Ammon's horn.

From the central nervous system, the virus soon spreads centrifugally, again mainly along nerve pathways, to invade specific organs, including the secretory glands and the eye. High virus titers are found in the salivary glands, where virus can usually be detected several days before initial symptoms appear. This means that infected animals pose a threat to their environment even before an outbreak is apparent.

Differential Diagnosis. All diseases associated with CNS signs must be excluded. Tetanus (sawhorse posture), listeriosis (very rare) and the non-European equine encephalomyelitides are distinguished by an absence of aggressive behavior or by high fever and high prevalence. Dysphagia is absent.

Borna disease may be difficult to differentiate from the 'dumb' form of rabies. This form may also be confused with subacute cases of botulism (incoordination; dysphagia with salivation; paralysis of tongue, lips and larynx!), though bite wounds and pruritus are absent. Staggers takes a slower and less dramatic course. Colic is unaccompanied by CNS signs.

In all cases a useful guide to differential diagnosis is the prevalence of rabies in the area and a history of potential exposure to rabid carnivores.

Diagnosis. A *clinical diagnosis of rabies* is based upon: (a) aggressive behavior, pruritus, dysphagia, bite wounds, later paralytic symptoms (= furious rabies); (b) depressed behavior, bite wounds, paralytic symptoms (= dumb rabies).

The 'cornea test' can sometimes confirm the presumptive clinical diagnosis. Cell smears are taken from the eye on a grease-free slide (rubber gloves, facial protection!) and tested in the laboratory for viral antigen. Experience is still lacking as to the validity of this test in domestic animals, although studies in experimentally infected lab animals (mice) indicate that the test is a valid one.

The only other laboratory method available for confirming the clinical diagnosis is the *demonstration of virus* in the brain of the killed animal. Compared to serologic methods, the immunofluorescent demonstration of aggregated viruses in impression

Fig. 2.2. — 11. Immunofluorescent demonstration of aggregated rabies viruses in a brain impression smear (Ammon's horn) from a mare that was suspected of rabies and destroyed. It had not been possible to demonstrate Negri bodies in stained preparations.

smears from the brain has assumed much importance owing to its sensitivity, specificity, and 'same-day' results (fig. 2.2. — 11). If the test is negative, the mouse intracerebral-inoculation test may be necessary due to the danger of human exposure.

Lesions. Disease-specific changes are confined to the CNS. There is extensive perivascular lymphocytic infiltration (nonpurulent encephalomyelitis) in nearly all parts of the brain. The presence of discrete glial-cell clusters resulting from cell proliferation (Babes nodules) and especially of round to oval, eosinophilic cytoplasmic ganglion-cell inclusions (Negri bodies) is considered pathognomonic for rabies. The latter bodies contain virus antigen and are viewed as 'large forms' of viral aggregates. Even in the early stage of a rabies infection, small viral aggregates, often in large numbers, can be demonstrated in ganglion cells by immunofluorescence (fig. 2.2. — 11).

Prognosis and Treatment. The prognosis is extremely grave when clinical signs are present, and the disease is invariably fatal. Symptomatic treatment is useless and is in fact contraindicated due to considerations of animal and public health.

Immunization. The pre-exposure active immunization of horses in regions where rabies is enzootic may be warranted. In the German Democratic Republic, prevailing health ordinances[1] make it permissible for approved live-virus vaccines (fixed virus) to be administered to horses. In the Federal Republic of Germany[2], only inactivated-virus vaccines may be used.

Attentuated live-virus vaccines, which usually are derived from cell culture (porcine or hamster kidney), afford 2 years' protection when administered in a single dose to horses over 4 years of age. Immunity is renewed for an additional 2 years by repeating the injection before the period of immunity has expired. Inactivated vaccines require higher doses and a booster injection after 3—4 weeks to give protection for 1 year.

[1] Ordinance for the Protection of Animal Populations from Epizootics, Parasitisms and Other Special Hazards, Animal Disease Ordinance (8-11-71); 1st Implementing Regulation (8-11-71); 2nd Imp. Reg. (8-3-73); Directive No. 4 for Animal Disease Ordinance, Prevention and Control of Rabies in Domestic Animals (10-24-74).

[2] Rabies Protection Ordinance of 5-10-77, Amended 7-1-80.

Comments and Control. Rabies is one of the most dreaded zoonoses. Rabid animals pose a grave threat to humans. When rabies is confirmed in horses, the post-exposure vaccination of stable personnel is mandatory.

In the GDR, citizens are required by law to report any suspected case of rabies in domestic animals. All countries have regulations requiring the destruction of rabid animals upon the order of the district veterinarian or health officials. Suspect animals must be isolated at once from contact with other domestic animals and attendants and placed under regular veterinary surveillance. Health ordinances will dictate the period of time for which suspect animals are to remain under observation (GDR: up to 4 months after the last occurrence of the disease; FRG: 6 months). Usage and pasturing during this time are permitted.

References

Eichwald, C.; Pitzschke, H.: Die Tollwut bei Mensch und Tier (VEB Gustav Fischer Verlag, Jena 1967).

Schneider, L. G.: The cornea test; a new method for the intra-vitam diagnosis of rabies. Zbl. Vet.-Med. *16:* 24 (1969).

Sikes, R. K.: Rabies vaccines. Arch. Environ Health *38:* 344 (1969).

Subcommittee on Rabies, Committee on Animal Health, Agricultural Board, National Research Council: Control of rabies. Nat. Acad. Sci., Washington 1973.

WHO-Techn. Rep. No. 523 (1973).

2.2.7. Infectious Diseases Involving Multiple Organ Systems

2.2.7.1. Equine Infectious Anemia

Definition. Equine infectious anemia (EIA) is a viral disease that affects horses, donkeys and mules. It is characterized by intermittent fever, loss of body weight, subcutaneous edema, and in some cases severe anemia.

Symptoms. After an incubation period of 6—38 days, the horse develops a high fever, usually above 40 °C. In acute cases the temperature remains elevated. The patient is profoundly depressed, the visible mucosae are dark red with a faint yellowish tinge, and hemorrhages in the mucosae may be apparent. If the temperature remains elevated, the patient will become visibly emaciated, and muscular pain (fidgety limb movements) and weakness will develop. The pulse rate also is elevated by the 4th day of the disease. If fever persists for more than a week and diarrhea develops, rapid emaciation follows, and the patient may die from cardiac failure within 8—14 days. In acute cases, hematologic studies are of little value, and the anemia is not pronounced. The white blood count, on the other hand, shows considerable leukopenia with a relative lymphocytosis. The ESR is increased by the 3rd or 4th day of illness. The ASAT values (aspartate amino transferase [SGOT]) are elevated. Urinalysis reveals a high specific gravity, a marked proteinuria, and frequently hemoglobinuria. The course may be relatively mild, in which case the temperature will return to normal in 4—8 days.

It is possible that no further febrile episodes will occur, and apparent recovery will ensue. However, the pulse rate remains markedly elevated for an additional 1—2 weeks, and proteinuria persists for several weeks. The acute disease may enter a subacute stage. After a transitory afebrile period lasting 4—6 days, there is a recurrence of fever, and then the temperature falls again several days later. The shorter the intervals between febrile episodes, the more severe the anemia. Subcutaneous edema appears on the lower chest, abdomen and limbs. Emaciation occurs despite a normal appetite. The pulse rate is markedly elevated during the febrile episodes. The patient may die during such an episode at any time from 30 to 60 days after the onset of the disease.

Laboratory tests show a marked hyperchromic anemia, a mild leukopenia with relative lymphocytosis, a marked increase in the ESR, and a slight rise of serum bilirubin values. A moderate proteinuria is present. The albumin-globulin ratio is shifted in favor of the globulin fraction (decreased A/G ratio). A chronic stage may be entered in which the febrile episodes become shorter in duration and spaced farther apart, perhaps by intervals of weeks or months. No significant systemic signs are present, although some loss of condition is noted. The horse tires easily during work. The pulse rate is always in the high-normal range even during afebrile periods. If the temperature is measured twice daily, an inverted pattern will be noted during both the febrile and afebrile periods, i.e., the temperature is higher in the morning than in the evening. Following exercise, the pulse rate rises above 60/min, and it often takes a half hour to return to resting values. The erythrocyte counts fall considerably during the febrile episodes. They may return to near-normal levels, however, if remissions are prolonged. The patient may die after a period of months or 1—2 years during an acute febrile episode. The episodes may become increasingly less frequent and last only 1—3 days, before finally ceasing altogether. This marks the latent stage of EIA. To all appearances the patient is clinically well. It regains lost weight, and its working capacity returns to normal. No hematologic abnormalities are noted, with the possible exception of the ESR, which remains in the high-normal range. These animals ultimately expire due to some other disease, though some may die from an acute recurrence of EIA after being asymptomatic for years.

The latent stage can develop from any of the aforementioned forms. However, it is significant from an epidemiologic standpoint that once a horse becomes infected, it remains a carrier for life.

Lesions. Patients that die with acute EIA show signs of acute septicemia, such as hemorrhages in serous membranes and parenchymatous organs (liver, renal cortex), hemorrhages in the skeletal muscles and edema of the muscle fasciae. The abdominal lymph nodes are markedly hyperplastic and are often permeated with hemorrhages. The spleen is markedly enlarged. The slower the course of the disease, the greater the changes that are seen at necropsy. A more or less pronounced degree of myocardial degeneration is apparent in nearly all cases, and areas of myocardial infarction may be seen. The spleen is hyperplastic with a marked increase of white pulp ('raspberry spleen'). The liver is likewise enlarged and shows a proliferation of interlobular tissue ('nutmeg liver'). The lymph nodes of the internal organs are enlarged and engorged with fluid. Histologically, lymphocytic and histiocytic infiltration is evident in practically all organs, most notably the liver, kidney and lung. There is also a considerable proliferation of Kupffer's cells in the liver, lung and spleen, which show a marked hemosiderosis.

Etiology. EIA was first described as a specific entity in 1843 [v. Hutyra, Marek and Manninger], and in 1904 a filtrable agent was identified as the cause [Vallée and Carré]. The virus is assigned to the group of oncornaviruses on the basis of various characteristic properties, such as ether susceptibility, size, morphology, group-specific antibodies, lack of hemagglutinizing ability, and an RNA that is dependent on a DNA polymerase in the early phase of proliferation [Ito et al., 1969; Kobayashi et al., 1969; Kono and Kobayashi, 1966; Kono et al., 1970, 1971; McGuire et al., 1971; Nakijama and Obar, 1964; Nowinski et al., 1970; Tajima et al., 1969]. Thus, the virus of EIA is included in the group of 'slow' viruses. Viruses of this group are characterized not only by long incubation periods, but also by the fact that the agent can remain in the host for a very long time without causing clinical symptoms. The EIA virus is cultivable in horse bone-marrow and leukocyte cultures [Ito et al., 1969; Kemeny et al., 1971; Kobayashi, 1961; Kobayashi and Kono, 1967]. Immunization experiments point to the existence of several varieties [Kono et al., 1970, 1971] which differ immunologically. Another peculiarity of the virus is that it can be demonstrated in the patient for a lifetime despite the formation of immune bodies [Banks et al., 1972; Kono et al., 1970, 1971; Stein et al., 1955]. The virus can be found in practically all organs as well as in the plasma and serum [Kono et al., 1970, 1971]. Viral titers are highest in the lymph nodes, spleen and liver. The agent is highly resistant to environmental influences [Stein et al., 1944]. It can withstand a moist heat of 100 °C for 15 minutes before being inactivated, and this must be taken into account when sterilizing instruments. The virus is also resistant to UV irradiation [Böhm, 1975].

Distribution of the Disease. EIA has a worldwide distribution, though its prevalence may show considerable regional variation within a given country [Steck, 1953]. The density of horse populations is clearly an important factor. With the increasing mechanization of agriculture and the associated decline in the number of work horses, the prevalence of EIA has decreased markedly. With the rise of equine sports and the congregation of horses at racetracks, the disease has again become prominent [Primus and Zettel, 1975]. All breeds and age groups of equidae are susceptible.

Epizootiology. Although the virus can be demonstrated in the discharges of affected animals [Kemeny et al., 1971], oral transmission in feed and drinking water appears to be of minor importance.

Evidence suggests that the virus is most commonly transmitted through the bites of blood-sucking insects, which are mainly important as purely mechanical vectors [Böhm, 1975; Ishitani, 1966]. However, the disease is also readily transmitted through improperly-disinfected needles and syringes, especially during vaccinations and the drawing of blood. Whether foals are infected *in utero* or by the mare's milk postnatally is not clear. It is also unclear whether infected stallions can transmit the disease to mares during coitus. However, the disease can be produced by injecting semen from an infected stallion subcutaneously into a susceptible horse [Stein and Mott, 1942].

Pathogenesis. Following an infection, the EIA virus can be demonstrated in practically all organs after only 6—38 days, being most prominent in the spleen, lymph nodes and liver. Titers are highest during the initial febrile episode [McGuire et al., 1971], fall considerably during afebrile periods, and then rise again with the recurrence of pyrexia [Kono et al., 1970, 1971; Nowinski et al., 1970]. The red cells are the principal local of attack, and their surfaces become coated with virus and antibodies [McGuire et al., 1971; McGuire et al., 1969]. This increases the osmotic fragility of the red cells, intensifies erythrocyte phagocytosis, and thus shortens the life span of the erythrocytes.

Energy metabolism is reduced during febrile periods. The plasma hemoglobin level rises, and so a hyperchronic anemia is usually present. Depression of the bone marrow contributes further to the anemic state. A viral-antibody complex is deposited on the renal glomeruli, causing a glomerulitis to develop [Banks et al., 1972]. In the liver there is a deposition of virus on Kupffer's cells, followed later by an infiltration of monocytes, particularly in the area of the portal veins and in the perisinusoidal spaces. The severity of hepatic changes varies with the frequency and severity of the febrile attacks. Hepatic lesions may largely regress during prolonged afebrile periods, only to recur when fever returns. The more frequent and severe the febrile episodes, the more severe the changes. The frequently chronic course of EIA and the life-long persistence of the viremia are attributed to an immune defect. Complement-fixing antibodies are detected serologically within 14—29 days after infection. The CF test is positive for several weeks, then becomes negative for a time [HENSON et al., 1969], and is alternatively positive and negative thereafter.

Precipitating antibodies appear within 14—38 days after exposure and can be demonstrated with the agar gel test (Coggins test) for the remainder of the animal's life [COGGINS and NORCROSS, 1970; COGGINS et al., 1972; HENSON et al., 1971].

Diagnosis. Today the diagnosis can be quickly confirmed with the aid of the Coggins test (agar gel-diffusion test [COGGINS and NORCROSS, 1970; COGGINS et al., 1972; HENSON and MCGUIRE, 1974]). Several countries now require a negative Coggins test before allowing the importation of horses. If this test cannot be done, then an antemortem diagnosis may prove difficult. It becomes necessary to make twice-daily temperature checks for a prolonged period, monitor changes in red blood status, and demonstrate the presence of monosiderocytes, whose peripheral blood levels are elevated during or immediately following a febrile episode. Minute sublingual hemorrhages can also assist the diagnosis. While such hemorrhages are not always detectable, significant sublingual bleeding is considered strong evidence of EIA [STECK, 1953].

Finally, the necropsy and histologic findings provide unmistakable evidence of the disease.

Differential Diagnosis. Abscesses of the internal organs can produce a clinical picture similar to subacute or chronic EIA. Besides the anemia, however, there will be a leukocytosis with a shift to the left. Blood parasitism, especially babesiosis, is characterized by hemoglobinuria, severe anemia and marked icterus in the early, acute stage. The causative parasite can also be demonstrated in the erythrocytes at this time. In chronic cases, however, serologic studies (CF test) often are the only means of differentiating between the two diseases. Viral arteritis shows similarities to acute EIA in its early stage but is distinguished by palpebral edema and photophobia with lacrimation. Deaths are rare. The disappearance of fever in 4—7 days is followed by rapid recovery. The diagnosis is confirmed by the neutralization test.

Prognosis. The prognosis is most unfavorable in terms of viral persistence, and an infected horse remains a carrier for life. The further course of the disease depends largely on the frequency of febrile episodes. The occurrence of significant myocardial damage, progressive anemia, and persistently high protein levels in the urine indicate an unfavorable prognosis.

Treatment. No specific treatment is available. Supportive treatment with antipyretics, cardiac glycosides and anabolics may be helpful, and nonspecific protein therapy is useful in stimulating resistance.

Prophylaxis. The destruction of infected horses is advantageous from a control standpoint. Infected animals should at least be kept in isolation, and large congregations like those at sporting events or sales barns should be avoided. Vaccinations, blood sampling and drug injections should be done with disposable needles and syringes, or the instruments should be boiled for at least 15 minutes after each use. Immersion in alcohol solution is not sufficient. In chronic enzootic areas where eradication is not possible, it is advantageous to replace removed horses with older animals. Vaccination is not feasible at present due to the different varieties of EIA virus with their different immunologic characteristics [KONO et al., 1970, 1971]. Only horses that are shown to be free of the disease by a negative Coggins test should be allowed access to sporting events [BÖHM, 1975; PRIMUS and ZETTEL, 1975].

References

Banks, K. L.; Henson, J. B.; Meljuise, T. C.: Immunological mediated glomerulitis of horses. I. Pathogenesis in persistent infection by equine infectious anemia virus. Lab. Invest. *26:* 701 (1972).

Böhm, H. O.: Neuere Ergebnisse bei der Forschung der ansteckenden Blutarmut der Einhufer. tierärztl. praxis *3:* 323 (1975).

Coggins, L., Norcross, N. L.: Immunodiffusion reaction in equine infectious anemia. Cornell Vet. *60:* 330 (1970).

Coggins, L.; Norcross, N. L.; Nusbaum, S. R.: Diagnosis of equine infectious anemia by immundiffusion test. Amer. J. vet. Res. *33:* 11 (1972).

Henson, J. B.; Gorham, J. R.; Kobayashi, K.; McGuire, T. C.: Immunity in equine infectious anemia. Amer. J. vet. med. Assoc. *155:* 336 (1969).

Henson, J. B.; McGuire, T. G.: Equine infectious anemia. Progr. med. Virol. *18:* 143 (1974).

Henson, J. B.; McGuire, T. C.; Gorbam, J. R.: The detection of precipitating antibodies in equine infectious anemia and partial purification of the antigen. Arch. ges. Virusforsch. *35:* 385 (1971).

Henson, J. B.; McGuire, T. C.; Kobayashi, K.; Banks, K. L.; Davis, W. C.; Gorham, J. R.: Recent research on the virology, serology and pathology of infectious anemia. Proc. 2nd Int. Conf. Equine Infectious Disease, p. 178 (Karger, Basel 1970).

Hutyra, F. v.; Marek, J.; Manninger, R.: Spezielle Pathologie und Therapie der Haustiere, 9. Aufl. (Gustav Fischer Verlag, Jena 1945).

Ishitani, R.: Research in Japan on control of equine infectious anemia. Proc. 1st. Int. Conf. Equine Inf. Disease, Stresa 1966.

Ito, Y.; Kono, Y.; Kobayashi, K.: Electron microscopic observations of equine infectious anemia (EJA) virus in cultivated horse leukocytes. Arch. ges. Virusforsch. *28:* 411 (1969).

Kemeny, L. J.; Mott, L. O.; Pearson, J. E.: Filtration of equine infectious anemia virus. Effect of dosage in incubation time and clinical signs. Cornell Vet. *61:* 687 (1971).

Kobayashi, K.: Studies on the cultivation of equine infectious anemia virus in vitro. II. Propagation of the virus in horse bone marrow culture. Virus *11:* 189 (1961).

Kobayashi, K.: Studies in the cultivation of equine infectious anemia virus in vitro. III. Propagation of the virus in leukocyte culture. Virus *11:* 249 (1961).

Kobayashi, K.; Henson, J. B.; Gorham, J. R.: Viral neutralizing antibodies in equine infectious anemia. Fed. Proc. *28:* 429 (1969).

Kobayashi, K.; Kono, Y.: Serial passage of equine infectious anemia virus in horses. Leukocyte culture. Nat. Inst. Anim. Hlth. Quart. *7:* 1 (1967).

Kono, Y.; Kobayashi, K.: Complement fixation test of equine infectious anemia. I. Specificity of the test. Nat. Inst. Anim. Hlth. Quart. *6:* 194 (1966).

Kono, Y.; Kobayashi, K.: Complement fixation test of equine infectious anemia. II. Relationship between CF antibody response and the disease. Nat. Inst. Anim. Hlth. Quart. *6:* 204 (1966).

Kono, Y.; Kobayashi, K., Fukunaga, Y.: Distribution of equine infectious anemia virus in horses infected with the virus. Nat. Inst. Anim. Hlth. Quart. *11:* 11 (1971).

Kono, Y.; Kobayashi, K.; Fukunaga, Y.: Serological comparison among various strains of equine infectious anemia virus. Arch. ges. Virusforsch. *34:* 202 (1971).

Kono, Y., Yoshino, T.; Fukunaga, Y.: Growth characteristics of equine infectious anemia virus in horse leukocyte culture. Arch. ges. Virusforsch. *30:* 252 (1970).

McGuire, T. C.; Crawford, T. B.; Henson, J. B.: Immunofluorescent localization of equine infectious anemia virus in tissues. Amer. J. Pathol. *62:* 283 (1971).

McGuire, T. C.; Henson, J. B.; Quist, S. E.: Viral induced hemolysis in equine infectious anemia. Amer. J. vet. Res. *30:* 2091 (1969).

McGuire, T. C.; Henson, J. B.; Quist, S. E.: Impaired bone marrow response in equine infectious anemia. Amer. J. vet. Res. *30:* 2099 (1969).

Moore, R. W.; Katada, M.; Redmond, H. E.; Wallace, M.: Clinical studies in equine infectious anemia. Proc. 19th. World Vet. Congr., Mexico City 1971.

Nakjiama, H.; Obar, J.: Ether susceptibility of equine infectious anemia virus. Nat. Inst. Anim. Hlth. Quart. *4:* 129 (1964).

Nowinski, R. C.; Old, L. J.; Sakar, N. H.; Moore, B. H.: Common properties of the oncogenic RNA virus (Oncornavirus). Virology *42:* 1152 (1970).

Primus, K.; Zettel, K.: Der Verlauf der ansteckenden Blutarmut der Einhufer. tierärztl. praxis *3:* 431 (1975).
Steck, W.: Studien über die infektiöse Anämie der Pferde. Schweiz. Arch. Tierheilk. *95:* 1—13 (1953).
Stein, C. D.; Mott, L. O.: Studies on congenital transmission of equine infectious anemia. Vet. Med. *37:* 370 (1942).
Stein, C. D.; Mott, L. O.; Gates, D. W.: Some observations on carriers of equine infectious anemia. Amer. J. vet. med. Assoc. *126:* 277 (1955).
Stein, C. D.; Osteen, O. L.; Mott, L. O.; Shahan, M. S.: Virus of equine infectious anemia. Amer. J. vet. Res. *5:* 291 (1944).
Tajima, M.; Nakajiama, H.; Ito, Y.: Electron microscopy of equine infectious anemia virus. J. Virol. *4:* 521 (1969).
Ushimi, C., Nakajiama, H.; Tanaka, S.: Demonstration of equine infectious anemia viral antigen by immunofluorescence. Nat. Inst. Anim. Hlth. Quart. *10:* 90 (1970).
Vallée, H.; Carré, H.: Nature infectieuse de l'anemie du cheval. C. R. Acad. Sci. *139:* 331 (1904),

2.2.7.2. Leptospirosis

Definition. Leptospirosis is a febrile, acute to chronic, often clinically inapparent infectious disease that is characterized by fever, anemia, icterus, CNS signs and ocular complications.

Occurrence and Epizootiology. Leptospiral infections in the horse have a worldwide distribution. Their epizootiology hinges upon various host animal species. *L. grippotyphosa* has been found mainly in field mice, swamp mice, hamsters and other rodents as well as in cattle, and *L. pomona* in pigs, striped field mice, and many other wild animal species that excrete the organism in the urine. Persistence of leptospires in the kidney marks the final stage of the disease and is responsible for the leptospiruria that maintains the chain of infection.

As a result of this, the prevalence of the disease shows a marked seasonal variation (highest in the pasturing season), is dependent upon the density and degree of infection of the host animal population, and is higher in older animals, in which reinfections with small numbers of leptospires can lead to allergic ocular complications (see Periodic Ophthalmia).

Transmission among horses is practically nonexistent, aside from the possibility of foal infections during the prenatal and perinatal period.

Owing to the low density of the horse population and to the excellent stabling hygiene that is generally maintained for sport horses, leptospirosis has only a sporadic occurrence. However, the possibility of a leptospiral infection is present at all times and in all locales.

Symptoms. The incubation period ranges from several days to 3 weeks. The course may be peracute to chronic. The relatively rare peracute form is characterized by depression, anorexia, impaired performance, tachycardia, rapid respiration, blood-tinged urine, pollakiuria, and pathologic changes in the blood. After the temperature falls to normal and subnormal levels, there is a sharp decline of erythrocyte counts and hemoglobin levels, leukocytosis and neutrophilia.

The acute form begins suddenly with a temperature rise to 40—40.5 °C, anorexia and impaired performance. Several days later, after fever has regressed, icterus may develop with a further deterioration of general condition. Other common symptoms are a stiff gait, paralysis and myalgia. Petechial hemorrhages appear on the icteric mucosae. Occasionally brief periods of diarrhea are observed, followed by severe constipation with colicky signs. Oliguria is present, and the urine is red-tinged and shows pathologic changes. Areas of necrosis are occasionally visible on the skin and mucosae. Acute leptospirosis lasts about 2 weeks.

In the chronic form, the most prominent symptoms are emaciation and weakness as well as intermittent febrile episodes that last 2—5 days and recur at intervals of several weeks. The recurrences are associated with subicterus, hemorrhages, and an accelerated heart rate.

A further clinical form, first described in France, is marked by meningoencephalitic signs. A hepatoencephalopathy syndrome known as Schweinsberg disease (see Sec. 2.1.5.11.1.) has been linked to leptospirosis, probably without justification.

Abortions, though less common than in other domestic animals, are entirely possible in the acute form of the disease. They occur during the third trimester.

Etiology and Pathogenesis. Infections in horses are caused mainly by *L. grippotyphosa* and *L. pomona*, which actually are serotypes of the single species *Leptospira interrogans*. However, most of the remaining 150 or so serotypes can infect horses that are at pasture and have contact with wild animals or other domestic species. The leptospires are fine, spirochaete-like microorganisms that grow best at 28 °C and a pH of 7.2—7.6. They are highly sensitive to pH values outside this range. This accounts for their poor survival in the environment, their high susceptibility to all disinfectants that shift the pH away from neutrality or mild alkalinity, and, consequently, the dependence of the infectious chain on the persistence of the organism in certain animal hosts. Under favorable conditions, however, leptospires can survive for several days or weeks outside the host. The enzyme activity of the organisms is also slight. Only lipases, hemotoxins and endotoxins are formed. Their pronounced antigenicity results in a high accuracy and specificity of antibody demonstrations with the microagglutination test, CF test, etc.

The organism enters the body actively using its own mechanisms and invades the blood stream. From there it passes to the liver, where it proliferates and causes disturbances of hepatic function.

The organism persists in the blood and liver for about 8 days after infection (septicemic phase), whereupon it either is destroyed by antibodies (toxic phase) or escapes into the convoluted tubules of the kidney, where it is safe from the body's defenses. Lipase production by the pathogen leads to the release of fatty acids, which in turn initiates hemolytic and cytotoxic processes. The hemotoxin from the pathogen causes a breakdown of erythrocytes, giving rise to hemoglobinemia, hemoglobinuria, anemia and icterus. The effect of the endotoxin is to damage the CNS, other organ cells and the blood vessels. These pathogenetic processes also determine the nature of necropsy findings.

Diagnosis and Differential Diagnosis. The diagnosis of leptospirosis requires complex clinical, epizootiologic, pathologic and laboratory investigations. Antibodies should be demonstrated in multiple serum samples obtained at 1-week intervals, due to the high nonspecific antibody titers that occasionally occur in the horse. Antibody titers of 800 in the microagglutination test (50% end-point titer) are diagnostic of infection. A rise of at least 2 titer levels within a week is indicative of a recent infection.

The organisms can be demonstrated directly in clinical specimens (urine, aqueous humor, etc.) with the aid of dark-field microscopy. The FA technique is also useful. Cultivation of the organisms is costly and requires special procedures and therefore should be attempted only in specially-equipped laboratories.

Differential diagnosis must be made from equine infectious anemia (Coggins test), Borna disease (virus isolation in experimental animals), listeriosis (bacteriologic and histologic examination) and babesiosis (direct microscopic examination).

Prognosis. The earlier antibiotic therapy is instituted, the better the prognosis. The mortality in peracute cases is as high as 100 %. Generally, however, the prognosis is favorable.

Treatment. Infected animals should be isolated and rested. Long-term antibiotic therapy is the treatment of choice. Daily doses of 5—10 mg/kg BW i. m. oxytetracycline or streptomycin, or corresponding depot preparations, are administered for at least 1 week.

Good results are also achieved with penicillin injected i.m. in doses of 10,000 to 15,000 I.U./kg BW. Penicillin cannot prevent invasion of the kidney, however. For that purpose streptomycin is the drug of choice.

Supportive treatment with laxatives, stimulants, diuretics or cardioactive drugs is indicated, depending on prevailing symptoms. Intravenous glucose therapy has also proved beneficial. Highly effective hyperimmune sera are available for use in some countries.

Prophylaxis and Control. All factors that promote the occurrence of infection (rodent infestation of stables, poor stabling and pasturing hygiene, contact with excreta of other animal species, stagnant water, etc.) should be eliminated.

Serial serologic studies in horse populations are indicated to ascertain the degree of exposure and the serotype involved. Whenever a performance decline is noted in an athletic horse, leptospirosis should be considered a a potential cause.

During the selling and purchasing of valuable horses, two serologic microagglutination tests should be performed 14 days apart. Animals with a rise of titers (at least 2 titer levels) may be started on antibiotic therapy. In districts where periodic ophthalmia is a problem, avoidance of pasturing and the implementation of intensive rodent control measures are advised. In special cases active immunization with a commercial leptospirosis vaccine that contains the serotypes most prevalent in a given area may be indicated.

References

Horsch, F.: Leptospirose, in Beer, Infektionskrankheiten der Haustiere; 2. Aufl. (VEB Gustav Fischer Verlag, Jena 1980).

Karimova, Z. Ch.: Vyjavlenne i likvidacija leptospiroza losadej v TASSR. Veterinarija (Moskva) *2:* 51 (1961).

Sosov, R. F.: Leptospirose; In Sosov, Epizootiologija (Kolos, Moskva 1974).

2.2.7.3. Tuberculosis

Definition. Tuberculosis is an insidious, infectious disease that is caused by mycobacteria and is associated with focal or infiltrative proliferations of a characteristic granulation tissue. The disease is relatively uncommon in horses, which show a high natural resistance.

Occurrence. Equine tuberculosis occurs in all countries in which tuberculous diseases of cattle, fowl and humans are widespread. Despite heavy exposure, the horse is not often affected. Abattoir statistics in various European countries indicate a morbidity rate among horses of well below 1 %, even during periods of heavy infection among cattle and poultry: GDR 1947—1950: 0.4 %; FRG 1956: 0.4 %; Denmark 1942: 0.14 % (out of 15,107 horses slaughtered); Sweden 1942: 0.09 %; Hungary 1942: 0.14 %, 1953—1960: 0.007 % (out of 131,817 horses slaughtered). The abandonment of small-farm practices with common stabling of horses and cattle and progress toward the eradication of tuberculosis among cattle and poultry have greatly limited the exposure of horses to the disease and thus have further reduced morbidity rates in recent years.

The horse, however, appears to experience a much stronger immune reaction to simple contact with the tubercle bacillus than do cattle, for tuberculin tests in enzootic areas produce skin swelling in a high percentage of horses (7—47 %) that show no visible tuberculous lesions upon necropsy.

Symptoms. In many cases, tuberculous lesions remain confined to the site of entry and/or the local lymph nodes, and they may cause no clinical symptoms for the rest of the animal's life.

Heavy proliferation of the tuberculous granulation tissue causes functional disturbances of varying severity, depending on location and extent. Disseminated tuberculosis of the lungs and pleura is manifested clinically by rapid, labored respiration, periodic coughing, a possible increase of abdominal respiration, and dullness on percussion. Lesions infiltrating the hepatic tissue can lead to cirrhotic changes and signs of hepatic dysfunction such as subicterus and even CNS symptoms ('hepato-encephalopathy syndrome'). The spread of tuberculous lesions to the skeletal system leads to corresponding locomotor disturbances with associated pain. Thus, tuberculous cervical spondylitis is manifested by stiffness of the neck, avoidance of neck movements, and obvious pain in response to side turns of the neck or rapid lifting of the head by the examiner. Skin tuberculosis is relatively common in horses. It is marked by the appearance of small, displaceable nodules under the skin that increase in size and may lead to considerable disfigurement of the head and other areas. The nodules may undergo purulent liquefaction at their centers and rupture, discharging a thick pus in which acid-fast rods can be demonstrated. The skin surrounding these fistulae exhibits pachydermia-like changes: It is dry, scaly, and the hairs stand erect and are shed. Lesions on the extremities have a greasy-heel appearance.

Tuberculosis of the udder is not too uncommon in mares and accounts for about 3—4% of tuberculosis cases. It may appear as a firm enlargement of one half of the udder, ranging to the size of a breadloaf, or it may take the form of multiple fluctuating nodules that rupture, heal, and reappear at a new site. A tense gait is apparent when lesions are extensive.

All organ and tissue manifestations of tuberculosis are accompanied by changes in the local lymph nodes. They are markedly enlarged, often to fist- or melon-size. Local cutaneous lymph nodes become visible to the eye, while altered lymph nodes in the abdominal cavity and pelvic area are palpable during rectal examination (!) as firm, nontender, tumorlike masses. The spleen is also palpable (i.e., enlarged and firm) in 50—90% of cases. Individual or multiple, discrete, coarsely-nodular elevations are often palpable on the visceral surface of the spleen.

Tuberculous lesions that remain localized generally do not impair the animal's general condition. On the other hand, disseminated organ tuberculosis, especially when generalized, leads to emaciation, roughening of the haircoat, and finally to cachexia. Working capacity is correspondingly reduced or abolished.

Specific hematologic changes do not accompany tuberculosis. However, as in other chronic inflammatory diseases, the ESR is significantly increased.

Etiology. Tuberculosis in horses is caused by mycobacteria of the species *M. tuberculosis*, *M. bovis*, and *M. avium*. *M. bovis* accounts for the great majority of tuberculous infections (80—90 %), with *M. avium* ranking second. Infections with *M. tuberculosis* are contracted from humans with 'open' tuberculosis, and in the horse they generally produce only localized tuberculous lesions with no tendency toward generalization.

Mycobacteria are straight or slightly curved, thin rods (0.2—0.5×1—5 μm) that can be cultivated on special media. Their speciation is determined by cultural features, biochemical reactions, and characteristic differences in pathogenicity toward laboratory animals (guinea pig, rabbit, chicken).

A common feature of the mycobacteria is their acid-fast staining property which derives from waxy substances (mycolic acids) contained in the bacterial wall. These soften upon heating and allow stain to penetrate into the bacterium, which retains the stain upon cooling and is not decolorized by acid, alcohol or alkali. This is the principle upon which the Ziehl-Neelsen staining method is based (acid-fast rods are stained red).

Pathogenesis. Infection in the horse usually occurs via the alimentary route, i.e., by the ingestion of feed contaminated with bacteria-laden secretions or excrement, and in foals by the feeding of milk from infected cows. Several cases of air-borne infection (inhalation tuberculosis) have also been confirmed. Often the 'primary complex', consisting of a circumscribed lesion at the site of entry and in the local lymph node, represents the limit of the animal's response. As a rule, however, the tuberculous lesion spreads within the organ of entry and leads to the development of coarsely-nodular, focal changes. At this time or somewhat later, the organisms are disseminated by the blood and lymph and cause new tuberculous lesions to form in other organs or tissues (protracted generalization, acute miliary tuberculosis), particularly the lung, liver, spleen, serous membranes, skin and udder, with simultaneous involvement of the local lymph nodes (tuberculous lymphadenitis). The granulation tissue that forms leads to the destruction of organ parenchyma and thus to symptoms of organ dysfunction. The myriad tuberculous lesions in the body lead to emaciation and debility and, when defensive mechanisms fail completely, to an unrestrained, lethal spread of the tuberculous growths.

Differential Diagnosis. Given the relatively low incidence of tuberculosis in horses, it is first necessary to exclude all other possible causes of isolated organ disease or poor general condition. These include endoparasitism and chronic infectious dieseases of other etiology (pneumonia, infectious anemia). Percussion can be used to differentiate between chronic obstructive pulmonary disease and tuberculosis of the lung (dullness on percussion). If coarsely-nodular masses are palpated rectally, neoplasms (lymphadenitis, carcinoma, sarcoma) must be considered; the coexistence of coarsely-nodular splenic changes will strengthen the suspicion of tuberculosis, however. Painless swellings of the udder may have a neoplastic origin. In the absence of obvious lymph node enlargement, biopsy may be needed to make the differentiation. Skin tuberculosis may be confused with nonspecific fistulizing, suppurating processes (cellulitis) or, in the area of the fetlock joint, with grease heel. Again, the local lymph nodes are important indicators of tuberculosis. Usually other lymph nodes will also be involved (rectal examination!).

Diagnosis. The diagnosis is based upon:

1. Clinical findings
2. Positive reaction in allergic test
3. Microscopic or bacteriologic demonstration of the causative organism.

1. Clinical findings: marked enlargement of lymph nodes, palpable spleen with nodular changes, nodular skin changes with possible fistulization and ulceration, possible cicatricial or ulcerous lesions of the nasal mucosa, wounds that fail to heal; poor general condition, pulmonary signs, weakness; exposure?

2. Allergic test: Of the allergic tests that are available (conjunctival or ophthalmic test, intrapalpebral test, thermal test, subcutaneous test, intradermal test, skin test), the (simultaneous) intradermal test with purified mammalian or avian tuberculin is today considered the best means of confirming the existence of a tuberculous process in the horse. Errors of interpretation based on nonspecific skin reactions, which are not unusual in the horse and have caused much uncertainty in the past, can be largely avoided by using the following criteria for a positive reaction:

a) Marked, very painful, doughy swelling of the skin at the site of injection, usually with associated swelling of local lymph nodes and lymphatics.

b) Anorexia and presence of systemic signs.

The degree of cutaneous swelling (increase in skin thickness) is not a reliable criterion in the horse! Assuming a careful injection technique and the use of a state-approved (tested) tuberculin, a negative reaction is considered proof that the animal is free of the disease (except in the general miliary form).

For the t.b. test, either mammalian or avian tuberculin is injected intradermally on one side of the neck, or, for comparative testing, both tuberculins are injected simultaneously on both sides of the neck. The prescribed dosage of tuberculin (0.1 ml) is injected with a special needle and syringe. The reaction is read 48—72 hours later and evaluated according to the criteria listed above. Possible anaphylactic reactions can be prevented by the prior injection of a tuberculin diluted 1: 3 with isotonic saline.

If the intradermal test is inconclusive, then the subcutaneous test should be performed for clarification.[1] A positive is declared if, 12 hours after the subcutaneous injection of 1 ml tuberculin, the body temperature of the animal rises by 1 °C over the previously measured value and remains at that level for more than 24 hours.

The hemagglutination test of Middlebrook and Dubos does not yield reliable results in the horse.

3. Demonstration of the organism: When chronic suppurative or ulcerous lesions are present on the skin or mucosae, the tubercle bacilli can be demonstrated microscopically as 'acid-fast rods' in suitably stained impression or smear preparations (Ziehl-Neelsen stain, etc.). The number of bacilli may be extremely low, however, and so often a direct identification cannot be made.

Biopsies (lymph nodes, udder) can be evaluated in the same way after being prepared for histologic examination. The demonstration of tuberculous granulation tissue provides additional confirmation. To determine speciation, bacteriologic studies using culture techniques and laboratory animals are necessary.

Lesions. Equine tuberculosis represents a productive, inflammatory tissue reaction in which caseation and calcification are not characteristic. The primary complex is generally located in the intestinal tract (alimentary infection) and consists of circumscribed, ulcerous mucosal lesions. In many cases the primary complex is incomplete, i.e., changes appear only in the mesenteric lymph nodes. The affected lymph nodes are markedly enlarged and may resemble extensive tumorous growths as a result of coalescence with adjacent nodes. The cut surface has a grayish-white, lardaceous appearance. Central caseation or calcification occurs only in patients with lowered resistance.

Dissemination of the bacilli in the blood and lymph leads to tuberculous involvement of other organs and tissues and their associated lymph nodes. The lung is most commonly affected by this dissemination and, besides coarsely-nodular, lardaceous foci, may develop the features of acute miliary tuberculosis. In this case the lung tissue is permeated extensively with minute, transparent nodules that later opacify. Coarsely-nodular foci tend to coalesce, and in this way entire pulmonary lobes can

[1] Directive No. 7, Appendix 1, to Animal Disease Ordinance, Prevention and Control of Bovine Tuberculosis, 7-29-75.

become infiltrated with lardaceous material. Coarsely-nodular lesions are a typical feature of tuberculosis in other organs as well (liver, spleen, renal cortex). Diffuse infiltration can also occur in exceptional cases, leading, for example, to cirrhotic changes in the liver. Serous surfaces, especially the pleura, are often covered by a thick, waxy layer of tuberculous granulation tissue. Tuberculous granulomas may occur in the skin and mucosae (nose) or in bony tissue (vertebral bodies, vertebral processes) and lead to liquefaction of the original tissue. In some cases all remaining organs may become involved (heart, udder, etc.) as a result of blood and lymph spread.

Histologically, the tubercle is a nonspecific granulation tissue consisting of lymphocytes, fibroblasts and histiocytes. It also contains variable numbers of specific cellular components in the form of epitheloid cells and Langhans-type giant cells.

Prognosis and Treatment. Clinically overt, generalized tuberculosis has a very poor prognosis. In most cases weakness and loss of condition are present early in the disease, and changes are irreversible. Progressive cachexia ensues.

Chemotherapy is possible in principle (streptomycin, paraaminosalicylic acid, isoniazid), but economic and epidemiologic considerations make it inadvisable to treat the disease in horses. The destruction of infected animals is indicated.

Comments and Control. Equine tuberculosis in itself is of minor economic importance, although individual cases in racehorses or show jumpers may entail considerable financial loss. Equine tuberculosis is mainly significant as it relates to the problem of eradication and especially to the maintenance of disease-free herds. Infected horses that are utilized for farming expose herds that have been freed from the disease to an acute risk of reinfection. While the horse generally represents a dead-end host for the tubercle bacillus, it has nevertheless been shown that certain forms of the disease (skin, pulmonary) are associated with a shedding of bacilli and thus pose a danger to the environment (including man). Therefore, an effective eradication program requires the disposal not only of clinically affected horses, but also of positive reactors to the tuberculin test.

References

Dietzmann, U.; Pitzschke, H.: Tuberkulose des Euters einer Stute. Mh. Vet.-Med. *14:* 543 (1961).

Kertay, N.; Vizy, L.; Jéger, S.: Zur Kasuistik der Pferdetuberkulose. Tierärztl. Umschau *20:* 276 (1965).

Nielsen, S. W.; Spratling, F. R.: Tuberculous spondylitis in a horse. Brit. Vet. J. *124:* 503 (1968).

Merritt, A. M., et al.: Case of avian tuberculosis of the intestinal tract of a horse. Amer. J. Dig. Dis. *20:* 598 (1975).

2.2.7.4. Anthrax

Definition. Anthrax is an acute infectious disease that is characterized by septicemia, splenomegaly, and a serosanguinous, gelatinous infiltration of the subcutaneous and subserous connective tissues.

Occurrence and Epizootiology. Anthrax occurs in all countries and can become widespread if control measures are inadequate. If good control is practiced, cases are sporadic. Nearly all mammalian species, including man, and other animal species are susceptible. Herbivores are particularly prone to infection. The disease is most common in sheep, goats, cattle and horses. Horses are especially susceptible to infection by the parenteral route. Among the solipeds, donkeys show a relatively high resistance to infection. The epidemiology of anthrax is based largely upon the ability of the organism to form highly resistant spores outside the body. While the vegetative forms of the organism are similar to other bacteria in their susceptibility to various environmental influences, the spores are among the most resistant in the bacterial kingdom. They cannot be destroyed by dessication. Spores have retained their viability in soil stored for 24 years, and it is likely that much longer survival times are possible. They can remain viable for months in discharges and manure, and for 11 years in putrefied blood. They can survive up to 100 hours' exposure to direct sunlight, and up to 3 hours' exposure to hot air at 120—140 °C. In manure stored in a sealed container and exposed to a temperature of 72—76.5 °C, the spores are killed in 4 days. They are not affected by gastric juices. The drying and salting of skins is also ineffective in killing the spores, which is why imported hides are often tested with the Ascolit reaction before further processing as a precaution against infections and dissemination of the bacillus by this route.

When sporulation occurs, the spore-contaminated materials become a permanent source of infection. The major sources of infection are the cadavers and discharges of animals with anthrax.

Infection occurs by the ingestion of food or water that is contaminated with anthrax spores, which generally originate from the soil. Contact transmission is uncommon.

The occurrence of infection depends upon the number of spores ingested. Resistance-lowering factors such as overexertion, cold, heat, starvation and thirst are predisposing. Epizootic outbreaks can occur in areas where heavy soil contamination is present. Pastured animals are primarily affected in such cases, although spores can also be picked up from hay or other feeds grown on infected soil.

Infection from spore-laden surface waters is also possible in anthrax districts. The spores contained in the mud of these waters can easily be ingested in numbers sufficient to produce infection, especially if water levels are low. Old carcass disposal sites still constitute a hazard in terms of new anthrax outbreaks.

In the GDR, isolated cases of anthrax have occurred in horses and other livestock following extensive land-improvement projects and in connection with the recultivation of strip-mined areas that apparently included carcass disposal sites. The discharges of animals infected with anthrax also contribute to soil contamination.

In cases that take a septicemic course, the bacillus is shed in the feces, urine and saliva. In localized anthrax of swine, characterized by ulcerative lesions of the bowel, the organism is excreted in the feces.

In anthrax districts, spores may be found even in the feces of healthy animals. Wildlife may carry the bacillus over large distances.

Contaminated bone meal that is used as fertilizer and the effluent from tanneries, etc. are additional causes of soil contamination. Imported feedstuffs of animal origin and other feedstuffs contaminated by them are yet another source of infection. Transmission by blood-sucking insects is a danger only if carcass disposal is inadequate. Anthrax shows a seasonal incidence, with the greatest number of cases occuring during pasturing periods.

Symptoms. The incubation period seldom exceeds 1 to 2 days. The course may be peracute, acute, subacute, atypical, septicemic, or characterized by a purely localized infection.

Anthrax in horses generally takes an acute, septicemic course. In peracute cases the animal dies before the appearance of clinical symptoms; often death occurs during work, but animals may also be found dead in the stable or at pasture.

The acute form is characterized by fever (up to 41—42 °C), rapid pulse (80—120/min), and respiratory distress. The mucosae are hyperemic and cyanotic. Colic is often present, and colicky episodes are accompanied by the passage of a liquid, bloody stool. Excitation states give way to general depression accompanied by weakness, staggering, and spasms of the limb muscles. Convulsive death from asphyxia occurs within 5—12 hours.

The subacute form takes a similar course but is marked by periods of clinical improvement. After several hours complications arise, and colicky periods lasting 2—3 days often occur. Frequently the infection takes an atypical course marked by intermittent colic, low-grade fever, abdominal respiration, and occasionally mandibular edema. The horse may recover, or it may die following a period of depression and colic. The course of illness may exceed 90 days.

The local form of anthrax is characterized by 'carbuncles' and edema of the skin and subcutaneous tissue. It frequently results from infection by blood-sucking insects. The carbuncles are initially circumscribed, hard and nontender. They contain a serosanguinous infiltrate with a necrotic center, occur mainly on the neck, chest, abdomen and limbs, and are considered a prognostically favorable sign.

Etiology and Pathogenesis. Anthrax is caused by *Bacillus anthracis*, an anaerobic, spore-forming, nonmotile rod 3—10 μm long and 1—1.3 μm in diameter. The organism grows well on ordinary media and forms characteristic asbestos-gray, dry colonies having a 'Medusa-head' appearance.

Horses generally become infected by ingesting food or water contaminated with spores. The spores enter the pharynx or, unaffected by gastric juice, reach the small intestine, where they germinate to vegetative forms. The bacilli enter the lymph spaces of the intestinal mucosa and begin to multiply. The further course of the infection depends upon the virulence of the bacillus and the resistance of the host. If the organism can surround itself in time with a protective capsule, thereby escaping the body's defenses, and is able to produce anthrax toxin (which consists of 3 fractions), then the bacilli will spread from the primary proliferation site to invade the lymphatics and blood stream and will propagate freely in the blood and later in the parenchymae and bone marrow. The result is a fulminating septicemia with a fatal outcome. The toxins and capsular substances released by lysis of the bacillus damage the vascular endothelium and lead to infiltrative hemorrhages, stasis, and exudation into the body cavities. Blood coagulation is simultaneously impaired.

If host resistance is high, the antibodies that are formed can neutralize the toxins and enable a recovery.

Diagnosis and Differential Diagnosis. Due to the hazards of antemortem specimen collection, a clinical diagnosis of anthrax should be confirmed only after death by accurate microbiologic studies. Such confirmation is necessary to justify the very costly prevention and control measures that must be implemented.

The causative organism can be demonstrated with the Ascoli test, which is highly accurate and specific, as well as by cultivation and the microscopic examination of stained specimens.

Materials suitable for examination are blood, pieces of the parenchymatous organs and membranes. Carcasses should not be opened in the field, however, because spores may form creating a focus of infection that can persist for decades.

Other spore-forming rods must be excluded in the laboratory. The result of the Ascolit test and microscopic examination should be reported by telephone immediately after the material has been received and processed. Identification in culture takes 24 hours.

Differential diagnosis must be made from anaerobic infections, the peracute form of equine infectious anemia, various parasites of the blood, poisoning, colic and petechial fever.

Lesions. The nature and severity of the lesions depend upon the form of the disease. Septicemic anthrax is characterized by hemorrhagic tendency, infiltration of the subserous and submucous tissue, and swelling of the lymph nodes, spleen, liver and kidneys. The splenic pulp shows a dark-red discoloration and has a mushy consistency. The intestinal mucosa is diffusely swollen and reddened or exhibits discrete swellings of a round (carbuncle) or elongated shape that may show ulcerous degeneration. The blood is dark, tarry, and may remain unclotted.

Prognosis. The prognosis depends upon the course but is usually unfavorable.

Treatment. Suspected animals must be placed in strict isolation, and all discharges and fomites safely disposed of.

Therapeutic measures are generally too late to be effective, owing to the extreme rarity of the disease among horses under European conditions and the consequent delay in making a presumptive diagnosis. In the GDR, the State Veterinary Authority may in special cases approve the use of antitoxic serum provided special precautions are taken. The serum is administered subcutaneously or, preferably, intravenously in a dose of 100—200 ml. If no antipyretic response is evident after 6 hours, the treatment is repeated. Because the serum neutralizes only the toxins, the concurrent administration of penicillin or other antibiotics in very large doses is recommended to stop proliferation of the bacilli.

Prophylaxis and Control. Prophylactic efforts are directed toward the prevention of oral infection by eliminating suspected pastures and feedstuffs, and on the safe disposal of established sources of infection. Contaminated pastures and meadows can be cleaned through drainage and multiple tilling. Diseased animals must be safely isolated. Contaminated feed, bedding and other fomites are best disposed of by burning. Hydrogen peroxide (3 % solution) and peracetic acid (0.4 % solution) make suitable disinfectants when contact with the solution is maintained for at least 30 minutes. Spores in feeds can be rendered incapable of germinating by exposure to pressurized steam at 131 °C for 2 hours.

The reliable destruction of all spores in a given focus of infection is an extremely difficult task. Therefore, active immunization is recommended in anthrax districts (prior approval of the State Veterinary Authority is required). The immunization may be done with spore vaccines or with the newer vaccines made from protective antigen (a natural component of anthrax toxin). Vaccinated animals may be released from isolation within one week after vaccination only on approval of the Veterinary Authority. Such approval is also required for slaughter, except in emergency situations.

Animals from a group in which anthrax has occurred should be passively immunized with 20 ml of serum and/or given prophylactic antibiotics. All treatments and vaccinations should be administered exclusively by veterinarians.

In Europe the law requires that all cases of anthrax be reported without delay.

An animal and material quarantine should be imposed on the affected premises until the last infected animal has recovered and until all designated prophylactic measures have been implemented.

References

Illner, F.: Milzbrand; In Beer, Infektionskrankheiten der Haustiere; 2. Aufl. (VEB Gustav Fischer Verlag, Jena 1980).

Jirina, K.: A case of atypical anthrax in the horse. Progress in Equine Pract., p. 148 (Amer. Vet. Public. Inc., Wheaton/Ill. 1966).

2.2.7.5. Tularemia

Definition. Tularemia is a contagious disease of rodents that may spread to horses, causing fever, swelling of the lymph nodes, and abortion.

Distribution and Epizootiology. Tularemia occurs between 35° north latitude and the polar circle. Within the various countries at these latitudes, the disease is confined to specific districts. The reservoir is recruited from rodents and blood-sucking Diptera.

Symptoms. The clinical picture of tularemia in the horse is variable and little-researched. The susceptibility of this species is low, and the course is usually mild and largely asymptomatic. Abortion may occur in pregnant mares.

Dorofeyev [1954] observed an outbreak on a stud farm in connection with an epizootic among rodents. The causative organism could be isolated from aborted fetuses and from necrotic placetal foci. The abortions occurred during the 4th to 5th month of gestation. No other clinical symptoms were observed.

Etiology and Pathogenesis. The causative organism, *Francisella tularensis,* is a bacterium that is cultivable only on special media. The organism proliferates at the portal of entry and from there invades the lymph nodes and blood. Septicemia may develop.

Diagnosis and Differential Diagnosis. The clinical diagnosis must be confirmed by demonstrating antibodies with the agglutination test or FA technique, by direct identification of the organism in specimens of lymph node, spleen, liver or lung from horses that die, or by guinea pig inoculation.

Titers of 25 determined in the slow agglutination test indicate exposure to the bacterium, with fresh infections producing a rise of titers in a 2nd test performed 1—2 weeks later. Cross-reactions with Brucella antibodies should be noted.

Differential Diagnosis. It is necessary to exclude anaplasmosis (by demonstrating the causative organism in the blood), tuberculosis (by demonstrating CF antibodies), and brucellosis (brucellosis serology and demonstration of organism in secretions).

Prognosis. Complete recovery may be expected in mild cases.

Treatment. Antibiotics are the therapy of choice. Streptomycin and oxytetracycline are administered in doses of 10 mg/kg BW/day for 8—10 days.

Prophylaxis and Control. Preventive measures must include the prevention of contact with rodents and their excreta, as well as a program of ectoparasite control, particularly in danger areas.

Reference

Petrenko, A. E.: In: Infekcionnye i invazionnye bolezni lošadej (Kolos, Moskva 1976).

2.2.7.6. Glanders (Farcy, Malleus, Morve, Pacin, Carn)

Definition. Glanders is an infectious disease, usually chronic, that is transmissible to humans and is characterized by nodules, ulcers or cicatrices in the skin, upper respiratory mucosa and lung.

Occurrence and Epizootiology. Though glanders was once widespread in horse populations, is has been eradicated in most countries through systematic control measures. Today it occurs only in a few Near Eastern countries and in Thailand.

The infection is introduced to healthy horse populations by clinically affected or carrier horses. Spread by direct contact is evidenced by the fact that the initial transmission is usually to the horse stabled next to the infected animal. Because primary infections often take a latent course, or disease symptoms are very mild and the horse shows little or no loss of working capacity, such animals can remain a source of infection within the group for some time. Frequent introductions to and removals from the group are conducive to spread, although the spreading tendency of the disease is relatively low. Communal feeding and watering troughs create particularly favorable conditions for spread.

Infection occurs by the ingestion of contaminated feed, water and bedding. Infection through skin lesions is also possible.

Transmission from mare to foal generally occurs postpartum via the alimentary tract. Glanders does not show a pronounced seasonal prevalence, though the bulk of cases tend to occur during the fall and winter.

Poor nutrition and stabling and heavy work loads are conducive to clinically overt infection with a severe course.

Symptoms. The incubation period is from 3 days to 3 weeks. The course of the infection may be acute, chronic or latent, the chronic form being the most frequent. A distinction may be made between nasal glanders, pulmonary glanders and cutaneous glanders, depending on the location of the pathologic process. The boundaries between these forms are indistinct, however.

Acute glanders is associated with a fever of 41—42 °C, nasal discharge (usually unilateral), and hyperemia of the ocular and nasal mucosae. The mandibular lymph nodes are inflamed. Diphtheritic membranes, nodules and ulcers form on the upper respiratory mucosa and skin and exhibit a strong tendency to spread. Dyspnea is present due to swelling of the nasal mucosa and edema of the glottis. Affected horses become badly emaciated and frequently die.

Chronic glanders is associated with less pronounced clinical signs and may persist for years. An irregular, recurring or intermittent fever, cough, and respiratory distress of varying frequency and severity are sometimes observed. The mandibular lymph nodes are painless, firm, nodular, and difficult to displace owing to the presence of adhesions.

The hind limbs may develop edematous thickenings extending down to the hocks.

Etiology and Pathogenesis. The causative organism of glanders, *Pseudomonas mallei* (*Actinobacillus mallei*, *Malleomyces mallei*, *Pfeifferella mallei*, *Loefflerella mallei*, etc.) is an aerobic, gram-negative, nonmotile, nonsporing rod with rounded ends that occurs in groups of two or more in the tissue. It grows slowly but well on ordinary laboratory media, and grows best when defibrinated horse blood or glycerol is added to the medium. The colonies have a slimy consistency and a hop-like odor.

The organism has the low resistance to environmental influences that is typical of non-spore-forming bacteria and is readily destroyed by common disinfectants. It is ingested with food or drinking water, invades regional lymph nodes by way of the pharyngeal and intestinal mucosae, and proliferates in the nodes. It can also enter the body through skin wounds, whereupon it invades the blood stream and is carried to various organs, in which nodules and ulcers are formed. The infectious process may terminate at that point, or the organism may invade other organs and tissues by metastatic spread.

Diagnosis and Differential Diagnosis. District veterinary health authorities must be notified whenever glanders is suspected, for complex epizootiologic and clinical investigations have to be instituted among the horses on the affected premises and in surrounding areas.

The mallein ophthalmic test and complement fixation test also should be performed. The subcutaneous or intradermopalpebral test may be used in special cases.

The CF test is positive by about 12 weeks after infection, or as early as 4 weeks in exceptional cases. It has a high accuracy and specificity (99 %). In the mallein ophthalmic test, a positive reaction is obtained by about 3 weeks after infection. It is reliable only in the absence of preexisting ocular changes. Approximately 0.1 ml of mallein (allergen from cultures of glanders bacillus) is instilled into the palpebral sac of one eye and distributed by gentle rubbing. The opposite eye serves as a control. The reaction is read after 8—12 hours and again after 18—24 hours. The positive reaction is a pronounced conjunctivitis and swelling of the palpebral conjunctiva accompanied by a purulent discharge from the medial canthus of the eye. The reaction is suspicious if lacrimation and mild reddening of the palpebral conjunctiva appear after 24 hours. A negative result is declared if the eye shows no change or only a slight reddening of the palpebral conjunctiva with lacrimation, which disappears within the first 24 hours.

In horses with glanders, the ophthalmic test has an accuracy of 95 %. It may not be reliable in advanced cases as a result of anergy.

Generally, differential diagnosis presents no problems owing to the characteristic clinical symptoms of the disease and the high reliability of the CF and mallein tests.

Lesions. Necropsy findings vary considerably with the form and duration of the infection.

The cutaneous lesions of glanders (cutaneous glanders, farcy) consist of pustules, nodules, ulcers, and characteristic scars. Changes in the respiratory organs are also present in most cases. Grayish-red or light-gray, glassy, miliary nodules surrounded by a reddened zone are found on the mucosa of the upper respiratory tract. These nodules degenerate rapidly through purulent liquefaction, leaving crater-shaped ulcers with a greasy base. The ulcers coalesce to form extensive ulcerous surfaces, and new nodules and small ulcers form in their vicinity. The ulcers may heal by second intention, as is usually the case, or complete tissue destruction may occur. The scars have a stellate shape and exhibit an ice-crystal-like pattern of fine, radially-oriented ridges. Typical glanders nodules or lobar pneumonitic foci are found in the lung. In chronic cases, fresh foci alternate with indurated or calcified nodules that are surrounded by a grayish-white, firm, fibrous capsule. They are easily distinguished from parasitic nodules.

The catarrhal-pneumonitic form is marked by the presence of reddish-brown, hepatized foci that tend toward central degeneration and liquefaction. A yellow, gelatinous infiltrate is seen in adjacent tissues.

Pulmonary glanders may also develop as a suppurative catarrhal pneumonia with induration.

Prognosis. The acute form of glanders is usually fatal within 2 weeks. Chronic cases can lead to prolonged illness and wasting with sudden death from general debility or pulmonary hemorrhage. Various stresses increase susceptibility to infection. Latent infections usually persist for years, but spontaneous recovery is possible.

Treatment. Treatment of glanders in horses is not advised. Clinically affected or carrier horses should be destroyed and safely disposed of.

Sulfonamides and certain antibiotics are the drugs of choice for treating the disease in humans.

Prophylaxis and Control. Prophylaxis includes the enforced restriction of importation of solipeds from infected areas and the diagnostic surveillance of horses in international traffic.

When a case of glanders is confirmed, the animal is destroyed without blood sampling, and the carcass safely disposed of. The affected premises are placed in quarantine, specific prophylactic measures are implemented, and testing is done in groups that have had contact with infected animals. The quarantined group should be kept under observation for 6 months. During this period clinical examinations should be performed at least once a weak, serologic studies (CF test) once per month, and the ophthalmic test every 3 months.

If all these tests are negative, the quarantine may be lifted. Disinfective measures should include the stables and stalls of all suspected solipeds as well as other objects that might be contaminated with the bacillus. Manure, bedding and feed residue that are encountered during clean-up are burned, disinfected, or stored in a hygienically safe place and plowed under after 3 weeks.

References

DHANDA, M. R.; GANGULEE, P. C.; BENERJI, T. P.: Effect of sulphonamides in experimental glanders. Indian vet. J. *35:* 342 (1958).

JARIMPIL, B.; JUDIN, G. A.: Diagnostika sapa lošadej. Veterinarija, Moskva *6:* 110 (1971).

LAZAREV, P. S.: Rotz. In: Infekcionnye i invazionnye bolezni lošadej, p. 156 (Kolos, Moskva 1976).

2.2.7.7. Melioidosis (Pseudoglanders, Pseudomalleus, Stanton's Disease)

Definition. Melioidosis is an infectious disease of animals and humans that is characterized by septicemia and by abscessation in the lung, liver, spleen, kidneys and other organs.

Occurrence and Epizootiology. The infection occurs principally in southeast Asia, and recently cases have been reported in France. Rats are the primary natural host. The disease mainly affects goats in Africa, and goats, sheep and horses in Australia.

Melioidosis occurs sporadically in horses. Infected rodents, domestic animals and their excreta are the most common sources of infection. Infection is acquired through ingestion of contaminated feed or water, inhalation, cutaneous abrasions, and insect bites. The organism can survive for 50 days in the rat flea and may be present in the feces.

Symptoms. The symptoms of melioidosis are similar to those of glanders. In horses the infection usually takes a benign course following an incubation period of 2—11 days. A cellulitis develops at the portal of entry. Other signs are transitory fever and a purulent nasal discharge. Septicemia, edema and abscessation in the internal organs are uncommon in the horse. The chronic form is predominant; acute cases are rare.

Etiology and Pathogenesis. The disease is caused by *Pseudomonas pseudomallei (Malleomyces pseudomallei, Bacterium whitmori, Loefflerella pseudomallei)*, a gram-negative rod that is similar in many respects to the glanders bacillus, but is different in that it is motile.

The disease usually takes an insidious course. Latent infections are predominant. The organism enters the lungs and other parenchymatous organs by way of the lymph and blood, where it precipitates an inflammatory process with local lymph node involvement. This process is characteristic of melioidosis and consists of an exudative inflammation and the formation of purulent nodules that tend toward caseous degeneration. Specific antibodies are formed, and an allergic state develops. Allergic reactivity appears 2—3 weeks after exposure and persists for a long time.

Diagnosis. Microbiologic studies (culture, guinea pig inoculation) are necessary to confirm the clinical diagnosis. No useful serologic or allergic tests have yet been developed.

Differential Diagnosis. Glanders, which does not affect ruminants, is excluded on the basis of clinical signs and by the ophthalmic test and CF reaction. Leptospirosis, salmonellosis, viral arteritis, and equine infectious anemia must also be excluded.

Prognosis. The prognosis is unfavorable, and the mortality rate of melioidosis is high.

Treatment. No specific therapy has been devised for horses. According to Chundanov et al. [1961], white mice infected experimentally with *P. pseudomallei* responded favorably to levomycetin, sulfadimetine and biomycin.

Prophylaxis and Control. The main emphasis of prophylaxis is on rodent control. Because the organism is excreted in large numbers by infected rodents, measures should be taken to prevent the contamination of food and drinking water, and good hygiene should be maintained.

Suspected cases should be isolated and subjected to bacteriologic testing. Premises should be disinfected, and rodent and insect control measures implemented. Under no circumstances should killed animals be processed for food. Competent medical authorities should be notified of any outbreak.

References

Chundanov, L. E.; Kupcevic, E. N.; Smirnova, M. A.; Skurko, E. D.: O kombinirovannoj terapii experimentalnogo melioidoza. Veterinarija, Moskva *10:* 55 (1961).

Desbrosse, F.; Dodin, M.; Galimand, M.: Bull. mens. Soc. vét. pract. *63:* 657 (1978).

Efimceva, E. P.; Ermoleva, Z. V.; Stösser, L.: Nekotoriye svedenija o vozbuditele melioidoza. Z. Mikrobiol., Moskva *2:* 38 (1974).

2.2.7.8. Listeriosis

Definition. Listeriosis is an acute to chronic infectious disease that occurs sporadically and is characterized by local pathologic processes or by septicemia.

Occurrence and Epizootiology. Listeriosis has a worldwide distribution. The Listeria organisms have low virulence, occur widely in dirt and soil, and may lead both a saprophytic and parasitic existence.

Soil, which is subject to contamination by carrier rodents, is the principal source of infection (e.g., through contamination of feedstuffs).

The relatively large concentrations of organisms required for infection are most commonly found in silages, where they are most abundant in the peripheral and surface layers.

Symptoms. The incubation period is 7—30 days. The course may be acute, subacute or chronic.

In horses, listeriosis generally present as an encephalitis. The earliest signs are a slight rise of body temperature (to 39.5 °C), unrest, motor incoordination, and paresis of the limbs. Foals have difficulty progressing or are unable to do so. Compulsive progression may be observed in some cases. Affected animals are depressed and apathetic and show a purulent conjunctivitis with icterus of the sclera. Food ingestion is impaired. The terminal stage of the disease is marked by paralysis and death.

In foals, SCHILADZE [1953] observed anorexia, somnolence, hyperemia of the mucosae, nasal discharge, fever (41.5 °C), increased pulse and respirations, edema of the limbs, shivering, spasms and incoordination. Death occurred within 1—3 days.

SVENKERND [1948] as well as PULST [1964] reported on a septicemic listeriosis in newborn foals in which death occurred after 3 days.

Etiology and Pathogenesis. Listeria monocytogenes is a nonfastidious bacterium that is easily demonstrated in the laboratory and occurs in several serotypes (at least 4). Spread from the site of infection may occur by the neurogenous, lymphogenous or hematogenous route, depending on the portal of entry, and leads to a local infection or, especially in foals, to septicemia. Organisms that enter the tissue reach peripheral nerve segments either directly or via the lymph. In the nerve they initiate an inflammatory process leading to an ascending neuritis. After one or more weeks, central nervous manifestations appear.

Diagnosis. The clinical diagnosis must be confirmed by demonstration of the causative organism.

In septicemic listeriosis, necropsy findings are a useful guide. The cerebral form is identified by the histologic demonstration of typical brain-stem encephalitic lesions. An antemortem diagnosis may be based upon repeated serum agglutination tests. High titers (320 or higher) indicate infection.

Differential Diagnosis. Encephalitides of viral etiology (e.g., Borna disease, equine encephalitides) must be excluded in the viral laboratory. Leptospirosis can be differentiated by serologic tests.

Prognosis. The prognosis is unfavorable, because veterinary help is usually summoned too late to be effective. Untreated, the septicemic and cerebral forms have a fatal outcome.

Treatment. Treatment with antibiotics and sulfonamides is indicated. Success depends upon the prompt initiation of treatment, however. For this reason, the mere clinical suspicion of listeriosis should be grounds for treatment in valuable horses. The advanced stage of cerebral listeriosis is incurable.

The recommended course of antibiotic therapy is 10—15 mg/kg BW oxytetracycline or 40,000 I.U./kg BW penicillin for 5 days.

Prophylaxis and Control. Prophylactic measures should include the prevention of alimentary infection by offering a non-contaminated feed, the control of harmful rodents, and the prevention of contact with infected animals. Horses with listeriosis should be safely isolated. Quarantine of the entire herd is not recommended due to the sporadic nature of the disease.

References

PULST, H.: Listeriose bei einem Fohlen. Mh. Vet.-Med. *19:* 742 (1964).

SCHILADZE, M. V.: Listerioz lošadej i svinej. Veterinarija, Moskva *9:* 23 (1953).

SVENKERND, R. R.: Listeriellainfektioner, spesielt med henblikk per deres forekomst hos hosten. Norsk Vet. Tidsskr. *60:* 321 (1948).

2.3. Parasitism

2.3.1. Protozoal Diseases

2.3.1.1. Coccidiosis

Coccidiosis in horses is relatively rare compared to other domestic species. The enzootic occurrence of an intestinal disease caused by coccidia, formerly called globidiosis, has occasionally been reported on stud farms, especially in ponies. Renal coccidiosis is even less common in horses and is largely sporadic in its occurrence.

Intestinal Coccidiosis

Causative Organism. Eimeria leuckarti. In the Soviet Union two additional species are recognized: *E. solipedum* and *E. uniungulati. E. leuckarti* oocysts: 70—85 × 50 to 65 μm; prominent micropyle.

Habitat: Lamina propria of the small intestinal villi.

Epizootiology. Infection is acquired orally through contaminated feeds or bedding in the stable or by the ingestion of sporulated oocysts in overcrowded yards, especially under breeding-farm conditions, where mares and foals are the source of infection. Oocyst sporulation in the environment requires about 20—40 days at 15—25 °C. Macro- and microgametocytes and oocysts have been demonstrated in the small intestine. Oocyst excretion starts on the 28th day after infection and continues for about 8—12 days.

Symptoms. Severe infestation leads to diarrhea, cachexia and ascites. Infection is most common in foals during the second half of the nursing period and shortly after weaning. In most cases oocyst excretion is not associated with overt symptoms.

Diagnosis is based on detection of the oocyst in the stool using the sedimentation technique; NaCl flotation is unsuitable.

Treatment. Anticoccidial drugs. Favorable results are seen following a 3-day course of sulfadimidine (sulfamethazine). Prevention in endangered populations is based upon regular cleaning and disinfection of stables, using a disinfectant known to be active against coccidial oocysts.

Renal Coccidiosis

Causative Organism. Klossiella equi. Oocysts 50—90 μm in diameter; each oocyst contains about 40 sporocysts, each with 8—12 sporozoites.

Habitat: Renal epithelium and endothelium; oocysts are excreted in the urine.

Epizootiology. Infection is oral; the sporozoites are probably carried in the blood stream from the intestine to the kidneys, where developmental stages have been detected in endothelial cells of Bowman's capsule and in epithelial cells of the proximal tubule and loop of Henle. The life cycle of *Kl. equi* is not yet fully understood.

Symptoms. Renal signs; most cases are clinically inapparent.

Diagnosis. Based on detection of oocysts or sporocysts in the urine. Suspected cases can be confirmed postmortem by microscopic or histologic examination of kidney tissue.

Treatment. See Intestinal Coccidiosis.

References

BARKER, I. K.; REMMLER, O.: The endogenous development of Eimeria leuckarti in ponies. J. Parasitol. *58:* 112 (1972).

BAUMANN, R.: Klossiella equi, ein neuer Parasit der Pferdeniere. Wiener tierärztl. Mschr. *33:* 257 (1946).

KITCHEN, D.; GAAFER, S. M.: Eimeria leuckarti in a horse from Indiana (a case report). Vet. Med. and Small Animal Clinician *69:* 408, 412 (1974).

KUTZER, E.: Eimeria leuckarti, ein seltener Parasit von Pferd und Esel. Dtsch. tierärztl. Wschr. *76:* 35 (1969).

LEE, C. G.; ROSS, A. D.: Renal coccidiosis of the horse associated with Klossiella equi. Austral. vet. J. *53:* 287 (1977).

ROBERTS, M. C.; COTCHIN, E.: Globidium leuckarti in the small intestine of three horses. Brit. vet. J. *129:* 146 (1973).

SHEAHAN, B. J.: Eimeria leuckarti infection in a thoroughbred foal. Vet. Rec. *99:* 213 (1976).

SNYDER, D.: Project Eimeria leuckarti. Speculum *23:* 19 (1971).

SUTOH, M.; SAHEKI, Y.; ISHITANI, R.; INUI, S.; NARITA, M.; HAMAZAKI, H.; YOKOTA, T.: Eimeria leuckarti infection in foals. Nat. Inst. Animal Health Quart. *16:* 59 (1976).

TODD, jr.; KENNETH, S.; GOSSER, H. S.; HAMILTON, H. S.: Klossiella equi Baumann 1946 (Sporozoa: Eucoccidiorida) from an Illinois horse. Vet. Med. Small Animal Clinician *72:* 443, 448 (1977).

WHEELDON, E. B.; GREIG, W. A.: Globidium leuckarti infection in a horse with diarrhoea. Vet. Rec. *100:* 102 (1977).

ZULINSKI, T.: Zwei Fälle von Nierenkokzidiose bei Pferden. Med. weteryn. *13:* 579 (1957).

2.3.1.2. Sarcosporidiosis

Sarcosporidiosis infections in the horse are relatively common but are notable mainly as an incidental finding during meat inspections rather than a disease-producing entity.

Causative Organisms. 1. *Sarcocystis equicanis;* 2. *Sarcocystis bertrami.* Cyst ranges to 350 μm in diameter.

Habitat: The muscles, especially the esophagus and masseter muscle.

Epizootiology. S. equicanis sporocysts are excreted in dog feces and ingested by horses in feed, contaminated bedding, etc. The sporozoites that are released in the intestine proliferate initially via a sarcocystemic phase and apparently are carried in the blood to predisposed muscle cells, where they form cysts. Little is known about the life cycle of *S. bertrami.*

Symptoms. A familiar symptom is generalized or focal myositis. It occurs sporadically and may cause locomotor disturbances.

Diagnosis. To date, sarcosporidial cysts have been detected only postmortem during the course of meat inspections. For antemortem diagnosis, a muscle biopsy is indicated if clinical suspicion is present. Indirect immunofluorescence offers a serologic means of diagnosis.

Treatment. So far no results are available on the treatment of muscular sarcosporidiosis. Prophylactic measures include the use of oocyst-active disinfectants, and removing horses from contact with dogs and other definitive hosts *(S. bertrami).*

References

BOGUŠ, A. A.; PIŠKO, I. I.: Rasširenie sarkocistoza u živetnich belorusskom SSR. Trud. Bjel. Nauk. iss. Minsk *12:* 130 (1974).
DOFLEIN, F.: Die Protozoen als Parasiten und Krankheitserreger (Gustav Fischer Verlag, Jena 1901).
ROMMEL, M.; GEISEL, O.: Untersuchungen über die Verbreitung und den Lebenszyklus einer Sarkosporidienart des Pferdes (Sarcocystis equicanis n. spec.). Berliner Münchener tierärztl. Wschr. *88:* 468 (1975).
SCHEBITZ, H.; HARTWIGK, H.: Myostitis sarcosporidica beim Pferd. Mh. Vet.-Med. *5:* 351 (1950).

2.3.1.3. Toxoplasmosis

Toxoplasmosis is a zoonosis that occurs mainly as a latent infection in horses. Studies in various countries indicate that an average of 10—25 % of the horse population harbors the organism. Clinically overt infections are rare. Presumably the horse is one of the few animal species susceptible to *T. gondii.*

Causative Organism. Toxoplasma gondii.

Habitat: Toxoplasma cysts and pseudocysts primarily in the brain, spinal cord and retina.

Epizootiology. The horse, like most other susceptible vertebrates, is an intermediate host for *T. gondii.* The oocysts are excreted in cat feces and ingested by the horse in contaminated feed or bedding.

Symptoms. Initial temperature rise to 40.8 °C, increased pulse and respirations, CNS signs (e.g., ataxia), retinal degeneration.

Diagnosis. Toxoplasmosis is difficult to differentiate clinically from other CNS diseases. The CF test and Sabin-Feldman test are indicated.

Treatment. No treatment methods have yet been described.

References

ALTAN, Y.; HEYDORN, A. O.; JANITSCHKE, K.: Zur Infektiosität von Toxoplasma-Oozysten für das Pferd. Berliner Münchener tierärztl. Wschr. *90:* 433 (1977).
CUSICK, P. K.; SELLS, D. M.; HAMILTON, D. P.; HARDENBROCK, H. J.: Toxoplasmosis in two horses. J. Amer. vet. med. Assoc. *164:* 77 (1974).
HILGENFELD, M.; HIEPE, TH.: Die Toxoplasmose beim Tier; in WILDFÜHR; WILDFÜHR, Toxoplasmose-Ratgeber für Ärzte und Tierärzte (VEB Gustav Fischer Verlag, Jena 1975).
MCDONALD, D. R.; CLEARY, D. J.: Toxoplasmosis in the equine. South West Vet. *23:* 213 (1970).
RIEMANN, H. P.; SMITH, A. T.; STORMONT, C.; RUPPANNER, R.; BEHYMER, D. E.; SUZUKI, Y.; FRANTI, C. E.; VERMA, B. B.: Equine toxoplasmosis: a survey for antibodies to Toxoplasma gondii in horses. Amer. J. vet. Res. *36:* 1797 (1975).
SEEMANN, J.: Possible role of horses in the epidemiology of toxoplasmosis. J. Hyg. Epidemiol. Microbiol. and Immunol., Prague *3:* 229 (1959).
SEYERL, F.: Untersuchungen über die Häufigkeit der Infektion mit Toxoplasma gondii bei Equiden. Tierärztl. Umschau *25:* 447 (1970).

2.3.1.4. Babesiosis (Piroplasmosis)

Definition. Equine babesiosis is a universally known, tick-borne parasite of the blood that is enzootic in warm climates and may be caused by two distinct *Babesia* species.

Causative Organism. 1. *Babesia equi* (formerly called *Nuttallia equi*). Zoites: smaller than 2 μm, round, amoeboid or pear-shaped, usually form 4 new parasites on division. Transmission: mainly by *Hyalomma dromedarii*; transmission by other tick species is possible. Distribution: Europe, Asia, Africa and South America. Host range: Equidae. 2. *Babesia caballi.* Zoites: either 1.5—3 μm, round disk-shaped or ring-shaped, or 2.5—4 × 2 μm, amoeboid or pear-shaped, dividing into 2 parasites that form an acute-angled figure within the erythrocyte. Transmission: mainly by *Hyalloma dromedarii* as well as other tick species of the genera *Rhipicephalus*, *Dermacentor*, *Amblyomma* and *Boophilus*. Distribution: Southern Europe, Asia, Africa, Central and North America.

Habitat: Intraerythrocytic.

Epizootiology. The parasite gains entry to the blood through tick bites. Tick larvae, nymphs and adults are potential vectors. A schizogonia and gametogonia take place within the vector. Horses with latent infection may remain carriers of the protozoan for up to 4 years.

Symptoms. Several days after infection a parasitemia develops, accompanied by high fever. Additional signs are an increased pulse and respiratory rate, reduction or loss of appetite, and swelling and dark-red discoloration of the palpebral conjunctivae. Colicky signs and hemoglobinuria are sometimes present; the latter is especially characteristic of *B. equi* infections. The peracute form of the disease is fatal within 2 days. The acute form lasts 6—12 days and is often accompanied by sweating, edema of the pastern area, and a dry, dark-brown stool. Chronic cases show gradual emaciation, hindquarter weakness and recumbency. All forms are associated with splenic enlargement. Generally, infections with *B. equi* take a more fulminating course and have a high mortality. Babesiae can also be demonstrated in aborted equine fetuses.

Diagnosis. If clinical signs raise suspicion of babesiosis, a blood smear should be obtained at once (peripheral blood is preferred). The parasite can be identified directly in stained blood smears during the first few days of the disease. Another method is to detect babesial antibodies in the serum by means of the CF test or indirect immunofluorescence. Speciation can be determined with the latter technique. The inoculation of a clinically healthy horse with 500 ml of blood from the suspected horse might be acceptable during an enzootic outbreak.

Differential diagnosis from infectious anemia is necessary.

Treatment. B. caballi infections can be treated causally with various drugs: phenamidine isothionate and aminocarbatide (9 mg/kg BW), diamidinodiazoaminobenzene (11 mg/kg BW) and imidocarb (2.2 mg/kg BW), each drug being administered intramuscularly on 2 consecutive days. So far only imidocarb administered in 4 doses of 10 mg/kg BW at 2-day intervals has proved effective against *B. equi.* Thus, besides the use of babecidal drugs, emphasis should be placed on supportive therapy.

Prophylactic efforts in enzootic areas center on the eradication or control of the vector tick with approved insecticides, either on an individual-animal or area basis. Many countries, such as the U.S., impose a 6- to 12-month quarantine on horses imported from danger areas.

References

Barnett, S. F.: Babesia of horses in Britain. Vet. Rec. *95:* 346 (1974).

Brock, W. E.: Comments on equine piroplasmosis. J. Amer. vet. med. Assoc. *155:* 460 (1969).

Bryant, J. E.; Anderson, J. B.; Willers, K. H.: Control of equine piroplasmosis in Florida. J. Amer. vet. med. Assoc. *154:* 1034 (1969).

DENNIG, H. K.: Die Beeinflussung der latenten Pferdepiroplasmose (Babesia equi Laveran) durch die Splenektomie. Berliner Münchener tierärztl. Wschr. *78:* 204 (1965).
FRERICHS, W. M.: Fine structure of Babesia equi: electron microscopy and phase-contrast microscopy. J. Parasitol. *56:* 108 (1970).
FRERICHS, W. E.; ALLEN, P. C.; HOLBROOK, A. A.: Equine piroplasmosis (Babesia equi): Therapeutic trials of imidocarb dihydrochloride in horses and donkeys. Vet. Rec. *93:* 73 (1973).
FRERICHS, W. M.; HOLBROCK, A. A.; JOHNSON, A. J.: Equine Babesiosis: complement-fixation titers of horses infected with Babesia caballi. Amer. J. vet. Res. *30:* 697 (1969).
GAINER, J. H.; AMSTER, R. L.; NEEDHAM, J. W.; SCHILLING, K. F.: Altered serum lipoproteins in equine infectious anemia; comparisons of values among normal horses and horses infected with Babesia caballi. Amer. J. vet. Res. *27:* 1611 (1966).
HOLBROOK, A. A.; JOHNSON, A. J.; MADDEN, P. A.: Equine piroplasmosis: intraerythrocytic development of Babesia caballi (Nuttall) and Babesia equi (Laveran). Amer. J. vet. Res. *29:* 297 (1968).
HOLBROOK, A. A.: Biology of equine piroplasmosis. J. Amer. vet. med. Assoc. *155:* 453 (1969).
KIRKHAM, W. W.: The treatment of equine babesiosis. J. Amer. vet. med. Assoc. *155:* 457 (1969).
MADDEN, P. A.; HOLBROOK, A. A.: Equine piroplasmosis: indirect fluorescent antibody test for Babesia caballi. Amer. J. vet. Res. *29:* 117 (1968).
NIKOL'SKIJ, S. N.; BATURINA, F. M.; LUCUK, S. N.: Piroplazmoz i nuttallioz losădej. Veterinarija, Moskva *9:* 40 (1979).
DU PLESSIS, J. L.; BASSON, P. A.: Babesiosis in aborted equine foetuses; a report on two cases in South Africa. J. South African vet. med. Assoc. *36:* 267 (1966).
RETIEF, G. P.: The diagnosis and treatment of biliary fever (babesiosis) in thoroughbreds. J. South African vet. med. Assoc. *34:* 601 (1964).
RETIEF, G. P.: A comparison of equine piroplasmosis in South Africa and the Unites States. J. Amer. vet. med. Assoc. *145:* 912 (1964).
RISTIC, M.; SIBINOVIC, S.: Equine babesiosis: diagnosis by a precipitation in gel and by a one-step-fluorescent inhibition test. Amer. J. vet. Res. *25:* 1519 (1964).
SIBINOVIC, K. H.; RISTIC, M.; SIBINOVIC, S.: Equine babesiosis: isolation and serologic characterization of a blood serum antigen from acutely infected horses. Amer. J. vet. Res. *26:* 147 (1965).
SIMPSON, C. F.: Electron microscopic comparison of Babesia spp. and hepatic changes in ponies and mice. Amer. J. vet. Res. *31:* 1763 (1970).
SIMPSON, C. F., KIRKHAM, W. W.; KLING, J. M.: Comparative morphologic features of Babesia caballi and Babesia equi. Amer. J. vet. Res. *28:* 1693 (1967).
TAYLOR, W. M.; BRYANT, J. E.; ANDERSON, J. B.; WILLERS, K. H.: Equine piroplasmosis in the United States. A review. J. Amer. vet. med. Assoc. *155:* 915 (1969).
THOMPSON, P. H.: Ticks as vectors of equine piroplasmosis. J. Amer. vet. med. Assoc. *155:* 454 (1969).

2.3.1.5. Trypanosomiasis

From a Central European standpoint, trypanosomal infections in horses may be divided into the indiginous dourine and the three exotic trypanosomiases, Mal de Caderas, surra and nagana. Each of the diseases has a unique clinical picture.

2.3.1.5.1. Dourine

Dourine is an often fatal, specific trypanosomiasis of horses that is transmitted primarily during coitus and is enzootic mainly in Asia, northern and southern Africa, and parts of Europe. It has been eradicated from Central Europe.

Causative Organism. Trypanosoma equiperdum, length 25—28 μm.

Habitat: The mucosae of the genital tract; there is also a transitory presence in the intercellular blood.

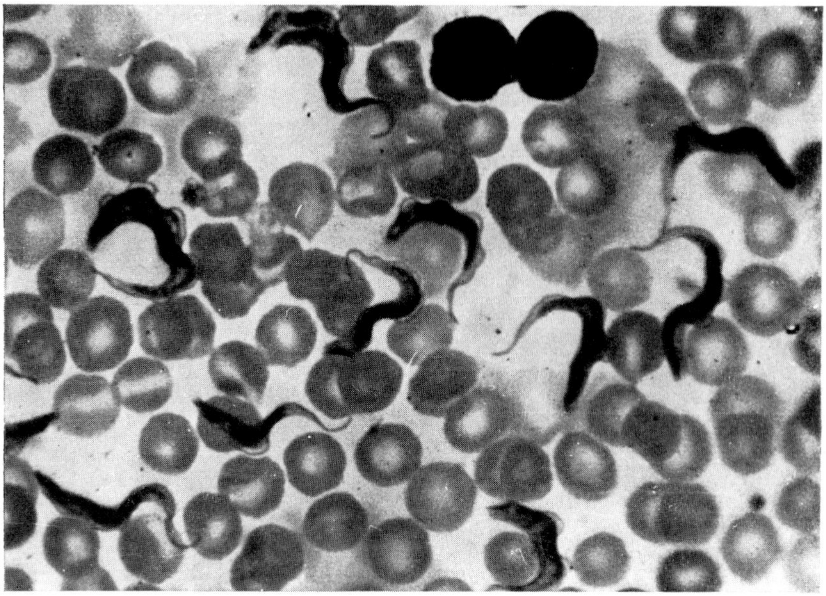

Fig. 2.3. — 1. Trypanosoma equiperdum.

Epizootiology. Transmission occurs primarily by coitus, and an infected stallion can transmit the *Tr. equiperdum* infection to a number of mares during the breeding season. The organisms multiply in the hyperemic genital mucosae. Rare, sporadic cases have been attributed to infected hands of attendants or transmission by blood-sucking arthropods.

Symptoms. The disease has three stages. (1) The *primary stage*, lasting 4—6 weeks. The trypanosomes invade the genital mucosa through minute lesions in its surface, reproduce by binary fission, and produce inflammatory changes in the form of edematous swellings and ulcers, mainly about the vulva and prepuce. Lesions heal leaving circumscribed white areas on the skin ('toad spots'). (2) The *secondary stage* is characterized by an intermittent trypanosomemia, and toxins from the organisms lead to swelling of the lymph nodes and vascular lesions, particularly in the skin. This creates a hemorrhagic tendency that causes wheals to form on the skin. Catarrhal signs sometimes develop as a complication. (3) The *tertiary stage* is characterized by nervous signs in the form of peripheral sensory and motor disturbances caused by endotoxins from the trypanosomes. The facial nerve (left-sided facial paralysis!), sciatic nerve, peroneal nerve, tibial nerve, infraorbital nerve and intercostal nerve are most commonly affected. The disease often proves fatal as a result of complications; the mortality is 50—75 %.

Diagnosis. The typical changes during the primary and secondary stages, combined with the intermittent fever and considerations on the prevalence of dourine in the area, should enable a clinical diagnosis to be made. Suitable serologic methods are the CF test, which gives useful results only by the 3rd week after infection, and the FA test (indirect fluorescent antibody test). Trypanosomes can be demonstrated directly in stained blood smears (fig. 2.3. — 1) only during febrile episodes. A useful method is to inoculate laboratory animals (especially white mice) with blood from infected or suspicious horses and then examine the blood for trypanosomes.

Treatment. Control measures must be implemented in accordance with prevailing laws. When dourine is detected, all breeding operations on the premises must be stopped at once; artificial insemination is an acceptable alternative. Affected horses are treated causally with neosalvarsan (2 doses of 2 g, administeres 10—14 days apart) or antrycide sulfate (5 mg/kg, repeated on 5th and 15th day). Supportive therapy is also given as needed. Animals that survive the disease should not be returned to breeding service, for a complete absence of parasite infestation cannot be ensured. Stallions should be castrated and, like infected mares, should be branded with a 'D' to indicate their breeding unsoundness.

2.3.1.5.2. Mal de Caderas

'Sacral lameness' is a trypanosomiasis caused by *Trypanosoma equinum* (size: 15—35 μm) which occurs in South America and is transmitted by biting flies and bats. Capybaras provide the animal reservoir. *Tr. equinum* infection is characterized by a chronic course, emaciation, edema, impaired performance, and in the final stage by irreversible hindquarter paralysis with high mortality.

2.3.1.5.3. Nagana

Nagana is an infectious protozoal disease that occurs in Africa and is caused by 3 different trypanosome species: *Tr. brucei* (the most important), *Tr. congolense* and *Tr. vivax*. The infection is transmitted by tsetse flies (*Glossina* species). Nagana can occur as a single or mixed infection and in the horse takes an acute or even peracute course with high mortality. All three trypanosome species can be detected in the plasma, and *Tr. brucei* can also be demonstrated in the cerebrospinal fluid. Good therapeutic results have been obtained with diamidine (3.5—7 mg/kg) and isometamidium (0.5—1 mg/kg). Eradication of the tsetse fly on a large-scale basis is a complex problem and calls for a highly organized control program based upon an accurate knowledge of the ecology of the fly.

2.3.1.5.4. Surra

Surra is a trypanosomiasis caused by *Tr. evansi*, a parasite with a broad host range that includes equidae, dogs, cats, camels, elephants, buffalo and oxen. The disease occurs in northern Africa, Asia, and in South and Central America and is transmitted by horse flies of the genus Tabanus. Its course is usually chronic and is characterized by intermittent fever, edema, and reduced performance. The recommended treatment agent is diamidine (3.5—7 mg/kg) or aminapyramine (12 mg/kg i.m.). Baited traps can assist in the control of the insect vector.

References

Anonym: Die Beschälseuche wurde in Marokko, Südafrika und UdSSR festgestellt. Aus: Berliner Münchener tierärztl. Wschr. *85:* 458 (1972); Internat. Tierseuchenbericht 1971.

Barrowman, P. R.: Observations on the transmission, immunology, clinical signs and chemotherapy of dourine Trypanosoma equiperdum infection in horses, with special reference to cerebrospinal fluid. Onderstepoort J. vet. Res. *43:* 55 (1976).

Brass, W.: Zum 'Mal de Cadeiras' der Equiden Südamerikas. Tierärztl. Umschau *18:* 353 (1963).
Gill, B. S.: Properties of soluble antigen of Trypanosoma evansi. J. genet. Microbiol. *38:* 357 (1965).
Holz, J.: Das Verhalten von Trypanosoma evansi unter Einfluß des Diadethyl-N^2-guanyl-N^2-(p-amidinophenyl)-dihydrazondihydrochlorid. Zbl. Vet.-Med. R. B. *12:* 67 (1965).
Neitz, W. O.; McCully, R. M.: Clinicopathological study on experimental Trypanosoma brucei infections in horses. Part 1. Development of clinically recognizable nervous symptoms in Nagana-infected horses treated with subcurative doses of Antrypol and Berenil. Onderstepoort J. vet. Res. *38:* 127 (1971).

2.3.1.6. Additional Protozoal Diseases

Three additional protozoal diseases — trichomoniasis, giardiasis and besnoitiosis — are listed in table 2.3. — 1. These are diseases that are rarely enzootic or have mainly a sporadic or subclinical occurrence. Details on these parasitisms may be found in textbooks and monographs on veterinary parasitology.

Table 2.3. — 1. Additional protozoal diseases (survey)

Disease	Causative organism	Distribution	Clinical findings	Diagnosis	Control	Remarks
Tricho-moniasis	*Tritrichomonas equi* habitat: cecum, colon	cosmopolitan	diarrhea, enteritis		metronida-zole; di-metridazole symptomatic: restoration of intestinal flora	commensalism, facultative parasitism?
	Trichomonas equibuccalis habitat: gingiva, oral mucosa	Yugoslavia	not described		causal therapy not available	
Giardiasis	*Giardia equi* habitat: small intestine	America, southern Africa	diarrhea	detection of cysts in feces; necropsy	causal therapy not available	
Besnoitiosis	*Besnoitia benneti* habitat: cysts in the skin and mucosae	southern and eastern Africa, France, U.S.	cutaneous syndrome: chronic pachydermia with nodulation; nasal and pharyngeal mucosae sometimes affected; acute febrile course with fatal outcome possible	detection of cysts in skin lesions and pharyngeal mucosa	causal therapy not available	

References

BEMRICK, W. J.: Giardia in North American horses. Vet. Med. and Small Animal Clinician *46:* 1 (1968).
BENNETT, S. P.; FRANCO, D. A.: Equine protozoan diarrhea (equine intestinal trichomoniasis) at Trinidad racetracks. J. Amer. vet. med. Assoc. *154:* 58 (1969).
BIGALKE, R. D.: Studies on equine besnoitiosis. J. Parasitol. *56:* 29 (1970).
DAMRON, G. W.: Gastrointestinal trichomonads in horses. Occurrence and identification. Amer. J. vet. Res. *37:* 25 (1976).
LAUFENSTEIN-DUFFY, H.: Equine intestinal trichomoniasis. J. Amer. vet. med. Assoc. *155:* 1835 (1969).
VARELA, J. C.; SALSAMENDI, R.: First account of a natural infection of our horses with Giardia equi Fantham, 1921. Ann. Fac. Vet. Uruguay *8:* 165 (1958).

2.3.2. Helminthiases

2.3.2.1. Fascioliasis

Liver fluke disease is somewhat rare in horses compared to its occurrence in cattle and sheep, but it can become enzootic among horses in heavily infested areas and during 'fluke years'.

Causative Organism. Fasciola hepatica, length about 20 mm in the horse.

Habitat: Adult flukes attach to the walls of the bile ducts with an oral and ventral sucker; young flukes migrate in the liver parenchyma.

Epizootiology. F. hepatica is a decidedly euryxenous parasite. Its intermediate host is the dwarf pond snail, *Lymnaea truncatula*. Horses are infected orally mainly by grazing common pastures with cattle and sheep and eating grass contaminated with encysted metacercariae. Moist, low-lying pastures and heavily-stocked permanent pastures are particularly dangerous. Horses are relatively resistant to *F. hepatica*.

The incidence of infection is highest during the late summer and early fall.

Symptoms. Characteristic symptoms are absent. With a mild infestation, the subclinical form is predominant. Heavier infestations cause general disturbances such as anorexia, dullness, reduced working capacity, anemia, hyperbilirubinemia and sometimes jaundice. Deaths are relatively rare. Strongyle infestations appear to promote infection with *F. hepatica*.

Necropsy findings in chronic cases consist mainly of cholangitic changes and interstitial hepatitis.

Diagnosis and Differential Diagnosis. Fluke eggs can be demonstrated in the feces by the sedimentation method, but a serologic demonstration by indirect immunofluorescence is more reliable. In heavily infested areas, a presumptive diagnosis of fasciolosis may be made on clinical grounds when hepatic diseases of other etiology have been excluded. Equine infectious anemia should also be considered.

Treatment. Treatment with hexachloroxylene (60 mg/kg), rafoxanide (3 mg/kg) or some other fasciolicide is recommended in conjunction with dietary measures.

Prophylaxis. In heavily fluke-infested areas and especially under stud conditions, horse pastures should be closed to cattle and sheep, and hygienic pasture management should be practiced. In areas where host snails are found, the use of molluscicides active against *Lymnaea truncatula* (niclosamide or triphenmorph) should be considered.

References

BREM, S.; WOJTEK, H.: Beitrag zum Wurmbefall der Pferde, insbesondere das Vorkommen des grossen Leberegels. Tierärztl. Umschau *27:* 264 (1972).

GRELCK, H.; HÖRCHNER, F.; WÖHRL, H.: Zur experimentellen Infektion des Pferdes mit Fasciola hepatica. Berliner Münchener tierärztl. Wschr. *90:* 371 (1977).

KRALJ, M.; SREBOCAN, V.; MARŽAN, B.; TURNER, V.; WIKERHAUSER, T.: Acute fascioliasis in horses with particular reference to the differential diagnosis of infectious anaemia. Veterin. Arh., Zagreb *30:* 192 (1960).

LABER, G.: Ein Fall von chronischer Fasziolose beim Pferd. Wiener tierärztl. Mschr. *58:* 432 (1971).

MIKLAUŠIĆ, B.; MIKAČIĆ, D.; PETROVIĆ, D.; VULINEC, M.; JUKIĆ, B.: Fascioliasis in horses in the Central Posavina, an enzootic area of equine infectious anaemia. Veterin Arh., Zagreb *41:* 38 (1971).

MOISANT, C.; JOLIVET, G.; PITRE, J.: La fasciolose des equidés. Observations en Normandie. Essais de traitement par le rafoxanide. Rec. Méd. Vét. École Alfort *148:* 443 (1972).

2.3.2.2. Dicroceliasis

Infection with the lancet fluke, *Dicrocoelium dendriticum*, represents an incidental finding in the horse. Little is known about enzootic or clinically-overt forms. *D. dendriticum* (8—12 mm long, 1.5—2.5 mm wide) resides in the bile ducts of the host. Infection is acquired at pasture by the ingestion of ants harboring the metacercariae.

The sedimentation method is suitable for demonstrating the characteristic *Dicrocoelium* eggs.

Treatment. Experience with causal therapy is not available. Hexachlorocylene (150 mg/kg) and thiabendazol (200 mg/kg) are recommended on the basis of experience in sheep.

The best prophylaxis in problem areas is to avoid grazing horses on pastures that are heavily used by sheep.

2.3.2.3. Tapeworm Infestation

Infestation with adult cestodes does not have the central importance of strongylosis and ascariasis in intestinal helminthiases of the horse, although enzootic occurrences are known.

Causative Organism. Several tapeworm species of the family Anoplocephalidae inhabit the small intestine of the horse as parasites:

Anoplocephala perfoliata: up to 25 cm long with wide, short proglottids.

Anoplocephala magna: up to 80 cm long and 2.5 cm wide.

Paranoplocephala mamillana: relatively short, only 1—5 cm long.

Habitat: Small intestine; *A. perfoliata* mainly in the ileum or ileocecal valve area.

Host range: Equidae.

Epizootiology. The intermediate hosts in the life cycle of the Anoplocephalidae are free-living mites *(Oribatidae)*, which eat the proglottids or encosphere-bearing eggs that are passed in the feces of the definitive host, the horse. Development of the cysticercoids in the intermediate host requires up to 16 weeks.

Horses pick up the parasite by ingesting infected mites while grazing at pasture.

Prepatent period: 6—7 weeks.

Symptoms. Pathogenicity varies from one tapeworm species to the next. Most *P. mamillana* infestations are benign. Infection with *A. magna*, on the other hand, causes digestive disturbances with intermittent anorexia, recurring colic, and diarrhea.

In heavy infestations, working capacity is reduced and emaciation becomes apparent. One case was reported in which a spontaneous, fatal rupture of the duodenum resulted from complete obstruction of the small bowel by adult worms. Anemia is sometimes reported as a sequel. *A. perfoliata* causes inflammation at the ileocecal orifice accompanied by severe colic due to spasm of the terminal ileum; peracute spastic ileus is a possible complication. A characteristic sign is the presence of tapeworm segments in the feces. At necropsy, signs of catarrhal enteritis are visible in addition to the obvious cestodes in the bowel lumen. Edematous areas are seen at the sites of tapeworm attachment to the mucosa. Sometimes hundreds of *A. perfoliata* are found about the ileocecal valve, where they cause the formation of granulomatous and polypous vegetations. Other possible complications are sporadic mechanical ileus and even peritonitis subsequent to intestinal rupture.

Diagnosis. Whenever tapeworm infestation is suspected, the feces should be examined grossly for the presence of proglottids. The microscopic examination of a fecal flotation may fail to disclose the typical cestode eggs, which have a rounded, polygonal shape, are embryonated, and vary from 50 to 80 μm in diameter, depending on species.

Treatment. Bithionol has proved effective at a dosage of 10 mg/kg BW, although a special diet must be maintained for 12 days before application. When bunamidine is used (25 mg/kg), its relatively long residual action (10 days) must be taken into account. The broad-spectrum antihelminthic drug mebendazole is recommended at a dose rate of 20 mg/kg BW. So far there are no reports on the use of the excellent cestodicide praciquantel in horses.

Prophylactic measures to eradicate oribatid mites on horse pastures through the use of insecticides appear entirely feasible under proper conditions. (This requires, of course, that the pasture be spelled for a designated interval.) With repeated outbreaks of tapeworm infestation, especially in breeding or racing animals, the prophylactic use of one of the aforementioned cestodicides in the late fall or early spring may be advised.

References

Böhm, L. K.; Supperer, R.: Beiträge zur Kenntnis tierischer Parasiten. Zbl. Bakteriol. Parasitenk. *172:* 298 (1958).

Christl, H., jr.: Darmruptur nach Massenbefall mit Anoplocephala perfoliata bei einer Stute. Berliner Münchener tierärztl. Wschr. *84:* 305 (1971).

Dorchies, Ph.; Amalric, M.: Traitement des helminthoses digestives et de la gastrophilose du cheval. Revue. Revue Méd. vét. *78:* 7 (1977).

Fukui, M.; Kaneko, C.; Ogawa, A.: Studies on equine tapeworms and their intermediate host. 2. Studies on removal effects of bithionol, bithionol acetate and dichlorophen for equine tapeworm, Anoplocephala perfoliata. Jap. J. Parasitol. *9:* 217 (1960).

Guilhon, J.; Graber, M.: Pouvoir anthelminthique du thio-bis-(hydroxychlorophényle) sur divers helminthes des équides. Bull. Acad. Vét. Franc. *38:* 23 (1965).

Oliver, D. F.; Jenkins, C. T.; Walding, P.: Duodenum rupture in a nine-month-old colt due to Anoplocephala magna. Vet. Rec. *101:* 80 (1977).

Safaev, Ja. S.: Effektivnost' fenasala pri anoplocefalidoze lošadej. Veterinarija *49:* 5, 68 (1972).

2.3.2.4. Hydatidosis

The horse serves as an intermediate host for several species of tapeworm. *Echinococcus hydatidosus*, the 2nd larval stage of *Echinococcus granulosus*, is found both sporadically and enzootically in the liver and lungs, as well as on the peritoneum and in the eyes. In Great Britain this helminthiasis was once a serious problem among horses that were exposed to proglottids or eggs shed at racetracks or on stud farms by dogs infected with *E. granulosus*. Infection is acquired by the ingestion of contaminated material. The presence of *E. hydatidosus* is usually diagnosed post-mortem. The echinococcus hydatids found in the horse are for the most part fertile, proving that this species is a true intermediate host. Prophylaxis includes the helminthologic surveillance and deworming of dogs that have contact with horses. Praciquantel is the drug of choice for infected horses.

The presence of *Cysticercus bovis* in the muscles (man is the definitive host and source of infection by passing *Taenia saginata* eggs in the stool) and *Coenurus cerebralis* in the CNS (larva of the dog tapeworm *Taenia multiceps*) are incidental findings in the horse.

On the other hand, it is not at all unusual to find *Cysticercus tenuicollis* (larva of the dog tapeworm *Taenia hydatigena*) on the serous surfaces of the abdominal organs during meat inspections.

The prevention of hydatidosis in the horse hinges upon regular parasitologic surveillance of the definitive hosts and their elimination as a source of infection.

References

Căpătînă, V.; Cristea, I.; Darie, I. M.; Ivascu, I.; Fodor, I.: Ein seltener Fall von orbitaler Echinokokkenkrankheit beim Pferd. Zbl. Vet.-Med. R. B. *16:* 77 (1969).

Dixon, J. B.; Baker-Smith, J. K.; Greatorex, J. C.: The incidence of hydated cysts in horses in Great Britain. Vet. Rec. *93:* 255 (1973).

Ronéus, O.: Förekomst och överlevnad av hydatidcystor till Echinococcus granulosus hos importerade hästar i Sverige. Nord. Vet.-Med. *27:* 49 (1975).

Thompson, R. C. A.; Smyth, J. D.: Potential danger of hydatid disease of horse/dog origin. Brit. med. J. *3:* 807 (1974).

Thompson, R. C.; Smyth, J. D.: Equine hydatidosis: a review of the current status in Great Britain and the results of an epidemiological survey. Vet. Parasitol. *1:* 107 (1975).

2.3.2.5. Dictyocaulosis

Reports of lungworm infestation in equids, while not frequent, are available from all parts of the world.

Causative Organism. Dictyocaulus arnfieldi; 3.5—7 cm long; eggs: embryonated, 85—100 × 50—60 μm.

Host range: horse, donkey, mule.

Epizootiology. The eggs laid by *Dictyocaulus* females pass via the pharynx or digestive tract of the host to the exterior. Within 6—24 hours the eggs hatch and release first-stage larvae, which, under pasture conditions, molt twice within 3 or more days to become infective larvae that exhibit a low tenacity and short life span. The larvae are capable of overwintering under Central European conditions.

The 3rd-stage larvae must be ingested to infest the primary host; foals are a particularly high-risk group. Only 5 days after infection the larvae pass to the lungs in the blood stream.

Prepatent period: 28—42 days.

The adult worms survive for about 6 months on the average, though many survive up to a year under favorable conditions. In the donkey, adult lungworms sometimes can survive for several years. As a result, donkeys that are stabled with horses represent an important source of infection, as they can shed *Dictyocaulus* eggs for a prolonged period.

Symptoms. The cardinal symptoms are coughing spells, transitory fever, and dyspnea with increased vesicular sounds or respiratory râles. Moderate and heavy infestations are associated with fever and systemic disturbances, combined with a reduced appetite and emaciation and also a bilateral seromucoid nasal discharge. Mixed infections with influenza virus and streptococci are not unusual and may lead to bronchopneumonia.

Necropsy reveals a frothy mucus in the bronchi and bronchial inflammation, in addition to the lungworms themselves.

Diagnosis. The characteristic eggs can be demonstrated in fresh fecal flotations (no more than 6 hours old). If fresh stool is unavailable, hatched larvae may be demonstrated by the migration technique. Clinical suspicion of dictyocaulosis is prompted by excessive coughing at pasture and the prior demonstration of *D. arnfieldi* in local fauna.

Differential diagnosis must be made from pneumonias of other etiology (viral, bacterial, *Strongyloides* and *Parascaris* infections).

Treatment. All animals in the affected group should be stabled. Cases of pneumonia or severe bronchitis are treated promptly with antibiotics or sulfonamides. Levamisole is effective against adult lungworms when given at a dosage of 15 mg/kg BW orally or 5 mg/kg intramuscularly; the medication is repeated after 3 weeks. During the treatment period, a diet of high-protein, dust-free feeds is maintained. From a *prophylactic* standpoint, horses should not graze the same pasture as donkeys, which are an important reservoir for *D. arnfieldi.* Pastures contaminated with *D. arnfieldi* larvae should be closed to equidae for a period of 3 months.

References

Campbell, E.; Gumbrell, R. C.; Murfitt, C. G.: The occurrence of Dictyocaulus arnfieldi in the lungs of horses. New Zealand vet. J. *19:* 217 (1971).

Dorchies, Ph.; Andrillon, C.: La dictyocaulose des équines: decouverte d'un foyer Pyrénéen. Revue Méd. vét. *125:* 233 (1974).

Enigk, K.; Weingärtner, E.: Zur Verbreitung und Behandlung der Dictyocaulose der Einhufer. Dtsch. tierärztl. Wschr. *80:* 145 (1973).

Jacob, E.: Lungenwurm-Fund beim Pferd. Berliner Münchener tierärztl. Wschr. *62:* 68 (1948).

Wetzel, R.; Enigk, K.: Zur Biologie von Dictyocaulus arnfieldi, dem Lungenwurm der Einhufer. Arch. Tierheilk. *73:* 83 (1938).

2.3.2.6. Strongyloidosis

Infestation with the dwarf threadworm is a typical breeding-farm disease that is especially common under stud conditions.

Causative Organism. Strongyloides westeri (from the Rhabditidae family of nematodes); geohelminth; only the parthenogenic female is parasitic, length 8—9 mm; eggs: 40—50 × 30—40 μm, ovoid, thin-shelled, embryonated.

Habitat: Small intestine, usually the duodenum or jejunum.

Epizootiology. Eggs hatch after being discharged with the feces, releasing larvae that become infective after 2 molts and may develop in the environment to free-living forms whose offspring are also infectious for equidae (fig. 2.3. — 2).

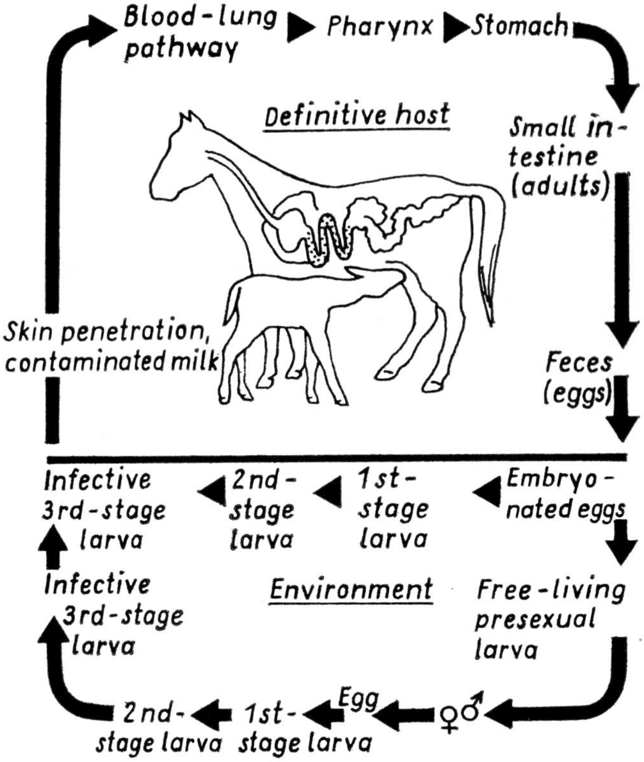

Fig. 2.3. — 2. Life cycle of *Strongyloides westeri.*

Infection is acquired either by skin penetration or orally via the milk.

Following skin penetration, the larvae travel to the lungs by way of the lymph and blood. In primary infections in foals, the larvae migrate from the alveoli to the bronchi, and thence to the trachea, pharynx, esophagus, stomach, and finally the small intestine, where they bore into the mucosa for a short time for molting and reach sexual maturity only 9 days after infection. In animals that are already infected with *Strongyloides*, the larvae do not enter the respiratory passages, but travel from the lungs to the muscles via the systemic circulation.

If infection occurs during pregnancy, *Strongyloides* larvae are discharged in the milk for about 50 days postpartum, and nursing foals can acquire a patent infection as early as the 10th day of life.

Symptoms. Strongyloidosis occurs mainly in nursing foals under stud-farm conditions. Massive primary infestations are characterized by the appearance of diarrhea between the 9th and 16th day of life, associated with intermittent anorexia, depression, and poor development. If a percutaneous *Strongyloides* infection supervenes during the nursing period, the larvae will tend to cause a dangerous pulmonary syndrome that can have severe and sometimes fatal consequences if secondary bacterial invasion occurs. The skin reactions caused by percutaneous infection are usually subclinical.

Diagnosis. Starting on the 10th day of life, the characteristic *Strongyloides* eggs containing a U-shaped embryo can be demonstrated in fecal flotations, assuming the specimen is examined immediately after collection. If this is not possible, the stool should be placed in an incubator for 12 hours at 20—25 °C and then examined for larvae by the migration technique. Due to the swimming ability of the *Strongyloides* larvae, it is advisable to examine the sediment no sooner than 24 hours after preparation of the specimen.

At necropsy the worms are easily overlooked, and so it is best to obtain a scraping of mucosa and examine it microscopically on a dark field. If bronchopneumonia develops during the nursing period, the lungs should be examined for *Strongyloides* larvae.

Treatment. Suitable drugs are thiabendazole (25—100 mg/kg), morantel tartrate (10 mg/kg), cambendazole (20 mg/kg), fenbendazole (50 mg/kg) and mebendazole (10 mg/kg). All the foals on the premises and their dams should be treated; medication should be repeated after 10—20 days. Galactogenic infection of the foals can be largely prevented by the daily administration of a cambendazole paste in a dose of 30 mg/kg to the dams from parturition to postpartum day 16.

On breeding farms where strongyloidosis has occurred enzootically, the meticulous cleaning and disinfection of stables before and after foaling has proved a useful hygienic and prophylactic measure. Peracetic acid is the preferred disinfectant.

References

Brglez, J.; Dolenc, M.; Rakovec, R.: Strongyloidosis of foals, a contribution to the knowledge of treatment and epizootiology. Veterinaria, Sarajevo *15:* 403 (1966).

Enigk, K.; Dey-Hazra, A.; Batke, J.: Zur klinischen Bedeutung und Behandlung des galaktogen erworbenen Strongyloides-Befalls der Fohlen. Dtsch. tierärztl. Wschr. *81:* 605 (1974).

Greer, G. J.; Bello, T. R.; Amborski, G. F.: Experimental infection of Strongyloides westeri in parasite-free ponies. J. Parasitol. *60:* 466 (1974).

Hiepe, Th.: Wirksamkeit von Moranteltartrat gegenüber Nematodenbefall bei Sportpferden. Schweizer Arch. Tierheilk. *114:* 613 (1972).

Hiepe, Th.; Nickel, S.; Siebeke, F.: Studies on the dynamics of strongyloides egg excretion under stud conditions. Folia Parasitol. *22:* 341 (1975).

Hiepe, Th.; Siebeke, F.; Nickel, S.: Thiabendazol gegen Strongyloidesbefall bei Fohlen. Angew. Parasitol. *12:* 65 (1971).

Lyons, E. T.; Drudge, J. H.; Tolliver, S. C.: On the life cycle of Strongyloides westeri in the equine. J. Parasitol. *59:* 780 (1973).

Lyons, E. T.; Drudge, J. H.; Tolliver, S. C.: Observations on development of Strongyloides westeri in foals nursing dams treated with cambendazole or thiabendazole. Amer. J. vet. Res. *38:* 889 (1977).

Ribbeck, R.; Kuller, H.-J.; Leonhard, I.: Einsatz von Mebendazol zur Bekämpfung des Magen-Darm-Nematoden-Befalls beim Pferd. medicamentum *17:* 352 (1976).

Siebeke, F.: Untersuchungen zur Dynamik der Helmintheneiausscheidung im Jahreszyklus bei Mutterstuten und Fohlen. Vet.-med. Diss., Berlin (1973).

2.3.2.7. Trichostrongylosis

Trichostrongylosis (stomach worm infestation) is a widespread but relatively seldom-diagnosed gastrointestinal helminthiasis of horses.

Causative Organism. Trichostrongylus axei, stomach worm; geohelminth; 3.5 to 5.5 mm long, threadlike, reddish-brown. Eggs: 70—90 × 40 μm, thin-shelled, ovoid, oviparous; segmented embryo with 8—16 segmentation spheres (blastomeres) in freshly voided stool.

Habitat: Gastric fundus, on and in the mucosa, and sometimes the anterior portion of the duodenum.

Host range: Horse, cattle, sheep, wild ruminants.

Epizootiology. Infection is acquired orally by the ingestion of 3rd-stage larvae during grazing, especially on small, heavily-stocked permanent pastures that are grazed concurrently or successively by horses, sheep, cattle or wild ruminants.

Prepatent period: 21—28 days; life span: 3—15 months. The oviparous, unsegmented *Trochostrongylus axei* eggs are passed in the feces and, under pastoral conditions and with a suitable ambient temperature (20—26 °C is optimum), will hatch in 2 days producing 1st-stage larvae that mature to an infective stage in 4—5 days. The *Trichostrongylus* larvae are highly resistant to the environment, can remain viable for nearly 12 months and can overwinter.

Symptoms. In moderate to heavy infestations, the main symptoms are digestive disturbances, diarrhea, constipation, mild spasmodic colic, reduced working capacity or dullness, emaciation, hypochromic anemia, and a protracted course. Light infestations take a subclinical course and cause a decrease in working capacity. At necropsy threadlike nematodes are found in the stomach and duodenum. Hyperemia and edema formation are evident in the early stage; later there is catarrhal inflammation of the mucosa, which exhibits erosive and necrotic lesions.

Diagnosis. The clinical picture is rather nonspecific. *T. axei* and strongyles cannot be reliably differentiated by microscopic inspection of the eggs in fecal flotations. To make an accurate differentiation, it is necessary to examine the 3rd-stage larvae following cultivation.

At necropsy it is possible to demonstrate the typical nematodes and their eggs as well as determine the worm burden and the extent of pathoanatomic changes.

Treatment. Suitable drugs are imidazole derivatives such as thiabendazole (50 to 100 mg/kg), mebendazole (10 mg/kg), fenbendazole and morantel tartrate (10 mg/kg), organophosphates (metriphonate), or other broad-spectrum anthelmintics. In areas where *T. axei* infections have been enzootic, it is imperative that potential definitive hosts, namely cattle, sheep and wild ruminants, be prohibited from grazing horse pastures. This is an effective means of preventing spread among the various host species.

References

Leland, S. E., jr.; Drudge, J. H.; Wyant, Z. N.; Elam, G. W.: Studies on Trichostrongylus axei (Cobbold, 1879). VII. Some quantitative and pathologic aspects of natural and experimental infections in the horse. Amer. J. vet. Res. *22:* 128 (1961).

Wetzel, R.: Parasitäre Erkrankungen des Magens. Magen-Trichostrongylose der Einhufer; in Joest, Handbuch der speziellen pathologischen Anatomie der Haustiere, 3. Aufl., Bd. VI, p. 500 (Parey, Berlin 1969).

2.3.2.8. Ascariasis

Ascarid infection is a relatively common equine parasitism that occurs in all countries and is especially damaging in foals and younger horses under stud conditions and in large herds.

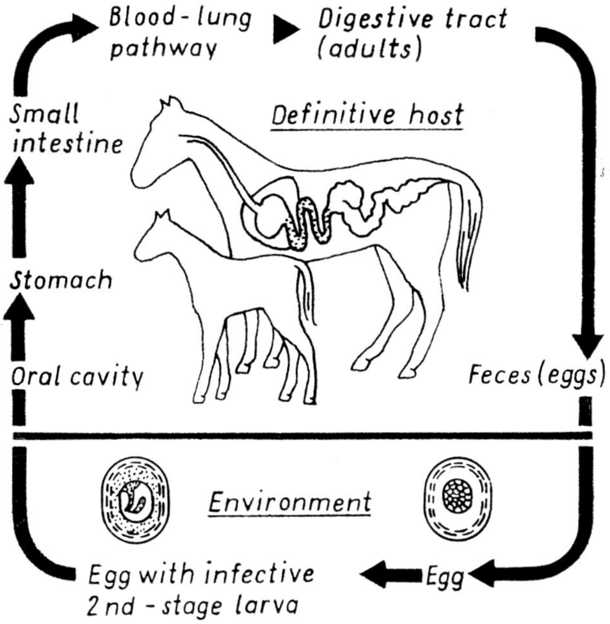

Fig. 2.3. — 3. Life cycle of *Parascaris equorum.*

Causative Organism. Parascaris equorum, approx. 10—40 cm long, straw-thick, pale yellow-gray in color. Eggs: 80—120 μm, thick-shelled, spheroid, oviparous; unsegmented embryo.

Habitat: Small intestine, usually the duodenum and jejunum. Adult ascarids tend to migrate and so are apt to inhabit hollow organs located adjacent to the duodenum (stomach, common bile duct), especially in heavy infestations.

Epizootiology. Stenoxenous geohelminth. The female ascarid lays more than 100,000 eggs per day, which pass in the feces to the exterior and develop to the infective stage in 20—40 days, the infective larvae being retained in the protective eggshell (fig. 2.3. — 3). Infection is acquired by ingesting the eggs in contaminated material; this usually occurs within the stable or in small foal yards. The eggs hatch in the small intestine, releasing larvae that penetrate the intestinal wall and reenter the small intestine via the 'blood-lung pathway', where they molt twice before reaching the adult stage. Ascarid eggs are highly tenacious in the environment. They can remain viable for more than 12 months in surface soil and in stables and are capable of overwintering.

Prepatent period: 6—12 weeks; patent period 8—10 months.

Symptoms. Ascariasis can occur as a clinically overt disease up to the age of about 2 years; mature horses generally show no symptoms, although mares in particular may shed eggs in significant numbers.

The clinical picture of ascariasis is variable, and the course is closely related to the degree of infestation:

— Intestinal syndrome (classic picture): Fluctuating, usually depressed appetite, diarrhea, passage of ascarids in the feces, poor development, emaciation, anemia, chronic recurring colic; 'chloroform' smell in stable; enzootic course.

— Ascarid ileus: Heavy infestations cause a mechanical ileus associated with a triad of anorexia, severe colic and constipation. A segment of small intestine that is impacted with a mass of ascarids may be easily palpated on rectal examination. In severe cases the small intestine may actually be ruptured by the massing of worms, allowing ascarids to enter the peritoneal cavity and cause a fatal peritonitis.
— Pulmonary syndrome: Following a massive *P. equorum* infestation, pulmonary manifestations may be expected from the migrating larvae. Secondary bacterial or viral invasion may complicate the picture, especially if much condition has been lost.
— CNS syndrome: Central nervous manifestations may be caused either by ascaridin, a metabolic product of ascarids that is toxic to the host (hypoglycemic encephalopathy is a sequela) or by the migration of ascarid larvae into the CNS.
— Subclinical form: This form is most common in adult horses but can also occur in foals and yearlings that have a light worm burden. The decline in working capacity may be substantial, especially in competitive performance horses. Subclinical cases often can be detected only by the microscopic identification of eggs in the stool.

Diagnosis. A clinical diagnosis is made difficult by the variable clinical picture and course. In suspected cases, the feces should be continually checked for the presence of voided ascarids, which are easily recognized. The characteristic eggs can be demonstrated in fecal flotations. Under stud conditions routine stool examinations should be performed at least three times a year.

Treatment. For more than 2 decades, piperazine compounds such as piperazine adipate, p. chlorohydrate, p. succinate and p. citrate have been successfully used at a dosage of 100—300 mg/kg for the control of ascarid infections. In the future the use of this vermifugal drug should be limited mainly to the treatment of patent ascarid infections. It acts by paralyzing the adult worms and has no larvicidal properties. Of the familiar broad-spectrum anthelmintics, morantel tartrate (10—15 mg/kg), thiabendazole (100—500 mg/kg), mebendazole (10 mg/kg) and fenbendazole (10 mg/kg), as well as the organophosphates metriphonate (50 mg/kg) and dichlorvos (30 mg/kg), have proved effective when given orally with special dosing devices or when administered in the feed. They have very good activity against adult worms as well as the juvenile stages. Under stud conditions, a program of regular fecal examinations should be maintained in mares, and anthelmintics given where necessary.

Prophylaxis. Stables should be regularly cleaned and then disinfected with a steam jet. Disinfectants with a cresol or peracetic acid base are only partially effective. Carbon disulfide is highly active against the relatively resistant, thick-shelled ascarid eggs. The careful heaping of manure (manure packing) has proved an effective control measure, retarding embryonic development within the eggs through heat generation.

References

Cornwell, R. L.; Jones, R. M.; Pott, J. M.: Critical trials with morantel tartrate against Parascaris equorum. Res. vet. Sci. *14:* 134 (1973).

Derkmann, K.: Untersuchungen über die askarizide Wirkung von Fenbendazol bei natürlich infizierten Pferden. Vet.-med. Diss., München (1976).

Derkmann, K.; Hasslinger, M.-A.: Zur Bekämpfung des Pferdespulwurmes, Parascaris equorum (Goeze, 1782) mit Panacur. Berliner Münchener tierärztl. Wschr. *90:* 95 (1977).

Gerber, H.; Hörning, B.; König, H.: Gastrointestinale Parasiten des Pferdes — Befallsfrequenz in Schweizer Beständen. Schweizer Arch. Tierheilk. *110:* 364 (1968).

HIEPE, TH.: Beiträge zur medikamentellen Askaridenbekämpfung I. Über die Anwendung von Piperazinchlorhydrat gegen Spulwurmbefall bei Equiden. Mh. Vet.-Med. *16:* 15 (1961).
HIEPE, TH.: Diskussionsbeitrag zum Vortrag 'Parasitenbekämpfung beim Pferd'. Wirksamkeit von Moranteltartrat gegenüber Nematodenbefall bei Sportpferden. Schweizer Arch. Tierheilk. *114:* 613 (1972).
RIBBECK, R.; KULLER, H.-J.; LEONHARD, I.: Einsatz von Mebendazol zur Bekämpfung des Magen-Darm-Nematoden-Befalls beim Pferd. medicamentum *17:* 352 (1976).
ROUND, M. C.: Experiences with thiabendazole as an anthelmintic for horses. Brit. vet. J. *124:* 248 (1968).
SIEBEKE, F.: Untersuchungen zur Dynamik der Helmintheneiausscheidung im Jahreszyklus bei Mutterstuten und Fohlen. Vet.-med. Diss., Berlin (1973).
VOSS, J. L.; HIBLER, C. P.: Critical tests of butonate as an ascaricide and boticide in horses. Amer. J. vet. Res. *32:* 2085 (1971).
VOSS, J. L.; HIBLER, C. P.: Critical tests of an orally administered butonate as an anthelmintic in horses. Amer. J. vet. Res. *34:* 1209 (1973).

2.3.2.9. Oxyuriasis

Infestation of the colon with oxyurids (pinworms) is a common disease of horses throughout the world. Mature horses are most frequently affected.

Causative Organism. Two different species occur:

Oxyuris equi; 1—18 cm in length with a long, pointed tail. Eggs: 80—100 × 40—45 μm, ovoid, relatively thick-shelled, operculated on the anterior end; ovoviviparous.

Probstmayria vivipara; relatively rare in Europe; ~ 2—4 mm long; viviparous type.

Habitat: Cecum, anterior portions of colon.

Epizootiology. After mating, the *Oxyuris equi* females migrate from the intestine to the perianal area for egg-laying. There they deposit large numbers of embryonated eggs (5000—6000) together with a rapidly-gelatinizing fluid that dries quickly. They then move back into the rectum and die shortly thereafter. Within a week the larvae molt twice to become infective 3rd-stage larvae, which drop off into the bedding while still contained within the egg. Infestation occurs by ingestion of these eggs. The larvae hatch in the small intestine and pass to the colon, where they attach by suction to the intestinal mucosa and mature to the adult stage.

Prepatent period: 4—5 months.

The *Probstmayria vivipara* females bear 1- to 2-cm-long larvae, which develop rapidly. The prepatent period is 16—18 days. A portion of the infective, poorly resistant 3rd-stage larvae are voided in the feces and create a source of infection for other horses, especially in warm stables with deep bedding.

Symptoms. Adult oxyurids are relatively harmless. Their main injurious effect is the severe pruritus that is stimulated when the *O. equi* females travel from the rectum to the perianal region, usually at night, to lay their eggs. Affected horses rub the base of the tail against hard objects, causing circumscribed loss of hair and sometimes eczema-like skin lesions.

Diagnosis. In horses that show unrest at night and hair loss about the base of the tail, the perianal region should be examined grossly for the presence of eggs, which will appear as yellow-gray or dark-gray filaments or crusts. With positive findings or in suspected cases, an anal smear should be obtained for microscopic examination. A Scotch tape slide preparation is best for this purpose. Oxyurid eggs are not always demonstrable in fecal flotations. Sometimes pinworms are seen during rectal examination or during the collection of feces.

Infection with *Probstmayris vivipara* is practically impossible to diagnose.

Differential Diagnosis. The changes associated with pruritus about the base of the tail serve to distinguish oxyuriasis from mange and from infestations with biting and sucking lice.

Treatment. Mebendazole at a dosage of 5—10 mg/kg has proved effective when mixed in the feed in granular form. Morantel tartrate (10—15 mg/kg) is also very effective. In horses engaged in shows and competitions that already are subject to meticulous daily grooming, regular washing of the anal region with cold or luke-warm soapy water followed by the application of a neutral fat or oil is indicated. Heavy powdering serves a similar purpose. These measures are effective in relieving pruritus and preventing egg deposition.

Prophylaxis. Frequent changes of bedding are a useful preventive measure.

References

Arundel, J. K.: Recent advances in anthelmintics. Austral. vet. J. *43:* 455 (1967).

Babaeva, M.: Probstmayria vivipara infection in horses and donkeys in the Uzbek SSR. Trudy Uzbek. Nauch.-Issl. Veterin. Inst. *20:* 43 (1972).

Cotteleer, C.; Joossens, G.: Les principales infestations parasitaires des équides en Belgique. III. L'oxyurose. Ann. Méd. vét., Bruxelles *118:* 239 (1974).

Enigk, K.: Zur Biologie und Bekämpfung von Oxyuris equi. Z. Tropenmed. Parasitol. *1:* 259 (1949).

Keller, H.: Oxyurenbefall bei Pferden. Berliner Münchener tierärztl. Wschr. *79:* 429 (1966).

2.3.2.10. Strongylosis

Strongyle infestations are the most common helminthiases of horses and are of major economic importance. It may be said that virtually every horse is a carrier of strongyles or has been infected with strongyles at some time during its life. While the adult strongyles, which inhabit the large intestine, have limited pathogenic capabilities, the larvae of the 'large strongyles', particularly *Strongylus vulgaris,* live a parasitic existence while migrating in the body and can inflict severe, sometimes irreversible tissue damage.

Causative Organisms. The equine strongyles belonging to the family Strongylidae encompasses nearly 60 species and are divided into two subfamilies: Strongylinae (includes the large strongyles) and Trichonematinae.

The large strongyle species include:

Strongylus vulgaris (Delafondia vulgatis); 1.0—2.5 cm long.

Strongylus equinus; 2.5—5.0 cm long;

Strongylus edentatus (Alfortia edentatus); 2.0—4.0 cm long.

Eggs: 70—95 μm $\times$ 40—55 μm; thin-shelled, ovoid; segmented embryo with 8—32 segmentation spheres.

A morphologic differentiation of these 3 species can be made from the buccal capsule of the adult, which is distinctive for a given species (fig. 2.3. — 4), as well as from distinguishing features of the 3rd-stage larva. The eggs, on the other hand, cannot always be differentiated by routine laboratory examinations.

The small strongyles include many species. Some belong to the subfamily Strongylinae and include the genera *Triodontophorus* (16—26 mm long), *Oesophagodontus* (15—22 mm long) and *Craterostomum* (4—8 mm long); the adults are blood-suckers.

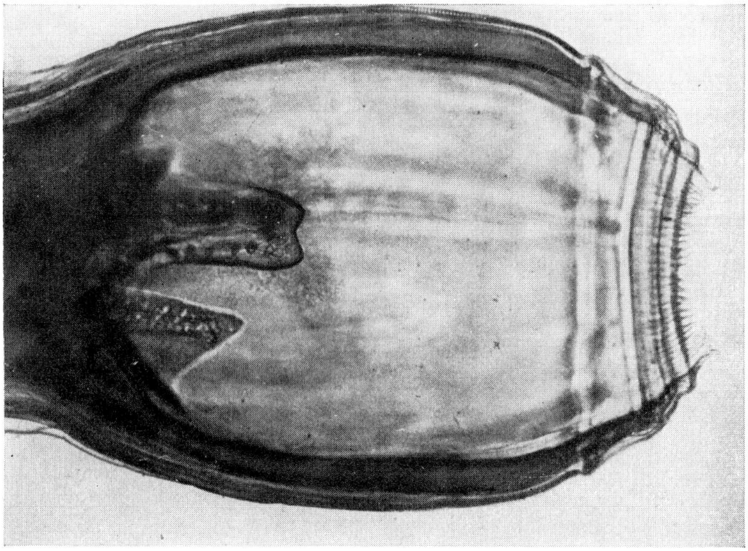

Fig. 2.3. — 4. Buccal capsule of *Strongylus equinus.*

Most, however, are from the subfamily Trichonematinae which includes the genera *Trichonema* (more than 30 species), *Poteriostomum, Cylicocercus, Cylicostephanus* and *Gyalocephalus;* the strongyles of this subfamily do not suck blood.

The eggs of the small strongyles have an elongated ovoid shape, are thin-shelled, and have a segmented embryo. They are well over 100 μm long and less than 40 μm wide, and thus appear longer but more slender than the 'robust'-looking eggs of the large strongyles. A differentiation between the large and small strongyles on the basis of egg morphology would seem to be possible, therefore.

Habitat: Adult strongyles inhabit the large intestine, especially the cecum and ventral colon, and, depending on species, attach firmly to the mucosa or live freely by embedding in mucus or bowel contents.

Epizootiology. All strongyles belong to the group of relatively stenoxenous geohelminths. While the environmental phase of the life cycle is similar in all species (see fig. 2.3. — 5), the endogenous phase varies from one species to the next, which accounts in large part for the differences in their pathogenic effects.

The embryonated eggs that are passed in the feces are not very resistant to environmental influences. Embryonic development is complete within 24 hours provided three requirements are met: abundant O_2, a relatively high ground and air moisture, and an ambient temperature around 18 °C. The rate of larval development depends largely on this triad of conditions. By 5 days at the earliest, the 1st-stage larvae hatch from the eggs and feed mainly on bacteria present in the feces. They then molt to 2nd-stage larvae and continue to feed in this stage. The infective 3rd-stage larvae are enclosed in a sheath and thus better protected from environmental influences. Although these larvae do not feed, they are quite active and are able to migrate upward on blades of grass. In heavily infested pastures, the larvae often congregate to form thick tufts atop the grass shafts. They are especially active in the early morning and evening or on overcast days when the grass is coated with a liquid

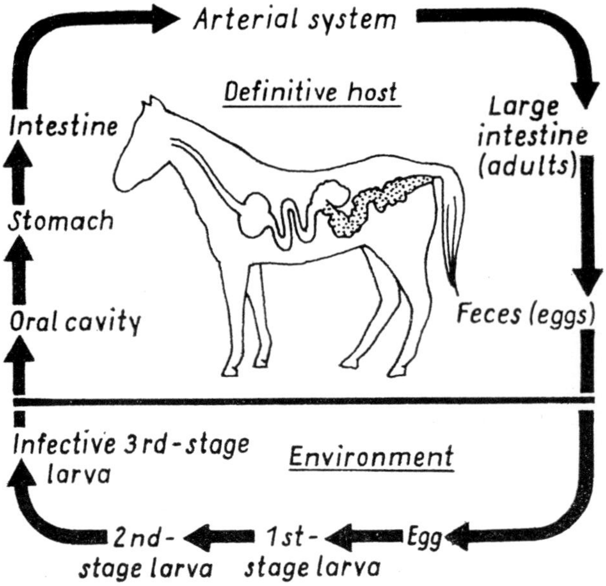

Fig. 2.3. — 5. Life cycle of *Strongylus vulgaris.*

film from dew, fog or rain. In bright daylight the larvae crawl down into the sheath of the blade or even into the soil to escape UV radiation and dessication (negative phototaxis). The 3rd-stage larvae can even migrate several centimeters into the ground, but in a vertical direction only. Frequent migrations at high ambient temperatures quickly exhaust energy and food reserves, and the larvae die. Conditions for larval development are also favorable in stables that maintain a constant temperature and a humid atmosphere that condenses on stable walls, creating a liquid film. Strongyle larvae are capable of climbing stable walls to a height of 1.5 meters.

Under pastoral conditions temperature changes, frost and dryness adversely affect the development of the larvae, which generally do not live longer than 4—6 weeks during the summer months. However, the overwintering of strongyle eggs and larvae has been demonstrated under Central European conditions, and so the pastures may still be infective in the spring.

Infection in horses is acquired by ingesting the 3rd-stage larvae either at pasture or in contaminated stables. Once in the small intestine, the larvae emerge from their sheaths, pass to the large intestine, and molt in the intestinal wall (histotropic phase) to become 4th-stage larvae. Further migration varies among different species.

— The 4th-stage larvae of *Strongylus vulgaris* penetrate into the arterioles of the submucosa by the shortest route available and migrate toward the blood stream along the intima of the small arteries, though this generally occurs only in massive primary infestations or as a result of immune reactions during the course of superinfections. This migration causes destruction of endothelial tissue, with the formation of threadlike ridges and thrombotic deposits. By about 8 days the larvae have reached the main arteries of the large intestine, and by 11 days they have entered the cranial mesenteric artery and aorta. Boring activity by the larvae produces arteritis and aneurysms of the vessel walls, although the internal elastic membrane is not perforated. By about 44 days most of the larvae have taken up residence in arteritis lesions and aneurysms of the cranial mesenteric artery, where they remain for 3—4 months. By 90 days at the earliest, the 4th-stage larvae molt and return via the blood stream to the wall of the large intestine, where they form nodules which later rupture, releasing the adults into the intestinal lumen.

Prepatent period: $6^1/_2$ months.

— The 4th-stage larvae of *Strongylus equinus* may migrate from the intestinal wall to the liver via the serosa and peritoneal cavity. By 6—7 weeks at the earliest, they move to the pancreas and finally return to the large intestine as 4th-stage larvae. Most likely the larvae leave the pancreas through its caudoventral surface, which borders on the base of the cecum and the colon (no serosa). Other 4th-stage *S. equinus* larvae apparently migrate aimlessly in the cecal wall for a period of 6 weeks.

Prepatent period: $8^1/_2$ to $9^1/_2$ months.

— The *Strongylus edentatus* larvae penetrate the wall of the large intestine and pass via the portal veins to the liver, where they molt to 4th-stage larvae following a migratory phase. By about 2 months they leave the liver and migrate to the intestinal wall, form verminous nodules there, and then return to the intestinal lumen, where they molt and develop to sexual maturity.

Prepatent period: 40—50 weeks.

— The small strongyle species penetrate the intestinal wall as 3rd-stage larvae and form black, yellow and red nodules in which they undergo 1 or 2 moltings. Then, as 4th-stage larvae or 'pre-adults', they return to the intestinal lumen.

Prepatent period: 6—12 weeks.

Symptoms. The larval migration of the large strongyles causes symptoms of varying severity, depending on the species concerned. *Strongylus vulgaris* migrations are associated with endarteritis, thromboembolitic colic, and aneurysms of the cranial mesenteric artery. Intermittent lameness, infarction of the bowel wall, and a fatal vascular rupture are possible complications. There are also reports of verminous encephalitis caused by aberrant *S. vulgaris* larvae, and of granulomatous lymphadenitis. *S. equinus* and *S. edentatus* larval migrations mainly cause intermittent fever, digestive disturbances, colic and poor development. Stray *S. edentatus* larvae are occasionally found postmortem in the testes and striated muscle. It would appear that the proneness of the horse to colic is closely related to infestation with strongyle larvae.

The harmful effects of adult strongyles depend largely upon the severity of the worm burden: Recurrent colic, diarrhea, intermittent anorexia, poor development, reduced working capacity, emaciation, poor coat and anemia syndrome (usually caused by members of the subfamily Strongylinae!) are frequently observed. Both the clinically overt form and the chronic, subclinical form lead to a significant decline of performance in athletic horses.

Diagnosis. An early diagnosis is extremely difficult owing to the long prepatent period of the strongyles. Patent infections can be diagnosed both quantitatively and qualitatively by the detection of eggs in fecal flotations. Under stud conditions a routine fecal examination is recommended in all dams and yearlings and in sport horses of all age groups.

If a strongylosis is suspected on clinical grounds, an effort should be made to determine speciation through larval cultivation and morphologic egg differentiation so that the potential significance of the infestation can be evaluated.

Differential Diagnosis. Equine infectious anemia of viral etiology should be excluded if anemia is present. In infected horses from large herds that die with the disease or are destroyed, a necropsy should be performed to evaluate for strongylosis so that conclusions with regard to herd infestation may be drawn.

Treatment. The cosmopolitan occurrence and high prevalence of strongyle infestations require well-organized control measures aimed at reducing the substantial economic losses caused by this helminthiasis. An essential aspect of control is the continual surveillance of stud-farm populations for strongyle infestation.

Strongyloses are treated causally with broad-spectrum anthelmintics that are active against both adult and immature forms. Among the imidazole and benzimidazole derivatives, the drugs thiabendazole (75—100 mg/kg), mebendazole (10 mg/kg), fenbendazole (10 mg/kg) and cambendazole (20 mg/kg) have proved most effective. Also effective are the organophosphates metriphonate (40—50 mg/kg) and dichlorvoj (30—40 mg/kg). Phenothiazine is no longer recommended in horses on account os its hepatotoxic side-effects and the existence of phenothiazine-resistant strains· Caution is advised in the use of tetramisole and levamisole.

Clinically affected horses should be stabled and temporarily rested from work or competition.

On breeding farms, the routine anthelmintic treatment of *all* dams is recommended at least twice a year — in the late fall after the end of the grazing season, and before or 3—4 weeks after the horses are turned out to pasture in the spring. Nursing foals in danger areas should be dewormed initially between about 4 and 8 weeks of life to remove pre-adult strongyles. Subtherapeutic doses of thiabendazole ($\sim$ 3.5 mg/kg/day for 30 days) have proved effective for this purpose. In racing animals, it appears that treatment at least once a year in the spring or late fall provides satisfactory control. Further treatments are guided by the results of fecal examinations.

When anthelmintics are being used, it is advisable to change medications after every 2 or 3 applications in order to remove drug-resistant strains or prevent their development.

Prophylaxis. Frequent changes of grazing areas using a rotational or apportionment method is a useful control measure; a given parcel should be grazed for no longer than 8 days and then spelled for at least 40 days before grazing is resumed. The application of ammonium nitrate, nitrophosphate or superphosphate fertilizers to pastures has proved effective against free-living strongyle larvae. Massive strongyle infestations in stables can be largely prevented through hygienic measures — low humidity, regular bedding changes, disinfection (e.g., with 0.4% peracetic acid), and the packing of manure.

References

Altaif, K. I.: Anthelmintic trial in arab horses with thiabendazole and tetramisole. Vet. Rec. *91:* 282 (1972).

Amborski, G. F.; Bello, T. R.; Torbert, B. J.: Host response to experimentally induced infections of Strongylus vulgaris in parasite-free and naturally infected ponies. Amer. J. vet. Res. *35:* 1181 (1974).

Ardans, A.; Walters, G. T.: Efficacy of a thiabendazole paste formulation to treat strongyle infections in horses. Amer. J. vet. Res. *34:* 1599 (1973).

Baird, J. D.; Hutchins, D. R.; Lepherd, E. E.: Phenothiazine poisoning in a thoroughbred horse. Austral. vet. J. *46:* 496 (1970).

Bello, Th. R.; Gordon, V. L.: Rapid concentration of strongyle eggs from equine feces for in vitro studies. Amer. J. vet. Res. *31:* 2285 (1970).

BOCH, J.; HÖRCHNER, F.: Zur Bekämpfung der Pferdestrongyliden. Tierärztl. Umschau *17:* 419 (1962).

CALLEAR, J. F. F.; NEAVE, R. M. S.: The clinical use of the anthelminitic mebendazole. Brit. vet. J. *127:* XLI (1971).

COFFMANN, J.; CARLSON, K.: Verminous arteritis in horses. J. Amer. vet. med. Assoc. *158:* 1358 (1971).

CORNWELL, R. L.; JONES, R. M.; POTT, J. M.: Critical trials of morantel tartrate in equine strongylosis. Vet. Rec. *93:* 94, 98 (1973).

COTTELEER, C. F.: Les principales infections parasitaires des equides en Belgique. I. Frequence des parasitoses. II. La strongylose. Ann. Méd. vét. *118:* 231 (1974).

DRUDGE, J. H.: The strongylides of equines. Internat. Congr. Parasitol., Proc. (München) *3:* 757 (1974).

DRUDGE, J. H.; LYONS, E. T.; TOLLIVER, S. C.: Resistance of equine strongyles to thiabendazole. Critical tests of two strains. Vet. Med. and Small Animal Clinican *72:* 433 (1977).

DUNCAN, J. L.: Strongylus vulgaris infection in the horse. Vet. Rec. *95:* 34 (1974).

DUNCAN, J. L.: Field studies on the epidemiology of mixed strongyle infection in the horse. Vet. Rec. *94:* 337 (1974).

DUNCAN, J. L.; PIRIE, H. M.: The life cycle of Strongylus vulgaris in the horse. Res. vet. Sci. *13:* 374 (1972).

ENDE, H.; STOYE, M.: Banminth-Paste zur planmäßigen Strongylidenbekämpfung beim Pferd. Dtsch. tierärztl. Wschr. *83:* 431 (1976).

ENIGK, K.; STOYE, M.: Versuche zur Behandlung des Strongylidenbefalls der Pferde mit Thiabendazol. Dtsch. tierärztl. Wschr. *70:* 257 (1963).

FAJZYEV, M.; KORNIENKO, Z. P.; DEMIDOV, N. V.: Dejstvie nekotorych mineral'nych udobrenij na jajca i ličinok strongiljat v konskom navoze (predyaritel'noe soobščenie). Bjull. vses. Inst. Gel'mintol. im. K. I. Skrjabina, Moskva *12:* 91 (1974).

GEORGI, J. R.: The Kikuchi-Enigk model of Strongylus vulgaris migrations in the horse. Cornell Vet. *63:* 220 (1973).

HASSLINGER, M.-A.: Untersuchungen über den Einfluß verschiedener Temperaturen auf Eier und Larven von Pferdestrongyliden unter Laboratoriumsbedingungen sowie das Verhalten dieser exogenen Stadien auf der Weide. Berliner Münchener tierärztl. Wschr. *94:* 1 (1981).

HIEPE, TH.: Parasitäre Erkrankungen des Peritoneums und der Peritonealhöhle; in JOEST, Handbuch der speziellen pathologischen Anatomie der Haustiere, 3. Aufl., 7, p. 517 (Parey, Berlin 1968).

HÖRCHNER, I.: Zur Differentialdiagnose ansteckender Blutarmut der Pferde und Strongylose. Tierärztl. Umschau *28:* 551 (1973).

JEGGO, M. H.; SEWELL, M. M. H.: Treatment of pre-patent equine strongyliasis. Vet. Rec. *101:* 187 (1977).

KESTER, W. O.: Strongylus vulgaris — the horse killer. Mod. vet. Pract. *56:* 569 (1975).

LINDBERG, R.: Överlevnad av infektiösa larver as hästens strongylida nematoderi betesgräs. Svensk Vet. Tidn. *28:* 509 (1976).

LITTLE, P. B.; LWIN, H. S.; FRETZ, P.: Verminous encephalitis of horses: experimental induction with Strongylus vulgaris larvae. Amer. J. vet. Res. *35:* 1501 (1974).

McCRAW, B. M.; SLOCOMBE, J. O. D.: Strongylus vulgaris in the horse: a review. Canad. vet. J. *17:* 150 (1976).

OGBOURNE, C. P.; DUNCAN, J. L.: Strongylus vulgaris in the horse: its biology and veterinary importance. Commonwealth Institute of Helminthology Miscellaneous Public. No. 4, Commonwealth Agric. Bureaux, Farnham Royal, Bucks (England) 1977.

RIZZOLI-STALDER, C.; PAULI, B.; LEUENBERGER, H.; HÖRNING, B.: Einfluß von Weidegang und Entwurmung auf den Befall mit Magendarmparasiten des Pferdes. II. Die Parasitenfauna zweier Testbestände. Schweizer Arch. Tierheilk. *118:* 367 (1976).

ROBERTS, S. J.; BENTINCK-SMITH, J.: Therapeutic results of the use of thiabendazole against strongyles in horses. Cornell Vet. *54:* 291 (1964).

ROHRBECK, E.: Strongylidenbefall und Rennleistung bei Traberpferden. Vet.-med. Diss., Berlin (1952).

SIEBEKE, F.: Behandlungsversuche mit dem Breitspektrum-Anthelminthikum Thiabendazol gegen Nematodenbefall in zwei Gestüten. Vet.-med. Dipl.-Arbeit, Berlin (1971).

Slocombe, J. O. D.; McCraw, B. M.: Suppression of the pathogenic effects of Strongylus edentatus larvae with thiabendazole. Canad. J. comp. Med. *39:* 256 (1975).
Slocombe, J. O. D.; Smart, J.: Evaluation of pyrantel pamoate against strongyles in horses. Canad. Vet. J. *16:* 310 (1975).
Smith, J. A.: The occurrence of larvae of Strongylus edentatus in the testicles of stallions. Vet. Rec. *93:* 1835 (1973).
Stoye, M.: Weitere Versuche zur planmäßigen Behandlung des Strongylidenbefalls der Pferde mit Thiabendazol. Dtsch. tierärztl. Wschr. *75:* 622 (1968).
Teredesai, A.: Granulomatöse Lymphadenitis beim Pferd, bedingt durch Strongylus-vulgaris-Larven. Berliner Münchener tierärztl. Wschr. *88:* 61 (1975).
Vibe-Petersen, G.; Nielsen, K.: Verminoes enteritis of tromboembolisk kolik hos hest. En beskrivelse af 36 tilfaelde. Nord. Vet.-Med. *31:* 385 (1979).
Violette, C.; Pistois, M.: Contribution à l'étude de l'activité anthelminthique de l'oxibendazole chez le cheval. Bull. mens Soc. vét. prat. Fr. *60:* 349 (1976).

2.3.2.11. Habronemiasis

Habronemiasis (stomach worm infestation) is caused by 3 species of *Habronema* that inhabit the gastric mucosa or stomach wall as adult heminths. It may occur in a gastric, pulmonary, cutaneous or conjunctival form. Cutaneous habronemiasis is also called 'summer sores'.

Causative Organisms. The *Habronema* species belong to the order Spiruridae ('spiral tail').

Haronema muscae, yellow-orange stomach worm; 8—33 mm long. Eggs: relatively large, 80—90 $\times$ 10—15 μm, sausage-shaped, ovoviviparous.

Habronema microstoma, large white stomach worm; 9—25 mm long. Eggs: relatively small, 45—50 $\times$ 15 μm, sausage-shaped, ovoviviparous.

Habronema megastoma, small white stomach worm; 7—13 mm long. Eggs: ovoviviparous; larvae hatch in the large intestine of the horse and so are not found in the feces.

Habitat: *H. muscae* and *H. microstoma* become embedded by their cranial ends in the gastric mucosa; *H. megastoma* lives in nodules in the stomach wall that range in size from a hazelnut to a hen's egg.

Epizootiology. The *Habronema* species are classified as biohelminths; their eggs and/or larvae are passed in the feces. The 1st-stage larvae of *H. muscae* and *H. megastoma* are ingested in the manure by housefly maggots *(Musca domestica)*, and the 1st-stage larvae of *H. microstoma* by stable fly maggots *(Stomoxys calcitrans)*. The larvae molt a second time in the abdomen and lipoid tissues of the fly, forming 3rd-stage larvae that migrate into the insect's proboscis. When the infected fly feeds on a horse, the larvae leave the proboscis and move toward the warm, moist stimulus.

Infection can be acquired in various ways. If the flies land on the lips, for example, the 3rd-stage *Habronema* larvae actively migrate from the proboscis, penetrate the oral mucosa and travel to the stomach.

Or: The horse may swallow an infected fly, allowing 3rd-stage larvae to enter the stomach directly. Only the young larvae that are swallowed complete their development in the stomach. 'Stray' larvae, on the other hand, can invade other tissues and lead to pathologic changes. For example, if 3rd-stage larvae are deposited on the nasal mucosa, they will migrate to the lungs and produce peribronchial nodules.

Or: Larvae deposited on the conjunctivae cause an ocular or conjunctival habronemiasis (granular conjunctivitis).

Or: Larvae deposited in wounds cause a cutaneous habronemiasis (summer sores).

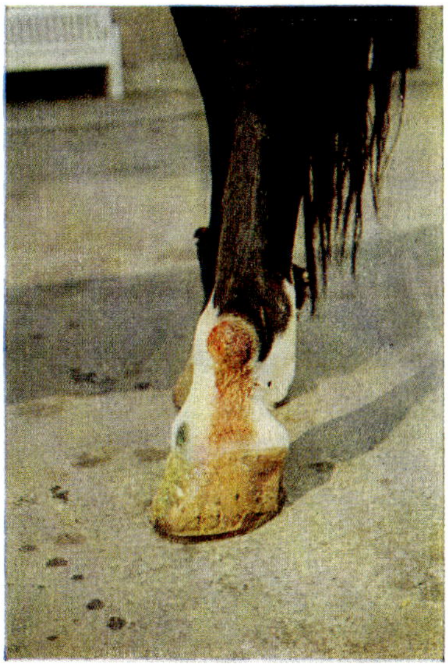

Fig. 2.3. — 6. Cutaneous habronemiasis (summer sores) of the distal limbs.

Symptoms. Habronema species and their developmental stages cause a variety of syndromes depending on the locus of infection:

— Gastrointestinal syndrome. *H. muscae* and *H. microstoma* sometimes cause ulceration and thickening of the gastric mucosa. The result is an intermittent colic that is especially marked during feeding.

H. megastoma forms nodules in the stomach wall. This can lead to various complications, including colic.

— Pulmonary syndrome. Peribronchial nodules as large as hazelnuts form in the lungs. This leads to the syndrome of pulmonary habronemiasis, marked by chronic coughing, dyspnea, impaired performance and emaciation.

— Cutaneous habronemiasis (summer sores). This form mainly affects the distal portions of the limbs but can also occur on the neck and under the harness or saddle (figs. 2.3. — 6 and — 7). It is marked by circumscribed skin lesions associated with heavy granulation and severe pruritus. The disease takes a chronic course and appears during warm weather without regard for age, breed or sex. The sores resist almost all forms of symptomatic treatment but heal with the onset of cold weather.

— Conjunctival habronemiasis. This syndrome is characterized by the clinical picture of granular conjunctivitis (fig. 2.3. — 8).

Diagnosis. The demonstration of *Habronema* eggs in the feces often proves difficult: The thin-shelled, embryonated, relatively small, elongated, sausage-shaped eggs are easily overlooked. *H. megastoma* larvae can be demonstrated only with the migration technique. Although the variable symptoms make a clinical diagnosis of habronemiasis difficult, the enzootic occurrence of poorly-healing summer sores and conjunctivitis in large groups of horses provides an important basis for evaluating the status of the herd.

Treatment. Habronemiases are treated causally with systemic organophosphates; metriphonate (50 mg/kg), dichlorvos (30 mg/kg) and fenchlorphos are suitable when administered orally. Of the imidazole derivatives, thiabendazole at 100 mg/kg and mebendazole at 10 mg/kg have proved effective.

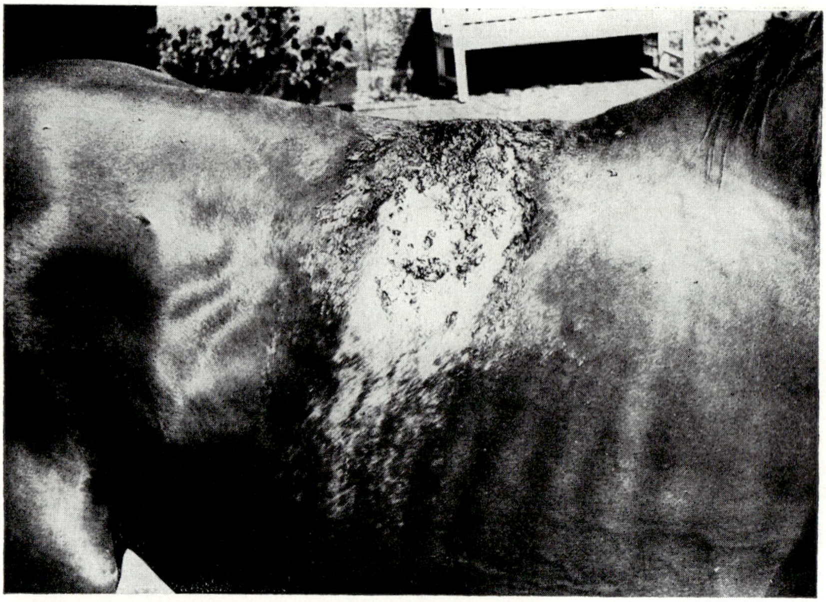

7

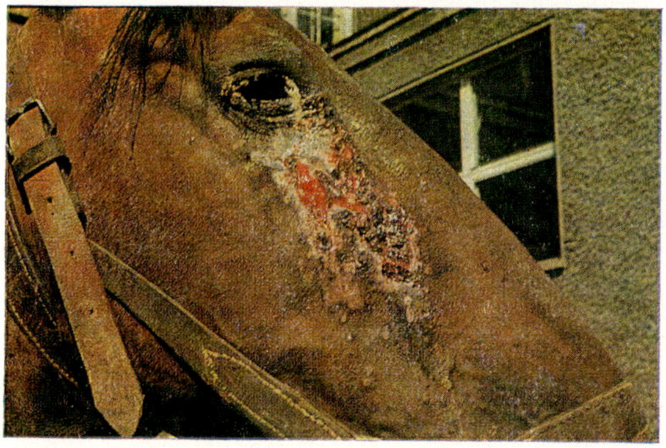

8

Fig. 2.3. — *7.* Cutaneous habronemiasis (summer sores) under the saddle.
Fig. 2.3. — *8.* Conjunctival habronemiasis.

Summer sores and habronema conjunctivitis are additionally treated topically with 2 % aqueous metriphonate solution (applied once daily for 3—5 consecutive days) and in accordance with the principles of surgical wound care.

Prophylaxis. Insecticides are recommended for systematic fly control in housing, and manure packing for the destruction of maggots and *Habronema* eggs.

References

CHABAUD, A. G.: Essai de classification des nématodes Habronematinae. Ann. Parasitol. Hum. Comp. *33:* 445 (1958).

JOYCE, J. R.; HANSELKA, D. W.; BOYD, C. L.: Treatment of habronemiasis of the adnexa of the equine eye. Vet. Med. and Small Animal Clinician *67:* 1008 (1972).

OWCZAREWICZ, A.; SOBIESZEWSKI, K.: Przypadki draszejozy żoładka konia. Med. weteryn. *24:* 737 (1968).
REID, C. H.: Habronemiasis and Corynebacterium 'chest' abscess in california horses. Vet. Med. and Small Animal Clinician *60:* 233 (1965).
WADDELL, A. H.: A survey of Habronema spp. and the identification of thirdstage larvae of H. megastoma and H. muscae in section. Aust. vet. J. *45:* 20 (1968).

23.2.12. Parafilariasis

Parafilariasis (summer bleeding, blood-sweats) is a cutaneous filiariasis that occurs enzootically during the summer in eastern and southern Europe and Iran.

Causative Organism. Parafilaria multipapillosa; 2.8—7 cm long; microfilaria ~ 150—200 μm long.

Habitat: Pea- to hazelnut-size nodules in the loose subcutaneous and intermuscular connective tissue.

Epizootiology. Parafilariasis is considered a vectoral disease. The vectors and intermediate hosts are blood-sucking insects, especially *Haematobia atripaltis.* The *P. multipapillosa* females lay eggs in superficial 'blood cysts' which rupture toward the exterior, releasing microfilariae that are ingested by the intermediate host with the blood. Within the vector they develop into infective 3rd-stage larvae in 10—14 days and are transmitted to other equidae (horses, donkeys, mules).

Symptoms. Parafilariasis appears on hot summer days, usually following heavy exertion (training, racing, etc.). The lesions consist of firm subcutaneous nodules that are palpable mainly about the chest and neck. These nodules rupture, discharging blood mixed with sweat that contains microfilariae and eggs. Affected horses snort and appear restless. The discharge of blood and sweat attracts hematophageous flying insects.

Diagnosis. Besides the typical clinical symptoms, microfilariae are often demonstrable in blood from the nodules (direct specimen or stained smear).

Treatment. The drugs of choice are the organophosphates metriphonate (50 mg/kg) and dichlorvos (30—40 mg/kg), administered orally or applied externally by dipping (2% aqueous trichlorphon solution), as well as diethylcarbamazine. In areas where parafilariasis is enzootic, it may be advisable to treat all horses with one of the foregoing organophosphates in the spring, preferably before the first cases appear.

References

BAUMANN, R.: Beobachtungen beim parasitären Sommerbluten der Pferde. Wien. tierärztl. Mschr. *33:* 52 (1946).
BERTA, S.; SZAÓ, J.: Über das Vorkommen der Parafilariose der Pferde in Ungarn und Beiträge zu ihrer Klinik. Magyar Allat. Lapja *15:* 270 (1960).
GIBSON, T. E.; PEPIN, J. A.; PINSENT, P. J. N.: Parafilaria multipapillosa in the horse. Vet. Rec. *76:* 774 (1964).
GNEDINA, M.; OSIPOW, A.: Zur Biologie der Nematode Parafilaria multipapillosa (Condaminaet Drouilly, 1878), die beim Pferde parasitiert. Helminthologica *2:* 13 (1960).
HEDJAZI; MIRZAYANS, A.: Parafilariose equine dans la region de Teheran (Iran). Aspect clinique et traitment. Rev. Méd. vét. *129:* 1685 (1978).
SCHANZEL, H.; ZARADIL, R.: Parafilarioza koni. Sb. rys. Sk. zemed. Brno *9:* 215 (1961).
SHARMA, K. M. L.; DEORANI, V. P.; DUTT, S. C.: Histopathology of parafilariosis in mules. Curr. Sci. *36:* 240 (1967).

2.3.2.13. Onchocerciasis

Onchocerciasis (worm nodule disease) is caused by parasites that infest the connective tissue and tendons. It is associated with various conditions such as lameness and fistulous withers.

Causative organisms. Two species of the genus *Onchocerca* are causative in the horse:

Onchocerca reticulata, whitish, long, thin, filarid nematode; 15—75 cm long, microfilariae 330—370 μm.

Habitat: Suspensory ligament and its insertion.

Onchocerca cervicalis, 6—50 cm long, microfilariae 210—240 μm.

Habitat: Ligamentum nuchae (adults); microfilariae in subcutaneous connective tissue, sometimes the eye (usually cornea or sclera).

Epizootiology. The life cycle of *O. reticulata* has not been elucidated. *O. cervicalis* on the other hand, deposits microfilariae in the area of the ligamentum nuchae, which then travel to the skin via the blood and lymph. There they are usually found in the papillary layer near the sweat glands. Transmission to other animals is through biting flies *(Culicoides nubeculosus)*, which act as active intermediate hosts. Within this host the microfilariae develop to an infective larval stage in 3—4 weeks, are transmitted to the new host by the blood-sucking fly, and then enter the connective tissue of the predilection sites listed above.

Symptoms. Infestation with *O. cervicalis* leads to necrotic lesions of the ligamentum nuchae that are about the size of a pigeon egg. After the parasites die, these lesions caseate and later partially calcify; at this point they tend to form fistulae, especially in riding horses (fistulous withers). The microfilariae produce pathologic changes in the eyes and lead to ocular changes that must be differentiated from periodic ophthalmia. *O. reticulata* adults produce painful, nodular swellings of the suspensory ligament and sesamoidean ligaments, which may lead to chronic sesamoid lameness.

Diagnosis. The typical changes in the ligamentum nuchae or sesamoidean ligaments offer an adequate basis for a clinical diagnosis. *Onchocerca* can be demonstrated only at necropsy or intraoperatively.

Treatment. Imidazole derivatives and organophosphates are effective in removing the microfilariae. No known drugs are effective against the adults. When the diagnosis is established, a clinical cure can be effected through surgical treatment followed by an often prolonged course of postoperative care.

References

Dimic, J.; Sibalic, J.; Tadic, M.: Periodische Augenentzündung und Augenfilariose der Pferde. Wien. tierärztl. Mschr. *46:* 374 (1959).

Enigk, K.: Die Bedeutung der Onchocerca reticulata (Filaroidea) für die Entstehung von Widerristfisteln beim Pferd. Dtsch. tierärztl. Wschr. *49:* 234 (1941).

Matov, K.; Vasilev, J.; Osikovski, E.; Jančev, J.: Bedeutung der Mikroonchocerken in der Ätiologie der Ophthalmia periodica beim Pferd. Helminthologia *1:* 257 (1959).

Mellor, P. S.: Studies on Onchocerca cervicalis Railliet and Henry, 1910: II. Pathology in the horse. J. Helminthol. *47:* 111 (1973).

Rabalais, F. C.; Eberhard, M. L.; Ashley, D. C.; Platt, T. R.: Survey for equine onchocerciasis in the midwestern United States. Amer. J. vet. Res. *35:* 125 (1974).

Rabalais, F. C.; Votava, C. L.: Cutaneous distribution of microfilariae of Onchocerca cervicalis in horses. Amer. J. vet. Res. *35:* 1369 (1974).

Sahu, S.: Intra-ocular parasite in horses: a report of live cases. Indian vet. J. *51:* 225 (1974).

Table 2.3. — 2. Additional helminthiases

Disease	Causative organism	Distribution	Clinical findings	Diagnosis	Control	Remarks
Schisto-somiasis	*Schistosoma spindale* *Schistosoma indicum*	subtropics, Africa, India	intestinal syndrome	fecal examination	praciquantel	
Micro-nemiasis	*Micronema deletrix*		CNS signs, disturbances of the urinary tract and lungs	postmortem (gross and histologic lesions)	unknown	
Pelodera dermatitis	*Pelodera strongyloides*		cutaneous syndrome	skin scrapings	thiabendazole	
Setariasis	*Setaris equina*		peritoneal cavity, peri-cardium, hepatic capsule, eye	incidental finding, usually after slaughter or at necropsy		vector: presumably mosquitoes
Elaeo-phoriasis	*Elaeophora boehmi*		lameness in the area of the pas-tern bone and cannon (vascular lesions)			
Theliaziasis	*Thelazia lacrymalis*	North America, northern Africa, Europe	ocular syndrome	direct de-monstration in conjunc-tival sac	imidazole preparations	vector: Musca autumnalis
Trichinosis	*Trichinella spiralis*	rare	muscular syndrome	serologic, trichino-scopy	meat in-spection; note horse as source of trichina in-fection!	transmitted by food con-taminated with intes-tinal or muscle trichinae
Diro-filariasis	*Dirofilaria immitis*	rare	cardiovascular syndrome	intra vitam, necropsy	—	only one case described to date

2.3.2.14. Additional Helminthiases

Eight additional diseases caused by helminth parasites are listed in table 2.3. — 2. These helminthiases are of relatively minor economic importance, relatively uncommon or occur enzootically outside of Central Europe, and, overall, appear to be of some importance in the differential diagnosis of diseases that take a similar course.

References

CSOKOR, J.: Experimentelle Infektion eines Pferdes mit Trichinen. Allg. Wiener med. Ztg. *29:* 248 (1884).
FARRINGTON, D. O.; LUNDVALL, R. L.; GREVE, J. H.: Pelodera strongyloides dermatitis in a horse in Iowa. Veterin. med. and Small Animal Clinician, Bonner Springer, Kansas *71:* 1199 (1976).
FRÉCHETTE, J. L.; MARCOUX, M.; PIERRE, H. S.: Presence de Thelazia sp. au Quebec chez le cheval et la vache. Canad. Vet. J. *17:* 114 (1976).
KLEIN, J. B.; STODDARD, E. D.: Dirofilaria immitis recovered from a horse. J. Amer. vet. med. Assoc. *171:* 354 (1977).
LYONS, E. T.; DRUDGE, J. H.; TOLLIVER, S. C.: Thelazia lacrymalis in horses in Kentucky and observations on the face fly (Musca autumnalis) as a probable intermediate host. J. Parasitol. *62:* 877 (1976).
LÖHRER, J.; HÖRNING, B.: Thelazia lacrymalis beim Pferd. Schweizer Arch. Tierheilk. *109:* 644 (1967).
ORTLEPP, R. J.: On a filaria worm from the eye of a horse. J. South African vet. med. Assoc. *33:* 43 (1962).
POHLENZ, J.; ECKERT, J.; MINDER, H. P.: Zentralnervöse Störungen beim Pferd, verursacht durch Nematoden der Gattung Nicronema (Rhabditida). Berliner Münchener tierärztl. Wschr. *94:* 216 (1981).
RUBIN, H. L.; WOODARD, J. C.: Equine infection with Micronema deletrix. J. Amer. vet. med. Assoc. *165:* 256 (1974).
SUPPERER, R.: Filariosen der Pferde in Österreich. Wien. tierärztl. Wschr. *40:* 193 (1953).
WÖHRL, H.; HÖRCHNER, F.; GRELCK, H.: Zur Trichinellose des Pferdes. Arch. Lebensmittelhyg. *28:* 198 (1977).

2.3.3. Diseases Caused by Arthropod Parasites

Parasitic arthropods, both insects and arachnids, are mainly important as causative agents of skin diseases. Many of them (ticks, flies, mosquitoes) can serve as vectors for the transmission of infections, while others cause annoyance and worry to horses and thus adversely affect their performance. Only the larvae of the botfly and nasal botfly live as true endoparasites. The continuing protection of horses from harmful arthropods has become an important veterinary responsibility.

2.3.3.1. Mange

Definition. Mange is a collective term for enzootic skin diseases, usually chronic, that are characterized by pruritus and hair loss. Mange in the horse is caused by three different species of mite, and its course is influenced by certain conditions of stabling and nutrion. According to the older literature, dangerous outbreaks of mange occurred during wartime among heavily-worked army horses, sometimes with devastating results. In recent decades relatively little has been reported about mange in horses. In the GDR and FRG, the reporting and control of sarcoptic and psoroptic mange are required by law.

Epizootiology. Infection is usually acquired by direct contact between horses; inanimate objects such as grooming tools and tack are a less frequent source of infestation. The causative mites of mange are all host-specific ectoparasites. After mating, the females lay 25 to 100 eggs in a relatively short time, which hatch into 6-legged larvae that mature to adults in 2—3 weeks via an 8-legged nymphal stage. The reproduction rate can increase dramatically in malnourished or cachexic animals, especially during minimal-daylight periods.

2.3.3.1.1. *Sarcoptic Mange*

Etiology. The causative mite is *Sarcoptes equi*, 0.2—0.45 mm long and the smallest of the mites that produce mange in horses. The body is turtle-shaped with a short head and short, thick legs.

Habitat: The sarcoptic mite lives in burrows in the epidermis of the stratum spinosum and stratum granulosum.

Symptoms. Sarcoptic mange usually commences on the head and spreads to the neck and shoulder area as well as to the skin below the harness and saddle. It tends to become generalized and within a week may involve the entire body except for the distal limbs. The lesions consist of cutaneous nodules, vesicles, scabs and crusts and are associated with intense pruritus, patchy hair loss, and thickening and wrinkling of the skin. Scratch wounds are commonly present. The skin lesions are accompanied by systemic effects, and death may occur in neglected cases. Sarcoptic mange is a zoonosis; in humans it produces the disease known as pseudoscabies.

2.3.3.1.2. *Psoroptic Mange*

Etiology. The causative mite is *Psoroptes equi*, 0.5—0.8 mm long with a long head and legs.

Habitat: The psoroptic mite lives on the skin, between and below the scabs, pierces the skin and feeds on lymph, tissue fluids, and sometimes blood.

Symptoms. The lesions usually start at the base of the mane or tail and may spread to involve the entire torso. There is severe pruritus with circumscribed hair loss, nodulation and thickening of the skin. The skin appears dry and parchment-like. If lesions become widespread, the animal will show systemic effects including emaciation.

2.3.3.1.3. *Chorioptic Mange (Foot Mange)*

Etiology. The causative mite is *Chorioptes equi*, 0.3—0.6 mm long, with a head as broad as it is long, and long legs.

Habitat: The chorioptic mite lives on the skin surface on the back of the pastern, especially in breeds with long fetlock hairs. The mites 'graze' the upper layer of epidermis, feeding on epidermal cells, inflammatory exudate and lymph.

Symptoms. Foot mange can be divided into three forms or stages: eczema crustosum, eczema madidans and eczema verrucosum. It usually commences with a circumscribed, serocellular infiltration, vesiculation, and the formation of scabs and crusts. This is followed by a loss of the upper epidermal layers, and the exposed corium presents a reddish, granulation-like, foul-smelling, weeping, greasy surface. The hairs become matted together due to the continuous sloughing of tissue. Secondary bacterial invasion of the skin lesions is already apparent at this stage. In protracted cases, multiple wartlike lesions ranging from several millimeters to several centimeters in diameter eventually appear. All three forms of foot mange are accompanied by a severe pruritus that is especially intense at night and in a warm, humid stable. Infested horses are restless and stomp their feet incessantly. Chain or rope injuries may result when a tied horse attempts to bite or lick the affected parts. Foot mange is most prevalent during the fall, winter and spring months.

Diagnosis. A tentative diagnosis of mange may be made on the basis of pruritus associated with the aforementioned skin lesions, after infestations with biting or sucking lice have been excluded. The tentative diagnosis is confirmed by microscopic demonstration of the causative mite. For this purpose skin scrapings are taken from the edges of the lesions and examined microscopically. A 'live' demonstration under the stereo microscope is recommended. Differentiation of the mites is readily made from morphologic features.

Treatment and Prophylaxis. Sarcoptic and psoroptic mange are treated with insecticides based on organophosphates, carbamates, or chlorinated hydrocarbons (though the latter are less often used because of their toxicity). A proven technique is to apply 2 % aqueous metriphonate or trichlorphon solution to the entire body as a spray or dip, using a maximum solution volume of 1200 ml for adult horses, 800 ml for yearlings, and 400 ml for foals. Given the relatively low therapeutic range of the organophosphates, these doses should not be exceeded. All horses on the premises should be treated, and treatment should be repeated after 5—10 days. Affected skin areas should be carefully washed with the insecticide, especially around the edges of lesions. If the aforementioned insecticides are unavailable or cannot be used, then dipping with a mixture of equal parts sodium thiosulfate (60 %) and hydrochloric acid (6 %) is acceptable. The liberated sulfur dioxide and sulfur ions will exert a miticidal action. Treatment is repeated twice at intervals of 5—10 days. There are also medicaments available for local application. One such preparation, called Helmerich mange ointment, is composed of precipitated sulfur, potassium carbonate and petrolatum in a ratio of 2 : 1 : 8. Another, called Viennese tar liniment, consists of equal parts of wood tar, sublimed sulfur and saponin potassium, to which propyl alcohol is added 1 : 1.

Exposure to sulfur dioxide gas in a closed chamber is effective, but it is relatively costly and time-consuming compared to other methods. The horse is placed into a hermetically-sealed cabinet that covers all but the animal's head, which is treated beforehand with a miticidal agent. Then the cabinet is filled with 4—5 vol.% SO_2 gas, and exposure is maintained for 60 minutes at a temperature of 25—30 °C. The treatment is 100 % efficient in killing mites when repeated after 8 days.

Treatment is supported by a high-protein diet, vitamin A supplementation and, following the initial insecticide treatment, by daily outdoor exercise. Tack items that come in contact with the skin are treated with insecticide solution or 2 % cresol.

Equine mange in the GDR is periodically made notifiable, and appropriate control measures are enforced. In danger areas, every new arrival should be examined clinically for mange, and skin scrapings should be examined in suspected cases. Stables are disinfected by spraying with a state-approved insecticide. Because the causative mites can live only a short time away from the host, the vacating of stables for a 3-week period is a sound control measure.

The *strategy for mange control* depends upon whether and to what degree skin lesions (crusts, weeping, verrucae) have developed. But regardless of the type of lesions present, a 4-step regimen of local therapy is followed.

- The limbs are cleaned from the coronary band up to the carpus or hock with a keratolytic soft-soap solution and allowed to dry, having first covered the coronary band with a bay ointment.
- The hairs at the fetlock are clipped.
- A contact insecticide is applied. Hexachlorocyclohexane γ-isomer (0.5—1 %) or metriphonate (2 %) is suitable for application by rubbing or dipping; treatment is repeated after 3, 5 and 10 days.

— Aftercare. In advanced cases the single application of a bactericidal sulfonamide or antibiotic spray is indicated.

If weeping or verrucous eczema is present, a dessicating, anti-inflammatory mixture of wood tar and zinc oxide should be applied at 2-day intervals. Advanced cases of eczema verrucosum are treated surgically. In heavy draft breeds, regular care of the long hairs at the fetlock is essential for the prevention of foot mange. In danger areas, all new arrivals should be examined for *Chorioptes equi* infestation, and all resident horses should be routinely examined once or twice yearly; insecticidal therapy (see Treatment) is then instituted if required.

References

Bochentin, R.: Die Bekämpfung der Pferderäude mit Hexachlorcyclohexan. Vet.-med. Diss. Berlin (1949).

Borchert, A.: Über Räudebehandlung mit Hexachlorcyclohexan. Mh. Vet.-Med. *4:* 153 (1949).

Franken, A.: Die Entwicklung der Räudebekämpfung der Haustiere mit besonderer Berücksichtigung der Begasung. Vet.-med. Diss., Hannover (1947).

Gaede, G. W.: Versuche und Beobachtungen bei der Bekämpfung der Pferderäude mit Schwefelsubstanzverbrennung. Vet.-med. Diss., Hannover (1947).

Kobulej, T.: Sarcoptes-Studien II. Beiträge zur Unterscheidung der an Haustieren schmarotzenden Vertreter der Gattung Sarcoptes. Acta vet. hung. *V:* 233 (1955).

Kurylo, P.: Die Behandlung von Räudepferden mit Wiener Teeröl. Vet.-med. Diss., Hannover (1947).

Kutzer, E.: Zur Wirtsspezifität der Gattung Sarcoptes. Z. Parasitenk. *28:* 60 (1966).

Kutzer, E.: Sarcoptes-Milben und Sarcoptesräude der Haustiere. Angew. Parasitol. *11:* Merkbl.-Nr. 17 (1970).

Mehls, H. J.: Eine seltene Form der Chorioptes-Räude beim Pferd. Berliner Münchener tierärztl. Wschr. *65:* 9 (1952).

Pecher, V.; Eichler, Wd.: Räudemilbentabelle der wichtigsten Haussäugetiere. Mh. Vet.-Med. *3:* 86 (1948).

Schikora, F.: Beiträge zur Morphologie von Sarcoptes equi Gerlach. Z. Infekt. Krankh. parasit. Krankh. Hyg. Haustiere *23:* 30 (1922).

2.3.3.2. Demodiciasis

Definition. Demodiciasis (follicular mite infestation, follicular mange) is a clinically inconspicuous skin disease that is relatively uncommon in horses.

Etiology. Demodex equi; 300—400 μm long, 40—50 μm wide; vermiform body with 4 pairs of stubby legs that terminate in claws; eggs: 60—80 × 40—50 μm, elliptical.

Epizootiology. Infection results from direct contact, and most transmissions probably are from dams to nursing foals. *Demodex equi* is strictly host-specific. Gravid females deposit eggs in the hair follicles, and these develop into sexually dimorphic adult mites within 3—4 weeks through two 6-legged larval stages and two nymphal stages. The *Demodex* mites and their developmental stages live in colonies in the hair follicles and cutaneous connective tissue. They form pinhead- to pea-size nodules in the skin.

Symptoms. Infestation with *Demodex* mites leads to circumscribed areas of hair loss on the head, usually about the eyes. In longstanding cases the infestation may spread to the shoulder, dorsum, flank, and sometimes the anterior and ventral thorax. Pruritus is absent. Solid, firmly-seated nodules are detected on palpation of affected areas.

Diagnosis. If clinical findings suggest infestation, either the nodules are biopsied, or skin scrapings are taken with a knife or curette and examined microscopically. Differentiation must be made from mange and enzootic skin diseases of other etiology.

Treatment and Prophylaxis. Localized cases are treated by sponging affected areas with 2% aqueous metriphonate or dichlorvos solution. If infestation is generalized, organophosphates are applied by a pour-on technique (e.g., 6% trichlorphon solution at 18 mg/kg BW). So far no prophylactic measure is known that will prevent *Demodex* nfections in foals.

References

Aries, L.: Über Demodikosis bei Pferden. Dtsch. tierärztl. Wschr. *58:* 102 (1951).

Künzel, K.: Die Behandlung der Räude der Einhufer in ihrer Abhängigkeit von der Biologie der Milben mit besonderer Berücksichtigung des Begasungsverfahrens. Vet.-med. Diss., Hannover (1947).

2.3.3.3. Tick Infestation

Definition. Ticks are important both as ectoparasites and as vectors for the transmission of equine babesiosis and various viral diseases. Tick infestations occur during the grazing season.

Etiology. The composition of the tick population varies from one climatic zone to the next. In Central Europe the common wood tick *(Ixodes ricinus)* is predominant; *Dermacentor marginatus, Dermacentor reticulatus* and *Haemaphysalis punctata* also occur. All are 3-host ticks belonging to the family Ixodidae (hard ticks).

Ixodes ricinus; 2.8—10 mm long, reddish-brown to bluish-gray in color, resembles a castor bean when engorged with blood; markedly euryxenous.

Epizootiology. Tick larvae, nymphs and adults attach to horses or other mammals solely for the purpose of sucking blood and spend the rest of their lives on vegetation, usually bushes and shrubbery. It is there that the females lay their eggs, about 3000 over a period of a month at an ambient temperature above 15—17 °C. If the relative humidity is high, the eggs hatch in 3—6 weeks into 6-legged larvae. These larvae attach to small mammals, suck blood, then drop to the ground where they molt after a month or more to become 8-legged nymphs, which again attach to a passing host, preferably a small to medium-size mammal, and suck blood. When engorged, the nymphs drop to the ground and, if environmental conditions are favorable (relatively high ambient temperature and humidity), develop in 10—12 weeks into adult ticks, which begin their search for a new host. At this time the horse, among other animals, may become infested. In Central Europe only the aforementioned *Dermacentor* species and *Haemaphysalis punctata* are important as vectors for the transmission of equine babesiosis.

Symptoms. In tick areas, horses at stud, nursery or racing-stable conditions should be examined regularly during the grazing season (especially in the spring) for tick infestation. Adult ticks are readily visible with the naked eye as they lie attached to their sites of predilection with their hypostome buried deep in the skin. For ascertaining genus and species in a parasitologic facility, the ticks are carefully removed from the body surface with the aid of a pipette. Before doing this, it is first necessary to daub the site with toluene, ether or strong alcohol solution in order to paralyze the tick's mouthparts; otherwise they will be left in the skin and create a persistent source of ulceration.

Differential diagnosis must be made from skin diseases of other etiology and from infestation with horse louse-flies.

Treatment and Prophylaxis. Infested horses are treated by the application of insecticides that are active against ticks. The organophosphate insecticides are most commonly used. In low-grade infestations, it is sufficient to wash infested areas locally with an insecticidal solution. If more than 50% of the horses in a group are infested with ticks, spraying of the entire group is recommended.

Prophylaxis on heavily-stocked grazing areas that are known to be tick-infested involves adherence to a program of hygienic pasture management and land improvement during and outside the vegetative period, with the object of minimizing the tick population. The spraying of pastures with insecticides for tick eradication presents real problems from an ecologic standpoint under Central European conditions and should be avoided if at all possible.

References

AESCHLIMANN, A.; BÜTHIKER, W.; ELBL, A.; HOOGSTRAAL, H.: A propos des tiques de Suisse (Arachnoidea, Acarina, Ixodidae). Rev. Suisse Zool. *72:* 577 (1965).

LIEBISCH, A.: Die Rolle einheimischer Zecken (Ixodidae) in der Epidemiologie des Q-Fiebers in Deutschland. Dtsch. tierärztl. Wschr. *83:* 274 (1976).

2.3.3.4. Infestation with Sucking Lice

Definition. Infestation with sucking lice leads to changes in the haircoat and a reduction of working capacity in horses of all ages. Anemia may develop in heavily-infested foals. This ectoparasitism is most common during the late winter and early spring and can spread extensively among stabled horses.

Etiology. Haematopinus asini, the sucking louse. 2.6—3.6 mm long; narrow, elongated head; thorax broader than head, brown with black spots; abdomen oval and at times yellow-gray; stationary, stenoxenous ectoparasite; blood-sucker.

Habitat: The haircoat, especially in protected areas.

Epizootiology. Infection is acquired by contact, either with other resident animals, new arrivals, or outside horses at competitive events. The adult lice have a life span of 30—40 days and seldom survive longer than 3—7 days when separated from the host. Gravid females deposit 25—300 barrel-shaped eggs about 1 mm in diameter on the hairs, from which adult lice develop in 3—6 weeks via 3 larval stages. The larvae (fig. 2.3. — 9) are also hematophagous. The louse population is strongly influenced by external factors: Dark, warm housing, high stocking densities, an unbalanced diet deficient in vitamin A, and a long, unkempt or dirty haircoat create favorable living conditions for the lice.

Symptoms. Restlessness and pruritus are caused by the active movements of the lice and by their piercing of the skin to suck blood. Infested horses rub against fixed objects, bite at affected areas and paw the ground. The haircoat appears scruffy and unkempt, and sometimes there is circumscribed alopecia with bloody crusts in the hairless areas. Heavy infestations lead to emacination and, in young horses, to anemia. The lice and their eggs ('nits'), which are cemented to the hairs, are visible on close inspection.

In addition to its pathogenic properties, the sucking louse is also capable of transmitting the causative organisms of various infectious diseases.

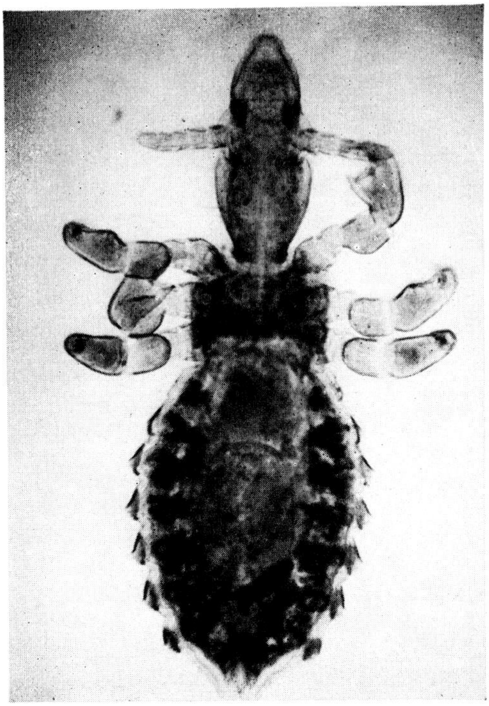

9

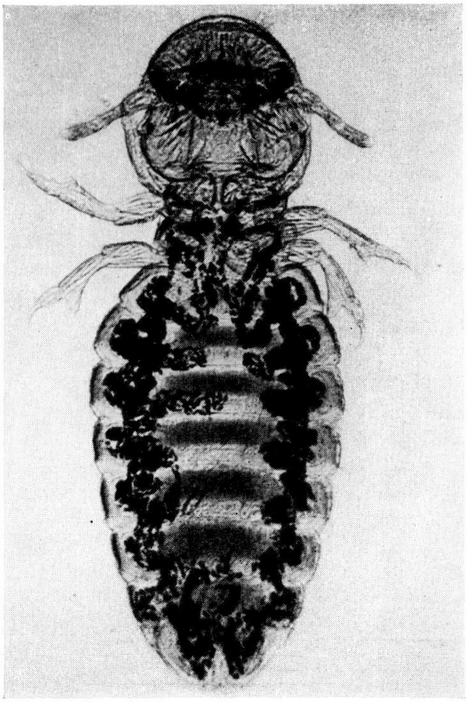

10

Fig. 2.3. — 9. Larva of the sucking louse, *Haematopinus asini macrocephalus*.
Fig. 2.3. — 10. The biting louse, *Werneckiella equi*.

Diagnosis. The foregoing clinical changes, combined with the direct demonstration of the lice with the aid of a loupe, enable a prompt diagnosis to be made.

Differential Diagnosis. Infestation with biting lice, sarcoptic and psoroptic mange (early stage), and skin diseases of other etiology most be excluded.

Treatment and Prophylaxis. Through the selective use of contact or systemic insecticides, it is possible to eradicate all sucking lice in a given horse population within a short time. *Haematopinus asini macrocephalus* has proved highly susceptible to chlorinated hydrocarbons (lindane) as well as to the less toxic organophosphates (metriphonate, butonate, coumaphos, dimethoate) and carbamates (carbaryl). Carbaryl has proved efficient when used as a whole-body spray, the insecticide being administered in 0.5—1% aqueous solution in a total volume not exceeding 1200 ml per adult horse. A simpler technique is the pour-on application of metriphonate, e.g. as a 6% solution. Because none of the aforementioned insecticides is definitely ovicidal, and their residual protection is of relatively short duration, it is necessary to *repeat the treatment after 5—10 days.* It is important that all the horses on the premises be treated. Stables are disinfected with the same insecticide used on the horses. All resident horses should be examined regularly for louse infestation, and introduced horses examined on arrival. If lice are found, a control program should be instituted with the object of eradicating all lice on the premises.

References

EICHLER, WD.: Grenzfälle der Parasitendifferenzierung. II. Esel- und Pferdelaus. Mh. Vet.-Med. *6:* 76 (1951).
HIEPE, TH.; RIBBECK, R.: Medikamentelle Bekämpfung der Parasitosen in Nutztierbeständen — eine Übersicht der in der DDR registrierten Antiparasitaria. medicamentum *17:* 327 (1976).
ZŁOTORZYCKA, J.; EICHLER, WD.; LUDWIG, H. W.: Taxonomie und Biologie der Mallophagen und Läuse mitteleuropäischer Haus- und Nutztiere. Parasitol. Schriftenreihe, Vol. 22 (VEB Gustav Fischer Verlag, Jena 1974).

2.3.3.5. Infestation with Biting Lice

Definition. This is an infestation with stationary, strictly host-specific insects of the order Mallophaga. It can occur as an enzootic skin disease, particularly in large, stabled horse populations.

Etiology. Werneckiella equi (Bovicola equi), the biting louse (fig. 2.3. — 10). 1.4 to 1.8 mm long, biting-chewing mouthparts; head reddish-brown, rounded, and broader than thorax; abdomen yellow-white, egg-shaped. The biting louse feeds mainly on cutaneous exudate and hairs.

Epizootiology. Infection spreads by contact among horses; *W. equi* is strictly stenoxenous. The louse is introduced into a clean herd mainly by new arrivals or by contact with outside horses at events. The entire life cycle of the biting louse takes place on the horse. *W. equi* females deposit a total of about 80—120 eggs on the hairs over a 2—3 month period. The eggs hatch in 7 days or more, producing larvae that mature to adults within 14 days through 2 further larval stages. The estimated life span of the adult is 60 days. *W. equi* males are not often found; reportedly, the ratio of females to males is greater than 10: 1. Some degree of parthenogenesis is presumed. Conditions for the life and development of biting lice are optimal during the winter months and in dimly-lit stables, and so the highest population densities and greatest damage occur in such settings. The biting louse is considered a vector for the virus of equine infectious anemia.

Symptoms. Movement and biting by the lice cause restlessness, pruritus, irritability and circumscribed alopecia. In heavy infestations the constant restlessness and rubbing of the skin can lead to local inflammatory lesions and denudation (fig. 2.3. — 11).

Diagnosis. Biting lice are demonstrated by inspection with the naked eye or with a loupe. Careful examination of the haircoat will reveal not only the adult lice and their developmental stages, but also the eggs glued to the hairs. These appear as whitish, pear-shaped objects about 0.8—1.2 mm in diameter.

Differential Diagnosis. The main condition to be differentiated is infestation with sucking lice. This is done by microscopic identification of the causative parasite in hair samples. Mixed infections with biting and sucking lice are not uncommon. Differentiation from infestations with other ectoparasites such as louse-flies, ticks and mites is easily made by examination of the causative parasite.

Treatment and Prophylaxis. Clinically overt infestations with biting lice are treated by spraying, dipping or dusting the animal with an organophosphate or carbamate insecticide. All horses on the premises should be treated, and treatment should be repeated after 8—10 days to kill newly-hatched larvae.

From a prophylactic standpoint, all new arrivals should be excluded as sources of infection by clinical examination and, if necessary, by the application of one of the aforementioned insecticides.

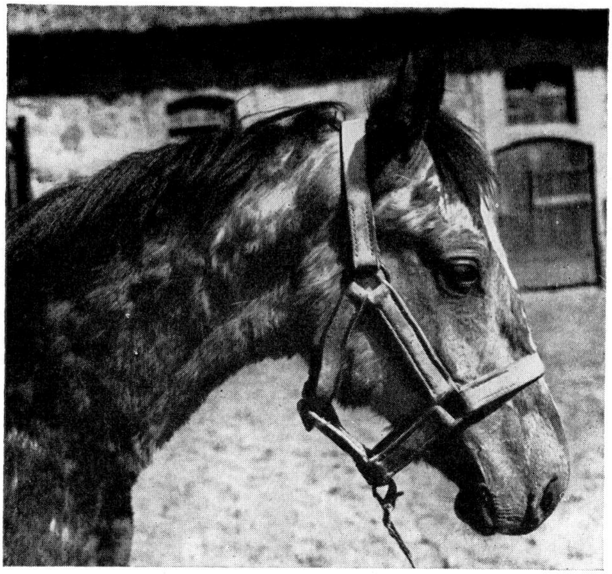

Fig. 2.3. — 11. Infestation with biting lice.

Reference

Złotorzycka, J.; Eichler, Wd.; Ludwig, H. W.: Taxonomie und Biologie der Mallophagen und Läuse mitteleuropäischer Haus- und Nutztiere. Parasitol. Schriftenreihe, Vol. 22 (VEB Gustav Fischer Verlag, Jena 1974).

2.3.3.6. Attack by Horseflies and Deerflies

Definition. Attacks by species of the family Tabanidae are included among the parasitism seen while at pasture. These buzzing and biting insects cause considerable worry and restlessness and, being blood-suckers, can cause loss of condition. The tabanids are also important as vectors of infectious diseases.

Etiology. In Central Europe, three genera of Tabanidae are of principal importance as ectoparasites. The following species are among the best known:

Tabanus bovinus, the bovine gadfly; about 2 cm long.

Tabanus fuscicostatus; about 2 cm long.

Haematopota pluvialis; 1.2—1.5 cm long.

Chrysops cecutiens, the small horsefly; about 1 cm long.

The three genera are distinguished from one another not only by their size but also by distinctive morphologic features and living habits.

Epizootiology. Tabanids live in warm, moist, muddy or marshy areas where water is abundant. They are transitory, decidedly euryxenous ectoparasites. Blood is sucked only by adult females. One female lays up to 3000 eggs, depositing them on plants growing in standing water. Puddles, moist ground and mud are favored, and so eggs are often laid in trampled fields and around watering troughs. They hatch into long, slender larvae that molt 7 or 8 times and are capable of overwintering.

The larval phase is followed by pupation and the adult stage. The female tabanids attack suitable hosts, which include the horse, and suck blood. One female horsefly can ingest 0.2—1 ml of blood at a time, defecating a portion of it onto the skin of the host while continuing to feed.

Symptoms. The buzzing and biting flies cause considerable worry and restlessness. Attacks can cause shying in working and riding horses, and severe attacks can lead to accidents. Loss of condition and impaired working capacity may be seen in performance and athletic horses. Tabanids sometimes pierce the skin repeatedly during one feeding, causing subsequent bleeding that attracts other flying pests which cause additional annoyance. The painful bites of the tabanids stimulate pruritus, and a toxin is excreted that causes wheals to form. The tabinids are also capable of transmitting pathogenic microorganisms (the EIA virus, among others) and filariae.

Diagnosis. Tabanids are readily distinguished from other flying insects by their characteristic appearance and behavior. Confusion with botflies is the most frequent error.

Treatment and Prophylaxis. Generally, treatment is not undertaken. The spraying of horses with insecticides is not recommended. Rellents are useful for prophylaxis, but their effect persists no longer than 3 days. The detection of development stages in breeding areas is often complicated and time-consuming, and the prophylactic control of larval stages presents the veterinarian with a difficult task. Reliance on nocturnal grazing to avoid the flies, which are active only during the day, cannot solve the problem.

The use of ‘horsefly traps’ is an effective biologic control measure on problem pastures. These traps consist of black-and-white, upright panels (75×75 cm) coated with a special glue that are set up at right angles to the wind about 50 cm above the ground in suitable locations. Experience with these traps to date has been promising.

References

Bauer, B.; Wetzel, H.: Versuche mit Fliegenfallen zur Tabanidenbekämpfung auf der Weide. Tierärztl. Umschau *29:* 206 (1974).

Hawkins, J. A.; Adams, W. V.; Cook, L.; Wilson, B. H.; Roth, E. E.: Role of horse fly (Tabanus fuscicostatus Hine) and stable fly (Stomoxys calcitrans L.) in transmission of equine infectious anemia to ponies in Louisiana. Amer. J. vet. Res. *34:* 1583 (1973).

Moucha, J.: Haematopota scutellata (Diptera, Tabanidae), auch in Deutschland festgestellt. Nachr.-Bl. Bayer. Ent. *15:* 72 (1966).

Tabuchi, E.; Yajima, A.; Shimoda, K.; Shibata, M.; Murakami, A.; Ito, K.: Control test of horse flies (Tabanidae) in the race course. equine health laboratory type in 1970. Exper. Rep. Equine Health Lab., 49 (1971).

2.3.3.7. Attack by Houseflies, Face Flies and Stable Flies

Definition. Attacks by these flies are frequent in larger horse populations during the warm months, both in the stable and at pasture. These insects are important both as direct ectoparasites and as vectors for the transmission of disease.

Etiology. Several of the many species of the family Muscidae (true flies) display a high affinity for the horse:

Musca domestica, the common housefly; about 0.7 cm long; cosmopolitan.

Musca autumnalis, the face fly.

Stomoxys calcitrans, the common stable fly; 0.6 cm long, blood-sucker.

Epizootiology. The foregoing fly species, of which *M. domestica* is the most common, are classed as transitory, euryxenous, partially facultative parasites. The life cycle of these species is tied to excrement or decaying organic matter; fresh horse manure is preferred. There the females lay several hundred eggs, from which adult insects develop in 1—3 weeks after passing through 3 larval stages and 1 pupal stage. In Central Europe as many as 6—10 generations can develop during the warm season. This can result in a very large fly population, especially in areas where livestock are highly concentrated. Horse manure provides the fly maggots with basic nutrients (carbohydrates, fats, proteins) as well as essential vitamins such as biotin, nicotinic acid, patothenic acid, pyridoxine, riboflavin, thiamine, folic acid and choline.

Symptoms. Houseflies and face flies cause considerable worry by their buzzing and mechanical irritation, especially when present in large numbers. Horses may become violent in their attempts to escape the flies. The insects are a particular problem on breeding farms during the nursing period, and on horses that have wounds or skin lesions caused by insect bites, since *M. domestica* and *M. autumnalis* have a strong affinity for blood and wound secretions, on which they feed with their licking-sucking mouthparts. *Stomoxys calcitrans* is a blood-sucker that can cause both worry and loss of condition due to blood loss. The importance of the flies as vectors of disease and intermediate hosts of pathogenic organisms should not be underestimated. *St. calcitrans* has been shown to be a vector for *Habronema microstoma* (summer sores) and the causative virus of equine infectious anemia; *M. domestica* for *Habronema muscae* and *H. megastoma* (summer sores); and *M. autumnalis* for rickettsiae (infectious keratoconjunctivitis) and *Thelazia lacrymalis* (eyeworm infestation).

Diagnosis. The flies should be caught and submitted to a parasitologic or entomologic facility for species identification. Fly populations should be regularly monitored, both quantitatively and qualitatively, on stud farms and around racing stables.

Treatment and Prophylaxis. The problem of fly control under pastoral conditions has not yet been adequately resolved. Fly attacks in stables can be controlled by spraying with insecticides that are active against the insects. The principal insecticides in current use are those having a phosphate base (metriophonate, bromophos and dimethoate) or pyrethrum base. During spraying, safety precautions such as removing feed residues and keeping the spray off the lower portions of walls are recommended. The density of fly populations can be effectively reduced by a program of three sprayings done in the early spring, midsummer and fall. The use of fly strips is also recommended in enclosed areas during the summer months. Another effective prophylactic measure is to eliminate breeding places by heaping manure (heat generation) and covering it with soil or 5 % chlorinated lime solution. The application of insecticides to breeding sites is not advised.

References

Derbeneva-Ukhova, V. P.; Lineva, V. A.: Poiski novykh sredstv unichtozhenija preimaginal'nykh faz razvitija mukh. Soobshenije 1. Predvaritel'nye ispytanija ammiachnykh udobrenij v kachestve larvicidov protiv Musca domestica L. Med. Parazitol. i parazitarnye Bolezni, Moskva *46:* 427 (1977).

Erbendruth, W.: Ein Beitrag zur Fliegenbekämpfung in Milchviehanlagen unter den tropischen Bedingungen der Republik Kuba bei besonderer Berücksichtigung tierhygienischer Maßnahmen und des Einsatzes von Flibol E. Vet.-med. Diss., Leipzig (1975).

Knobloch, H.; Ribbeck, R.; Hiepe, Th.: Untersuchungen zur Entwicklung von Musca domestica Linné, 1758, und Fannia canicularis Linné, 1761, in verschiedenen Brutsubstraten. Mh. Vet.-Med. *32:* 905 (1977).

2.3.3.8. Gasterophilosis

Definition. Gasterophilosis (bot infestation) is an intestinal and cutaneous myiasis specific for equidae that is caused by the prolonged residence of *Gasterophilus* larvae in the gastrointestinal tract and by the subdermal migration of the 1st-stage larvae.

Etiology. The causative organisms belong to the family Gasterophilidae (botflies, bots). The horse is parasitized only by species of the genus *Gasterophilus*, whose 2nd- and 3rd-stage larvae (L 2 and L 3) inhabit various portions of the intestinal tract. Six species are important in the Palearctic region:

Gasterophilus intestinalis	Habitat: gastric mucosa (L 2 and 3)
G. inermis	Habitat: gastric mucosa
G. haemorrhoidalis	Habitat: L 2 in stomach, sometimes pharynx, esophagus, duodenum; L 3 in rectum.
G. nasalis	Habitat: duodenum
G. nigricornis	Habitat: duodenum
G. pecorum	Habitat: duodenum

The adult flies are 8—18 mm long, hairy, and resemble a bumble bee. Their life span does not exceed 2—3 weeks. Their rudimentary mouthparts prohibit them from feeding, and the flies must rely on energy stores accumulated during the larval and pupal period. The parasitic 3rd-stage larvae remain in the intestinal tract for 8 to 9 months, ultimately reaching a length of 2 cm. Data on the reproductive characteristics of the parasites are presented in table 2.3. — 3.

Epizootiology. The fly is active only during the warm season, the exact period of fly activity varying from one species to the next. Flying and mating take place on sunny, windless days. The females lay from 150 to 2,500 eggs, depending on species. The eggs are highly resistant to environmental influences and usually are laid on the horse's coat (fig. 2.3. — 12) or on vegetation (overwintering possible!).

Infection is acquired orally at pasture (fig. 2.3. — 13), in the case of *G. pecorum* by the ingestion of eggs containing infective larvae, and in the other species by active migration of the 1st-stage larvae. The larvae develop further in the oral

Table 2.3. — 3. Reproductive characteristics of the *Gasterophilus* species

Species	Number of eggs laid by one female	Sites of egg deposition	Duration of embryonic development in days	Survival time of 1st-stage larvae in the egg
G. intestinalis	1,000—1,500	forelimbs, shoulders, flanks and mane of the horse	7—16	90 days
G. inermis	330—360	cheeks of the horse	uncertain	relatively short
G. haemorrhoidalis	160—200	lip hairs of the horse	uncertain	relatively short
G. nasalis	480—520	intermandibular area of the horse	uncertain	relatively short
G. nigricornis	330—350	cheeks of the horse	3—5	relatively short
G. pecorum	1,300—2,650	forage plants	5—8	9 months

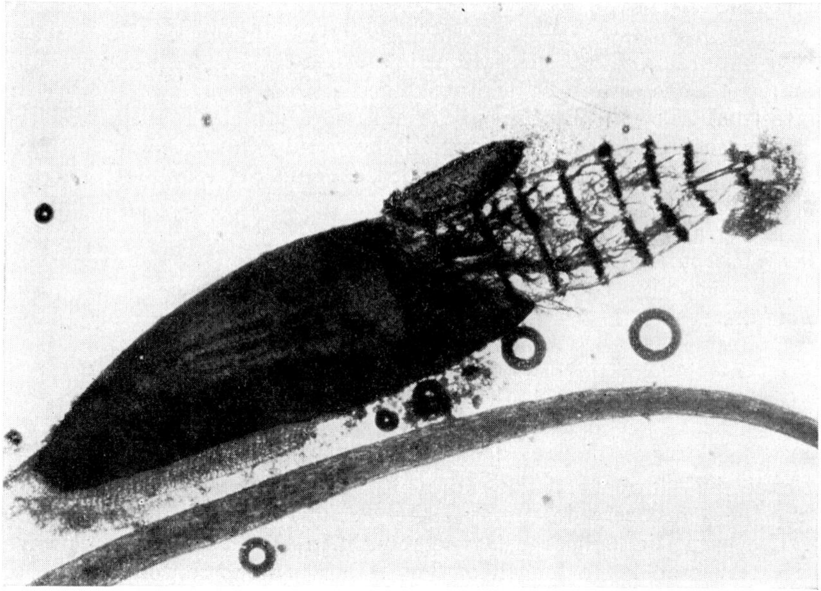

12

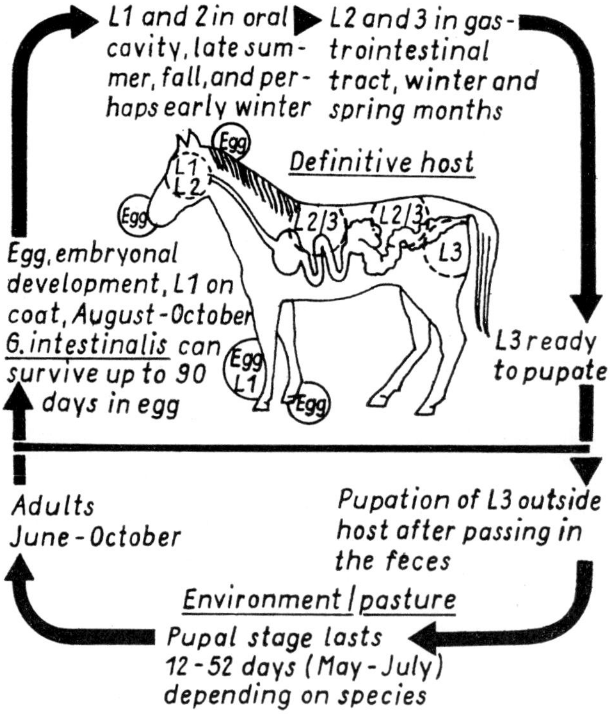

13

Fig. 2.3. — 12. *Gasterophilus intestinalis* (larva hatching from egg) on a horse hair.
Fig. 2.3. — 13. Life cycle of *Gasterophilus* spp. (Central European conditions).

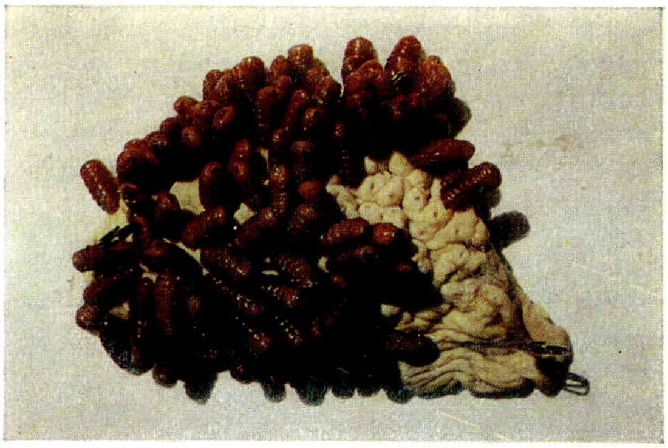

Fig. 2.3. — 14. Gasterophilus intestinalis larvae (3rd-stage) in the equine stomach.

mucosa and molt to 2nd-stage larvae, which move to the definitive site of attachment. By the following spring or summer the brown 3rd-stage larvae (fig. 2.3. — 14) are ready to pupate. They leave the intestinal tract with the feces and migrate into the upper layer of soil (typical mode of pastoral infestation). The pupal stage reportedly lasts an average of 3—4 weeks, depending on temperature, climate and soil structure.

Symptoms. The clinical picture is variable. Gastrointestinal symptoms are predominant, but often the course is subclinical. Fly-worry is evident during the period of egg deposition on the coat. The horses attempt to escape the flies, stand in shallow water or congregate in groups during periods of fly activity (midday sun!). 'Summer streak eczema' is caused by migrating 1st-stage larvae of *G. inermis*, which burrow in the skin of the buccal region toward the angle of the mouth. Residence of the 1st-stage bot larvae in the oral cavity may cause stomatitis, gingivitis, glossitis, masticatory difficulties and dysphagia. Dilatation and stenosis of the esophagus are also sometimes observed. The greatest damage is inflicted by the 2nd- and 3rd-stage larvae in the gastrointestinal tract: erosions, ulcerous lesions, papillomatous vegetations, digestive disturbances, colic. Uusually the clusters of bot larvae are easily seen at necropsy. Anemia, emaciation, and even death in young animals are not unusual complications. Gastric rupture and peritonitis are relatively uncommon, as is the presence of larvae in the liver, brain and ovaries and on the peritoneum.

The earlier theories of bot infestations as a cause of precancerous lesions of the stomach are no longer considered valid.

G. intestinalis and *G. haemorrhoidalis* are a cause of 'creeping eruption' (larva migrans) in humans. Attendants and other persons in close contact with horses are most susceptible. Creeping disease is characterized by the formation of centimeter-long, horizontal ducts in the stratum corneum, which are clearly visible as red streaks.

Diagnosis. The syndromes produced by bot larvae present no pathognomonic signs, aside from the eggs in the coat during the summer months and the spontaneous passage of 3rd-stage larvae in the feces. It remains to be determined whether immunologic processes following a bot infection can be utilized for early diagnosis.

Treatment and Prophylaxis. Organophosphates are available for internal use in the treatment of bot infections. Dichlorvos (20—40 mg/kg) and metriphonate (35 to 50 mg/kg) are highly effective against all 3 larval stages when administered in the feed or applied directly into the oral cavity in gel or paste form. The mode of administration remains problematic under herd conditions. The administration of bot-removing agents by nasogastric tube is feasible only on an individual-animal basis. Under Central European conditions the best time for treatment is between October and March, preferably in the late fall after the end of the grazing season. All horses within the problem area should be treated. A second prophylactic treatment should be administered no later than 4 weeks before the end of the stabling period. If a regimen of this type is maintained for at least 3 years, it is possible to achieve eradication on a regional basis. Effective control of adults with insecticides or repellents during the season of fly activity, though sound in theory, is difficult in practice. On the other hand, good result have been achieved by washing egg-infested body areas with insecticides during the summer and fall months. This will kill the hatching 1st-stage larvae.

References

Azimov, Sh. A.; Enileeva, N. Kh.; Ishmirzaev, B. R.: Gastrofilez loshadij i mery borby s nim. Selekcija i Semenovodstvo, Kiev *7:* 56 (1977).

Belli, P.; Cevrey, J.: Localisations erratiqué de gastrophiles chez un cheval. Rev. Méd. vét. *132:* 265 (1981).

Bello, Th. R.; Seger, C. L.: Antiparasitic efficacy of dichlorvos paste formulation against first-instar Gasteriphilus intestinalis in the tongues of Shetland pony foals. Amer. J. vet. Res. *33:* 39 (1972).

Delak, M.; Mijatovic, I.: Die Anwendung von Neguvon zur Behandlung der Gasterophilose beim Pferd (III). Vet.-med. Nachr. *1968*, p. 115.

Dorchies, Ph.; Amalric, M.: Traitement des helminthoses digestives et de la gastrophilose du cheval revue. Revue Méd. vét. *128:* 7 (1977).

Drudge, J. H.; Lyons, E. T.: Activity of dichlorvos against horse bots. Mod. vet. Pract. *51:* 45 (1970).

Drudge, J. H.; Lyons, E. T.; Swerczek, T. W.: Activity of gel and paste formulations of dichlorvos against first instars of Gasterophilus spp. Amer. J. vet. Res. *33:* 2191 (1972).

Drudge, J. H.; Lyons, E. T.; Tolliver, S. C.: Activity of organophosphorus compounds against oral stages of Gasterophilus intestinalis and Gasterophilus nasalis. Amer. J. vet. Res. *36:* 251 (1975).

Graber, M.; Pitois, M.; Dancer, M.; Euzéby, J.: Activité du phosphate de 2-2 dichlorovinyl-diméthyle (dichlorvos) absorbé sur trame solide sur les larves de gastrophiles parasites du tractus gastrointestinal des équidés. Bull. Soc. Sci. vét. Méd. comp., Lyon *73:* 597 (1971).

Hass, D. K.; Marsland, W. P.; Fogg, T. J.; Collins, J. A.: New concepts in the pathogenesis of Gastrophilus sp. in the horse. Internat. Congr. Parasitol., Proc. München *3:* 1013 (1974).

Hasslinger, M.-A.; Jonas, D.: Zur gebietsmässigen therapeutischen Beeinflussung des Magen-dasselbefalles bei Pferden. Fortschritte Vet.-Med., p. 265 (1974).

Hasslinger, M.-A.; Jonas, D.: Control of Gasterophilus intestinalis (De Geer, 1776) with dichlorvos. Brit. vet. J. *131:* 89 (1975).

Jonas, D.; Hasslinger, M.-A.: Erfolgsaussichten einer planmäßigen Gasterophilus-Bekämpfung bei Pferden. Dtsch. tierärztl. Wschr. *80:* 369 (1973).

Schulz, J. A.; Wujanz, G.; Wick, R.: Versuche zur Anwendung von Bubulin bei Pferden. Ein Beitrag zur Bekämpfung der III. Larven von Gasterophilus intestinalis und des Askaridenbefalls. Mh. Vet.-Med. *17:* 450 (1962).

Tadmer, A.; Perl, S.; Weinberg, H.: Infestation of a mare's liver with Gasterophilus intestinalis. Vet. Med. and Small Animal Clinician *76:* 85 (1981).

Waddell, A. H.: The pathogenicity of Gasterophilus intestinalis larvae in the stomach of the horse. Aust. vet. J. *48:* 332 (1972).

2.3.3.9. Rhinoestrus Infestation

Definition. Infestation with *Rhinoestrus* (nasal bots) is caused by fly larvae that live as parasites in the nasopharynx during the fall, winter and spring months and harm the working capacity of the host. The importance of this parasitism varies.

Etiology. Rhinoestrus purpureus, the horse nasal botfly; 8—12 mm long, purple, viviparous flying insect of the family Oestridae.

Epizootiology. The female *Rg. purpureus* fly, which lives only a few days, deposits up to 800 1st-stage larvae in batches around the nostrils of the horse. This occurs mainly in the late summer. In the area of the choanae, ethmoid bone and pharynx the larvae gradually grow until, by the following spring or summer, they leave the nasopharynx and pupate on the ground. The adult fly emerges in 15—30 days.

Symptoms. Fly-worry with a flight response is typical, and complications such as injuries and fractures are a danger. The freshly deposited larvae provoke severe pruritus, snorting and sneezing as they migrate into the nasal passages. The 1st-through 3rd-stage larvae cause inflammatory reactions and stenoses at their definitive habitats (the choanae, ethmoid, anterior pharynx), leading to head-shaking, a sustained bilateral nasal discharge, stenotic respiratory sounds, 'laryngeal' coughing and dyspnea, depressed appetite, emaciation, and impaired performance. The severity of symptoms is related to the larval burden. Heavy infestations can lead to death.

Rh. purpureus sometimes attacks humans (stud-farm workers, riders, attendants) and deposits larvae in the area of the conjunctivae. The growing larvae cause painful, protracted conjunctivitis.

Diagnosis. A tentative diagnosis of nasal bots is readily made in problem areas on the basis of epidemiologic and practical experience. Suspected cases should always be confirmed by direct demonstration of the larvae with a laryngoscope. Differentiation must be made from infectious diseases of the upper respiratory tract and sinuses of other etiology.

Treatment and Prophylaxis. Treatment with organophosphates (metriphonate in 6 % pour-on preparation at 18 mg/kg BW) or rafoxanide (7.5—10 mg/kg BW orally) is recommended. Prophylactic treatments should be given in the fall immediately after the grazing season. Nasal botfly populations in problem areas can be significantly reduced by maintaining a control program for several years that encompasses all horses in the area.

References

GRUNIK, K. J.: 64a. Gasterophilidae; in LINDNER, Die Fliegen der palaearktischen Region (Schweizerbartsche Verl.-Buchh., Stuttgart 1969).

HIEPE, TH.: Parasitäre Erkrankungen der Nasenhöhlen und der Nasennebenhöhlen; in JOEST, Handbuch der speziellen pathologischen Anatomie der Haustiere, 7, p. 59 (Parey, Berlin 1968).

2.3.3.10. Additional Parasitisms Caused by Arthropods

(See table 2.3. — 4)

Table 2.3. — 4. Additional parasitisms caused by arthropods

Parasitism	Causal agent	Clinical findings	Control	Remarks or source
Louse fly infestation	*Hippobosca equina*	Restlessness from bites	Carbamate and phosphate preparations; repellents	Holometabolic, pupiparous life cycle
Cutaneous myiasis	*Hypoderma bovis*	Cutaneous swellings	Phosphate preparations; surgical treatment indicated in certain cases	Rec. Med. vet. *151:* 423 (1975)
Myiasis of the CNS	*Hypoderma bovis* *Hypoderma lineatum*	Paralysis Encephalomalacia	Individual cases, prognosis unfavorable Individual cases, prognosis unfavorable	Cornell Vet. *67:* 272 (1977); Pathol. Vet. *4:* 477 (1967)
Black fly infestation	*Wilhelmia equina Boophthora erythrocephala Odagmia ornata, etc.*	Pastoral parasitism. With massive infestation: flight reactions, cutaneous syndrome, cardiovascular syndrome	Ca infusion; antihistamines, cardiovascular agents, insecticide use at gathering places	Parasitologia *11:* 77 (1969); GRÄFNER, G.: Nat.-Diss. B, HU Berlin (1977)
Sweet itch	[*Onchocerca* microfilariae] *Culicoides pulicaris*	Circumscribed dermatitis in withers area (parasitism of pasture)	Antihistamines, corticosteroids, phosphates, repellents	Vet. Rec. *95:* 411 (1974)
Trombidiiasis	*Neotrombicula autumnalis* larvae	Cutaneous syndrome (in late summer and early fall), blood loss, pruritus	Whole-body insecticide spray	Tierärztl. Umschau *5:* 187 (1950)
Infestation with red bird mite	*Dermanyssus gallinae*	Nocturnal restlessness, blood loss, cutaneous syndrome (pruritus, petechial hemorrhages in the skin)	Spraying of stables with insecticide (walls, ceilings, fixtures), or fumigation	Very common when poultry are housed in horse stables
Infestation with free-living mites	*Leiodinychus krameri* lives in bedding and on moldy organic matter	Skin lesions in area of mane and base of tail, pruritus	Insecticide dip	Incidental finding? Wien. tierärztl. Monatschr. *52:* 858 (1965)

2.3.4. Antiparasitic Management

Parasitism in horse populations requires constant veterinary surveillance, especially under stud conditions and in racing and riding stables. The economically important parasitisms that cause heavy losses are of main diagnostic concern. It is a basic assumption that high levels of performance can be expected only from horses

Table 2.3. — 5. Yearly treatment program for controlling strongyles, strongyloids, ascarids, oxyurids and bots in horses (after STOYE [1975])
Important prerequisites: accurate herd diagnosis
veterinary supervision of measures
treatment of all animals in the herd

	Time	Foals Measures	Time	Mares, yearlings, etc. Measures
January				
February		1st treatment against *Strongyloides* at 10 days. Treatment repeated at weekly intervals. 1st treatment against ascarids and strongyles at 8 weeks. Treatments repeated in accordance with herd treatment schedule		Treatment against strongyles, oxyurids and bots
March				
April				Treatment against strongyles and oxyurids 3 days before pasturing
May				
June		Treatment against ascarids and strongyles		Treatment against strongyles and oxyurids
July				
August		Treatment against ascarids and strongyles		Treatment against strongyles and oxyurids
September				
October		Treatment against ascarids and strongyles		Treatment against strongyles and oxyurids
November				
December		Treatment against ascarids, strongyles and bots		Treatment against strongyles, oxyurids and bots

that are either free of parasites or have a low level of infestation — for, with few exceptions, the adverse effects of parasitisms on the host tend to be general in nature.

The objectives of a parasite control program are three-fold:

1. The eradication of dangerous parasitism: acute, highly contagious diseases and zoonoses such as sarcoptic and psoroptic mange and dourine. Horse populations must be kept free of these parasitisms or protected against their occurrence.
2. The prevention of clinically-overt outbreaks of parasitic disease.
3. The control of chronic, subclinical, performance-hampering parasitism.

Specific therapeutic and prophylactic measures have already been outlined in the sections dealing with specific parasitic diseases. In the present section, our objective is to set up a yearly schedule for the implementation of control measures on a month-by-month basis. (Recommendations are based on clinical experience and prevailing climatic and geographic conditions in Central Europe.)

STOYLE [1975] has devised a control program for strongyloid, strongyle, ascarid, oxyurid and bot infections in horses which gives recommendations for the timing of antiparasitic treatments (table 2.3. — 5). The primary objective of the program

Table 2.3. — 6. Efficacy of commonly used anthelmintics against adult and intestinal stages of common endoparasites of the horse (modif. from Stoye [1975])

Anthelmintic agent	Dose mg/kg BW	Efficacy								
		Strongyloides westeri	*Parascaris equorum*	*Strongylus* *vulg.*	*Strongylus* *equi.*	*Strongylus* *eden.*	Small strongyles	*Trichostrongylus axei*	*Oxyuris equi*	*Gasterophilus* spp.
Piperazine compounds (various salts: phosphate, citrate, hydrate)	200	—	+++	+	—	—	++	—	+++	—
Pyrantel tartrate	20	+	+++	+++	+++	+++	+++	+++	+++	—
Morantel tartrate	10	+++	+++	+++	+++	+++	+++	+++	+++	—
Thiabendazole	75	+++	++	+++	+++	+++	+++	+++	+++	
Mebendazole	10	+	+++	+++	+++	+++	+++	+	+++	—
Fenbendazole	8	—	+++	+++	+++	+++	+++	?	+++	—
Metriphonate	50	—	++	++	++	+	++	—	+++	+++
Dichlorvos	40	—	+++	++	++	++	+++	—	++	+++

— = < 50 %
\+ = 50—80 %
++ = 80—90 %
+++ = > 95 %

is to limit the possibilities for parasitic infection in the horse's environment, for antiparasitic treatments are supplemented with intensive measures to promote and maintain hygiene in pastures and stables.

Table 2.3. — 6 presents data on the efficacy of numerous antiparasitic and athelmintic agents that have been tested in the horse. From these agents, a suitable antiparasitic regimen is pieced together on the basis of diagnostic findings. When putting this program into practice, care should be taken that the economic costs of the control measures are in proper relation to the anticipated benefit. It should also be noted that the repeated, frequent use of a single antiparasitic agent can lead to the development of drug-resistant parasites. It is essential, therefore, that treatment response be assessed periodically during the control program.

In our experience, the systematic control of strongyles and ascarids is aided best by the deworming of all dams and yearlings at the end of the grazing season in the late fall, and again immediately before the animals are put to pasture in the spring. We do not recommend the routine anthelmintic treatment of dams against these parasites during the grazing season. However, if examination of the stool points to an increase in the level of infestation, as is often the case in highly-susceptible yearlings, strategic treatments during the grazing period are indicated.

In nursing foals, it is essential that an initial anthelmintic treatment be given on the 10th day of life, and that prophylactic treatment against ascarids and strongyles be given between the 8th and 12th week. The control of bot infestation should aim a eradication of the disease in an affected area within a 3-year period. Treatment with dichlorvos-base organophosphates is favored at the present time (see the section on Gasterophilosis for details).

The mode of administering antiparasitic agents is a problem that has not yet been entirely resolved. Anthelmintics and boticides should be administered in the feed if at all possible. In foals, drenching with a dosing device or with a Janet or Buhner syringe is suitable. Insecticides are applied mainly as a spray or by dusting, depending on the time of year. In Thoroughbreds and breeding stallions, which tend to be extremely noise-sensitive, insecticides may be applied by dipping or, for louse infestation, by a pour-on technique.

Every parasite control program should be founded upon a well-defined set of objectives.

References

Andersen, F. L.; Wright, P. D.; Walters, G. T.: Palatability and efficacy of a powder formulation of thiabendazole and trichlorfon for horses. J. Amer. vet. med. Assoc. *162:* 206 (1973).

Bennett, D. G.; Bickford, A. A.: Efficacy of dichlorvos paste against parasites of horses. Vet. Med. and Small Animal Clinician *66:* 441 (1971).

Bennett, D. G., jr.: Efficacy of mebendazole as an anthelmintic in horses. Vet. Med. and Small Animal Clinician *68:* 604, 607, 609 (1973).

Bussiéras, J.: Essai de traitment des helminthoses digestives des equides par le pamoate de pyrantel. Revue Méd. vét. *128:* 343 (1977).

Commergnat, J.: Essais d'utilisation du levamisole comme anthelminthique chez le cheval. Bull. mens. Soc. vét. prat. *58:* 339 (1974).

De Vries, J. P.: Eens makelijk vormmiddel voor paarden. Tijdschr. Diergeneesk. *96:* 693 (1971).

Drugge, J. H.; Lyons, E. T.: Critical tests of a resin-pellet formulation of dichlorvos against internal parasites of the horse. Amer. J. vet. Res. *33:* 1365 (1972).

Drudge, J. H.; Lyons, E. T.; Swerczek, T. W.: Critical tests and safety studies on a levamisole-piperazine mixture as an anthelmintic in the horse. Amer. J. vet. Res. *35:* 67 (1974).

DRUDGE, J. H.; LYONS, E. T.; TAYLOR, E. L.: Critical tests and safety studies on trichlorfon as an antiparasitic agent in the horse. Amer. J. vet. Res. *37:* 139 (1976).

DRUDGE, J. H.; LYONS, E. T.; TOLLIVER, S. C.: Critical test of the benzimidazole anthelmintic, fenbendazole in the horse. Vet. Med. and Small Animal Clinician *70:* 537 (1975).

DUNCAN, J. L.: The anthelmintic treatment of horses. Vet. Rec. *98:* 233 (1976).

ENIGK, K.: Zur Vorbeuge des Parasitenbefalles beim Pferd. Lohmann Inform., Cuxhaven 1972, Nov., p. 6.

FOLZ, S. D.: Control of parasites in equines. J. Parasitol. *56:* No. 4, part 2, No. 1, p. 103 (1970).

FORSTNER, M. J.; HASSLINGER, M.-A.: Untersuchungen über die Wirkung des Anthelminthikums Fenbendazol an Pferden. Berliner Münchener tierärztl. Wschr. *87:* 325—327 (1974).

HASS, D. K.; ALBERT, J. R.; PILLOW, B. G.; BROWN, L. F.: Dichlorvos gel-formulation as an equine anthelmintic. Amer. J. vet. Res. *34:* 41 (1973).

HIEPE, TH.: Wirksamkeit von Moranteltartrat gegenüber Nematodenbefall bei Sportpferden. Schweizer Arch. Tierheilk. *114:* 613 (1972).

HIEPE, TH.; RIBBEK, R.: Medikamentelle Bekämpfung der Parasitosen in Nutztierbeständen — eine Übersicht der in der DDR registrierten Antiparasitaria. medicamentum *17:* 327 (1976).

JONAS, D.; HASSLINGER, M.-A.; WOLPERT, E.: Neue Aspekte zur Endoparasitenbekämpfung beim Pferd. Prakt. Tierarzt *53:* 427 (1972).

KATES, K. C.; COLGLAZIER, M. L.; ENZIE, F. D.: Oxibendazole: Critical anthelmintic trials in equids. Vet. Rec. *97:* 442 (1975).

LANG, K.; GRASSLER, R.: Feldversuche mit Cambenzole®, einem neuen Wurmmittel für Pferde. Tierärztl. Umschau *30:* 392 (1975).

LANGE, E.; TOMSEN, K.: Erfahrungen mit Fenbendazol bei der Behandlung des Helminthenbefalls der Pferde unter Bedingungen der tierärztlichen Praxis. Tierärztl. Umschau *31:* 441 (1976).

LYONS, E. T.; DRUDGE, J. H.; TOLLIVER, S. C.: Critical tests of three salts of pyrantel against internal parasites of the horse. Amer. J. vet. Res. *35:* 1515 (1974).

LYONS, E. T.; DRUDGE, J. H.; TOLLIVER, S. C.: Field tests of three salts of pyrantel against internal parasites of the horse. Amer. J. vet. Res. *36:* 161 (1975).

RIBBECK, R.; KULLER, H.-J.; LEONHARD, I.: Einsatz von Mebendazol zur Bekämpfung des Magen-Darm-Nematodenbefalls beim Pferd. medicamentum *17:* 352 (1976).

RIZZOLI-STADLER, C.; PAULI, B.; LEUENBERGER, H.; HÖRNING, B.: Einfluss von Weidegang und Entwurmung auf den Befall mit Magendarmparasiten des Pferdes. 1. Eine vergleichende Untersuchung in zwei Beständen mit unterschiedlichen Haltungsbedingungen. Schweizer Arch. Tierheilk. *118:* 341 (1976).

SOMMER, W.: Bekämpfung des Helminthenbefalles beim Pferd. Prakt. Tierarzt *56:* 141 (1975).

STOYE, M.: Parasitenbekämpfung beim Pferd. Schweizer Arch. Tierheilk. *114:* 601 (1972).

STOYE, M.: Möglichkeiten und Grenzen der planmässigen Parasitenbekämpfung beim Pferd. Dtsch. tierärztl. Wschr. *82:* 328 (1975).

WALKER, D.; KNIGHT, D.: The anthelmintic activity of 'Mebendazole'. A field trial in borses. Vet. Rec. *90:* 58 (1972).

2.4. Metabolic Disorders

2.4.1. Deficiencies of Inorganic Substances

Besides organic compounds, living protoplasm contains a number of elements that are of mineral origin. Some of these elements are bound to organic matter, but most occur in inorganic form, either as fixed, poorly-soluble salts or as free ions dissolved in the body fluid, depending on their function. Inorganic compounds make up approximately 2.5 % of the total body weight. About four-fifths of these are contained in the bone and about one-tenth in the muscle. The quantity of each of these elements is highly variable, and their concentrations tend to increase with age. The only exception to this rule is sodium, which is far more plentiful in newborn animals than in adults. Elements that make up more than 0.01 % of the body weight are called 'minerals', while those occurring in smaller amounts are called 'trace elements'.

2.4.1.1. Minerals

Calcium, phosphorus, magnesium, sodium, potassium and chlorine are among the most important mineral nutrients. They play an important role in regulating the osmotic pressure in cells and tissues and maintaining the colloidal structure of living matter. They help to produce electrical potentials and currents at cell membranes that are essential for nerve impulse conduction and other vital functions. Minerals are also important in the synthesis and action of hormones and enzymes and assist in maintaining an optimum pH for biochemical reactions. Finally, they are important as structural components of certain tissues such as bone, cartilage and teeth.

Improper soil treatment practices lead not only to an absolute deficiency of one or more essential elements in the plants and thus in the animals that graze on them, but also to an imbalanced mineral intake. Mineral supplementation of the ration is necessary in such cases to prevent the occurrence of deficiency symptoms.

In the German Democratic Republic (GDR), a mineral supplement with the following composition (in g/kg) is available for horses:

64.00 phosphorus
276.00 calcium
77.00 sodium
1.22 manganese
0.37 copper
0.02 cobalt
1.23 zinc.

The recommended feeding rates for this supplement are 100 g/day for foals and 150 g/day for mature horses. For the total mineral requirements of horses see Sec. 1.3.2.4. Foals require at least 0.23 % Ca and 0.21 % P based on the dry matter content of their ration.

Minor defects of mineral nutrition frequently lead to nonspecific, generalized behavioral disturbances or simply to a heightened susceptibility to clinical disease. For this reason it is important that defects of mineral metabolism be recognized promptly. While this is by no means a simple task, evidence for the existence of such defects can be found in:

1. the gross and chemical composition of the feed;
2. clinical signs, including performance changes;
3. the mineral content of the blood or serum;
4. the mineral content of the hair, liver and bone;
5. the mineral balance, or level of mineral excretion in the urine;
6. the response to treatment.

2.4.1.1.1. Calcium and Phosphorus

About 99 % of the calcium in the animal body is contained in the bone and teeth. Calcium has a plasma concentration of about 2.25—2.99 mmol/l (9—12 mg%) and accounts for 1.2—2% of the adult body weight. The general requirement for agricultural animals is 0.8—1.2 % of the ration dry matter. The metabolism of calcium is closely linked to that of phosphorus. As a result of this, a dietary excess of calcium interferes with phosphorus utilization, leading indirectly to deficiency symptoms. Calcium absorption takes place mainly in the small intestine and is dependent upon the calcium content of the feed, the Ca : P ratio in the feed (1 : 1 to 2 : 1 is considered optimum for the horse), the requirement of the animal, its age, and its vitamin D intake. Calcium absorption decreases with increasing calcium intake and with age. The higher the requirement, the greater the absorption. Vitamin D promotes calcium uptake through the synthesis of a calcium-binding transport protein in the intestinal mucosa.

When the Ca : P ratio exceeds 1: 2.9, clinical signs of metabolic disease will develop within a few months. A constant serum calcium level is maintained by:

1. hormonal regulation (parathormone, calcitonin);
2. an equilibrium between bone tissue and extracellular fluid;
3. the action of vitamin D (an excess of vitamin D_3 increases the blood calcium level, while vitamin D_2 has little if any effect);
4. calcium intake.

Phosphorus, in the form of tricalcium phosphate, makes up about 0.8—1.0 % of the body weight. Seventy-five to 80 percent is contained in the bones and teeth. Of the rest, most is bound to intracellular organic substances (proteins, nucleic acids, phospholipids). Tricalcium phosphate is also a constituent of many substrates and enzymes of the intermediary metabolism. Phosphorus occurs in the serum as a free phosphate, where its concentration ranges from 0.97 to 2.58 mmol/l (3—8 mg%) and is influenced by parathormone. Phosphorus absorption takes place in the proximal part of the small intestine.

All questions relating to calcium and phosphate imbalance must take into account the interrelationship of these minerals and the effect of vitamin D on their metabolism. In young animals, the earliest signs of defects in the calcium and phosphorus metabolism are digestive disturbances, followed later by poor growth, cachexia, and deficient bone mineralization and growth leading to bony deformities (osteomalacia). In severe cases there is a failure of bone calcification leading to generalized osteodystrophia fibrosa. The pathogenesis of such diseases depends largely on the fact that the mineralization and to some extent the growth of bones are basically a function of mineral supply (disregarding the rare primary endocrine or renal causes). According to reports in the literature, calcium and phosphorus imbalance combined with a vitamin D deficiency leads to what has been called rickets, while malnutrition that stimulates parathyroid activity leads to osteodystrophia fibrosa. The two diseases can be differentiated only by histologic examination of the bone.

In mature animals, calcium and phosphorus imbalance leads to demineralization of the bone (osteoporosis, oeteomalacia) and to disturbances of reproductive function. Additional effects are a general impairment of performance, deficient intrauterine growth, rapid fatigability during work, and reduced gastrointestinal motility. Deformities of the head, pelvis and mandible are commonly present, and lameness with eventual paralysis of the limbs is common in older animals. Paresis and recumbency are seen in extreme cases. Parturient paresis is rare and is discussed in the section on Magnesium.

Diagnosis. Subclinical phosphorus deficiency is extremely difficult to diagnose. It may be expected to occur when the phosphorus content of the ration falls below 0.14 % by dry matter. (The average content in hay, for example, is 0.21 %, compared to a desired level of 0.3 %; the content is grain seeds, on the other hand, usually exceeds 0.3 %.)

Special attention should be given to highly conditioned horses in this regard, for such animals are especially likely to have an improper Ca : P ratio in their ration. Blood studies done in suspected cases should show a serum phosphate level of at least 0.97 mmol/l (3 mg%). The typical bony changes are readily demonstrated by radiographic examination.

Treatment. In animals with so-called 'rickets', modification of the diet should be followed by treatment with vitamin D, which may be combined with vitamin A if desired. The first priority, however, is to correct the phosphorus deficit. In this regard, it should be noted that a protein-rich diet is more favorable for calcium utilization than a low-protein diet. On the other hand, the oxalic acid that is present in certain feedstuffs, such as turnip leaves, forms poorly-soluble calcium salts in the monogastric animal, and these can pass through the digestive tract practically unchanged.

The treatment for osteomalacia is similar to that for rickets.

Prophylaxis consists in providing an adequate mineral supply in the ration. Because grain seeds, milling residues, and the residues from oil production contain relatively large amounts of phosphorus, mineral supplements for horses that receive suitable amounts of a feed concentrate need not contain as much phosphate as those for cattle, for example. Thus, a supplement containing 6.4% phosphorus is entirely adequate for horses that are fed concentrate at a rate of 100—200 g/500—700 kg BW/day (bovine mineral supplements in the GDR contain between 6.6 and 16.1% phosphorus).

2.4.1.1.2. Magnesium

The animal body is approximately 0.03—0.04 % magnesium, of which 62% is contained in the bones, 37% in tissue cells and 1% in the extracellular fluid. With a normal magnesium intake, the serum levels in most animals are between 741 and 1,440 μmol/l (1.8 and 3.5 mg%). A magnesium deficiency is reflected not only in serum levels, but also in the magnesium content of the bone ash, which in severe cases can fall to about 40 % of normal (~0.7 %). Magnesium serves as an activator of the phosphorylating and phosphorus-transferring enzymes. Also, as a component of other enzymes, it plays a role in the energy metabolism, glycolysis, the citric acid cycle and other processes. Magnesium also influences calcium metabolism by inhibiting the calcification of certain tissues. If the diet is high in calcium and phosphorus but low in magnesium, calcium builds up in the kidneys, cardiovascular system and other organs, leading to severe tissue calcifications. Presumably the eucolloidal state of the cells is disrupted if the Ca : Mg ratio is too high. This results in the degeneration and necrosis of certain cell constituents, and calcium salt deposits form on these structures; this calcium binding is apparently due to a buildup of substrates from the disrupted citric acid cycle. The inhibitory effect of magnesium on tissue calcification derives from its ability to promote the excretion of excess calcium and inhibit calcium absorption.

Magnesium appears to be a calcium antagonist with regard to blood coagulation. However, the most pronounced symptoms of an acute magnesium deficiency relate to disturbances of neurologic function.

The magnesium content of the body, and especially the magnesium level in the serum, are determined almost exclusively by the level of magnesium absorption and excretion. The skeletal reserves are small. Magnesium is absorbed chiefly in the proximal portion of the small intestine. Generally speaking, magnesium ingested with the feed is utilized better by monograstric animals than by ruminants. A high calcium and phytin content in the ration interferes with magnesium utilization, while phosphate improves magnesium absorption to some degree. The average apparent digestibility of magnesium in the horse varies between 12 and 52 %. Assuming a digestibility of 25 %, a working horse has a magnesium requirement of about 10 g/day, and a lactating mare, about 16—18 g/day.

Magnesium deficiency in the horse is characterized by eclampsia and transit tetany; but, like other monograstric animals, the horse is very rarely affected. In parturient paresis, which is thought to relate to a calcium deficiency, the blood calcium level may be entirely normal or may fall below 1.0 mmol/l (4 mg%). The magnesium level in such cases is below 0.37 mmol/l (0.9 mg%). As in other species, lactation is a predisposing factor, i.e., heavily lactating mares are at greatest risk. The mortality rate may exceed 60% in some instances.

Symptoms. The cardinal symptoms of magnesium deficiency are profuse sweating, incoordination, stiffness of the limbs, and rapid breathing with flaring of the nostrils. Spastic contractions of the diaphragm lead to a 'thumping' respiration (synchronous diaphragmatic flutter). Trismus of the masseter and shoulder muscles is occasionally seen. The body temperature and pulse are usually normal. Urination and defecation are reduced. Tetanic convulsions appear within 24 hours, and death may follow within 48 hours.

Treatment. The intravenous injection of calcium solutions similar to those used to treat parturient paresis leads to a rapid and complete recovery, manifested by increased diuresis. It must be borne in mind that mares respond more sensitively to calcium injections than do cows. A heart block can easily develop if solutions are administered too rapidly.

2.4.1.1.3. Potassium, Sodium and Chloride

These three elements are closely interrelated in terms of their metabolism and their biochemical, biophysical and physiologic functions, and so it is natural to discuss them together. They also tend to occur together in feedstuffs. Besides their specific physiologic actions, these elements are of general importance in maintaining the osmotic and ionic structure of the body fluids. Potassium, sodium and chloride are

Table 2.4. — 1. Average potassium and sodium content of the blood, serum and erythrocytes (after KOLB [1962], modified from WIESNER [1970])

Animal species	Potassium			Sodium			Units
	Blood	Serum	Erythro-cytes	Blood	Serum	Erythro-cytes	
Cow	10	4	20	113	142	74	mmol/l
	40	17	80	260	325	170	mg/100 ml
Sheep	9	5	20	122	144	89	mmol/l
	35	18	80	280	330	205	mg/100 ml
Goat	22	5	51	109	139	52	mmol/l
	85	18	200	250	320	120	mg/100 ml
Horse	44	5	92	87	139	24	mmol/l
	170	18	360	200	320	55	mg/100 ml
Pig	44	5	95	94	146	11	mmol/l
	170	20	370	215	335	25	mg/100 ml
Chicken	49	6	98	106	163	26	mmol/l
	190	22	390	245	375	60	mg/100 ml

considerably less abundant in the body than are calcium and phosphorus and, unlike the latter elements, are localized in the soft tissues, where they are distributed in accordance with their functional significance in a particular region. Only about one-third of the sodium is contained in the cartilage and skeleton, and about 18% in the skin. Potassium is most plentiful in the intracellular fluid. In young animals the K : Na ratio is shifted throughout the body in favor of sodium; the relative abundance of sodium decreases with age.

The content of potassium, sodium and chlorine in the whole blood varies greatly among different animal species, while their concentration in the blood plasma is fairly constant. The interspecies differences relate mainly to differences in the potassium content of the erythrocytes (see table 2.4. — 1).

The absorption of all three ions from the intestine is very rapid and complete; chloride is especially mobile.

The animal body possesses no significant depots for the three elements that might serve as a buffer in the event of dietary deficiencies or excesses. However, it does possess efficient regulatory systems that enable the ion balance to be adjusted in accordance with physiologic demands.

Symptoms. No cases of clinical disease due to a dietary *deficiency* of potassium and chloride have yet been reported in veterinary practice. Deficiency symptoms have been observed only under experimental conditions. The earliest signs of potassium deficiency are a general deterioration of health, poor appetite, muscular weakness and a fall of blood pressure. Death occurs within a few weeks due to severe tissue degeneration in various organs. The effects of an isolated chloride deficiency are very difficult to produce experimentally. Pronounced, clinically overt symptoms of sodium deficiency appear only after the animal has been on a low-sodium diet for some months. These consist mainly in a noticeable deterioration of performance in many areas. LEHR [1961] reports the following signs, which are the same in the horse as in other animal species:

1. poor growth due to impaired protein utilization,
2. poor appetite,

3. fertility disturbances,
4. reduced milk output,
5. neurologic disturbances.

Disturbances of reproductive function are especially likely to develop in cases where the K : Na ratio is greater than 10, but this probably will occur only in cases where the diet is sodium-deficient from the outset.

Diseases caused by a *dietary excess* of potassium, sodium and chloride, or by poisoning with these elements, are based almost exclusively on errors of feeding or management. They are especially common in herbivorous animals, which often develop a physiologic 'salt hunger' due to a dietary sodium deficiency. This may prompt the animal to consume excessive amounts of salt that are either offered in the ration itself or are made accessible through negligence (e.g., mineral fertilizers). As a rule, however, sodium chloride ('salt') poisoning is rare in horses. Signs include anorexia, excessive thirst, apathy, redness of the oral mucosa, salivation, polyuria, profuse diarrhea, and possibly rectal prolapse. The pulse and respiratory rates are elevated. Neurologic signs include hyperesthesia of the skin, an unsteady gait, abnormal excitability of the motor nerves, teeth gnashing, and finally extreme excitement with rabies-like episodes.

Lesions. Necropsy findings are fairly nonspecific. Inflammation of the gastric and intestinal mucosae is usually the most prominent finding.

Diagnosis. The history, clinical picture and necropsy findings do not always provide an adequate basis for diagnosing sodium chloride poisoning. Moreover, determination of the salt content of the feed and ingesta may be misleading. In animals with a chronic dietary salt excess, for example, even a relatively small dose can lead to a fatal intoxication. The histologic examination of necropsy material is the most reliable method. The histologic demonstration of edema, heavy eosinophilic leukocyte infiltration and glial cell proliferation in the central nervous system enables sodium-ion poisoning to be diagnosed with a high degree of confidence (assuming that infectious diseases have been excluded).

Treatment. Calcium preparations have given good results in the treatment of sodium chloride poisoning. Symptomatic treatment should also be given to improve circulation and relieve gastroenteric symptoms. This should be followed by protective liver therapy aimed at promoting the regeneration of damaged parenchyma. Giving copious amounts of drinking water is not advised, as this is usually too late to be of value and may actually exacerbate symptoms.

2.4.1.2. Trace Elements

Besides the minerals discussed above, the organs and tissues also contain about 40 additional elements, most of which occur in minute amounts. Taken together, they make up about 0.25% of the total body mass. Only a few of these elements are absolutely essential for life (copper, zinc, selenium, manganese, iodine, iron, cobalt). Others, such as fluorine and molybdenum, are not considered essential under all circumstances.

In most feedstuffs the trace elements occur in milligram or microgram quantities (10^{-3} or 10^{-6} g), but even so, the normal diet usually provides amounts sufficient to meet requirements.

Trace element deficiencies may result from a dietary lack of the element as well as from endogenous causes such as:

Table 2.4. — 2. Occurence of essential trace elements in the major organs

	Fe	Cu	Co	Mn	Zn	J	Se	F	Mo
Liver		+	+		+		+		+
Heart				+					
Muscle						+	+		
Blood	+								
Kidney							+	+	
Spleen	+								+
Bone								+	

1. intestinal diseases that interfere with digestion and absorption;
2. impaired assimilation in the tissues due to an absence or deficiency of enzymes or of vitamins that constitute the enzymes;
3. damage to certain vitamin-forming microorganisms due to a deficiency of trace elements in the ration [Halama, 1955].

The deficiency symptoms resulting from an inadequate intake or uptake of trace elements are both general and specific in nature. Disturbances of metabolism, digestion, reproduction and locomotion lead to a decline in all areas of performance. General deficiency symptoms consist mainly of growth disturbances, anemia, reproductive disorders, emaciation to the point of cachexia, and in some cases death. Disturbances relating to loss of the deficient factor are also observed.

The demonstration of a trace element deficiency is done in the manner previously described for mineral deficiencies.

The amounts of essential trace elements contained in the tissues vary from one organ to the next, as shown in table 2.4. — 2. It should be noted, however, that the predominance of a given element in an organ or tissue does not always denote a specific function of that element at that location.

2.4.1.2.1. Iron

Iron is a relatively abundant trace element, making up 0.007 % of the body weight. More than half the iron in the body is contained in hemoglobin, which has an iron content of 4.47 %. Iron is also contained in myoglobin, the oxygen-binding pigment that occurs in muscle, and in a number of important enzymes. Part of the iron in the body is bound in ferritin, the principal storage form of iron in the tissues. This form is most abundant in the intestinal mucosa, spleen, liver and bone marrow.

The normal ration contains much more iron than the animal can utilize. This is why the mineral supplement for horses mentioned earlier in this chapter contains no iron. Iron deficiency diseases generally occur only in young animals whose hepatic iron stores become depleted during the first weeks of life, and which do not receive adequate iron replacement via the milk. As yet, however, the literature contains no reports of iron deficiency anemias occurring naturally in foals.

On the other hand, a dietary excess of iron can bind excessive amounts of phosphorus, leading to metabolic bone disease [Beeson, 1966]. The oral administration of iron rarely causes disease, however, because the 'mucosal barrier' acts to protect the body from an iron overload [Behrens, 1957]. This protective mechanism is inoperative, of course, when iron is administered parenterally.

2.4.1.2.2. Copper

The trace element copper also performs functions that are essential for life, and it occurs in almost every organ of the body. The total copper content of an adult animal makes up about 0.0002 % of its body weight; newborns have from 2 to 3 times this amount [Chou and Adolph, 1935]. The highest absolute copper levels occur in the skin and hair, and about 36% of all the copper in the body is contained in these tissues [Brenner, 1953]. Cunningham et al. [1966] report the following dry-matter copper levels for various organs in the horse:

liver	15.0 mg/kg,
heart	17.5 mg/kg,
lung	7.0 mg/kg,
spleen	3.0 mg/kg,
kidney	29.0 mg/kg.

The most important effect of copper is its influence on erythropoiesis, specifically on the formation and maturation of erythrocytes. Copper performs a specific, probably biocatalytic function in the synthesis of hemoglobin and other hemin proteins [Elvehjem and Sherman, 1932] by activating iron [Brenner, 1953] or by mediating its incorporation into the hemoglobin molecule [Underwood, 1977]. In addition, it exerts a mobilizing and activating effect on the remainder of the iron metabolism and promotes the absorption of iron from the food [Seelemann and von Baudissin, 1953/54]. Copper plays an important role in the catalysis of essential enzymes, hormones and vitamins. Copper also has marked effects on the carbohydrate metabolism owing to its role as a mediator for the action of vitamin B_1. The absorption of copper ingested with the feed takes place only in the acid milieu of the cranial portions of the small intestine [Tompsett, 1934].

Ruminants are particularly susceptible to copper deficiency. The copper requirement of agricultural work animals is very low, and so copper deficiencies are apt to occur only in areas where there is a marked deficiency in the soil and thus in the plants grown on the soil. The minimum daily requirement for horses is 60 mg, and this is satisfied by only a few kilograms of good grass. As a result, no clinical cases of copper deficiency have been reported in horses, particularly since the mineral supplement for horses in itself provides about 60 mg of copper when fed at a rate of 150 g/day.

2.4.1.2.3. Manganese

Manganese is important for endocrine function and fertility. Its main importance, however, is as a constituent and activator of essential enzymes. Blood levels of managanese tend to be somewhat low, though this varies from one species to the next. The numerous metabolic functions of manganese account for the importance of this trace element for skeletal development, muscular function, and the development and function of the genital organs in both sexes. Manganese is most abundant in the thymus, kidneys, adrenals and heart.

Symptoms. The cardinal signs of manganese deficiency relate to disturbances in the growth of the long bones. Frequently there is a disturbance of endochondral ossification, resulting in curvatures of the forelimbs and lameness. The hock joints and the distal ends of the radius and ulna are enlarged. In stallions, spermatogenesis may cease and testicular degeneration may develop. Mares may experience a delay of sexual maturation and fertility disturbances.

On the other hand, a very high level of manganese in the ration (1,000—2,000 mg/kg dry matter) can cause a delay of hemoglobin formation, probably through the inhibition of iron absorption.

Treatment. Under more or less natural feeding conditions, manganese deficiency is a relatively rare disease. It is assumed, however, that hay must contain at least 50 mg/kg manganese in order to prevent deficiency symptoms. 150 g of the customary mineral supplement for horses supplies about 180 mg of manganese. It should be noted that an excess of calcium in the diet can adversely affect the manganese supply, because each element influences the retention of the other.

2.4.1.2.4. Zinc

Zinc is a relatively abundant trace element in the animal body, occurring in a concentration of about 30—50 mg/kg. It is a constituent of many enzymes and thus plays a part in essential reactions of the intermediary metabolism. The zinc content of the organs is approximately 5 to 6 times that of copper.

Zinc levels are highest in the eye, in cell nuclei, and in the liver, skin, genital organs and semen. Of the zinc present in the blood, about 75% is contained in the erythrocytes, 22 % in the plasma, and 3% in the leukocytes.

Symptoms. Symptoms of zinc deficiency are most common in swine (dietetic parakeratosis) and are occasionally seen in cattle and poultry. No clinical cases have yet been diagnosed in the horse. Moreover, it is unlikely that such deficiencies will be diagnosed in the future, inasmuch as 150 g of mineral supplement supplies about 180 mg of zinc (close to the daily requirement), and natural feedstuffs contain considerable amounts of the element (grain 30—50 mg/kg, pasture hay 35 mg/kg, meals 20—180 mg/kg).

2.4.1.2.5. Cobalt

Cobalt is an essential trace element that is required in very minute amounts, yet performs an extremely important function. The requirement in non-ruminants is very much lower than in ruminants and in fact cobalt is essential for life in ruminants owing to its participation in the synthesis of vitamin B_{12} in the rumen and intestinal tract. Cobalt deficiency symptoms are unknown in the horse, particularly since ordinary feedstuffs have a certain natural cobalt content, and cobalt is provided in the mineral supplement.

2.4.1.2.6. Selenium

For at least 20 years selenium has been known to be an essential trace element for chicks, pigs, calves and lambs. The importance of the element was realized when the liver necrosis that ordinarily occurred in rats maintained on a vitamin E-free diet failed to occur in rats fed selenium compounds. Thus, it is clear that a close interrelationship exists between the two nutrients, although they are by no means interchangeable in all deficiency states. Typical signs of selenium deficiency are an exudative diathesis, encephalomalacia and muscular dystrophy in chicks; hepatosis diatetica and skeletal muscle degeneration (white muscle disease) in swine; and white muscle disease in calves and lambs.

Nutritional muscular dystrophies in foals were first described by Jones and Reed in 1948. White muscle disease (WMD) is most commonly observed on soils treated with sulfate-containing fertilizers, because sulfate ions may inhibit soil selenium uptake by plants. Similarly, it appears that WMD is caused not only by a primary dietary deficiency of selenium, but also by certain dietary constituents (including sulfur) that interfere with selenium metabolism.

Symptoms. WMD has been observed for some time in many countries with intensive horse-bredding programs, occurring both sporadically and in outbreaks. The myopathy mainly affects nursing and weaned foals from birth up to about 12 months of age. For example, in the district served by the Institute for Veterinary Pathology of the University of Munich, von Sandersleben and Schlotke [1977] saw a total of 46 cases of muscular dystrophy in foals during the period from 1973 to 1976, with most cases occurring during the latter part of that period. The 46 cases represented 32 % of all necropsied foals up to 1 year of age. Sixty-five percent of the foals were 1 week old or less, 30 % were 2—8 weeks old, and 5% were older than 8 weeks. The signs of WMD are degeneration of the muscles of locomotion, the muscles in the pectoral, intercostal and diaphragmatic region, the muscles in the upper portion of the digestive tract, or the myocardium [Bostedt, 1977]. Affected newborn foals are dull, cannot stand without assistance, and, when on their feet, assume a crooked or bowlegged stance. Swelling of the gluteal and neck muscles is apparent. Pounding, irregular heart sounds are sometimes heard on auscultation. This early form occurring in newborns contrasts with the late form, which has a more protracted course. Affected animals show a stiff, clumsy gait with a particular unsteadiness of hindquarter movements. The croup muscles feel abnormally tense and hard and appear to be overdeveloped in relation to surrounding muscles. The animal lies down frequently, and decubital lesions are common. A dark discoloration of the urine may be noted. With involvement of the intercostal and diaphragmatic muscles, the respiration becomes rapid and shallow. The mouth is difficult to open due to swelling of the masseters (differential diagnosis: tetanus). Unable to eat, untreated animals become emaciated within 5—7 days. The terminal stage is marked by advanced cachexia and recumbency.

Diagnosis and Differential Diagnosis. The degenerative, lytic and necrotic processes in the muscles lead to increased blood levels of muscle enzymes: creatine phosphokinase (CPK), aspartate aminotransferase (formerly called glutamic oxalacetic transaminase [GOT]), alanine aminotransferase (formerly called glutamic pyruvic transaminase [GPT]), as well as certain dehydrogenases such as lactate dehydrogenase (LDH) and malate dehydrogenase (MDH), and possibly aldolase [Gerber, 1964, 1969]. The behavior of these enzymes in the blood serum can be detected in the laboratory. For example, while the CPK activity in healthy foals is approximately 1.08 μkat/l (65 mU/ml), clinical manifestations appear at about 8.34 μkat/l (500 mU/ml). Levels up to 23.34 μkat/l (14,000 mU/ml) have been observed in foals dying with the disease [Bostedt, 1977].

The uncoordinated movements of affected foals are similar clinically to neuropathogenic states, and the respiratory disturbances may be confused with symptoms of bronchopneumonia or pleuritis. Differentiation from tetanus on the basis of masseter swelling has already been mentioned.

Pathogenesis. Along with PUFA-containing phospholipids, triglycerides and cholesterol, vitamin E forms a major structural component of cellular membranes: by binding to free peroxide radicals, vitamin E protects the membranes from their destructive action. Glutathione peroxidase, whose synthesis depends on dietary selenium, is a key enzyme in various tissues. It acts as an antioxidant, preventing oxidative damage by breaking down lipid peroxides. On the one hand, selenium can reduce the consumption of vitamin E, while vitamin E and sulfur-bearing amino acids provide a certain safety margin in the event of a selenium deficiency. In the absence of these substances, cellular peroxidation proceeds unchecked, and tissue destruction follows.

Lesions. Besides subcutaneous edema, the most obvious change is a generalized pallor of the affected muscle tissue, interrupted by white streaks or flecks. The histologic picture is one of hyaline muscular degeneration, frequently combined with lytic or necrotic processes. The degenerated muscle fibers may already be replaced by fibrous tissue, depending on the duration of the disease.

Treatment. Because the body requires both vitamin E and selenium to protect against oxidative cell damage, and the response of a nutritional muscular dystrophy to doses of vitamin E and/or selenium cannot be predicted with certainty, it is recommended that a combination of vitamin E and selenium be used in treatment, and that treatment be initiated as soon as possible. Clinical symptoms already represent the final stage of WMD! Treatment in foals should begin with the parenteral administration of 2.5 mg selenium and 750 mg vitamin E. Then 700—1,000 mg/day vitamin E is given orally for 5 days. The parenteral therapy should be repeated after a week. In defficient areas, selenium and vitamin E should be administered to newborn foals as soon after birth as possible. At present it is unclear whether the treatment of pregnant mares is worthwhile, for it is not known whether the selenium and vitamin E injection can pass the placental barrier.

2.4.1.2.7. Iodine

The physiologic role of iodine probably relates exclusively to the synthesis and function of thyroid hormones, principally in the thyroid gland itself. Some 20—40 % of all the iodine in the body is contained in the thyroid gland.

Symptoms. An iodine deficiency and inhibition of thyroid hormone synthesis lead to a compensatory hypertrophy of the thyroid gland, and thus to the development of a goiter. A decrease in hormone production like that associated with iodine deficiency leads to a fall of the basal metabolic rate, while hyperfunction of the thyroid increases this rate, possibly by as much as 100 %. This increase is not associated with an increase in working capacity, however; in fact, working capacity in the hyperthyroid animal generally is reduced. Mature horses show loss of condition and loss of libido or prolonged anestrous periods. Prolonged gestation also has been observed. Foals show an exaggerated flexion of the forelimbs and extreme extension of the hindlimbs.

The dietary requirement of iodine is quite low. Moreover, the occurrence of iodine deficiency symptoms is confined to specific regions in which the drinking water and forage plants are highly iodine-deficient. However, iodine deficiency symptoms can appear despite an adequate iodine intake in animals that are fed an excess of calcium, because calcium inhibits iodine absorption. Iodine metabolism is also inhibited by the excessive feeding of plants of the *Brassica* species or peanut oil meal.

Diagnosis. The presence of a goiter is the most obvious symptom of an iodine deficiency. The normal iodine content of the plasma varies between 189 and 315 nmol/l (2.4—4.0 μg/100 ml).

Lesions. Gross enlargement of the thyroid, with a histologic picture of thyroid hyperplasia.

Treatment. Generally the iodine content of green plant matter is considerably higher than that of roots, fruits and seeds. The iodine content of the green plant matter can be increased significantly through the use of iodine fertilizers. Thus, the iodine fertilization of pastures offers an effective alternative to the direct feeding of iodized salt as a means of correcting iodine deficiency. For feed supplementation, iodized salt can be prepared by sprinkling 100 kg of salt with 1 kg of water in which 1—3 g of potassium iodide has been dissolved. This is fed to horses at a rate of 15 to 70 g/day.

References

Beeson, W. M.: Spurenelementbedarf der Haustiere. Tierzüchter *18:* 495 (1966).

Behrens, H.: Die Parakeratose des Schweines. Tierärztl. Umschau *12:* 6 (1957).

Bostedt, H.: Zur Klinik der ernährungsbedingten Muskeldegenerationen bei Fohlen. Dtsch. tierärztl. Wschr. *84:* 293 (1977).

Brenner, W.: XIII. Die Bedeutung des Kupfers in Biologie und Pathologie unter besonderer Berücksichtigung des wachsenden Organismus. Erg. inn. Med. (N. F.) *4:* 806 (1953).

Chou, T. P.; Adolph, W. H.: Copper metabolism in man. Biochem. J. *29:* 476 (1935).

Cunningham, G. N.; Wise, M. B.; Barrick, E. R.: Effect of high dietary levels of manganese on the performance and blood constituents of calves. J. Animal Sci. *25:* 532 (1966).

Elvehjem, C. A.; Sherman, W. C.: The action of copper in iron metabolism. J. biol. Chemistry *98:* 309 (1932).

Gerber, H.: Aktivitätsbestimmungen von Serumenzymen in der Veterinärmedizin. III. Bestimmung der GOT-, GPT- und CPK-Aktivität in einigen Organen des Pferdes als Grundlage für die klinische Verwendung von Serumenzym-Aktivitätbestimmungen. Schweizer Arch. Tierheilkd. *106:* 410 (1964).

Gerber, H.: Serum enzyme determination in equine medicine. Equine vet. J. *1:* 129 (1969).

Halama, A. K.: Die Bedeutung der Spurenelemente für die Ernährung der Haustiere. Wiener tierärztl. Mschr. *42:* 430 (1955).

Jones, T. C.; Reed, W. O.: Muscular dystrophy in a foal. J. Amer. vet. med. Assoc. *113:* 170 (1948).

Kolb, E.: Lehrbuch der Physiologie der Haustiere (VEB Gustav Fischer Verlag, Jena 1980).

Lehr, J. J.: Verschinselen van natriumarmoede bij het dier, alsmede de gefolgen van een te ruime dosering van keukenzout. Tijdschr. Diergeneesk. *86:* 729 (1961).

Sandersleben, J. von; Schlotke, B.: Die Muskeldystrophie (Weissmuskelkrankheit) bei Fohlen, eine offensichtlich im Zunehmen begriffene Erkrankung. Dtsch. tierärztl. Wschr. *84:* 105 (1977).

Seelemann, M.; Baudissin, F. von: Experimentelle Untersuchungen über die Wirkung von Kupfer-Verbindungen, insbesondere auf das hämatopoetische System. Zbl. Vet.-Med. *1:* 354 (1953/54).

Tompsett, S. L.: The copper content of blood. Biochem. J. *28:* 1544 (1934).

Underwood, E.: Trace Elements and Human and Animal Nutrition; 4th ed. (Academic Press, New York 1977).

Wiesner, E.: Ernährungsschäden der landwirtschaftlichen Nutztiere; 2. Aufl. (VEB Gustav Fischer Verlag, Jena 1970).

2.4.2. Vitamin Deficiencies

Vitamins are organic substances which exert specific physiologic actions in very minute amounts. Some can exert true pharmacologic actions when administered in larger doses. Vitamins are formed almost exclusively by higher plants and microorganisms. In some cases, however, the animal organism is capable of synthesizing vitamins from specific precursors (provitamins). Some substances are vitamins in one animal species but not in another. For example, vitamin C (ascorbic acid) can be metabolically synthesized by most domestic animals and so does not represent a 'true' vitamin for these species. A great many vitamins are synthesized by intestinal and ruminal flora and then absorbed by the animal. This is why ruminants are far less dependent on the dietary intake of certain vitamins than are monogastric animals.

The following vitamins are necessary in the diet of the horse: A, D, E, K, B_1, B_2, pantothenic acid, folic acid, B_6, choline, niacin and B_{12}.

Vitamins are of fundamental importance for growth and reproduction as well as for good general health and condition. In addition, some vitamins exert very specific actions.

2.4.2.1. Vitamin A (Retinol)

Vitamin A surpasses all other vitamins in its practical and economic importance to the nutrition of domestic animals. Optimum breeding, maintenance and performance depend in large measure on an adequate supply of this vitamin. Vitamin A is essential for the horse, and the requirement is met largely by ingestion of its precursor carotene, β-carotene being the most important form. From 75 to 90% of the body's vitamin A reserves are stored in the liver.

Symptoms. Vitamin A deficiency can lead to infertility, nerve degeneration, night blindness, abnormal hoof development, susceptibility to respiratory infection, incoordination, corneal keratinization, and various skeletal changes. In malnourished draft horses that were made to perform heavy work, Fehér [1966] observed anorexia, progressive weakness, alopecia and hemeralopia as a consequence of vitamin A deficiency. The symptoms increased until late winter, and at spring shedding the animals lost their entire haircoat, including the hair roots. Hypoactivity of the sweat, sebaceous, salivary and lacrimal glands led to extreme drying of the epithelial layer of the skin, mucosa and conjunctivae. Cornification, extensive depilation, clouding of the cornea and pigmentation of the nictating membrane were observed. Photosensitivity and photophobia were also apparent.

Diagnosis. Symptoms of vitamin A deficiency appear when the blood level falls below about 40 I.U./100 ml plasma.

Treatment. According to Pearson et al. [1949], 10 mg of carotene (= 3,000—4,000 I.U. vit. A) per 100 kg body weight is necessary for the maintenance of all physiologic processes, especially those associated with reproduction and lactation. Sager [1950], on the other hand, recommends 8,000—12,000 I.U. vit A/100 kg BW. Based on our own experience, horses with vitamin A deficiency respond well and quickly to the administration of 200 g/day irradiated yeast for 5 days, the topical application of cod-liver oil to the hairless skin, and the injection of vitamin A.

2.4.2.2. Vitamin D Group (Calciferols)

Like most classic vitamin deficiency diseases, metabolic bone disease due to vitamin D deficiency has been known for many centuries. Only two components of the vitamin D group, vitamin D_2 (ergocalciferol) and vitamin D_3 (cholecalciferol), are of real biological, medical and nutritional importance. Calciferols are important in the mobilization of calcium reserves and the promotion of calcification processes in the growth zone of bones, leading indirectly to an increase in calcium absorption.

Under conditions of an unphysiologic calcium and phosphorus supply (cf. Sec. 2.4.1.1.1.), calciferol continues to regulate normal bone growth but is unable to effect a complete mineralization. With a deficiency of these elements, calciferol enables a normal calcification of the epiphyseal growth zone by mobilizing calcium and phosphorus from the diaphyses. The result of this is a decalcification of the diaphysis, which increases the susceptibility of the bone to fracture. Vitamin D promotes mineral deposition in the skeleton regardless of the level of the mineral supply and the Ca : P ratio (hypermineralization) but has little effect on the growth of the organic matrix. The result is a narrowing of the ratio of inorganic matter to fat-free organic matter in the bone. It should be stressed, however, that the absolute level of mineralization depends basically on the calcium and phosphorus content of the feed and on the Ca : P ratio. Vitamin D acts to maintain the cartilaginous growth and ossification zones of the skeleton within normal limits, regardless of the degree of mineralization. It is extremely capable in this action and maintains it in the face of a highly unphysiologic mineral supply — even to the point of death [GÜNTHER, 1966).

Symptoms. Diseases due to vitamin D deficiency are especially common in animals that are housed in a dark stall and fed a poor-quality diet. Impaired mineralization of the bony tissue leads to a proliferation of the organic matrix of the bones (osteoid), which become calcium-depleted, soft and pliable. The clinical picture of 'rickets' appears as the bones subjected to the highest mechanical loads develop characteristic curvatures (bowlegs, knock knees, sickle hocks, spinal curvature, pelvic contraction). There are also marked enlargements of the epiphyses (joint enlargements) and costochondral junctions (rachitic beads). Enlargements of the carpal, stifle, tarsal and fetlock joints are highly characteristic and frequently lead to the appearance of a 'double joint'. Longitudinal bone growth ceases (rachitic ramification), and the cranial sutures either remain open or are very slow to close. In severe cases the tendons, especially those of the Achilles complex, become torn from their sites of attachment. Usually the rachitic syndrome develops over a period of 1—4 months. The corresponding deficiency disease in mature animals is osteomalacia (see Sec. 2.4.1.1.1.).

Diagnosis. The diagnosis is made from the history (stabling and feeding conditions, exposure to sunlight) and the characteristic clinical symptoms. The serum levels of calcium and phosphate show no change in either 'rickets' or osteomalacia. *Often values are normal.* In disease due to a calcium excess, however, the phosphate levels are strongly depressed. Conversely, rickets and osteomalacia of acidotic origin are associated with very high phosphate levels (3.2—4.2 mmol/l = 10—13 mg/100 ml) and reduced calcium levels. The determination of alkaline phosphatase, however, offers the most reliable means of detecting a rachitic metabolic state prior to the appearance of clinical symptoms. Even in the early stage of rickets, there is a 2- to 3-fold increase in the activity of this enzyme. Characteristic radiographic changes serve to confirm the diagnosis.

Lesions. The lesions correspond to the pathophysiologic and clinical changes.

Treatment. The calciferol requirement of an animal increases with its level of work. While foals up to 8 months of age do well on increasing vitamin D_3 doses of 1,000 to 1,800 I.U./day, working and riding horses require 2,500—3,000 I.U./day. This is why the effects of a vitamin D deficiency in hypovitaminotic herds are felt first by in the fastest-growing, hardest-working members of the group. Thus, increasing use is being made of calciferol-containing mixed feeds in countries with intensive livestock breeding programs.

Generally it is assumed that the requirement of 7-dehydrocholesterol (cholecalciferol) can be adequately met by a half-day's exposure to sunlight each day. However, if sunlight is lacking due to clouds, fog or atmospheric pollution, the level of ultraviolet irradiation is not sufficient to meet the demand. Animals with rickets or osteomalacia have a very good chance of recovery when treated promptly with vitamin D_2 given parenterally or orally (1,000 I.U./100 kg BW/day), and with oral calcium and phosphorus compounds. However, successful treatment is possible only if all contributing factors are controlled. It should also be noted that unlike other vitamins, calciferol can have toxic effects if administered in excessive amounts. A vitamin D overdose has an effect opposite to its therapeutic effect in that it causes a demineralization of the bone, similar to excessive amounts of parathormone. In contrast to the hormone effect, however, the mineral loss from the bone is not replaced by osteoid tissue, and an osteoporotic syndrome develops. Acute calciferol poisoning, which can result from a 200- to 1,000-fold excess, also causes general health disturbances such as anorexia and diarrhea.

2.4.2.3. Vitamin E (Tocopherols)

So far researchers have been unable to determine the site of action of α-tocopherol in the intermediary metabolism or to demonstrate its direct involvement in specific enzyme reactions. The varied nature of the clinical and biochemical deficiency symptoms suggests that vitamin E possesses several biochemical sites of action. The ribonucleic and deoxyribonucleic acid content of the skeletal muscle and bone marrow is elevated in animals with vitamin E deficiency. Another important function of vitamin E is its antioxidant effect on tissue lipoids, which relates to its synergistic effect on other vitamins. Its relationships to vitamin A and carotene are well known. Animals maintained on a vitamin A-free diet show a greater survival rate when fed an adequate supply of vitamin E.

Symptoms. Given the biochemical function of vitamin E, its depletion from tissues has the effect of increasing peroxide formation. The importance of vitamin E as a biological peroxidant and the consequences of its absence were detailed in the section on Selenium (2.4.1.2.6.).

2.4.2.4. Vitamin K

Vitamin K, like the group-B vitamins, is a substance that is active in all phases of cellular metabolism and therefore is vital to the formation and existence of cells. On the whole, the properties of vitamin K may be characterized as growth-promoting. Vitamin K also has antihemorrhagic activity. It occurs naturally in two chemical forms: vitamin K_1, which is formed in higher plants, and vitamin K_2, which is synthesized by numerous microorganisms that inhabit the rumen and large intestine. Both are derivatives of 2-methyl-1,4-naphthoquinone (menadione).

Vitamin K deficiencies are nonexistent under ordinary circumstances because of the high content of the substance in plants feedstuffs and its substantial synthesis by microbial activity in the digestive tract.

Symptoms. Vitamin K deficiency symptoms in the horse occur only in the form of sweet clover poisoning (cf. Sec. 2.5.1.3.). This condition, also known as dicoumarin poisoning, is caused by the ingestion of moldy, moisture-damaged hay or moldy sweet clover silage (*Melilotus* spp.).

Treatment. In acute vitamin K deficiency, the administration of 100—400 mg menadione within 24 hours is recommended. The exact dose level depends on the size of the animal and its condition.

2.4.2.5. Vitamin B_1 (Thiamine, Aneurin)

The principal action of thiamine is on the carbohydrate metabolism. It also influences other reactions in the intermediary metabolism. Only small amounts of vitamin B_1 are stored in the body. It is most plentiful in the liver, kidneys, heart and brain, i.e., in organs with a high metabolic activity.

Symptoms. The effects of a deficient thiamine intake relate mainly to its function in the general metabolism and neurologic processes. The clinical symptoms of thiamine deficiency are highly complex and often nonspecific. Vitamin B_1 deficiencies are relatively uncommon in horses, because the requirement is partially satisfied by cecal flora. Deficiencies are most commonly observed when the overall plane of nutrition is poor [BRONSCH, 1957]. They are manifested by growth disturbances and in most cases by emaciation, despite a good appetite, and a dull haircoat. These are followed by neurologic manifestations in the form of increased central excitability, incoordination and unphysiologic gaits.

The body temperature is usually unchanged, and the pulse varies with the clinical picture. A relationship exists in horses between thiamine deficiency and paralytic myoglobinemia.

Lesions. Necropsy reveals hemorrhages in the stomach and myocardium, yellowish spots on the liver, and stagnant blood in the kidneys.

Treatment. Horses that are fed a high-carbohydrate diet and perform heavy work should receive prophylactic vitamin B_1 in the form of 1—2% yeast added to the ration. Under normal circumstances the requirement is adequately met by grain, green feed and good-quality hay. About 2—4 mg thiamine should be fed per kg digestible non-fat raw nutrients (crude protein, crude fiber, N-free extracts).

2.4.2.6. Vitamin B_2 (Riboflavin, Lactoflavin)

The biochemical action of riboflavin is based upon its binding to the flavin enzymes, which function as hydrogen transfer agents in the tissues during substrate oxidation.

Symptoms. Because riboflavin is involved in fundamental metabolic processes, a lack of this vitamin leads to general, relatively nonspecific deficiency symptoms. Young animals manifest a retardation or cessation of growth. Skin changes appear, and a sustained B_2 deficiency leads to nerve damage, testicular atrophy, impaired fertility, and changes in the thyroid and adrenals. Diarrhea, increased salivation and lacrimation, and hair loss are also observed. Riboflavin deficiency is also incriminated in various ocular diseases and is considered a cause of 'moon blindness' (periodic ophthalmia).

Diagnosis. Riboflavin deficiency is extremely difficult to diagnose. Generally the clinical changes and reduced blood values will provide the only basis for diagnosis.

Treatment. Riboflavin deficiency is unlikely to occur in horses that receive green feed. The daily requirement is about 4—8 mg/100 kg BW. Riboflavin is effective in preventing periodic ophthalmia when administered at a rate of 40 mg/day.

2.4.2.7. Pantothenic Acid

The ubiquitous occurrence of pantothenic acid in all living systems is based upon its binding to coenzyme A (CoA), which is involved in the transfer and transformation of acid esters. It occurs in practically all cells. Also important is its compound with succinic acid, called succinyl coenzyme A, which is the primary substrate for the breakdown of the amino acid glycine. It is understandable, therefore, that a deficiency of pantothenic acid leads to profound metabolic derangements.

Pantothenic acid is a dietary essential for horses. A pantothenic acid deficiency is most likely to develop in animals that are fed a riboflavin-deficient diet. The highest levels of pantothenic acid are found in yeast, molasses, peanut oil meal, milk and milk byproducts, and in green feed. The substance can also be produced synthetically. Pantothenic acid usually occurs as calcium pantothenate, is highly unstable at a high pH, and is destroyed by heat.

Symptoms and Lesions. Experimentally induced pantothenic acid deficiency (a spontaneous deficiency is unlikely in the horse under natural feeding conditions) is manifested by a rough haircoat, alopecia, growth disturbances, secondary pneumonia, and adrenal insufficiency.

Diagnosis. A diagnosis of pantothenic acid deficiency is made from the history, an analysis of the diet, and possibly from symptoms of adrenocortical insufficiency.

Treatment. The daily pantothenic acid requirement of the horse is between 200 and 400 μg/100 kg BW. Reports by U.S. authors indicate that about 400 μg/kg (!)/day is an effective therapeutic dose.

2.4.2.8. Folic Acid Group

Folic acid (pteroylglutamic acid) plays a central role in the metabolism of C_1 fragments, which undergo complicated, enzyme-mediated reactions involved, for example, in the synthesis of choline, methionine and thymine. It is believed that folic acid is essential for the maintenance of normal splenic function.

In nature, folic acid is most abundant in yeast, wheat and green feed and is probably also synthesized in the digestive tract.

Symptoms. Naturally-occurring folic acid deficiencies have not been diagnosed in the horse. Deficiency symptoms appear only after the prolonged administration of sulfonamides, or if the vitamin has been destroyed by heating the feed. Disturbances of erythropoiesis are observed in such cases.

Treatment. Animals with a suspected folic acid deficiency should be given foods that are rich in folic acid. About 100 mg sodium foliate/horse/day may be administered orally or parenterally, distributed in several daily doses over a period of 4—7 days.

2.4.2.9. Choline

In a strict sense choline is not a true vitamin, because it can be synthesized within the body. In recent years it has often been assigned to the B group of vitamins because of its close metabolic relationships with other B-complex vitamins, and because endogenous production is insufficient in many animals to meet the requirement. Thus, liver diseases can lead to vitamin losses, or dietary deficiencies can arise if certain essential amino acids, such as methionine or betaine, are lacking in the diet.

As a component of the phospholipids, choline plays an important role in fat metabolism. Besides its lipotropic activity, choline is important, together with methionine, as a supplier of methyl groups. It is through the mobilization of these methyl groups, and presumably their subsequent oxidation, that betaine is formed. Choline is a constituent of lecithin and occurs in high concentrations in most animal tissues as well as in wheat and soybeans.

Symptoms. The major symptoms of a choline deficiency are fatty degeneration of the liver, renal hemorrhages and a reduced growth rate.

Treatment. The choline requirement generally is satisfied by the natural choline content of the ration, presuming a reasonably well-balanced diet. The choline requirement is influenced to some extent by the pantothenic acid content of the feed, although a choline deficit cannot be offset even by a very high intake of pantothenic acid. Choline dehydrogen citrate or choline gluconate may be administered therapeutically; horses tolerate relatively large doses owing to the extremely low toxicity of choline. Fatty degeneration, fatty infiltration and other liver diseases should be treated with large doses of choline salts combined with a soybean oil meal.

2.4.2.10. Vitamin B_6 (Pyridoxine)

The metabolically-active form of these compounds is pyridoxal, which serves as a coenzyme for numerous reactions in the amino acid metabolism. It participates in reactions that enable the body to transform, degrade and synthesize amino acids. Besides its function in the protein metabolism, pyridoxal also has relationships with the carbohydrate metabolism. It is also thought to influence the metabolism of vitamin B_{12}.

Symptoms. A deficiency of pyridoxine is relatively rare under natural conditions. Experimental vitamin B_6 deficiency causes a variety of fairly nonspecific symptoms such as growth retardation, anorexia and neurologic signs. These are frequently accompanied by a hypochromic anemia, which may be attributed to a disturbance of protein metabolism in the bone marrow and a reduced synthesis of δ-aminolevulinic acid. Pyridoxine hydrochloride, incidentally, is a specific antidote for an overdose of the anthelmintic drug cyanacethydrazide.

Lesions. Fatty degeneration of the liver, thickening of the skin, pallor of the kidneys.

Treatment. The pyridoxine content of ordinary mixed feed rations, together with the yet-unknown quantity of the vitamin produced by biosynthesis, are sufficient to satisfy at least the minimum requirement (see above). If a deficiency is suspected, 50 mg of pyridoxine hydrochloride may be given by injection 2—3 times weekly.

2.4.2.11. Niacin (Antipellagra Vitamin, PP Factor)

The substance in niacin with true vitamin activity is nicotinic acid amide. Nicotinic acid has an equivalent activity, for it is readily transformed into the amide within the body. Both compounds are pyridine derivatives and often are collectively termed 'niacin'. Nicotinic acid amide is the chemically active component of the codehydrases (NAD, NADP). Nicotinic acid, like choline, is not considered an essential nutrient in all cases. If supplies of vitamin B_6 and tryptophan are adequate, the vitamin is capable of synthesizing nicotinic acid from tryptophan. Yeast, legumes and soybeans are naturally rich in niacin.

Symptoms. Niacin deficiency has not yet been observed in horses.

2.4.2.12. Vitamin B_{12} (Cyanocobalamin)

Research into the function of the cobalt-containing vitamin B_{12} in the metabolism is not yet complete. It has been learned that vitamin B_{12}, like folic acid (q.v.), plays a significant role in the metabolism of the C_1 group. The requirement of vitamin B_{12} for ruminants and horses is completely satisfied by microbial synthesis under normal feeding conditions (cobalt-containing feedstuffs). Supplemental feeding of the vitamin is unnecessary, therefore, if the cobalt supply is adequate.

Vitamin B_{12} is essential for the synthesis of nucleoproteins as well as for the maintenance of a normal sulfhydryl level in the blood. It is important for normal hematopoiesis.

Symptoms. Deficiency symptoms include fertility disturbances, loss of condition, muscular weakness and anemia.

Diagnosis. A vitamin B_{12} deficiency should be presumed whenever a cobalt deficiency and erythrocyte deficit are present.

Treatment. The oral administration of cobalt or parenteral administration of vitamin B_{12} will relieve deficiency symptoms. Thoroughbred horses should receive 1,000 to 2,000 μg of vitamin B_{12} routinely at weekly intervals. In South African racehorses with an unfavorable blood status apparently stemming from a cobalt deficiency, SIMPSON [1961] was able to improve performance by treating the animals with vitamin B_{12} and iron preparations. Within 4 weeks the hematocrit rose from 0.49 to 0.61 (49 to 61 vol.%), the hemoglobin level from 11.17 to 13.22 mmol/l (18.0 to 21.3 g%), and the erythrocyte count from 10.1 to $14.1 \cdot 10^{12}$/l (!). Nursing animals receive an adequate supply via the milk.

References

BRONSCH, K.: Zur Ursachenermittlung von Mangelkrankheiten durch den praktizierenden Tierarzt. Vet.-med. Nachr. p. 1 (1957).

FEHÉR, T.: Idös lovak A-avitaminosisa. Magyar Allat. Lapja *21:* 511 (1966).

GÜNTHER, K.: Über die Wirkungsweise der D-Vitamine und ihre Bedeutung für die Tierernährung. 1. Mitt. Z. Tierphysiol., Tierernähr. Futtermittelkunde *21:* 361 (1966).

PEARSON, P. B., WINCHESTER, C. F.; HARVEY, A. L.: Recommended nutrient allowances for horses. National Res. Council Publ. (1949).

SAGER, F. C.: Feeding Horses. Stud Managers Handbook, Lexington, Ky. 1950.

SIMPSON, L. A.: A note on the effect of vitamin B_{12} on the haematological picture of the race horse. J. South African Vet. Med. Assoc. *32:* 95 (1961).

2.4.3. Nutritional Limb Abnormalities

Among Thoroughbred horses in southern Africa, two different limb abnormalities of nutritional origin have repeatedly been described in yearlings.

2.4.3.1. 'Open Knees'

This disease generally appears between the first and second year of life and is more common in male foals than in females. Affected animals tend to have an above-average rate of growth, and the changes are most pronounced when there is an excess of energy in the diet. Affected foals, moreover, are always the offspring of large, heavy horses. Bone growth in these foals apparently outstrips bone mineralization, especially in magnesium-deficient areas. The clinical severity of the disease varies from transitory mild forms to forms in which there is considerable enlargement of the distal radial epiphysis and carpometacarpal joint, and the carpal bones are clearly visible from the front.

2.4.3.2. Block Hoof Syndrome

Block hoof syndrome is most common in horses about 3 months of age or older and is characterized by a knuckling-over of the fetlock as a result of tendon shortening. The syndrome tends to be associated with a high dietary intake of protein and calcium, combined with a phosphorus deficiency. It can occur, for example, in horses fed an exclusive diet of lucerne hay, which contains about 18% crude protein, 1.8% calcium, and only 0.22% phosphorus. Affected horses may still be able to perform light work for a limited time. Severe acute cases are usually seen during the weaning period; the occurrence of congenital cases has also been reported.

Reference

Boyazoglu, P. A.; Barrett, E. L.; Du Toit, J. de V.: Nutritional limb abnormalities in yearling horses. World veterin. Congr., Proc., Thessaloniki *20:* 3, 2095 (1975).

2.4.4. Diabetes Insipidus

Diabetes insipidus is most common during the summer months and tends to affect horses that perform heavy work.

Symptoms. The disease is characterized by excessive thirst, poor appetite, and colicky signs or bloating. Eating of the bedding is not unusual. The urine is clear and increased in volume. Affected horses have a weak, emaciated appearance and a rough, dull haircoat. Fever is rarely present.

Etiology. Feeding errors or nutritional deficiencies are the most frequent cause. These include the feeding of spoiled grain, green feeds containing poisonous plants (e.g., meadow saffron), or the overfeeding of potassium-rich molasses. The disease generally lasts 1—2 months, and recovery is complete if suitable care is given.

Treatment. Feeding errors are corrected, and the animal is given 6—100 g of calcium carbonate daily, combined with a mixture of *Nux vomica,* gentian, quinine and iron carbonate.

2.4.5. Hyperlipemia in Ponies

Definittion. Hyperlipemia is an often fatal metabolic disease that mainly affects pony mares in the third trimester of pregnancy and is characterized by an elevation of blood lipids, fatty infiltration of the liver, and the cardiac changes of Hegglin's syndrome.

Symptoms. The disease, which has been described since about 1960, affects ponies exclusively and is most common in the Shetland breed. The initial signs are a reduced appetite or complete anorexia with a normal water intake, depression, a temperature rise to 38.5—40.4 °C, reduced defecation or a watery, malodorous diarrhea, and a fetid odor to the breath. The mortality is about 65 %. The disease occurs mainly in late pregancy or shortly after foaling or abortion. The blood of affected ponies has an opalescent sheen, and the serum shows a milky cloudiness that is especially marked in the supernatant layer. The heart rate is increased to 60—80/min. 'Hegglin's syndrome' appears to be a typical finding in the electrocardiogram or phonocardiogram. The QT interval is prolonged (electrical systole), and the interval from the start of the Q wave to the 2nd heart sound is shortened (mechanical systole), so that the 2nd heart sound appears before the end of the T wave. This finding is more pronounced in moribund patients than in patients that recover.

Etiology. Hyperlipemia in ponies is not thought to be a separate disease entity, but rather a clinical manifestation of other diseases such as parasitism, enteritides, respiratory diseases, etc.

Diagnosis. The aforementioned ECG changes are in themselves suggestive of hyperlipemia. Blood studies show elevated levels of total fat, total and free cholesterol, phospholipids, neutral lipids, fatty acid esters and free fatty acids. Serum electrophoresis shows an elevation of β-lipoproteins with a depression of the α-fraction. An acidosis is present, and alkaline phosphatase values are increased. Clotting time is shortened, and the bromsulphalein test shows decreased values as evidence of liver damage. If the blood sample is left to stand for only 1—2 minutes, a milky-white layer will form on its surface. Hypercalcemia tends to develop in animals with low blood sugar values. With a normal or elevated blood sugar, calcium levels are normal, but magnesium levels are somewhat low. The serum values of ASAT, SGPT, LDH and SDH are elevated, ASAT and LDH showing approximately a 10-fold increase above normal.

Lesions. There is extensive fatty infiltration of the liver and most other organs, especially the kidneys.

Treatment. Treatment is directed in many fronts and relies mainly on the administration of glucose and glucocorticoids. The underlying disease may warrant the use of special drugs such as anthelmintics for parasites or antibiotics for the control of diarrhea or respiratory infection. SCHOTMAN and WAGENAAR [1969] administered 20,000—50,000 units/day heparin i.v., distributed in two daily doses, for several days, administering physiologic saline to patients with a low hematocrit. The acidosis is neutralized with 2% sodium bicarbonate solution. To date, however, the results of treatment have not been encouraging. It is recommended, therefore, that ponies be examined prophylactically for hyperlipemia whenever anorexia is present, and that the transporting of ponies in late pregnancy be avoided in order to minimize unnecessary stresses.

Prognosis. The prognosis varies with the nature of the underlying disease. Generally the prognosis is guarded, but a grave prognosis is indicated if there is fatty infiltration of the liver and kidneys, or if the difference between electrical and mechanical systole is less than 50 ms.

References

DEEGEN, E.: Die prognostische Bedeutung des 'Hegglin-Syndroms' bei der Hyperlipämie der Ponys. Dtsch. tierärztl. Wschr. *79:* 297 (1972).

ERIKSEN, L.; SIMESEN, M. G.: Hyperlipaemi hos ponier. Nord. Vet.-Med. *22:* 273 (1970).

SCHOTMAN, A. J. H.; WAGENAAR, G.: Hyperlipemia in ponies. Zbl. Vet.-Med. R. A *16:* 1 (1969).

2.4.6. Digestive Disturbances

The anatomic and physiologic peculiarities of the equine digestive system predispose this species to certain digestive disturbances that can arise just as suddenly and unexpectedly as colic. Moreover, the horse appears especially prone to microbial disturbances leading to diarrhea, degenerative liver disease, allergic symptoms, laminitis and myoglobinuria (q.v).

Traditional feedstuffs that are high in crude fiber carry a significant risk of causing intestinal impaction with associated colic. This is quickly relieved by the ingestion of granulated mixed feeds, which hasten the passage of food through the digestive tract [Wolter, 1975]. For example, grain straw (33 % crude fiber) takes 27 hours to traverse the equine digestive tract when ingested in the long, uncut form, 26 hours when chopped, and 31 hours [sic] when granulated [Wolter, 1976]. While the large amounts of carbohydrates and proteins normally present in the digestive tract are readily broken down by intestinal microflora, the presence of excessive amounts of cellulose in the alimentary tract can lead to microbial disturbances. Thus, large amounts of starch in the cecum can lower the pH sufficiently to cause excessive lactic acid fermentation leading to diarrhea, dehydration and diuresis. Heart and liver disease may also result.

Conversely, the lack of crude fiber in many commercial feeds adversely affects large bowel motility and can lead to stasis and other problems. The exclusive use of pelleted feeds, moreover, can cause spasmodic colic.

Finally, *Clostridia* spp. can be an important factor in digestive disturbances, for their endotoxins hamper bowel motility and can cause necrosis in various parenchymatous organs. *Cl. perfringens* is especially important in this regard.

All these digestive disturbances are treated initially by a careful modification of the ration, followed by symptomatic therapy (see under specific disease headings).

References

Wolter, R.: Désordres nutritionnels chez les cheveaux. World veterin. Congr., Proc. Thessaloniki *20:* 3, 2091 (1975).

Wolter, R.: Quelques actualites a propos troubles alimentaires chez le cheval. Rev. Méd. vét. *126:* 1249 (1975).

Wolter, R.: Alimentation et pathologie chez le cheval. Rec. Méd. vét. *152:* 377 (1976).

2.5. Poisonings

Poisons can be classified in various ways:

1. by their effect on the animal (e.g., drugs, stimulants, protoplasmic and parenchymal poisons. narcotics);
2. by their chemical or physical properties (e.g., organic poisons such as alkaloids and glycosides, inorganic poisons, gaseous poisons, etc.);
3. by their analytical behavior (e.g., volatile, acid-soluble, metals);
4. by their origin or usage.

For practical purposes, it appears most useful to classify the most common poisons according to the group or class of substances from which they originated. This approach is usually best from the standpoint of history-taking, and an accurate history is essential for identifying at least the group to which the poison belongs and thus for instituting specific treatment.

The statistics of recent years indicate that the importance of specific toxins as causes of animal poisonings has changed dramatically during the course of the century. The burgeoning use of chemicals in agriculture has significantly increased the risk of poisoning from pesticides, herbicides, fertilizers and industrial emissions, while poisonings caused by toxic plants or drugs have assumed a minor role. Even today, of course, all effective drugs may be regarded as poisons with a selective action. The effects of a given drug depend greatly on the dose administered per kilogram body weight and per unit time. Besides absolute and relative overdoses, idiosyncrasies also play a role. Thus, as HAPKE [1975] points out, proteins (e.g., ACTH), procaine, salicylates, organic iodine compounds, certain antibiotics (penicillin, streptomycin) and nitrofurazone have a strong tendency to provoke allergic reactions, while other drugs such as coal tar products, chlorpromazine, griseofulvin, sulfonamides and many plant constituents have a tendency to cause photosensitization. Finally, drug toxicities are a function of species-specific responses, and these do not play a dominant role in the horse. Thus, drug poisonings in this species will not be discussed separately, as the principles valid for other species will also apply to the horse.

Reference

HAPKE, H.-J.: Toxikologie für Veterinärmediziner (Enke, Stuttgart 1975).

Food poisonings are disturbances in normal vital processes that are caused directly or indirectly by feedstuffs. Any number of animals in a group may be affected, from one to a great many. The main categories of food poisoning, such as those caused by poisonous plants, industrial emissions, agrochemicals, bacteria-contaminated feedstuffs, etc., are discussed separately. In addition to these, there are a number of other conditions that can result from improper feeding of the horse.

Feedstuffs may in themselves be entirely safe, yet, for physiologic reasons, may not be suitable for feeding to a particular species. In other cases, normally safe feedstuffs may be rendered harmful by improper preparation or storage (e.g., mold or mite contamination). Vegetable feeds may spoil as a result of prolonged soaking in water. Molasses-containing mixed feeds tend to undergo alcoholic or acetic fermentation, leading to disturbances of bowel motility.

Feedstuffs with a high sand content cause enteritis in horses ('sand colic'). Unwashed turnips and hay that have been covered by flood water are common sources.

Some feeds, such as corn stalks, can cause mechanical injury to the oral and lingual mucosa unless cut into very small pieces before feeding. Injuries of this type can provoke complete feed refusal in the affecred animal.

Special care should be taken in the feeding of very dry feeds, such as chopped turnips, which have a tendency to swell within the stomach, especially if the animal is watered immediately after feeding. This volume increase may be great enough to cause gastric rupture. Finally, a special risk is associated with the feeding of frozen feeds.

2.5.1. Nitrates and Nitrites

Horses are susceptible to nitrate and nitrite poisoning, though far less so than pigs, cattle and sheep. The main causes of these poisonings are:

1. the ingestion of nitrate-containing forage plants or weeds;
2. the ingestion of other nitrate- or nitrite-containing feedstuffs, such as silage and especially the juices draining from silos;
3. the ingestion of nitrate-containing mixtures, such as various mineral fertilizers or ensiling aids;
4. the ingestion of nitrate- or nitrite-containing water or effluent.

Other less common poisoning sources are nitrate- and nitrite-rich drugs and saltpeter, as well as collections of nitrate- or nitrite-containing water in stall drainage pipes.

The nitrate level in plants in which nitrate represents an intermediate stage of protein synthesis is influenced both by the species of the plant and by various ecologic factors.

Assuming equal conditions of growth and fertilization, common plants may be classified as follows according to their ability to accumulate nitrates, based on the enzyme complement of the plants and their synthesis activity:

1. Plants that accumulate high nitrate levels: green oats, sunflowers, corn, rape and mustard (as stubble crops), turnips, turnip tops, potato tops, and various weeds (orache, galinsoga, thistle, wild lettuce, foxtail, chickweek, bindweed, nightshade [6—10 % NO_3], goosefoot spp.). The difference in the nitrate content of turnips and potatoes derives from the fact that turnips have a natural tendency to accumulate univalent ions, mainly in the body of the turnip, while potatoes accumulate very low nitrate levels even in nitrogen-rich soils. Similarly, nitrate levels tend to be low in sugar-beet roots but high in sugar-beet tops.
2. Plants that accumulate moderate nitrate levels: most forage grasses and green rye.
3. Plants that accumulate low nitrate levels: orchard grass, legumes (clover, lucerne, vetch, etc.).

Factors the can reduce nitrate accumulation in plants include heat and cold, light reduction due to clouds or fog, drought, soil acidity, unbalanced fertilization, plant diseases, metabolic disturbances caused by hormone weed killers (e.g., dichlorophenoxyacetic acid products), as well as primary and secondary trace element deficiencies. One interesting effect of trace elements is the inhibitory effect of manganese- and molybdenum-containing fertilizers on the uptake of nitrates by plants. Copper tends to negate this effect, apparently by acting as a molybdenum antagonist.

Care must be taken in the use of ensiling aids, which contain 0.1% nitrites and up to 0.5% nitrates. Nitrites in the silage do not pose a serious hazard, for within 18 days they are reduced to nitrous gases, ammonia or nitrogen in reactions that are catalyzed by microbial enzymes (e.g., ammonia formed by nitrite reductase from *E. coli*) and possibly by plant enzymes. Given this fact, nitrite poisoning is unlikely in herbivores as a result of nitrite use in silage. Nitrates, on the other hand, are reduced very slowly and incompletely in ensiled material. As a result, about 70% of the nitrate added to the silage is still present when the feed is removed from the silo, and the nitrate may be consumed in amounts sufficient to cause poisoning.

Finally, drinking water may contain high levels of nitrates and nitrites and is a significant factor in the etiology of nitrate and nitrite poisonings. Spring water, for example, may become contaminated by liquid manure fertilizers or nitrogenous mineral fertilizers, or by the effluent from silos, stables and food processing plants. An even more common source is surface water that has become contaminated as a result of heavy rainfall or the runoff from fast-melting snow.

In the GDR, green feeds and their byproducts are classified as 'low-nitrate' if their nitrate content is less than or equal to 1.0% by dry matter. Feedstuffs with a content higher than 1.0% are classified as 'high-nitrate'.

The diagnosis of acute nitrate poisoning in itself presents few difficulties. The clinical signs are the product of three mechanisms:

1. vasodilatation
2. methemoglobin formation
3. local irritation of the gastrointestinal mucosa.

The earliest signs are sudden anorexia, colic, salivation, vomiting, diarrhea, polyuria and heightened excitability. The cardinal symptoms are a subnormal temperature, weakness, muscle tremor, dyspnea, cyanosis, tachycardia, ataxia, tonic-clonic convulsions, coma and death within 1—4 hours, although a 2- to 3-day course is occasionally observed. In peracute cases characteristic changes are usually absent, and pigs with nitrate poisoning may die without showing any symptoms. Late symptoms consist of pulmonary emphysema and abortion.

The most prominent finding at necropsy is a dark, tarry blood. The gatrointestinal mucosae show a cherry-red to reddish-purple discoloration; the intestinal contents are sanguineous or brown. The mucosae of the kidneys, urinary bladder and trachea also show hemorrhagic inflammation.

Laboratory analysis of the methemoglobin level in the blood and the nitrate and nitrite content of the plasma provides important evidence as to the nature of the poisoning. Whole blood is unsuitable for analysis, because both anions are unstable in the presence of blood cells. Results are meaningful only if blood is drawn while the animal is still alive or immediately after its death, and laboratory tests are done the same day the blood is drawn. Any delay in sampling or analysis will reduce the chance of detection. Hence, negative findings in the ingesta or clotted blood from a dead animal do not necessarily preclude poisoning. If fresh samples cannot be obtained and promptly analyzed, then an analysis of the feed is the best procedure.

In the treatment of nitrate and nitrite poisoning, the main goal is the reconversion of methemoglobin to hemoglobin, i.e., the reduction of the trivalent iron in methemoglobin to a divalent form that can carry oxygen. Artificial respiration is useless, therefore, before this reduction has been accomplished. The intravenous administration of methylene blue in a 0.1—1.0% solution (1—2 mg/kg BW) has proved useful for this purpose. The subcutaneous injection of epinephrine and cardiotonin® is also beneficial.

The diagnosis of chronic nitrate poisoning, which is of potentially greater significance than acute poisoning, is considerably more difficult than in acute cases. Symptoms in the horse include growth retardation, poor food utilization, fertility disorders in the form of low conception rates and abortions. There is also carotenase inhibition, increased vitamin A and vitamin E consumption with consequent deficiency symptoms, a disturbance of thyroid iodine utilization with an associated deficit of thyroid hormone production and goiter formation. There may even be sudden death without premonitory symptoms. The vitamin A disturbance is especially severe in monogastric animals. Hepatic reserves may be decreased by up to 50% following the prolonged ingestion of nitrates or nitrites, because nitrites create an acidic pH that is destructive to carotene and vitamin A. The vitamin A deficiency is obviously to blame for the fertility disturbances observed in poisoned animals, as well as for hyperkeratosis and the occurrence of epithelial defects in the respiratory and digestive tract that predispose to infection. Nitrites are also destructive to vitamin B_6 and thiamine.

References

Wiesner, E.: Ernährungsschäden der landwirtschaftlichen Nutztiere; 2. Aufl. (VEB Gustav Fischer Verlag, Jena 1970).

Wiesner, E.: Chronische Nitratbelastung bei Wiederkäuern. Mh. Vet.-Med. *33:* 834 (1978).

Wiesner, E.; Berschneider, F.; Neuffer, K.; Willer, S.; Waldeck, B.: Zur Frage der Nitrattoleranz bei Milchkühen. Mh. Vet.-Med. *34:* 487 (1979).

Zaribnicky, F.: Fütterungslehre und Futterschädlichkeiten. Münchener Tierärztl. Wschr. *80:* 124 (1929).

2.5.2. Poisonous Plants

Livestock poisonings resulting from the ingestion of natural plant constituents are by no means as common today as they once were. Plants deemed to be 'poisonous' have become scarce in livestock operations owing to modern techniques of pasture and grassland management, and it is rare for their constituents to appear in the feed of agricultural animals. Nevertheless, it is still common to make a catch-all diagnosis of 'plant poisoning' whenever a horse dies suddenly and a specific cause cannot be ascertained. Such a diagnosis cannot be considered established, however, until it has been verified by laboratory tests, postmortem examination, of feeding trials in experimental animals. While hundreds of plants may be suspect in any given case, only a few produce clinical symptoms, and few of these symptoms are pathognomonic for plant poisoning. Moreover, only a few plants cause lesions that are visible at necropsy. This does not reflect a lack of toxicity, however, for many poisonous plants can cause death without producing clinical signs or demonstrable lesions. Finally, a number of plants are poisonous only at specific times or under certain conditions. Thus, a plant may be poisonous when freshly picked or cut, but not after it is dried.

By and large, poisonous plants are not palatable, and horses will eat them only if normal forage is insufficient or the plant has become mixed with the ration. Sometimes a mineral deficiency will provoke a horse to eat toxic plants. As a rule, horses must consume at least 1—3 % of their own body weight in poisonous plants before toxicity symptoms appear.

The effects of plant poisonings are most apparent in the nervous system, gastrointestinal tract and liver. General signs include anorexia, dehydration, depression, emaciation and dyspnea. The body temperature usually is normal or slightly below normal. Signs indicative of gastrointestinal disease include diarrhea, salivation and colic. The diarrhea may be thin, malodorous or bloody, but diarrhea in itself is not pathognomonic for plant poisoning. Salivation from stomatitis is not as common as diarrhea, while colic is generally present. Signs indicative of central nervous system involvement include hyperexcitability, muscular twitching, incoordination, paresis, coma, convulsions, abnormal movements, and the assumption of peculiar positions. Of course these signs are not pathognomonic of poisoning, either, and may be caused by rabies, meningitis, liver disease, certain drugs, etc.

It is seldom possible to render a specific therapy for plant poisonings. Most cases are managed with general therapy supported by symptomatic treatment with sedatives, tranquilizers, electrolyte solutions, etc. After the diet has been checked and changed as needed, an attempt is made to remove the toxic material from the digestive tract the aid of a laxative. A 500-kg horse should be given about 1—3 liters of mineral oil, 500 g of magnesium sulfate, or an injection of lentin. Poison remaining in the body should be inactivated by administering activated charcoal, Fuller's earth, bentonite or tannic acid, which act as adsorbents. Nonspecific detoxicants that may be given orally include calcium gluconate (20 %, 100—500 ml), dextrose (10—50 %, 500 to 1,000 ml), or a 25 % sodium thiosulfate solution (150—500 ml). Calcium gluconate and dextrose are additionally useful as sources of energy.

2.5.2.1. Horsetail

Of the many known species of horsetail, *Equisetum palustre*, the swamp horsetail (fig. 2.5. — 1), is considered the most poisonous. Its toxic principles are silicic acid and a mixture of amine-like bases that includes the principal alkaloid palustrin (formerly called equisetin). Other alkaloids (palustridin, nicotine, etc.), aconitic acid, flavequisetin and volatile oils are present in much smaller amounts. The plant also contains a thiaminase.

Symptoms. The horse is by far the most susceptible of the domestic animal species to equisetum poisoning. Four to five weeks after ingestion of the horsetail, the thiaminase in the plants causes a thiamine deficiency syndrome in which neurologic signs are predominant. In acute cases a basic distinction is made between a syndrome of general hypersensitivity and a syndrome of ataxia. The former is characterized by psychic excitability, anxiety, hypersensitvity of the higher senses, and a heightened peripheral nerve excitability that mainly affects the sensory fibers, leading to cutaneous hyperesthesia, abnormal pressure sensitivity of the peripheral nerve trunks and exaggerated reflexes. The stage of increased excitability is followed later by signs of motor unrest: fibrillary twitching of the facial muscles and extensor muscles of the forelimbs. Apparently the toxins produce mixed sensory-motor lesions that initially cause a sensory and motor excitation, followed later by neurologic losses. The ataxic syndrome is characterized by disturbances of motor coordination. Presumably a concurrent peripheral and cerebellar ataxia is involved. The late stage is marked

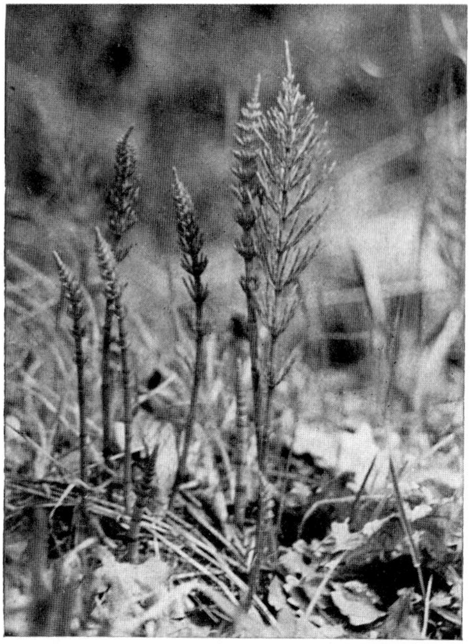
1

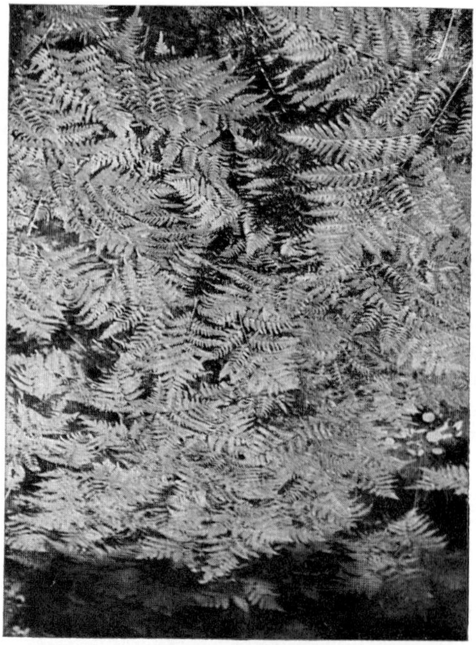
2

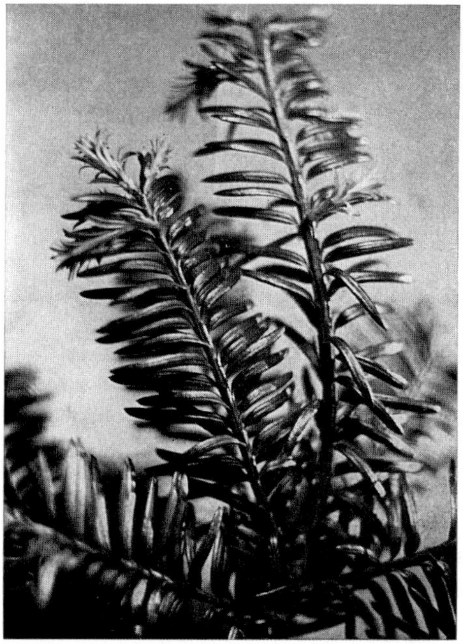
3

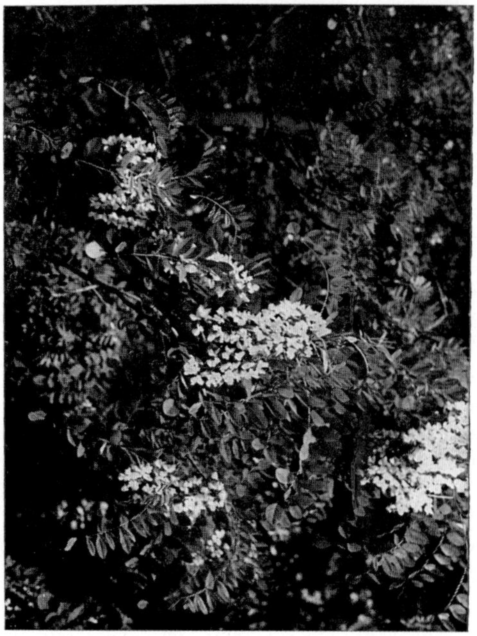
4

Fig. 2.5. — *1.* Swamp horsetail.
Fig. 2.5. — *2.* Bracken fern.
Fig. 2.5. — *3.* Yew.
Fig. 2.5. — *4.* Locust.

by regular convulsions, though in some cases the ataxia gives way to a paresis or complete paralysis of the hindquarters. While most animals show no sensory losses, blindness develops in some instances Eventually the animal goes down, becomes exhausted, and dies in a comatose state. As in most poisonings, the severity of symptoms depends upon individual predisposition, the animal's nutritional status, and the presence or absence of preexisting diseases such as gastrointestinal catarrh.

The thiamine deficiency in horsetail poisoning leads to disturbances of the intermediary carbohydrate metabolism. Autonomic disturbances may also be apparent: sinus bradycardia (18—30/min), hypothermia (35.5—37.5 °C) and hypotension (pressure in abdominal aorta 60—80 mm systolic, 48—65 mm diastolic). Other frequent symptoms are mydriasis, hypotonia of the gastrointestinal tract, and a proneness to intestinal obstruction. Rapid, shallow respiration and oliguria are less frequently seen. Signs of liver parenchymal disease are absent. The duration of the illness is about 12—14 days; chronic cases are unusual.

Lesions. The major lesions are a serous inflammation of the meninges and an infiltration of the brain and spinal cord. Exudate is present in body cavities. The myocardium is flaccid and has a grayish color. The liver parenchyma is clay-colored, and the kidneys show indistinct boundaries between cortex and medulla. The gastric and intestinal mucosae are inflamed. Histologically, atrophic and degenerative changes are evident in the ganglion cells of the cerebral cortex and caudate nucleus, and to a lesser degree in the quadrigeminal bodies. Hyperemia of the parenchymatous organs also is generally present.

Treatment. Besides a ration change, horsetail poisoning is treated primarily with laxatives, cardiac and nerve stimulants (caffeine, strychnine, veratrin), and by giving 100—200 g dried brewer's yeast orally or 250—500 mg thiamine parenterally to correct the B_1 deficiency.

2.5.2.2. Bracken Fern

The bracken fern (*Pteridium aquilinum;* fig. 2.5. — 2) is a plant that grows in deciduous and coniferous forests, in forest clearings, barren timberlands, meadows, peat bogs and similar areas that are exposed to sunlight and are poor in calcium. Bracken poisoning is most common following a dry spring or summer. The toxic principle of the plant is different for monogastric animals than for ruminants. The substance affecting the horse is thought to be a thermolabile thiaminase, as in equisetum poisoning, that is present during certain growth stages of the plant.

Symptoms. The clinical symptoms of bracken poisoning in the horse resemble those of equisetum poisoning, because certain horsetails contain a similar thiaminase. As a constituent of carboxylase, thiamine performs important metabolic functions. In its absence, the breakdown of carbohydrates is greatly hampered. Pyruvic acid and α-ketoglutaric acid accumulate in the tissues, because they are no longer broken down into acetic acid and succinic acid, respectively. In turn, these metabolic derangements quickly lead to profound disturbances of central nervous system function that resemble those seen in thiamine-deficient animals (cf. Horsetail Poisoning).

Treatment. Most horses respond well to the prompt administration of thiamine (0.25—0.5 mg/kg thiamine hydrochloride i.m.; this would be about 0.12—0.25 g for a 500-kg horse). The best regimen is to give two 100-mg doses in the morning and evening of the first day, followed by single daily doses of 100 mg each for 7 additional days; 200 mg/day for 14 days may be necessary in severe cases.

2.5.2.3. Yew

The yew (*Taxus baccata;* fig. 2.5. — 3) is a decorative tree that is common in gardens, parks and cemeteries. Its needles, branches and berries contain a highly poisonous alkaloid, taxine, which is a specific respiratory and cardiac toxin. The yew also contains taxicatine, milossine, and relatively large amounts of formic acid, which also have cardiotoxic properties. The most poisonous parts of the yew tree are the needles, especially the old, soft, dark-green needles of fall and winter.

Symptoms. The yew is one of the few poisonous plants that are palatable to animals. Horses are the most susceptible to yew poisoning, and 100—200 g of needles may be lethal. In cattle, by comparison, the lethal dose is five times that amount. The effects and clinical signs of yew poisoning are variable on account of the various toxic factors contained in the plant. The ingestion of large amounts of yew is generally followed by sudden death without apparent clinical signs. If a small amount is consumed, or if the local irritating effect of taxine becomes evident as a result of slow absorption, a more complicated picture emerges. The earliest symptom is excitation, accompanied by a rise of body temperature. This is followed by colic, diarrhea and gross hematuria, as well as muscle tremors, muscle contractions and motor incoordination (ataxia). Pregnant mares may abort. There is a gradual failure of respiration and circulation, the animal becomes increasingly depressed, and death from diastolic cardiac arrest occurs within a few hours.

Lesions. There may be no visible changes at necropsy, especially in cases that take an apoplectiform course. Some dilatation of the stomach may be evident. In animals that do not die suddenly, there will be pallor of the mucous membranes, a bloody froth in the oral cavity, a violet-red inflammation of the gastric mucosa, and a brownish-black liver. Nephritis is sometimes present. The spleen and lungs are engorged with dark blood, and evidence of asphyxia is apparent. The left heart is empty, while the right heart contains dark, sticky blood. The brain is hyperemic and edematous. In most cases yew needles can be recovered from the stomach. Histologic examination shows multiple necrotic foci in the gastric mucosa. Small collections of lymphocytes are visible in some places. Dilated, engorged blood vessels are found throughout the liver. There is extensive disruption of the liver cell trabeculae, and the Disse spaces are dilated and filled with edematous fluid. The protoplasm of the liver cells is turbid and shows a honeycomb-like pattern in some areas. In the kidneys, the glomeruli are engorged with blood, the protoplasm of the tubular epithelial cells is turbid and swollen, especially in the area of the convoluted tubules. The lumina of the tubules are narrowed. The protoplasm also contains small numbers of fine fat droplets, which are most numerous in proximity to the basement membrane. The protoplasm of the myocardial fibers is turbid, and the cross-striation is apparent. As in the renal tubular epithelium, the myocardial protoplasm is diffusely infiltrated with fine fat droplets.

Treatment. In cases that take a rapid course, treatment generally is too late to be of value. In less fulminating cases, treatment with cardiac stimulants and respiratory analeptics (nicethamide, lobeline), animal charcoal, purgatives and coating agents is indicated. In addition, symptomatic treatment is given for neurologic signs.

2.5.2.4. Crowfoot

Three species of the genus *Ranunculus* are of toxicologic importance: the poisonous crowfoot *(Ranunculus scleratus)*, the rough crowfoot *(R. acris)*, and the globe crowfoot *(R. bulbosus)*. All parts of these plants contain large amounts of protoanemonin and anemonin, as well as saponins and other toxic compounds. Protoanemonin has a very strong local irritating effect on the skin and mucous membranes. When absorbed, both protoanemonin and anemonin lead first to excitation and then paralysis of the central nervous system. They also cause skin and mucosal changes, nephritis, and urinary tract inflammation.

Symptoms. Crowfoot poisoning usually affects animals at pasture, because drying converts protoanemonin to inactive compounds. Generally, however, the danger of crowfoot poisoning is minimal because animals tend to avoid the plant. Clinical signs of poisoning include inflammation of the oral mucosae, salivation and obstructive colic, followed by hematuria and the passage of a black, evil-smelling stool. Th ingestion of large amounts of the plant may lead to convulsions, muscle tremors, mydriasis and blindness. Lethal doses cause death from cardiac and respiratory paralysis.

Lesions. Usually the only visible change is an inflammatory swelling of the gastrointestinal mucosae, which show numerous hemorrhagic foci. Signs of a hemorrhagic nephritis are sometimes apparent.

Treatment. The treatment of crowfoot poisoning is entirely symptomatic and relies on the use of mild laxatives, diuretics and stimulants. The i.v. administration of 150—250 ml of a 10% sodium thiosulfate solution is recommended twice daily for the first three days.

2.5.2.5. Locust

The white locust tree (*Robinia pseudoacacia;* fig. 2.5. — 4), often mistaken for the acacia, contains robin, a highly poisonous toxalbumin that may reach concentrations of 1.6% in the bark of the trunk. The locust also contains the toxalbumin phasin (also present in the kidney bean) as well as the harmless glycoside syringin (also present in lilac bark), tannins and resins. Trace amounts of robin and phasin are also contained in the locust seeds. The glycosides contained in the flowers and leaves are of no toxicologic importance.

Symptoms. Locust poisonings in animals occur almost exclusively in horses and are nearly always caused by ingestion of the locust bark, which appears to be especially toxic in the fall. Robin and phasin, like other toxalbumins, are true antigens and, as such, they agglutinate red blood cells and are destructive to animal tissues. The earliest signs of locust poisoning in the horse are a rapid heart rate, weak pulse, mydriasis, salivation, polyuria, and colicky signs either in the form of a profuse, watery diarrhea or impaction due to paralysis of the large intestine. Cerebral irritation signs may also appear and dominate the clinical picture. Initially there may be episodes of frenzy, spasmodic twitching, masticatory spasms and circling, to be followed later by drowsiness, apathy, staggering, weakness and paralysis. The initial acceleration of heart rate is gradually replaced by a condition of myocardial asthenia and cardiac failure. Toxic laminitis of all four feet is not uncommon. The first obvious disease symptoms appear about 3—5 hours after ingestion of the plant, and the crisis comes at about 10 hours post-ingestion.

Lesions. Signs of diphtheritic and hemorrhagic enteritis are the principal findings at necropsy.

Treatment. Appropriate symptomatic treatment is given. It is recommended that this be preceded by gastric lavage with animal charcoal.

Prognosis. With suitable treatment, horses with locust poisoning should recover within hours and regain full working capacity after a few days' rest.

2.5.2.6. Beech Nut

The nuts of the red beech *(Fagus silvatica)*, which is common in Central Europe, contain a palatable oil that occurs in concentrations up to 17 %. Residues from beech-nut extraction contain degradation products of choline, fumaric acid and various phenolcarboxylic acids, as well as two thiamine-splitting substances that are responsible for toxic effects in animals.

Symptoms. Horses are highly susceptible to poisoning from the beech nut or its residues. Quantities as small as 1 kg can cause severe colicky episodes to the point of frenzy and self-mutilation. Additional signs are hyperexcitability, tetanic spasms, staggering, trembling, dyspnea and hindquarter paresis. Death from asphyxia may occur. The poisoning usually takes an acute course, and the outcome is decided within 12 hours.

Lesions. Necropsy findings are fairly nonspecific. Usually one finds only circumscribed inflammations of the gastrointestinal mucosae. Pronounced edema or even fluid collections are sometimes found in the brain and spinal cord. There may also be small necrotic foci in the liver and intimal reddening of the aorta and pulmonary artery.

Treatment. Beech-nut poisoning is treated with purgatives, tannin-containing preparations, thiamine, and purely symptomatic measures.

2.5.2.7. Ground Ivy

Ground ivy *(Glechoma hederacea)* grows in forests, in shrubbery and on meadows and is a significant cause of poisoning in horses when ingested in the fresh or wilted state. It also remains toxic for some time after drying, but is completely safe when ingested as fodder that is several months old. The toxic effect of ground ivy is attributed mainly to the presence of glechomin, a 'bitter' whose chemistry has not been elucidated.

Symptoms. Symptoms appear within 4—6 days after the horse has begun feeding on the plants. Severe cases are marked by mydriasis, profuse sweating, a very rapid (70—100), rattling, gasping respiration that is accompanied by trembling of the whole body, a weak, rapid pulse (40—60), cardiac arrythmias, and cyanosis of the visible mucosae. The second heart sound is accentuated and often is as strong as the first. A reddish-yellow, frothy fluid is discharged from the widely-dilated nostrils, and a viscid mucus is discharged from the mouth. A painful, wet cough is present in some cases, and loud rales may be audible over the lungs and airways. The body temperature is elevated, and the appetite is depressed. Affected horses refuse to drink water, have colicky pains and constipation, and tend to assume a straddle-legged stance. After a while the clinical picture is dominated by signs of cardiac insufficiency leading to hyperemia, pulmonary edema and bronchitis. A leuko- and lymphocytosis is present. Death may occur within hours or days in severe cases.

Lesions. Myocardial degeneration, pulmonary emphysema, splenic enlargement, hepatic congestion, cecal dilation and acute gastroenteritis are found at necropsy.

Treatment. Beech-nut poisoning is treated with laxatives (castor oil, arecoline), the injection of 50—150 ml camphor oil as a circulatory and respiratory analeptic, and with calcium preparations and glucose.

Prognosis. Ground ivy poisonings in the horse usually occur after the feeding of alfalfa that has been freshly harvested from wet lowlands in which the ivy grows as a weed. The prognosis, therefore, depends on the amount of ivy growing in the harvested area and thus on the quantity ingested.

2.5.2.8. Thorn Apple

The white thorn apple *(Datura stramonium)* grows at dump sites and along paths and is well known for its toxic and pharmaceutical properties. In former times the horse traders often used its seeds for deceptive purposes as a means of suppressing emphysema symptoms in horses to be sold. The active principles of the thorn apple are alkaloids from the tropine group: hyoscyamine, atropine and scopolamine. Reports in the veterinary literature deal mainly with poisonings in horses and cattle.

Symptoms. Clinical signs include mydriasis with visual disturbances, anorexia, polyuria (possibly associated with hematuria), intermittent muscle spasms and shivering. In feeding experiments, horses survived after ingesting 0.5 kg of fresh leaves or 1 kg of wilted plants but manifested characteristic poisoning symptoms; 1,250 g of ripe seeds was lethal.

Lesions. The cerebral vessels of poisoned horses were engorged with blood, and the liver had a spotted appearance, with some degeneration of the liver cells.

Treatment. Treatment is given in the form of gastric lavage with animal charcoal. Pilocarpine hydrochloride is an effective parasympathetic antidote for peripheral symptoms when injected subcutaneously in a dose of 0.2—0.5 g. A 0.1 % solution of picrotoxin may be tried in severe cases. Circulatory agents are also beneficial.

2.5.2.9. Ragwort

The ragwort (*Senecio jacobaea;* fig. 2.5. — 5) is the most important poisonous plant of the genus *Senecio.* Its principal alkaloid is jacobine, but it also contains the alkaloids jaconine and jacodine, the flavone quercetin, and the associated flavone glycoside. Poisonings by *Senecio* species ('senecioses') are mainly seen in the horse and are most common during the blooming season of the plants.

Symptoms. In the horse, frequent yawning is one of the first symptoms of ragwort poisoning. The appetite is reduced, there is profound dullness and depression, and the animal stands with the head lowered. These signs are followed later by unrest, excitation, an unsteady gait with foot-dragging ('sleepy staggers'), and partial blindness that causes the horse to run into walls or fall over obstacles and possibly sustain serious injuries. The respiratory and pulse rates are increased (100—120), the body temperature is elevated to 39.5—40.0 °C, and there is a persistent, bloody diarrhea that may be accompanied by rectal prolapse. Convulsions may appear in acute poisonings, and jaundice is always present in both the acute and subacute forms. As a result the mucous membranes are pale and icteric, becoming bright yellow toward the end of the disease. Serum bilirubin levels are elevated as a sign of profound parenchymal liver damage as soon as clinical symptoms appear. Hypertrophic cirrhosis of the liver results in an enlarged area of hepatic dullness that is easily demonstrated on percussion. Apparently the toxic substances cannot pass the placental barrier.

Differential Diagnosis. In the absence of icteric discoloration of the visible mucosae, a differentiation must be made from staggers and Borna disease, and from aflatoxicosis on the basis of necropsy findings.

Lesions. The poisonous substances in ragwort are hepatotoxic and cause a hypertrophic hepatic cirrhosis. At necropsy the liver appears markedly enlarged and firm, and it presents a 'nutmeg liver' appearance when cut (dilatation of the central veins and grayish to yellowish discoloration at the periphery of the lobules). Other common findings are inflammation and edema of the gastric mucosa, and gastric rupture is occasionally seen. The peritoneal fluid may be blood-tinged and greatly increased in

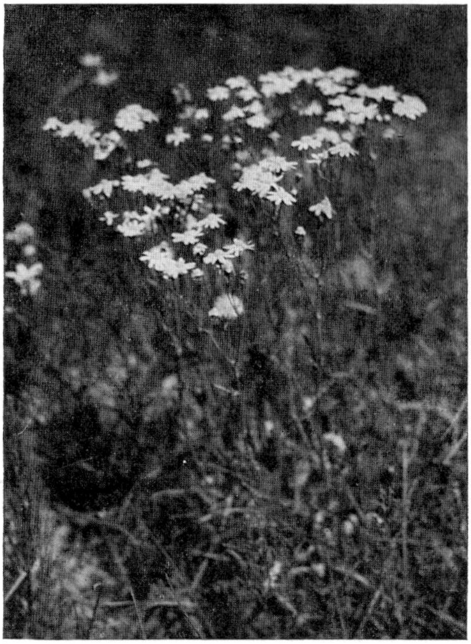

Fig. 2.5. — 5. Ragwort.

volume. There is hemorrhagic inflammation of the small intestine, and hyperplastic splenic enlargement is occasionally present. A fatty degeneration of the kidneys is apparent. In acute cases petechiae are found in the subcutaneous tissue and on most internal organs. Histologic examination of the liver shows parenchymal degeneration and varying degrees of necrotic fatty infiltration, vacuolization and cellular atrophy in the liver cell trabeculae surrounding the dilatated central veins. Round-cell infiltration and bile-duct proliferation are apparent in later stages. The central nervous system disturbances are believed to be due to the destruction of ganglion cells and the atrophy of medullary sheaths.

Prognosis and Treatment. Treatment is of no value in ragwort poisoning. Fatalities can occur even months after removal of the contaminated feed.

2.5.3. Mycotoxicoses

Mycotoxicoses, or poisonings by fungi, are an increasingly common cause of serious disease in domestic animals. The horse is particularly susceptible to poisoning by a variety of fungal toxins. As a rule, mycotoxicoses are caused by feedstuffs that have become contaminated by fungi.

In the hygienic evaluation of feedstuffs, it is recognized that virtually all feeds harbor microorganisms, and that vegetable products tend to have a higher microflora content than do animal products. A particular product becomes injurious to health or performance only when its microflora content is significantly abnormal both in qualitative and quantitative terms.

The contamination of feedstuffs with spoilage-causing microorganisms may occur either before the feed is harvested or when the feed is stored, in which case various environmental factors determine the degree of infestation.

The most important fungi that infest feedstuffs are the molds, which live a saprophytic existence. The molds and their spores have a ubiquitous distribution, and molds can grow on practically any stored feed. As they grow, the molds produce a variety of mycotoxins which are either excreted into the substrate on which the mold is growing, or are stored in the cells and are not released until the mycelium breaks apart. Mold spores contain only trace amounts of toxin.

Because the only effective means for the control of mycotoxicoses is to prevent the fungal contamination of feeds, it is important to know the *conditions of growth* of the fungi. Foodstuffs form an ideal substrate for most species of mold: Carbohydrates, animal and vegetable fats, organic or inorganic nitrogen compounds, trace elements and a minimum amount of usable water are among the most important factors that contribute to optimum fungal growth.

The water content of a substrate as well as the relative humidity of the surrounding air have a critical influence on the growth of molds. 'Field molds', which grow on forage in the field, require substrates with a moisture content of about 22 %, while 'storage molds', which infest feedstuffs only during transportation and storage, require a moisture content of about 13—18 %. These circumstances can create diagnostic problems, as in the case of a stored feed that contains toxins even though the fungi that produced them have long since died and can no longer be demonstrated.

Molds have become adapted to almost all habitable regions on earth and thus to a very wide range of temperatures (0—60 °C). This makes them a potential problem throughout the year in many locations, and for most of the year in many others. It must be borne in mind, however, that the optimum temperature for fungal growth does not coincide with that for toxin production.

Molds require an adequate supply of atmospheric oxygen for good growth. The growth of *Aspergillus flavus*, for example, is greatly inhibited when the CO_2 concentration exceeds 20 % or when the O_2 content is less than 5 %.

Finally, the species of molds that are known to be toxinogenic (about 240 were known by 1970) show genetic differences with regard to their ability to produce toxins. For example, some strains of *Aspergillus flavus* are unable to form aflatoxin, while many other strains can produce several different aflatoxins at one time.

The microfloral composition of a feedstuff changes during harvesting, transport, storage and processing in accordance with the aforementioned factors. The fungae inhabiting the original feedstuff may even change while the material is being analyzed in the laboratory. The microflora content of a mixed feed is dependent on the microflora of the individual components used in its manufacture, additional microflora picked up during processing, and the physical conditions that prevail during manufacture, transport and storage. Quantitative shifts in the individual components of a mixed feed can cause significant shifts in the composition of its microflora. Moreover, toxin production by the microorganisms is strongly influenced by the composition of the substrate. For example, amino acids such as glutamine and proline appear to stimulate the formation of toxic metabolic products, as do the protein sources provided by wheat, oats, rice and millet.

In addition, if wheat husks, corn husks, peanut shells or the like become damaged by insects or mechanical stresses during harvesting or are destroyed by excessive heat during drying, then the kernel or nut becomes highly susceptible to invasion by germinating fungal spores.

Grains and mixed feeds are not the only substrates for the growth of toxin-producing fungi. Basic feedstuffs such as lucerne, hay, straw, silage (cf. Sec. 2.4.2.4.) and pasture grass can also be spoiled by fungal infestation.

As mentioned earlier, horses appear to be more susceptible to myoctoxicoses than any other animal species. Depending on the mode of introduction of the toxin (ingestion or inhalation), the *clinical signs* of mycotoxicoses can be classified into three main groups: gastrointestinal and urinary tract symptoms, neurologic symptoms, and allergic symptoms. The first of these groups is the most important. In mild cases that are associated with only a mild enteritis, no treatment is necessary other than removal of the offending feed. Occasionally, however, fungal poisonings produce severe colic with tympany of the cecum and colon, or with extremely dense impactions mainly affecting the left ventral colon. A hemorrhagic gastroenteritis may also develop in acute cases. A peracute gastroenteritis of this type was seen among troop horses in the Bielefeld-Paderborn area of Germany during the mid-1930's.

Neurologic symptoms, including paralyses, do not occur as separate entities in mycotoxicoses, but always represent complications of a gastroenteritis. Hindquarter paralysis, spastic movements of the hind limbs (stringhalt) and esophageal spasms have been described. Encephalitides manifested by episodes of frenzy have also been observed.

Allergic symptoms in mycotoxicoses are apparently the result of a specific action of the fungal spores (which may enter the animal's respiratory system with hay dust) and are due mainly to irritation of the oral and respiratory mucosae. The spores of rust and smut are more important than mold spores in the pathogenesis of these symptoms.

The most common and dangerous mold poisonings are caused by *Aspergillus* species. The degree of infestation of a feed may be so slight that the mold goes unnoticed or can be detected only with a magnifying glass. Roughages and bedding are commonly affected. Hay bales infested with *Aspergillus* usually have a noticeable dank, musty odor. When broken open, the bale may be found to be moldy throughout, or the mold growth may be patchy. In the latter case an attempt is frequently made to salvage the bale by 'shaking out' the moldy portions, but this serves only to disseminate the mold spores over a broad area and increases the risk of respiratory tract irritation by air-borne spores. The various grain feeds rank second to roughages as a source of mold poisonings. The residues from oil production are also highly susceptible to mold infestation and can be hazardous when ingested.

The aflatoxins are hepatotoxins produced by certain strains of *Aspergillus*. The main source is peanuts and their residues, though various other feedstuffs may also contain the toxin. Evidence to date indicates that the aflatoxins are of only minor importance in horses, however.

On the other hand, several representatives of the 'imperfect' fungi appear to be an important cause of mycotoxicoses in horses. The first reports on the occurrence of a disease known as stachybotrytoxicosis, caused primarily by *Stachybotrys alternans*, come from the Soviet Union, where thousands of horses were affected in the early 1930 s. Most poisonings occurred after the ingestion of infected roughage, and two forms of the disease were observed: the acute, atypical form occurring after short-term ingestion of the toxin and characterized by fever, cardiac insufficiency and neurologic signs (hypersensitivity or depression); and the more common chronic form, which shows three stages: (1) inflammation of the oral and nasal mucosae, palpebral conjunctivitis and facial edema occurring 2—3 days after toxin ingestion and persisting 1—4 weeks; (2) signs of impaired hematopoiesis (leukopenia, agranulocytosis, thrombocytopenia), which persist about 5—10 days; and (3) a final stage characterized by a rise of body temperature, rapid pulse and respiration, dehydration and a fall of the leukocyte count to 200—800/mm^3. Secondary bacterial infection finally complicates the condition, which generally has a fatal outcome.

Poisoning by *Fusarium* has become increasingly common in recent years. The clinical picture of fusariotoxicosis is highly variable, because the disease can be caused by several *Fusarium* species, which produce a variety of toxins. The occurrence of the disease is closely related to the increased growing of late-ripening hybrid corn, which is highly susceptible to fusariosis. *Fusarium* is also capable of infesting other types of grain. The most familiar of the 12 known *Fusarium* toxins is T2, which causes necrosis of skin and mucosal surfaces that come in contact with it. When absorbed, the toxin attacks the hematopoietic system. Another *Fusarium* toxin, ceralenon, exerts an estrogenic effect.

The mycotoxicosis caused by eating grain or hay infected with *Fusarium sporotrichioides* leads to an unsteady, staggering gait, profuse sweating and muscle spasms in horses. Terminally the animal goes down and often makes running movements with the limbs before death occurs. In Egypt, southern Africa and America, the feeding of corn infested with *Fusarium moniliforme* has led to hemorrhagic encephalitis and leukoencephalomalacia. In Japan, spasms, circling, respiratory distress and cardiac arrhythmias have been observed in horses fed bean pods infected with *Fusarium solani*.

The *detection* of mycotoxins in feedstuffs is a complex problem. Several biologic tests are available for this purpose, such as the rabbit skin test (e.g., for *Stachybotrys* toxins), the use of experimental animals, chick embryos, parasitic larvae or tissue cultures, and testing the antibacterial effect of certain plant toxins. Physicochemical techniques, such as thin-layer chromatography, are also available.

The *treatment* of mycotoxicoses is made extremely difficult by a lack of specific medications. Gastric lavage is recommended in acute cases, and this may be supplemented by symptomatic treatment. The surest *prophylaxis* is the prevention of food and bedding contamination by the measures outlined earlier.

References

Christensen, C. M.; Nelson, G. H.: Mycotoxins and Mycotoxicoses. Modern vet. Pract. *57:* 367, 529 (1976).

Gedek, B.: Zur Bedeutung von Mykotoxinen. Die Blauen Hefte für den Tierarzt Nr. 41, p. 32 (1969).

Gedek, B.: Futtermittelverderb durch Bakterien und Pilze und seine nachteiligen Folgen. Übers. Tierernährung *1:* 45 (1973).

Gedeck, B.: Kompendium der medizinischen Mykologie (Parey, Berlin 1980).

Palyusik, M.: Mykotoxikosen. Wien. tierärztl. Mschr. *64:* 211 (1977).

Sahliger, S.: Dünnschichtchromatographische Trennverfahren zum Nachweis von Mykotoxinen. Milchwirtschaftl. Ber. *43:* 107 (1975).

Shreeve, B. J.; Patterson, D. S. P.: Mycotoxicoses. Vet. Rec. *97:* 279 (1975).

Wiesner, E.: Ernährungsschäden der landwirtschaftlichen Nutztiere; 2. Aufl., p. 273ff. (VEB Gustav Fischer Verlag, Jena 1970).

2.5.4. Animal Toxins

2.5.4.1. Mites

Infestation with mites, mostly tyroglyphids, is not unusual in feedstuffs that have been improperly stored. Brans and mixed feeds are most commonly affected. The presence of mites is an indicator of the incipient decomposition of a feed. The natural defenses of a food material are very quickly lost under improper storage conditions. The infestation of stored grains can be prevented by storing the material in an airy place, preferably when it is fully ripe, turning it at regular intervals, and by disinfecting prior to storage. It may also be necessary to keep acidity levels to a minimum (e.g., for certain meal extracts from oil-yielding crops).

Opinions vary widely with regard to the adverse health effects of mite-infested feeds. Pigs are the most commonly affected species. In horses fed material heavily contaminated with live mites, EGGEBRECHT [1928] observed several days of anorexia followed by swaying of the hindquarters and finally hindquarter paralysis. The limbs were swollen, and within a week two animals were no longer able to stand. Symptoms improved within 8—10 days after the contaminated feed was withdrawn. HÖVE and FIEDLER [1932] observed colic, hindquarter paralysis, and three fatalities in horses given feed mixes containing large numbers of the meal mite *Tyroglyphus farinae* [L., 1758]. VON LENGERKEN [1931] observed two deaths in horses fed imported La Plata corn that had been infested in the country of origin with *Thyroglyphus farinae* [L., 1758], *Glyciphagus domesticus* [De GEER, 1771] and *Cheyletus eruditus* [SCHRANK, 1781]. SIDKI [1934] reported illness and one death in horses that had received a mixed feed whose bran component was heavily infested with live mites.

The mechanism by which mite-infested feeds produce disease in animals remains unclear. It is not known whether lesions are caused by live or dead mites, by metabolic products excreted by the mites, or as a result of decomposition of the organic substrate by the mites. For this reason, one should be hesitant to give mite-infested feeds to horses, which, like pigs, appear to be unusually susceptible to their effects. Under no circumstances should a feed be given that shows more than a mild degree of mite contamination.

References

EGGEBRECHT, H.: Tiererkrankungen durch gesundheitsschädliche Futtermittel. Dtsch. Landw. Presse, p. 464 (1928).

HÖVE, K. R.; FIEDLER, K.: Beitrag zur Schädlichkeit milbenbefallener Futtermittel. Tierärztl. Rundschau *38:* 584 (1932).

SIDKI, B.: Ein Beitrag zur Kenntnis von Futtermittelschädlichkeiten bei den Haustieren. Vet.-med. Diss., Berlin (1934).

2.5.4.2. Aphids

Aphids, which are plant lice belonging to the order Hemiptera, are believed to contain an unknown toxin that causes irritation of the skin and mucous membranes. Adverse effects from the ingestion of aphids are described only in the older literature. There are reports, for example, of circumscribed inflammatory swelling of unpigmented skin areas in horses that ate lucerne and green vetch heavily infested with aphids. In gray and dappled horses, inflammatory skin swellings appeared over large portions of the head and legs. Similar changes were noted in the oral and conjunctival mucosae. It is possible, of course, that these changes were caused by substances present in certain leguminous feeds.

Additional symptoms were colic, tympany and convulsions. A hemorrhagic gastroenteritis was found at necropsy.

2.5.4.3. Caterpillars

Poisonings have been observed in several domestic animal species, including horses, following the ingestion of caterpillars in significant numbers. Such poisonings are especially common in areas and during years in which certain moth and butterfly species, like those from the family Thaumetopolidae and Pieridae, are present in unusually large numbers. Horses manifest severe colicky symptoms, enteritis and hindquarter weakness, with death occurring in some instances. Enteritis and petechiae on the heart and kidneys are seen at necropsy.

2.5.4.4. Bees, Wasps and Hornets

Animals at pasture are especially vulnerable to attacks by stinging insects. Severe disease symptoms can result from multiple stings in sensitive areas. Female bees, wasps and hornets have a stinger, actually a modified ovipositor, located at the posterior tip of the abdomen. In the bee this stinger is equipped with barbs that cause it to remain in the wound after stinging. Besides histamine, hyaluronidase and phospholipase A, bee venom contains mellitin, which is considered the true toxin. The overall effect of bee venom may be characterized as hemolytic. Mellitin stimulates smooth muscle contraction, induces a fall of blood pressure after an initial rise, and blocks neuromuscular transmission. Wasp venom contains kinin-like peptides; histamine, 5-hydroxytryptamine and acetylcholine have been found in hornet venom.

Insect stings cause local swelling as well as systemic effects manifested by a sharp rise of body temperature, hematuria, excitation, spasms and paralysis. Stings are treated first by extracting the stinger from the wound and then dabbing or washing the affected area with soap solutions or a weak ammonia solution. The concurrent administration of antihistamine may also be beneficial.

2.5.4.5. Poisonous Snakes

The only poisonous snake native to Central Europe is the adder or European viper (*Vipera berus*), which is brown or grayish-brown with dark zig-zag markings commencing at the back of the head. Although its venom, a high-molecular polypeptide with an enzymatic character, is not very toxic compared to that of other poisonous snakes, the adder can be dangerous even to large animals. Horses seem particularly susceptible. Most bites occur at pasture on warm spring days, with the legs being the most frequent target; bites about the mouth are less common. Severe inflammation quickly appears about the bite area, the pulse becomes weak and rapid, and breathing becomes labored. Paralysis and collapse occur in severe cases, and a few bitten horses may die. The effects of the snakebite depend on many factors, including the location of the bite and the degree of perfusion of the affected tissue.

In the treatment of snakebites, an attempt must be made to prevent absorption of the venom by applying a tourniquet above the bite or by excising or cauterizing the wound. Local potassium permanganate injections can destroy the venom. If possible, systemic treatment should be given by administering the specific antivenom serum.

As a rule, bitten animals will recover within a few days.

2.5.5. Botulism

Of the anaerobic microorganisms that cause food poisoning, certain *Clostridium* species are the most important. These bacteria tend to occur wherever organic matter is undergoing hydrolysis in the absence of oxygen, and they are common in various soils, in manure heaps, in mud, in the digestive tract of animals, and in a number of feedstuffs that are stored under anaerobic conditions. The foremost toxin-producing species are *Cl. perfringens* and *Cl. botulinum.* The type-B toxin of *Cl. botulinum* is the cause of botulism in man, chickens and horses and is most commonly detected in preserved meats.

The natural infection of horses with *Cl. botulinum* results from the ingestion of feed or drinking water contaminated by the bacteria or their toxins. In agricultural settings the main sources of *Cl. botulinum* are improperly-packaged sweet pelleted feeds, moldy silage (mangels, sugar-beet tops, turnip slices), spoiled potatoes, spoiled hay and grain, and damp, moldy straw. Rats and mice play an important mediating role by contaminating feedstuffs with their feces and cadavers; the carrion of herbivorous animals on pasture also represents an important source of infection, even if the animals themselves did not die of botulism (infection of forage plants). Carrion contamination of this type sometimes accounts for significant outbreaks on pastures and in stables. Oats, oat straw, hay and silage contaminated by chicken manure have frequently been identified as a cause of botulism in horses [Zaribnicky, 1924; Bürgi, 1931]. *Clostridium* contamination of wheat and rye brans has also been reported [Hiltner, 1887].

Botulism is manifested clinically by dysphagia, protrusion of the tongue, ptosis, general weakness, and inability to stand. Fever is not present. In most cases paralysis worsens and ends in death. Necropsy reveals mild inflammation of the small and large intestine, slight hemorrhaging in the myocardium and kidneys, and impaired blood coagulation. In Denmark, Müller [1963] has shown that a syndrome in horses long known as 'spinal typhus' is actually a form of botulism intoxication. In this form as in others, infection occurs by the ingestion of feed that has been contaminated by the infected carrion of rodents or cats. The disease could be produced experimentally by feeding contaminated material. The peracute or subacute course of the disease is determined by the amount of toxic material ingested. A mere 50—100 g of hay taken from the vicinity of an infected cadaver is sufficient to kill a horse.

A mortality rate of 90% is reported for horses. The toxin or bacterium can be demonstrated bacteriologically in liver tissue samples in about 66% of suspected cases; the reliability of this method is about 90%.

In the prevention of botulism, it must be recognized that the botulism toxin is an exotoxin that is not completely destroyed by short-term exposure to heat. At least 20 minutes' boiling is necessary to inactivate the toxin.

References

Bürgi, O.: Beobachtungen über Futterschädigungen beim Pferd. Tierärztl. Rundschau, p. 489 (1931).

Hiltner, L.: Die Bakterien der Futtermittel und Samen. Landwirtschaftl. Versuchsstat. *34:* 390 (1887).

Müller, J.: Equine and borvine botulism in Denmark. Bull. Office internat. Epizooties *59:* 1379 (1963).

Zaribnicky, F.: Fütterungslehre und Futterschädlichkeiten. Münchener tierärztl. Wschr. *80:* 124 (1929).

2.5.6. Ensiling Aids

In the ensilage of low-carbohydrate (and thus high-protein) feedstuffs, such as grass, clover and alfalfa, proper fermentation can be ensured only by the addition of 'ensiling aids'. which generally contain calcium formiate and sodium nitrate. If excessive amounts of the ensiling salt are used, poisoning from the nitrite component may result (see p. 378).

2.5.7. Fertilizers

Efforts to increase crop yields have led to growing reliance on the use of mineral fertilizers in agriculture. During the period from 1950 to 1970, for example, the production of nitrogen, phosphorus and potassium fertilizers was increased approximately four-fold on a worldwide scale. Although a large percentage of these fertilizers are potentially harmful to animals, and the careless or improper transport, storage and use of these materials can lead to poisonings in livestock, fertilizer poisonings have been a relatively minor problem in horses. They only require a brief discussion.

Most fertilizers can be classified into one of several groups, depending on whether they are composed of nitrogen, phosphate, potassium or calcium compounds. Fertilizers containing mixtures of these compounds are also available. As a rule, fertilizer poisonings result from oral ingestion of the toxic materials, although poisonings due to inhalation (of ammonia, for example) are also possible. While the clinical picture and corresponding treatment usually are determined by one or more of the principal constituents of the fertilizer, it is possible for fertilizers to become contaminated by other toxic materials. Phosphate fertilizers, for example, are frequently contaminated by fluorine and arsenic compounds.

Symptoms. Among the *nitrogen fertilizers*, sodium nitrate and calcium nitrate cause severe gastroenteritis, paralytic symptoms, methemoglobin formation, collapse, and in some cases death. Potassium nitrate additionally causes cardiac paralysis (cf. Sec. 2.5.1.).

Ammonium sulfate and urea cause pulmonary edema, severe colic, muscle tremors, petechial hemorrhages of the mucosae, tonic-clonic convulsions, slowing of the respiration, cardiac arrhythmias and urinary retention. Calcium cyanamide causes local irritation and vasomotor disturbances.

Phosphate fertilizers are not very toxic as a rule. High concentrations lead to irritation of the mucosae, and the absorption of large amounts can result in hypocalcemic symptoms.

The various *potassium fertilizers*, such as kainite powder, magnesia potash and potassium sulfate, mainly cause myocardial lesions. In addition, kainite powder, owing to its high salt content (up to 80 %), can cause symptoms of salt poisoning (cf. Sec. 2.4.1.1.3.).

The *calcium fertilizers*, such as lime marl, burnt lime (caustic lime = white lime), slaked lime and defecation mud, cause local skin lesions, and when ingested can cause chemical burns with their attendant consequences.

Lesions. In *nitrate* poisonings, a reddish-brown, violet or cherry-red discoloration of the gastric and small intestinal mucosae is visible at necropsy. An acute gastroenteritis, sometimes hemorrhagic and ulcerative, is also apparent. There is hemorrhagic inflammation of the kidneys and the bladder mucosa, and the blood is chocolate-colored if methemoglobin formation has occurred. In poisonings with *ammonia fertilizers* and *urea*, the gastrointestinal mucosae are severely ulcerated and edematous and contain large hemorrhagic areas. The ingestion of *phosphate fertilizers* usually causes only mucosal inflammation and chemical lesions of the esophagus, stomach and bowel; similar effects are observed in poisonings with *potassium* and *calcium fertilizers*.

Treatment. Poisonings with *nitrate-containing fertilizers* are treated as described in Sec. 2.5.1. In *ammonia poisoning*, like that caused by the ingestion of excessive amounts of *urea*, treatment is essentially symptomatic (cf. Sec. 2.5.1.). *Phosphorus poisoning* is also treated symptomatically by administering animal charcoal and sodium sulfate or mineral oil. Fats and animal oils are contraindicated in the treatment of phosphorus poisoning. In poisonings with *potassium fertilizers*, symptomatic treatment should be supported with large doses of vitamin C. For *calcium fertilizer* poisonings, weak solutions of acetic or citric acid should be administered as quickly as possible to neutralize the toxins. Symptomatic therapy is also indicated.

2.5.8. Pesticides

A variety of chemical products are used in agriculture to protect plants and harvested crops from damage by plant and animal pests. The improper storage and use of pesticides, or the contamination of food and drinking water with these chemicals, can create a serious health risk both for humans and animals. In statistical terms, pesticide poisonings in horses account for only about 3% of all such poisonings, owing to the relatively small horse populations compared to other livestock. The diagnosis of pesticide poisonings is often a difficult problem, because symptoms tend to be nonspecific, and a number of other diseases must be excluded. In treating a poisoning, it is necessary to determine which substance the animal may have ingested, and whether the ingested dose is sufficient to produce the symptoms observed. It is not necessary to identify the specific agent responsible for the poisoning; it is sufficient to ascertain the class of substance to which the poison belongs.

2.5.8.1. Insecticides

The majority of insecticides are applied in the form of a spray, fog or dust. They kill insects through simple contact (contact poisons) or following oral ingestion (stomach poisons). Organophosphate compounds, chlorinated hydrocarbons and a number of carbamates are the insecticides most commonly used in modern agriculture.

Organophosphate Compounds

These highly toxic compounds act by inhibiting cholinesterase, thereby creating a postsynaptic acetylcholine excess that interferes with nerve impulse transmission. The individual organophosphates differ in both the intensity and duration of their inhibitory effect. Malathion (dicarboxyethoxyethyldimethyldithiophosphate), for example, is not thought to be particularly toxic for horses under most conditions. The organophosphates are rapidly absorbed in the digestive tract and can be detected in the blood only 30 minutes after ingestion. They are broken down relatively quickly in the gastrointestinal tract and, except for phosdrin = 0,0-dimethyl(2-methoxycarbonyl-1-methylvinyl)phosphate, are stored in the body in very small amounts. The most widely used products include chlorthion (chloronitrophenyl-0), dichlorvos (dimethyl-dichlorovinyl-phosphate), trichlorphon (0,0-dimethyl-2,2,2-trichloro-1-hydroxyethylphosphate), malathion (see above), parathion (0,0-diethyl-p-nitro-phenylthiophosphate) and coumaphos (3-chloro-4-methyl-7-cumarinyl-diethylphosphothionate).

Symptoms. The general symptoms of organophosphate poisoning are bradycardia, dyspnea due to bronchospasm, increased bronchial secretions, impaired diaphragmatic contraction, and a slowing of respiration due to paralysis of the respiratory center. There is also vomiting, diarrhea and colic due to smooth muscle irritation in the bowel, along with excessive salivation and lacrimation, and increased gastric juice secretion. Muscle tremors, convulsions, unrest, impaired equilibrium, hindquarter paralysis with the adoption of a 'sawhorse' stance, and severe miosis also occur.

Lesions. Necropsy findings are fairly nonspecific and include pulmonary edema, congestion of the enteric blood vessels, and petechial hemorrhages at various sites including the epicardium and endocardium.

Treatment. To counter the effects of the increased acetylcholine, atropine sulfate is given by i.v. injection every 8—12 hours in a dose of about 0.15 mg/kg BW (up to 0.5 mg in severe cases) until symptoms disappear. Various oximes (hydroxylamine derivatives) are most effective in reactivating the blocked cholinesterase. For example, the oxime PAM (2-pyridinaldoxime methylhydroxide) is administered in 1% solution in a dose of 30—60 mg/kg. However, this drug is inadequate in severe poisonings because it does not relieve central nervous symptoms. Morine (pentahydroxyflavone) has proved most useful in suppressing acetylcholine synthesis by inhibiting choline acetyltransferase. Muscle tremors can be treated symptomatically with barbiturates. Morphine, theobromine and nicethamide are contraindicated.

Prognosis. The prognosis is favorable for animals that survive the first day.

Chlorinated Hydrocarbons

With few exceptions, the chlorinated hydrocarbons are far less acutely toxic than the organophosphate insecticides. However, their cumulative effects and tendency to accumulate in fat depots make them no less dangerous than the organophosphates. The mobilization of depot fat as a result of malnutrition, infection or the action of certain drugs may result in liberation of the compounds into the blood stream and the appearance of toxicity symptoms, even if the toxin has not been recently ingested. This is one reason why the use of one of the best-known chlorinated hydrocarbon insecticides, DDT, has been banned or restricted in many countries.

The main effect of the chlorinated hydrocarbons is probably based on the inhibition of certain enzyme systems. Compounds that are absorbed but not stored are rapidly excreted via the urine, bile and milk, either unchanged or in the form of their degradation products.

The best-known representatives of the chlorinated hydrocarbon insecticides are, in order of decreasing storage tendency, dieldrin (hexachloro-epoxy-octahydro-dimethano-naphthalene), aldrin (hexachloro-hexahydro(endo,exo)-dimethano-naphthalene), DDT (p-p′-dichloro-diphenyl-trichloroethane, lethal oral dose for horses > 300 mg/kg BW), HCH (γ-hexachlorocyclohexane, lethal oral dose for horses 50 mg/kg BW), endrin (stereoisomer of dieldrin), chlordane (octachloromethylene-tetrahydrohydringen), heptachlor (heptachloro-endomethylene-tetrahydroindene), toxaphene (polychlorocamphene) and methoxychlor.

Symptoms. Animals with little depot fat (foals, for example) are particularly susceptible to the toxic effects of halogenated hydrocarbons. Nevertheless, acute poisonings from the ingestion of contaminated feedstuffs are practically unknown· This route is more likely to be a cause of chronic intoxications. Acute poisonings are most common in circumstances where animals have direct access to the toxic product. The symptoms of chlorinated hydrocarbon poisoning are referable mainly to central nervous excitation. A latent period of about 4—5 hours is followed by hypersensitivity and convulsions. A high fever is characteristic of toxaphene poisonings, and blindness may occur in chlordane poisonings. Exhaustion and paralysis are seen in advanced stages, and muscle tremors may appear, especially with HCH and aldrin poisoning. In animals that die, the terminal stage may be marked by respiratory failure (HCH), coma (DDT) or convulsions (aldrin, dieldrin).

Lesions. Necropsy findings are nonspecific. The digestive tract is pale and swollen, and small hemorrhagic foci are seen, especially on the heart. The lungs show a dark discoloration and are engorged with blood; pulmonary edema may be present. Hemorrhagic edema of the brain and spinal cord is usually apparent. In chronic poisonings the foregoing changes are accompanied by degenerative lesions of the liver and kidneys.

Treatment. The main goal of symptomatic treatment is to control the excitation state. This may be attempted with short-acting barbiturates and various thiobarbiturates, though the use of these drugs should not be repeated. Here the use of chloralhydrate appears to be indicated, as well as 20.0 g of 10 % calcium borogluconate i.v., preferably combined with a glucose-saline solution to avoid liver damage. Bradycardia is controlled with atropine sulfate (1 : 1,000) given by subcutaneous injection in a dose of 0.01—0.08 mg/kg BW. In all cases the animal should be rested and shielded from unnecessary stimuli (noise!). In the early stage of acute poisonings, treatment with mineral laxatives may be attempted; oils and fats are contraindicated.

Prognosis. Generally a long convalescence is required. Hence, treatment should not be discontinued on initial disappearance of symptoms. The prognosis for acute poisonings varies with the causative toxin. The following prognostic rules apply for common insecticides:

DDT:	Death or recovery within 24 hours.
Aldrin:	Death within 24 hours is the rule, though fatalities may occur up to 8 days after ingestion of the poison.
Dieldrin:	Death after 4—10 days is common.
Chlordane:	Death after 2 weeks is common.
Toxaphene:	Death or recovery within 24—36 hours.

Carbamates

In recent years a number of carbamate insecticides have come onto the market, of which sevin (carbaryl, 1-naphthyl-N-methylcarbamate) is the best known. Other carbamates are pyrolane (1-phenyl-3-methylpyrazolyl-5-dimethylcarbamate) and IPC = agermine = tixite (0-isopropyl-N-phenylcarbamate). Like the organophosphates (q.v.), carbamates lead to a reversible inhibition of cholinesterase. Thus, the clinical and necropsy findings correspond to those of organophosphate poisoning. Treatment differs in that oxime (PAM) is not recommended.

2.5.8.2. Herbicides

Herbicides have various uses in agriculture: weed and fungus control, defoliation (e.g., to remove potato tops prior to harvesting), and to speed the ripening of legumes. Especially in the latter case, heavy residues may be expected to occur on the harvested crop. The most important products are dinitrophenol derivatives: DNOC (4,6-dinitro-orthocresol) and dinoseb (4,6-dinitro-2-*sec*-butylphenol). The remaining herbicides, such as phenol acetate derivatives, sodium monochloroacetate, etc. are less toxic than the dinitrophenol compounds. Also, because they are usually applied to food crops in the spring, poisonings from the ingestion of feeds contaminated by these herbicides are very rare. However, because the toxicity of the dinitro compounds is a function of ambient temperature, it appears that dinitro sprays pose a hazard only when used during the hot months of the year.

Symptoms. Dinitro compounds are readily absorbed through the lungs, intestine and intact skin and remain in the body for some time before being excreted. The dinitrophenols act on the intermediary metabolism. They increase cellular respiration while inhibiting the synthesis of ATP. The result is an increase in the metabolic rate, with the liberated energy being converted mainly to heat.

After a latent period of 1—2 days, the internal body temperature rises by 3—4 °C, and the animal becomes dull, anorexic and lethargic. Additional signs are profuse sweating, excessive thirst, rapid pulse, deep, rapid respiration, cyanosis, staggering, vomiting, colic, oliguria and albuminuria. Often there is a yellow discoloration about the mouth ('yellow sprays'), and permanent yellow staining of the haircoat is not uncommon. Some of the breakdown products of the dinitro compounds are red in color, and this accounts for the reddish to reddish-brown discoloration of the urine.

Lesions. In many cases a yellowish discoloration of all the visceral mucosae, the pleura and the subcutaneous connective tissue is apparent. The rapid development of rigor mortis is believed to be characteristic.

Treatment. No specific antidote is available, and treatment is symptomatic only.

Prognosis. Affected animals may die in a deep coma within 4—6 hours after the appearance of initial symptoms, depending on the severity of the intoxication. With each hour of survival the prognosis improves, and animals surviving longer than 12—24 hours have a good chance of recovery.

2.5.8.3. Fungicides

The fungicides used in agriculture include a number of highly diverse chemical compounds: copper compounds, sulfur compounds, inorganic and organic mercury compounds, and various other organic compounds. The principal source of fungicide poisonings in farm animals is seed grains that have been treated with antifungal agents before sowing in order to protect the seedlings and mature plants from infestation with parasitic fungi, or treated with a combination fungicide and insecticide. If the treated grain is accidentally fed to livestock, illness may result.

The most potent fungicidal chemicals, and those that are the most toxic to animals, are the organic mercury compounds such as phenylmercuric acetate or phenylmercuric pyrocatechol. Other fungicides pose no serious threat to livestock.

Symptoms. Mercurial fungicide poisonings have a two-stage clinical course. First the complete compound exerts a specific action that is manifested by CNS disturbances owing to the affinity of organic mercury compounds for nervous tissue. After the organic constituents of the molecule have been broken down, the inorganic mercury causes additional effects. Horses are among the animals most susceptible to mercury poisoning. The ingestion of grain treated with organic mercury compounds is followed by anorexia, refusal to feed, weight loss, diarrhea, profuse salivation, general weakness and locomotor disturbances (especially of the hindquarters), incoordination, lameness, muscle tremors and spasms. The toxicity of the treated grain depends not only on the specific compound ingested, the concentration of the compound and the duration of its toxic effect, but also on the age of the animal and the composition of the ration.

Lesions. In acute cases there is severe gastroenteritis and acute parenchymatous nephritis. Chronic poisonings do not produce characteristic gross changes. Histologically, however, there is necrosis of the renal convoluted tubules and the nerve cells of the brain.

Treatment. Because mercury is absorbed very rapidly after ingestion, treatment in acute cases is of value only if the stomach can be evacuated within 10—15 minutes after the poison is consumed. This may be followed by antidotal treatment with dimercaprol (dithioglycerine) given by intramuscular injection. This substance binds metals and metalloids and can remove metals bound to the SH groups of proteins and enzymes, thereby reactivating enzymes that have been inactivated by heavy metals.

2.5.8.4. Rodenticides

Rodents are controlled with smoke cartridges, traps, baits and poisons. Classic rodent poisons include arsenic, barium and thallium compounds, as well as phosphorus, zinc phosphide and strychnine. Newer rodenticides include the thiourea derivatives, fluoroacetate, the indandione derivatives, red squill preparations, and the coumarine derivatives. The rodenticides most widely used in the GDR are hydrogen phosphide, polychlorocamphene and zinc phosphide derivatives, and to some extent indandione derivatives. Warfarin, a coumarine derivative, is considered the most potent rat poison, and it is the preferred agent for eradicating this pest. It is not harmful to farm animals unless ingested repeatedly and in large amounts.

Symptoms. Warfarin is an anticoagulant and acts by slowing the rate of blood coagulation. Even minor capillary trauma or vascular lesions can lead to fatal hemorrhaging in poisoned animals. Lameness can occur as a result of hemorrhages over bony prominences on the limbs. A bloody diarrhea is observed in many cases. Sudden deaths without premonitory signs have been reported.

Lesions. At necropsy multiple hemorrhages are seen in the muscles, especially over bony prominences on the limbs and thorax. Varying degrees of internal hemorrhaging are also apparent.

Treatment. Poisonings with coumarine derivatives are treated by administering vitamin K or an analog. Blood transfusions are also indicated in severe cases.

2.5.8.5. Acaricides

Acaricides are used to control mites and lice in agriculture (grain, fruit trees, vegetables, hops, vineyards) and in veterinary medicine. The acaricides used agriculturally include several products already discussed under Insecticides, most notably HCH, aldrin and dieldrin (q.v.). The remaining acaricides consist mainly of chlorinated hydrocarbons, organophosphates and carbamates. Thus, the clinical picture and treatment correspond to statements made in the section on Insecticides.

In veterinary medicine, the acaricide benzyl benzoate is used to control sarcoptic and otodectic mites, and tetmosol for other mites. These acaricides are among the least toxic to livestock. Poisonings are manifested by vomiting, diarrhea, hepatomegaly, and respiratory and circulatory difficulties.

2.5.9. Wood Preservatives and Other Toxic Compounds Used in Construction

Many materials used in the construction, weatherproofing and fireproofing of barns, stables, storehouses and other farm buildings can pose a hazard to livestock if carelessly stored or improperly used. These materials include wood preservatives and finishes, various floor coatings, concrete hardening agents, protective coatings for silos and silo paper, burnt lime, slaked lime and various paints.

Acute poisonings from *wood preservatives*, such as sodium fluoride on telephone poles, are rare in horses and other domestic animals. Chronic intoxications by water-soluble fluorides, chromium salts, arsenic salts, sodium chlorphenolate, etc. are more frequent, although the incidence of such poisonings in horses is relatively low.

Poisonings may also result from asphalt-like *floor coatings*. The toxicity of these coatings depends on their content of phenol components, which are absorbed through the skin and are highly hepatotoxic. Poisonings can also result from oral ingestion. Coal-tar and bitumen poisonings are treated with vitamin A and therapy to aid liver function.

Poisonings by *concrete hardening agents*, such as magnesium silicofluoride, zinc silicofluoride and fluorosilicic acid, and poisonings by *protective coatings for silos* and *silo paper*, which also are attributed to the bitumen component, are extremely rare in horses.

Burnt lime and *slaked lime* (calcium oxide and calcium hydroxide, respectively) are used by builders in the form of lime mortar or white lime. Poisonings are usually the result of carelessness in transport, storage or use (e.g., failure to remove livestock when whitewashing stables). Both kinds of lime cause local skin lesions through the precipitation of proteins (coagulative necrosis). Oral ingestion leads to severe chemical burns of the esophagus and gastrointestinal mucosae, followed by painful gastroenteritis. Poisonings are treated at once by giving large amounts of water to dilute the lime. External contact is treated by applying weak solutions of acetic, tartaric or citric acid to neutralize the irritant. Symptomatic treatment is given as needed. Coating agents and medicinal carbon are given orally.

Most poisonings by *paints* used as protective coatings are lead poisonings caused chiefly by minium (lead tetroxoplumbate) and white lead (lead carbonate). Lead and its salts are absorbed very slowly and only in small amounts, however. Acute lead poisonings are practically nonexistant and would require the ingestion of extremely large amounts of lead. The lethal dose of lead acetate for the horse is about 500—750 g. Chronic lead poisoning in horses is far less pronounced than in other species. Sometimes a recurrent nerve paralysis occurs, leading to roaring (laryngeal hemiplegia). Generally, however, paints are a less important cause of lead poisonings than are industrial emissions (see below).

2.5.10. Industrial Emissions

The degree of atmospheric contamination by industrial emissions has increased steadily with the development of industry. 'Air pollution' is the term commonly applied to atmospheric contaminants present in levels sufficient to cause direct or indirect adverse health effects in humans, animals or plants. The principal polluting elements in urban and industrial centers take the form of:

a) corpuscular,
b) gaseous,
c) vaporous emissions.

All three forms can occur simultaneously, of course. In the GDR, the Orders of 28 June, 1968 (BG. II, 1968, p. 640) and the 5th Implementing Degree subsequent to the issuance of those orders contain regulations which specify maximum allowable concentrations (MAC values) for atmospheric contaminants. Analogous regulatory standards have been adopted in other countries.

The MAC values of particular interest are those pertaining to contaminant levels near the ground in the open air, or to the amounts of dust settled on the ground, that may be considered generally safe for humans, animals and plants in the light of previous experience.

The contaminants may have a direct adverse effect on the animal body, or they may be indirectly harmful by damaging and altering plants on which the animals feed. In addition, they may cause disturbances of vitamin metabolism, enzyme actions and hormone balance, they can alter the pH in the digestive tract, leading to changes in the intestinal flora, and they can precipitate allergic responses. General clinical manifestations include digestive disturbances, colic, diarrhea, emaciation or cachexia, anemia, infertility, abortion or the birth of weak foals, alopecia and eczema. These general effects, moreover, increase the animal's susceptibility to other diseases.

Illness due to atmospheric pollutants may take an acute, subacute, subchronic or chronic course. When high concentrations of the injurious substance are absorbed and produce acute effects, these usually consist of the general symptoms listed above. Repeated exposure to lower levels of the pollutant lead gradually to the development of a subchronic or chronic intoxication. The variable clinical picture in such cases is based partly on variations in the concentration of the toxic substance, climatic factors, and on the resistance and general health of the affected animal.

Relatively few industrial emissions have been found to cause disease in the horse. Alopecia has been observed in horses exposed to *arsenic* emissions. An oral dose of 10—45 g arsenic acid or 5—10 g water-soluble potassium arsenite is lethal for horses. *Fluorine* is emitted primarily by superphosphate factories and aluminum works, with lesser amounts emitted by steelworks and metal works, iron foundries, brick-works, enamelling plants, etc. The processing of fluorine-containing materials creates a health risk through emissions of gases, vapors and dusts into the atmosphere. Highly toxic gases are hydrogen fluoride (HF, H_2F_2) and silicon tetrafluoride (SiF_4), which are converted by atmospheric humidity into toxic clouds of hydrofluoric acid (HF) and fluorosilicic acid (hexafluorosilicic acid, H_2SiF_6). Emitted dusts also contain poorly-soluble materials (cryolith) that are moderately hazardous.

Poisonings from fluorine pollutants may result both from the inhalation of fluorine-containing gases and from the ingestion of fluorine in the feed and drinking water. About 2 mg of fluorine per kg BW must be ingested before symptoms appear in horses. In foals, acute and chronic disease symptoms have been observed only 8 days after the animals were turned out to pasture. Chronic fluorine poisoning, or fluorisis, is characterized by moderate emaciation, bony swellings, discoloration of the teeth, and eventual lameness.

Factory emissions containing *lead* can also cause disease in animals. Symptoms in horses include colic, stomatitis, muscle tremors and paresis. A 50% mortality rate has been recorded in horses grazing on pasture near a lead factory. In horses that were experimentally given a feed containing 4.0—9.8 mg% lead, a lead level of 0.02—2.28 mg% was found in the liver.

Other industrial emissions, such as *copper, molybdenum, zinc, selenium, sulfur dioxide* and *phenol-containing emissions*, as well as *soot* and *particulate matter*, have not yet caused observable illness in horses and so need not be discussed here.

2.6. Thermal, Electrical and Radiation Injuries

2.6.1. Sunstroke

Definition. Sunstroke is an irritation and hyperemia of the meninges, leading to serous meningitis. It results from excessive exposure to the sun.

Symptoms. A horse that has been exposed too long to direct sunlight appears lethargic, sweats heavily, and may stagger and even collapse. Consciousness is impaired, often to the point where the animal is indifferent to stimuli. In contrast to heat stroke, the rectal temperature usually is normal in sunstroke and may even be subnormal. The pulse and respiratory rates are increased, however. The skin surface feels warm to the touch, especially about the cranium. In extreme cases there may be involvement of the medulla oblongata, and death can occur.

Etiology. Sunstroke is relatively uncommon in horses, because much of the cranial roof is covered with long hairs that shield it from insulation, and the anterior portion of the cranial roof is protected by relatively large frontal sinuses. Nevertheless, if a horse is exposed to direct sunlight for too long, as may occur in horses that pull harvesting machines or in racing and show horses that work on outdoor tracks and arenas, the meninges of the brain may become overheated, irritated and hyperemic.

Prognosis and Treatment. Most cases of sunstroke in horses respond well to early treatment. The horse should be moved to a cool, shady spot away from the sun. If possible the cranium should be sprayed with cold water, or ice packs applied to the recumbent animal. Up to 200 mg of glucocorticoids are given i.v. to reduce vascular permeability and minimize brain edema. Diuretics are also beneficial when given intravenously. If the animal is unconscious, central-acting circulatory agents are indicated. Spasmodic or convulsive episodes are treated with the appropriate drugs.

2.6.2. Heat Stroke

Definition. Heat stroke is a condition of deficient heat loss that is usually combined with excessive heat production. The result is an accumulation of heat within the body. Heat stroke in horses most commonly occurs on hot, humid, windless days.

Symptoms. The horse suddenly begins to stagger and sway, and it may collapse and enter a stuporous state like that seen in general anesthesia. Convulsions may also occur at this time. Respiration becomes rapid and shallow. The pulse is very rapid and weak, and the heart sounds are faint and irregular. The mucosae appear cyanotic as a result of venous congestion and deficient oxygen exchange. The body temperature rises to 42 °C. Sweating is virtually absent, and the skin is dry and hot. In extreme cases death occurs immediately or within several hours.

Etiology. Heat stroke occurs when the atmospheric humidity is high and heat loss by evaporation is impaired. These conditions are often encountered in poorly-ventilated, overheated stables with narrow stalls and low ceilings. Another cause of heat stroke is prolonged transportation in railway cars and trucks or confinement in sheds and tents on hot, humid days. The heat buildup within such enclosures can becomes unbearable.

Heat storage within the body and the consequent rise of body temperature lead to an acceleration of tissue metabolism and thus to a further temperature rise. Eventually the local circulation becomes inadequate to meet demands, and tissue hypoxia develops followed by metabolic acidosis. Cellular damage, in turn, can lead to changes in the CNS (e.g., brain edema) and to petechial hemorrhages in the hypothalamus and the major parenchymatous organs. These changes are accompanied by clinically apparent disturbances in the water and electrolyte balance and clotting mechanisms. At this point sweat secretion ceases. However, a resumption of sweat secretion often has been observed in racing horses that became recumbent and delerious after developing heat stroke during workouts on very hot, humid days.

Differential Diagnosis. Heat stroke must be differentiated from sunstroke and, in some cases, from colic. A differentiation between sunstroke and heat stroke is easily made on the basis of weather and other environmental conditions. Sunstroke requires direct exposure to the sun's rays, especially of the cranium, while heat stroke is associated with a high atmospheric humidity and diminished heat loss. Clinically, heat stroke is distinguished by a marked rise of body temperature, as opposed to the very slight elevation that typically accompanies sunstroke. Spasmodic colic, which may occasionally occur on hot, humid days when rain is threatening, is easily exluded by rectal examination.

Diagnosis. The diagnosis is obvious from the history and clinical signs. If necessary, the shifts in the water and electrolyte balance and the metabolic acidosis that accompany heat stroke can be demonstrated biochemically with the appropriate blood tests.

Prognosis and Treatment. If the horse is comatose, a guarded prognosis is indicated. However, recovery can usually be expected in such cases if intensive treatment is rendered.

The horse should be moved at once to a cool, shady place where there is a breeze. Massage with a cold water spray has proven highly effective in reinitiating cutaneous thermoregulation and lowering the body temperature. The bursts of cold water are applied to the entire body surface for about 5 minutes, and the procedure is repeated after 30 minutes to an hour. The body temperature is measured periodically to guard against excessive heat loss. At the time the first cold-water massage is given, central-acting circulatory agents are administered together with agents that improve myocardial action and tone; glucose solutions and the cardiac stimulant strophanthin are suitable for this purpose. If the animal is conscious, tepid drinking water may be offered. The ingestion of water will stimulate sweat secretion and assist heat dissipation. If the animal is in a deep coma, it should additionally be treated for shock. Prednisolone is administered i.v. in a dose of 200—400 mg. If urine secretion is impaired, osmotic diuresing agents should be given in the form of a sorbitol or mannitol solution (5—20 %) administered by continuous i.v. drip. Hypertonic solutions of this type, as well as hypertonic dextrose solutions, help to prevent edema formation in the brain and subcutaneous tissues. In comatose animals that are convulsing and hyperventilating, a 10 % calcium gluconate solution should be injected in a dose of 200—250 ml to control respiratory alkalosis. Injections of neuroleptics are contraindicated in heat stroke.

Comments. All symptoms in horses with heat stroke should be carefully monitored and controlled. Treatment must be as intensive as possible, especially in the presence of convulsions and coma.

2.6.3. Burns

Definition. A burn, or thermal injury, is a reversible or irreversible tissue lesion caused by the action of intense heat. Temperatures of 50—75 °C cause an increase of microvascular permeability in the affected area, while temperatures in excess of 75 °C cause the skin to undergo coagulation necrosis. The local lesions, moreover, may be accompanied by a variety of systemic disturbances ('burn sickness').

Symptoms. In the horse as in man, four degress of clinical burn severity are recognized:

With a *first-degree burn* there is skin inflammation with hyperemia, edema and burning pain. The skin feels warm to the touch, is thickened, tense and shiny. The hairs are always singed. In this type of burn, the thermal injury is confined mainly to the stratum corneum. From about the 5th day on, superficial portions of the stratum corneum are sloughed. Generally this is followed by spontaneous healing.

In the *second-degree burn*, blistering and marked skin edema appear within 24 hours. As the blisters form, the epidermis becomes separated from the dermis, creating a dead space that fills with a serous, yellowish fluid. Very large blisters sometimes become loculated by fibrinous septae, and their contents become jelly-like. Burn blisters are always very painful. Cutaneous sensation is fully preserved. The further course of the burn wound is variable. Burn blisters of small size tend to dry up, and if the epidermal defect is epithelialized, the dry blister wall will be sloughed. Large, fluid-filled blisters, on the other hand, tend to rupture as a result of movement, contact, rubbing or scratching. The contents drain, and the blister membrane is partly or completely lost. As a result, the base of the blister becomes exposed, and weeping, painful dermal wounds develop that are slow to heal and susceptible to infection.

The inhalation of hot fumes or gases can lead to a diphtheritic inflammation of the mucosae that corresponds to a 2nd-degree burn ('inhalation injury').

In *third-degree burns*, or full-thickness burns, an eschar is formed by the action of the intense heat. An eschar consists of a crust of devitalized skin whose blood vessels are thrombosed. In rare cases the necrotic tissues are moist and undergo ulceration. Most 3rd-degree burns produce a dry necrosis in the form of a burn eschar that retains its elasticity for several days. Exudate may seep through the eschar and form beads on its surface. Usually the eschar hardens within 8—10 days, becoming dark-brown and leathery.

Third-degree burns of this type have been produced in the horse by firing for therapeutic purposes. They also occur when the skin is branded with a hot iron. The blood supply to the skin is interrupted in the affected area, and the burned tissue is insensitive to pain. 1st- and 2nd-degree lesions are always found in the vicinity of a 3rd-degree burn.

With 3rd-degree burns that cover a large area, severe edema and exudation may be the only visible changes during the first few hours, whereupon the skin gradually becomes devitalized over the next 8—10 days. At that time a hard, hairless, armor-like eschar forms that remains firmly adherent to the subcutaneous connective tissue, which is permeated with a gelatinous material. Subeschar healing will occur in such cases, but the delicate, new epithelium that forms beneath the eschar often is sloughed by desquamation. Complete demarcation requires up to six weeks.

A *fourth-degree burn* is a type of full-thickness burn in which the tissues are charred by extreme heat. The sites most commonly affected in the horse are the ears, eyelids and tail. The charred areas are black, dessicated and friable.

The systemic changes occurring subsequent to thermal injuries are manifested in the horse by the following signs: The animal is restless or has colicky episodes.

The body temperature and pulse rate are markedly elevated. Restlessness and pain increase further during subsequent hours. Within 12—24 hours the rectal temperature starts to fall below normal due to excessive heat loss in the burned area. The loss of plasma volume causes excessive thirst. The pulse becomes progressively weaker, and breathing progressively more rapid. The palpebral conjunctivae and all other visible mucosae become markedly cyanotic. Hemoglobinuria is also observed. Finally the horse may become stuporous and lapse into unconsciousness. Death from cardiac failure and circulatory collapse occurs in extreme cases. Death is attributed to intoxication by protein degradation products with damage to the major parenchymatous organs, a massive loss of body fluids and blood plasma, hemolysis and severe renal damage.

Functionally, the systemic effects of burns involve significant shifts of blood and lymph. Edema results from an increase in capillary permeability. Shifts in the electrolyte balance occur as extracellular sodium moves into the intracellular space, removing potassium and phosphorus from the tissues. A loss of nitrogenous substances also occurs. The circulatory collapse that may develop subsequent to thermal injuries, with its associated fall of blood pressure, leads to a failure of glomerular filtration in the kidney. Also, the plasma losses and dehydration of the blood impair the elimination of urea. Finally, the protein breakdown products cause an interstitial nephritis with destruction of the tubule epithelial cells.

Etiology. Stable fires are the most common cause of burns in horses. Local 1st-, 2nd- and 3rd-degree burns are inflicted in such cases by proximity to flames and by contact with hot objects (red-hot metal, glowing cinders, hot ash). Contact with very hot liquids and hot vapors can cause scalding and diphtheritic inflammation of the mucous membranes. Burns on the limbs and ventral abdomen are usually caused by straw burning on the stable floor. Burns on the back are generally caused by burning debris falling from the ceiling. It should be noted that heat sensitivity varies among different tissues, depending on the consistency of the tissue and its blood flow.

Differential Diagnosis. Fagopyrism is occasionally seen in horses but is easily distinguished from thermal burns if an adequate history is obtained.

Diagnosis. The diagnosis is based on local changes. If any systemic changes are present, the animal should be treated for burn sickness as described below.

Prognosis. With 1st- and 2nd-degree burns covering no more than a third of the body surface area, a complete recovery may be expected. Even small 3rd-degree burns will heal, though with considerable scar formation. The survival rate is poor for burns covering more than one-third of the total body area, regardless of the degree of the injury. Extensive skin grafting similar to that practiced in human patients is rarely done in horses. Moreover, large burns are almost always associated with very severe systemic effects leading to a mortality rate of about 25 %.

Treatment. First-degree burns are treated with drying or cooling ointments and powders or with greasy medicaments that exert an analgesic effect (talcum, dermatol, iodoform, pellidol-cod liver oil-benzocaine ointment). Glucocorticoid ointments are widely used in the treatment of 1st-degree burns and some 2nd-degree burns; dexamethasone has proved most effective. A cooling and analgesic effect is also obtained with antihistamine gels, which are applied to the erythematous areas. Bismuth burn dressings are suitable for burns on the limbs of the horse and may be left in place for 6—7 days.

Second-degree burns with vesicle formation are likewise covered and treated with drying powders or ointments, especially zinc ointments. Blisters are extremely painful during the first few hours after the burn. Blisters that rupture due to mechanical influences or their own size lose their membrane, and the resulting wounds are easily infected. At this stage, Stahl's burn liniment (linseed oil, calcium hydroxide solution) has proved beneficial. Larger blisters are incised or punctured so that contact between the epidermis and dermis will be restored when the dressing is applied. This will enable an eschar to form within a few days. The burn is further treated with ointments that promote demarcation, and finally with epithelializing ointments. Cod-liver oil ointments containing a sulfonamide or antibiotic are recommended for this purpose.

With *third-degree burns*, the object is to achieve subeschar healing. This presents no difficulties in burns of the skin. If the burn involves deeper tissues, however, healing takes place by inflammation involving a considerable degree of wound exudation and suppuration. The formation of a brick-red granulation tissue takes 4 to 6 weeks. Epitheliazation proceeds from the margins of the wound and from intact epithelial islets. As the granulation tissue is converted to connective tissue, it undergoes a large degree of scar retraction. It is common for scar retractions of this type in the flank-stifle region of the horse to become torn apart during strenuous exercise, creating new bleeding and granulating wound surfaces. Complete healing will require about 3—5 months. Third-degree burns are treated initially with dessicating powders, but greasy ointments or oils should be applied starting the 2nd or 3rd week. If the skin is ischemic as a result of charring, it must be removed with scissors and forceps. With the appearance of healthy granulation tissue, especially on the limbs, skin grafting should be given consideration as a means of preventing severe scar contraction.

With *fourth-degree burns*, debridement is the only viable option.

The *systemic effects of burns* require treatment for circulatory collapse if present, and measures to correct metabolic disturbances. The horse is placed in a warm, well-ventilated stall and blanketed if necessary. Caffeine, strophanthin and 20 % glucose solution are administered i.v. This is combined with the administration of antihistamines and glucocorticoids, and essential amino acids, with the aim of neutralizing protein breakdown products and preventing fatty degeneration of the major organs. The fluid loss is corrected by giving plasma or a whole blood transfusion. If plasma and whole blood are unavailable, dextran may be given as a blood substitute. Complete electrolyte solutions are also infused to regulate the water balance, and this may be supplemented by frequent drinking. If metabolic acidosis is present, sodium bicarbonate solution is administered with the intravenous solutions. For renal failure, sorbitol or mannitol solutions are administered by continuous i.v. drip. Metapyrine or phenylbutazone should be given if analgesic therapy is required. Finally, in animals with extensive burns, a prolonged course of antibiotic therapy (8 or 10 days) should be considered as a means of preventing septicemia. If systemic changes are complicated by diphtheritic inflammation of the respiratory tract (inhalation injury), oxygen therapy is recommended.

Phosphorus Burns

Definition. Because phosphorus burns at 60 °C, the thermal lesions it produces take the form of 1st- and 2nd-degree burns. Phosphorus residues present in the skin or in the wound are transformed by oxidation into phosphorus pentoxide. This compound reacts with tissue fluids to form an acid that produces chemical burns which complicate the thermal injury.

Symptoms. Circumscribed 1st- or 2nd-degree burns are visible on the affected skin. In addition, the burned area gives off pungent vapors that smell of phosphorus. Residual phosphorus remaining in the skin or wounds will glow visibly in a darkened room. The extent and depth of the acid burn vary with the amount of available oxygen. The skin becomes necrotic and dry. In severe thermochemical burns, deeper tissue layers may also be destroyed.

Prognosis and Treatment. The prognosis is good if treatment is commenced early. Phosphorus particles that are grossly visible on the skin are brushed off as quickly as possible or are painstakingly removed with forceps, after first clipping the hairs if necessary. Oxygen must be denied access to the wound in order to prevent additional phosphoric acid formation. Wounds already present are flushed copiously with water as quickly as possible, and the acid is neutralized by prolonged irrigation with 5% sodium bicarbonate solution. An absence of phosphorescence in darkness is considered evidence that the acid has been neutralized. Alternative neutralizing agents are silver nitrate, ammonia soda, 5% potassium permanganate solution, and 10% tannin spirit. Such treatment is indicated only after all phosphorus residues have been removed. Treatment then follows the principles of burn care.

2.6.4. Frostbite

Definition. Frostbite is the damage to cells and tissues resulting from exposure to low environmental temperatures. Three degrees are recognized, which correspond essentially to the categories of burn but are more intensive:

— First-degree or mild frostbite, characterized by erythema of the affected skin.
— Second-degree or moderate frostbite, characterized by blistering.
— Third-degree or severe frostbite, characterized by eschar, necrosis and gangrene.

Symptoms. In death due to freezing, the body temperature falls below 20 °C (hypothermia), and all vital processes cease. Initial signs in the horse are fatigue and a sluggishness of movements. Even intestinal peristalsis ceases. The hypothermia always starts at the periphery of the body and gradually spreads inward. Deep unconsciousness and convulsive movements mark the terminal stage, which is also characterized by cerebral anoxia, cardiac failure, and hemolysis. In more chronic cases of hypothermia, death from cardiac and circulatory failure may occur weeks after the actual cold injury.

Localized cold injury, or frostbite, leads to vasoconstriction and thus to ischemia of the affected part. Further cooling causes cell damage and cell death. The affected parts are numb, and they feel hard and cold to the touch. Extremities that are completely frozen may break off.

The further course varies with the degree of the injury: In 1st-degree frostbite, sensation returns with rewarming, and the tissues become reddened, hot and very painful. The previous vasoconstriction gives way to a marked vasodilation with subsequent vasoparalysis, resulting in passive hyperemia of the part. Blood serum leaks through the damaged vessel walls, producing the edema that is characteristic of mild frostbite. The edema and hyperemia persist for about 10—14 days and then gradually subside. At this time the thickened skin begins to desquamate, and superficial epithelial layers are sloughed until a normal skin thickness is gradually restored.

In 2nd-degree frostbite, serum transudes through the stasis or thrombus in the damaged and paralyzed vessels, passing into the cold-injured tissues and causing separation of the epidermis and dermis. A severe dark-red to violet, glassy edema develops, accompanied by vesiculation. The red, laky, serous blister fluid gradually dries, and the epidermis desquamates. The frostbite blisters sometimes rupture when touched. As in 2nd-degree burns, ulceration may occur.

Third-degree frostbite in the horse most commonly affects the ears and tail, though the penis (when paralyzed) and the prepuce are also vulnerable. In severe frostbite the tissue cells rupture, and all blood flow to the tissues is suspended. As a result, tissue vitality does not return with rewarming. The frostbitten parts are deep red to deep violet in color, have a glassy appearance, are strongly fluid-congested and friable. A pale red transudate oozes through the skin. Even after rewarming, the tissue remains cold and insensitive and gradually acquires a rubbery appearance and consistency. After a few days the entire skin is cast off, producing a slimy, necrotic slough. Dry necrosis occurs only in very small parts, such as the tips of the ears.

Etiology and Occurrence. Frostbite in the horse affects only hairless areas or places where the skin or hair is wet. Generalized cold injury leading to death from freezing occurs only in severely overworked or emaciated animals. Horses are highly resistant to the effects of dry cold. Local 1st-degree cold injuries are observed in the lower part of the prepuce, while all three degrees of frostbite can occur in the prolapsed penis. Prolonged exposure to very low temperatures can cause frostbite of the perioplic band, the heel bulbs, or 1st-degree frostbite at the tips of the ears.

Diagnosis and differential diagnosis should present no difficulties. Usually it is easiest to assess the degree of cold injury after rewarming the affected part.

Prognosis and Treatment. The prognosis is good for 1st- and 2nd-degree frostbite. Generalized cold injuries have a poor prognosis. Local 3rd-degree injuries must be carefully evaluated, for extensive necrosis is usually present. Whatever the degree of the injury, it is important that the affected part be rewarmed slowly. The horse is placed in a cool or moderately warm room. The affected parts are rubbed with snow or wrapped in cold, wet towels. Once a gradual rewarming has been achieved, the part is dried and very gently massaged. In parts that are to be bandaged, especially the limbs and perioplic band, thick layers of cotton should be applied over the affected area to help prevent secondary infection. Larger blisters are incised and removed with a scissors. This is followed by open wound treatment with dessicating powders. Areas that cannot be bandaged should be covered with boric-acid ointment, vaseline or cod-liver oil ointment. The paralyzed, frostbitten penis is dressed with a splinted bandage.

The treatment for generalized cold injury is the same as that for shock. The cardiac stimulant Strophanthin as well as 20—30% glucose solutions are administered i.v. The room containing the animal is heated very gradually. The body surface is vigorously massaged or brushed to stimulate peripheral blood flow. Prednisolone is administered i.v. or i.m. in a dose of 200—400 mg. Tepid fluids should also be administered by mouth (stomach tube).

2.6.5. Electric Shock

2.6.5.1. Injuries from Power Lines and Electrical Wiring

Definition. Injuries from such sources may involve contact with electricity at low voltages (100—1,000 V) or in the high-voltage range (20,000—100,000 V).

Symptoms. As a rule, horses are highly susceptible to electric shock. Contact with low voltages from 100 to 1,000 V can cause immediate central respiratory arrest, ventricular fibrillation and consequent death. In other cases the animal may show convulsive symptoms, collapse, and enter a coma-like state in which respirations are slow and deep. This state lasts from several minutes to several hours, whereupon the horse slowly rises to its feet and remains dazed for some time. Burning may also occur in shocks caused by high voltages of 20,000—100,000 V. A damp haircoat and moist skin increase conductivity. All degrees of burn severity may occur. Thermal heat is produced in areas where the current passing through the body meets points of increased resistance, and the generation of extremely high temperatures in such cases is not unusual. The surface resistance at the spot where the current enters the body causes local burning and scorching of the skin. Spark discharges also cause small burn wounds, the breakthrough of current through the skin, and localized charring.

Etiology. Electrical transmission wires or electrically charged objects (feed troughs, hay racks, hanging wires) can cause shocks in horses due to contact with the head or, less frequently, the limbs. Horses may also take electric wires playfully in their mouth or even chew the insulating material from the wire and expose the bare metal. Often in such cases the current flows from the head longitudinally through the body, cerebrum and heart to the limbs. Resistance is lowest in the blood vessels and muscles. Where resistance is high, the energy is converted to heat, and temperatures of 2,000 to 3,000 °C may be generated in these areas.

Currents at lower voltages tend to pass along the body surface, causing burns in their wake.

Prognosis. In shocks causing transitory unconsciousness and mild burns, the prognosis is good. Deaths are more frequent from low-voltage shocks than from high-voltage injuries. Currents with an amperage of 100 mA or more are always lethal.

Treatment. Because respiratory and metabolic acidosis can develop very rapidly during unconsciousness, a continuous intravenous drip of sodium bicarbonate should be started without delay. This is also of value in controlling ventricular fibrillation. Burns are treated according to the rules outlined under that heading.

2.6.5.2. Lightning Stroke

Definition. The lightning channel is the path traveled by the principal discharge from the earth to a cloud. During this process, a potential difference of approximately 25—50 million V is equalized in about 1/1,000 of a second.

Symptoms. A lightning stroke causes extensive burns, violent molecular jarring with concussion of the brain, shock, and possibly death. A characteristic feature is the finding of zig-zag lines of scorched skin and singed hairs ('lightning figures') at the points of entry and exit of the lightning stroke. The skin may be deeply perforated and torn, even down to the muscles. Residual peripheral nerve paralysis often persists in animals that survive.

Etiology and Occurrence. Lightning occurs in connection with thunderstorms and is most common in the afternoon and evening of the summer months. Horses usually are struck under trees while at pasture. Even at distances up to 10 meters from the tree, there is a danger of electrocution. Closed horse trailers provide the safest environment.

Prognosis. In horses that survive, the prognosis depends upon the severity of burn injuries.

Treatment. The animal is treated for shock, with special emphasis placed on the use of alkalizing agents. Thermal burns are treated using methods recommended above.

2.6.6. Radiation Injury

Definition. This type of injury is caused by electromagnetic rays or radioactive materials. Electromagnetic waves (e.g., x-rays) propagate at the speed of light and, like simple light, can be reflected. During nuclear fission or nuclear fusion, large amounts of energy are released in various forms. Besides the initial burst of deeply-penetrating γ-rays, neutrons and α- and β-rays, additional energy is released in the form of heat and pressure waves. 'Radiation sickness' results from whole-body exposure to γ-rays and includes all the symptoms induced by the initial burst of radiation. Neutrons liberated by nuclear fission produce radioactivity only upon entering the body. The corpuscular α- and β-rays have considerably less penetrating power. However, their relative biologic activity is 10—20 times higher than that of γ-radiation. Beta rays mainly cause external radiation injury corresponding to the various degrees of thermal burn. Residual radiation is emitted by the fission products of radioactive fallout.

Symptoms. The general clinical manifestations of radiation exposure are collectivized under the term 'radiation sickness'. The first clinical symptoms of radiation sickness appear between 30 minutes and 2—3 hours following a whole-body exposure. Initial signs in the horse include apathy, swaying and diarrhea. The breakdown of tissue protein is increased. Partial-body exposure is followed by a temperature elevation up to 40 °C. This may subside in 2—3 days. The effects of radiation exposure in the horse are most pronounced in the hematopoietic system, followed by the germinal tissue, glands, mucosae, skin, lungs, kidneys and liver. In the first hours after exposure the leukocyte and lymphocyte counts are reduced by as much as 90 % for about 3 hours [Bolz, 1964]. On the 2nd or 3rd day following whole-body exposure, the horse exhibits behavioral disturbances, inflammation of the mucosae and corneal ulceration. If the animal was exposed to a lethal dose, death occurs during the initial phase of radiation sickness, with shock developing within 3—5 days. Otherwise a second phase will be reached between the 5th and 10th day. This is a latent period of apparent normality, although diarrhea and hemorrhagic enteritis are often present.

The third phase of radiation sickness is marked by a reappearance of apathy, depression, ataxia and hindquarter paralysis, alopecia, anorexia, dyspnea and diarrhea. Hemorrhages occur in the major organs as well as in the skin and subcutaneous tissues, and edema later becomes the predominant feature. Finally, extensive damage causes a failure of the body's immune mechanisms, and death from secondary systemic infection usually occurs in the 3rd week after exposure.

If only part of the body has been irradiated, or if the whole-body dose is sublethal, the symptoms of radiation sickness are less pronounced. Horses so affected generally will reach the 4th phase — a long period of convalescence that leads to permanent recovery only in some cases. In many animals, long-term effects become evident only after a period of years. These may take the form of neoplasms, liver degeneration, cataracts, and atrophy of the hematopoietic tissues.

Fission products are yet another source of radiation injury, leading to additional α- and β-irradiation of varying duration and itensity.

The *local* effects of radiation exposure, especially exposure to γ-rays, have been studied in the horse in some detail. Partial-body irradiation is rapidly followed by erythema. Epilation occurs shortly thereafter. 'Soft' irradiation at a dose of 1,080 to 1,200 r leads to erythema and hair loss, the epilation being followed by the regrowth of white hairs. An exudative eczema was produced by 2,400 r under equivalent exposure conditions. At higher doses, skin necrosis occurs. This necrotic skin is sloughed, leaving poorly-healing ulcerous wounds. Hypertrophic, keloid-like scars form later.

The relatively low sensitivity of horses to radiation exposure is based upon the anatomic structure of the equine skin — especially its relatively low degree of innervation and vascularization per unit skin area.

All reaction stages in the horse are long-lasting and slow to regress. Long-term effects from 1st- and 2nd-degree exposures are associated with a temporary or permanent regrowth of unpigmented hairs. Third- and fourth-degree reactions are characterized by pigmentary changes, permanent hair loss, and atrophy and necrosis of the skin.

Prognosis. The prognosis depends on the nature of the radiation and on whether a partial- or whole-body exposure was involved. The heat generated by nuclear fission or nuclear fusion causes 1st- through 3rd-degree burns. Nuclear explosions, moreover, create a destructive shock wave that can cause fatal internal injuries.

Treatment. First- through third-degree burns are managed according to the rules discussed above. The damage to hematopoietic tissues requires that whole-blood transfusions be administered; this is also useful in terms of platelet replenishment. Glucocorticoids and central-acting circulatory agents are also beneficial. A high plane of nutrition should be maintained during therapy. Antibiotics and sulfonamides are given for infection prophylaxis.

Radioactive fallout is removed by prolonged, repeated irrigation.

Comments. In the event of a disaster, treatment should be given only to horses that are mildly affected and are expected to live.

References

BOLZ, W.; DIETZ, O.: Lehrbuch der Allgemeinen Chirurgie für Tierärzte; 4. Aufl. (VEB Gustav Fischer Verlag, Jena 1970).

KARAVAEV, V. M.; KOLJAKOW, V. L.; KORSHEVENKO, G. N.; ILJIN, V. G.: Schutz landwirtschaftlicher Tierbestände vor Kernstrahlung (VEB Deutscher Landwirtschaftsverlag, Berlin 1973).

SCHEBITZ, H.; BRASS, W.: Allgemeine Chirurgie für Tierärzte und Studierende (Parey, Berlin 1975).

WEGENER, H. K. V.: Radioaktivität und Veterinärmedizin (Parey, Berlin 1966).

2.7. Diseases of Newborn Foals

2.7.1. Hypoxemia

Definition and Occurrence. Hypoxemia is a deficient oxygenation of the erythrocytes that often is observed perinatally in foals. It is associated with a mortality rate of 3—4 %. It occurs in horses of all breeds, ponies being affected somewhat more frequently than large horses.

Symptoms. Immediately after birth, mildly affected foals show a cyanotic, bluish discoloration of the mucosae, rapid pulse, sluggish palpebral and anal reflexes, diminished muscle tone, increased intestinal peristalsis and spontaneous meconium excretion.

Severe hypoxemia is manifested by a gasping respiration, the aspiration of amnionic fluid, pale, white mucosae and porcelain-colored sclerae. All reflexes are absent, the body is completely limp, and the tongue is anemic and pale and hangs from the side of the mouth. The anus is patent and stained with meconium.

Etiology and Pathogenesis. The problem lies in a delayed or incomplete establishment of respiration with normal cardiac activity. This may result from premature separation of the placenta, anemia of the dam and/or the foal, premature division of the umbilical cord, intrauterine or intrapartum strangulation of the cord, or a premature onset of respiratory activity. It may also be caused by delivery in an unbreached amnionic sac, causing amnionic fluid to be aspirated following division of the cord. In all these cases, an early buildup of CO_2 in the fetal blood prematurely stimulates the respiratory center, thus causing a premature initiation of respiratory excursions. It is common in such cases for large amounts of amnionic fluid to be aspirated. Moreover, if the intrauterine oxygen deficiency arises during the expulsion stage, then expansion of the lungs will be hampered for mechanical reasons. The premature perfusion of the lung with blood, together with the preexisting oxygen deficiency and increasing buildup of CO_2, soon exhaust the initially heightened functional activity of the respiratory center.

Diagnosis. The course of the delivery and the clinical picture provide the basis for diagnosis. A differentiation must be made from weak-foal syndrome, prenatal hypovitaminoses and intrauterine infections (e.g., with *Salmonella abortus equi*).

The prognosis depends largely on the degree of hypoxemia present, the amount of fluid that has been aspirated, and the time at which treatment is instituted. With mild hypoxemia and minimal fluid aspiration, the prognosis is favorable. With moderate hypoxemia the prognosis is very guarded, and with severe hypoxemia it is often grave.

Treatment and Prophylaxis. Given the etiology of the condition, prophylaxis begins with the monitoring of parturition and the provision of obstetric assistance and intervention where needed. The first therapeutic measure is to lift the hypoxemic foal by its hind legs so that the aspirated amnionic fluid can drain. This is aided by opening the foal's mouth, pulling the tongue forward, and attempting to express fluid in the nostrils by stroking firmly down the dorsum of the nose with the hand. Respiration and circulation can be stimulated by brushing the skin and by spraying the occiput and chest with cold water. Ventilatory assistance can be rendered by grasping the left metacarpus with the left hand and the humerus above the elbow with the right hand, and then making gentle, rhythmical, circular movements with the limb so that the scapula is alternately elevated and lowered somewhat. These resuscitative measures are frequently successful when continued for a period of 5—15 minutes. In moderate and severe cases, the administration of oxygen from pressurized cylinders is always indicated. The supply hose is either inserted into the nasal passages or placed endotracheally via the nose or mouth. Intubation and artificial respiration are the optimal procedure in many cases.

Pharmacologic therapy consists in:
— stimulation of the respiratory and circulatory center,
— circulatory support, and
— the early care of aspiration pneumonia.

Drugs that have proved efficaceous include:
— lobeline hydrochloride (0.02 g i.m.)
— pentamethylenetetrazol (0.1 g i.m.)
— caffeine and sodium benzoate or salicylate (0.5—1.0 g i.m.)
— dimethylamide N-crotonylethylaminobutyric acid (0.3 g)
— dimethylamide N-crotonylpropylaminobutyric acid (0.3 g in cheek or nostril).

2.7.2. Weak Foals

Definition and Occurrence. The terms 'weak foal', 'failure to thrive' and 'physiologically immature' have all been used to describe this condition of congenital weakness in horses. Affected foals show little vitality postpartum (p. p.) and one hour after birth are either unable to stand without assistance or have extreme difficulty doing do. Cases occur sporadically, and most are born to mares that received poor nutritional support during pregnancy.

Symptoms
— a birthweight that is significantly below average for the breed;
— inability to stand within 60 min p. p.;
— absence of sucking reflex 30 min p. p.;
— failure to seek the dam;
— sparseness of hair around the mouth and eyes;
— weak palpebral and anal reflex;
— erythrocyte count $<$ 11 million/ml blood;
— heightened susceptibility to neonatal infections.

Etiology and Pathogenesis. The cause of congenital weakness in foals lies partly in a maternal dietary deficiency of energy, fat-soluble vitamins (especially vitamin A), minerals and trace elements during pregnancy. Other possible causes are problems of maternal acclimatization to stable changes during pregnancy, as well as genetic factors. A significant percentage of cases are causally related to acute and especially to chronic diseases of the dam, such as rhinopneumonitis, *Salmonella abortus equi* infection, influenza, intestinal parasitisms, etc.

Diagnosis. The diagnosis is based upon direct clinical and laboratory examination, an analysis of prenatal care, and the routine examination of all pregnant mares for infectious diseases and parasitisms.

The prognosis depends on the severity of the syndrome. In most cases it is guarded.

Treatment and Prophylaxis. The birth of weak foals can be largely prevented through prophylactic measures. The foremost of these relate to sound prenatal care. The approximate nutritional requirements of a mare weighing 550 kg are as follows, starting in the 5th month of gestation (cf. Sec. 1.3.3.1.) and increasing as term approaches:
— 4.5—5.5 kEFr (11,250—13,750 kcal),
— 480—630 g digestible crude protein
— 40,000 I.U. vitamin A,
— 80 I.U. vitamin E,
— 6,000 I.U. vitamin D_2.

It is essential that these requirements be safely met. Pregnant mares should if possible be moved to the intended foaling facility by the 6th month of gestation. The health status of all the broodmares on a farm should be continually monitored through routine serologic and fecal examinations, and specific prophylactic and therapeutic measures instituted promptly whenever an infectious process is detected (cf. Sec. 2.2.).

In addition, all broodmares should be treated with 10 mg of mebendazole or 50 mg of thibendazole per kg BW at 8-week intervals for an entire year, and in 3-month intervals thereafter. Introduced broodmares should always be treated at 8-week intervals during the first year after their introduction to the herd.

2.7.3. Neonatal Jaundice

(See Sec. 2.1.3.2.2.)

2.7.4. Pervious Urachus

Definition and Occurrence. In this condition the canal within the umbilical cord that joins the fetal bladder with the allantois (the urachus) fails to close at the time the cord is severed. This allows urine to be discharged through the urachal opening at the umbilicus. The condition is more common in foals than in other domestic animals.

Symptoms. A dribbling of urine from the umbilicus is observed either at birth or two to three days afterward. Generally the urethra is still patent, however. The constant wetting of the umbilical stump with urine can lead to omphalitis, which in turn may progress to septicemia and bacteremia (see Sec. 2.7.14.).

Etiology and Pathogenesis. Pervious urachus sometimes represents a defect, or cleft-type malformation, of hereditary origin. Avulsion of the umbilical stump or other trauma to the stump can also be the cause.

The *diagnosis* is made from clinical findings.

Treatment. Assuming the urethra is patent, surgical closure of the urachus should be undertaken without delay. A common method of treatment is to first cleanse the umbilicus and then cauterize it with heat or caustic chemicals (silver nitrate or strong tinctures) to produce swelling and closure of the urachus. An alternative method is to ligate the urachus with catgut, either before inflammatory symptoms appear or after they have subsided.

2.7.5. Meconium Retention

(cf. Sec. 2.1.5.10.7.)

Definition and Occurrence. In this condition the spontaneous passage of meconium fails to occur during the first 36 hours of life despite an initially regular nursing routine. Among farm animals, this neonatal disease is most commonly seen in foals. Males are affected more often than females by virtue of their narrower pelvis.

Symptoms. Affected foals show a reluctance to nurse that usually is first noticed on the 2nd day of life. The foal strains frequently and makes repeated abortive attempts at defecation. Soon the foal becomes reluctant to move and may lie down frequently. In the next stage of the disease colicky symptoms become apparent. The animal lies down, assumes unusual positions, stretches, strains, and may start to roll. The conjunctivae show signs of congestion and the pulse rate is elevated.

Etiology and Pathogenesis. There are two main causes of meconium retention in the foal. On the one hand, the wide lumen of the foal's intestinal tract facilitates the collection of large amounts of meconium anterior to the pelvic inlet. On the other hand, the explusion of meconium may be inhibited by reduced peristalsis, maternal malnutrition during pregnancy, and incipient neonatal infections. If these problems are compounded by an inadequate or delayed ingestion of colostrum by the foal, initial symptoms often will appear on the 2nd postpartum day.

Diagnosis. The diagnosis is based upon the general clinical examination and digital rectal palpation. Meconium retention must be distinguished from the less-common atresia coli (cf. Sec. 2.8.4.2.). On digital rectal examination, some dark, brownish-green mucus mixed with fecal material will adhere to the examining finger when meconium retention is present. In atresia coli, pure mucus will be obtained. The prognosis is favorable given a prompt diagnosis and immediate therapy.

Treatment. The prophylaxis of meconium retention centers on sound prenatal nutrition in the mare and on ensuring the timely ingestion of colostrum by the foal. The passage of meconium should be carefully noted on the 1st and 2nd postpartum days. Treatment should be commenced at once if no meconium has been passed within 12 hours after birth. Meconium located in the rectal ampulla can be removed in pieces with the finger. At the same time, mineral oil enemas should be given by means of a rubber catheter (maximum diameter about 1.4 cm) and Janet syringe. In severe cases the enemas should be repeated three times daily. No more than about 150 ml of mineral oil should be administered per treatment. Even in stubborn cases, the last traces of meconium should be removed within 2—3 days under this regimen, and rarely will operative intervention, with manual propulsion of the impacted meconium, prove necessary.

2.7.6. Diarrhea due to Noninfectious Causes

Definition and Occurrence. Inflammation and functional disorders of the gastro-intestinal tract that are manifested clinically by diarrhea are relatively common in suckling foals. The primary causes of these disorders are injurious factors that are unrelated to bacterial or viral infection. However, these noninfectious changes of the gastrointestinal tract often create conditions that are conducive to the spread and propagation of pathogenic microorganisms.

Symptoms. The course of the illness may be acute, subacute or chronic; a subacute course is the rule. The feces usually have a thin to watery consistency, although this is subject to much variation, as are the fecal odor and color. A grayish-green color is very common. Mucus and blood are rarely present in the stool. Soon the foal becomes lethargic and anorexic, develops a fever, loses weight, and shows increasing signs of dehydration and general debility. Severely affected foals less than about 3 weeks of age may die from circulatory failure within a matter of days unless prompt treatment is given. Older foals, too, may die within a few weeks following a period of progressive debility. In chronic cases some degree of growth retardation is usually seen.

Etiology and Pathogenesis. The causes of diarrhea are highly varied. Severe diarrhea is common in foals during the 'foal heat' period of the mare. Other factors that contribute to diarrhea in newborn foals are vitamin deficiencies in the mare or the heavy feeding of legumes or very young grass, coprophagy or drinking from puddles by the foal, and stresses such as exposure to heat or cold. It is not unusual for a primary noninfectious diarrhea to become complicated by secondary bacterial infection (*E. coli*, salmonellae, micrococci, clostridia, etc.), leading to infectious gastroenteritis. Infestation with strongyles, strongyloids or ascarids (see Sec. 2.3.2.) should always be suspected in foals with intermittent, subacute to chronic diarrhea, and these helminthiases must be excluded.

Diagnosis. First, an infectious etiology for the diarrhea is excluded by bacteriologic and parasitologic examinations. Then the cause is determined on the basis of a comprehensive history, the age of the affected foal, and a systematic analysis of environmental factors that might be predisposing (see above).

Control. Major factors in control are:
— optimum prenatal care,
— routine cleaning and disinfection of foaling stalls,
— helminth control in broodmares,
— administration of vitamin A to pregnant mares (50,000 I.U. per day) and to foals (12,000 I.U. per day),
— omission of laxative feedstuffs from the ration during the first weeks of nursing,
— early introduction of coarse feeds into the foal's diet.

Treatment. For younger foals, the subcutaneous administration of electrolyte solutions containing energy is always indicated (e.g., 100.0 glucose, 8.5 NaCl, 3.0 KCl, distilled water to 1,000.0). At the onset of the illness, 1 million I.U. of vitamin A in water should be given by mouth. In severe cases, thin black tea, sassafras tea or camomile tea containing 5 g NaCl/1,000 ml should be given by nasogastric tube. Blood flow is promoted by repeated parenteral injections of caffeine and sodium benzoate (or salicylate) in doses of 0.5—1.0 g per foal. Styptics suitable for oral use include humic acic preparations, medicinal charcoal, opium tincture (1 × 30—40 drops daily per foal) and thiocyanate hydracid preparations (1—3 g). Specific sulfonamides or antibiotics should be administered orally or parenterally as needed, depending on bacteriologic findings, the drug sensitivity of the infecting organisms, and the clinical picture.

2.7.7. Colic in Foals

Definition and Occurrence. The forms of colic discussed in Sec. 2.1.5.10.6. also occur in foals. However, the prevalence of the various forms differs considerably from that in adult horses. The forms of colic affecting foals are listed below in order of frequency:
— acute and subacute enteritis,
— inflammatory intestinal pain associated with spasmodic colic,

— spastic impaction,
— primary intestinal tympany,
— impaction of the large colon,
— cecal torsion,
— colonic torsion.

Inflammatory intestinal pain frequently arises during the course of subacute to chronic diarrhea, and any of the above forms of colic may supervene during its course.

Symptoms. Colicky symptoms in the foal are often preceded by several days of diarrhea and appear suddenly. The pain is intermittent, recurring at intervals of several minutes, and is accompanied by sweating and a rapid pulse. During attacks the animal falls to the ground, stands up, presses against the walls of its stall, or lies in unusual positions in the corner of the stall. The scleral vessels are deeply congested. Intestinal sounds often disappear for a short time and then reappear with a metallic, clinking sound that is best heard just behind the costal arch on the right side.

Etiology and Pathogenesis. Frequent causes of foal colic are a very high-carbohydrate diet, primary digestive disorders in the form of diarrhea, vitamin deficiencies, and the ingestion of unsuitable feeds or puddle water leading to fermentative processes in the digestive tract. Blood flow disturbances and bowel motility disorders can also be causative and may result from stresses such as heat or cold exposure and overexertion.

Diagnosis. The diagnosis is made from the history, an analysis of the animal's environment, and a careful clinical examination to ascertain current status.

Treatment. Easily-digested carbohydrates should be fed in minimal amounts during the first three months of the foal's life. From the time the foal is weaned, small amounts of hay should always be made available during feeding. Ample fresh water also should be offered to discourage the foal from drinking dirty water in the stable or drinking from puddles outdoors. Green feeds should not be too cold, too moist or wilted when eaten. Intestinal parasitism should be prevented by adopting a systematic parasite control program on the breeding farm. In acutely ill animals, the parenteral administration of spasmolytics, atropine sulfate, analgesics and caffeine is indicated. Vitamin A (1 million I.U. in water), linseed gruel and tea should be given orally, and oral doses of mineral oil (about 150 ml) plus 1—2 liters of Na_2SO_4 solution (2—5 %) are of value in some cases.

2.7.8. Actinobacillus equuli Infection (Shigellosis, Sleepy Foal Disease, Pyosepticum Infection)

Definition and Occurrence. A. equuli infection is a widespread bacterial disease of horses. The organism inhabits the nasopharynx and intestinal tract of the dam, and the foal is highly susceptible to infection by the organism during the first days of life. An infection during the first 4—5 days very often leads to septicemia with secondary localization in the kidneys (glomerulonephritis) and joints (polyarthritis). After streptococcal infection, which generally occurs in foals that are several days older, infection with *A. equuli* is the most common cause of neonatal septicemia in foals. From 10 to 15% of all neonatal deaths in foals due to infectious disease are caused by actinobacillosis.

Symptoms. The foal is healthy and vigorous at birth. Clinical observations indicate that the disease takes either a peracute or acute course. In peracute cases, extreme apathy and drowsiness appear suddenly 12—24 hours after birth. There are muscle tremors, a high fever (41 °C or more), a yellow-gray discoloration of the oral mucosa, and marked congestion of the conjunctival and scleral vessels. Soon the foal becomes severely dyspneic and goes down, unable to rise. The eyes become sunken, and the face acquires a drawn, pinched appearance. Death within a few hours is usual. In acute cases, the foal becomes dull, weak, and reluctant to suck about 24—72 hours post-partum. The temperature remains at about 40 °C for some time. The conjunctivae are deeply congested and reddened. The haircoat is rough and may have a urine-like odor as a result of purulent glomerulonephritis. The animal stands with the back slightly arched and shows no inclination to move. Lameness is frequently present as a result of metastatic infectious arthritis (gonitis and tarsitis are common). Diarrhea, incipient dehydration, and even a serous to mucopurulent nasal discharge may appear as the illness progresses. Inflammation of the atlanto-occipital joint is frequently present and accounts for the rigid extension and slight drooping of the head that are typical of the disease.

Etiology and Pathogenesis. The causative organism, *Actinobacillus equuli*, is a gram-negative rod that is killed by ordinary disinfectants. It is ubiquitous, and many mares harbor it. This, as well as equine hospital environment, are the sources of infection in foals. The congenital hypogammaglobulinemia of foals makes these animals highly susceptible to *A. equuli* before sufficient colostral antibodies have been ingested. Infections are mainly acquired via the umbilical and oral route. While infections *in utero* have been reported, the course and epidemiology of the disease suggest that this is minimal. Invasion by the organism leads very rapidly to septicemia with focal necrosis of the liver and other organs, minute pulmonary abscesses, purulent glomerulonephritis (which is pathognomonic for the disease), and clinically overt arthritides. Endocarditis may also occur.

Diagnosis. The diagnosis usually is obvious from clinical findings, for the symptoms are highly characteristic. In addition, the causative organism should be identified as soon as possible from urine samples and its resistance determined so that specific chemotherapy and antibiotic treatment can be instituted without delay. The necropsy findings are characteristic, especially the presence of a purulent glomerulonephritis and multiple microabscesses and necrotic foci in various organs combined with arthritic changes.

Differential diagnosis must be made from *E. coli* septicemia, Klebsiella sepsis, septicemic salmonellosis, and early infections with *Streptococcus zooepidemicus*.

Control. Control of the disease centers on health surveillance in pregnant mares and the maintenance of optimum nutrition and stabling hygiene during pregnancy. A sound diet that is high in vitamin A, sufficient exercise, and the hygienic stabling of pregnant mares in meticulously cleaned and disinfected box stalls are prerequisites. These factors will ensure a normal onset of lactation, good passive colostral immunization, and freedom from infection by bacteria in the immediate environment. The goal of these measures is to prevent exposure to large numbers of microorganisms while ensuring a high humoral immunity level in day-old foals. If at all possible, intervention should be avoided at parturition, and the umbilical cord should be allowed to sever spontaneously; ligation of the cord is seldom necessary. If the cord is left alone, it frequently will remain intact for 2—5 minutes after expulsion of the fetus, and approximately 800 ml more placental blood will drain into the foal than if the cord is manually severed immediately. This, of course, increases the foal's natural resistance to infection through phagocytosis, because more polymorphonuclear cells are available for defense against infections. In all cases the umbilical stump should be treated with a suitable antiseptic, preferably iodine, as soon as the cord is severed. Care must be taken not to squeeze the umbilical stump when applying the antiseptic (hemorrhage, infection, pervious urachus!). Sometimes in central Europe pregnant mares between the 7th and 10th months are vaccinated 2 or 3 times at about 21-day intervals with relatively high doses (20, 20, 10 ml) of a commercial or stable-specific *Actinobacillus equuli* vaccine (e.g., Dessau-brand *Pyosepticum viscosum* vaccine) to raise the specific antibody content of the colostrum.

At the same time, foals should receive 50.0 ml of *A. equuli* serum or 150—200 ml of fresh blood from the dam by subcutaneous injection. The injection of maternal blood, once widely employed in earlier years, is increasingly being advocated. In large herds in which 'sleepy foal' disease is a problem, the administration of 1—2 g streptomycin, 1 g streptomycin plus 1 million I.U. penicillin, 1 g chloramphenicol, or 1 g chlortetracycline for a 3- to 5-day period is often recommended.

In foals with overt *A. equuli* infection, the very rapid institution of pharmacologic therapy will critically influence the course of illness. The main priorities are:
- control of inflammation,
- supply of energy and electrolytes,
- control of bacterial infection.

A sample scheme of treatment, which always requires individual modification, is outlined below:
- 50 ml serum by slow i.v. injection,
- 50 ml serum by s.c. injection,
- combination analgesic and antipyretic parenterally,
- 8-day course of antibacterial therapy with i.m. antibiotics, possibly combined with i.v. sulfonamides,
- parenteral glucocorticoids at 50—150 mg/day,
- electrolyte solutions with sorbitol by i.v. or s.c. infusion.

It is important that immune therapy and antibacterial measures be supplemented by treatment with analgesics, antipyretics and glucocorticoid preparations. This is necessary because the foal still lacks a localized response to stimuli and, like all young mammals, manifests an exaggerated, generalized response that leads to severe inflammatory conditions. If arthritis and tenosynovitis are already present, simultaneous external and/or internal treatment with anti-inflammatory and antibacterial drugs is indicated. For external treatment in the early stage, dimethylsulfoxide is recommended for no more than 3—4 days. Glucocorticoids and aqueous antibiotic preparations are recommended for internal use.

The response to treatment and the convalescent course in sleepy foal disease depend greatly on the animal's status at the time treatment is commenced. Prophylaxis and early treatment are the foundation for the control of this serious foal disease.

2.7.9. Escherichia coli Infection

Definition and Occurrence. Two types of *E. coli* infection (colibacillosis) occur in foals: the septicemic form and the less common enteric form. They are caused by different groups of *E. coli* serotypes. The β-hemolytic *E. coli* bacteria are the most common infectious agents and cause a fulminating septicemia in newborn foals. Colibacillosis without involvement of *Proteus vulgaris*, *Klebsiella pneumoniae* and *Actinobacillus equuli* is less common in foals, however, than in calves and piglets. Hypogalactia in the dam and poor stabling hygiene are predisposing factors.

Symptoms. Foal septicemia caused by *E. coli* tends to appear within 3—4 days after birth. The course is hyperacute during the first 2 days of life. Foals that are still nursing at 6 : 00 a.m. may no longer be able to stand by 9 : 00 or 10 : 00 a.m.

The major signs at this time are respiratory distress, dry cornea, mydriasis, a progressively weakening pulse, a tense abdominal wall, colic, and agonal death within a short time. The early stage of the disease is marked by a transitory temperature peak that may exceed 41 °C but very soon the temperature falls below normal. Subnormal temperatures are more commonly seen than fever, because only very attentive and experienced breeders will recognize the fulminating disease in its prodromal stage, before the foal goes down. In foals that are 3—5 days old, the disease may occasionally take a 1- to 2-day course. It is in these cases that treatment is likely to be of value. Septicemic collibacillosis of foals is most commonly observed on breeding farms that have a high foaling density, as well as in the foals of primiparous mares that resist nursing or are poor milk producers. The disease is also observed in the foals of wild horses and zebras in zoos.

Enteric collibacillosis in foals, unlike the disease in calves, may occur up to 3 weeks after birth or even up to 4 weeks in some cases. The disease has an acute onset. Systemic effects are mild initially, and the temperature is subfebrile. Soon a watery, yellow-green diarrhea appears; the watery feces are often blood-streaked and may even contain fibrin. The foal rapidly becomes lethargic and dehydrated. Its nutritional status deteriorates, and its eyes become deeply sunken. Breathing is labored, the abdominal wall is tense, and tenesmus is present. In foals, the disease is more likely to take a subacute to chronic course than in calves, and so clinical symptoms are likely to be more protracted. The feces vary in consistency from thin to pasty. Overall development is retarded.

Infectious arthritis is also observed in some cases but is not typical of colibacilloses in foals, and tends to reflect the presence of a mixed infection.

Etiology and Pathogenesis. Following infection by the oral or nasal route, the bacteria enter the blood and lymph via the nasopharynx or gastrointestinal tract. Infection may also be acquired through the umbilicus, but the intrauterine infections frequently described in the literature are of minor importance. Newborn foals, which are born hypo- or agammaglobulinemic, must ingest immunoglobulins via the colostrum. If ingestion of the colostral immunoglobulins is delayed or insufficient, a fulminating, often fatal bacteremia and septicemia can develop without hours after birth. Contributing factors include poor nutrition of the pregnant mare, vitamin A deficiency, and the late transfer of the pregnant mare to the foaling stall. An insufficient intake of colostrum during the first hours of life, and the presence of a yet-unidentified defect that blocks the absorption of colostral antibodies in some foals, also contribute.

In enteric colibacillosis, there is a massive proliferation of enteropathogenic *E. coli* strains in the small intestine. Given the markedly enteritic course of the illness, all cases cannot be ascribed to the action of enterotoxins.

The lower incidence of enteric colibacillosis in foals is attributable to the high nursing frequency of newborn foals, which ensures a constant supply of immunoglobulins A and M for local defense. In somewhat older foals, disturbances of the intestinal flora with an overproliferation of certain *E. coli* strains can occur. This is due to the unlikely consumption of easily-digested and often highly-fermentable maternal feeds (carrots, molasses) or to licking and drinking from puddles on the way to the paddock. These are probably the major causes of the more subacute forms of diarrhea that are not easily assigned to the *E. coli* disease complex.

Diagnosis. Clinically, *E. coli* infections are very difficult to distinguish from other infectious diseases of foals. The septicemic form must be differentiated from *Actinobacillus equuli* infection and other neonatal septicemias. The enteritic form must be distinguished from diarrhea of noninfectious etiology, salmonellosis, and gastroenteritides caused by other organisms. The presumptive clinical diagnosis is confirmed by demonstrating the causative organism in the urine and rectal smears as well as in the intestine and parenchymatous organs of necropsied foals. This should also involve identifying the serotype of the *E. coli* that is found. In all cases of foal septicemia, the possibility of a pure *E. coli* infection should be considered. This is especially important if the mares are housed together with cattle and pigs. Severe *E. coli* infections in foals are especially common under such conditions.

Control. The same measures apply as in the control of sleepy foal disease. Any program for colibacillosis control must start with prophylaxis in the form of optimum prenatal care and meticulous sanitation in foaling stalls. This will ensure that healthy vigorous foals will be delivered into an environment that is as free of infectious organisms as possible. This will help to ensure that adequate amounts of colostrum are ingested on the first day of life to afford humoral antibody protection against septicemic *E. coli* strains and other bacteria or viruses, and that the initial infecting dose of microorganisms is kept to a minimum. In areas where septicemic colibacillosis is a problem, it is also recommended that foals be given horse gamma globulin (up to 100 ml). Some advocate fresh maternal blood (up to 200 ml) intramuscularly or subcutaneously (fresh blood) on the first day of life. Infected animals should receive parenteral antibacterial treatment as soon as possible, taking into account the antibiotic sensitivity of the infecting organism. The trimethoprim-sulfonamide combinations generally have high activity against gram-negative organisms, and their bactericidal action makes them excellent for use in young animals as well as those that are just entering training. Also, recent evidence indicates that the resistance of the various *E. coli* serotypes to the combinations containing trimethoprim is still relatively low. When antibiotics are used, the resistance of the causative organisms must always be given careful attention, because the resistance rate of *E. coli* to conventional antibiotics has increased alarmingly in recent years, often making it difficult to select a drug that will have efficacy.

The administration of electrolytes, analgesics, antipyretics and glucocorticoids follows the same rules outlined for the treatment of *Actinobacillus equuli* infections.

The *prophylaxis* of enteric colibacillosis involves basically the same pre-, peri- and postnatal precautions that were advocated for septicemic colibacillosis and sleepy foal disease. It is especially important that foals during the first three weeks of life be given every opportunity to exercise their natural desire to nurse (50 to 70 nursings per day are normal) in order to ensure a continuous supply of the colostral immunoglobulins A and M, which become active upon reaching the small intestine of the foal. In herds that are known to be at high risk for infection, foals may be given maternal serum, mare's milk or horse gamma globulin orally twice a day during the first week of life. Early therapy centers on the oral administration of sulfonamide-trimethoprim combinations or, based on the results of sensitivity tests, other highly active sulfonamides or antibiotics. Due to the ever-present danger of dehydration in enteric colibacillosis with diarrhea, a regimen of intravenous or subcutaneous electrolyte solutions containing energy is always indicated. Repeated subcutaneous depots of 100—200 ml are absorbed slowly. They do not alter the energy status of the foal as suddenly as doses administered i.v. or intra-abdominally, and hence are preferred. The energy concentration of these solutions should not exceed 5—10 %. Solutions containing more than 10 % invertose or sorbitol are readily tolerated by well-nourished foals, but in hypoglycemic foals they can produce life-threatening hyperglycemic shock and are therefore contraindicated. The foremost measure for the control of enteric colibacillosis is the reduction of microorganism levels in the foaling environment.

2.7.10. Klebsiella pneumoniae Infection

Definition and Occurrence. The genus *Klebsiella* belongs to the family Enterobacteriaceae. The klebsiellae are gram-negative, nonmotile, plump rods that may occur singly but usually are found in pairs or chains. They are encapsulated and form mucoid cultures on ordinary media. Eighty serotypes have been identified by capsular-swelling or agglutinizing reactions with the aid of K and O antigens. The species *Klebsiella pneumoniae* is highly resistant to environmental factors and chemotherapeutic agents. It occurs ubiquitously in nature. It is especially common in horses, dogs, cattle, monkeys and humans. The major clinical diseases produced in horses are purulent endometritis, foal septicemia and foal diarrhea. Generally these conditions occur sporadically, though outbreaks are possible.

Symptoms. Symptoms appear suddenly during the first week of life and consist of profound apathy, fever (40—41 °C), a mucopurulent nasal discharge, dyspnea, and increased bronchial sounds. In some cases rales, anorexia, arthritis, tendovaginitis and prostration occur. Signs of meningitis appear in a small percentage of cases.

Etiology and Pathogenesis. Kl. pneumoniae occurs universally and has a strong affinity for the horse. Many mares harbor the organism, and mares with a latent infection are considered the main source of infection in foals. Hospitalization may also be a contributing factor on some farms.

Diagnosis. A mucopurulent, gray-yellow nasal discharge and the bacteriologic demonstration of *Kl. pneumoniae* confirm the presumptive diagnosis.

Control. Control centers on the bacteriologic surveillance of broodmares and the routine cleaning and disinfection of foaling stalls prior to foaling, combined with appropriate cleaning between foalings. Prompt bacteriologic examinations in suspicious cases that include a test of drug sensitivities are a necessity. In our experience, *Klebsiella* spp. proved most susceptible to tetracycline, chloramphenicol, polymyxin B and sulmycin, and good results were achieved with all four drugs.

2.7.11. Salmonellosis (Infection with Salmonella abortus, S. typhimurium, S. enteritidis)

Definition and Occurrence. The specific equine salmonellosis, or *Salmonella abortus equi* infection (salmonella abortion in mares, paratyphus abortion), is discussed in Sec. 2.1.11.7. Infections with *S. abortus equi*, *S. typhimurium* or *S. enteritidis* can occur both in newborn foals and in foals 2—3 weeks old, sometimes causing a severe septicemic-pyemic or enteritic syndrome. Pulmonary metastases may occur.

Symptoms. Mares infected with *S. abortus equi* may abort, as described in Sec. 2.1.11.7., or they may deliver a live, weak foal. The mare frequently develops an intrauterine or perinatal infection which leads to a fulminating septicemia in the foal within 2—3 days after birth. The infected foals lie down much of the time and are reluctant to nurse. Dyspnea, arthritis, tendovaginitis and a blood-tinged diarrhea are also present. The animals often die before effective treatment can be implemented.

In infections with *S. typhimurium* or *S. enteritidis*, the foals generally appear normal for the first 2—3 weeks of life or even longer, but then show depression, fever, reluctance to nurse, and persistent diarrhea. The feces are gray-green in color and may contain blood. Soon dyspnea, polyarthritis and tendovaginitis also appear. In some cases abscesses may form subcutaneously in the thoracic region as well as in the lungs. The infection may become quickly generalized in very young foals, causing death from circulatory collapse within a matter of hours after symptoms first appear. In older, well-developed foals the course tends to be more protracted, although death may still occur in some instances following a 2- to 3-week period of illness. Meningitis is also observed in a few cases. At one time these forms of salmonellosis were assigned to the 'foal septicemia' complex. Today they are viewed as separate entities caused by specific organisms that generally can be isolated in pure culture.

Etiology and Pathogenesis. The infections are caused by one or more of the aforementioned *Salmonella* species. Passive colostral immunization, infective dose and natural resistance are the major factors governing the clinical manifestations of infection. Thus, aside from aborting mares, clinically overt salmonellosis is observed most frequently in foals. Infection may be acquired *in utero* or by the umbilical, oral or nasal route. The incubation period is several hours for highly toxic types and several days for others. The primary lesion is caused by bacterially-produced endotoxins. These cause further damage to the intestinal wall which enables additional orally-ingested bacteria to invade the blood stream via the bowel. While *S. abortus equi* forms a more or less closed chain of infection within the horse population, *S. typhimurium* and *S. enteritidis* are more ubiquitous, occurring in rodents, effluent, man, cattle, contaminated feeds and a number of other hosts and media.

Diagnosis. The clinical diagnosis of salmonellosis is very difficult and must rely on culture of the causative organism from tendon-sheath aspirate, nasal secretions, rectal smears or necropsy material. Maternal serologic examinations are also indicated. The serologic examination of blood from affected foals is meaningful only when done in conjunction with the mare or as a follow-up study, due to the possible presence of serum antibodies that have been passively acquired via the colostrum. Splenic enlargement, cholecystitis, and necrotic foci and granulomas in the liver, spleen, kidneys and lungs are typical findings at necropsy, but a definitive diagnosis may be accomplished only by isolation of the causative organism.

Control. Control relies mainly on measures aimed at preventing the spread of infection. Above all, these include the meticulous disinfection of buildings, the prevention of *Salmonella* introduction by rodents, humans and other animals or vectors, and the identification and isolation of infected animals. Infected mares that deliver or abort are always a reservoir for *S. abortus equi.* On farms where salmonellosis in foals has been a problem, a salmonella anti-serum that is specific for the problem serotype should be administered prophylactically to newborn foals (up to 100 ml i.v. or i.m.). The foals should be actively immunized at 2 weeks of age, the vaccination being repeated once or twice at 3-week intervals. The administration of antibacterial drugs must be preceded by isolation of the organism and a determination of its sensitivity. Drugs commonly recommended for salmonellosis include chloramphenicol, neomycin, sulfamerazine-trimethoprim combinations and polymyxin B parenterally or orally depending on the course of the disease and indications.

2.7.12. Streptococcus zooepidemicus Infection

Definition and Occurrence. Streptococci are important causes of disease in the horse. Infection with *Streptococcus zooepidemicus (Str. pyogenes animalis C)* is the most widespread disease of foals and is synonymous with 'classic' foal septicemia. Concurrent infection with *Str. equi* may also occur. The disease often is enzootic within large groups of horses. Clinically, *Str. zooepidemicus* infection is manifested by a metastatic, often fatal bacteremia.

Symptoms. Except for isolated peracute cases, symptoms generally do not appear before 1 week after birth, with most foals becoming ill during the 2nd week. The initial symptoms are a reluctance to move and lameness due to a painful polyarthritis affecting the carpus, hock, and especially the stifle, elbow and shoulder joints. Although horse breeders know of this insidious foal disease, many will report that the foal has been kicked or stepped on by the dam. Such accidents are extremely rare. The temperature rises as high as 40 °C. Affected foals lie down a great deal, stand about idly and rarely nurse. As the disease progresses, there is moderate diarrhea and pulmonary metastases with a mucopurulent nasal discharge, swelling of the mandibular and retropharyngeal lymph nodes, and an abnormal carriage of the head due to meningitis. In younger foals the infection takes an acute to subacute course. Even in older, more resistant foals, the disease often takes a subacute to chronic, metastasizing course unless appropriate drug therapy is started early. The *prognosis* in such cases is guarded.

Etiology and Pathogenesis. The causative organism, *Streptococcus zooepidemicus*, is widely distributed in horse populations. In many mares that present with fertility problems, β-hemolytic streptococci can be recovered from uterine secretions. Abortion or intrauterine infection of the fetus is possible in such cases. The great majority of infections, however, are acquired postnatally through the umbilical, oral or nasal route. Old animals that harbor purulent, discharging lesions are also a major source of infection. *Str. zooepidemicus* infections are especially common when stabling hygiene is poor. In infections acquired through the umbilicus, the bacteria invade the blood stream by way of the hepatic and portal veins, leading to bacteremia and, through metastasis, to fibrinopurulent polyarthritis, bronchopneumonia, pleuritis, and abscess formation in the liver, kidneys, brain and even the lymph nodes.

Diagnosis. The time of onset of the disease and the pathognomonic clinical picture enable a clinical diagnosis to be made. However, the bacteriologic examination of nasal or conjunctival secretions, throat swabs, urine, feces, or fluid aspirated from tendon sheaths or joints is necessary from the standpoint of specific antibacterial therapy and herd prophylaxis. In foals that die, a necropsy should be performed that includes a bacteriologic and if possible a virologic examination. Every bacteriologic examination should include a test of the organism's drug sensitivity to provide a basis for specific antibacterial treatment.

Treatment. A well-organized program of health surveillance in broodmares is of primary importance, with particular emphasis placed on the control of endometritis, infections of the upper respiratory tract and other pyogenic processes. Equally important is the rigorous cleaning and disinfection of buildings to maintain a low level of environmental contamination. Because a large percentage of overt *Str. zooepidemicus* infections in foals are acquired through the umbilicus, it is essential that the umbilical stump be atraumatically handled and disinfected, and that dry bedding be provided for the foal to lie upon. Maternal vaccination with equine *streptotoccus* vaccine in late pregnancy, combined with the subcutaneous injection of about 50 ml of streptococcus anti-serum, may be indicated. As in other infections, the old method of administering about 200 ml of fresh maternal blood to the foal by subcutaneous injection has proved effective. When overt infection is present, the time at which treatment is commenced has a critical bearing on the outcome. Besides the local treatment of existing omphalophlebitis, parenteral antibacterial therapy should be started without delay. Various drugs are recommended for this purpose: penicillin (1.0—1.5 million I.U. twice daily), streptomycin (1 g twice daily), a combination product containing both antibiotics, tetracyclines (750 mg twice daily), sulfonamides (30 mg/kg BW twice daily), or a sulfonamide-trimethoprim combination. Tendovaginitis and arthritis require local therapy as well. The need for the intra-articular or intratendovaginal injection of nonirritating antibacterial preparations must be decided on an individual basis.

2.7.13. Streptococcal Pharyngitis

Definition and Occurrence. Streptococcal pharyngitis is an infection with *Str. zooepidemicus* in older foals that frequently occurs when foals mix with other foals or with mares, or when foals are moved to a new herd. The disease is also common in weanlings or young horses that have just embarked upon a hard training regimen or have just run their first race.

Symptoms. The initial symptoms are transient anorexia and a persistent fever of 40—41 °C. This is followed by a serous, increasingly mucopurulent nasal discharge, a hacking cough, and a yellowish discoloration of the sclerae. The mandibular lymph nodes are swollen but not abscessed. Increased salivation is apparent in some animals. Depression and dyspnea are always present, and bronchopneumonia invariably develops in protracted cases.

Etiology and Pathogenesis. Streptococci introduced orally or nasally may not cause clinical infection until the animal is exposed to unaccustomed stress, such as hard training. In other cases the animal may contract a primary overt infection with *Str. zooepidemicus*, having been exposed to an infecting dose high enough to precipitate a severe, acute reaction. Initially it is limited to the pharynx. The importance of viral infections in the pathogenesis of the disease remains unclear. The course, severity and duration of the disease depend largely on the animal's resistance and on the infecting dose.

Diagnosis. The diagnosis is made from the clinical picture and by culturing the organism from nasopharyngeal swabs. The clinical features of the infection are highly characteristic. The abscence of abscess formation is the most important feature that distinguishes *Str. zooepidemicus* infection from strangles. The early stage is dominated by symptoms of a certain degree of obstruction of the upper respiratory tract, and these account for the characteristic extension of the head.

Prophylaxis and Treatment. Antibacterial hygiene and minimizing overtraining in young horses form the basis for prophylaxis. Vaccinations are indicated in problem areas, and overt cases are treated early with large doses of streptococcal anti-serum (50—100 ml). Antibacterial treatment is basically the same as that recommended for classic foal septicemia (p. 424).

2.7.14. Navel Infections

Definition and Occurrence. Navel infections are infections in which the umbilical stump forms the portal of entry for the infecting organisms. Not infrequently, their occurrence in foals results from an adhesion between the umbilical vessels and the amnionic sheath. The infection may remain confined to the umbilicus, or it may take a septicemic course. An unhygienic foaling environment contributes to the incidence of navel infections. The umbilical vein, umbilical artery or urachus may be affected.

Symptoms. Symptoms appear within a few days after birth. The umbilical cord is thickened, a palm-size area of inflammatory edema appears around the navel, and the amnionic sheath is moist and shows signs of necrosis. Pus or a reddish-brown exudate is discharged when pressure is applied. With further localization of the process, periumbilical abscessation becomes apparent. The initially local naval infection will develop into a neonatal bacteremia if the infectious organisms pass into the hepatic vein or systemic circulation. In that event, the course and clinical picture will be similar to that of *Str. zooepidemicus* infections. With omphalophlebitis, the infection will metastasize to the liver. With omphaloarteritis, the thickened cord will deviate in a caudal direction.

Etiology and Pathogenesis. Most navel infections are caused by streptococci, especially *Str. zooepidemicus*, as well as *Str. equi*, *Corynebacterium pyogenes*, *C. equi*, micrococci and *E. coli*. *Fusobacteria* spp. may also be the cause in stalls bedded with damp or wet straw. Poor stable hygiene, heavy bacterial contamination of the environment, and improper care of the umbilical stump are the major predisposing factors for a clinically overt navel infection. The infection may be confined to the umbilical vessels, the tissue of the umbilical stump and its surroundings, or it may ascend via the umbilical vessels to produce a systemic infection with metastatic lesions in the liver, kidneys, lungs and synovial spaces.

Diagnosis. Generally the diagnosis is obvious from the clinical picture. Isolation of the causative organism and the determination of its antibiotic sensitivity may be attempted.

Prophylaxis and Treatment. The rigorous cleaning and disinfection of foaling facilities prior to winter stabling contribute greatly to the prevention of umbilical infections and ascending omphalophlebitis. Care should be taken not to raise any dust in the foaling stall. At parturition, the spontaneous severance of the umbilical cord should not be done by surgical division. This usually is done one to several minutes prematurely. The umbilical stump should be treated at once with a suitable antiseptic. Iodine is recommended for this purpose, for it not only has a good antiseptic effect, but also exerts a highly desirable astringent action. Streptococcus hyperimmune serum may be administered. In all cases it is important that drying of the umbilical stump be checked daily and perhaps hastened by the application of sulfonamide powder. In the face of overt infection, immediate local surgical and antibacterial treatment is indicated. Systemic treatment with sulfonamides or antibiotics also should be started as soon as possible.

2.7.15. Streptococcus equi Infection (Strangles)

Definition and Occurrence. Strangles is an acute infectious disease of both foals and mature horses that has a world-wide distribution. It is characterized by a purulent, catarrhal inflammation of the upper respiratory tract and suppuration and abscessation of the adjacent lymph nodes. In previous decades it was of major importance in breeding farms due to the greater density of horse populations. Today its prevalence appears to be increasing once more, and even older horses are being affected.

Symptoms. Following an incubation period of 2—5 days, infected foals generally become acutely or hyperacutely ill. They are profoundly depressed, have a fever of 40.0—41.5 °C, are extremely reluctant to nurse, eat or drink, have a dry cough, and stand with the head extended. Other signs are an initially serous and later purulent nasal discharge, slight salivation, and increasing swelling of the mandibular and especially the retropharyngeal and subparotid lymph nodes with inflammatory edema of surrounding tissues. Drainage of the retropharyngeal abscesses into the pharyngeal space or guttural pouches in foals frequently leads to an ascending or metastatic spread of the infection, resulting in pneumonia or acute bacteremia with up to 30 % mortality in foals under 3 months of age. In older horses the disease takes a more chronic course.

Etiology and Pathogenesis. Str. equi occurs almost exclusively in the horse. The susceptibility of horses is generally high, especially in very young foals. The presence of acutely infected horses in foaling areas is certain to cause a high morbidity among the foals. The virulence of the organisms, and thus the infective dose for other animals, increases until the morbidity among adult animals is also high.

Diagnosis. The typically high morbidity rate in the herd and the enzootic course of the disease generally enable a presumptive diagnosis of *Str. equi* infection to be made. *Differential diagnosis* must be made from the foal septicemia complex, viral pharyngitis (e.g., Herpes II), *Corynebacterium equi* and rhinovirus infections, the enzootic bronchopneumonias, and the pyemic form of salmonellosis. This is easily done by demonstrating *Str. equi* in purulent nasal or lymph-node discharges.

As the course of the infection progresses, an enzootic abscessation of the involved lymph nodes usually becomes apparent. Moreover, it is common for many dams to fall ill, more or less acutely, with the same apparent symptoms. Enzootic strangles may also develop in racehorse populations.

Treatment. The introduction of strangles by new arrivals to the herd or by 'visiting' broodmares or stallions can be largely prevented by thorough, conscientious examination. Routine disinfection should be done to keep environmental contamination low. Foals should receive very large doses of penicillin (4 million I.U. twice daily) and/or sulfonamides (4 g twice daily) as soon after birth as possible to avoid abscessation and the danger of metastasis, which is significantly higher in foals than in mature horses. Often the antibiotics are administered in the form of 'combination' products. These contain a protein component which produces concurrent, nonspecific stimulation therapy. Generally, treatment for adult animals follows the same principles. If abscess formation is already advanced, the abscesses should be treated locally with warm compresses and, when mature, surgically opened and drained. Active and passive immunization may be indicated in threatened herds and in districts where the disease is a problem; this must be decided on a herd-by-herd basis. In mature horses, large doses of streptomycin (5.0—6.0 g/animal/day) have proved to be of value.

2.7.16. Diplococcus lanceolatus Infection (Pneumococcal Infection, Diplococcal Septicemia)

Definition and Occurrence. This infection most commonly affects young animals and produces a clinical syndrome of pulmonary septicemia. It occurs both sporadically and enzootically but does not have a wide distribution.

Symptoms. Foals infected during the first days of life usually die quickly with a fulminating septicemia. Foals infected after the first week of life generally develop a primary bronchopneumonia, but this may also progress to septicemia in some cases. The main symptoms are lethargy, weakness, reluctance to nurse, fever, coughing, dyspnea, polyarthritis, and convulsions due to meningitis.

Etiology and Pathogenesis. Most infections are acquired *in utero* or by inhalation. Infection by the oral or umbilical route is also possible. Transmission from humans has been recorded in calves. The generally hyperacute course of the infection is attributed to potent endotoxins produced by the bacteria. Vitamin deficiencies and mucosal damage due to irritants or thermal injury are believed to predispose to infection.

Diagnosis. A diagnosis is difficult to make on clinical grounds alone and must rely on necropsy findings and bacteriologic methods.

Prophylaxis and Treatment. Prophylaxis centers on the elimination of carrier mares and rigorous hygienic precautions. The examination of nasal secretions from persons with chronic inflammation of the upper respiratory tract to identify possible sources of infection, and the adoption of immunization procedures in herds or districts that are threatened by the disease are also recommended. Immunization may be done with ordinary commercial vaccines or with stable- or type-specific vaccines and anti-sera. Foals already infected with diplococci should be treated at once with a penicillin-streptomycin combination, sulfonamides, or a sulfonamide-trimethoprim given i.v. or i.m. in the doses stated previously for streptococcal infections. Due to the fulminating course of the disease, the prognosis in younger foals is not favorable.

2.7.17. Corynebacterium equi Infection (Focal Bronchopneumonia, Foal Pneumonia)

Definition and Occurrence. This infection occurs as a bacteremic disease in foals less than about 6 weeks of age, and as a very chronic, focal bronchopneumonia in older foals. Its occurrence in a given herd is always enzootic and is associated with a high morbidity.

Symptoms. In very young foals the infection often takes a peracute course with high mortality. Without warning the foal suddenly becomes acutely ill, showing anxiety, severe dyspnea, purulent conjunctivitis, a viscous, purulent nasal discharge and pumping respiration. Arthritis and subcutaneous abscessation are also commonly seen in foals less than about 6 weeks old. In older foals the disease usually takes the form of a suppurating, subacute to chronic pneumonia with marked involvement of the regional lymph nodes. Initially, systemic signs are often mild or absent, but coughing and dyspnea soon appear. As the disease progresses, abscesses develop in the lungs and lymph nodes as well as subcutaneously. *C. equi* infection often is restricted to particular districts, recurring annually in some herds while sparing others for years at a time.

Etiology and Pathogenesis. C. equi is highly adapted to the horse. Old horses and stables previously used for sick horses are considered the prime sources of infection in foals. The pathogenicity of the organism is high in foals, given a sufficient infecting dose. Oral, nasal or intrauterine infection in very young foals leads rapidly to an acute, life-threatening pyemia with principal localization in the lung. However, in foals older than about 6 weeks, a focal pneumonia with abscessation develops. This usually proves fatal after several weeks.

Diagnosis. C. equi infection must be differentiated from other bacterial diseases of foals. This is very difficult to do clinically, and a definitive diagnosis can be made only by culturing the organism from nasopharyngeal secretions or abscesses. Once the disease has occurred in a particular area, the chance of a renewed outbreak in that area is high. Extensive abscess formation in the lungs is a characteristic feature of *C. equi* infection.

Prophylaxis and Treatment. A key factor in prophylaxis is the surveillance of all horses on the stud farm with attention to suppurative processes as well as the population of pathogenic organisms present in the herd. Also, it is essential that foaling stalls and paddocks be disinfected regularly, and that optimum pasture hygiene be maintained. The response to treatment in infected foals depends largely on the stage of the disease at the time treatment is initiated. If the lungs have already developed multiple abscesses, or even one or two abscesses of large size, then the *prognosis* is very poor. Recovery is possible only if treatment is commenced during the prodromal stage of the illness. In enzootic outbreaks, sulfonamides and/or antibiotics should be administered as dictated by sensitivity findings. Foals requiring immediate treatment, before sensitivity testing is complete, should be given large parenteral doses of products containing neomycin, chloramphenicol or chlortetracycline, or sulfonamide-trimethoprim combinations. The intramuscular use of tylosin (200—500 mg/animal/day) is efficaceous if treatment is started early.

2.7.18. Herpesvirus Infection (Equine Viral Abortion)

(cf. Sec. 2.1.11.7.)

Definition and Occurrence. Rhinopneumonitis is not exclusive to foals and therefore has already been discussed under a separate heading (Sec. 2.2.3.4.). In acutely affected herds, foals acquiring sufficient colostral antibodies are adequately protected against manifestations of this disease. But if the virus is introduced into a clean herd that includes foals, very severe rhinopneumonitic symptoms generally will develop in foals challenged with equine herpesvirus type 1 or 2 (EHV 1 or 2) for which they lack colostral antibodies.

Symptoms. The initial symptom is conjunctivitis. In foals this is soon followed by fever, rhinitis, icterus, pharyngitis, dyspnea and follicular catarrh. Very young animals are prone to pulmonary edema and bronchopneumonia, possibly associated with edema of the limbs.

Etiology and Pathogenesis. EHV 1 and 2 are widely distributed in horse populations throughout the world. Once introduced into a herd, the virus is transmitted mainly by droplet inhalation.

Diagnosis. A clinical diagnosis is difficult to make based on examination of the foals alone. A presumptive diagnosis of EHV infection can be made from the status of the herd and the typical occurrence of abortions in mares. Serologic, virologic and pathologic studies provide confirmation.

Prophylaxis and Treatment. Prophylaxis is based primarily on hygienic procedures to avoid spread of the disease, which in turn rely on the systematic surveillance of all foals and breeding stock to keep abreast of herd status. Vaccinations with killed vaccines have traditionally been ineffective against EVH. However, in central Europe good results have been obtained by vaccinating animals twice yearly (in July and October) with a hamster-adapted live virus, or by vaccinating all horses older than 3 months twice with an attenuated vaccine (available commercially), and then giving a yearly booster to all mares in early pregnancy. The foals of vaccinated mares show a good colostral antibody titer up to the age of 3 months. Besides vaccination, traditional hygienic procedures on the pasture, in the stable and at parturition are of paramount importance.

2.7.19. Parainfluenza 3 Virus Infection

Virus isolation and serologic studies in foals with respiratory tract disease have confirmed the occurrence of parainfluenza in foals. A pure infection with myxovirus parainfluenza 3 generally produces a mild, self-limiting disease. The main symptoms are a transient high temperature, marked conjunctivitis and lacrimation, a seromucous nasal discharge, moderate anorexia and dyspnea. Secondary bacterial infection often leads to serious complications in the form of suppurative bronchopneumonia, pleuropneumonia and bacteremia.

2.7.20. Rhinovirus Infection (Equine Respiratory Viruses)

Definition and Occurrence. This is a widely-distributed infectious disease of the upper respiratory tract that occurs enzootically on many farms.

Symptoms. An incubation period of 3—7 days is followed by apathy, fever, anorexia, pharyngitis, swelling of the regional lymph nodes, nasal discharge and coughing. Symptoms are the same in both natural and experimental infections. Mild cases of bronchitis and complications from secondary bacterial infection are also observed. It is not uncommon for the pharyngitis to persist for several weeks, even with treatment.

Etiology and Pathogenesis. The causative agents are rhinoviruses belonging to the picornavirus group. They colonize mainly the upper respiratory tract of horses, humans, and especially cattle and cats. So far two serotypes, equine rhinovirus 1 and 2 (ERV 1 and 2), have been identified in the horse, while more than 90 are recognized in man. High levels of environmental contamination have been demonstrated for the rhinoviruses, and the infections have a world-wide distribution. The equine serotypes are transmissible to humans, and the reverse may also be true. In the horse as in man, immunity after a rhinovirus infection is serotype-specific, and so recurrences are possible. Infection is acquired mainly by droplet inhalation.

Diagnosis. A presumptive diagnosis of rhinovirus infection can be made on clinical grounds but should be confirmed by serologic studies and isolation of the causative virus. The ERV types identified to date are not very specific with regard to the origin of tissue cultures. They can be cultivated in cell cultures from horses, monkeys, humans, dogs and rabbits. Moreover, they have been found to be pathogenic for monkeys, rabbits and guinea pigs. Because these viruses enter the blood and stimulate antibody formation, animal inoculation is a potentially useful diagnostic aid.

Prophylaxis and Treatment. Control relies mainly on preventing the introduction of rhinovirus into clean herds by infected or carrier animals. Because the rhinoviruses are acid-sensitive, stalls should be routinely disinfected with solutions having a pH less than 4. If the horse is indeed affected only by the few viral serotypes that have been identified to date, it should be possible to provide temporary immunity by intranasal inoculation with a stable- or serotype-specific vaccine. Therapeutic measures include the nonspecific activation of immune system and stimulus response, the administration of antibacterial agents to prevent secondary infection, and epithelial protection by vitamin A administration. Expectorants such as mistura pectoralis or potassium iodate have also been used.

2.7.21. Adenovirus Infection

There is only one known adenovirus serotype that causes respiratory and intestinal symptoms in foals similar to those occurring in calves. It produces a primary inflammation of the respiratory and intestinal mucosae. Severe bronchopneumonia and bacteremia may develop subsequently as a result of secondary bacterial infection. Further studies are needed to clarify the importance and spread of adenovirus infections in foals.

2.7.22. Chlamydia Infection

It is unclear whether chlamydiae are of etiologic importance in the clinical effects of bronchopneumonias or polyarthritides in foals. Horses have been found to be seropositive for Chlamydia, but this means little in view of the ubiquitous nature of the organism.

2.7.23. Mycoplasma Infection

Individual *Mycoplasma* species have been isolated from the nasal discharges of horses with pneumonia, as well as from horses free of respiratory disease. Thus, it cannot be said whether and to what degree *Mycoplasma* spp. contribute to the etiology of diseases in foals, especially diseases of the respiratory organs and locomotor system.

2.7.24. Enzootic Bronchopneumonia (Enzootic Nasal Discharge in Foals)

Definition and Occurrence. This is a mixed infection that is enzootic on many breeding farms, where it recurs annually. On some farms it occurs each year after mares with foals are congregated in groups after being individually housed. It leads to a high rate of direct and indirect losses among foals due to outright death or failure to thrive.

Symptoms. The disease most commonly affects nursing foals about 8 weeks old, although the weaned foals of that year's crop may also contract the disease. Yearlings may also be affected in heavy outbreaks, but this is rare. Enzootic bronchopneumonia is basically a disease of foals between the ages of 2 and 6 months.

The course of the disease is very protracted within a herd, and persistence for several weeks or months is not unusual. The biphasic clinical course that usually is seen at the start of an outbreak indicates a primary viral infection. Initially there is apathy, reluctance to nurse, lacrimation, a serous nasal discharge, and a dry cough that is most pronounced after standing up or exercising. Peaks of high fever (up to 41 °C) are characteristic of this stage. After 3—5 days the nasal discharge becomes mucopurulent and viscous. This is particularly evident during drinking, and large flakes of purulent nasal exudate may be found floating in the watering trough or bucket. Marked symptoms of bronchitis or bronchopneumonia may also appear at this time. The mandibular and retropharyngeal lymph nodes become swollen, coughing increases, bronchial respiration intensifies, and loud, crackling rales may be heard on auscultation. The dyspnea is characterized by difficult inspiration with some stridor. Diarrhea may also be present. The visible mucosae usually are pale gray or slightly cyanotic. The disease always takes an enzootic course, with morbidity approaching 100% within a given band of foals. The severity and course of the disease vary markedly from one animal to the next. The animals affected first usually have somewhat milder symptoms than those affected later on, apparently due to an increase in virulence and infecting dose. The mortality varies from one herd to the next, depending on the degree of secondary bacterial invasion, the resistance of the host, and environmental conditions.

Etiology and Pathogenesis. Herpesvirus and rhinovirus are considered the main causative agents. The role of parainfluenza 3 and adenoviruses is not clear. The major secondary bacterial invaders are *Streptotoccus zooepidemicus*, *Str. haemolyticus*, *Corynebacterium equi* and coliforms. Infection is transmitted chiefly by droplet inhalation and by contact with infected discharges. Recent evidence also indicates that both endogenous and exogenous predisposing factors must be present in order for a clinically overt mixed infection to occur, thus placing the syndrome in the category of 'multifactorial' diseases. At the age of about 6 weeks, passive colostral immunity to the foregoing viral infections diminishes. At this time it is not uncommon for the foals of poor milkers to experience a retardation of growth. In foals infected with *Strongyloides*, the migrating larvae cause severe lesions of the pulmonary mucosae which facilitate the development of overt viral and bacterial infection.

Additional factors such as unfavorable stable temperatures, a relative air humidity above 75 or below 60%, high winds, transportation, unaccustomed stresses such as sudden chills, mucosal irritation, etc. can cause organisms present in the airways to produce disease symptoms. Moreover, a buildup of organisms can occur on many breeding farms, and this can lead to massive infection with highly virulent viruses or bacteria. Outbreaks of this kind will involve virtually all foals on the premises, even those whose resistance is high.

Diagnosis. Based on the clinical picture, the age of the foals and the enzootic course of the disease, a clinical diagnosis of enzootic bronchopneumonia may be made after specific viral infections have been excluded by serologic and virologic methods.

Prophylaxis and Treatment. Optimum prenatal care in the form of sound nutrition, routine dewormings and rigorous stable hygiene are the main prerequisites for the birth of healthy foals. Good milk output by the mare, and a colostrum rich in antibodies and nutrients are also neccessary. All mares with chronic respiratory disease represent a potential source of infection for foals. On return from pasture, the mares should be placed in clean, disinfected foaling stalls and treated intensively until their latent infection has been cured. It is equally important that foals be protected from sudden overexertion, undue heat or cold, and irritation of the respiratory mucosae by toxic gases or an indoor relative air humidity that is outside the optimum range. Weather permitting, the foals should be put in the paddocks with their dams at a relatively early age, as they will benefit from brief exposure to sunlight and fresh air. Exposure to wind or to damp, cold weather should be avoided, however.

In herds threatened by the disease, the parenteral administration of nonspecific protein preparations or polyvalent vaccines is indicated. The continuous oral administration of expectorants such as mistura pectoralis or bromhexine hydrochloride (about 10—20 mg/day) or potassium iodate is strongly recommended. Also, about 200,000 I.U. of vitamin A in water should be given once weekly for the first 12 weeks. For treatment in infected foals, a sulfonamide or sulfonamide-trimethoprim combination is given intravenously, or a penicillin-streptomycin combination, chloramphenicol or tetracycline is given parenterally in the doses previously indicated for other foal diseases. In all cases the drug of choice is determined by the spectrum of organisms cultured from nasopharyngeal secretions and the results of sensitivity tests. The possible presence of a herpesvirus or rhinovirus infection should always be taken into account.

2.7.25. Care of Orphaned Foals

(cf. Sec. 1.3.3.2.)

Foals whose dams had to be euthanized due to complications during or after parturition, and foals that relieve little or no milk by natural nursing need not be hampered in their growth and development as long as they are given proper care and nutrition.

Physiology of Nursing. The successful care of orphaned foals requires a knowledge of the physiology of natural nursing, especially with regard to:

— milk composition,
— milk quantity,
— duration of nursing period,
— nursing frequency,
— rate of weight gain.

Composition of mare's milk: Mare's milk generally contains less dry matter, protein, fat and minerals than cow's milk, but is richer in lactose. The following mean values are useful for comparison:

	Mare's milk	Cow's milk
Dry matter	10.0 %	12.4 %
Protein	2.1 %	3.5 %
Fat	1.2 %	3.5 %
Lactose	6.3 %	4.6 %
Minerals	0.4 %	0.8 %

Protein: While mare's milk has roughly the same percentage content of amino acids as cow's milk, it must be noted that only about 65% of the total protein in mare's milk ('albumin milk') is present in the form of casein, as opposed to about 85 % in cow's milk ('casein milk').

The high casein content of cow's milk can lead to indigestion if cow's milk is fed to newborn foals or piglets as a milk substitute, particularly since 'foreign' casein is not precipitated as finely in the newborn's stomach as casein from a like species, but tends to form viscous clumps.

Fat: The milk fat of mare's milk contains more unsaturated fatty acids than that of cow's milk. It also contains more volatile, water-soluble fatty acids. Consequently it is more fluid.

Vitamin A: During periods when green feeds are offered (May and June), mare's milk contains about twice as much vitamin A and carotene as cow's milk (e.g., 2,700 I.U./l vs. 1,400 I.U./l).

Colostral period: Generally the mare continues to secrete colostrum for only about 24—48 hours after parturition.

During this period the lactose content remains below that of normal milk, while the content of dry matter, protein, fat and minerals is increased, causing the nutrient content of mare's colostrum to approach that of normal cow's milk.

Unlike cow's milk, however, only about 15% of the protein in mare's colostrum is present as casein, while more than 80 % is in the form of albumin and globulin (antibodies!).

Of particular interest is the high vitamin A content of mare's colostrum, which reportedly is 6 to even 20 times that of normal milk.

Quantity of milk, duration of nursing period, nursing frequency and rate of weight gain: On average, a mare produces between 10 and 12 liters of milk daily, though many will produce 20 liters or more. The nursing period of the foal lasts about 5—6 months.

Nursing frequency: Foals nurse more frequently than is generally assumed. About 3 nursings per hour, or 60 to 70 per day, are usual. At the start of lactation about 0.2 liters of milk are consumed at each nursing.

Rate of weight gain: The following data characterize a normal rate of weight gain in the foal: The average foal weighs about 40—50 kg at birth (varies with breed!). The birthweight equals about 10% of the dam's weight and of the adult body weight.

The foal should double its birthweight in 60 days.

Body weight at end of 1st year: 50—70 % of adult weight.

Body weight at end of 2nd year: 90 % of adult weight.

Composition of formula and its feeding: Cow's milk provides the base for most simulated mare's milk formulas. Whole cow's milk or 2% milk may be used. Even a 2 % fat content is unnecessary, however, and so the milk should be skimmed once again before feeding. To reduce the casein content, the cow's milk should be diluted with water (about 0.2 liters water per liter milk) for about the first week of feeding. During the 1st and 2nd weeks of life, it is advisable to increase energy intake by adding:

20 g of lactose/liter cow's milk, or 20 g of glucose, or 30 g (70 %) or about 20 ml invertose.

Saccharose (cane or beet sugar) should not be fed during the first 4 weeks of life, because the enzyme saccharase [β-(h)-fructosidase] is slow to break down in the neonate. The vitamin A content of the cow's milk should definitely be increased by adding about 50,000 I.U. vitamin A daily (cf. Sec. 1.3.3.1.).

Volume, technique, frequency and timing of feedings: Orphaned foals should not be fed too much formula, especially during the first two weeks of life, due to the high content of foreign casein. Starting with 200 ml per feeding, the foal is fed every 1—2 hours about 10—12 times daily during the first days of life (= only about $^1/_6$ of natural nursing frequency!), e.g., at 6:00, 7:00, 8:00, 9:00, 10:00, 12:00 noon, 2:00, 4:00, 6:00, 7:00, 10:00 and 11:00 (1st day), for a total of about 2 liters.

At first the foal is fed using a bottle and long nipple, taking strict care that the foal does not gulp the formula too quickly. After about a week the foal may be fed from a bucket.

Depending on the foal's appetite, the feeding volume may be increased daily or every other day by 100 ml to a volume of 1 liter per feeding.

After the 5th week of life, the frequency of feedings is gradually reduced to 8/day as larger amounts of dry feed are consumed, and to 4—6/day by the end of the 9th week.

We have found that 10 liters of formula/day is the most that should be fed through the end of the nursing period if the foal can be given its fill of concentrated feeds and tepid drinking water. Free access to concentrates and water significantly shortens the breaks in food and water consumption that ordinarily occur when foals are raised naturally with their dams and enables orphaned foals to ingest small amounts of feed at frequent intervals.

After about the 5th week of life, an increasingly larger proportion of skim milk (fresh or evaporated) may be added to the formula.

Concentrates, Hay. There is an old rule that nursing foals should receive 'as many pounds of concentrate as they are months old, but not more than 4 kg'.

Orphaned foals generally ingest dry feed at a very early age. This feed must be highly digestible and contain little crude fiber.

A concentrate with the following composition is recommended in the literature:

Oats, crushed	approx. 50 %
Wheat bran	approx. 15 %
Barley, rough-ground	approx. 10 %
Linseed oil meal or oil cake Beans, rough-ground Fish meal (max. 8 %)	approx. 15 %
Vegetable shavings, dry or mixed with molasses	approx. 10 %
and 20 g mineral supplement per day.	

Hygienic Care of Orphaned Foals. The umbilical stump should be disinfected immediately after birth, and the foal placed into a box stall. A 2×2-meter stall may be adequate during the first days of life, but foals more than 2 weeks old require a stall area of about 10×15 m² so that they can move about more freely.

Before the stall is occupied, it must be thoroughly cleaned and scoured (hot soda solution, 2% Stallosept or 4% Virex solution). Feces should be removed from the stall daily. The disinfection is repeated as necessary, depending on local bacterial and parasitic contamination. Feeding bottles and buckets should be cleaned thoroughly after each feeding to prevent the acidification of milk residues. Buckets should be raised somewhat while the foal is feeding. A trough containing concentrated feed should be placed on the stall floor or hung on the wall no higher than about 30 cm from the floor.

Dry cold is not harmful to foals. Drafts and damp cold should be avoided.

Foals born in January through March may become accustomed to the outdoors by putting them in the paddock for 5- to 15-minute periods on windless days, starting at about 3—4 weeks. Foals born during the pasturing season may be put in a paddock or pasture during the first days of life to hasten their acclimatization. If the paddock is separate from the stall, 15 minutes in the paddock on warm, windless days is sufficient for the first few days. Soon this is increased until the foal is able to be pastured for several hours daily. On many alpine studs, the mares foal directly on the pasture, and the foals are immediately accustomed to spending the entire day outdoors (the foaling season in such regions begins in late April).

When an orphaned foal is first turned out into a yard, paddock or pasture, accidents can be prevented if the attendant accompanies the foal until it is familiar with its new surroundings.

Foals should be pastured on good meadow with young, protein-rich grass. Pasturing is not just important as a source of nutrition; it also provides an opportunity for the foals to exercise and to develop good gaits from an early age.

Regular brushing of the haircoat is strongly recommended for orphaned foals. It promotes skin circulation and invigorates the foal. Foot care should begin at the age of 4—6 weeks and be repeated at about 8-week intervals. It is far easier to correct faults of foot and limb confirmation while the animal is still a foal than when it is more mature. By the same token, poor foot care during this period can cause errors of confirmation that persist for a lifetime.

References

Beer, J.: Epidemiologie der Salmonellen in veterinärmedizinischer seuchenhygienischer Sicht. Mh. Vet.-Med. *22:* 204 (1967).

Bone, J. F., et al.: Equine medicine and surgery. A text and reference work; 1st ed. (Amer. Veterin. Public., Wheaton/Ill. 1963).

Buening, G. M.; Perryman, L. E.; McGuire, T. C.: Practical methods of determining serum immunglobulin M and immunglobulin G concentrations in foals. J. Amer. vet. med. Assoc. *171:* 455 (1977).

Bürki, F.: Ein kombinierter Impfplan für Vollblutpferde gegen Influenza, Equine Rhinopneumonitis und Tetanus. Dtsch. tierärztl. Wschr. *83:* 89 (1976).

Bürki, F.; Lorin, D.; Sibalin, M.; Ruttner, O.; Arbeiter, K.: Experimentelle genitale und nasale Infektion von Pferden mit dem Virus des equinen Coitalexanthems. Zbl. Vet.-Med. R. B *21:* 362 (1974).

Coggins, L.; Kemen, M. J.: Viral respiratory infections of horses. Some specific viruses affecting the horse. J. Amer. vet. med. Assoc. *166:* 80 (1975).

Cosgroce, J. S. M.: The veterinary surgeon and the new-born foal. Vet. Rec. *67:* 961 (1955).

Elze, K.; Meyer, H.; Steinbach, G.: Jungtierkrankheiten (VEB Gustav Fischer Verlag, Jena 1973).

Elze, K.; Bührdel, P.; Eulenberger, K.; Seifert, S.; Kronberger, H.; Bergmann, A.: Klebsiella-pneumoniae-Infektion bei Orang Utans (Pongo pygmaeus), in: Erkrankungen der Zootiere. Verhandlungsber. des XVIII. Internat. Symp. 4.—8. 6. 1975 in Tunis, p. 285 (Akademie Verlag, Berlin 1975).

Fitzer, H.: Untersuchungen über das Vorkommen von Serumantikörpern gegen Influenza-Rhinopneumonitis-, Rhino- und Parainfluenza-3-Virus bei Pferden. Vet.-med. Diss., München (1972).

Floer, W.: Zum Vorkommen von Klebsiellen in Geschlechtsorganen und Feten von Vollblutpferden. Dtsch. tierärztl. Wschr. *81:* 20 (1974).

Floer, W.; Schmidt, R.; Petzoldt, K.: Mikrobiologische Untersuchungen zur Frage von Herpesvirusinfektionen des oberen Respirationstraktes des Pferdes. Dtsch. tierärztl. Wschr. *79:* 49 (1972).

Green, R. H.: The role of viral infection in the etiology and pathogenesis of chronic bronchitis and emphysema, with consideration of a naturally occuring animal model. J. Biol. Med. *40:* 462 (1968).

Hammer, D.: Die Verteilung von Pneumokokkentypen bei Mensch und Kalb unter Berücksichtigung der Übertragungsmöglichkeit. Zbl. Vet.-Med. *2:* 218 (1955).

Hurtienne, H.: Akute Atemwegserkrankungen des Pferdes. Tierärztl. Umschau *31:* 112 (1976).

Jaksch, W.: Diagnose und Therapie der Koliken des Pferdes in der Landpraxis. Wiener tierärztl. Mschr. *65:* 161 (1978).

Jeffcott, L. B.: Übertragung der passiven Immunität beim neugeborenen Fohlen. Prakt. Tierarzt *57:* 158 (1976).

Kemen, M. J.: Clinical aspects of viral respiratory infections of horses. J. Amer. vet. med. Assoc. *166:* 85 (1975).

Kielstein, P.; Kötsche, W.: Untersuchungen zur biochemischen und serologischen Abgrenzung von Corynebakterien tierischer und menschlicher Herkunft. Mh. Vet.-Med. *21:* 20 (1966).

Kirchhoff, H.; Deegen, E.; Zeller, R.; Floer, W.: Nachweis von Mykoplasmen in Luftsack und Pharynx von Pferden mit akuten Erkrankungen der Respirationsorgane. Dtsch. tierärztl. Wschr. *79:* 465 (1972).

Lepel, J. D. von: Aufzuchtkrankheiten bei Fohlen (Erhebungen über Fohlenverluste in der westdeutschen Vollblutzucht). Berliner Münchener Tierärztl. Wschr. *83:* 429 (1970).

Lütje, F.: Aufzuchtkrankheiten; in Stang; Wirth, Tierheilkunde und Tierzucht, vol. 1, p. 711 (Urban & Schwarzenberg, Berlin 1926).

Mahnel, H.; Herlyn, M.: Stabilität von Teschen-, HCC-, ND- und Vacciniavirus gegenüber 5 Desinfektionswirkstoffen. Zbl. Vet.-Med. R. B, *23:* 403 (1976).

Mayr, A.: Schutzimpfung der Pferde gegen Virusabort. Tierärztl. Umschau *25:* 111 (1970).

McChesney, A. E.; England, J. J.: Adenoviral infection in foals. J. Amer. vet. med. Assoc. *166:* 83 (1975).

McChesney, A. E.; England, J. J.; Rich, L. J.: Adenoviral infection in foals. J. Amer. vet. med. Assoc. *162:* 545 (1973).

McGuire, T. C.; Poppie, M. J.; Banks, K. L.: Combined (B- and T-lymphocyte) immunodeficiency: A fatal genetic disease in Arabian foals. J. Amer. vet. med. Assoc. *164:* 70 (1974).

Merkt, H.: Säuglingsinfektionen (Fohlen); in Richter; Götze, Tiergeburtshilfe; 2. Aufl., p. 834 (Parey, Berlin 1960).

Meyer, O.: Fohlenaufzucht — Fohlenkrankheiten; 2. Aufl. (Schaper, Hannover 1948).

Miessner, H.: Bekämpfung der Aufzuchtkrankheiten. Dtsch. tierärztl. Wschr. *31:* 126 (1923).

Miessner, H.: Die Bekämpfung der Fohlenkrankheiten. Dtsch. tierärztl. Wschr. *31:* 348 (1923).

Moorthy, A. R. S.; Spradbrow, P. B.: Isolation of mycoplasmas from the respiratory tract of horses in Australia. Vet. Rec. *98:* 235 (1976).

Parry, H. B.; Day, F. T.; Growhurst, R. C.: Diseases of newborn foals. Vet. Rec. *61:* 435 (1949).

Petzoldt, K.: Equines Coital-Exanthem. Berliner Münchener Tierärztl. Wschr. *83:* 93 (1970).

Petzoldt, K.: Equine Herpesvirusinfektionen (Infektionskrankheiten und ihre Erreger, *15*) (VEB Gustav Fischer Verlag, Jena 1974).

Poppie, M. H.; McGuire, T. C.: Combined immunodeficiency with failure of colostral immunoglobulins transfer in foals. Vet. Rec. *99:* 44 (1976).

POWELL, D. G.: Equine infectious respiratory disease. Vet. Rec. *96:* 30 (1975).

PROCTOR, L. D.: Comments on streptococcic infections. J. Amer. vet. med. Assoc. *155:* 414 (1969).

REINISCH, F.; ELZE, K.: Leitfaden für die mutterlose Fohlenaufzucht. Lehrmaterial der Ambulatorischen und Geburtshilflichen Tierklinik der Karl-Marx-Universität Leipzig, 1966.

REISSINGER, H.: β-hämolysierende Streptokokken im Puerperalgeschehen bei der Stute. Berliner Münchener Tierärztl. Wschr. *87:* 445 (1974).

RICHTER, J.; GÖTZE, R.: Tiergeburtshilfe; 2. Aufl. (Parey, Berlin 1960).

ROSSDALE, P. D.: Das Pferd, Fortpflanzung und Entwicklung. Deutsche Ausgabe, übersetzt und bearbeitet von H. GERBER (Karger, Basel 1975).

RUMBAUGH, G. E.: Disseminated septic meningitis in a mare. J. Amer. vet. med. Assoc. *171:* 452 (1977).

SATTERFIELD, W. C.; BISHOP, G. L.: Application of intermittent positive pressure breathing in a neonatal tarpan horse with acute pulmonary edema. J. Amer. vet. med. Assoc. *169:* 894 (1976).

SCHMATZ, H.-D.; SCHMATZ, S.; WEBER, A.; SAILER, J.: Seroepidemiologische Untersuchungen zum Vorkommen von Chlamydien bei Haus- und Wildtieren. Berliner Münchener Tierärztl. Wschr. *90:* 74 (1977).

SZÉKY, A.: Zur Histopathologie der vom Bacterium pyosepticum verursachten Erkrankungen der Pferde und Schweine. Acta Vet. Hung. *12:* 145 (1962).

THEIN, P.; HÄRTL, G.: Isolierung eines Reovirus aus einem respiratorisch erkrankten Pferd. Zbl. Vet.-Med. R. B *23:* 698 (1976).

THEIN, P.; MAYR, A.: Untersuchungen über die Bedeutung von Reovirus-Infektionen für respiratorische Erkrankungen beim Pferd. Zbl. Vet.-Med. R. B *21:* 219 (1974).

TILLMANN, H.: Die Genitalinfektionen des Pferdes unter Hinweis auf Paarungsinfektionen mit Beta-Streptokokken und Klebsiellen. Vollblut, Zucht und Rennen *56:* 476 (1973).

TODD, J. D.: Comments on rhinoviruses and parainfluenza viruses of horses. J. Amer. vet. med. Assoc. *155:* 387 (1969).

WEBER, A.; NEUMEIER, U.; SCHLIESSER, TH.: Untersuchungen über das biochemische Verhalten und die Antibiotikaempfindlichkeit von Keimen der Gattung Klebsiella, isoliert aus Untersuchungsmaterial von Pferden. Berliner Münchener Tierärztl. Wschr. *88:* 121 (1975).

WEISS, R.; BÖHM, K. H.; MERKT, H.; KLUG, E.: Untersuchungen zur Besiedelung der Genital- und Nasenschleimhaut des Pferdes, speziell des Hengstes mit in der Pferdezucht bedeutsamen bakteriellen Infektionserregern, unter besonderer Berücksichtigung der Klebsiellen. I. Epidemiologische Erhebungen. Berliner Münchener Tierärztl. Wschr. *88:* 436, 445 (1975).

WEISS, R.; BÖHM, K. H.; MERKT, H.; KLUG, E.; HEUSER, H.: Untersuchungen zur Besiedelung der Genital- und Nasenschleimhaut des Pferdes, insbesondere des Hengstes mit in der Pferdezucht bedeutsamen bakteriellen Infektionserregern, unter besonderer Berücksichtigung der Klebsiellen. III. Serologische Untersuchungen an Klebsiellen. Berliner Münchener Tierärztl. Wschr. *89:* 193 (1976).

WITTIG, W.: Neue Erkenntnisse zur Pathogenese und Prophylaxe der Escherichia-coli-Infektion der Schweine. Mh. Vet.-Med. *26:* 74 (1971).

ZAKOPA, J.; NESVATBA, J.: Actinobacilläre Septikämie als Massenerkrankung in einer Zuchtstutenherde. Zbl. Vet.-Med. R. A *15:* 41 (1968).

2.8. Inherited Defects

2.8.1. General

The horse, like other animals, is subject to a number of inherited, genetically-determined diseases and defects, as well as diseases that are based upon an inherited disposition. Both are the product of mutations, or alterations in the structure of the germinal cells:
— alterations of a single gene (genic mutation),
— alterations in the structure of one or more chromosomes (chromosomal mutation),
— alterations in the number of chromosomes (genomic mutation),
— alterations of genetic material within the cytoplasm (extrachromosomal mutation).

Possible causes of mutations include chemical irritants, mechanical insults and radiation exposure.

Most inherited diseases are transmitted as a *simple recessive* trait, i.e., the defect is expressed phenotypically only if both parents carry the same mutated character. If this occurs, the previously heterozygous state of the recessive character (acquired from the father or mother) becomes homozygous, 25 % of the offspring acquire a 'double dose' of the character (from the father *and* mother), and the recessive trait is expressed.

Besides recessive mutations, a number of *simple dominant* mutations are known in which the trait in one parent is observed to predominate over the corresponding trait in the other.

A third possible mode of inheritance is by *factor coupling*, in which the mutated gene is coupled with another genetic factor, and both are always inherited together as a recessive or dominant, possibly sex-linked trait.

In practice, recognizing the cause of a particular defect as being hereditary is made extremely difficult by the occurrence of noninherited *phenocopies*. These are phenotypes which mimic traits usually recognized as inherited, and which result from the action of nonspecific injurious agents in the environment.

Lethal factors are mendelian units which lead to death of the zygote or of the individual before sexual maturity is attained.

In the presence of dominant lethal factors, a chromosomal factor causes the death of the carrier while still in the heterozygous state. Dominant lethal mutations are always isolated events, because the carrier of a completely dominant lethal factor dies before its traits can be genetically transmitted.

In the presence of dominant lethal factors with a recessive lethal effect, a developmental abnormality occurs in the heterozygous state that generally is compatible with life. However, these mutations become lethal factors when no longer matched with a normal allele.

Autosomal recessive lethal factors are those whose carriers do not differ phenotypically from normal individuals in the heterozygous state. Death occurs only in homozygosis.

Sex-linked lethal factors produce a shift in the normal sex ratio.

The known lethal factors in domestic animals have been assembled into an internationally recognized list, in which the horse is designated with the letter B:

Lethal factor	Name of condition	Phenotype	Mode of inheritance
B_1	atresia coli	closure of colon, often associated with gliomas of brain; foals are born alive	simple recessive
B_2	Frederiksborg lethal factor	sterility in Frederiksborg grays; pleiotropic effect of a dominant lethal factor with recessive, early embryonic mortality	dominant
B_3	antimasculine lethal factor	sex ratio approximately 100 ♀♀ : 90 ♂♂ in foals	sex-linked recessive
B_4	epitheliogenesis imperfecta	irregular defects in skin	simple recessive
B_5	arthrogryposis of the forelimbs	flexion deformity of carpal, fetlock and pastern joints	simple recessive or dominant
B_6	Oldenburg foal ataxia	cerebellar ataxia; foals are born live, ataxia appears in 3rd to 4th week, with paralysis and death 5—6 days later	recessive
B_7	anophthalmia	absence of the eyes	unknown
B_8	abrachia	absence of forelimbs	recessive
B_9	torticollis	stillbirths, twisting of the neck combined with cranial scoliosis	probably recessive
B_{10}	umbilical hernia	cherry- to melon-size hernia at umb. opening	simple recessive

In addition to these lethal factors, a number of other inherited defects are important in the horse. In the sections that follow, both types will be discussed according to the organ systems involved.

Reference

Wiesner, E.; Willer, S.: Veterinärmedizinische Pathogenetik (VEB Gustav Fischer Verlag, Jena 1974).

2.8.2. Inherited Defects of the Facial Bones

Inferior Brachygnathia (Micrognathia)

Definition and Occurrence. Inferior brachygnathia (parrot mouth, overbite) is a jaw deformity of domestic animals in which the upper and lower incisors do not appose due to an abnormal shortness of the lower jaw. The defect is not uncommon in horses.

Symptoms. The upper incisors project over the lower incisors, destroying the normal alignment of these teeth. If the deformity is not severe and the upper and lower incisors still touch, the teeth will be eroded in chisel-like fashion (fig. 2.8. — 1), and

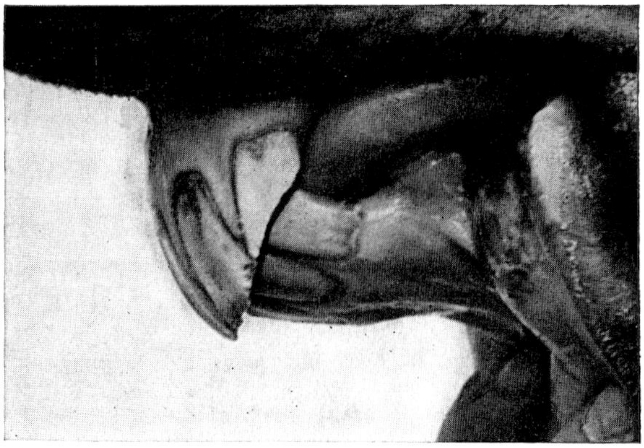

Fig. 2.8. — 1. Inferior brachygnathia (after SCHOOP [1953]).

the pulp cavity of some teeth may become exposed. If the deformity is so extreme that the upper and lower incisors do not touch at all, the teeth may become greatly elongated due to an absence of occlusal wear, even to the point of causing injury and inflammation of the hard palate. Eating becomes extremely difficult, and foals with the condition will have difficulty nursing.

Etiology. In most cases inferior brachygnathia is an inherited defect that probably is transmitted as a simple recessive trait, although many have considered it to be a dominant trait.

Treatment and Prognosis. No treatment is possible. In many cases, especially those in which the mandibular arch is narrowed and there is concomitant hypoplasia of the tongue, death from starvation is possible. On the other hand, inferior brachygnathia is sometimes a benign condition that is of no real importance in mild cases.

References

GÖBEL, F.; SCHUMANN, H.; HEERLEIN, R.: Tierärztl. Umschau, Konstanz *15:* 71 (1960).
GÖTZE, R.: Tierärztl. Umschau *7:* 466 (1952).
HAMORI, D.: Magyar Allat. Lapja *9:* 57 (1941).
SCHOOP, P.-G.: Die Vererbung von Zahnstellungs- und Bissanomalien beim Pferd. Vet.-med. Diss., Berlin (1953).
SPANU, P.: Bull. Méd. Vét. *50:* 141 (1938).

2.8.3. Inherited Defects of the Eye

2.8.3.1. Microphthalmia and Anophthalmia

Definition and Occurrence. Microphthalmia denotes an abnormal smallness of the eye. Even in extreme cases, the orbit will contain at least some remnants of the globe. Vision in the small eye is impaired or absent.

Anophthalmia refers to the complete absence of one or both eyes. Both defects have been described in all domestic and laboratory animals.

Symptoms. Microphthalmia is observed more frequently in domestic animals than is anophthalmia. The small but mobile eye is recessed within its orbit, and the finger can be inserted some distance into the orbit past the small globe. Often microphthalmia is associated with other ocular deformities such as colobomas, or with cataracts, orbital cysts or tumors. Severe cases are recognized by the narrowness of the palpebral fissure. In anophthalmia the palpebral fissure is very narrow, and the eyelashes curl inward. The condition is often associated with cyst formation in the lower lid. The orbit is abnormally small and usually contains only fatty and connective tissue, though occasionally a spherical structure composed of glia and individual ganglion cells may be found. Anophthalmia tends to be bilateral.

Etiology. Both abnormalities can be inherited, although their exact mode of inheritance remains unclear.

Anophthalmia in the horse is designated as B_7 in the international list of lethal factors. In most cases, however, both anophthalmia and microphthalmia are dependent to some degree on exogenous factors — particularly a vitamin A deficiency in the pregnant mare.

Lesions. Besides the changes in the globe itself, *microphthalmia* is always associated with atrophy of the optic nerve. This may involve hypoplasia, secondary atrophy, or both. A true vitreous body is absent, and in many cases the vitreous chamber is occupied by a vascularized connective tissue. In other cases a rudimentary vitreous body may be found in the superior half of the globe. The poor development of the vitreous body, which normally is formed from the retina, has its cause in a malformation of the retina, which may be completely devoid of structure. In *anophthalmia*, the intraorbital glial structure mentioned above usually is connected to the brain by a pedicle that passes through the optic foramen. The optic nerve is absent.

Pathogenesis. Böhler [1929] states that there are three possible groups of etiologic mechanisms for inherited microphthalmia: (1) malformations of structures derived from the embryonic brain (retina, optic nerve, vitreous body), (2) absence or abnormal development of the mesodermal parts of the globe (middle and outer tunics), and (3) maldevelopment of components arising directly from the ectoderm (e.g., aphakia).

Treatment and Prognosis. Neither defect is treatable. If an inherited etiology has been established, the defect should be eliminated through breeding procedures.

References

Baier, W.: Mikrophthalmus congenitus bei einem zwei Tage alten Fohlen. Vet.-med. Diss., München (1927).

Böhler, H.: Ein rechtsseitiger Mikro- und Kryptophthalmus congenitus beim Hund. Vet.-med. Diss., Zürich (1929).

Eckhardt, H.; Ostertag, B.: Körperliche Erbkrankheiten (J. A. Barth, Leipzig 1940).

2.8.3.2. Hydrophthalmos (Hydrops oculi, Secondary Glaucoma)

Definition, Occurrence and Etiology. This condition is characterized by a 2- to 4-fold enlargement of the globe due to an excessive collection of fluid within the eye. It may occur during the course of inflammations or as a direct sequel to inflammatory processes in the interior of the eye. Congenital cases also occur and are an hereditary cause of blindness. The condition is rare in foals, and its mode of inheritance remains unknown.

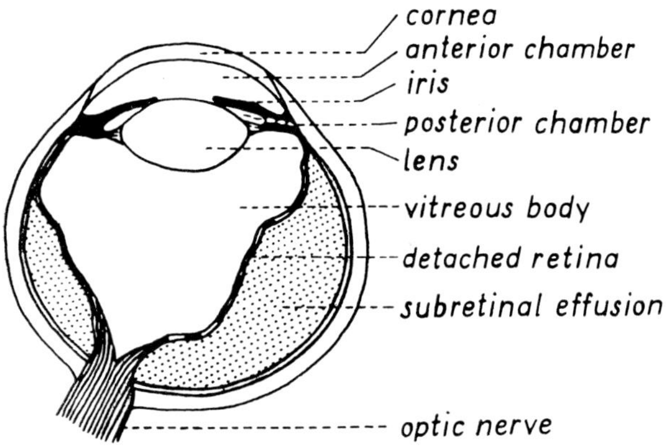

Fig. 2.8. — 2. Advanced retinal detachment (schematic).

Symptoms. The eyeball is markedly enlarged and often protrudes through the palpebral aperture, preventing complete closure of the lids. Clouding of the cornea and keratitis soon result. Inherited hydrophthalmos usually involves both eyes, whereas the acquired form tends to be unilateral.

Lesions. When the enlarged globe is opened, a clear but slightly flocculent fluid is discharged. The lens may also be discharged at this time; it is clouded and may be either swollen or shrunken. In many cases hydrophthalmos is accompanied by other ocular changes of varying degree, such as subluxation of the lens, retinal detachment, cataract, aniridia, etc.

Pathogenesis. Congenital hydrophthalmos is based upon a rise of intraocular tension during fetal development, at a time when the cornea and sclera are still highly distensible. Due to an absence or very poor development of the ciliary venous plexus, normal filtration of the internal ocular fluid is hampered or its outflow is prevented altogether.

2.8.3.3. Retinal Detachment

Definition and Occurrence. Retinal detachment is a separation of the retina from the choroid in its nonadherent portions. It is observed in various animal species and is especially common in the horse.

Symptoms. Foals with complete retinal detachment are born blind. With partial detachment, the eye is reduced in size. The cornea and anterior chamber are unchanged, the iris appears small, and the pupil is large and oval or circular in shape. The lens is clear or granular with cloudy opacities. Vitreous opacities also are evident in the form of streaks or flakes. The optic fundus appears translucent or hazy and opaque, and the optic disc (where the optic nerve pierces the retina) is indistinct. The pupillary response to light is absent or very sluggish. While smaller retinal detachments near the periphery cause only minimal vision impairment, more extensive detachments lead to more severe vision loss or blindness.

Etiology. The primary form of retinal detachment in the horse is congenital and, in some cases, an inherited, multifactorial disease. It was first observed in horses by Schnelle in 1939, and was described further on breeding farms in the Hannover area in 1950.

Lesions. The cornea, anterior chamber and iris appear normal, but the funnel-like separation of the retina from the choroid is very obvious (fig. 2.8. — 2). A large, protein-rich effusion collects between the detached retina and the pigmented epithelium remaining on the choroid. There will be some liquefaction of the vitreous body, depending on the size of the effusion. All other parts of the eye and the optic nerve itself are unchanged. The layer of rods and cones in the stratum neuroepithelium of the retina is lost.

Treatment and Prognosis. The operative treatment of retinal detachment in the horse (which tends to be complete) is extremely difficult and rarely successful. The most that can be done is to promote reabsorption of the subretinal fluid or aspirate it with a needle. The prognosis of retinal detachment is unfavorable, because normal function cannot be restored to the separated parts of the retina.

References

Brandenburg, W.: Tierärztl. Umschau *7:* 48 (1952).
Koch, P.: Berliner Münchener tierärztl. Wschr. *68:* 43 (1955).
Koch, P.; Fischer, H.: Tierärztl. Umschau *7:* 46 (1952).
Schnelle, W.: Dtsch. tierärztl. Wschr. *58:* 325 (1951).

2.8.3.4. Glass Eye

Definition and Occurrence. 'Glass eye', known also as wall eye, blue eye and spotted eye, is an inherited defect based upon a pigmentary deficiency in the stroma of the iris. Glass eye is most frequently observed in horses that are spotted, although there is no absolute correlation between the two traits. The condition is also observed in bays, in which the partial albinism is often marked by large white areas on the face and extremities (fig. 2.8. — 3).

Symptoms. The iris of affected horses usually is white at its periphery and rarely bluish, owing to the relatively thick and strong iridal connective tissue in this species. The condition may be present in one or both eyes, and part or all of the iris may be involved (fig. 2.8. — 4).

The pigmentary deficiency affects the ventral side of the iris in about 50 % of cases and the medial side in about 30 %. The dorsal, lateral and circular forms are relatively uncommon. The defect causes little or no impairment of vision or light perception.

Etiology. Glass eye is usually inherited as a simple recessive trait and is equally common in both sexes. A dominant mode of inheritance has been reported in some cases.

Lesions. In the glass eye, in contrast to the albinotic eye, the innermost layer of the iris (stratum iridis or pars iridica retinae) has normal pigmentation. However, the stromal pigment cells exterior to this layer show a more or less pronounced pigmentary deficiency.

Treatment and Prognosis. Glass eye is untreatable. Because the condition does not interfere with vision and represents not a constitutional weakness but simply a cosmetic blemish, there should be no hesitancy in breeding affected animals, provided the defect is not associated with any other serious abnormality.

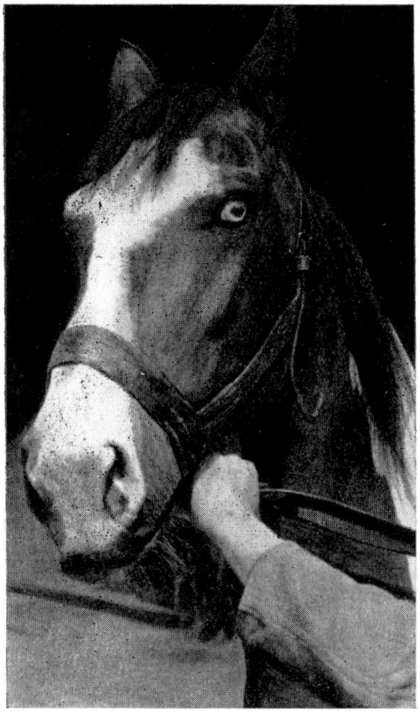
3

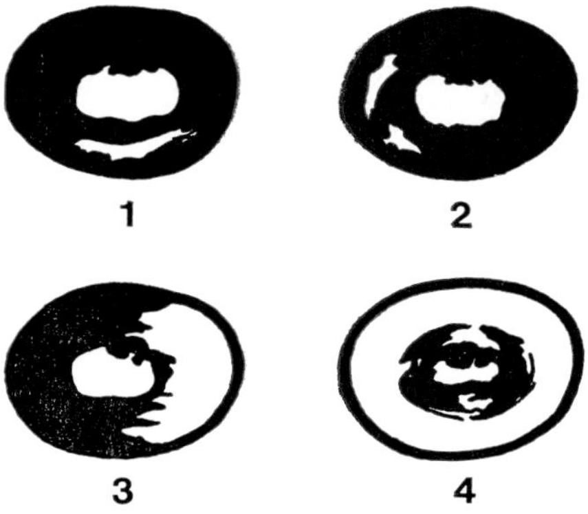

4

Fig. 2.8. — 3. Glass eye.
Fig. 2.8. — 4. Forms of glass eye (schematic).
1: ventral form; 2: medial or lateral form; 3: medial or lateral form; 4: circular form

References

HAECHER, V.: Dtsch. landw. Tierzucht *29:* 209 (1925).
KLEMOLA, V.: Tierzücht. Züchtungsbiol. *20:* 24 (1931).
KLEMOLA, V.: J. Heredity *24:* 65 (1935).

2.8.3.5. Ocular Albinism

Definition and Occurrence. Ocular albinism refers to a failure of pigmentary development in the eye. It has been described in most domestic and laboratory animals. Among horses, gray, white, bay, light-brown, spotted and dun-colored animals are most commonly affected.

Symptoms. The absence or deficiency of pigmentation in the iridic stroma and retinal iridic epithelium alters light passage through ocular tissues whose purpose is to filter and screen incoming light. As a result of this, light rays are able to enter the eye freely from all directions. Consequently the pupil dilates even in ordinary daylight (red fundus reflex), and the iris shows an abnormally high transparency. Excessive illumination of the retina leads to photophobia. The pigmentary defect may affect the eye alone, or it may be one manifestation of a general albinism. It is likely that the area centralis of the retina also is poorly developed in the albinotic eye, contributing further to poor vision.

Etiology. Ocular albinism is recognized as an inherited disorder, usually being transmitted as a simple recessive trait.

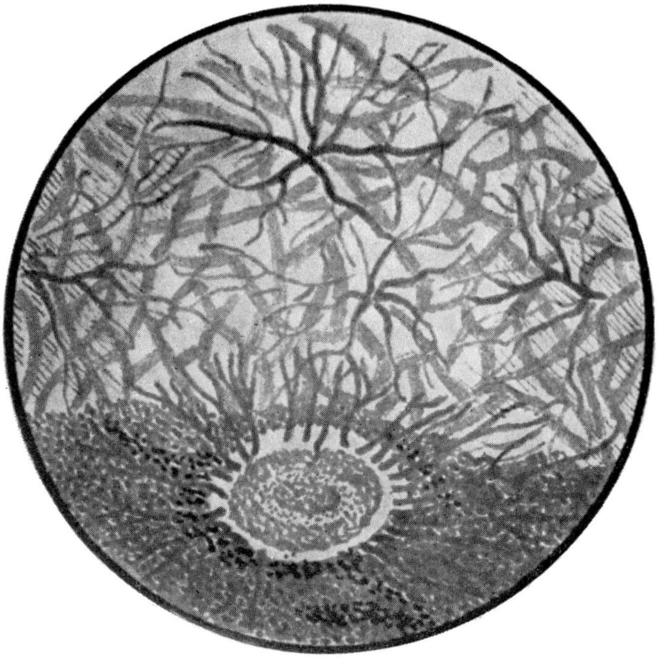

Fig. 2.8. — 5. Fundus of an albinotic equine eye (schematic).

Lesions. Histologically, ocular albinism is characterized by a lack of pigmentation in ocular structures that normally contain pigment, i.e., the pigmentary epithelium of the outermost layer of the optic cup, and the uveal pigment, which is tied to the chromatophores. The chromatophores, which arise from the ectodermal neural crest and resemble connective-tissue cells, also are reduced in number (fig. 2.8. — 5).

Pathogenesis. With regard to the timing of the teratogenesis, it is apparent that the defect leading to the albinism must arise in a very early stage of embryonic development, for pigmentation of the optic vesicle is a very early process.

2.8.3.6. Cataract

Definition and Occurrence. Cataract is the term applied to any opacity of the lens. Cataracts appear gray or white under oblique illumination, and dark or black on transillumination. They have been observed in various species of domestic, wild and laboratory animals, the horse included.

Symptoms. The opacity of the lens (fig. 2.8. — 6) may be partial or complete. A 'central cataract' is one in which the opacity is confined to the nucleus of the lens, while in a 'lamellar cataract' the opacity affects only certain layers between the cortex and nucleus. In both forms the peripheral layers of the lens that border on the opaque zone are unchanged or show only isolated, circumscribed opacities. Nystagmus is sometimes present.

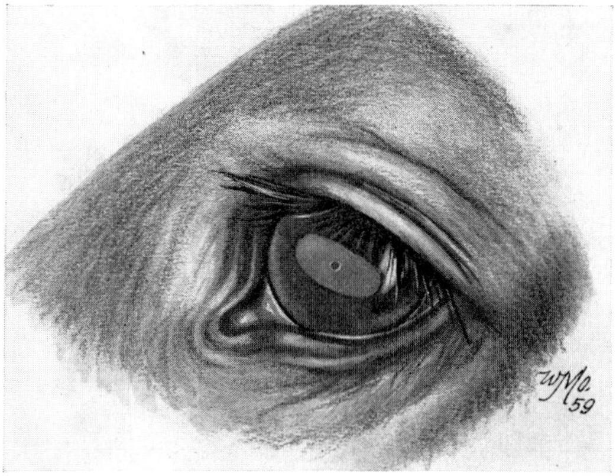

Fig. 2.8. — 6. Cataract.

Etiology. Cataracts may result from environmental causes, or they may be congenital and inherited. Hereditary cataracts in the horse are transmitted as a recessive trait according to WEBER [1974], and as a dominant trait according to ERIKSSON [1955].

Lesions. Opacity of the lens and pupillary dilation are usually the only visible changes. In some cases the globe may be slightly reduced in size as a result of disuse atrophy.

Pathogenesis. Congenital cataract is based upon a disturbance in the separation of the lens vesicle from the ectoblast — analogous, apparently, to the more familiar processes occurring in the human embryo during the 4th—5th week of development.

Prognosis. Congenital blindness due to cataract limits the animal's usefulness.

References

DIECKERHOFF, W.: Z. Veterinärkunde *14:* 53 (1902).
ERIKSSON, K.: Nord. Vet.-Med. *7:* 773 (1955).
SMALL, C. P.: Amer. J. Ophthalmol. *2:* 681 (1919).
ÜBERREITER, O.: Wiener tierärztl. Wschr. *26:* 135 (1939).
WEBER, W.: Schweiz. Arch. Tierheilkunde *89:* 397 (1947).
YOUNG, J. S.: Austral. vet. J. *45:* 574 (1969).

2.8.4. Inherited Defects of the Digestive System

2.8.4.1. Dental Defects

Dental defects may involve entire rows of teeth or tooth buds, or they may be limited to individual teeth. Defects of the first group result from disturbances in the development of the maxillary or alveolar processes. Inferior brachygnathia, described under abnormalities of the facial bones, is one such defect. Here we shall discuss only congenital abnormalities that involve individual teeth. These include alterations in the normal number of teeth as well as abnormalities of position, form and structure. Defects of this type are responsible for a great many disease symptoms in the horse. In addition, by interfering with mastication, they impair feed utilization and thus reduce the animal's working capacity. BECKER [1937] estimates that an average of

0.5 kg of oats per animal per day are wasted as a result of dental defects and disease. In a horse with dental disease or abnormal dentition, approximately 40,000 oat grains pass undigested through the gastrointestinal tract each day.

Abnormalities in the number of teeth may take the form of polyodontia (presence of extra teeth) or oligodontia (absence of teeth). Polyodontia can occur in two forms. Typically the condition is characterized by supernumerary teeth within the dental arch and, in the case of the wolf tooth, is considered almost physiologic in the horse. The second form is the 'atypical' form, characterized by an irregular polyodontia. Oligodontia is based upon a defect in the tooth bud or maldevelopment of the dental germ. Both polyodontia and oligodontia are observed in horses. The question of their inheritance in this species has not yet been resolved.

Abnormalities of dental position include torsion (rotation of a tooth about its long axis), deviation (rotation about the transverse axis), inversion (rotation by 180°), diastema (abnormally wide gap between teeth), and mandibula angusta (crowding together of the teeth).

Rupprecht [1938] found diastemas of the cheek teeth in 4.7 % of all horses examined, Gnädinger [1947] in 13 %, and Grigorescu et al. [1955/56] in 17 %. Schoop [1953] describes a diastema between the upper and lower central incisors. Diastemas, especially those involving the cheek teeth, frequently cause food particles and foreign bodies to become lodged between the teeth, which in turn cause injury to the tooth and gum. The gaps may measure up to 6—12 mm without interfering with the remaining dentition. As is humans, diastema of the incisors is most common in females. This led Schoop [1953] to postulate an X-chromosome-linked dominant inheritance in the horse, though this is disputed by Göbel et al. [1960]. Schoop [1953] also states that crowding (mandibula angusta) of the lower incisors in the horse is probably inherited as a simple recessive trait. While the remaining teeth in this condition are entirely normal in number and arrangement, the incisors are crowded together and rotated about their long axis.

References

Becker, E.: Dtsch. Tierärzteblatt *4:* 465 (1937).

Berge, E.: Berliner Münchener tierärztl. Wschr. *73:* 462 (1960).

Gnädinger, F.: Erhebungen über die Häufigkeit von Zahnfehlern beim Pferd. Vet.-med. Diss., Hannover (1947).

Göbel, F.; Schumann, H.; Heerlein, R.: Tierärztl. Umschau *15:* 71 (1960).

Grigorescu, I.; Chitescu, St.; Meisescu, M.; Voicu, Ch.: Communicari Stiintifice Fac. Med. Vet. Arad (Rumänien) 1955/56, S. 9.

Heinze, W.: Mh. Vet.-Med. *19:* 592 (1964).

Lundh, T.: Tierärztl. Umschau *16:* 255 (1961).

Rupprecht, K.: Statistische Erhebungen über die Häufigkeit von Gebissanomalien beim Pferd. Vet.-med. Diss., Leipzig (1938).

Schoop, P.-G.: Die Vererbung von Zahnstellungs- und Bissanomalien beim Pferd. Vet.-med. Diss., Berlin (1953).

Vos, N. de: Vlaams diergeneesk. Tijdschr. *30:* 93 (1961).

2.8.4.2. Atresia coli

Definition and Occurrence. This is a congenital deformity in which the large intestine terminates in a blind, club-shaped pouch. The horse is the species most commonly affected. The defect was first recognized by Nusshag in the Saxony-Anhalt region

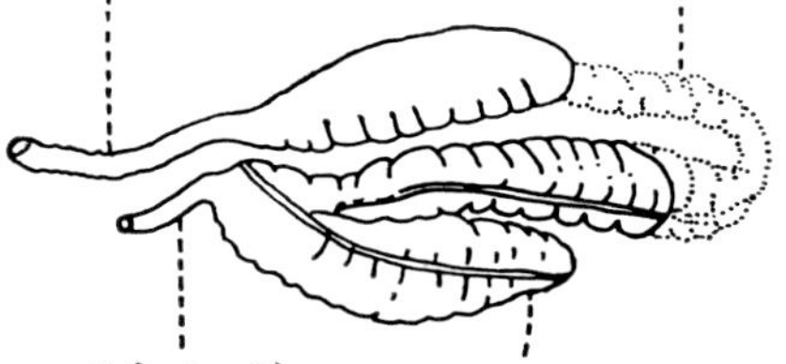

Fig. 2.8. — 7. Atresia coli (schematic).

of Germany in 1925 in several warm-blooded foals of Eastern Frisian ancestry, and in 1928 YAMANE described it in 25 descendants of a Percheron stallion (heavy French breed) that had been imported to Japan from Ohio in 1886.

Symptoms. Affected foals appear healthy when born but show little interest in nursing and do not defecate. Meconium is not expelled, and response to laxative therapy is futile. Most of the foals die on the 3rd day of life with severe colicky symptoms.

Etiology. YAMANE [1928] demonstrated the hereditary nature of the deformity, pointing to a simple recessive mode of inheritance. Atresia coli is designated as lethal factor B_1.

Lesions. The large intestine ends in a dilated, blind pouch. Its surface is grayish-red back to the cecum, which is unchanged. Anterior to the rectum, the descending colon also terminates blindly in the area of its adherence to the duodenum and does not connect with the transverse colon (fig. 2.8. — 7). Cerebral glioma is a frequent coexisting lesion.

Pathogenesis. The deformity is attributed either to a defect in the formation of the rudimentary bowel or to an inhibition of development during fetal growth.

References

NUSSHAG, W.: Berliner tierärztl. Wschr. *41:* 646 (1925).
YAMANE, J.: Z. indukt. Abstamm.- und Vererbungslehre *46:* 188 (1928).

2.8.4.3. Atresia ani

(cf. Sec. 2.1.5.10.7.)

Definition and Occurrence. Atresia ani, or imperforate anus, occurs in three principal forms:

1. Atresia ani simplex: The anal membrane is intact, the anal opening is absent, the proctodeal pit is present, and the well-developed rectum ends blindly beneath the skin.
2. Atresia recti simplex: The rectum is not fully developed, ends blindly, and is connected to the proctodeum and a pouch-like skin invagination only by a cord of fibrous tissue.
3. Atresia ani et recti: The anus and rectum are imperforate, there is no proctodeal pit, and the rectum ends blindly 5—20 cm from the skin.

The deformity occurs in humans and in many animal species, especially swine. Various authors have reported its occurrence in the horse.

Symptoms. In male animals the intestinal obstruction causes a marked distension of the abdomen that increases steadily over the next 2—3 weeks until death occurs. Death results from autointoxication due to a failure of intestinal absorption. In females with atresia ani, the rectum frequently communicates with the urogenital sinus, thus providing an outlet for bowel contents. The condition may, in fact, go undetected in some females. The deformity can become lethal only if there are large defects of the urorectal septum and complete persistence of the cloaca.

Etiology. The defect is inherited as a simple recessive trait. It is most common in Rhenish German cold-bloods and their descendants.

Lesions. The lesions in the various forms are described above. Life-saving cloacal formation in females may result from the creation of various fistulae: rectovaginal, vestibular rectovaginal, rectourethral or rectovesical.

Pathogenesis. During early embryonic development, a patch of endoderm becomes closely applied to the ectoderm at the caudal end of the embryo to form the purely epithelial cloacal membrane, the endoderm also forming the start of a primordial hindgut at this time. The anus attains its final position following regression of the caudal end of the hindgut during subsequent development of the postumbilical abdominal wall and elongation of the torso. After breakdown of the cloacal membrane into an anal and genital part with formation of the genital tubercle and perineum, the anal orifice comes to be directed posteriorally. The various forms of atresia ani result from disturbances in the separation of the cloaca into the rectum and urogenital sinus or in the formation of the cloacal membrane [LEIBBRANDT, 1939].

Treatment and Prognosis. If the defect is not too severe, it may be possible to keep the animal alive by the surgical creation of an artificial anus. However, if the distance between the rectum and skin opening is more than 1 cm, the two cannot be connected by suture, and scarring with renewed closure of the anal orifice will eventually occur. Inoperable cases have a poor prognosis in males, while females have some chance of surviving if spontaneous cloacal formation occurs.

Reference

LEIBBRANDT, H.: Gehäuftes Auftreten von Afterlosigkeit in Zuchten des hannoverschen veredelten Landschweines. Vet.-med. Diss., Hannover (1939).

2.8.5. Inherited Defects of the Nervous System

Ataxia

Definition and Occurrence. This is mainly a disease of the spinocerebellar system that is manifested by impaired locomotor coordination. Many domestic species are susceptible. 'Oldenburg foal ataxia' is a well-known form that occurs in the G line of Oldenburg light horses in all areas where these animals are bred.

Symptoms. A foal with Oldenburg ataxia appears healthy but experiences a paroxysmal 'collapse' of the hindquarters that causes it to fall over backward. Senses are unimpaired and the foal remains on the ground for several minutes before it recovers and is able to stand. A mild form of the disease, characterized only by a clumsy gait, is easily overlooked. The first signs of Oldenburg foal ataxia usually appear during the 3rd to 4th week of life. Within a week or two the attacks of falling become in-

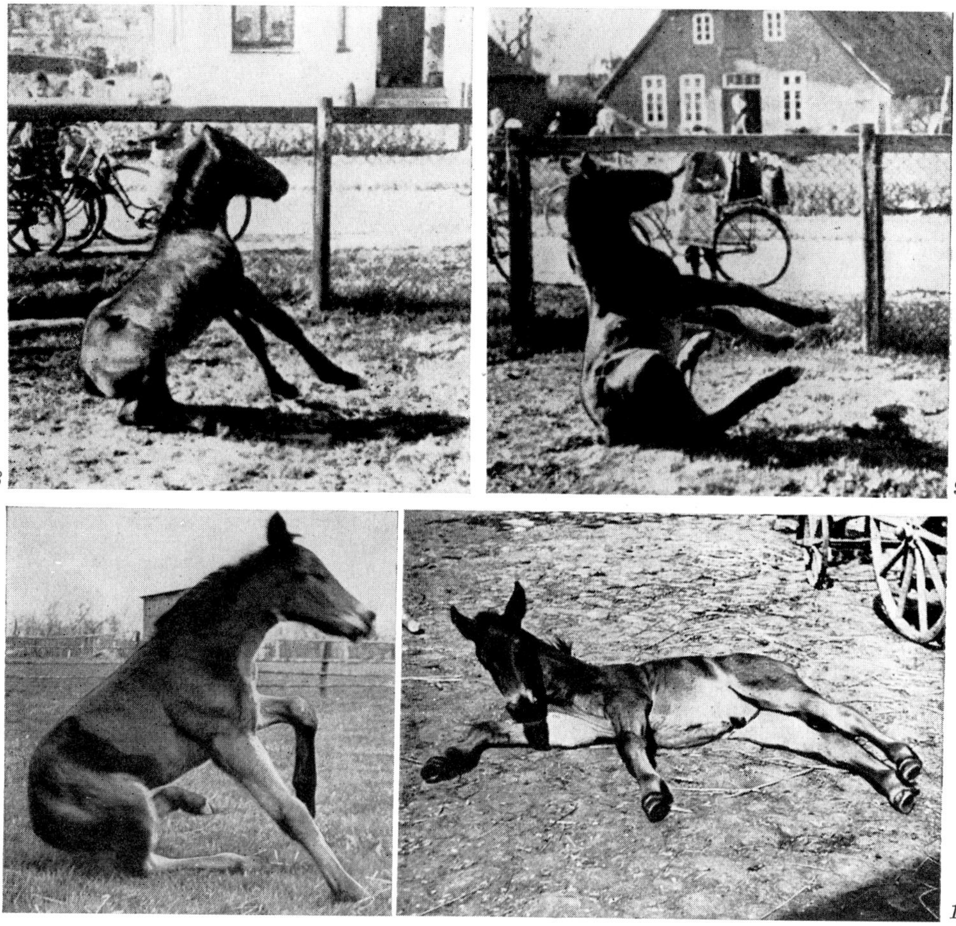

8 9 10 11

Fig. 2.8. — 8. through — 11. Foal with Oldenburg foal ataxia collapsing in the hindquarters (2.8. — 8) and falling over backward (2.8. — 9). The foal stands up again after the attack (2.8. — 10) or stays recumbent where it fell, exhausted (2.8. — 11) (after FISCHER).

creasingly frequent and severe. Paralysis gradually develops, and foals that do not die spontaneously must be destroyed (figs. 2.8. — 8 through — 11). Hence, the disease has not yet been observed in older foals or yearlings.

Etiology. Oldenburg foal ataxia is inherited as a recessive trait and is designated as lethal factor B_6.

Lesions. Gross examination of the cerebellum reveals circumscribed reddish-gray areas, which on histologic examination are found to be malacic foci.

References

HIPPEN, F.: Erbbiologische Untersuchungen der Fohlenataxie im Oldenburger Zuchtgebiet. Vet.-med. Diss., Hannover (1949).

KOCH, P.; FISCHER, H.: Tierärztl. Umschau *5:* 317 (1950); *6:* 158 (1951).

2.8.6. Inherited Defects of the Spine

Torticollis

Definition. Torticollis is a collective term for various diseases that are manifested clinically by a twisting of the neck and head.

Symptoms. Besides loss of the foal, the deformity carries a high risk of injury to the foaling mare. A normal delivery is impossible when the fetal head and neck are retracted to one side, and the mare may die if, through ignorance, the foal is forcibly delivered without veterinary assistance. Only small fetuses can be delivered in the wryneck position [Mauderer, 1939].

Etiology. Besides forms acquired due to spastic or traumatic causes, torticollis may also be congenital and inherited, occurring either as a solitary deformity or in connection with other inherited defects such as arthrogryposis. Wryneck in foals is due to the inheritance of a factor, probably recessive, that is designated as lethal factor B_9.

Lesions. A distinction is made between muscular torticollis caused by a unilateral traumatic, inflammatory or nervous lesion of the shoulder muscles inserting on the head, and osseous torticollis, which is associated with a secondary asymmetry of the skull (cranial scoliosis).

Reference

Mauderer, H.: Abrachie und Torticollis, rezessive Letalfaktoren in der Pferdezucht. Vet.-med. Diss., Hannover (1939).

2.8.7. Inherited Defects of the Limbs

2.8.7.1. Abrachia (Anterior Amelia)

Definition and Occurrence. The congenital abscence of the forelimbs has been known in various domestic animal species since medieval times and has been particularly well researched in the horse [Fröhner, 1932].

Symptoms. Both forelimbs are absent (fig. 2.8. — 12). Affected foals are vigorous at birth, but being unable to stand and nurse independently, they die within a short time or have to be destroyed.

Etiology. Abrachia is due to the inheritance of a recessive lethal factor, B_8. Its occurrence in one area of Germany where cold-blooded horses are bred has been documented for more than 100 years.

Lesions. A scapula is always present in foals with abrachia but often is rudimentary and cartilaginous. Sometimes a walnut-size rudiment of the humerus is found caudoventral to the distal end of the scapula, embedded within a mass of muscular tissue.

References

Fröhner, R.: Dtsch. tierärztl. Wschr. *50:* 504 (1932).

Mauderer, H.: Abrachie und Torticollis, rezessive Letalfaktoren in der Pferdezucht. Vet.-med. Diss., Hannover (1939).

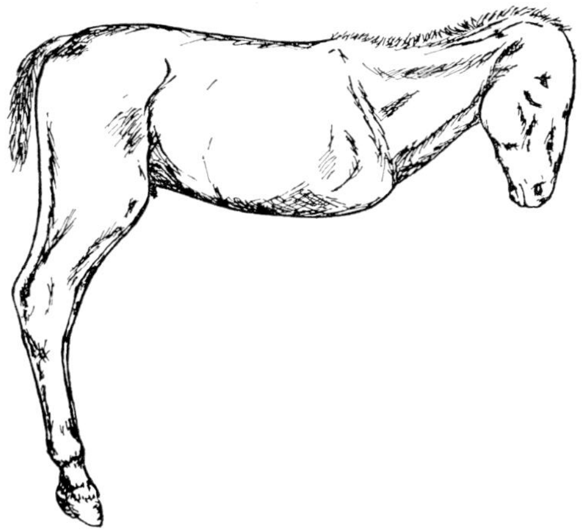

12

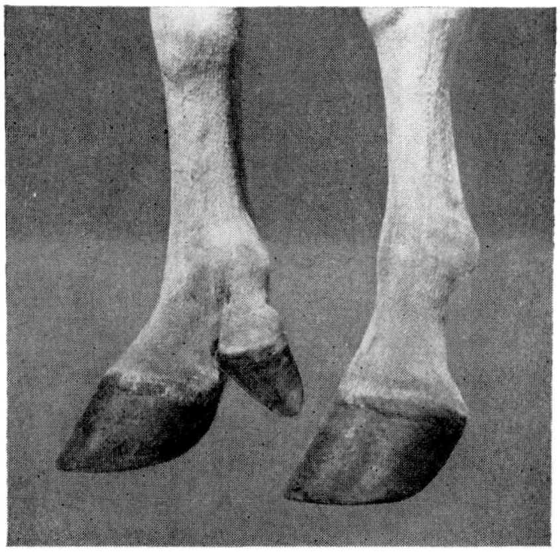

13

Fig. 2.8. — 12. Abrachia (after MAUDERER [1939]).
Fig. 2.8. — 13. Polydactyly (after GEBERT).

2.8.7.2. Polydactyly

Definition and Occurrence. Polydactyly, characterized by the presence of more than the normal number of fingers or toes, has been documented in man and almost all domestic animals. In the horse, in which polydactyly is most frequently observed, one form of the anomaly is considered a throwback to an early phylogenic stage, while the teratogenic form, involving a true redundancy of the foot or individual digits, usually has developmental causes.

Symptoms. The defect is most commonly seen in one of the forelimbs and usually involves the presence of an extra digit. A third digit may be present in rare cases. The distal phalanx of the extra digit generally bears a hoof wall, and the digit itself tends to be less well developed than the principal digit, although they may be of comparable size (figs. 2.8. — 13 through — 17).

Etiology. One form of polydactyly is usually inherited, though the exact mode is unknown. The teratogenic form is based upon a displacement or splitting of the carpal or tarsal bones to form supernumerary rays ('schistodactyly').

Lesions. The extra digit may arise from the carpus or tarsus, the metacarpus or megacarpus, or from the phalanges themselves. Redundancy of the phalanges is most common in the teratogenic form.

Treatment and Prognosis. The atavistic form of polydactyly can be treated surgically by disarticulation of the extra digit at the splint bone. Given the inherited etiology of the defect, animals thus treated should be clearly branded as being unfit for breeding, because signs of the genetic defect are no longer apparent following surgery.

References

BICKMEIER, K.: Dtsch. tierärztl. Wschr. *47:* 161 (1939).
DRAHN, F.: Berliner tierärztl. Wschr. *37:* 75 (1921).
DUBOIS, J.: De la polydactylie des solipèdes. Vet.-med. Diss., Lyon (1931).

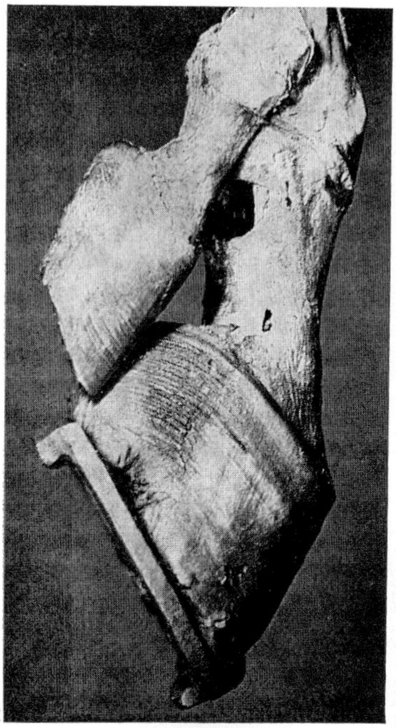
14

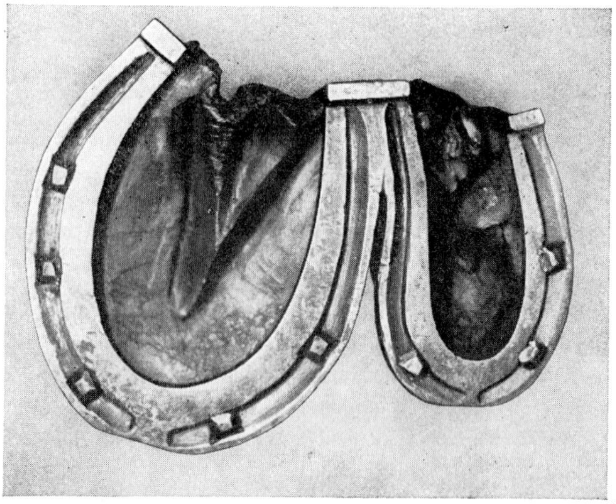
15

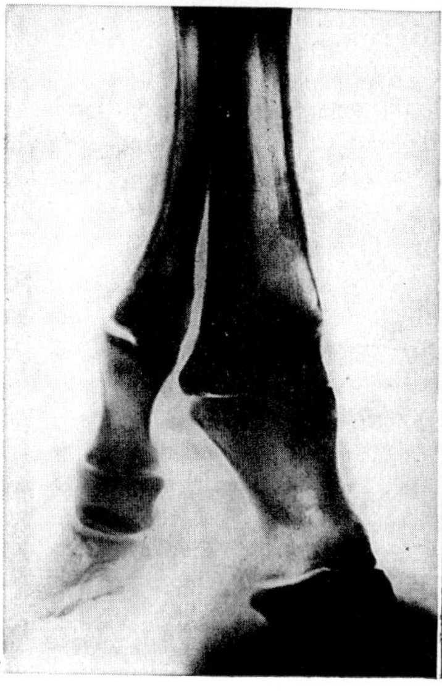
16

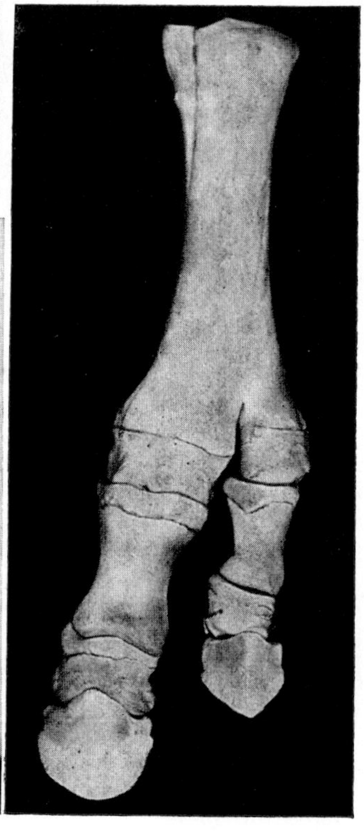
17

Fig. 2.8. — *14.* Polydactyly (after KNEZEVIC).
Fig. 2.8. — *15.* Polydactyly, both hooves shod (after KNEZEVIC).
Fig. 2.8. — *16.* Polydactyly (radiograph).
Fig. 2.8. — *17.* Polydactyly (skeletal specimen).

2.8.7.3. Luxation of the Patella

Definition and Occurrence. Dislocation of the patella is most common in cattle and horses, and less so in dogs.

Symptoms. Stifle lameness is apparent in affected foals. Many become lame while still sucklings or weanings. Weight is borne on the forelimbs only, while the stifle joints are flexed and cannot be extended. The laterally dislocated patella is easily palpated. The animal will be able to stand if the luxations are manually reduced, but the patellae will redislocate as soon as the hands are removed, and the animal will collapse.

Etiology. Most luxations of this type are caused by trauma (see Sec. 2.1.19.2.5.). However, patellar luxations have been described in both warm- and cold-blooded horse breeds that reportedly are inherited as a recessive trait.

Lesions. Traumatic patellar luxations are usually the result of ligamentous sprains and ruptures. The patella may luxate in a dorsal, lateral or medial direction. Even inherited forms are always associated with a unilateral or bilateral stretching of the patellar ligaments.

Treatment and Prognosis. See Sec. 2.1.19.2.5.

References

Butz, H.; Sonnenbrodt, A.: Dtsch. Warmblut *35:* 107 (1940).
Fischer, H.; Helbig, K.: Tierzucht *5:* 105 (1951).

2.8.7.4. Arthrogryposes of the Forelimbs

Definition and Occurrence. Arthrogryposis ('crooked joint') is the term applied to a persistent flexure of one or more joints. Arthrogryposes of the forelimbs are most common in the horse.

Symptoms. The carpal, fetlock and pastern joints are rigidly flexed, and there is a marked shortening of the digital flexor tendons. In severe cases the animal cannot put the sole of the foot on the ground and knuckles over if it attempts to rise. Sometimes the flexion is associated with varying degrees of lateral rotation of the limb from the carpal joint downward (knock-knees; fig. 2.8. — 18).

Etiology. Arthrogryposis in the horse may be an inherited condition. Keller [1937] described a simple recessive form, and Pravochenski [1936] a dominant form that is now classified as lethal factor B_5.

Treatment and Prognosis. In some cases gradual improvement can be achieved by orthopedic treatment with splint-reinforced extension bandages.

References

Keller, K.: Wiener tierärztl. Mschr. *24:* 289 (1937).
Pravochenski, R.: J. Heredity *27:* 411 (1936).

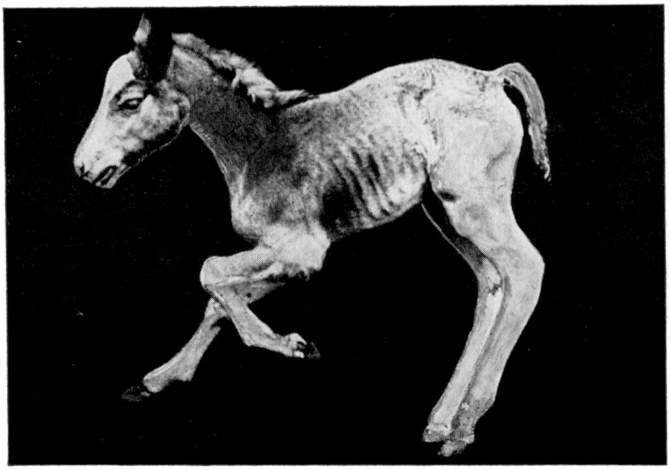

Fig. 2.8. — 18. Arthrogryposis of the left forelimb.

2.8.8. Abdominal Hernias

Umbilical Hernia

Definition and Occurrence. An umbilical hernia is a protrusion of omentum and intestinal loops through the umbilical ring due to a failure of this opening to close during embryonic development. It is observed in almost all domestic mammals and is relatively common in the horse, affecting warm- and cold-blood breeds equally.

Symptoms. Clinically the umbilical hernia presents as a soft, elastic, painless mass ranging from about 2 to 15 cm in diameter. The hernial ring is palpable following reduction. Except in incarcerations, the hernial contents are easily reduced (fig. 2.8. — 19).

Etiology. Umbilical hernia may be congenital and inherited, or it may be acquired postnatally. The umbilical hernia is the most prevalent of the inherited hernias and is identified as a simple recessive lethal factor, B_{10}. The extent to which the disposition for umbilical hernia is inherited is not known.

Lesions. The hernial ring is a circular or slit-like opening in the abdominal wall at the umbilicus and is large enough to accommodate 3—4 fingers. The hernial sac is formed by the outpouching peritoneum (internal sac) and the outer abdominal wall (external sac). The sac contains parts of the small intestine, cecum, colon, omentum or, in neonates, the urachus and umbilical vein. Incarceration of the herniated tissues can lead to intestinal obstruction.

Pathogenesis. The embryo begins as a flattened disc which changes to a more cylindrical shape during the course of early embryonic development. Through infolding and convergent growth of the embryonic disc at its sides and ends, the embryo becomes well-defined relative to the blastocyst and soon surpasses it in size. The umbilical vessels and urachus enter the body cavity at the umbilical ring. If closure of the body walls is inhibited, then clefts (the future hernial openings) will remain on the ventral surface of the embryo, constituting a defect whose formal cause is a delay in the latitudinal growth of the primordial vertebrae.

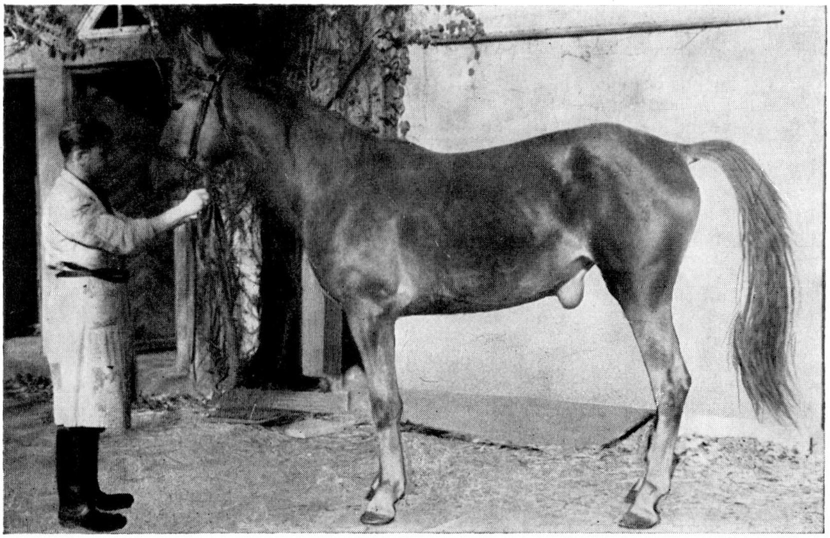

Fig. 2.8. — 19. Umbilical hernia.

Treatment and Prognosis. Umbilical hernia may be treated by either the closed or open method. The former more risky method involves the use of blisters (e.g., potassium bichromate, biiodate) or alcohol or hypertonic saline injections. Other less antiquated techniques are based on the use of ligatures, sutures, skewers and clamps. The preferred open method involves radical surgical correction and is of particular value in fillies. Unincarcerated umbilical hernias have a favorable prognosis, provided the hernial ring is not too large. A spontaneous, permanent reduction is often observed.

References

AURICH, R.: Berliner Münchener tierärztl. Wschr. *72:* 420 (1959).
SCHLAAK, F.: Untersuchungen über die Vererbung von Nabelbrüchen in einem Pferdezuchtgebiet. Vet.-med. Diss., Hannover (1941).

2.8.9. Inherited Defects of the Circulatory System

Hemorrhagic Diathesis
The subject of hemorrhagic diathesis in the horse is discussed in Sec. 2.1.3.2.3.

2.8.10. Inherited Defects of the Skin

Epitheliogenesis imperfecta neonatorum
Definition and Occurrence. Incomplete skin formation in neonates, also variously called perodermia or 'frog skin', has been recorded mainly in calves, pigs and foals but may also occur in other species.

Symptoms. The size and distribution of the areas devoid of epithelium are extremely variable. Sites of predilection are the head, neck, torso, and portions of the limbs distal to the carpal or tarsal joint. In some cases the hoof wall is absent, or the horn of the hoof separates from the corium shortly after birth. For these cases, WIEDEKING [1969] proposes the term 'epitheliogenesis et keratogenesis imperfecta neonatorum equi'. Affected foals are born live but generally die within a few hours to 2 weeks after birth.

Etiology. Inheritance of the defect in horses (lethal factor B_4) is conditioned by a single recessive gene. The defect was introduced to German breeding areas from Belgium via the Netherlands and is especially prevalent in the Brin d'Or — Indigene du Fosteau — Laboureur d'Isaac — Lion de Flandre line.

Lesions. Skin lesions are characterized by absence of the epidermis. The exposed corium has a pearly appearance or presents a velvety, blood-red surface. Often the superficial blood vessels, muscles and tendons are clearly visible beneath the corium, as in an anatomic preparation. Histologically, the epidermis in affected areas is replaced by a thin, stretchy, highly-cellular connective tissue layer. Longitudinal, oblique and transverse sections of hair follicles are visible in the deeper layers of the corium. Some of these follicles undergo a cystic degeneration and become filled with horny lamellae, horny scales and hair residue.

References

BOLLE, A.: Tierzüchter *9:* 139 (1957).

BUTZ, H.; MEYER, H.: Dtsch. tierärztl. Wschr. *64:* 555 (1957).

SONNEK, A.: Die Vererbung der Epitheliogenesis imperfecta neonatorum equi (unvollständige Hautbildung bei Fohlen). Vet.-med. Diss., Hannover (1944).

SONNENBRODT, A.: Dtsch. tierärztl. Wschr. *60:* 225 (1953).

SPIEGL, A.: Dtsch. tierärztl. Wschr. *45:* 42 (1937).

2.8.11. Inherited Defects of the Reproductive System

2.8.11.1. Cryptorchidism

Definition and Occurrence. Cryptorchidism is a partial or complete failure of the testicles to descend into the scrotum. One or both testicles may be involved, and the retained testicle may be in the inguinal canal or in the abdomen. Among domestic animals, cryptorchidism is particularly common in horses, sheep, swine and dogs; it is less frequent in cattle.

Symptoms. Abdominal cryptorchidism is present if the testicle and epididymis is retained in the abdominal cavity (usually near the vaginal ring), and inguinal cryptorchidism if it is retained in the inguinal canal. Any number of transitional forms may also be present. Cryptorchidism in the stallion may be difficult to diagnose clinically. In the inguinal form, the retained testicle can be palpated (if the horse is not too fat) by inserting the fingers upward and backward into the inguinal space. Abdominal cryptorchidism can be diagnosed only by rectal examination. Specific diagnostic techniques are discussed in Sec. 2.1.8.1.

Etiology. In the majority of observations in domestic animals, cryptorchidism has proved to be an inherited defect. The mode of inheritance in the horse still remains something of a mystery, however. In the literature the condition is variously attributed to a recessive, sex-linked recessive, dominant and partial dominant inheritance.

Lesions. In most cases the retained testicle is located just medial to the internal inguinal ring, although other intra-abdominal and even juxtaspinal locations have been reported.

Pathogenesis. Opinions vary as to the pathogenesis of the defect, and a combination of mechanical and humoral factors appears to be involved.

Various mechanical factors have been implicated: a too-short vascular pedicle (internal spermatic artery) or vas deferens, poor development of the scrotum, premature fusion of the peritoneal layers, a superficial inguinal pocket, or a coexisting hernial sac that hampers testicular descent (bibliography in PANZNER and SCHOBER [1961]).

The gonadotropic hormones play an important role in the physiologic descent of the testicles. Most authorities now believe that unilateral cases of cryptorchidism are due mainly to mechanical causes, while bilateral retentions usually have a hormonal etiology.

Treatment and Prognosis. Because cryptorchid stallions tend to be poor breeders and may transmit the defect to offspring, they should be eliminated from breeding service. The impairment of spermatogenesis in the retained testicles derives both from the poor development of the testicles themselves and from the temperatures to which they are exposed.

FLECHSIG [1952] offers a striking example of the potential economic impact of cryptorchidism in horse breeding. The stallion Albonin, born in Trakehnen in 1936 and descended from English and Arabian Thoroughbreds, was a right-sided abdominal cryptorchid. From 1946 to 1949 the stallion did service on several breeding farms of the Mark Brandenburg, sired 46 live foals out of 250 covers (17.7 %), and achieved only about 40 % of the reproductive efficiency that was average for other stallions on the same farms. Of the 24 stallions sired by Alboin, 8 were themselves cryptorchids.

References

BÖTSCHI, A.: Untersuchungen über den Kryptorchismus beim Pferd, Schwein, Hund und bei der Katze unter besonderer Berücksichtigung der mikroskopischen Anatomie. Vet.-med. Diss., Zürich (1929).

FLECHSIG, J.: Einseitiger, abdominaler Kryptorchismus bei einem Landbeschäler und seine genetische Analyse. Vet.-med. Diss., Berlin-Dahlem (1952).

KRAUSE, G.: Literarische Studien über Kryptorchismus bei Mensch und Tier mit Untersuchungen über Vererblichkeit desselben bei Schaf und Pferd. Vet.-med. Diss., Hannover (1942).

PANZNER, R.; SCHOBER, K. L.: Zbl. Chirurgie *86:* 2459 (1961).

VOGEL, G.: Tierärztl. Umschau *7:* 189 (1952).

WINTER, F.: Die Kryptorchiden und deren Kastration mit besonderem Hinblick auf das Pferd (Schoetz, Berlin 1923).

2.8.11.2. Frederiksborg Lethal Factor

Definition, Occurrence and Etiology. An impressive example of the adverse effects of poor fertility is provided by horses of the Danish Frederiksborg stud. There, in 1672, Christian V bred the stallion Jomfruen, imported from Oldenburg, to light-colored and white mares to produce a breed that later was crossed with oriental Thoroughbreds. As long as the white and gray-white stallions of the stud were not inbred, conception rates within the white herd remained high. But when the white herd was inbred during the 18th Century, there were seasons in the late 1800' s during which a band of 12 or 13 mares produced only one foal. Today it is thought that the fertility disorder is based upon the pleiotropic effect of a dominant factor with a recessive, early-embryonic lethality [PULOS and HUTT, 1969]. The causative lethal factor has been designated B_2.

References

KISSLOWSKY, D.: Z. Tierzücht. Züchtungsbiol. *7:* 58 (1932).
PULOS, W. L.; HUTT, F. B.: J. Heredity *60:* 59 (1969).
WRIEDT, CHR.: Z. Tierzücht. Züchtungsbiol. *1:* 231 (1924).

2.9. Vices of the Horse

During the last three decades, the changes in the way that horses are used have brought corresponding changes in the way horses are managed and in the attributes their owners wish them to possess. At the same time, attitudes have changed with regard to what constitutes a vice in the horse. The classic vice of wind sucking, for example, may be entirely acceptable in a good jumping horse or a simple pleasure horse, particularly since the habit poses no healthy threat in horses that are well fed and cared for. On the other hand, tongue lolling, which would be unimportant in a work horse, is a serious vice in show horses and can render them worthless.

2.9.1. Wind Sucking

Wind sucking is a habit in which the horse retracts the larynx, arches the neck and swallows air, sometimes audibly. The horse may do this while standing freely, or it may place the upper incisors over the edge of the feed trough or some other fixed object ('cribbing') before swallowing the air. The vice can reach the proportions of a true mania, with the horse even interrupting its feeding in order to 'suck wind'. Older references state that the habit causes gas to accumulate in the stomach and bowel, leading to colic. The fact that such complaints are seldom observed today suggests that feeding errors were partially to blame. Wind sucking usually starts as a playful habit in young horses, and the youthful habit of licking and nuzzling objects often progresses to wind sucking and cribbing.

Vices of this type are almost always a result of boredom, and care should be taken to avoid undue isolation, especially in young horses, and to provide opportunities for adequate exercise and normal herd behavior. Wind sucking also may be learned through imitation.

In some countries the vice constitutes grounds for the return of a purchased horse, based upon a warranty period of 14 days — for experience has shown that horses do not crib right away when placed in a new stall, but require several days' acclimatization before resuming the habit. The working soundness of a wind-sucking horse that is adequately fed and free of disease is practically unimpaired. The vice can be prevented by the use of a cribbing strap that presses tightly against the tendons of insertion of the neck muscles and thus keeps them from contracting. However, the horse will resume the vice once the strap is removed. Another measure is to string an electric-fence wire over all projecting objects in the stall that could be used for cribbing. Various operative methods have also been devised which prevent wind sucking by surgical removal of the sternocephalicus, sternohyoid, sternothyroid an omohyoid muscles in the upper third of the neck. In central Europe, the most widely-used methods are the Peterson technique, in which the muscles are approached through three incisions, and the Forssell technique, which uses a single incision. Myectomy of the sternocephalicus muscle may be replaced by a neurectomy of the ventral branch of the spinal accessory nerve. This has the advantage of preserving the degenerated muscle as a fibrous cord to maintain the ventral line of the neck, and thus avoiding the often poor cosmetic results of myectomy. Details on operative technique may be found in the literature [Firth, 1980; Huskamp et al., 1981]

References

Firth, E. C.: Bilateral ventral accessory neurectomy in windsucking horses. Vet. Rec. *106:* 30 (1980).

Huskamp, B.; Henschel, E.; Arenhoevel: Technik und Ergebnisse einer modernen Kopperoperation. IV. Tagung über Pferdekrankheiten, Equitana, Essen 1981.

2.9.2. Refractoriness

Refractoriness denotes an habitual disobedience and defiance during ordinary use which *substantially* reduces the serviceability of the animal.

In the show horse, for example, 'ordinary use' would mean submission to tying, transporation and riding under a variety of conditions. A pleasure horse or saddle horse should submit to riding in terrain, either alone or in groups. A riding horse that strenuously resists tying, shoeing or saddling is considered to be refractory. Resistance to harnessing, driving and load-pulling constitutes refractoriness only in horses that are sold expressly as draft animals.

2.9.3. Weaving

Weaving is a vice that apparently stems from the natural love of movement that characterizes the horse. It consists of a rhythmical shifting of the weight from one front foot to the other, accompanied by a swaying of the upper body and head. Many horses weave only when excited or disturbed by a change of stable, feeding, the introduction of new stable-mates, or extended idleness or isolation. Others weave almost constantly during the intervals between feedings, or even during feeding in rare instances. Many 'cures' have been prescribed over the years (e.g., tying the legs together, mounting colorful pictures at eye level, cross-tying the head), but none are really effective. Weaving horses should be given an opportunity to exercise adequately and develop a normal social behavior. Fully-enclosed box stalls and prolonged standing in stocks without contact with other horses should be avoided. If pasturing is not possible, the animals should be exercised several times daily.

2.9.4. Shying

(See Sec. 2.1.15.3.)

Subject Index

Ducharme

Diseases of the Horse, Part 2/I

Diseases of the Horse

A Handbook for Science and Practice

Part 2/I

Edited by

Prof. Dr. sc. med. vet. Olof Dietz, Berlin

Prof. Dr. sc. med. vet. Ekkehard Wiesner, Berlin

English translation edited by

Dr. A. S. Turner, Fort Collins, Colo.

227 figures (partly in color), 1 table, 1984

KARGER

S. Karger · Basel · München · Paris · London · New York · Tokyo · Sydney

Translated from the original German edition by Terry C. Telger, Marina, Calif.

National Library of Medicine. Cataloging in Publication

Handbuch der Pferdekrankheiten für Wissenschaft und Praxis. English.
Diseases of the horse: a handbook for science and practice / edited by Olof Dietz, Ekkehard Wiesner; English translation edited by A. S. Turner. Basel; New York: Karger, 1984. Translation of: Handbuch der Pferdekrankheiten für Wissenschaft und Praxis.
1. Horse Diseases I. Dietz, Olof II. Turner, A. Simon III. Wiesner, Ekkehard
ISBN 3-8055-3497-3
SF 951 H 236

Printed in the German Democratic Republic
ISBN 3-8055-3497-3

Contents of the Present Volume

Part 2/I Special Part

Contents of the Complete Work

Part 2/II Special Part (Continuation)

2. Special Part

2.1. Organic Diseases

2.1.1. Diseases of the Skin

2.1.1.1. Diseases of the Haircoat

2.1.1.1.1. Loss of Hair and Lack of Hair (Alopecia, Hypotrichosis)

Definition. Alopecia refers to a generalized or circumscribed abnormal hair loss in which the skin itself shows no other demonstrable lesions. The term alopecia adnata, denoting a congenital absence of hair, is no longer the preferred term and hypotrichosis or atrichosis (atrichia) is used in order to distinguish this condition from the alopecia acquired in postnatal life.

Symptoms. The generalized form (alopecia universalis) is more common in the horse, with hair loss affecting the entire body but usually sparing the mane, tail and pastern region. Initially there is an intensive hair loss resembling that of heavy seasonal shedding. Soon irregular hairless areas may appear scattered over the entire body. If the alopecia is secondary to an exogenous cause, it appears only in the area where the animal has come in contact with the offending agent.

Less frequently the disease is manifested as *alopecia areata* which is circumscribed hair loss occurring in an irregular or symmetrical pattern. These bare patches may gradually enlarge and join to form larger alopecic areas.

The hair loss is sometimes preceded by transient, nonspecific reactions such as gastrointestinal disorders, pruritus or sensitivity, and swelling of the skin. These symptoms disappear by the time the hair loss begins, leaving no visible skin changes other than occasional hyper- or hypopigmentation.

Etiology. The causes are so varied that alopecia may be viewed as a disease *symptom* rather than a separate disease entity. The acquired form usually occurs secondary to chronic digestive and metabolic disorders, febrile diseases or the ingestion of certain toxic substances such as selenium or mercury.

Reportedly, alopecia can also result from the long-term feeding of steamed potatoes, turnips and raw sugar, and cases have been observed in horses fed alfalfa (lucerne) hay and certain plants such as the jumbey *(Leucaena glauca)*.

Endocrine factors are thought to play a minor causative role in the horse, though occasional cases have occurred in late pregnancy or during lactation that allow no other explanation. In very rare instances, psychosomatic alopecia can occur in anxious or excitable horses [Guilhon, 1962]. One outbreak of alopecia was the result of contact with stalls that had been freshly painted with an oil-base paint. The action of the paint or solvent as a depilatory, was confirmed experimentally.

Differential Diagnosis. A number of skin diseases such as parasitism, dermatomycoses and many inflammatory conditions are also associated with hair loss and must be differentiated from alopecia on the basis of specific findings. It must also be considered that lesions such as extensive skin wounds, burns, radiation damage, and deep-seated pyodermas can form scar tissue that is devoid of hair follicles. In doubtful cases these forms of hair loss can be differentiated by the histologic examination of biopsy material. Physiologic hair loss associated with aging is of little importance in the horse and may be excluded.

Extreme brittleness of the hairs (trichorrhexis nodosa) may be of differential diagnostic importance. This condition causes the hairs to break off just above the skin and affects mainly the mane and tail. The remaining stubs fray, thus creating a brush-like appearance.

The *diagnosis* is established by hair loss in the absence of any other significant skin changes.

The *prognosis* is far better in generalized alopecia than in the very rare circumscribed form (alopecia areata).

Treatment. No specific therapy is known. Every effort must be made to isolate and remove the immediate cause. Special attention should be given to sound nutrition and regular skin care. Multivitamin preparations and trace-element mixtures are recommended to promote healing. Local applications of ointments based on resorcin, Peruvian balsam, salicylic acid, naphthalane, etc. are reported to be of benefit in stimulating hair regrowth.

2.1.1.1.2. Excessive Hair Growth (Hypertrichosis)

Excessive hair growth can be congenital or acquired, generalized or localized. Hypertrichosis affecting only the mane and tail is rare. A long, dense haircoat may simply be a response to climatic extremes and is common in horses that are kept outdoors the year round. Circumscribed hypertrichosis sometimes develops in areas underlying the harness or saddle as a response to sustained skin irritation. This condition does not impair performance and treatment is not recommended.

When present together with polydipsia and polyuria, hypertrichosis is symptomatic of Cushing's syndrome and is called *hirsutism.* It is caused by tumors of the pituitary or adrenal gland, for which no therapy is available.

2.1.1.1.3. Pigmentary Disorders

Disorders of pigmentation usually affect the skin and coat and rarely affect the hairs alone.

Hyperpigmentation, characterized by excessive amounts of melanin, is of no practical importance in the horse. Kral and Schwartzman [1964] report a single case of circumscribed hyperpigmentation, which they identify as nevi pigmentosi. Sometimes pigmentation is increased in skin areas previously affected with trichophytosis or other lesions.

Hypopigmentation, either congenital or acquired, is considerably more common in horses. Some forms are clinically unimportant. The main types are albinism, leukoderma, vitiligo and canities (graying of the hair, see below).

Albinism refers to a congenital absence of melanin that also affects the hooves and eyes. The occurrence of true equine albinism is disputed, however, for the majority of horses classified as 'albinos' have pigmented irides. Albinism is considered the result of a genetic defect (see chap. 2.8.3.5.).

Leukoderma is a localized depigmentation that occurs as a sequel to skin diseases or other noxious influences (liniments, wound or nasal secretions, etc.). Usually the pigmentation returns a short time after the primary symptoms have passed. On the other hand, some skin injuries lead to the destruction of melanocytes, resulting in permanent depigmentation; this usually occurs in areas where pressure is exerted by a saddle, harness or collar.

Vitiligo refers to an acquired loss of pigmentation. Here the affected sites are circumscribed and show no other signs of disease, although some local sensory loss has been described in humans. Often the depigmented areas are encircled by a hyperpigmented border that similarly contrasts with the surrounding skin.

The disorder is attributed to endocrine and neurogenic abnormality. A relationship between thyroid and pituitary abnormalities has not been confirmed. The prevalence of vitiligo in certain breeds must be viewed as evidence of genetic influences.

Canities is a grayish discoloration of the hair that may be associated with aging (canities senilis) or may occur at a younger age (canities prematura). It is especially prominent in the craniofacial region, about the eyes, on the forehead and around the lips, as well as on the limbs.

Loss of pigmentation (leukotrichia) in the hairs can also result from nervous influences, deficiency states, and exposure to x-rays or other irritants. If generalized leukotrichia appears, it may represent nothing more than the natural 'coming into color' of a gray or white horse.

No specific treatment for these disorders is known or necessary, for they generally do not cause ill health or affect performance. However, the depigmented areas are relatively sensitive to solar radiation, and so care should be taken when exposing the animal to sunlight or other UV radiation sources.

2.1.1.2. Diseases of the Cutaneous Glands

2.1.1.2.1. Inflammation of the Hair Follicles and Sebaceous Glands (Folliculitis, Acne, Furunculosis)

Definition. Suppurative inflammation of the hair follicles due to bacterial infection is called folliculitis (sycosis). When it spreads to the sebaceous glands, it is called acne. If the process penetrates into the deeper layers of the corium to the subcutis, accompanied by tissue destruction, skin abscesses or furuncles will form; the presence of multiple furuncles is termed furunculosis.

Symptoms. The changes usually appear in relatively dry areas where the harness or saddle can cause small skin lesions to form. Thus, areas of predilection include the lateral chest wall to the lumbar region (area below the saddle), the croup to the root of the tail, and the area between the neck and thoracic inlet (collar, breastpiece).

Initially, large skin areas become hot, swollen and painful. The overlying hairs are dull, erect, and can be easily plucked out. If a fold of skin is taken up and squeezed, a yellowish, blood-tinged fluid will exude from the follicular orifices (folliculitis). Often the exudate will cause sticking together of the hairs and crust formation. Meanwhile, nodules gradually form that vary in size and are firm on palpation; the hairs overlying these lesions are soon shed (acne). The nodules rupture, and a purulent, bloody material is extruded when pressure is applied. Crater-like ulcers form in the skin from the spontaneous rupture and coalescence of the individual lesions. The ulcers heal, but the hairless areas persist for some time. Eventually eczematous changes, heavy scaling or keratinization appear over the entire affected area.

Etiology. Staphylococcus aureus is the main causative agent. However, skin lesions must be present to create a portal of entry for the organism. Chafing tack can actually massage the organisms into the skin. Soiling and heavy sweating also predispose to infection. Even in the absence of bacterial invasion, sweat combined with the accumulation of dirt or dust can cause skin irritation and the blocking of follicular orifices and sebaceous glands. These forms have been described by such terms as 'summer rash', 'sweat eczema' and 'saddle mange'.

The same effect (clogging of the sebaceous gland, skin irritation) is occasionally produced by the application of liniments. A symptomatic folliculitis is sometimes seen in strangles.

Differential Diagnosis. Folliculitis and furunculosis must be differentiated from parasitic skin diseases, which can be identified by the examination of skin scrapings. They must also be distinguished from the various types of eczema. Otherwise the clinical picture is definite.

Course and Prognosis. If lesions are mild, spontaneous healing will be fairly rapid once the causes have been eliminated. If this is not done, the disease takes a chronic course, and the prognosis is poor. Furunculoses can prove highly resistant to treatment. Healing may take weeks or months, and recurrences and reinfections are possible.

Treatment. It is important that the skin be protected from further irritants. Thorough antiseptic washings are also indicated, during which time any loose hairs are removed. Complete removal of the hair is often recommended.

Local treatment consists in the application of ointments, powders or tinctures which contain coal tar, sulfur, iodine, formalin sulfonamides or antibiotics. The results are often unsatisfactory unless every focus has been eliminated. For this each infected focus must be expressed, probed or incised and then individually treated with a disinfectant medication. These measures should be repeated every 3—4 days. Cauterization has also been employed with success.

The therapeutic use of UV radiation and in particular of X-irradiation is also promising. Treatment should consist of 3 to 4 exposures repeated at 3- to 4-day ntervals, using dose levels of 200 R.

Vitamins are indicated to assist natural defenses. The disease is also an indication for nonspecific stimulation therapy. In unresponsive cases an autogenous vaccine may have to be prepared and administered in order to effect a cure.

Finally, treatment includes the thorough cleansing and disinfection of all parts of the harness, saddle and grooming utensils in order to prevent reinfection.

Prophylaxis consists in the use of clean, well-fitting equipment and in proper skin care.

2.1.1.2.2. Disturbances of Sweat Secretion

The sweat glands of the horse are well developed in comparison with other domestic species. Sweat secretion is extremely important for temperature regulation in the horse. Disturbances in a quantitative sense are present only if sweat production does not correspond to the demands of thermoregulation. Excessive sweating is called hyperhidrosis, and an abnormal deficiency of sweat is termed hypohidrosis or anhidrosis. The sweat may also be altered in its composition, as in hematidrosis (the excretion of bloody sweat).

Hyperhidrosis

Definition. In hyperhidrosis there is a functional disturbance of the sweat glands in which the animal sweats without apparent cause or for reasons unrelated to temperature regulation. The sweating may occur all over the body (h. universalis) or be confined to certain areas (h. localis) or one half of the body (h. unilateralis). Sweating is especially profuse on the insides of the thighs, the sides of the neck, at the base of the ears, as well as around the eyes and nostrils.

Symptoms. The affected areas appear darker, the animal literally 'steams' in cold surroundings, and sweat drips from the body. The hairs cling to the body surface, and lather forms where body areas come in contact with each other. The skin is wet. In local hyperhidrosis the affected area contrasts sharply with the surrounding skin. Such sweating can often continue unabated for several days.

Etiology. Excessive sweating is regarded not as a disease entity, but as a clinical manifestation of various syndromes. These include conditions that are associated with severe dyspnea and inadequate oxygen delivery. Painful conditions (severe colics) as well as certain stages of febrile diseases may also be accompanied by profuse sweating. Untrained and obese horses and animals weakened by acute or chronic illness sweat on even the slightest exertion. Hyperhidrosis has been observed as a separate entity in connection with the overfeeding of raw sugar and pumpkin, although the pathogenesis remains unclear.

Localized or unilateral sweating is the result of nervous system pathology. The most common causes are traumatic peripheral nerve damage, diseases of the spinal cord, and central excitation of the autonomic nervous system.

Circumscribed sweating may also occur at sites where epinephrine or other drugs have been administered by injection.

Treatment. Emphasis is on identifying the cause and treating the primary disorder. Sponging with 2—5% vinegar water, a 5—10% alcohol salicylic acid solution or, for local sweating, with 0.1% formalin can afford symptomatic relief only. In addition, potassium iodide may be given orally (5.0 g) or an iodine preparation intravenously. Subcutaneous atropine injections are less frequently justified and also represent a form of symptomatic treatment.

Anhidrosis

Definition. Anhidrosis refers to a state in which the ability to sweat is partially or completely lost. The disease chiefly affects horses that have been raised in temperate climates and subsequently imported to countries with hot, humid climates. It is widespread in parts of India, Indonesia, Sri Lanka, the Philippines, etc., affecting up to 15% of imported horses. Indiginous horses are not affected.

Symptoms. The signs usually appear within a year after the horse has arrived. Initially there is increasing dyspnea on exertion, and sweating is restricted to the neck, the base of the ears, between the thighs, and under the saddle. Later the areas in which sweating occurs gradually diminish in size, the skin becomes dry and rough, and hair is shed. Finally sweating ceases altogether, even during exercise, although the skin is noticeably warm.

While various transitional forms are encountered, temperature regulation is always impaired to some degree. As a result, the internal body temperature rises markedly during exertion. There may be damage to the renal parenchyma, as evidenced by urinary findings (proteinuria, cylindruria), and there is a potential danger of acute cardiovascular failure during exercise.

Etiology and Pathogenesis. Formerly it was thought that anhidrosis was caused by infectious organisms, toxic agents or vitamin deficiencies. More recent research points to a complex situation involving electrolyte imbalances, endocrine factors and functional abnormalities of the sweat glands themselves. Horses with anhidrosis have abnormally low blood chloride and sodium levels. The favorable effect of iodine compounds or thyroid extract is evidence for involvement of the thyroid glands, although hypothyroidism has not been clearly demonstrated in anhidrotic horses. It is interesting to note that horses in tropical countries have much higher epinephrine levels than horses living in the temperate zones. In many cases the sweat glands become refractory to stimulation by epinephrine. A partial blockage of the sweat gland ducts has also been demonstrated, but this may be a result of the gland's functional alteration.

Treatment. No sure treatment is known. The primary step is to correct any electrolyte imbalance by dietary salt supplementation or by infusing electrolyte solutions. Good results have also been achieved with the oral administration of iodinated casein or thyroid extract. Vitamin therapy (especially vitamin E) has not been proved to be of definite benefit. The only sure prophylactic measure is to return the animal to its country (or climate) of origin.

2.1.1.2.3. Disturbances of Sebaceous Secretion

Of the abnormalities of sebaceous secretion, only hypersecretion, or seborrhea, is important in the horse. Diminished or absent sebaceous secretion (asteatosis) is extremely rare. Sebaceous cysts (atheromas) are also uncommon in horses.

Seborrhea

Definition. Seborrhea is the term applied to excessive secretion of sebum by the sebaceous glands of the skin. The principal forms are seborrhea oleosa, which produces an oily film, and seborrhea sicca, which leads to scaling and crusting. A third form is seborrheic dermatitis. The dry form of seborrhea is most common in the horse.

Symptoms. The changes develop gradually and may be confined to certain aresa, such as the mane and root of the tail (seborrhea localis), or may affect the entire body (seborrhea universalis).

The affected areas give off an unpleasant odor like rancid fat. Among the hairs are many grayish-white clumps of greasy material, creating a bran-like coating. In serious cases the skin may be covered with a greasy crust from 1 to 1.5 cm thick in which the hairs are embedded. The haircoat becomes thin and dull, as if covered with dust. The skin itself is unchanged beneath the scales and crusts. In seborrheic dermatitis there is little or no pruritis, but the skin under the coatings is moist, somewhat thickened in places, and is reddened in unpigmented areas.

Etiology. The etiology of the disease is not clear. Clinical observations suggest a causal relation with endocrine dysfunctions, digestive and metabolic disorders such as hypoproteinemia, vitamin deficiency or excessive carbohydrate intake, as well as anemic and wasting diseases. Other authors cite climatic factors and external irritants as possible causes, noting a predisposition in horses exposed for long periods to cold, rainy weather or, formerly, to the dust-laden atmosphere of coal mines. Recent findings rule out infectious factors while lending support to genetic factors.

In most cases, however, neither the history nor clinical findings are sufficient to clarify the cause and pathogenesis.

Of main *differential diagnostic importance* are the various forms of mange, which themselves are distinguished by severe pruritus and the presence of parasites in skin scrapings. It is more difficult to differentiate seborrheic dermatitis from seborrhea sicca or crustosa, because there are no clear dividing lines. The histologic picture always shows hyperplasia of the epidermis, corium and sebaceous glands, as well as enlargement of the glandular orifices.

The *prognosis* is guarded. The disease is chronic in character and usually persists for life. There is a gradual deterioration of the horse's nutritional status and working capacity, and often the only recourse after futile attempts at treatment, is euthanasia.

Treatment. No specific therapy is known. The standard treatment is to wash affected areas with antiseborrheic shampoos. Further local treatments include the application of products that contain sulfur, salicylic acid, coal tar derivatives, etc. The result of these washings and baths should be closely followed, for the removal of crusts and cleansing of the skin sometimes exacerbates scaling, causing a return to the initial situation within a few days.

Attempts have been made to treat seborrhea by the oral or parenteral administration of vitamins (A, E, B_6, B_{12}, etc.) and of iodine, bromine, selenium and arsenic compounds, as well as by the infusion of sodium thiosulfate and procaine (Novocain) solutions. If the skin is inflamed, glucocorticoids may be beneficial, but their effect is at best, temporary.

Because connections have been reported between an excess or deficiency of estrogens or testosterone and sebaceous gland activity, hormone injections as well as castration have been tried, but have proved unsuccessful in the majority of cases.

2.1.1.3. Inflammations of the Skin

2.1.1.3.1. Eczemas

Definition. Eczemas, called also idiopathic exanthemas, are primary, superficial skin inflammations that are confined mainly to the epidermis. They may also involve the upper layers of the cutis to some degree. The precipitating causes are varied, but every case involves a specific inflammatory reaction of the sensitized skin. The clinical manifestations of eczema are extremely diverse, and various stages and degrees of inflammation may be present at any given time. Eczemas may take an acute or chronic course. They are classified according to their predominent signs, nature of onset, localization or precipitating cause, if known.

In the horse as in other domestic species, eczemas are among the most common skin diseases. Some forms are already regarded as separate disease entities by virtue of their typical localization or established etiology.

Symptoms. The inflammatory process goes through various well-defined stages. However, the excematous changes seldom progress through all the changes but tend to halt at a particular stage and then regress. Meanwhile, the process can start anew in adjacent or more distant areas.

The major stages of eczematous change are as follows:

1. Erythematous stage: Erythema with slight epidermal damage as a sign of hyperemia of the superficial skin layers with weak serous infiltration.
2. Papular stage: Nodules develop as an expression of circumscribed cellular proliferation.
3. Vesicular stage: Serous exudation increases, leading to the formation of vesicles filled with clear fluid.
4. Weeping stage: The vesicles rupture and, if they have coalesced, produce diffuse weeping. The stratum corneum is disrupted and detached at many points, resulting in a weeping, highly erythematous surface.
5. Pustular stage: Usually pustule formation is due to secondary bacterial invasion.
6. Crusting stage (fig. 2.1.1. — 1): The exudate of the vesicles or pustules dries, forming concretions. These crusts may overlie a layer of pus.

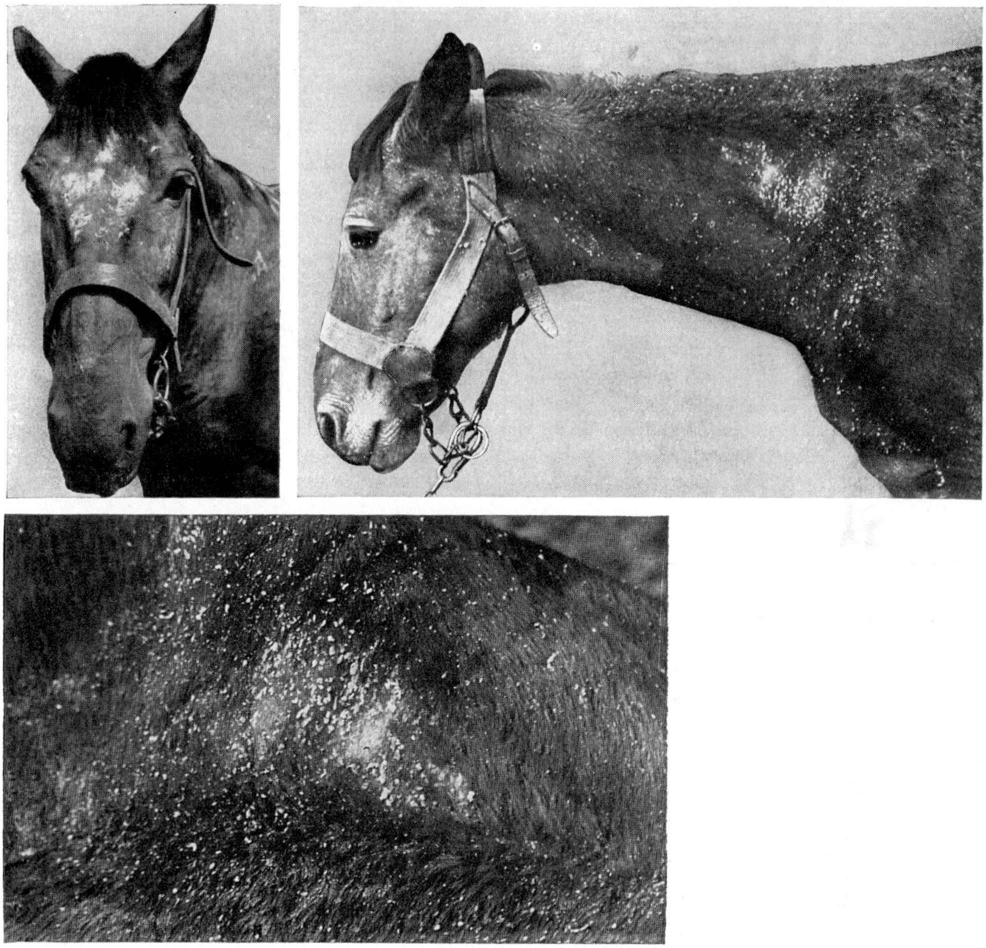
1 2 3

Fig. 2.1.1. — 1. Eczema with crusting on the forehead and dorsum of the nose.
Fig. 2.1.1. — 2–3. Diffuse eczematous skin lesions with heavy scaling (squamous eczema).

7. Scaling stage (fig. 2.1.1. — 2 and — 3): The skin surface is covered with scales of varying size as a manifestation of hyper- or parakeratosis.

Acute eczemas typically begin with erythema, then their progression halts at one of the above stages. It may skip the remaining stages and heal with scaling. In chronic eczemas the early stages are less pronounced, and erythema is usually absent. The major signs are localized thickenings of the skin as a result of cell proliferation and heavy keratinization of the epidermis with scaling. The skin itself feels dry due to the absence of sebaceous and sweat secretion.

In the horse, certain eczemas have characteristic localizations and symptoms. Chronic eczemas are the most common.

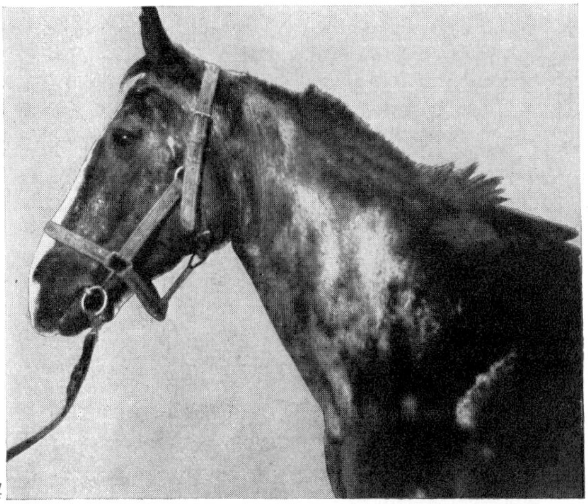

4

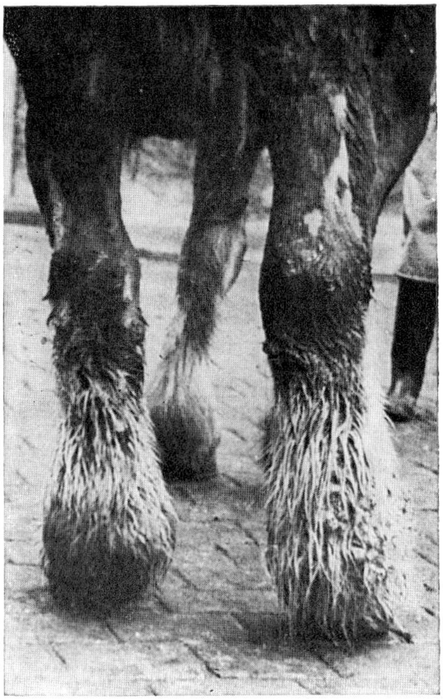

6

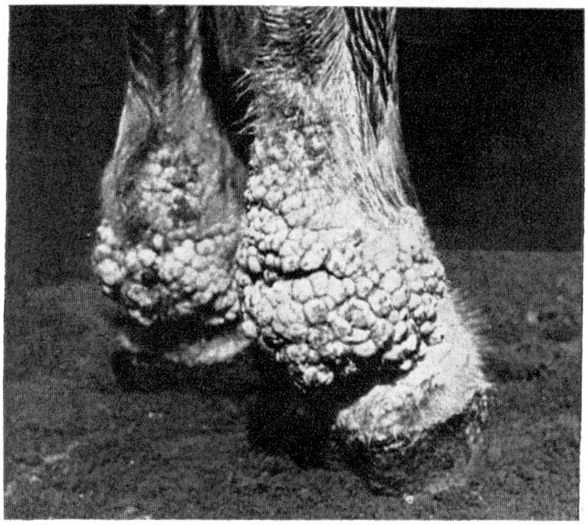

5

Fig. 2.1.1. — 4. Chronic squamous eczema (psoriasis, hunger mange).
Fig. 2.1.1. — 5–6. Greasy heel (dermatitis verrucosa).

1. *Chronic squamous eczema (psoriasis, hunger mange)* (fig. 2.1.1. — 4) is most often seen in horses with tender skin that have been improperly fed or cared for. The primary lesions appear as nodules and vesicles about the eyes or on the neck, shoulder, root of the tail or hindlimbs and have a tendency to spread to other areas. The vesicles rupture, forming crusts. When these exfoliate, the embedded hairs are also shed, producing small areas of alopecia that gradually become larger by coalescing. At this stage the skin is already thickened and covered with scales. Most animals show signs of severe pruritus. This form of eczema may persist for years, usually showing improvement during the colder months.

2. *Summer eczema* is a skin disease that appears with the onset of warm weather. Areas affected are the ears, neck, mane, withers, back, and root of the tail. The skin changes, which consist initially of papulation are later marked by scaling and alopecia. They may be accompanied by a violent pruritus, which is the most striking and unpleasant symptom of the disease. Summer eczema is unknown in yearlings but is observed with increasing frequency as the horse matures. It seems especially common

after the age of ten. It is very similar clinically to the skin reactions known as 'Queensland itch' in Australia, 'allergic dermatitis' in the Northeastern U.S., and 'sweet itch' in England, all of which are recognized as an allergic response to insect bites. In cases of average severity the lesions are confined to the withers.

3. *Aural plaques.* This disease with its peculiar lesions involving the inner surface of the pinna and occasionally the anus and vulva, has been described mainly by American authors. There are reports from Europe on the occurrence of eczemas in these areas. Foals are not affected. Outbreaks in the remaining age groups are limited to the summer months.

The lesions consist initially of papules from 1 mm to 2 cm in diameter that appear on the inner surface of the pinna. Later they are covered by a gray or white crust, or plaque. In severe cases over half of the pinna may be affected. Pruritus may not be present.

4. *Mane and tail eczema* is a chronic, impetigo-like eczema of the long-haired body regions (mane and base of tail) that sometimes also involves portions of the head down to the lips. The initial skin reactions are unknown, and so the disease often escapes detection until severe pruritus and irritation are noticed. As a result of exudation and the accumulation of dirt, the hairs stick together, becoming matted and tangled. Beneath the layer of dirt and impetigo-like crusts is a weeping, reddened, partially suppurative surface. The skin is thickened, wrinkled and tender and has an unpleasant odor. Itching is intense and prompts constant rubbing, which can cause further irritation and promote secondary infection. A frequent result is extensive folliculitis (eczema sycosiforme), with associated alopecia. Even after the suppurative inflammation has subsided, a noticeable thinness of the hair remains, especially in the tail, producing a ragged or 'rat-tail' appearance.

Most cases are recorded in the spring and summer months, with a particularly high incidence observed in certain geographical locations.

5. *Grease heel* is the term given to eczema involving the posterior aspect of the pastern, usually of the hindlimbs. Horses with long hair are predisposed. Grease heel is chiefly a disease of the fall and winter months.

The disease begins with erythema, followed by the formation of nodules and vesicles. Soon the fetlock consists of a weeping, tender surface covered by a greasy, foul-smelling coating. Drying of the secretions, together with dirt accumulation, can cause thick, friable crusts to form (figs. 2.1.1. — 5 and — 6).

In more chronic cases, the skin thickens and fissures develop. These lesions are very painful and restrict normal movement of the joint. Movement can cause cracks (rhagades) to form, and a bloody exudate often oozes from these cracks, leading to further crust formation on drying. The hairs are often bristly ('hedgehog foot') and are eventually shed. Scars or projections may form due to progressive thickening of the skin, further altering the appearance of the fetlock. In the skin folds, the decomposing, greasy, malodorous secretion mixed with sebum, epidermal cells and dirt perpetuates the inflammatory process.

Wartlike elevations may appear in circumscribed areas, where thick, knobby epidermal thickenings form, accompanied by hyperplasia of the skin and subcutaneous tissue (dermatitis verrucosa).

6. Chronic eczema of a predominantly squamous character occurring on the posterior aspect of the carpal and tarsal joints is called *rasp*. This condition is similar to grease heel in its onset and course, because it is characterized by periodic acute flareups.

Eczemas can develop in other areas as well, depending on the animal's care and susceptibility to precipitating causes. They may occur under the saddle in riding

7 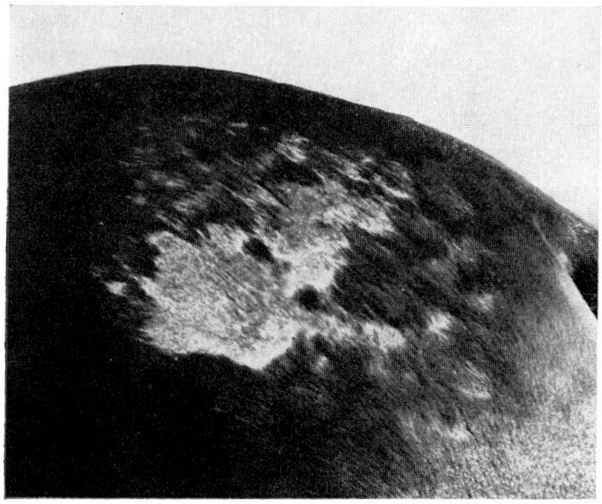 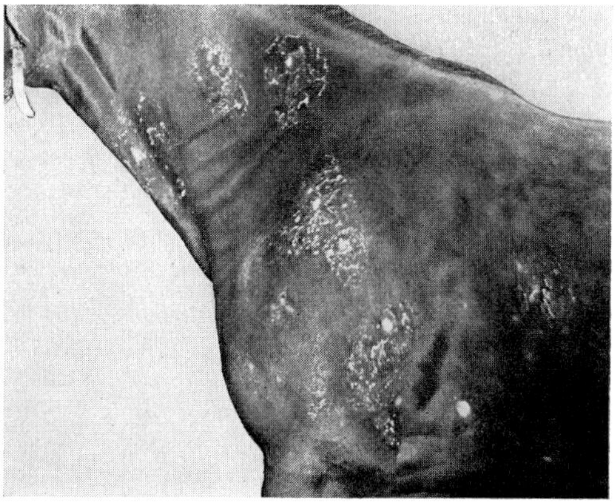 8

Fig. 2.1.1. — 7. Dirt eczema in the region of the croup.
Fig. 2.1.1. — 8. Blistering following the topical application of isothiocyanate.

horses, or on the limbs and ventral body surface of animals housed under wet, unsanitary conditions. A special form of eczema is seborrheic dermatitis (see Seborrhea).

Etiology and Pathogenesis. Despite uncertainties that exist regarding the etiology of this class of skin diseases, it is now generally agreed that eczemas represent an allergic skin reaction. Eczemas understandably can seldom be related to the direct action of a particular agent. Alternatively such an action may bear no obvious relation to the lesions.

Eczemas are allergic phenomena of the delayed type, meaning that there must be direct contact with an allergen to which the skin has become sensitized. Predisposition also must exist for a delayed allergic response to occur. Passive transmission via the blood serum is impossible. The serum itself contains no antibodies, and the allergic response is related to immune cells.

There are any number of external causes that are capable of triggering an allergic reaction. The causal agents need not meet the requirements of a complete antigen, for once in contact with the skin, low-molecular weight substances (haptenes) are conjugated to skin proteins to form the antigen.

Eczemas are very often associated with poor skin care. Dirt particles (fig. 2.1.1. — 7), exfoliated epidermal cells, loose hairs, and sweat and sebum decompose on the skin, and the decomposition products lead to sensitization. Frequent wetting of the skin predisposes to eczematous change.

These factors explain why certain eczemas have a predilection for areas that are easily accessible to dirt and moisture (long-haired areas, the back, the fetlock). The same applies to areas that are constantly moist as a result of ocular or nasal discharge or chronic diarrhea. Mechanical irritations, such as rubbing by tack items or body parts (insides of the thighs, base of the tail), are another frequent cause of superficial skin inflammation. Mechanical factors can also initiate grease heel. The common practice of clipping the fetlock hairs very short, supposedly to keep this area cleaner and facilitate care, produces a course stubble that can severely chafe the skin.

According to a number of recent studies, ectoparasites (fleas, flies, lice, etc.) and their excretion products are important in the etiology of many eczemas. In the past there was a tendency to view the mechanical irritating effect of the ectoparasites as the cause. When the same changes were produced with extracts from the parasites or with their products, the allergic origin of these eczemas became obvious. Queensland itch has been associated with sensitization to sandflies of the species *Culicoides robertsoni*, sweet itch in Great Britain with *Culicoides pulicaris*, and allergic dermatitis in the U.S.A. with *Culicoides variipennis* as well as with mosquitoes of the genus *Aedes (Aedes triseriatus)*. Similarly, summer eczema has been related to flying insects of the order Diptera, especially black flies (*Simulium* spp.). These species also cause eczemas that are localized in the ear (e.g., *Simulium maculatum*).

Any number of other substances can act as causative agents, provided they come in contact with the skin. These include soaps, liniments, topical medications, preservatives or impregnating agents used in tack items, as well as plastics and rubber parts (fig. 2.1.1. — 8). Occasionally it is possible to identify the allergen by careful observation and a process of elimination but in most cases the precise etiology remains unknown.

Bacteria, especially pyogenic types, also contribute to the development of eczema. However, they are considered more important as secondary pathogens than as direct causes.

The factors that predispose the animal to eczema are usually referred to as endogenous causes. These are just as diverse as the exogenous causes but in most cases are even more difficult to identify and control.

It is known from human medicine and has been demonstrated in domestic animals, including horses, that predisposition to eczema is inheritable and increases with age. On the other hand eczema may be related to nutrition and metabolism. A number of orally ingested substances have an affinity for the skin and are capable of causing eruptions (exanthema). A high protein content in the ration as well as overfeeding (obesity) predispose to allergic reactions. On the other hand, it appears that deficiencies of fats, vitamins (A, C, B) and minerals may also be related to skin diseases.

Subclinical digestive disorders can also have adverse effects. In horses with mane and tail eczema, the feces were found to have an abnormally high pH, and a disproportionate colonization of the intestine with coliform organisms [Mansson and Niléhn, 1958; Nilsson, 1958].

Increased susceptibility has also been associated with lesions of internal organs (liver, kidney). In addition, there is evidence that points to endocrine disturbances as a predisposing factor. This particularly applies to the pancreas, thyroid gland, sex glands and pituitary. The bulk of this evidence comes from small animal practice. The importance of disturbances of nervous regulation in the pathogenesis of eczema has been demonstrated both by clinical observations and experimental research.

The *differential diagnosis* can be quite involved due to the diversity of clinical manifestations. It is especially important that eczema be differentiated from infectious skin diseases of parasitic (mange) and mycotic origin. Their exclusion is based upon the course, the clinical picture, and by the presence or absence of organisms in skin scrapings. In acne, the skin shows nodular lesions, while in alopecia there is hair loss without damage to the skin itself. In dermatitis the inflammation involves both the dermis and the epidermis, and the lesions are homogeneous. They are closely related to the severity of the causal agent. In photosensitization the skin changes are confined to unpigmented areas.

The *diagnosis* is established by the history and clinical findings. These allow the condition to be subdivided into special categories on the basis of further characteristics.

Prognosis. Acute eczemas usually have a good prognosis even when the causal agent is unknown, provided prompt treatment is given. The prognosis is poor in cases that have become chronic. Chronic eczemas can persist indefinitely and often are refractory to all forms of treatment. Recurrences are always possible, and so caution should be exercised when making a prognosis.

Treatment. Eczemas vary widely in their reponse to therapeutic measures. Many are among the most refractory conditions known to medicine. Eczema treatment is often expensive and time-consuming, demanding patience and persistence. The initial goal is to identify the cause and eliminating it if possible. This may include the use of insecticides or temporarily stabling the animals during the times when suspected insects are swarming. If tack items are suspected, they should be changed. Any suspected medications or liniments should be discontinued.

In recent decades glucocorticoids have gained key importance in the treatment of eczema. They are mainly used topically in ointment or spray form. To control or prevent secondary bacterial infections, the glucocorticoids should be combined with antibiotics. Usually they are not given orally or parenterally, as this can cause unwanted side-effects. Glucocorticoid therapy is not directed to the cause, and its effects are only temporary, assuming the etiological agent is still present. Therefore, measures should be taken to reduce or eliminate predisposition or sensitization. Primary attention is given to the feed. Every effort is made to ensure an ample vitamin supply (A, B, E, etc.) and calcium intake, if necessary by parenteral supplementation. Trace elements should also be given. Sometimes potassium arsenite solution (Fowler's solution) is prescribed, to be given daily with the ration; the dose is increased from one to six tablespoons per day and then reduced daily back to one tablespoon. Antihistamines are also a standard part of eczema therapy.

In addition, the animal should also be treated for any demonstrable organ dysfunction (liver, kidney). Horses with mane eczema and abnormal bacterial flora in the intestine, may respond to administration of *E. coli* cultures or a fecal suspension from a healthy horse administerd via nasogastric tube.

Local adjunctive treatment is often indicated, and for this to be effective, the affected skin must be accessible to the medication and must be mechanically cleansed. It is often enough to just clip the hair in and around the affected area. Frequent washing or spraying with water, on the other hand, is not well tolerated by the eczematous skin. The area should be washed with lukewarm water and neutral soaps, at the start of treatment. In many cases it is best to use a 3% solution of H_2O_2 or other mild antiseptic solution.

In other respects the local treatment differs for acute and chronic eczemas. In acute forms a variety of drying agents and anti-inflammatory drugs are used, including oily emulsions; pastes and ointments containing zinc, cod-liver oil and vitamins; astringent preparations and drying tinctures. For suppurative eczemas, antibiotics or sulfonamides are also recommended. Because secondary bacterial infection may be present in other forms of eczema, combined preparations of this type are suitable.

The treatment of chronic eczemas on the other hand relies more on the use of preparations that act as irritants. The most popular local agents are coal-tar derivatives, but sulfur, salicylic acid, iodine, and other substances are also used.

Physiotherapeutic measures, especially the use of UV radiation and X-irradiation, have also proved effective in the treatment of eczema.

2.1.1.3.2. Dermatitis

Definition. Dermatitis is an inflammation of all the skin layers and is usually caused by the direct action of noxious agents. Dermatitis may take an acute or chronic course. The severity of the inflammatory process varies considerably from one form to another, ranging from mild erythema to necrosis.

Symptoms. All lesions are usually at the same stage of development. However, the degree of inflammation varies widely according to the severity and duration of action of the etiologic agent, as well as the sensitivity of the individual skin areas.

In acute cases all the signs of inflammation are present — erythema, swelling, increased warmth and pain. Pruritus is not always present but is usually manifested in the early stage as well as during the later healing stage. When inflammation is severe or extensive, there is impairment of general health with fever, rapid pulse and depression.

The following forms or stages of dermatitis can be distinguished according to the lesions that develop:

1. Erythematous dermatitis. This mildest form is characterized only by erythema; the affected areas show increased warmth as a further expression of hyperemia and pain. As inflammation progresses, scaling becomes the predominant feature.

2. Erysipelatous dermatitis. The signs of inflammation are more severe. There is an extensive, inflammatory cell infiltration of the skin, and the inflamed region is painful.

3. Vesicular and bullous dermatitis. Vesicles and bullae filled with clear fluid appear.

4. Pustular dermatitis. The clear fluid in the vesicles is replaced with purulent material.

5. Weeping dermatitis. The epidermis is broken and the vesicles or pustules rupture, producing a reddened, weeping skin surface.

6. Crusty dermatitis. The exudate dries and hardens, forming crusts. Often violent itching is triggered by these lesions. Exudation is promoted by rubbing, and crusting is increased accordingly. Secondary infection can also be introduced in this manner.

7. Phlegmonous dermatitis. There is suppurative inflammation of the cutis and subcutaneous connective tissue. Such inflammation of the skin always has marked effects on general health.

8. Escharotic and gangrenous dermatitis. This form is marked by tissue necrosis; the necrotic skin assumes a brown to brownish-black color, loses its sensation and feels noticably colder than the surrounding healthy skin. The dead skin becomes demarcated as a foul-smelling mass (moist gangrene) and is sloughed.

The specific precipitating cause is important in determining the degree of inflammation as well as the course of the inflammatory response. For example, in dermatitis due to radiation exposure, the latency period is much longer than in skin inflammation of other causes. Horses are very sensitive to burns of the skin. Shock develops rapidly and can easily take a fatal course. Even with a more favorable course, renal function is often seriously impaired.

In chronic forms of dermatitis, the predominent feature is tissue infiltration, rather than hyperemia with vasodilatation. The skin is rough, has lost part or most of its elasticity, and is more heavily pigmented. It tends to become hypertrophic, developing marked thickenings or wartlike proliferations.

Etiology. Dermatitis can be caused by the action of physical or chemical agents on the skin. A number of pathogens can subsequently enter the skin via the blood or lymph route. Often skin inflammation is the result of mechanical trauma or irritation (traumatic dermatitis). Horses that are restrained, have colic episodes, or CNS diseases, boney prominences, such as the zygomatic arch and supraorbital region, tuber coxae, elbow, etc. are highly susceptible to trauma. Grain stubble and thorny plants can irritate the skin on the limbs, as can close-clipped hairs in the fetlock area. The resulting irritation may not remain superficial and can cause deeper inflammation. Pressure or constriction from tack items must also be considered. 'Interfering', which is observed mainly in the hindlimbs, can also cause abrasion with inflammation as well as a more severe skin injury.

The term toxic dermatitis is often applied when the causal agents are chemical in nature. This form of contact dermatitis has a diverse pathogenesis, because not all offending substances damage the skin directly. This implies that sensitization of the skin may play an etiologic role. Acids, lyes, quicklime, various fertilizers, etc. can cause severe skin changes. Substances such as lubricating oils, soaps, antiseptic and antiparasitic ointments, mustard packs, etc. are probably of greater practical significance. Close contact with the spurge plant *(Euphorbia)* has been cited as a cause of limb dermatitis in horses.

Thermal changes can cause skin inflammation (caloric dermatitis) of varying degrees. Dermatitis due to frostbite is rare at our latitudes. Cold burns with liquid nitrogen are a more likely cause of inflammatory reactions. Scalds or thermal burns may occur as a result of accident or negligence.

Actinic dermatitis is caused by excessive exposure to radiant energy. Solar radiation rarely causes true sunburn in horses. Usually photosensitization must be present for an inflammatory reaction to occur. On excessive exposure to therapeutic UV radiation, dermatitis lesions usually appear within 12 h. Dermatitis due to X-irradiation on the other hand, takes two to three weeks to appear.

Ectoparasites can also cause skin inflammation, which generally takes a more chronic course. Dermatophytes, or skin fungi, are included in this category. Cutaneous streptotrichosis or dermatophilosis caused by *Dermatophilus congolensis* is manifested as a stubborn exudative dermatitis with scale and crust formation.

Of *differential diagnostic* importance are eczema and exanthema. In the case of eczema, unlike dermatitis, the clinical severity is not related to the severity of the cause. The boundary between healthy and affected skin is often indistinct and itching is more intense, therefore there is less pain in eczema.

In the case of exanthema, or skin rash, the inflammatory changes may be similar to those of dermatitis or may remain superficial. The latter more closely resembles eczema. Unlike dermatitis, exanthematous lesions are usually the product of endogenous factors, such as infections (e.g. strangles), poisonings (e.g. selenium, mercury) or allergic reactions. Parasitic and mycotic causes can be excluded by the examination of skin scrapings, especially in chronic cases.

The *diagnosis* is based on the history and clinical examination. The goal is to go beyond a simple diagnosis of dermatitis, because an etiologic diagnosis can almost always be made.

Prognosis. Mild cases heal completely in 8—14 days with suitable treatment, whereas severe inflammatory lesions are very slow to heal. Very severe inflammation may take a fatal course if extensive. Chronic cases are often refractory to treatment.

Treatment. The primary goal of treatment is to identify the causative agent and remove it from the horse's environment.

Early stages require cold packs with Burow's solution, aluminium acetate solution, or alcohol, or the application of commercially available cold cream. For vesiculation or weeping, Stahl's liniment (aqua calcis, oleum lini āā) is the medicament of choice. If secondary infections are present, the ointments or liniments should contain effective antibiotics or sulfonamides. Corticosteroids for relief of inflammation, should be used only in combination with antibiotics.

In phlegmonous dermatitis as well as other severe skin inflammation with systemic signs, parenteral antibiotics are indicated. Circulatory disturbances should be

9 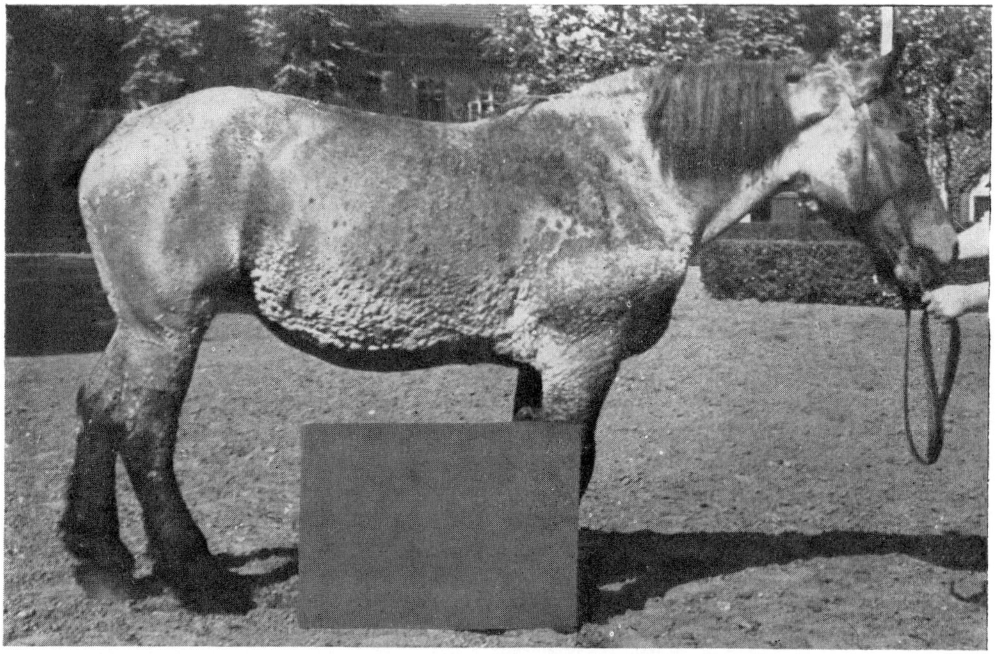

10 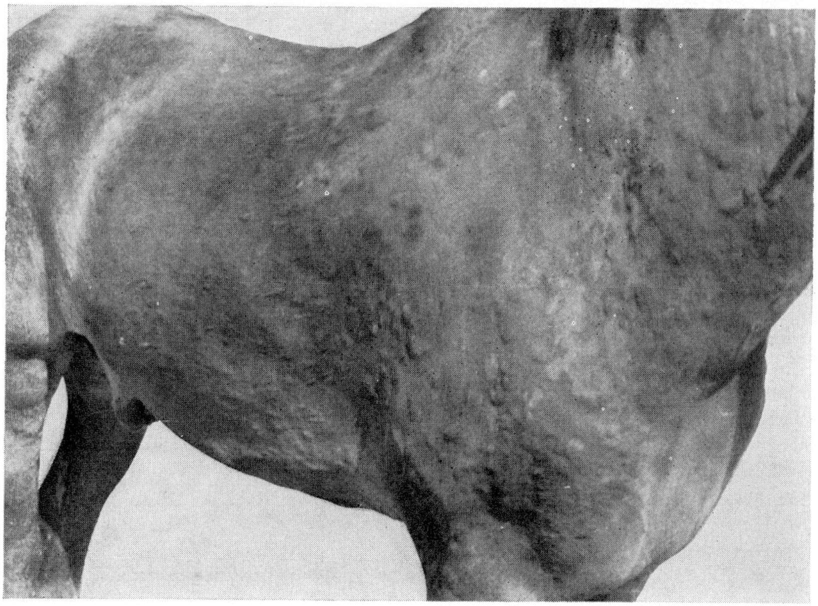

Fig. 2.1.1. — *9.* Urticaria with numerous round wheals in the abdominal region.

Fig. 2.1.1. — *10.* Urticaria, rare form with large, flat welts on the neck and lateral chest and abdominal wall.

corrected if present. Surgery may be indicated in some cases. Crusting and severe drying of inflamed areas can be effectively treated with ointments of cod-liver oil, cod-liver oil and zinc, or boric acid.

Prevention of dermatitis is based upon strict adherence to various work-safety rules as well as to dose recommendations for drug therapy. In doubtful cases, tolerance may be tested by first applying the agent to a small patch of skin.

2.1.1.3.3. Urticaria (Hives, Nettle Rash)

Definition. Urticaria, or nettle rash, refers to the sudden appearance of sharply circumscribed elevations of various shapes on the skin surface. It is caused by a serous infiltration of the skin into the stratum papillare and stratum germinativum (Malpighian layer).

Symptoms. Urticaria is characterized by the sudden appearance of skin wheals, most of which are initially round (fig. 2.1.1. — 9).

Within a few minutes to an hour, the first few lesions may spread to cover the entire trunk. Later the wheals may further change their appearance by becoming confluent, thus forming elevations of varying contour.

The hairs stand erect, especially over the smaller wheals (fig. 2.1.1. — 10). Initial redness is observed only in unpigmented areas. The redness passes quickly, however, and the affected skin tends to be pale at the height of the eruption.

In rare cases exudation of the skin is so massive that the epidermis becomes raised in spots, and vesicles form. In these cases pruritus occurs. With rupture of the vesicles moist skin areas appear, and the secretions dry to form crusts.

An unusual form of nettle rash has been reported in which the wheals appear as parallel, pencil-thick striae on the chest or abdomen (fig. 2.1.1. — 11). On rare occasions this manifestation of the disease is preceded by a short prodromal stage with weakness and fever. Usually it is absent or is too mild to be noticed. Neither is the further course accompanied by significant systemic effects, except in cases where the serous infiltration spreads to the mucous membranes of the eyes, nose, larynx, mouth, vagina and rectum. This severe form is unusual in horses, and if accompanied by pruritus is pathognomonic of an anaphylactic reaction following serum therapy (serum sickness). Primary urticaria caused by contact with stinging nettles may be marked by unrest, tetanic muscle spasms, weak pulse and dyspnea. Finally, urticaria may occur as a sequel to other diseases, such as leptospirosis, requiring that the primary disease symptoms be differentiated.

A special form is dermatographia (urticaria latens or urticaria factitia), in which stroking the skin with a finger or blunt instrument or tapping it with a crop produces immediate localized swelling and redness of the skin. This phenomenon is attributed to vasomotor disturbances. In a cow with this disease, Stöber and Trautwein [1971] were able to demonstrate a marked proliferation of mast cells in the skin.

Etiology. Wheal formation can be triggered by the action of external agents, such as insect bites (bees, wasps, horseflies) or from contact with stinging nettles. The lesions in such cases, are caused by histamine, which may be present in relatively high concentration (up to 0.1 % in stinging nettles). Most cases of urticaria are based on an allergic reaction, usually to an unknown antigen. It may be ingested with the feed or is formed during subsequent digestion, especially when a digestive disturbance is present.

The administration of hyperimmune serum for prophylactic or therapeutic purposes can lead to serum sickness, whose most prominent clinical sign is urticaria.

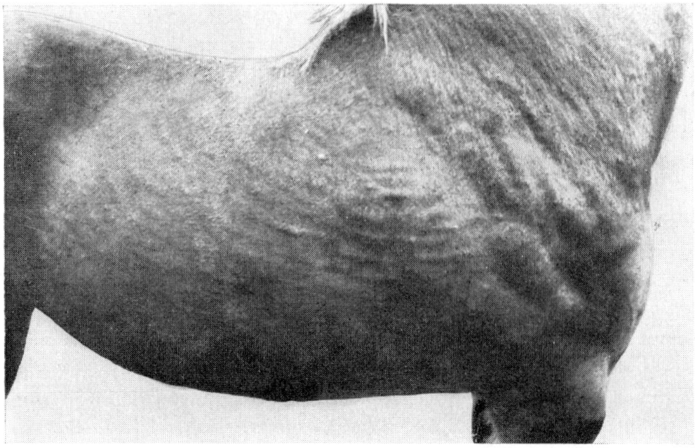

Fig. 2.1.1. — 11. Urticaria with striate wheal pattern.

The term 'serum sickness' is not applied to every type of anaphylactic reaction, only to those that occur some 6—12 days following a single serum injection. The pathogenesis is due to the response by the organism to relatively large serum injections by forming antibodies against the antigenic stimulus. By the time the antibodies are mobilized, there is still enough antigen present that violent antigen-antibody reactions can occur.

Of greater practical importance is urticaria due to the administration of antibiotics and glucocorticoids. Cases of milk allergy (autoallergy) associated with premature weaning as well as cold allergy have also been described in the horse.

Urticaria is also observed as a sequel to bacterial, parasitic and viral infections such as strangles or rhinopneumonitis.

Of greatest *differential diagnostic* importance is hemorrhagic diathesis. In this disease the lesions consist of firm, well-demarcated swellings on the head, abdomen and limbs and may coexist with urticaria. It is also marked by localized swelling and bleeding of the mucous membranes.

The *diagnosis* is readily established by the clinical signs.

Prognosis. As a rule the lesions disappear completely within 12—48 h. In rare cases they may persist for 2—3 weeks; recurrences are rare.

Treatment is usually unnecessary, as the disease is self-limiting. Recovery can be hastened if desired by the infusion of calcium preparations, vitamin C, or the injection of antihistamines or glucocorticoids.

Specific *prophylaxis* is possible only if the antigen is known thereby avoiding further contacts.

2.1.1.3.4. Photosensitization (Solar Dermatitis)

Definition. Photosensitivity is an abnormal cutaneous sensitivity to sunlight. It results from various causes and can lead to severe skin reactions or even a necrotizing dermatitis in extreme cases. Photosensitization occurs only sporadically in the horse.

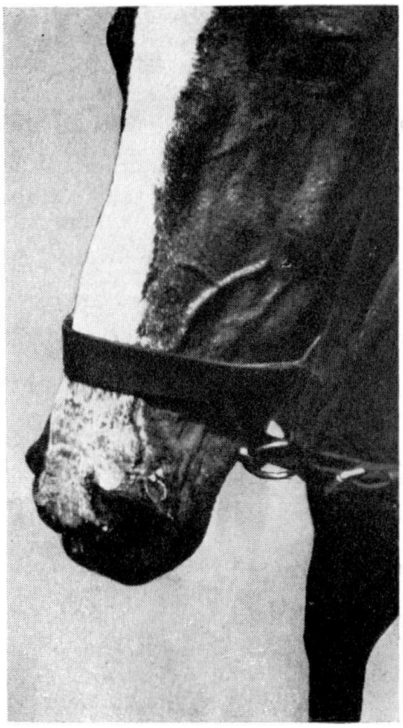

12

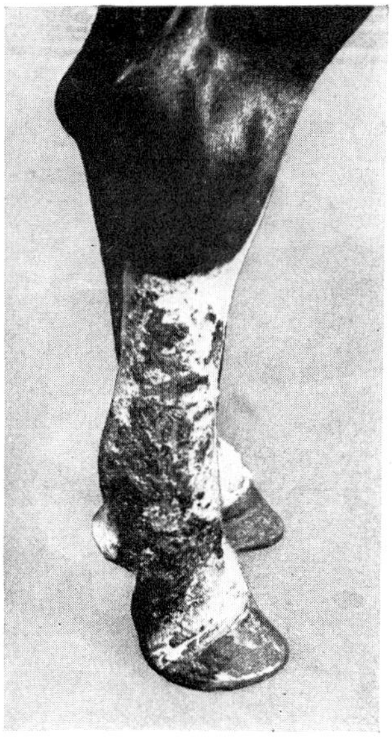

13

Fig. 2.1.1. — 12. Necrotizing dermatitis from photosensitization of the unpigmented skin of the head.

Fig. 2.1.1. — 13. Necrotizing dermatitis from photosensitization of the unpigmented skin of the extremities.

Symptoms. Symptoms develop only in animals that have been exposed to direct sunlight. The first sign is erythematous dermatitis with marked redness, edema and pain. These and all other reactions are restricted to unpigmented skin. The lesions stop abruptly at the boundary between pigmented and unpigmented areas, creating a demarcation between inflamed and normal skin. There are no predilection sites. The typical involvement of parts of the head and limbs in the horse is due to the prevalence of white markings in these regions. In mild cases the erythema, which is also associated with heat and pruritus, persists for several days. After the inflammation has passed there is a period of increased scaling and brownish discoloration.

In severe cases there is an immediate dark-red to bluish-red discoloration of the skin, pronounced swelling, and pain in the affected areas. There is rapid progression to a severe dermatitis, with the formation of vesicles and pustules. These may rupture to form a weeping, greasy surface. Secondary bacterial infection is likely at this stage, and the clinical picture of pyoderma can result.

Often, however, the reaction is so intense that regression of the erythema leaves the skin hard, parchment-like, cool and desensitized. This can also affect the unpigmented skin (figs. 2.1.1. — 12 and — 13). The lesions become demarcated at their edges and are eventually sloughed. This is a very slow process, and consequently there is a long period during which secondary infection can occur. Severe inflammation and bacterial infections involving the lymphatic vessels provoke multiple abscess formation, resulting in septicemia and other systemic signs of varying degrees. Often there is conjunctivitis with mucous membrane involvement. Transitory excitement and disequilibrium are sometimes observed as well.

The abnormalities of liver function may be an extension of the disease process to the liver as well as the primary condition responsible for the photosensitization.

Etiology and Pathogenesis. For a reaction to occur, a photosensitizing substance, either exogenous or endogenous, must be present within the skin. The majority of cases are due to the direct action of a phototoxic substance; a few are caused by a photoallergic agent to which the animal has become sensitized via immunologic mechanisms. The photodynamic agent, which is typically a fluorescent compound, enters the corium. By causing oxidation of the amino acids histidine, tryptophan and tyrosine, it alters the structure and permeability of the cells.

Four basic types of photosensitization can be distinguished according to the source of the photodynamic agent:

1. Primary photosensitization results from the ingestion of plants containing phototoxic compounds. The red fluorescent dye, hypericin, which occurs in St. John's wort *(Hypericum perforatum, H. crispum, H. maculatum, H. pulchrum),* is particularly dangerous for horses. Other phototoxic agents are fagopyrin in buckwheat *(Fagopyrum esculentum)* and phenothiazine, which is converted to phenothiazine sulfoxide in the digestive tract.

2. In hepatogenous or secondary photosensitization, the photodynamic agent is phylloerythrin, a breakdown product of chlorophyll that is formed by bacterial action in the digestive tract. A portion of the phylloerythrin is absorbed by the portal system and subsequently returned to the intestine with the bile. If liver function is impaired, however, the phylloerythrin accumulates in the tissues and may reach levels in the skin which cause the skin to become light-sensitive.

3. Photosensitization of uncertain etiology has been observed in animals fed on legimunous plants, especially lucerne, Swedish clover, vetch, etc., as well as Sudan grass. The photodynamic agent is unknown. Some cases of the disease, also known as trifoliosis, have been attributed to infestation of the green feed with fungi or certain species of aphid.

4. Photosensitization due to aberrant pigment synthesis has been demonstrated in cattle with porphyria but has not been described in horses.

Photosensitivity reactions cannot occur, however, unless the animal is exposed to direct sunlight and certain wavelengths of light strike the photosensitized skin. The wavelengths vary for the different photosensitizing compounds but for the most part occupy the visible range.

Differential diagnosis presents no difficulties as long as the dermatitis is restricted to unpigmented skin areas.

The *diagnosis* can be made from the history and clinical signs. For an etiologic diagnosis, however, it is often necessary to examine the feed for its plant content, perform liver function studies, and question the owner or attendant as to prior drug treatments.

Treatment. Regardless of the precipitating cause, the animals must be placed in a stall, away from direct sunlight, at the first sign of the disease. Plants suspected of causing the photosensitization must be eliminated from the ration. If liver disease is established as the cause, appropriate treatment is initiated.

Corticosteroids and antihistamines should be given parenterally to reduce inflammation and relieve pruritus.

Local treatment is similar for other forms of dermatitis. It should consist of protective ointments, astringents and topical antibiotics. The parenteral administration of antibiotics may be indicated if severe secondary infection is present.

Specific *prophylaxis* is possible only in primary photosensitization. Green feed containing significant amounts of St. John's wort should not be fed, and pastures containing the plant should not be grazed. If this is not possible, measures should at least be taken to shield the animal from direct sunlight during this time.

References

AUSTIN, V. H.: Atopic skin disease. If other treatments fail is hyposensitization the answer. Mod. vet. Pract. *57:* 355 (1976).

BECKER, W.: Über Vorkommen, Ursachen und Behandlung des sogenannten „Sommerekzems" bei Ponys. Ergebnis einer Umfrage. Berliner Münchener tierärztl. Wschr. *77:* 120 (1964).

BELL, T. G.; FARRELL, R. K.: Polarization stress analysis — a method for detecting cryogenic fraud in the horse. Vet. Med. and Small Animal Clinician. *64:* 968 (1969).

BERRY, J. M.; MERRIAM jun., J. G.: Phototoxic dermatitis in a horse. A case report. Veterin. Med. and Small Animal Clinician *65:* 251 (1970).

BINNINGER, C. E.; PIPER, R. C.: Hyperplastic dermatitis of the equine ear. J. Amer. vet. med. Assoc. *153:* 69 (1968).

BREUER, D.: Indikationen und Nebenwirkungen der Corticoidtherapie beim Pferd. Tierärztl. Umschau *28:* 15 (1973).

BRUDNJAK, Z.; ZELENKA, P.; SIBALIN, M.: Prilog poznavanju leptospiroze konja. Vet. Arh. *26:* 165 (1956).

CORREA, J. E.; CALDERIN, G. G.: Anhidrosis, dry coat syndrome in the Thoroughbred. J. Amer. veterin. med. Assoc. *149:* 1556 (1966).

DAM, A.: Om behandling med colikultur of heste mid dermatiter og hudkløe. Medlemsbl. danske Dyrlaegeforen *42:* 300 (1959).

DOM, J.; MORTIMER, P. H.; TAYLOR, A.: Some observations on field of facial eczema. Pathology and determinations of serum bilirubin, cholesterol, transaminase and alkaline phosphatase. Res. Vet. Sci. *1:* 76 (1960).

EKWALL, P.: Hydrocortalsalva mot eksem pa häst med ovanlig lokalisering. Medlemsbl. Sveriges Veterinaerförb. *10:* 68 (1958).

FOWLER, M. E.: Clinical manifestations of promerary hepatic insufficiency in the horse. J. Amer. vet. Med. Assoc. *147:* 55 (1965).

GERBER, H.: Nebenwirkungen von Kortikosteroid-Behandlungen beim Grosstier. Schweiz. Arch. Tierheilk. *112:* 51 (1970).

GUILHON, J.: Alopecie psycho-somatique des animaux domestiques. Rec. Méd. Vét. *138:* 839 (1962).

HALLIWELL, R. E. W.: Pathogenesis and treatment of pruritis. J. Amer. veterin. med. Assoc. *164:* 793 (1974).

KAPLAN, W.; JOHNSTON, W. J.: Equine dermatophilosis (cutaneous streptotrichosis) in Georgia. J. Amer. veterin. med. Assoc. *149:* 1162 (1966).

KELLEY, D. C.; KNAPPENBERGER, T. E.: Cutaneous streptotrichosis (equine dermatophilosis) in Kansas horses. Vet. Med. and Small Animal Clinician *63:* 1055 (1968).

KOETSVELD, E. E. VAN; HAMININK, A. J. B.; ZEGWAARD, A.: Een onderzock naar de corzaken van het manenen staart eczem bij paarden. II. Analyse van bloed, urine, faeces en manen. Tijdschr. Diergeneeskd. *85:* 381 (1960).

KOETSVELD, E. E. VAN; LEHR, J. J.; GRASHNIS, J.: Een onderzock naar de corzaken van het manenen staarteczem bij paarden. I. Gronden gewasonderzock. Tijdschr. Diergeneeskd. *85:* 246 (1960).

KRÁL, F.: Grundsätze der Behandlung der Hautkrankheiten bei Haustieren. Kleintier-Praxis *5:* 1 (1960).

KRÁL, F.; SCHWARTZMAN, R. M.: Veterinary and comparative dermatology, 2nd ed. (Lippincott, Philadelphia 1964).

LANG, E.; SENDIL, C.: Hypericum crispum, die Ursache einer bei Pflanzenfressern in der Türkei beobachteten Lichtkrankheit. Tierärztl. Umschau *26:* 73 (1971).

MANSSON, J.; NILÉHN, P.-O.: Tarmfloran hos tva fall av man — ocj svansskorv hos häst. Nord. Vet.-Med. *10:* 709 (1958).

MAPLESDEN, D. C.; COTE, J. F.; MITCHELL, D.: Allergy in a horse. J. Amer. vet. med. Assoc. *128:* 152 (1956).

MCCAIG, J.: A survey to establish the incidence of sweet itch in ponies in the United Kingdom. Vet. Rec. *93:* 444 (1973).

MEIJER, W. C.: Vitiligo bij paarden en runderen. Tijdschr. Diergeneeskd. *87:* 411 (1962).

MEIJER, W. C.: Verkregen en aangeboren depigmentaties bij de huisdieren gezien in het licht van de recente stand der humane dermatologie. Tijdschr. Diergeneeskd. *87:* 1305 (1962).
MEIJER, W. C.: Dermatological diagnosis in horse and cattle judging. Vet. Rec. *77:* 1046 (1965).
MEIJER, W. C.: Pigmentverlust des Integumentes und die dermatologische Diagnose bei der Beurteilung von Pferden und Rindern. Dtsch. tierärztl. Wschr. *73:* 85 (1966).
MELLOR, P. S.; MCCAIG, J.: The propable cause of 'sweet itch' in England. Vet. Rec. *95:* 411 (1974).
MODRAKOWSKI, A.: Powstawanie tzw. grudy u koni. Med. Weteryn. *11:* 161 (1962).
NILSSON, S. A.: Om behandling med kolikultur av man-och svanskorv och andra dermatoser hos häst. Nord. Vet.-Med. *10:* 82 (1958).
NORDSTRÖM, G.: Man-och svansklada hos häst. Medlemsbl. Sveriges Veterinaerförb. *7:* 95 (1955).
PASCOE, R. R.: The nature and treatment of skin conditions observed in horses in Queensland. Austral. vet. J. *49:* 35 (1973).
RAGHAVAN, R. S.; SUDHIR CHANDRA REDDY, V.; AHMED KHAN, N.: Clinical trials of 'Ekzebrol' in the treatment of eczema and eczematoid conditions in animals. Indian vet. J. *45:* 603 (1968).
RUSCH, K.; LATORRE, G.: Photosensibilitätsreaktion beim Pferd. Tierärztl. Umschau *28:* 436 (1973).
SAFER, E. D.; JONES, H. L.; ZIMMERMANN, O.: Management of dermatologic condition in animals. A review. Vet. Med. and Small Animal Clinician *60:* 1028 (1965).
SCHAAF, A. VAN DER: Geografische verbreiding van enkele huidziekten bij landbouwhuisdieren on de hiervoor verantwoordelijke omgeringsfactoren. Tijdschr. Diergeneeskd. *92:* 1139 (1967).
SCHUKLIN, N. F.: Patogeneticeskaja terapija seborrejnych ekzem n losadej. Veterinarija *35:* 11, 45 (1958).
STANKIEWICZ, S.: Choroby powloki skörnej uzwierzat. Warszawa 1966.
STANNARD, A. A.: Some important dermatoses in the horse. Mod. vet. Pract. *53:* 8, 31 (1972).
STÖBER, M.; TRAUTWEIN, G.: Dermographismus (Urticaria factica) bei einer Kuh. Dtsch. tierärztl. Wschr. *78:* 55 (1971).
VIND, R.: Et tilfaelde af hypericismus hos hest. Nord. Vet.-Med. *9:* 322 (1957).
WALTON, G. S.: Skin diseases of domestic animals. I. Skin manifestations of allergic response in domestic animals. Vet. Res. *82:* 204 (1968).

2.1.1.4. Tumors and Neoplasms

2.1.1.4.1. Disturbances of Keratinization (Hyper- and Parakeratosis)

Definition. Two forms of abnormal keratinization occur in the horse. Excessive keratinization, usually associated with a thickening of the skin and connective tissue proliferation, is called hyperkeratosis. Incomplete keratinization is called parakeratosis. It occurs in pigs as a result of dietary zinc deficiency but does not affect horses.

Symptoms and Occurrence. Hyperkeratosis in the horse tends to occur at sites that are continually subjected to pressure from tack or over boney prominences. The affected area may range from a few centimeters to palm-size and is devoid of hair. The skin surface appears horny, and if the keratinized surface is not smooth, cracks or fissures may form. The skin in these areas always shows a four- to five-fold increase in thickness. Very small, circumscribed, hyperkeratinized areas resemble a callus and are called tylomas. The surface of the hyperkeratosis, scleroderma or tyloma lesion (fig. 2.1.1. — 14) is usually grayish-black in color. Hyperkeratoses and tylomas are not usually hot or painful. Their sensation is apparently reduced as a result of the heavy keratinization. No systemic signs occur. Such lesions are regarded as cosmetic defects.

Etiology. Hyperkeratosis develops at sites that are continually subjected to moderate pressure. Grossly there is no extravasation of blood. Hyperkeratosis is most frequently observed below the harness and occasionally on the anterior aspect of the carpal joint, and medial aspect of the fetlock joint (where it forms scarlike fibrous thickenings involving the skin and subcutis). In standardbreds it occurs on the medial surface of the third metacarpal (cannon) bone and carpal joint. Sclerodermatous and hyperkeratotic changes of the skin and subcutis are occasionally found over shoe boils and on the posterior surface of the tuber calcis. Repeated mild contusions are also the cause.

Diagnosis and Differential Diagnosis. The diagnosis is easily made on the basis of symptoms. Neoplasms occurring at atypical sites may be mistaken for hyperkeratosis.

Treatment and Prognosis. Because most forms of hyperkeratosis are cosmetic defects, surgical excision is indicated only if inflammation or infection is present. Many lesions heal promptly once their stimulus has been safely and permanently removed. Removal of the inciting cause is also indicated in cases of extensive hyperkeratosis, where excision would necessitate skin grafting to cover the wound.

Prophylaxis. Hyperkeratoses of the fetlock and carpal joints in athletic horses can be prevented by the use of suitable protective gear made of soft leather, especially if interfering is the cause. Hyperkeratoses at the olecranon are best prevented by providing soft bedding and, if necessary, by shortening the branches of the offending shoe.

2.1.1.4.2. Cutaneous Horns, Keratoma (Cornu Cutaneum)

Definition. Cutaneous horns are malformations of the skin that are generally acquired. On rare occasions they may be congenital. These growths are 'horns' in name only. The keratoma consists of a small, fibrous papillary body. The overlying epithelium undergoes marked proliferation, becomes keratinized and forms clawlike or hornlike processes. Keratomas are extremely rare in the horse.

Symptoms. Bulbous or hornlike growths appear on the skin of the head, neck or limbs. They may attain a length of up to 20 cm in some cases. They may be firmly anchored to their bed or may hang pendulously in a skin fold, depending on their internal structure. Cutaneous horns of the head occur most frequently on the dorsum of the nose, eyelids, lips, ears, intermaxillary area and lower neck.

The internal hemispherical or conical keratomous portion has a firm fibrous consistency. It shows no villi or laminae like those occurring, for example, in layers of the hoof. The heavily keratinized epidermal portion is elastic, sometimes scaly, friable, and shows varying degrees of thickening.

Prognosis and Treatment. The prognosis is always good. Cutaneous horns are cosmetic defects. They are surgically removed from their subcutaneous bed by making a circular or elliptical skin incision about the growth. The resulting skin wound is sutured. Skin grafts or relaxing incisions are rarely necessary.

2.1.1.4.3. Cutaneous Neoplasms

Definition. Neoplasm of the skin and subcutaneous tissue may be benign, semimalignant or malignant in nature. Tumors may be caused by infections agents, such as papillomatosis and possibly equine sarcoid.

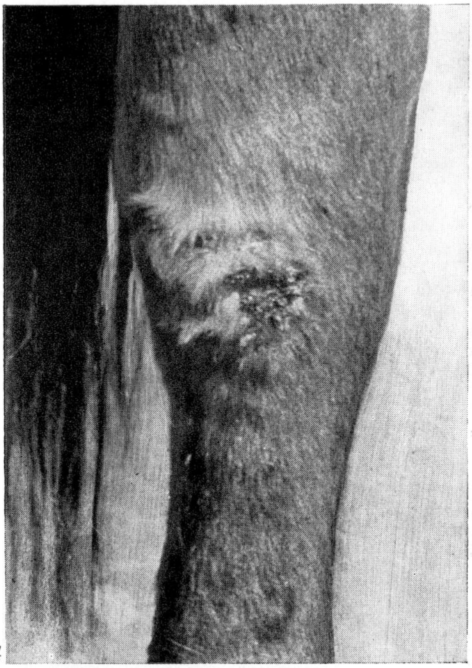
14

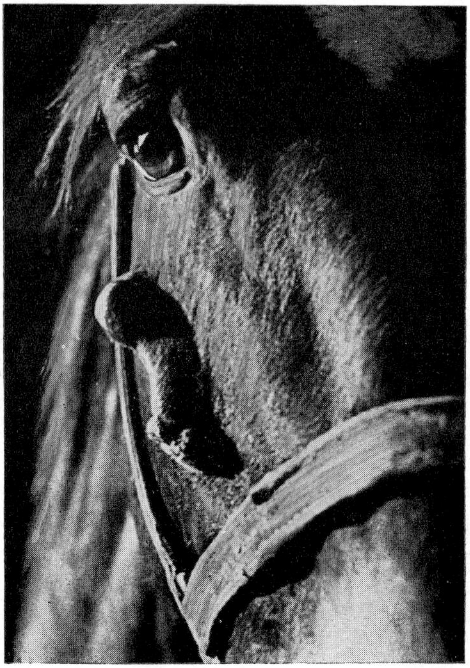
15

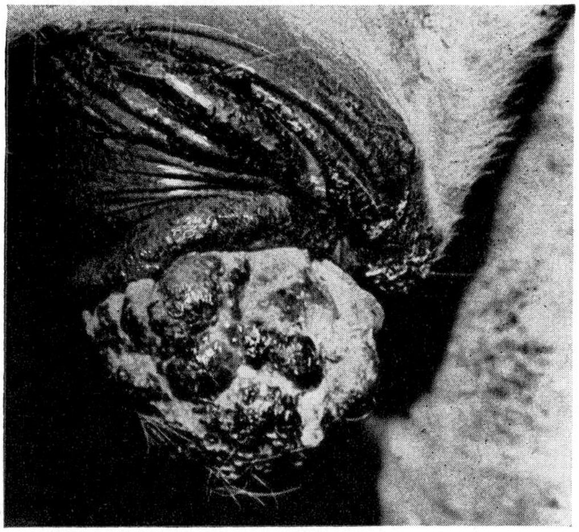
16

Fig. 2.1.1. — 14. Tyloma (rasp).
Fig. 2.1.1. — 15. Papilloma on the zygomatic arch.
Fig. 2.1.1. — 16. Papilloma of the penis.

Papilloma

Symptoms. Solitary papillomas are comprised of a fibrous papillary base with a hoodlike covering of dense, keratinized epithelial layers. The surface is very often cracked and fissured. There are also cases in which the conical papillae are individually covered by epithelium. The resulting mass has an irregular surface resembling a raspberry, cauliflower or bunch of grapes. Such papillomas may have either a broad or pedunculated attachment.

The keratoma or cutaneous horn is comprised of a small fibrous papillary body. The overlying epithelium shows marked proliferation, is keratinized and forms claw-like or hornlike processes. Such growths are found in older horses on the dorsum of the nose, upper eyelid, and sometimes on the lips, the ear (where they hang from the border of the pinna), the intermaxillary area and the neck.

Papillomas and cutaneous horns can be moved about in the skin. Sometimes they are pigmented. They vary greatly in size; papillomas may be as small as a pea or twice the size of a fist (figs. 2.1.1. — 15 and — 16). External trauma can cause the epithelium of the papilloma (or wart, as the case may be) to become detached, forming ulcerated wounds covered with a foul-smelling pus. Solitary papillomas, warts and cutaneous horns grow slowly. If they are forcibly avulsed, their rich vascularization will result in bleeding. Papillomas may show a more rapid growth (and be mistaken fo r malignant tumors) if they are partially removed, when these growths are tied off, twisted off and superficially cauterized.

Treatment and Prognosis. Warts, papillomas and cutaneous horns have a generally good prognosis. The tumors are excised under local or general anesthesia by cutting around their base and extirpating them. Skin grafting may be necessary in some instances to achieve adequate wound repair. Primary healing should be the goal and ntention in every case.

Fibroma

Definition. The fibroma is a tumor that arises from the subcutaneous tissue. It is composed of maturing connective-tissue cells and a fibrillary intercellular substance.

Symptoms. Fibromas in the horse occur in many forms (fig. 2.1.1. — 7). They can arise in the subcutaneous tissue anywhere on the body. They grow slowly, displacing the surrounding tissue, and vary greatly in size. Some fibromas are no bigger than a pea, while others are as large as a man's head. The tumor may be rounded, nodular or tuberous in appearance. It is rarely pedunculated but may be lobulated. It is always well circumscribed and seldom shows a diffuse growth pattern. Even on clinical examination variations in tumor consistency may be noted. Fibromas that are uniformly hard and firm are designated by the term *fibroma durum*, or hard fibroma. Other fibromas are very soft, lipoma-like and edematous; these are called *fibroma molle*, or soft fibroma. Fibromas are painless when palpated. Unlike the papilloma, the surface of the fibroma is always smooth. The haircoat over the fibroma appears intact, though individual hairs may be shed. At operation the neoplasm is found to be walled off from the remaining loose connective tissue by a firm fibrous capsule. When cut, the fibroma durum presents a grayish-white surface with a filamentous, sinewy tecture, a dull or lard-like luster, and is poorly vascularized. There are also fibromas which, when cut, show individual closely-packed nodules of varying size that are held together by more loose, healthy fibrous tissue. These are easily shelled out of their capsule. Sometimes the tumor tissue has a gritty texture whencut. The fibroma molle is also grayish-white on its cut surface but is gelatinous and very moist. Tissue fluid escapes from the network of fluid-filled lacunae and drips from the cut surface. There are also solitary fibromas of the skin that are attached by a long cutaneous pedicle (fibroma pendulans). In the horse they occur on the head, the eyelids, the prepuce, in the stifle fold, and on the medial and anterior surface of the thigh.

Treatment and Prognosis. The prognosis is always good. The excision must be carried deep into the subcutaneous tissue. With a wide, deep excision, the chances of recurrence should be minimized and primary healing should result.

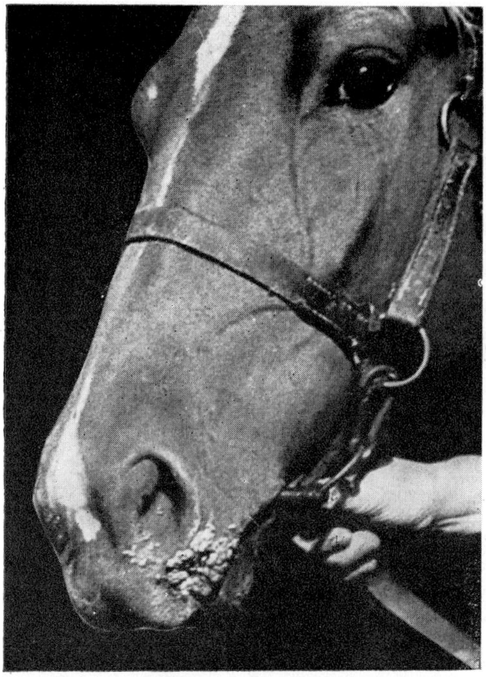
17

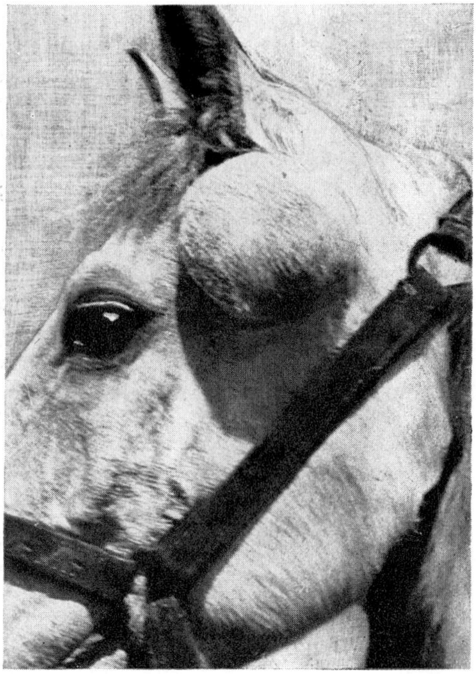
18

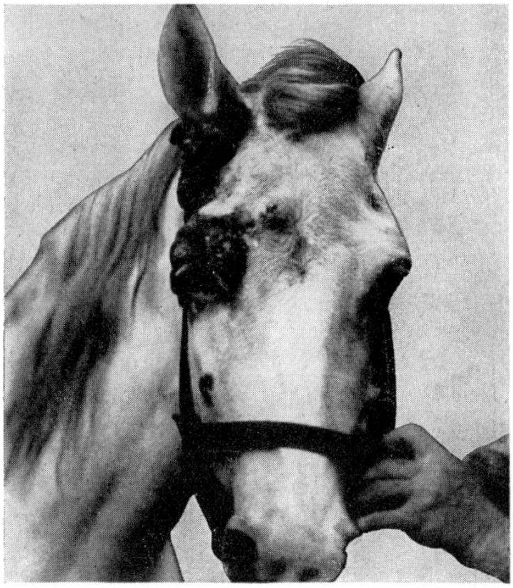
19

Fig. 2.1.1. — 17. Juvenile fibromatosis.
Fig. 2.1.1. — 18. Melanoma at the base of the ear.
Fig. 2.1.1. — 19. Melanoma of the ear.

Semimalignant and Malignant Tumors of the Skin

Melanoma

Definition. A melanoma is a neoplasm of melanocytes (melanin-containing cells). The tumor may follow a benign or malignant course depending on its degree of differentiation.

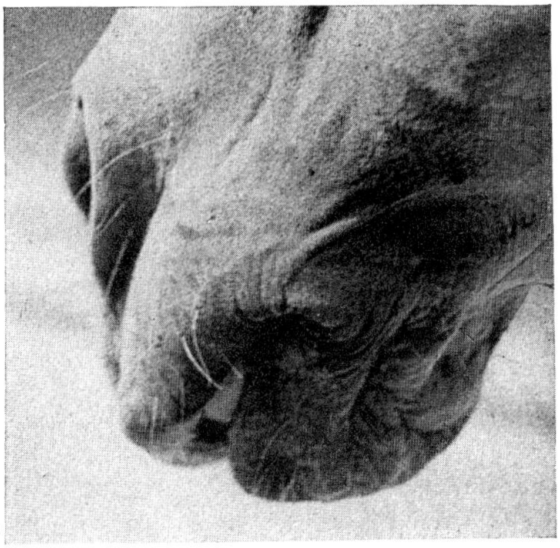

20

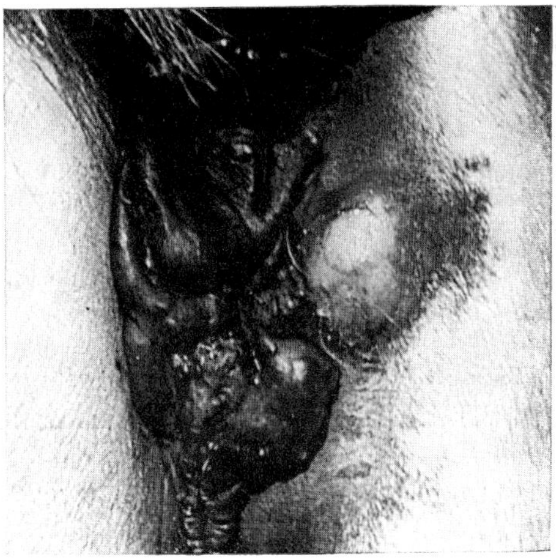

21

Fig. 2.1.1. — 20. Melanosarcoma of the lip.
Fig. 2.1.1. — 21. Melanosarcoma of the perineal region.

Symptoms. Melanomas occur most frequently in gray horses. Occasionally they are found in horses of other hair color (bay, brown, black). Melanomas are extremely rare in horses less than 5 or 6 years of age. The older gray or black and white (piebald) horse is the most likely to develope melanomas. It is reported that up to 80% of gray horses more than 15 years old develop melanomas. Also interesting is the absence of breed predilection; i.e., grays of the English Thoroughbred breed, grays of the American, French and Russian trotting breeds, and cold-blooded grays are at equal risk for the disease. No sex predilection has been observed.

Benign and malignant melanomas can occur anywhere on the body. However, there are sites of predilection. The most frequent sites are the undersurface of the tail near its root, the perineal and perianal regions, and on the head below the entrance to the outer ear and on the ear margin (figs. 2.1.1. — 18 and — 19). The parotid region is another common site.

Melanomas are usually solitary in their early stage. Initially they appear as small lumps, and the overlying skin is blackened but intact. Soon, small metastases arise near the primary one. All appear to lie within the skin, and the overlying cutis appears intact. These tumors, which reach the size of a cherry or walnut, may remain quiescent for months or even years, representing little more than cosmetic defects. They may be troublesome if situated around the anus or under the halter.

Pedunculated melanomas are usually benign and should be removed only if absolutely necessary. Such melanomas can suddenly start to grow after months or years of quiescence, erupting through the skin surface. Some fluctuation is sometimes present prior to such eruption. Rupture of these lesions, either spontaneous or artificial, liberates a brownish-black, odorless fluid. This leaves ulcerated skin areas which histologically appear as malignant melanomas or melanosarcomas (figs. 2.1.2. — 20 and — 21).

Solitary melanomas occurring in the perineal region or on the head may remain quiescent for years, showing no metastases, while other apparently benign melanomas may suddenly become malignant especially when subjected to slight mechanical irritation. Finally, there is a third pattern of development in which the melanoma

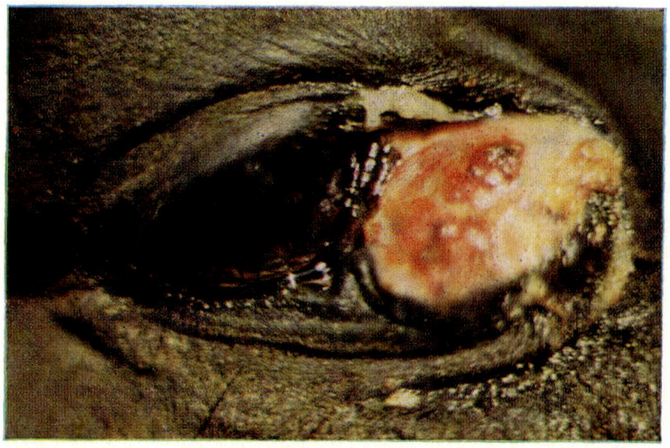

Fig. 2.1.1. — 22. Squamous-cell carcinoma of the nictating membrane.

is obviously malignant from the start. These melanomas spread quickly via the lymphatics to the reginal lymph nodes. Countless small growths arise along the lymph channels. These lead to very rapid metastasis, with growths occurring on serosal surfaces (especially on the peritoneum but also on the pleura), in the lymph nodes of the gastrointestinal tract, and in the liver, lungs and spleen. The metastatic growths are usually much larger than the primary tumor and always have a soft consistency. Even with such metastases, general weakness and cachexia do not develop until late in the course of the disease. Death results from general debility associated with the widespread metastases.

Treatment and Prognosis. The prognosis is good for solitary melanomas in the perineal or head region, provided they have remained quiescent for some years and there is no irritation at or near the tumor site. Such growths in the horse should be left alone.

If the overlying skin has been disrupted and there is ulceration, radical surgical treatment is recommended. However, radical surgery is generally effective only in the case of solitary melanomas. With multiple melanomas involving the anal, vaginal, ear or parotid region that are associated with edematous swelling and discoloration, surgery should not be attempted. The horse can be kept alive until signs of general metastasis and cachexia appear. In radical operations for the removal of a solitary but irritating melanoma, it is always wise to remove the regional lymph nodes as well. A survival time of 3—5 years can be obtained in this way. When metastases have occurred, melanosarcoma is often diagnosed histopathologically. Treatment with cytotoxic drugs has not proved effective for either solitary melanomas or ones with metastases.

Carcinoma

Definition. The carcinoma is a malignant, highly infiltrative neoplasm of epithelial origin. The parenchyma of such tumors consist of epithelial cells of the skin, mucous membrane or glands, or of embryonic rests of epithelialized cysts. A scirrhous carcinoma is one in which the stroma is dense and fibrous. A medullary carcinoma is soft and mainly parenchymal with little stroma. Carcinomas may be described according to their epithelial origin as squamous-cell carcinomas, cylindrical-cell carcinomas or adenocarcinomas. These types often can be distinguished clinically. The columnar-cell carcinoma arises from the epithelium of the mucous membranes or from the rests of columnar epithelial cells. Because these epithelial cells are often still capable of forming mucus, such neoplasms are also called mucinous or colloid carcinomas.

Symptoms. All carcinomas grow by infiltration. In the horse as in other species, they are most frequent in the third quarter of life, becoming less common in old age. They may arise on the head, neck, back, penis, clitoris, prepuce, scrotum, anal region and undersurface of the tail. Carcinomas of the mucous membranes are observed on the tongue, on the lips, in the pharynx, and on the preputial mucosa. Squamous-cell carcinomas of the nictating membrane are not infrequent in the horse (fig. 2.1.1. — 22). These tumors can spread quickly to the cornea, the rest of the globe and the orbit. Carcinomas of the maxillary sinus of the horse may arise from the gingiva, the hard palate, or the epithelial rests of the embryonic enamel organ located in the periodontium.

Like other tumors, the carcinoma begins as a nodule. These nodules feel hard when the stroma is dense, and soft when the neoplasm is of the medullary type. In the typical rapidly-growing carcinoma there is a constant alternation between growth and degeneration. The surface becomes ulcerated and may resemble exuberant granulation. Two types of skin cancer may be distinguished. The first is raised, granulation-tissue-like growths that widely infiltrates and adheres to the skin with a broad base or pedicle projecting above the skin surface. The other type of skin tumor appears as pitted or craterlike ulcerous lesions. They secrete a malodorous fluid. The tissue shows a bluish-red discoloration and bleeds easily. Decomposition occurs readily. The edges of such carcinomas are undermined and eroded. Carcinomas of the hard palate or maxillary sinus form fistulas extending into the bone. The removal of biopsy material provokes bleeding that may be difficult to control. With skin cancers there is usually involvement of the regional lymph nodes. Carcinomas spread mainly via the lymphatics, although blood spread also occurs. The primary sites of metastases are the lung, liver, spleen, kidneys, adrenal glands, ovaries and their lymph nodes. Later, metastases may spread to the pleura, peritoneum, omentum, stomach, intestine, bone and other skin sites. Involvement of the brain and spinal cord is also possible. Interestingly, squamous cell carcinomas of the third eyelid and penis rarely metastasize. 'Contact tumors' arise in areas that are in prolonged contact with a skin or mucous-membrane carcinoma and occur most commonly between the thighs and on the eyelids, lips, vulva and preputial mucosa.

Cancer cachexia has a very slow onset in the horse. There is a gradual weight loss over a period of weeks or months, accompanied by a corresponding loss of working capacity. When cachexia is advanced, the animal must be destroyed.

Diagnosis. Only the histologic examination of biopsy material obtained pre- or intraoperatively provides an accurate diagnosis.

Prognosis. The prognosis is generally poor. In the case of a squamous-cell carcinoma of the third eyelid, surgical excision is possible in the early stage. For carcinomas in other sites, surgery can afford improvement and prolong life, but only until there is a recurrence or metastasis.

Treatment. Wide surgical excision is preferred. Where local anatomy permits, concurrent removal of the regional lymph nodes is also indicated. Compared with man, radiation therapy has received relatively little attention in the horse. Chemotherapy or the use of cytotoxic drugs has failed to produce a breakthrough in the treatment of equine carcinomas.

Lymphosarcoma

Definition. Lymphosarcomas arise from lymphatic tissue and can develop anywhere on the body where such tissue occurs. They are composed of lymphocytic cells in a vascularized network. In the horse lymphosarcoma can grow from subcutaneous

23 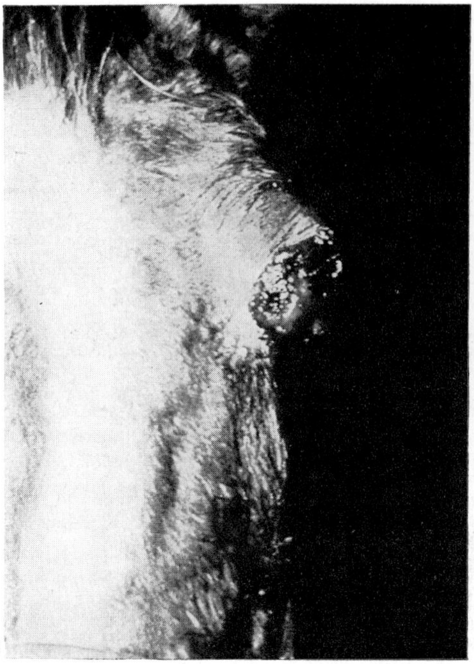

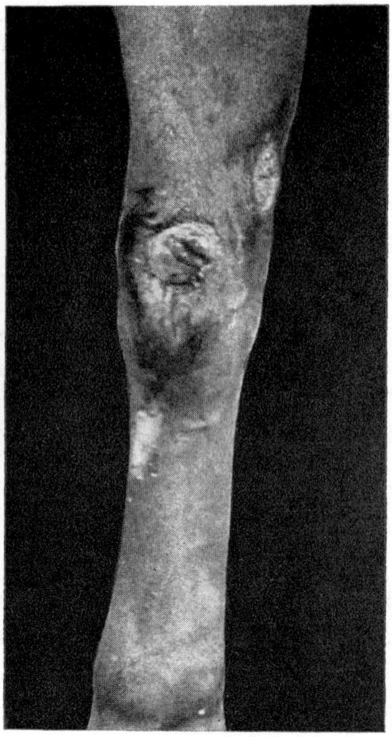 24

Fig. 2.1.1. — 23. Lymphosarcoma of the orbit.
Fig. 2.1.1. — 24. Sarcoma of the carpus (healed).

lymph nodes or other lymphatic tissue and spread rapidly by nodular or diffuse infiltration. Horses more than 5 years old are usually affected.

Symptoms. The lesions consist of one or more varying-sized subcutaneous nodules, sometimes occurring as broad swellings that show diffuse or multiple nodular infiltration. Initially there are no systemic effects, but anorexia, weight loss and depression gradually ensue. The nodules usually are fairly generalized, appearing on the head, neck, shoulder, lateral thorax, flank, and subcutaneous tissue of the croup and thigh (figs. 2.1.1. — 23 and — 24).

Diagnosis. Diagnosis is based on the histologic examination of biopsy material. The hemogram may show atypical lymphocytes in the peripheral blood.

Prognosis and Treatment. The prognosis is poor. Although chemotherapy has afforded good results in the treatment of lymphosarcoma in man and lab animals, such treatment is unprofitable in the horse and cannot be recommended. Theoretically it may prolong life, but it cannot produce a permanent cure. Affected horses should be destroyed.

References

Bolz, W.; Dietz, O.: Lehrbuch der Allgemeinen Chirurgie für Tierärzte (VEB Gustav Fischer Verlag, Jena 1970).

Cardeihac, P. T.: Recent approaches to the treatment of neoplastic disease in animals. J. Amer. vet. med. Assoc. *156* (1970).

CONROY, J. D.: Melanotic tumors of domestic animals. Arch. Dermatol. *96:* 372 (1967).
COTCHIN, E.: Tumors of farm animals. Vet. Rec. *72:* 816 (1960).
MANKRULKAR, M. Y.: Melanomata in domesticated animals. Indian J. Vet. Med. *14:* 178 (1944).
MCFADYAN, J.: Equine melanomatosis. J. Comp. Pathol. *46:* 186 (1933).
MOSTAFA, M. S. E.: A case of malignant melanoma in a bay horse. Brit. Vet. J. *109:* 201 (1953).
MOULTON, J. E.: Tumors in Domestic Animals (University of California Press, Berkeley 1961).
RUNNELLS, R. A.; BENBROOK, E. A.: Malignant melanomas of horses and mules. Amer. J. Vet. Res. *2:* 340 (1941).
RUNNELLS, R. A.; BENBROCK, E. A.: Epithelial tumors of horse. Amer. J. Vet. Res. *3:* 176 (1942).
RUNNELLS, R. A.; BENBROCK, E. A.: Malignant lymphoid tumors in horses. J. Amer. vet. med. Assoc. *104:* 148 (1944).
SCHEBITZ, H.; BRASS, W.: Allgemeine Chirurgie für Tierärzte und Studierende (Parey, Berlin 1975).
THEILEN, G. H.; FOWLER, A. E.: Lymphosarcoma (lymphocytic leukemia) in the horse. J. Amer. Vet. Med. Assoc. *140:* 923 (1962).
ÜBERREITER, O.: Über das Vorkommen und Behandlungserfolge von Neubildungen bei Tieren (Hund, Katze, Pferd). Zbl. Vet.-Med. R. A. *12:* 711 (1965).
ÜBERREITER, O.: Klinische Krebsforschung bei Tieren. Fortschritte der Veterinärmedizin, Heft 27 (Parey, Berlin 1977).

2.1.1.5. Diseases of the Subcutaneous Tissue

2.1.1.5.1. Subcutaneous Emphysema

Definition. This term denotes the accumulation of air in the subcutaneous connective tissue.

Symptoms. A small puncture or incised wound that communicates with a large wound cavity can allow air to enter the loose subcutaneous connective tissue and accumulate. Such small wounds are sealed rapidly by blood or exudate, and the air that has entered the subcutaneous connective tissue is displaced into the adjacent loose subcutaneous and intermuscular tissue. Owing to the spaces in the subcutaneous connective tissue, the entrapped air causes the skin to balloon outward, forming obvious swelling.

Subcutaneous emphysema can spread over a large area within a matter of hours. This results in a loss of normal body contours, and affected areas take on a bloated appearance. Natural depressions are obliterated. From the loose skin in the area of the elbow joint or stifle fold, the air can spread beneath the skin of the lateral thoracic wall or flank region. Even small wounds in the submaxillary region can cause air accumulation in the lateral and lower neck area and jugular furrow. On palpation the swellings feel soft, elastic and puffy; they are crepitant when stroked. The entrapped air moves about when pressure is applied. There is generally no pain. The swollen areas feel cold to the touch. Percussion of the skin elicits a dull, tympanitic sound. Emphysema in the horse usually occurs in areas where the skin is freely mobile owing to very loose connective tissue. Small wounds can alternately open and close as the skin is stretched and relaxed, sporadically aspirating additional air. If such wounds are located on the limbs, neck, head or thorax, extensive emphysema can rapidly develop. Wounds in the inguinal region can lead to emphysema of the ventral abdomen.

Emphysema of the head can also result from trephination of the maxillary, nasal or frontal sinus. Similarly, subcutaneous emphysema can develop on the side of the neck following surgery of the guttural pouch.

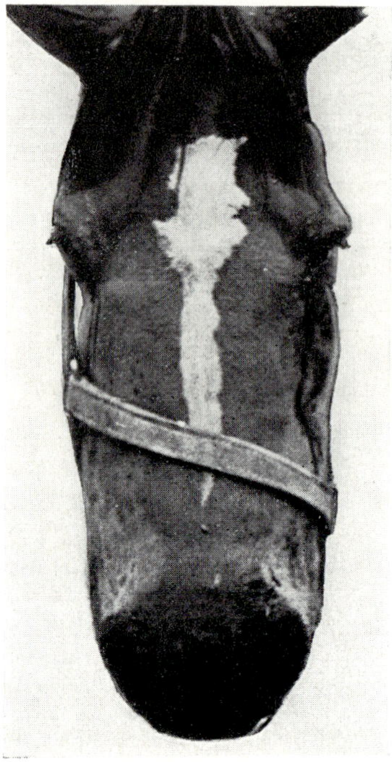

25

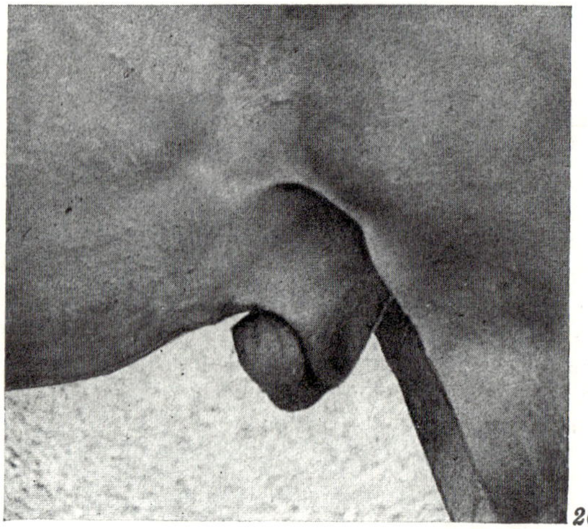

26

Fig. 2.1.1. — 25. Edema of the head ('hippopotamus head').
Fig. 2.1.1. — 26. Preputial edema.

Subcutaneous emphysema is usually not accompanied by systemic signs. The layman often considers emphysema as a grave condition because it is so disfiguring. As a rule, subcutaneous emphysema develops during the first 3 to 4 days following a puncture wound or laceration. Once the wound has closed or the wound cavity has become fully granulated, further emphysema formation ceases.

Etiology. The primary cause of subcutaneous emphysema is invariably a wound inflicted by a sharp object. The wound may be surgical or accidental.

Differential Diagnosis. The possibility of a clostridial infection (gas gangrene) must always be considered. In contrast to subcutaneous emphysema, gas gangrene produces severe systemic signs with fever, localized pain and increased warmth. In addition, a clostridial infection spreads much more rapidly than the emphysema.

Prognosis. The prognosis of subcutanous emphysema is generally good. The entrapped air causes no tissue damage and will be absorbed once the access wound is closed.

Treatment. Small puncture or incised wounds are extended to allow the entrapped air to escape, if anatomic circumstances permit. If not, the wounds should be securely closed by suturing or by packing and suturing. We do not recommended incising swollen skin areas with the object of releasing the entrapped air, as this predisposes to infection. Rarely is the swelling so severe as to interfere with the local blood supply and cause circumscribed skin necrosis. If this occurs, one should administer antibiotics while awaiting demarcation of the ischemic area. If emphysema cannot be distinguished from an infection with a gas producing organism the administration of polyvalent clostridial antiserum is indicated as a precaution.

2.1.1.5.2. Subcutaneous Edema

Definition. Subcutaneous edema is an accumulation of serous fluid in the subcutaneous connective tissue.

Symptoms. Subcutaneous edema is marked by visible swelling. The limbs, for example, show a cylindrical thickening with a loss of articular contours. In edema of the ventral abdomen there is a patchy swelling from the sternum to the prepuce or udder. In preputial edema the internal layer of the prepuce is swollen and prolapsed. Edema of the head (fig. 2.1.1. — 25) is characterized by enlargement of facial contours. Edematous swellings (except for the inflammatory type) are painless, cold and pit easily on pressure. The edematous fluid can be massaged about in the subcutaneous tissue. Early edema of the back is sometimes 'mushy', mimicking a fluctuant swelling. If the skin over an edema is ruptured or incised, a yellow to white fluid oozes from the cut surface, or light-yellow to colorless beads of secretion are exuded. Sometimes the fluid spurts from the congested lymph vessels in a thin stream. The tapping of an edema usually yields only a few drops of fluid.

Systemic signs are absent in most cases of subcutaneous edema.

Etiology. It is useful to distinguish three basic types of subcutaneous edema:

Obstructive edema is caused by either venous stasis or obstructed lymph drainage and affects, for example, the limbs and prepuce (fig. 2.1.1. — 26). Subcutaneous edema of the ventral abdomen is also of the obstructive type. It occurs in horses with chronic myocardial disease or, less commonly, renal disease. Obstructive edema may also affect the vulva, limbs, ventral abdomen and udder of mares that are about to foal. Obstructive edema of the limbs is a frequent result of excessivly tight bandages. 'Autumn legs' or 'winter legs' is a term applied to obstructive edema of the hindlimbs of the horse; it, too, results from venous stasis or lymphatic obstruction. Edema of the head develops rapidly as a sequel to fractures or dislocations of the cervical spine. This form of obstructive edema is caused by drooping of the head in response to the injury, with consequent venous compression. Edema of the mucus membranes has an etiology similar to subcutaneous edema. For example the surgical treatment of laryngeal hemiplegia (roaring) is occasionally followed by obstructive edema in the region of the epiglottis, leading to respiratory distress.

Inflammatory edema occurs at the periphery of an inflammatory process. This form of edema is caused by hyperemia, whereby the healthy tissues surrounding a traumatic or surgical wound become engorged with fluid. Inflammatory edema is devoid of inflammatory cells, however, and so should not be confused with the inflammatory process itself. If the inflammatory edema is located close to a wound or abscess, the term 'collateral edema' is also employed.

Traumatic edema occurs as a sequel to blunt trauma in which minute blood or lymphatic vessels are crushed or torn.

A *neuropathic edema* can also occur in the horse. This is seen in neurectomy in which the vasoconstrictors accompanying the sensory nerves have also been severed. It may also occur secondary to paralyses of motor nerves of the extremities (radial nerve, fibular nerve, etc.). Such edema is always located peripheral to the surgical site or injury. Sometimes there is transudation through the intact skin, producing a weeping eczema. The edema of the deeper tissues may predispose to tendon, ligament and muscle tears.

Subcutaneous edema will gradually gravitate to the lowest point. This pooling is called dependent edema. Obstructive edema in the limbs of the horse will migrate from the thigh to the cannon region, where it is gradually mobilized. Obstructive edema of the back will migrate to the ventral abdomen. Edema of the inguinal region migrates to the umbilical area and is mobilized there. This takes place slowly and only after the initiating cause has been eliminated. Persistent edema, in the connective tissue, can stimulate fibrous tissue within the connective tissue itself. As a result, the swellings no longer pit easily on pressure, and the tissue becomes harder. Gradually a chronic condition develops which may progress to fibrous hyperplastic thickening especially in the limbs.

Diagnosis. The subcutaneous connective tissue arising from mesenchymal tissue plays a crucial role in the overall water balance. Fluid exchange must obey the laws of filtration, diffusion, osmosis and imbibition. Disturbances of this circulation result from the causes cited above. As fluid increases and accumulates in the subcutaneous tissue, edema develops. This may be inter- or intracellular and may result from fluid leakage through blood vessel walls or, in the case of lymphedema, from a general or local failure of lymphatic drainage. The following causes may underlie subcutaneous edema and must be considered during diagnosis:

a) Increased hydrostatic pressure in the capillaries, due, for example, to constriction or ligation of the draining vessels or to arterial hypertension.

b) Decreased hydrostatic pressure in the subcutaneous connective tissue space.

c) Obstructed lymph drainage due to venous stasis.

d) Increased permeability of the lymph capillary walls or cell membranes (the most frequent cause).

e) Obstructed lymph drainage due, for example, to compression of the lymphatics or narrowing or blocking of the drainage channels.

f) Renal sodium retention; the adrenal gland responds to increased fluid extravasation by releasing aldosterone, which in turn increases sodium retention.

g) Estrogenic effects, especially during late pregnancy.

Treatment and Prognosis. The treatment and prognosis depend on the inciting cause. Obstructive edema has a good prognosis if the primary condition can be successfully treated. Inflammatory and traumatic edemas very often regress spontaneously and require no treatment. In obstructive edema, cardiovascular agents may be indicated to improve the stroke volume and circulatory status. Absorption can be hastened by withholding fluids and administering diuretics and laxatives. Pressure bandages on the limbs will prevent spreading of the subcutaneous edema while promoting its mobilization. Astringents must be used with care, especially if applied in high contentrations. Massage and exercise have proved favorable in promoting edema mobilization, particularly in edema of the hindlimbs that is seen in the fall and winter months. Incisions of edematous areas are contraindicated.

The use of modern saluretics, such as hydrochlorothiazide, has proved beneficial in certain types of subcutaneous edema. Such drugs inhibit the reabsorption of sodium and chloride in the renal tubules, resulting in increased fluid excretion. Hence, saluretics are used with equal success in edema of the udder, severe wound edema, preputial edema and postpuerperal edema in mares. Salt should be withheld during the treatment period.

Summary. Subcutaneous edemas are always secondary in nature. The primary condition must be ascertained. The circulatory status must be improved in all cases.

2.1.1.5.3. Cellulitis (Phlegmon)

Definition. Cellulitis is an inflammation of the connective tissue and lymph vessels. It is classically located in the subcutaneous tissue, and is usually caused by bacteria. Cellulitis in the horse may be serous or purulent, depending on the kind of inflammatory

27 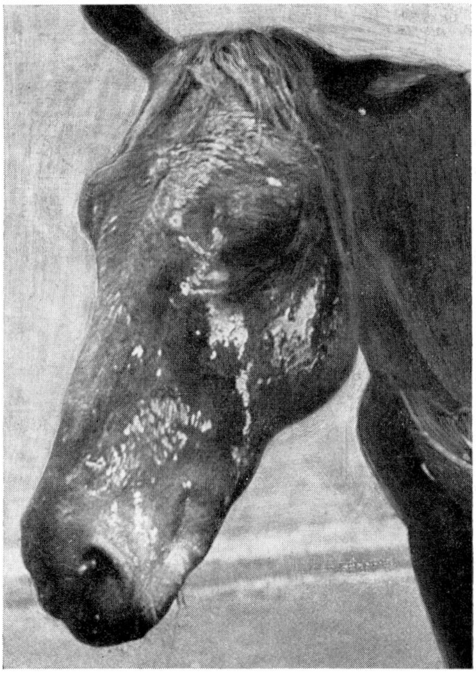 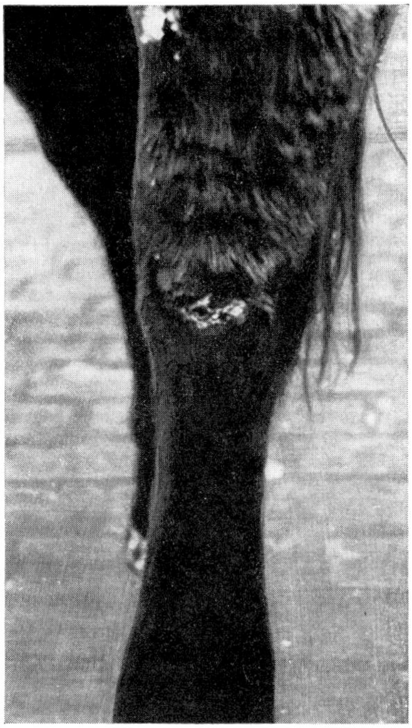 28

Fig. 2.1.1. — 27. Subcutaneous cellulitis of the head ('hippopotamus head').
Fig. 2.1.1. — 28. Cellulitis of the gaskin.

product formed. The subcutaneous cellulitis caused by *Staphylococci* and *Streptococci* in the horse is purulent in nature. The subcutaneous infection always leads to concurrent inflammation of the lymphatic vessels and lymph nodes and sometimes the blood vessels. Cellulitis may assume more serous character if chlostridial organisms are present.

Occurrence. Cellulitis in the horse may affect the head, neck, limbs, as well as the ventral abdomen and lower chest (figs. 2.1.1. — 27 to — 30). In theory it can occur practically anywhere in the subcutaneous connective tissue.

Cellulitis may be circumscribed or diffuse. Circumscribed cellulitis may affect the lips, cheeks, prepuce, withers, or udder. The cellulitis of the coronary band region is due to a bacterial infection of the subcutaneous connective tissue above the hoof wall.

Symptoms. Cellulitis may develop within a few hours. Streptococcal infections in the horse usually cause severe, rapidly progressive infections with marked systemic effects. With staphylococcal infections the systemic effects are mild, with low-grade fever, depression and anorexia. A serous cellulitis may be difficult to distinguish clinically from a purulent cellulitis in the early stages of their development. Later the purulent form is distinguished by liquefaction and abscess formation.

Initially cellulitis appears as a circumscribed, patchy swelling. The lymphatic vessels are often very prominent, especially on the limbs. This is most obvious in thin-skinned horses. The regional lymph node is enlarged and painful. There is increased warmth in the affected area, and the animal resents the site being touched.

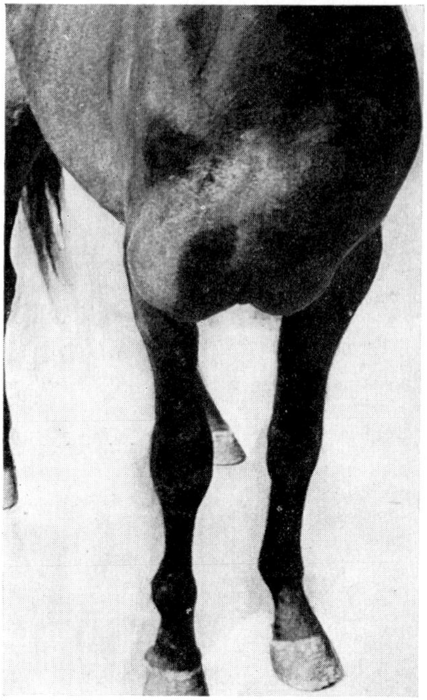
29

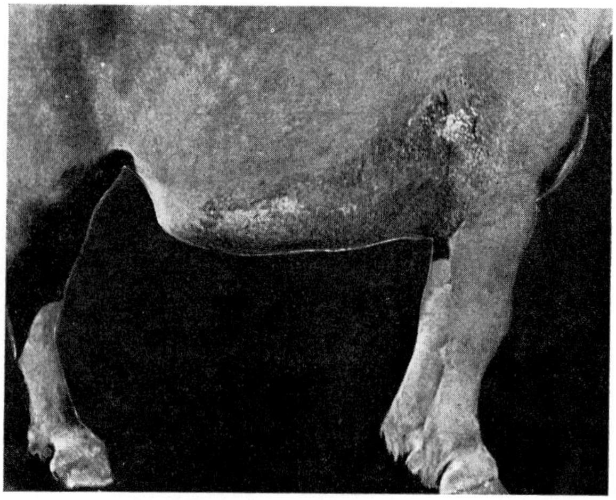
30

Fig. 2.1.1. — 29. Cellulitis of the pectoral region (before abscessation).
Fig. 2.1.1. — 30. Cellulitis of the ventral thorax.

A diffuse cellulitis of the limbs invariably causes lameness. This may be severe if the lesion is suppurative. If liquefaction of the tissues is present, exercise of the affected limb is contraindicated. The swelling does not pit easily on pressure, and the pit, once formed, persists for some time. The eventual course of a cellulitis of the head, neck, limbs, prepuce, etc. will show considerable variation. In many cases healing occurs by absorption and resolution. As the inflammatory products in the subcutaneous connective tissue are absorbed, clinical symptoms improve, and complete recovery ensues. This course of healing is the most rapid, and treatment in the horse is generally directed towards such a goal.

On the other hand, abscessation may take place within 10 to 14 days. This occurs in areas where connective tissue is abundant or at the site of the primary wound infection. The associated lymph node may also undergo abscessation. The abscess must drain before healing can occur (fig. 2.1.1. — 31). A cellulitis that has abscessed is always accompanied by severe systemic signs. When drainage occurs, the body temperature returns to normal and the horse's appetite improves. A serous cellulitis usually leads to generalized infection, and death generally follows within a few days.

Prognosis. It is always favorable for cellulitis, regardless of whether there is abscessation or it is absorbed. However, a longstanding pyogenic, serous cellulitis can lead to fibrous tissue proliferation in the subcutis, producing irreversible thickening of the extremities.

Treatment. Because cellulitis represents a bacterial infection of the subcutaneous tissue, systemic treatment with antibiotics or sulfonamides active against streptococcal and staphylococcal organisms should be instituted. An effective blood level should be maintained for a period of 6 to 7 days, or longer if fever persists. Local heat application is also recommended. The purpose of local heat is to induce an intensive

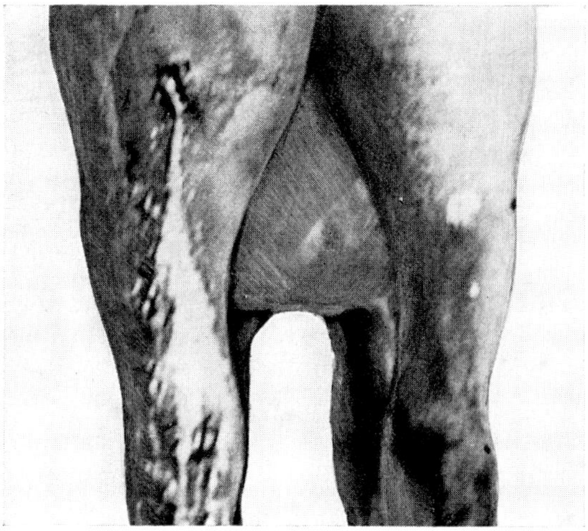

31

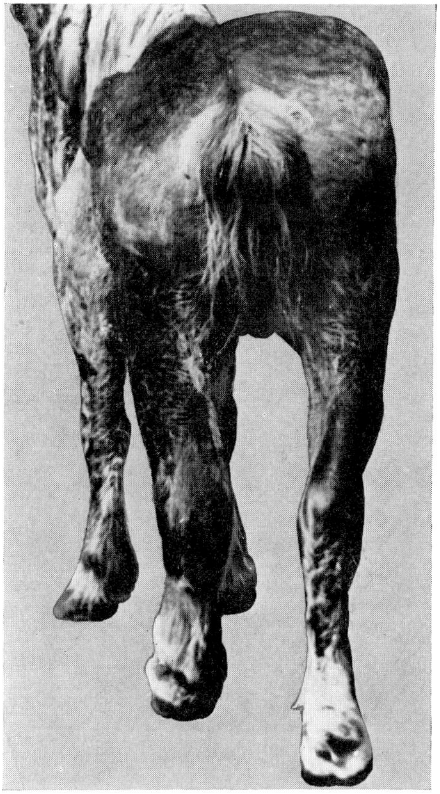

32

Fig. 2.1.1. — 31. Abscessed cellulitis of the thigh with drainage.

Fig. 2.1.1. — 32. Chronic fibrous thickening of the left hindlimb.

hyperemia that will either promote the absorption of inflammatory products or hasten abscessation. In addition, heat serves to alleviate pain. Although time-consuming, warm baths and warm-water hosing are very beneficial. Warm water should be just hot enough to tolerate. Alternatively, the affected area may be wrapped with a well-padded bandage that is soaked every 2 to 3 h in hot water (45—50 °C), preferably containing a suitable antiseptic. Moist heat is applied most frequently to the limbs. Other areas may be heated by infrared radiation.

For cellulitis of the ventral abdomen, lower chest, and sometimes the head, treatment with topical ointments is indicated. Deep-acting rubefacients such as 10—20 % camphor ointment, 5—10 % iodoform ointment, or gray mercurial ointment are preferred. Alternatively, camphor spirit has proved excellent in the treatment of cellulitis. This solution can be poured onto well-padded cotton bandages, or it can be repeatedly rubbed into the surface of the limb by the owner or attendant. Care must be taken not to massage the area too vigorously, or bacteria may be actually massaged into neighboring tissues.

In areas that cannot be bandaged, one may apply poultices containing anti-inflammatory drugs or similar medicaments. Such poultices must be changed daily and kept moist.

Areas of cellulitis that show fluctuation (pointing) should be incised. One should not await spontaneous abscessation, otherwise this may allow infection to break through into a tendon sheath or the joints. Alternatively it may allow a septicemia to develop with an accompanying high fever. Cellulitis in the head that is about to abscess must usually be incised in the intermaxillary area. Cellulitis in the neck with concurrent jugular thrombophlebitis should be incised just before spontaneous rupture of the abscess, taking care to avoid injury to the jugular vein. Cellulitis of the lower chest or ventral abdomen must be incised at the first sign of fluctuation. Cellulitis in the thigh region can lead to abscessation in the region of the stifle joint. In such cases the cellulitis can become subfascial so incision must not be delayed.

In cellulitis of the limbs, mild exercise to improve circulation and promote absorption of the inflammatory products is indicated, provided the animal is afebrile. Once lameness has subsided, the animal may be worked for short periods. Cold should never be applied to a cellulitis, as this may worsen the condition.

2.1.1.5.4. Subcutaneous Abscess

Definition. This is a collection of pus accompanied by cavity formation in the subcutaneous connective tissue.

Symptoms. The lesion presents as a fluctuating, painful, hot, dome-like swelling of varying size and extent and can occur practically anywhere on the body. Hairs may be shed over the mass. Systemic signs may vary in intensity, depending on the size and extent of the developing abscess. There may be considerable temperature elevation before drainage occurs. When the abscess ruptures or is incised, a grayish-yellow, malodorous fluid is discharged in amounts up to 10 l; usually this is streptococcal or staphylococcal pus. With drainage of the abscess, the animal's general condition usually improves within a few hours, and the body temperature returns to normal.

Abscesses in the horse occur most frequently in the intermaxillary area, pectoral region, lateral cervical regions, ventral abdomen, inguinal region, forearm, gaskin, and portions of the limb below the carpal and tarsal joints.

Etiology. Subcutaneous abscesses in the horse are most often caused by infected puncture wounds. They can also arise from cellulitis (see 2.1.1.5.3.). The abscesses are the product of pus or gas producing organisms.

Prognosis and Treatment. Every infected puncture wound initially forms a hard, painful, circumscribed swelling. Until the abscess points, the area is treated with rubefacients or with heat in any form. Fluctuating abscesses should be incised. In some instances two adjacent incisions are made to allow spontaneous, continuous drainage of the abscess cavity. The abscess capsule is usually thin in the horse; it is unnecessary to shell it out. The surgically opened abscess cavity should be irrigated with antiseptic solutions. If two openings are present, a drain may be employed. The wound usually heals by granulation, and thus the prognosis for subcutaneous abscesses is generally good.

2.1.1.5.5. Scleroderma, Elephantiasis

Definition. Subcutaneous connective tissue proliferation that follows chronic subcutaneous edema or longstanding cellulitis may be accompanied by a thickening of the skin and subcutis. This is called scleroderma or elephantiasis (pachydermia).

Symptoms. Scleroderma or elephantiasis in the horse most commonly affects the limbs, especially the hindlimbs (fig. 2.1.1. — 32). Occasionaly the ear, penis or prepuce may be affected. Other areas are rarely involved. The thickening of the skin and subcutaneous tissue is usually preceded by a chronic subcutaneous obstructive edema or a cellulitis that was inadequately treated. The affected limb or body region is enlarged, and the skin feels tough and inelastic. Thick, persistent skin folds form, especially on the limbs, and especially near joints and on flexor surfaces. The skin can no longer be easily moved over underlying tissue. The thickened body parts are not hot or painful. The skin surface is sometimes covered with crusts which, if scraped off by the animal, leave behind a bleeding surface. Some hairs are shed in the affected area while others stand erect. Mild cases of scleroderma or elephantiasis are not disabling, while more severe cases can lead to extreme disfigurement and lameness. Scleroderma of the penis or prepuce causes these structures to become greatly enlarged and pendulous; the same applies to scleroderma of the ear. Scleroderma of the hindlimbs of the horse often leads to eczema in the transverse furrows of the skin ('rasp') as well as to cracks and fissures in the skin called rhagades. Wounds in such areas heal very poorly or leave behind hypertrophic scars and keloid-like thickenings.

Scleroderma does not affect general health.

Etiology. The proliferation and thickening in the subcutaneous connective tissue are the result of irritation from inflammatory products that have stagnated in the tissue. It may also be a response to the action of bacterial toxins such as occurs in cellulitis. There are probably many contributing factors. The veins in the subcutis lose their elasticity and are widely dilated, causing their valves to become nonfunctional. The serum or plasma of the blood in the dilated veins escapes through the damaged vessel wall into the subcutaneous connective tissue. This chronic irritation leads to fibrous tissue proliferation. Combined with the increased exudation and transudation is an impairment of lymphatic drainage. The lymph vessels are also thrombosed or obliterated by inflammatory endothelial proliferation in response to the bacterial irritation, resulting in lymph stasis.

Prognosis and Treatment. The prognosis is always poor. Animals with scleroderma of the limbs may continue to be used for breeding and in many cases can do light work. Very rarely does the swelling subside to any degree; complete remission is unknown. Treatment is limited to applying compression or pressure dressings, which can decrease swelling over a period of weeks. Long-term corticosteroid therapy can be a useful adjunct, though the risks and possible complications of such therapy must be understood. Some success has been achieved with mud paraffin packs. Treatment with pungent ointments is useless, as is any form of cauterization. Adequate exercise should be provided. The limbs may be bandaged when the animal is not being exercised.

2.1.2. Diseases of the Lymphatic System (Lymphadenitis)

Definition. Lymph nodes serve as filtering organs for the lymph. Lymphadenitis is an aseptic or infectious inflammation of the lymph node.

Symptoms. The inflammation of a palpable lymph node is manifested by pain, enlargement, and a change in contour. The enlargement may cause a subcutaneous node to become visible as a distinct lump or bulge. In the horse the mandibular, parotid, prescapular and popliteal lymph nodes may be affected. In some situations, the enlarged lymph nodes may be painless and present a hard, knobby surface. This latter sign is more indicative of involvement in tumor metastasis than of inflammation. Fluctuation in a lymph node is a signal of impending abscessation. Often the lymph vessels supplying the enlarged, inflamed lymph node are engorged and prominent ('cording' of the lymphatics). Sometimes swelling due to cellulitis is present in the vicinity of the inflamed node. If the node becomes abscessed, systemic signs (fever etc.) may be present.

Such abscessation commonly affects the intermaxillary lymph nodes. Numerous bacterial diseases occur in the regions drained by these nodes, e.g., the teeth and the maxillary and nasal sinuses. The retropharyngeal lymph nodes may also be affected following an infection of the pharynx and nasopharyngeal area. The inferior superficial lymph node lying anterior to the shoulder joint is usually affected in abscesses of the brachiocephalic muscle. The inguinal lymph nodes become abscessed during the course of cellulitis of the hindlimbs. This is preceded by a gradual swelling in the inguinal space. Large amounts of pus may be discharged from the abscess cavity, in these cases.

Etiology. Ideally, pathogenic organisms are destroyed and tumor metastases arrested in the inflamed lymph node. If infectious organisms or tumor cells overcome this barrier, they are carried into the bloodstream, producing a systemic bacterial infection (bacteremia) or metastatic tumor spread. Toxic products from bacterial organisms lead to inflammation of the parenchyma of the lymph node. If local defense mechanisms fail to halt this process, necrosis and abscess formation ensue. In chronic lymphadenitis, the lymph node acquires a dense consistency owing to the increase of fibrous connective tissue in the node itself. Defense mechanisms evoke a hyperplasia of the lymphoreticular tissue. In all cases the lymph vessels draining into the node may be also involved or at least markedly congested. In lymphadenitis of bacterial origin, the glandular tissue becomes infiltrated with polymorphonuclear leukocytes.

Prognosis and Treatment. The prognosis depends upon the nature and cause of the lymphadenitis. With noninfectious lymphadenitis the prognosis is always good, provided the lymph node enlargement is not the result of tumor metastases. In lymphadenitis due to pyogenic bacteria, the prognosis is good if the node becomes abscessed, and the precipitating cause can be permanently removed. The prognosis is poor if tumor metastases are present.

The treatment of lymphadenitis should be directed at stopping the influx of bacteria and their toxins into the node. In the head region, this is achieved by appropriate treatment of the infected focus that may be present in the maxillary or nasal sinus, pharynx or larynx. When the primary focus is eliminated, the lymph node swelling will subside. If abscessation is anticipated, pointing of the abscess should be encouraged. This is done in the same way as in the treatment of cellulitis and subcutaneous abscesses. We particularly recommend heat in the form of infrared radiation or rubefacient ointments, especially iodine preparations. If definite fluctuation and pointing are present, the node should be lanced. Early incision is contraindicated due to the heavy bleeding that may result. Sometimes a cluster of small abscesses will form in the lymph node; each must be separately incised. In cases of neoplasia, operative removal of the entire lymph node metastases is recommended.

References

Bolz, W.; Dietz, O.: Lehrbuch der Allgemeinen Chirurgie für Tierärzte, 4. Aufl. (VEB Gustav Fischer Verlag, Jena 1970).

Schebitz, H.; Brass, W.: Allgemeine Chirurgie für Tierärzte und Studierende (Parey, Berlin 1975).

2.1.3. Diseases of the Cardiovascular System, Blood and Blood-Forming Organs

2.1.3.1. Diseases of the Cardiovascular System

The functional state of the cardiovascular system and its degree of development have a profound effect on the physical performance ability of the horse. This system is frequently subjected to such large loads that its function can be very seriously impaired. In a relatively high percentage of cases, cardiovascular lesions occur concurrently with other diseases of the horse. The recognition of such lesions demands close attention to the major symptoms of cardiac and circulatory failure, such as cardiac arrhythmia, dyspnea, cyanosis and edema. When cardiovascular lesions are severe, additional symptoms such as tachycardia, premature beats, atrioventricular blocks and other cardiac arrhythmias may be present. Dyspnea, or labored breathing, results from stimulation of the respiratory center in the medulla oblongata by carbon dioxide and other metabolic products. Cyanosis is a bluish discoloration of the visible mucous membranes that is caused by the accumulation of reduced hemoglobin in the blood. It is associated with inadequate oxygenation of the blood in the lung as well as increased tissue oxygen consumption with a slowing of the blood flow. Edema is mainly of the cardiac or obstructive type. It is usually a result of congestion and increased pressure in the veins and capillaries. Edema formation is also promoted by a slowing of the blood flow and a rise in capillary permeability. The cardiac edemas are characteristically limited to dependent or ventral body areas. In such cases the transudate accumulates in the subcutaneous tissues and may effuse into body cavities. Obstructive edemas, unlike edemas of other origin, are always symmetrically arranged, have a doughy consistency (pit on pressure), and are neither warm nor painful.

Vascular edemas may be generalized or local; the local forms are asymmetrical.

The cardiovascular diseases that most frequently affect the athletic horse are diseases of the myocardium — myocarditis, myocardial fibrosis, and cardiac hypertrophy and dilatation. Diseases of the endocardium, pericardium and blood vessels are less common.

2.1.3.1.1. Diseases of the Heart and Pericardium

Diseases of the pericardium are most frequently manifested as pericarditis and hydropericardium.

Pericarditis

Definition. Pericarditis is an inflammatory condition of the pericardial sac.

Symptoms. Dry pericarditis is characterized by fever, accelerated pulse, and varying degrees of weakness and anorexia. Affected horses are reluctant to lie down. The cardiac impulse is increased. Pain is evidenced on palpation and especially percussion of the cardiac area. In the early stage of the disease the heart sounds are intensified. At the same time, friction sounds are audible and grow louder when pressure is applied to the cardiac area with the stethoscope or phonendoscope.

Exudative pericarditis on the other hand is associated with more pronounced disturbances of circulation and overall health in general. Incomplete filling of the arteries results in a small and sometimes irregular pulse. The apex beat is decreased, diffuse, and is shifted upward, backward and to the right. When large amounts of exudate are present, the area of cardiac dullness is increased and there is a merging of absolute and relative dullness. Pain is evident on percussion of the cardiac area. The heart sounds are soft and muffled as if in the distance; with a purulent exudate, they are accompanied by pericardial splashing sounds. In these cases a gas bubble may give a tympanitic sound on percussion in the upper part of the cardiac area. The ensuing cardiac tamponade leads to congestion in the jugular veins and increased pressure. Often there is inflammatory and obstructive edema with enlargement of the regional lymph nodes. The EKG is characterized by low voltages in all waves (especially in limb lead I). Premature beats and other arrhythmias are also present.

Often a neutrophilic leukocytosis with a regenerative or degenerative left shift is detectable. Urinalysis may show proteinuria and albuminuria.

The disease may be accompanied by disturbances of hepatic and pulmonary function; other organ functions may also be impaired.

Etiology. Pericarditis in athletic horses may be primary or secondary, fibrinous or exudative. Primary pericarditis has been associated with exposure to certain viral agents, while the more common secondary form develops as a complication of infectious or noninfectious diseases. Occasionally, trauma to the cardiac area of the chest wall is a cause of primary pericarditis in horses.

Pathogenesis and Lesions. Dry pericarditis is characterized by a fibrinous inflammation of the epicardium and pericardium, with fibrin deposits on both layers. This leads to a decrease or loss of pericardial elasticity and thus to an impairment of cardiac action. In later stages, adhesions may form between the pericardium and epicardium.

In wet or exudative pericarditis there is an effusion of liquid exudate into the pericardial cavity, which restricts diastolic filling of the heart. The result is a decrease in the myocardial contractile force and systolic volume. The excessive accumulation of pericardial fluid leads to cardiac tamponade, causing venous congestion in the lungs and liver. Venous pressure rises, and obstructive edema develops. The arterial blood pressure falls, and the velocity of blood flow is reduced. Inflammatory products entering the blood stream cause septacemia, fever, disturbances of hematopoiesis, and functional disturbances in other organs and body systems.

At necropsy, exudate is found in the pericardial cavity. The pericardium is thickened and hyperemic, and hemorrhages are sometimes noted. There may be calcification of the pericardium. Myocardial atrophy is often apparent. In secondary pericarditis one also finds the changes characteristic of the primary disorder.

Diagnosis. Acute dry (fibrinous) pericarditis is marked by pain and pericardial friction sounds, an increased cardiac impulse and tachycardia. Exudative pericarditis is characterized by a shifting, and weakening of the cardiac impulse, an enlargement of the area of cardiac percussion with a merging of absolute and relative dullness. In addition there are weak and dull heart sounds, tachycardia, pericardial friction and splashing sounds, and edema. Radiographic examination reveals an enlarged, cardiac shadow; a small poorly defined heart-diaphragm triangle; and, if gas is present in the pericardium, zones of radiolucency in the upper part of the cardiac area.

In contrast to 'dry' pleuritis, the friction sounds in dry pericarditis are not synchronous with respiration. Exudative pericarditis is distinguished from hydropericardium by presence of cardiac pain and fever. It is distinguished from exudative pleuritis by the absence of a horizontally limited dullness in the region of the lung field.

Prognosis. The prognosis is usually poor. In many cases it depends on the nature and severity of the primary illness. In suppurative and especially in purulent pericarditis, the prognosis is unfavorable.

Treatment and Prophylaxis. In the early stage of aseptic pericarditis symptomatic treatment with cold compresses applied to the cardiac area may be of value. Further treatment of secondary pericarditis consists of parenteral administration of sulfonamides, antibiotics, iodine preparations, and diuretics. Caffeine and glucose have also been used.

A suitable iodinated preparation is calcium iodine (2—10 g administered orally, 1—3 times daily). Caffeine and sodium benzoate or caffeine and sodium salicylate is given in doses of 2—5 g s.c. or 3—8 g orally. Glucose is best administered as a 30—40 % i.v. solution in amounts of 30—150 g per dose.

Hydropericardium

Definition. Hydropericardium is an accumulation of transudate in the pericardial cavity.

Symptoms. The main symptoms are those of congestive heart failure: irregular rhythm, dyspnea, cyanosis, edema. There may also be congestion and protrusion of the jugular veins, a weak and diffuse cardiac impulse, enlargement of the cardiac percussion field, and weak and dull heart sounds. Splashing sounds may be detectable in some instances. The arterial blood pressure is low while venous pressure is elevated, and the blood flow velocity is decreased. The EKG shows low-amplitude waves, particularly in limb lead I.

Etiology. Hydropericardium is usually secondary to chronic heart and circulatory failure associated with various diseases.

Pathogenesis and Lesions. Circulatory failure gives rise to congestion in the venous system, which in turn leads to increased hydrostatic pressure on the venous side of the capillaries, and in lymphatic vessels, increased vessel-wall permeability, and thus to a leakage of fluid into the tissues and body cavities. Such leakage can occur into the pericardial sac. The pericardial fluid accumulation exerts compression on the heart, seriously impairing cardiac action and disrupting the circulation as a whole.

At necropsy a considerable amount of colorless or yellowpink fluid is found in the pericardial cavity. This is usually combined with atrophy and degeneration of the myocardium.

Diagnosis. In contrast to pericarditis, hydropericardium does not produce fever and nor is there pain in the cardiac area of the chest wall. In many cases, the diagnosis can be confirmed by paracentesis of the pericardial sac. In hydropericardium this will yield a *transudate* that differs from the *exudate* of pericarditis in its lower density (less than 1.016) and low protein content (1—3 %).

The *prognosis* is guarded. It is unfavorable in severe cases.

Treatment and Prophylaxis. Emphasis is on treatment of the underlying disease. The proportion of bulk feeds and salt in the ration should be reduced, and water intake should be limited. Cardiotropic drugs and diuretics can be given. Infusions of calcium chloride and glucose have proved beneficial.

As a diuretic we give theobromine orally in a dose of 5—10 g 2—3 times daily.

Calcium chlorate is infused slowly as a 10 % i.v. solution with 10—30 g of drug administered per dose. It may also be given orally in a dose of 20—60 g. As an alternative, calcium gluconate may be given in approximately the same dosage and concentration. Carbonic anhydrase diuretics have proven very useful.

The *prophylaxis* of hydropericardium consists in the prompt recognition of heart failure in a variety of illnesses as well as in its prevention and treatment.

Cardiac Arrhythmias and Diseases of the Myocardium

Arrhythmias are abnormalities in the rhythm of cardiac activity that occur usually in association with myocardial diseases or disturbances of the impulse conduction system. Highly detailed studies on arrhythmias in the horse have been conducted by DOMRAČEV, ZAJCEV, SCHARABRIN, FILATOV and SUDAKOV. Equine cardiac arrhythmias have also been described by SPORRI and LEEMANN, DETWEILER, WIRTH, NAGORSKI, SEVESTRE and BARON, LIGHTOWLER and GRISOLIA, DEEGEN and others.

The prompt diagnosis of cardiac arrhythmias is essential for the successful treatment and prophylaxis of a variety of cardiovascular diseases that affect the athletic horse. The electrocardiogram (EKG) is of crucial importance in the diagnosis of cardiac arrhythmias. It is also essential for accurately interpreting the findings of the clinical examination.

Following the classification of DOMRAČEV, which has been refined by the work of FILATOV, SUDAKOV and others, we recognize four classes of cardiac arrhythmia in the horse:

1. arrhythmias due to disturbances of cardiac autorhythmicity,
2. arrhythmias due to impulse formation disturbances,
3. arrhythmias due to impulse conduction disturbances,
4. arrhythmias due to contractility disturbances.

Class 1 includes sinus tachycardia, sinus bradycardia, sinus arrhythmias in the form of respiratory and nonrespiratory arrhythmia or sinoatrial block, and ectopic rhythms in the form of nodal rhythm or idioventricular rhythm.

Sinus tachycardia may occur with excitation of the sympathetic nervous system (excitement, fear, pain, hyperthyroidism, intense psychological stress) or as a compensatory mechanism in response to anemia or circulatory failure. The EKG in sinus tachycardia shows a shortening of the PQ, QT and especially the TP intervals. The wave forms and amplitudes may appear normal. Occasionally a voltage increase is seen in the P, R and T waves.

Sinus bradycardia is associated with a preponderance of parasympathetic tone (during rest, sleep, hypothyroidism, liver disease, etc.). There is a lengthening of the PQ, QT and TP intervals in the EKG. The amplitudes of the P and T waves are often markedly low. Occasionally there is a slight broadening of these waves and of the QRS complex.

Respiratory arrhythmia is the term applied to the increase and decrease in the heart rate that occurs during inspiration and expiration, respectively. It is caused by stimulation of vagus nerve branches in the intercostal muscles, diaphragm and lung at the level of inspiration, resulting in a periodic waxing and waning of the heart rate with the respiratory cycle. This arrhythmia is abolished by exercise or atropine injection. Respiratory arrhythmia is somewhat rare in horses.

Nonrespiratory arrhythmia is manifested by diastolic periods of varying duration, unassociated with respiration. The EKG shows irregular cardiac cycles (RR intervals of varying duration). This arrhythmia, too, is associated with a preponderance of parasympathetic tone and is relatively rare in the horse.

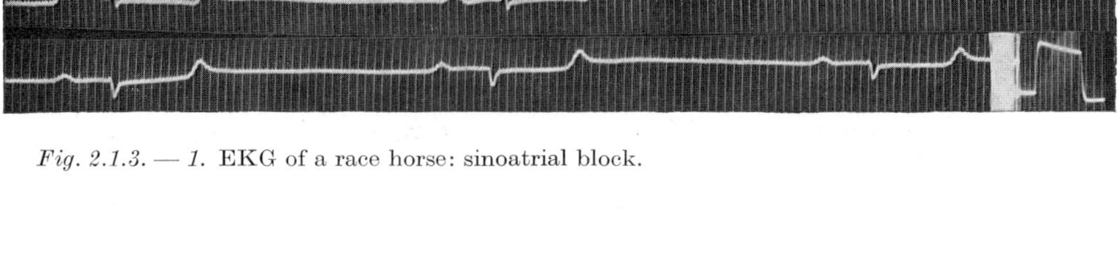

Fig. 2.1.3. — 1. EKG of a race horse: sinoatrial block.

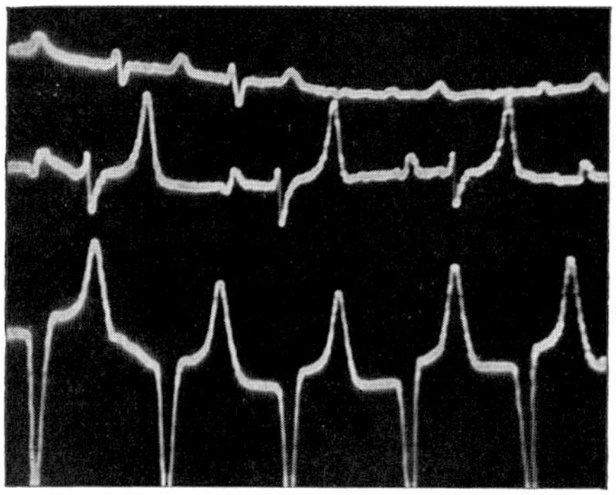

2

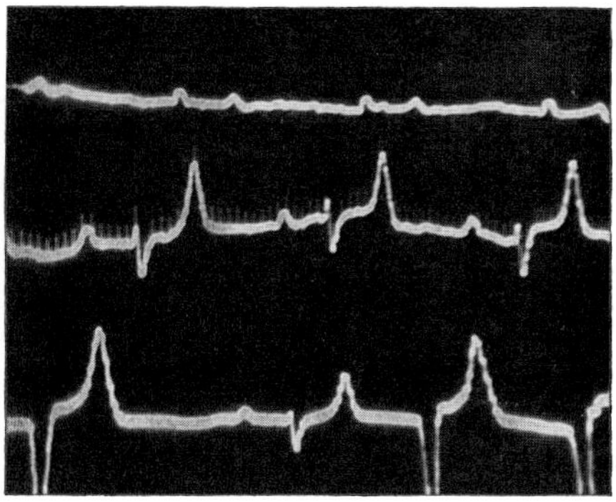

3

Fig. 2.1.3. — 2. EKG in acute myocarditis: two limited extrasystoles in lead I, all complexes in lead III; extrasystoles arise from the right ventricle.

Fig. 2.1.3. — 3. EKG in acute myocarditis: extrasystoles arising from the right ventricle in lead III.

Sinoatrial block is characterized by the occurrence of pauses in which one or more beats are lost (fig. 2.1.3. — 1). These pauses disappear after exercise or subcutaneous atropine injection. The absence of atrial sounds (P waves) during the pauses distinguishes sinoatrial block from the partial AV block. Sinoatrial block is relatively common in horses, especially athletic horses. In most cases the disturbance is an indication of excessive vagal tone with resulting impairment of impulse formation in the sinoatrial node.

Nodal rhythm can be diagnosed only by electrocardiography. It is associated with fusing together of the sinoatrial node (Keith-Flack node), with the atrioventricular node (Aschoff-Tawara node) and assuming the pacemaker function. In this ectopic rhythm the ventricles usually are excited first, followed by the atria. Due to the retrograde flow of impulses from the AV node to the atria, negative P waves appear in the EKG. The P waves may appear before, after, or within the QRS complex, depending on the origin of the impulses. The first location indicates a high nodal rhythm, the second a middle nodal rhythm, and the third a low nodal rhythm. Especially in the middle nodal rhythm, when the atria and ventricles contract simultaneously, very loud heart sounds ('cannon sounds') are frequently heard on ausculation. Nodal rhythm is generally a sign of advanced toxemia.

Idioventricular rhythm occurs when the bundle of His or bundle branches assume the pacemaker function. Idioventricular rhythm is distinguished by a lower rate than nodal rhythm, because the bundle of His is a tertiary center and as such is relatively refractory to impulses. The EKG features of idioventricular rhythm resemble those of low nodal rhythm, when the impulse arises from the lower part of the node near the bundle of His. In idioventricular rhythm the negative P wave appears between the QRS complex and the T wave.

Class 2 of cardiac arrhythmias, involving disturbances of impulse formation, includes premature beats, paroxysmal tachycardia, absolute arrhythmia and dissociation with interference.

Premature beats are characterized by the occurrence of extrasystoles, or premature contractions of the heart or any of its parts. Premature beats arise under the influence of ectopic impulses and are classified according to their site of origin as sinus, atrial, atrioventricular, ventricular or polytopic. Etiologically they may be classified as

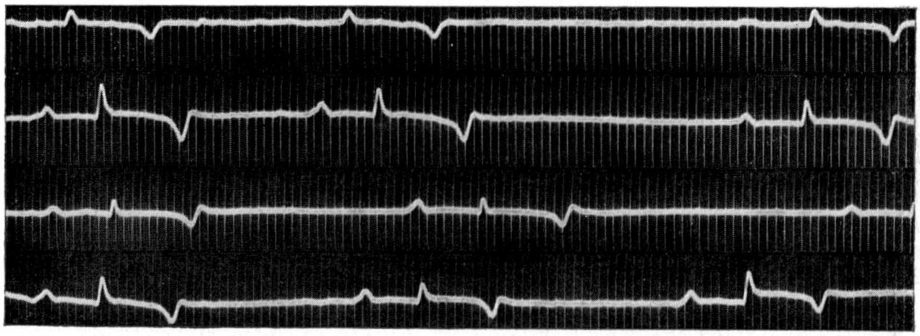

Fig. 2.1.3. — 4. EKG of a race horse. Leads I, II and III and lead II after fast gait: neurogenic atrial extrasystoles (after FILATOV).

neurogenic (in functional disturbances of the nervous system), dynamic (in decompensated valvular defects, cardiac dilatation, or from significant blood pressure changes in the cardiac chambers), and myocardial (in myocardial diseases, especially myocarditis).

Auscultation or EKG reveals premature beats followed by compensatory pauses. Sinus premature beats are generally unaccompanied by compensatory pauses, owing to the high lability of the sinus node. Premature beats are associated with a pulse deficit due to the periodic occurrence of 'empty' ventricular contractions. In these cases the pulse rate and heart rate do not coincide. To illustrate this, the EKG recording of a horse with acute myocarditis is shown (figs. 2.1.3. — 2 and — 3). Also shown is the EKG of an athletic horse with atrial premature beats of neurogenic origin (fig. 2.1.3. — 4).

Paroxysmal tachycardia usually takes the form of rapidly recurring premature beats. The impulse may arise in the atrium, AV node or ventricle. Paroxysmal tachycardia arising from the sinus node cannot be distinguished from sinus tachycardia, even in the EKG. The etiology of this arrhythmia coincides largely with that of premature beats.

Absolute arrhythmia is a flutter or fibrillation of the atria that can occur in the horse in both a rapid (tachyarrhythmic) and slow (bradyarrhythmic) form. It is associated with the presence of multiple foci of excitation in the atria, leading to incomplete, chaotic atrial contractions in the form of a fibrillation or flutter. The ventricular rhythm is also irregular and depends upon the impulses transmitted from the atria. In general there is a marked pulse deficit, for many ventricular contractions occur after diastoles that are too short to produce a palpable pulse. On auscultation a chaotic sequence of heart sounds is heard ('delirium cordis'). The serious disruption of ventricular rhythm may be apparent in the EKG, and the P waves are replaced with small undulations whose frequency and character depend on the nature and severity of the arrhythmia (cf. fig. 2.1.3. — 8). The arrhythmia is best recognized in the precordial lead, especially when a unipolar or augmented unipolar lead is used. The prognosis is better for the slow form than the rapid form. The major causes of atrial fibrillation in horses are acute and chronic toxicoses or infectious diseases.

Dissociation with interference is an arrhythmia in which two centers of impulse formation coexist, representing a combination of the nodal and sinus rhythms (fig. 2.1.3. — 5). In most cases the ventricles are excited first and so contract before the atria. In contrast to nodal and idioventricular rhythm, the P wave is always positive (the impulse to the atrium arises from the sinus node). It is not unusual for atrial

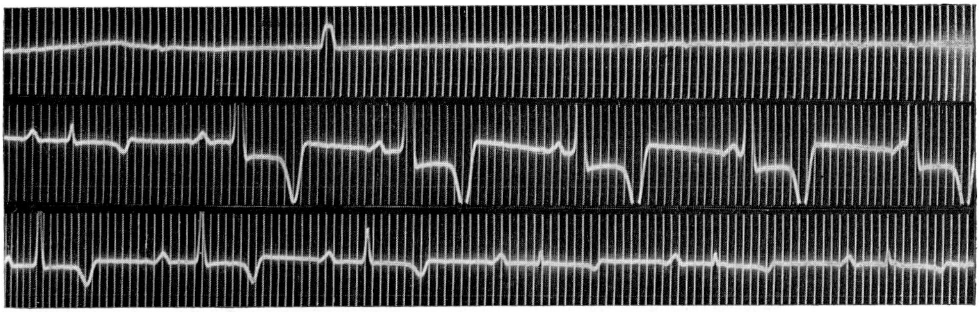

5

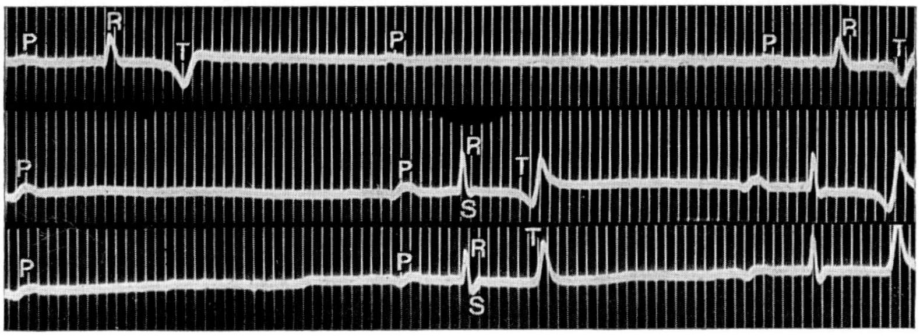

6

Fig. 2.1.3. — 5. EKG: dissociation with interference (after FILATOV).
Fig. 2.1.3. — 6. EKG of a race horse: intermittent partial atrioventricular block.

and ventricular contractions to occur simultaneously, in which case 'cannon' sounds become audible. This pararrhythmia occurs when fused foci arise in the sinus and AV nodes. It usually signifies a severe coronary flow disturbance and myocardial damage.

Class 3 of arrhythmia based on disturbances of impulse conduction includes sinoatrial block (SA block), atrioventricular block (AV block) and intraventricular block (IV block).

Sinoatrial block can be diagnosed only by electrocardiography. A broad, distorted P wave of abnormal amplitude is characteristic. The fusion of foci in the atria are considered the main cause of this arrhythmia.

Atrioventricular block is relatively common in horses, including athletic horses. It is characterized by the periodic occurrence of pauses with dropped ventricular beats. In partial AV block, soft ventricular sounds can be auscultated during the pauses. The intermittent partial block, which is commonly seen in fit horses (fig. 2.1.3. — 6), is abolished by exercise or atropine injection, whereas the stable partial block persists (fig. 2.1.3. — 7). In complete AV block (fig. 2.1.3. — 8) the atria and ventricles beat independently of each other. Ventricular contractions are infrequent and arrhythmic, with long pauses between beats. Stokes-Adams seizures with cannon sounds and fainting spells are typical of complete AV block. Fainting occurs during the long pauses between ventricular beats. These pauses may amount to 12—13 s in the horse. Fainting is due to insufficient oxygen delivery to the brain.

According to Russian authors, the causes of AV block lie in the formation of fused foci in the region of the atrioventricular node and bundle of His. The block may be of the partial intermittent, partial stable, or complete type, depending on the stage of the fusion (transformational, paradoxical or inhibitory).

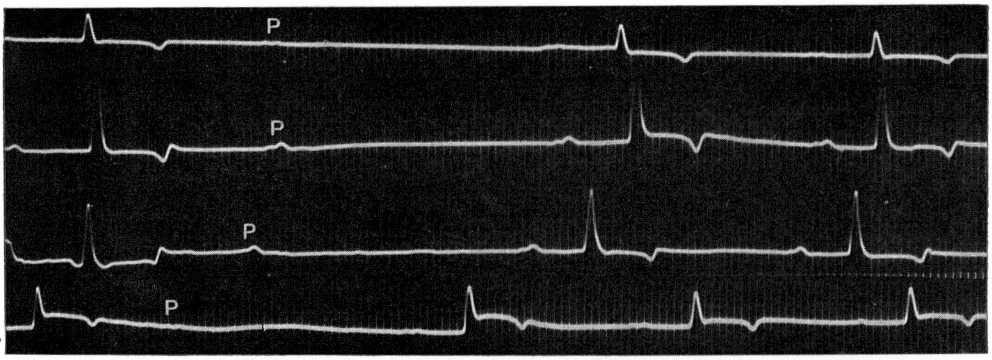

7

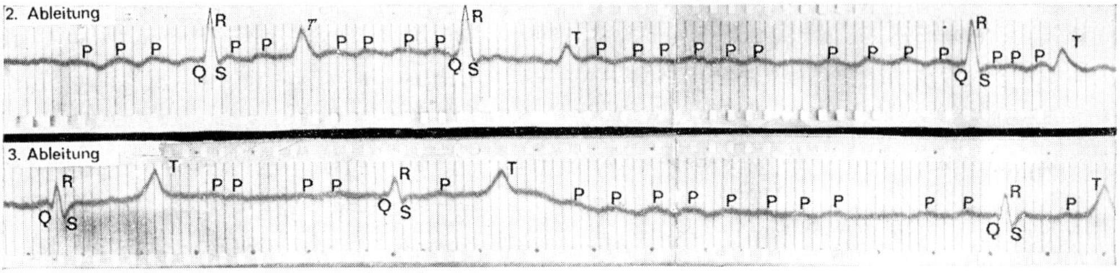

8

Fig. 2.1.3. — 7. EKG of a race horse. Leads I, II and III and additional lead II after fast gait: stable partial atrioventricular block.

Fig. 2.1.3. — 8. EKG, leads II and III: complete atrioventricular block and atrial fibrillation.

An *intraventricular block* can be diagnosed only by evaluation of the EKG record. Changes in the duration and form of the QRS complex are characteristic. Bundle branch block is further characterized by an abnormal direction of the electrical axis. A block of the Purkinje fibers is marked by a very low-amplitude QRS complex.

The arrhythmia is attributed to the occurrence of separate foci in the region of the bundle branches and Purkinje fibers.

Class 4 of cardiac arrhythmia based on contractility disturbances includes an arrhythmia known as pulsus alternans. This disturbance is characterized by an alternation of weak and strong pulse waves that are easily seen if the blood pressure is monitored. It is indicative of partial cardiac asystole. The presence of this change is usually a sign of severe dystrophic or degenerative myocardial damage.

Myocardosis

Definition. Myocardosis is a general term for noninflammatory myocardial disease that is accompanied by impaired myocardial contractility due to various disturbances in the cardiac muscle [Domračev, 1950; Kedrov, 1963].

Symptoms. The clinical picture of myocardosis depends on the stage of the disease. Myocardial dystrophy is characterized by a moderately accelerated pulse, weakening of the cardiac impulse, accentuation, splitting or duplication of the first heart sound and weakening of the second sound. One may also see disturbances in impulse formation and conduction, a lowered arterial and elevated venous blood pressure, and a reduction of the blood flow velocity. In the early stage of myocardial dystrophy the EKG may show a broad, abnormally shaped T wave. This is accompanied by a

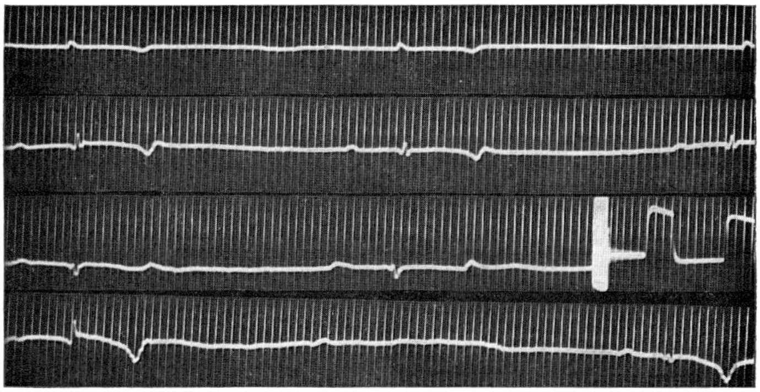

Fig. 2.1.3. — 9. EKG in myocardosis. Leads I, II and III and lead II after fast gait: partial atrioventricular block and coronary blood flow disturbances after exercise.

lengthening of the PQ and QR intervals, displacement and distortion of the ST segment, and a voltage decrease in all waves, especially the QRS complex (fig. 2.1.3. — 9). In myocardial degeneration, the heart rate is higher than in myocardial dystrophy. The disturbances of impulse conduction are much more pronounced and are exacerbated by exercise. In addition, the cardiac impulse is weak and usually diffuse, and the heart sounds are soft and muffled. The blood pressure changes are also more severe. This applies both to the fall of arterial pressure and the rise of venous pressure, as well as to the slowing of the blood flow. In the EKG there is low amplitude in all waves, the QRS complex is broadened and abnormally shaped, and the PQ and QT intervals are prolonged. AV, SA and IV blocks are frequent.

According to Urazaev [1965], the phonocardiogram (PCG) in myocardosis shows a prolongation of the first heart sound as well as a decrease in myocardial contractility and tone. This is based upon a lengthening of the interval from the start of the first heart sound to the start of the second, a decrease in the frequency of the first sound, and the occurrence of a third and fifth sound.

Myocardosis is almost always associated with disturbances of the respiratory and digestive systems. The disease is usually accompanied by symptoms of severe heart and circulatory failure with abnormalities of heart rate, dyspnea, cyanosis and edema. The edema of myocardosis is slower to develop than that of acute myocarditis; it often worsens when the horse stands quietly, and disappears when the animal is exercised.

Etiology. Myocardosis usually develops as a secondary lesion following other diseases. It may also result from a poor diet leading to metabolic disturbances. Additional causes are overexertion, anemic states, 'autointoxication' in intestinal disease, intoxications in chronic infectious and parasitic diseases, mycoses and mycotoxicoses.

Pathogenesis and Lesions. The aforementioned etiologic factors produce changes in the myocardium, leading to disturbances of biochemical processes in the heart muscle. This causes changes in the colloidal chemical structure of the muscle fibers, which in turn leads to impairment of myocardial contractility. Similar changes can occur in the impulse formation and conduction system of the heart.

In the initial stage of myocardosis (the dystrophic stage), the myocardium is free of demonstrable gross and histologic lesions. The disturbances of biochemical processes at this stage can be detected only by histochemical analysis. In the second stage of myocardosis (the degenerative stage) the myocardium is markedly pale and flabby. Histologic study often reveals hyaline and fatty degeneration.

The *diagnosis* is established by the characteristic symptoms of the various disease stages, taking into account the findings obtained by electrocardiography, phonocardiography, arterio- and phlebotonometry, as well as the determination of blood flow velocity.

Differential Diagnosis. The disease must be differentiated from myocarditis and myocardial fibrosis. Myocardosis has less severe systemic signs than myocarditis, and its course is afebrile. In addition, there is less elevation of the heart rate, which may be in the high normal range. Above all, myocardosis is characterized by arrhythmias due to conduction disturbances, while arrhythmias due to impulse formation disturbances are more indicative of myocarditis.

The *prognosis* is guarded and depends on the stage of the myocardosis as well as the nature and severity of the primary disease.

Treatment and Prophylaxis. The prime concern is the elimination of the etiologic factors responsible for the disease. Rest or very light work is indicated. The ration should contain all basic nutrients, vitamins and trace elements in the correct amounts and proportions. In addition, glucose, caffeine, ascorbic acid, nicethamide and pentetrazol may be indicated. A special 20% injection solution of camphor oil is administered s.c. in a dose of 20—40 ml. Nicethamide is also administered in a dose of 15—20 ml s.c. or 10—15 ml i.v. The single dose for pentetrazol is 0.5—2.0 g s.c. or 0.5—1.0 g i.v.

At one time preparations made from foxglove *(Digitalis purpurea)*, lily of the valley *(Convallaria majalis)*, helleboraster *(Adonis vernalis)*, *Strophanthus* spp. and hedge mustard *(Raphanus raphanistrum)* were frequently prescribed. Strophanthin is administered in a dose of 0.005—0.015 g i.v. together with 10—40% glucose solution or isotonic saline. In the presence of functional disturbances of other organs and systems, corresponding symptomatic treatment is also indicated.

Prophylaxis is based on the prompt treatment of poisonings and on providing a well-balanced diet, regular exercise, and a scientifically-based training program for athletic horses.

Myocarditis

Definition. Myocarditis refers to an inflammatory condition of the myocardium.

Symptoms. Body temperature is elevated, the horse is depressed, and feed intake is markedly reduced, even to the point of complete anorexia. The early stage of acute myocarditis is marked by tachycardia, extrasystoles, large pulse waves and a full pulse as well as pain in the cardiac area, and an increased or 'pounding' cardiac impulse. There is an accentuation of the heart sounds affecting mainly the first sound. The arterial blood pressure is elevated, and the blood flow velocity is increased. According to reports by DOMRAČEV, SCHARABRIN, FILATOV, SUDAKOV and others, the equine EKG at this stage shows a significant amplitude increase in the P, R and especially the T waves, shortening of the PQ and QT intervals, and ST segment displacement. Extrasystoles frequently appear (figs. 2.1.3. — 10 and — 11).

In the second stage of myocarditis, when dystrophic and degenerative lesions are present in the myocardium, all the symptoms of severe heart failure such as dyspnea, cyanosis, edema and arrhythmia are observed. When vascular filling is deficient, the pulse becomes small and the cardiac impulse weak. The first heart sound is intensified and is often split or reduplicated, while the second heart sound is weakened. Gallop rhythm, similarly sounding first and second heart sounds (embryocardia), and functional endocardial murmurs can develop in severe cases. The arterial blood

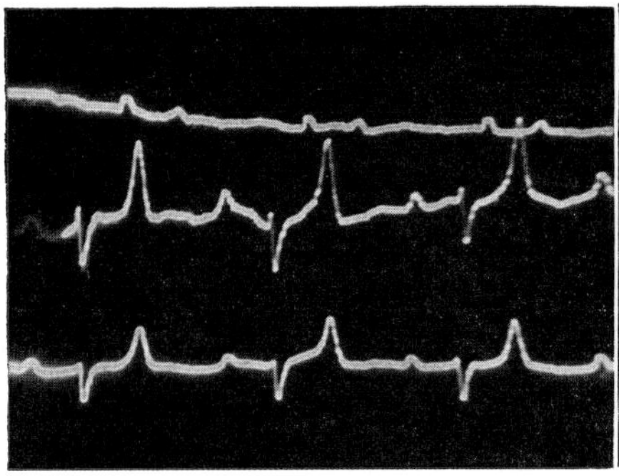
10

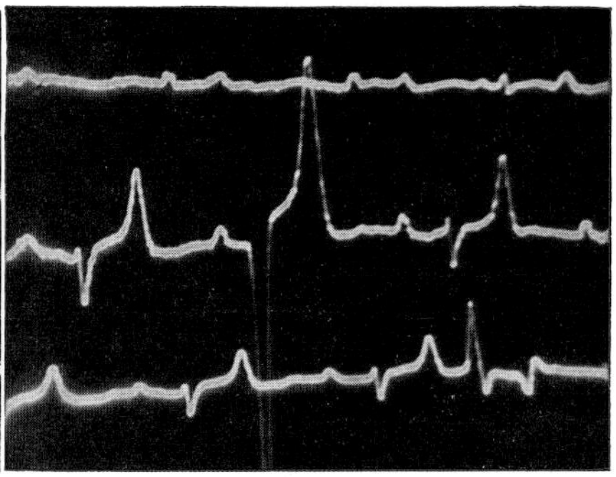
11

Fig. 2.1.3. — 10. EKG in acute myocarditis.

Fig. 2.1.3. — 11. EKG in acute myocarditis: left ventricular extrasystole in lead II, limited extrasystole in lead III.

pressure falls, the venous pressure rises, and the blood flow becomes more sluggish. In this second stage of myocarditis the EKG is marked by low amplitudes in all waves, widening of the QRS complex and lengthening of the PQ and QT intervals.

Myocarditis is usually associated with some degree of dysfunction of the lungs, liver, kidneys, digestive tract and nervous system. Blood tests usually demonstrate leukocytosis with neutrophilia and a regenerative or degenerative shift.

Etiology. Myocarditis is usually secondary in nature, occurring as a complication of infectious, noninfectious and parasitic diseases (influenza, rhinopneumonitis, equine infectious anemia, strangles, piroplasmosis, pericarditis, endocarditis, etc.). Acute myocarditis also frequently complicates mycoses and mycotoxicoses.

Pathogenesis and Lesions. The myocardial inflammation develops as a result of toxins produced by the causal agents of the primary disease. According to Davidovskij [1956], Rapoport [1960] and Skvorcov [1949], the general pathogenesis is based upon a prior sensitization of the myocardium to repeated exposure to an infectious agent, following the pattern of an allergic response. The early stage of the disease is marked by exudative processes and swelling of the myocardial fibers; in later stages alterations and proliferations become predominent. The toxins and inflammatory products stimulate the cardiac receptor system, precipitating tachycardia, extrasystoles and other arrhythmias. Later the impulse conduction system of the heart may also become involved in the pathologic process. The nature of the myocardial damage depends on the severity of the primary disease and on the initial state of the heart and organism as a whole.

Domračev [1950] describes two stages in the development of acute myocarditis. In the first stage there are no destructive myocardial changes, and there is a rapid rise in the strength of cardiac contractions. This leads to a significant rise of the arterial blood pressure and acceleration of the blood flow. In the second stage, dystrophic and degenerative lesions develop and the myocardial contractions become weaker, resulting in a fall of arterial blood pressure and blood flow velocity. The characteristic signs of heart failure appear — pronounced abnormalities of heart rate and rhythm, dyspnea, cyanosis and edema.

Necropsy findings depend on the stage and severity of the myocarditis as well as on the primary disease. In the initial stage of myocarditis the myocardium appears swollen. The cut surface is red in color and is occasionally spotted by hemorrhages.

In the second stage the myocardium appears lighter in color and may have a 'boiled' look in severe cases; it is also flaccid and friable. Histologic examination usually reveals hyaline or fatty degeneration of the myocardial fibers. Edema, accumulations of lymphocytes, macrophages and granulocytes are observed in the connective tissue. Examination of the vessels reveals extravascular infiltrates, hyalinization of the vascular walls, and occasionally intravascular thrombi.

Diagnosis. Myocarditis can be diagnosed on the basis of the symptoms characteristic of the two stages, paying attention to EKG findings and blood pressure measurements. A simple function test may be carried out by exercising the animal briefly and then assessing the pulse changes in response to the stress. If myocarditis is present, the pulse rate will continue to rise during the first 2—5 min after exercise, reflecting the abnormal excitability of the heart.

Differential Diagnosis. Myocarditis must be differentiated from pericarditis, endocarditis and myocardosis. Fibrinous pericarditis is distinguished from myocarditis by the presence of pericardial friction sounds, and exudative pericarditis by the syndrome of cardiac tamponade and by splashing sounds. In endocarditis, endocardial murmurs of organic origin are audible. The differential diagnosis of myocarditis and myocardosis relies chiefly on the findings of clinical and electrocardiographic examination (see Myocardosis).

The *prognosis* depends largely on the nature and severity of the primary disease that is responsible for the myocarditis. In the absence of prompt treatment, myocarditis may take a fatal course or become complicated by myocardial fibrosis.

Treatment and Prophylaxis. Complete rest is mandatory. In the early stage symptomatic treatment with cold compresses applied to the cardiac area may be of benefit. The use of glucose and anti-inflammatory drugs may be justified. In severe cases oxygen administered by inhalation, antibacterial agents (sulfonamides, antibiotics), caffeine, camphor, nicethamide and pentetrazol are recommended. Digitalis preparations are contraindicated in myocarditis.

The principal anti-inflammatory drugs are sodium salicylate, aminophenazone, calcium chlorate or calcium gluconate, and hormonal preparations (ACTH, cortisone and other glucocorticoids). Corticotropin (ACTH) is administered i.m. in a dose of 0.08—0.13 I.U. per kg BW, dissolved in isotonic saline. The athletic horse should receive 30—50 I.U. 3 to 4 times daily for several days. Alternatively, ACTH zinc phosphate may be given in the same dose, but only once a day or 2—3 times per week.

Camphor may be given orally in doses of 5—10 g or subcutaneously as a 20% solution in a dose of 20—40 ml. Nicethamide and pentetrazol are administered subcutaneously or intravenously (see Treatment of Myocardosis).

The *prophylaxis* of myocarditis relies on prompt treatment of the primary disease with anti-inflammatory agents.

Myocardial Fibrosis

Definition. Myocardial fibrosis is a disease caused by the proliferation of fibrous connective tissue among the myocardial fibers.

Symptoms. In mild cases affected horses appear normal while standing, but even the slightest physical exertion is sufficient to produce signs of cardiac failure. In severe cases signs of heart failure may be apparent even at rest. The first heart sound is muffled, weak and often prolonged, split or duplicated; the second sound is also weak and dull, but may be increased if arterial hypertension is present. The venous pressure is usually elevated, and the blood velocity is reduced. The EKG shows low voltages in all waves. The PQ and QT segments are lengthened, and the QRS complex is widened and abnormally shaped (fig. 2.1.3. — 12). Functional disorders of other

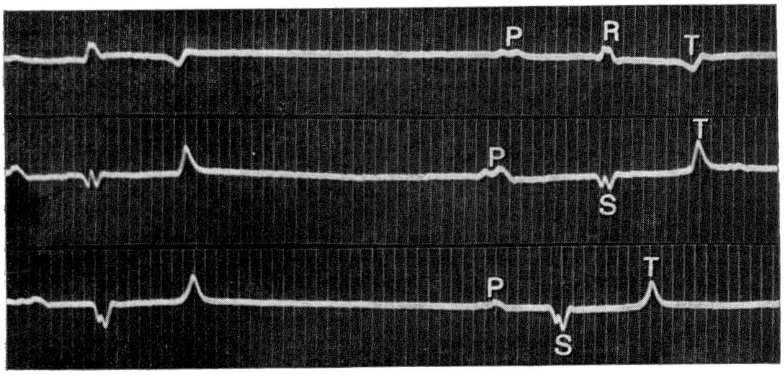

Fig. 2.1.3. — 12. EKG of a race horse: myocardial fibrosis.

organs and systems are typical in this disease. Exudation of the bronchi frequently develops.

Etiology. The disease usually develops as a complication of myocarditis or myocardosis. It may also arise independently in connection with longstanding disturbances of the myocardium associated with coronary heart disease. The illness appears to be age-related in many cases.

Pathogenesis and Lesions. The formation of fibrous tissue in the heart is usually the result of inflammatory or degenerative processes in the myocardium. Fibrous tissue formation among the heart muscle fibers leads to compression of healthy areas of the myocardium and coronary vessels, which in turn leads to localized nutritional disturbances in these areas with subsequent dystrophy and degeneration. The degenerated myocardial areas, in turn, are replaced by additional fibrous tissue. In severe cases calcium deposits can form in certain areas of the myocardium, especially the papillary muscles. The induration of the myocardium impairs its contractile ability, leading to circulatory disturbances, producing symptoms of heart failure. This may be exacerbated by exercise. Myocardial fibrosis associated with aging or arteriosclerosis is accompanied by arterial hypertension.

At necropsy grayish-white streaks of fibrous tissue are found in the muscle. The myocardium and coronary vessels are indurated, and the latter show luminal narrowing. In severe cases focal calcium deposits may be present in the myocardium.

The *diagnosis* is based on the results of the clinical examination, EKG and cardiac function tests. Affected horses show a marked increase in heart rate after 10 min exercise, and the heart rate returns to the resting value much more slowly than in normal animals.

The *prognosis* is poor in most cases and is grave in severe cases.

Treatment and Prophylaxis. A balanced diet, good nursing care and regular exercise should be maintained. Further treatment is with cardiac glycosides, glucose, camphor, nicethamide, pentetrazol, diuretics, as well as limb massage. Sound nutrition and a well-planned conditioning program are regarded as the main prophylactic measures. The prompt treatment of myocarditis and myocardosis also contributes to minimizing the effects the disease.

Cardiac Dilatation

Definition. Cardiac dilatation is a disease characterized by enlargement of the chambers of the heart.

Symptoms. The cardiac impulse is diffuse, increased (or occasionally weakened) and short, and the pulse is small, weak and usually shows an abnormal rhythm. The area of relative cardiac dullness and especially of absolute dullness is increased. The heart sounds are muffled. The first heart sound is increased, prolonged, split or duplicated, and the second heart sound is weakened. Functional endocardial murmurs are frequently audible. Occasionally gallop rhythm and similar sounding first and second heart sound embryocardia are also noted. The EKG shows extrasystoles, widening of the QRS complex and ST segment shifts. Cardiac dilatation is often accompanied by ataxia, dulled reflexes and pulmonary edema.

Etiology. Cardiac dilatation usually develops as a complication of myocarditis, myocardosis, chronic obstructive pulmonary disease (COPD), nephritis or other diseases.

Pathogenesis and Lesions. Enlargement of the heart leads to serious disturbances of blood flow. The cardiac stroke volume is decreased, as is the volume of circulating blood. This in turn leads to a fall of the arterial blood pressure. Collapse and cardiac standstill can occur in severe cases. A state of venous reflux develops in the organs and tissues, accompanied by signs of edema. Occasionally, a coma-like state develops as a result of venous congestion in the brain. The heart is markedly enlarged and somewhat spherical in shape. The walls of the dilated parts are thin and flabby. Venous congestion appears in the other organs.

The *diagnosis* is based on the clinical picture. The disease needs to be differentiated from myocardial hypertrophy. In the latter case the cardiac impulse is more prolonged, and no serious circulatory disturbances are present.

The *prognosis* is poor. In severe cases it is grave, and sudden death may occur as a result of cardiac arrest.

Treatment and Prophylaxis. Affected horses require complete rest, easily-digested feed and good nursing care. Oxygen inhalation is indicated in severe cases. Intravenous glucose and NaCl solutions may also be administered.

Prophylaxis includes prompt treatment of the primary disease and attention to correct nutrition, and overall care.

Endocarditis

Definition. Endocarditis is an inflammation, usually chronic, of the inner lining of the heart.

Symptoms. Profound depression, anorexia, fever, tachycardia, dyspnea and other symptoms of heart failure characterize the disease. In acute endocarditis the cardiac impulse is increased and the heart sounds are intensified, especially the first, in the early stage. Later the heart sounds become weaker, muffled, and are often accompanied by murmurs. These murmurs, having a fluctuating character and intensity, are characteristic of endocarditis. The alterations of blood flow lead to functional disturbances in other organs. In some cases of endocarditis hemorrhages can be seen on the skin and visible mucous membranes, and there may be lesions in the brain and meninges.

In the EKG, the amplitudes of the P, R and T waves are increased, the PQ and QT intervals are shortened, and the ST segment is displaced. Extrasystoles often appear. Blood tests reveal a neutrophilic leukocytosis and often changes that are indicative of septicemia.

Etiology. Most cases of endocarditis are secondary to infectious or toxic conditions.

Pathogenesis and Lesions. Inflammatory, necrotic and degenerative lesions develop during the course of the disease, affecting mainly the valvular portion of the endocardium. In verrucous endocarditis there is superficial inflammation with endothelial degeneration and necrosis. Fibrin, leukocytes and platelets are deposited on the valvular surface. These deposits become organized to form round, wartlike vegetations which distort the valve and interfere with its function. Disturbances of the general circulation result. So called 'ulcerative' endocarditis is characterized by necrosis which leads to the destruction of the valves. Ulcerative endocarditis generally takes an insidious course, causing emboli that can result in sudden death. Heart defects with corresponding circulatory disturbances are a common sequel to endocarditis.

Murmurs develop as a result of valvular lesions. In verrucous endocarditis, reddish-gray deposits are found on the valves or mural endocardium, and the valve leaflets show distortion and adhesion formation. In ulcerative endocarditis, there are erosions of the valves or mural endocardium that are covered with loose, fibrinous thrombi. Occasionally valvular perforations, vascular emboli and changes indicative of septicemia can be observed.

The *diagnosis* is based on the presence of characteristic symptoms and consideration of the primary disease. The *prognosis* is usually poor in ulcerative forms.

Treatment and Prophylaxis. The main emphasis is on treatment of the causative disease. Sulfonamides and antibiotics are used. If the endocarditis is immune mediated (antigen/antibody), treatment with anti-inflammatory drugs is indicated (see Treatment of Myocarditis). Prophylaxis consists in the prevention of complications of the primary disease.

Heart Defects

Definition and Etiology; Occurrence. Heart defects (valvular defects) in the horse most commonly occur as a complication of endocarditis. The majority are acquired. Far less common are congenital defects due to developmental abnormalities such as septal defects, patent ductus arteriosus or valvular stenoses. The cardinal sign of the heart defect is usually a persistent endocardial murmur. The murmur may be described as blowing, buzzing, harsh or sighing, depending on the degree and nature of the valvular lesion (deformity, thickening, perforation, adhesion, cusp tear, neoplasia). Frequently murmurs are accompanied by a palpable vibration of the chest wall, called a fremitus or thrill. The sensation is similar to that of stroking a purring cat.

Eight heart defects are recognized in association with the four cardiac valves and four orifices. A complicated defect is one in which stenosis of the orifice is combined with an insufficiency of the corresponding valve. A combined heart defect is characterized by multiple valvular lesions coexisting in various parts of the heart.

The *diagnosis* of heart defects in the horse has been discussed at length by DOMRAČEV [1950] and ZAJCEV [1971]. It depends largely on the detection of a murmur, its duration, its relation to a particular phase of the cardiac cycle, and its site of maximum audibility.

The heart defect is said to be compensated if it is unaccompanied by major signs of cardiac failure such as arrhythmia, dyspnea, cyanosis or edema.

Clinical Signs of Heart Defects

Mitral Stenosis. The blood flows from the left atrium into the left ventricle through a narrowed orifice, creating a presystolic murmur that is audible before ventricular systole. It is best heard at the area of maximal audibility of the bicuspid valve (left 5th intercostal space, 3 fingerbreadths below the level of the shoulder joint). Occasionally a thrill is felt on palpation of the cardiac area. As a result of constant overfilling of the left atrium and reflux into the pulmonary circulation, the left atrium and right ventricle gradually become dilatated and then hypertrophied. Auscultation reveals a sharp first sound. This valvular defect cannot be compensated for adequately. With decompensation there is dilatation of the left atrium and pulmonary edema. Dyspnea, cyanosis and other symptoms of heart failure appear.

Tricuspid Stenosis. When the blood flows from the right atrium into the right ventricle through the narrowed orifice, a presystolic murmur is produced that is best heard at the area of maximum audibility of the tricuspid valve (right 4th intercostal space, 3 fingerbreadths below the level of the shoulder joint). Overfilling of the right atrium and reflux leads to dilatation with subsequent hypertrophy of the right atrium and left ventricle. Due to inadequate filling of the right ventricle, a loud first heart sound is audible. With decompensation, comes dilatation of the right atrium and venous engorgement, leading to edema, cyanosis, passive congestion of the liver along with other disturbances.

Mitral Insufficiency. Mitral insufficiency allows blood to regurgitate from the left ventricle into the left atrium, producing a systolic murmur that is most intense at the area of maximum audibility of the mitral valve (left 5th intercostal space). Sometimes a thrill is palpable. The overfilling of the left atrium and increased blood volume in the left ventricle lead to the dilatation and subsequent hypertrophy of both chambers. The right atrium also becomes dilatated and hypertrophied due to the pulmonary congestion that occurs. Decompensation leads to passive hyperemia in the pulmonary circulation, dyspnea, cyanosis and other signs of cardiac failure.

Tricuspid Insufficiency. In tricuspid insufficiency blood leaks back into the right atrium during right ventricular systole. This creates a systolic murmur that is most audible in the area of the tricuspid valve (right 4th intercostal space). The stasis of blood in the right atrium and ventricle leads to dilatation and hypertrophy of these chambers. This, in turn, may lead to left ventricular dilatation and hypertrophy. Tricuspid insufficiency is poorly compensated. Decompensation is accompanied most notably by passive hyperemia in the general circulatory system. A characteristic sign of this valvular defect is a positive venous pulse.

Aortic Stenosis. The blood, as it exits the left ventricle and traverses the narrowed aortic opening, produces a systolic murmur heard best at the area of the aortic valve (left 4th intercostal space, 2 fingerbreadths below the level of the shoulder joint). Occasionally a thrill is noted. The stasis of blood in the left ventricle causes that chamber to become dilatated and then hypertrophied, providing permanent compensation for the valvular defect. The cardiac impulse is increased, and the arterial pulse is small and slow. Decompensation is manifested chiefly by left ventricular dilatation, cerebral ischemia, ataxia and fainting spells.

Pulmonary Valve Stenosis. The blood flowing from the right ventricle through the narrowed pulmonary valve produces a systolic murmur that is best heard at the area of the pulmonary valve (left 3rd intercostal space, 4 fingerbreadths below the level of the shoulder joint). The obstruction to flow causes dilatation of the right ventricle and hypertrophy. The cardiac impulse is increased on the right side, as is the first heart sound at the tricuspid valve. Compensation is difficult to achieve. Decompensation is manifest as dilatation of the right ventricle and passive venous congestion in the general circulation.

Aortic Insufficiency. An insufficient aortic valve allows blood to regurgitate into the left ventricle during diastole, producing a diastolic murmur heard best in the area of the aortic valve (left 4th intercostal space). Phonographic and EKG studies [Spörri and Leemann, 1972] have revealed two forms of aortic insufficiency in the horse: the first is accompanied by one diastolic murmur, and the second by two diastolic murmurs, one faint and one loud.

The increased load of blood causes dilatation and subsequent hypertrophy of the left ventricle. The systolic pressure is elevated, the diastolic pressure is reduced, and consequently the pulse pressure is greatly increased. The arterial pulse is large, full and rapid. The defect is usually well compensated. Decompensation is accompanied by left ventricular dilatation. The overfilling of this chamber makes it difficult for the left atrium to empty. This is followed by passive hyperemia in the pulmonary circulation, leading to dyspnea and cyanosis.

Pulmonary Valve Insufficiency. In pulmonary valve insufficiency blood is regurgitated into the right ventricle, producing a diastolic murmur that is most intense in the area of the pulmonary valve (left 3rd intercostal space). This regurgitation causes the right ventricle to become dilatated and hypertrophied. Compensation is difficult. Decompensation is attended by right ventricular dilatation, dyspnea and cyanosis.

Prognosis of Heart Defects: The prognosis depends upon the severity of the defect and the degree of compensation. Horses with well-compensated defects have much the same working capacity as normal horses, though they often require close veterinary observation. Defects that are compensated by left ventricular hypertrophy carry the best prognosis.

For congenital heart defects, which mainly affect stallions, the prognosis is usually poor.

Treatment and Prophylaxis. The aim of treatment is to promote and maintain a state of compensation. Care is taken to ensure good nutrition, general care and sensible use of the horse. Regular exercise and fresh air are essential. Drug treatment is indicated only if decompensation has occurred. Rest is prescribed. Glucose and cardiac glycosides may be indicated. If disturbances arise in other organ systems, appropriate symptomatic treatment is indicated.

Prophylaxis consists in the prevention and prompt treatment of diseases that can predispose to endocarditis and the development of valvular disease.

2.1.3.1.2. Diseases of the Blood Vessels

Arteriosclerosis

Definition. Arteriosclerosis is a lesion characterized by the massive growth of fibrous tissue in the arterial walls. The disease usually begins as atherosclerosis, in which deposits of cholesterol are formed within the vascular intima, leading to degeneration and plaque formation in the vessel walls.

Symptoms. The clinical picture is often subtle owing to the insidious onset of the disease. Affected animals show a decline of working capacity and fatigue easity. In addition, there is a noticeable decrease in skin elasticity, reflex activity and neuromuscular tone. The first heart sound is muffled and prolonged, while the second is increased and often accentuated at the aortic valve. The arterial blood pressure is elevated.

Etiology. In rare cases arteriosclerosis occurs as a primary condition in old animals. Usually, however, the disease is secondary to metabolic disorders or arises as a complication of prolonged toxcemic states. Pauli [1973] found marked sclerosis of the coronary vessels in 8- to 12-year-old horses with chronic respiratory and digestive disease. Overexertion and the overfeeding of large amounts of bulk feeds may predispose to arteriosclerosis.

Pathogenesis and Lesions. The lesions of arteriosclerosis form gradually. The disease begins with fatty, hyaline degeneration and necrosis of the intima (atheromatosis). Next the vessel wall becomes permeated with fibrous tissue (arteriosclerosis).

In severe cases, calcium may be deposited in the vessel wall. These lesions interfere with blood flow and have the effect of raising the arterial blood pressure and increasing cardiac work. The most severe hemodynamic changes occur with damage to the coronary vessels, aorta and cerebral arteries.

At necropsy a hardening and thickening of the arterial walls are seen as a result of fibrous tissue proliferation. Occasionally the vessel walls are found to be calcified and hemorrhage when ruptured.

The *diagnosis* is made from clinical findings and from blood pressure measurements, and the patient's history.

Prognosis. It is poor in severe cases.

Treatment and Prophylaxis. In advanced cases treatment is unrewarding. The animal should be limited to light work. Early cases may respond to dietary changes as well as iodine preparations and cardiovascular drugs.

Thrombosis

Definition. Vascular thrombosis is characterized by the partial or complete occlusion of blood vessels by thrombi.

Symptoms. The symptoms depend on where the thrombus is located and the caliber of the affected vessel. Thrombosis of the coronary vessels can lead to myocardial infarction with the attendant symptoms. Thrombosis of the renal artery can cause renal colic, hypertension, proteinuria and hematuria. With thrombosis of arteries of the extremities, the affected limb tends to collapse when load is applied. The limb feels cold, and its sensation is impaired. Thrombosis of the cranial vena cava is accompanied by venous congestion in the region of the head, neck and forelimbs. Hydrothorax may develop. Thrombosis of the caudal vena cava leads to venous congestion in the caudal body regions and occasionally to ascites. Portal vein thrombosis produces signs of congestion in the gastrointestinal tract.

The thrombosis of large veins in the horse is manifested by anxiety, muscular tremor, sweating, dyspnea and tachycardia. The thrombosis of small veins, in contrast, may cause no obvious clinical symptoms. Thrombosis of the anterior mesenteric artery is discussed unter Thromboembolic Colic (2.1.5.10.6.).

Etiology. Primary thromboses can occur as a result of mechanical or parasitic irritation or vascular inflammation. Secondary thromboses can arise from endocarditis or arteriosclerosis. Predisposing factors are myocardial weakness or asthenia, decreased vascular tone and increased coagulability of the blood. Venous thromboses are more common than arterial thromboses in the horse.

Pathogenesis and Lesions. Vascular thromboses often lead to serious functional disturbances of the affected organs and tissues. The thrombosis of large vessels, such as the abdominal aorta, iliac artery or hypogastric artery, can have grave consequences. The large vessels typically contain white laminar and mural thrombi that are composed of fibrin and cellular blood constituents.

The *diagnosis* is made on the basis of characteristic local symptoms and the patient's history.

The *prognosis* is always questionable. Lesions of larger vessels invariably have a poor prognosis.

Treatment and Prophylaxis. Early cases of thrombosis can be treated with fibrinolysin, heparin and sodium gluconate, 500—600 mg/kg BW, 20 % i.v. In addition, complete rest and treatment with suitable cardiovascular drugs are indicated. In infectious thrombophlebitis, heat is applied locally to induce hyperemia and promote abscessation, while systemic treatment with sulfonamides and antibiotics is indicated. Prophylaxis centers on the prevention and prompt treatment of endocarditis, arteriosclerosis and strongylosis. As well, strict adherence to the correct techniques of venipuncture and the intravenous administration of drug solutions, is important in prophylaxis.

2.1.3.1.3. Functional Changes and Disturbances of the Cardiovascular System during Training

The working capacity (speed, endurance) of a horse depends primarily on its state of training and on the functional state of the organ systems, especially the cardiovascular system. If alterations in the function of this system are promptly recognized, it is possible to prevent various types of cardiovascular damage, as well as damage to other organs. Assessment of the cardiovascular system is important in evaluating the animal's state of training. Studies by Sudakov, Bobylev [1968], and Laskov [1973] indicate that the results of the clinical examination are good indicators of the state of training of the equine athlete. According to Sudakov, untrained horses have weaker heart sounds and lower-amplitude pulse waves at rest (before exercise) than do well-trained horses. In well-trained athletic horses, the first heart sound is generally increased, prolonged and muffled. The increased intensity and duration are the result of physiologic hypertrophy of the heart, particularly of the left ventricle, as evidenced by clinical and EKG examination. The muffling of the first heart sound in well-trained horses is attributable to an increase in vagal tone. Signs of increased vagal tone are exhibited by the majority of fit horses. According to Fogelson [1961] and others, the rate of the blood pressure rise within the ventricles is reduced in animals with increased vagal tone thereby slowing the closure of the atrioventricular valves and causing a muffling of the first heart sound. The veterinarian must be careful not to confuse this muffling with weakening of the first sound, for the two are entirely different. Weakening combined with muffling is usually a sign of severe dystrophic-degenerative myocardial changes.

During auscultation of the heart in athletic horses, it must be remembered that healthy, well-trained horses at rest may show a splitting of the first heart sound which disappears with exercise. For example, of the horses entered in the Tenth World Championships of the Modern Pentathlon in Moscow, 31 % had a split first heart sound at rest before the start. Clinical and EKG examination indicated that the causes of these alterations lay either in a temporary slowing of atrioventricular impulse conduction (prolongation of the PQ interval to 0.50—0.60 s), with the atrial sounds occurring separately from the first heart sound; or in a delayed excitation of one of the ventricles, usually the left, as a consequence of myocardial hypertrophy.

Persistence of the change after exercise indicates a significant delay in the excitation of one of the ventricles in connection with insufficient blood delivery to its myocardium. It can also indicate a permanent disturbance of atrioventricular conduction associated with a two foci in the region of the AV node or bundle of His. Such horses should be removed from work or training and placed under veterinary supervision.

Splitting of the second heart sound may be heard at rest and after exercise in untrained horses as well as in animals that have been overworked in training. It generally denotes a functional weakness of one of the ventricles and significant blood pressure elevation in the pulmonary or systemic circulation. Splitting of the second heart sound is usually found in connection with exaggerated closure of the pulmonary valve in horses with symptoms of chronic obstructive pulmonary disease (COPD).

When the functional state of the cardiovascular system in the horse is severely reduced after strenuous exertion, abnormal heart sounds in the form of gallop rhythms or similarities in the sound of the sound of the first and second heart sound (embryocardia) are sometimes heard. Gallop rhythm must not be confused with a splitting of the first heart sound like that commonly occurring in the fit horse with excessive vagal tone. Unlike gallop rhythm, splitting of the first heart sound in such cases occurs when the heart rate is slow. Gallop rhythm is characterized by a sequence of three beats spaced at approximately equal intervals. The first beat is often accentuated, and pronounced tachycardia is always present. Most cardiologists feel that gallop rhythm is based on a reduplication of the first heart sound associated with functional weakness of one of the ventricles (dilatation or dystrophic-degenerative myocardial lesions) or a functional disturbance of the impulse conduction system (bundle of His or its branches).

Embryocardia refers to evenly-spaced heart sounds that vary little in quality and intensity, i.e. the first and second heart sounds are similar. Phono- and electrocardiographic studies have shown that embryocardia is due to an extreme weakening or loss of the second heart sound resulting from a strong fall of the arterial blood pressure. The examiner hears only the first heart sound, as during auscultation of the fetal heart, in which the aorta still communicates with the pulmonary artery via the ductus arteriosus. Hence, the blood pressure in these vessels is so low that closure of the semilunar valves is almost inaudible.

The veterinarian must be aware that the appearance of a gallop rhythm or embryocardia in the horse after exercise signifies the heart is in trouble and warrants immediate therapy. Abnormalities of this type have been observed in untrained horses after strenuous exercise, as well as in fit horses that are overworked in training or have been subjected to maximal loads during competition.

During the clinical examination it is important not only to detect qualitative changes in the heart sounds at rest and after exercise, e.g. during the training period, but also to assess the heart rate. The respiratory rate should also be determined. As an example, consider the observations made on changes in the heart and respiratory rates of standardbreds at the Central Moscow Hippodrome during a training period. On the average, the heart rate of well-trained horses increased after slow trotting (6 rounds) by a factor of 1.5 and returned to the resting value within 20—30 min. In horses with less training, the heart rate rose by a factor of 2 or more after the same exercise and took 40—50 min to normalize.

After a fast trot (2 heats), the heart rate of the well-trained horses rose by an factor of 2.5 on the average and normalized in 50—60 min. The less fit horses responded to the same exercise with a 3-fold or greater increase, and normalization took 70—80 min.

The respiratory rate of the well-trained horses increased after a slow trot (6 rounds) by an average factor of 2 and normalized in 10—15 min. The animals with less training showed a 2.5-fold increase, with normalization after 15—20 min.

After a fast trot (2 heats) the respiratory rate of the well-trained horses increased by a factor of 4 and normalized in 25—30 min, compared to a factor of 5 or more and 35—40 min in the animals with less training.

Similar but even more pronounced changes in heart and respiratory rate were observed in Thoroughbreds during the 1973 European Three Day Event Championship in Kiev. In horses in top condition, the heart rate following the cross-country phase did not exceed 100—110 beats/min, and the respiratory rate did not exceed the heart rate.

These findings are of obvious practical value in that they allow a horse's state of training to be assessed and permit conclusions to be drawn regarding the duration of post-exercise rest periods necessary for recovery.

Besides assessment of the pulse rate and quality of the heart sounds, the detection of arrhythmias and murmurs forms an important part of the clinical examination of the equine athlete. 'Functional' murmurs are not unusual in such animals and represent a transitory disturbance of hemodynamics in the heart.

The major causes of systolic functional murmurs in horses are as follows:

— relative insufficiency of the left or right atrioventricular valve with dilatation of the corresponding ventricle;
— excess tension of the papillary muscles;
— lack of tension of the papillary muscles;
— acceleration of the blood flow in anemic states;
— rapid change in the blood flow velocity.

The main causes of diastolic functional murmurs are:

— relative insufficiency of the aortic valve due to loss of tone and dilatation of the muscular aortic ring;
— relative insufficiency of the pulmonary artery valves with loss of tone and dilatation of the muscular ring of the pulmonary artery;
— spasm of the left atrioventricular musculofibrous ring;
— spasm of the right atrioventricular musculofibrous ring.

Our own observations indicate that fit horses are affected mainly by systolic functional murmurs of a blowing quality that can arise in the following situations:

— excess tension in the papillary muscles, when the chordae tendineae are tense and the valve leaflets cannot adequately seal the atrioventricular orifice; such murmurs have often been demonstrated in excited horses prior to a race;
— lack of tension of the papillary muscles, when during systole the leaflets of the left and right atrioventricular valves are bowed in toward the atria due to laxness of the papillary muscles and chordae tendineae;
— a strong increase in the blood velocity. This is a common pre-race condition in fit horses during training, and particularly during performance trials and competitions;
— relative insufficiency of the bicuspid valve due to dilatation of the left ventricle due to increased tone;
— relative insufficiency of the tricuspid valve due to dilatation of the right ventricle.

Functional murmurs need to be distinguished from organic endocardial murmurs associated with valvular defects. Functional murmurs are caused by excessive tension of the papillary muscles and disappear after exercise. Those associated with lack of papillary muscle tone or accompanying the transient increase in blood flow velocity just before a race are also abolished by exercise. However, if the papillary hypotension is a result of dystrophic myocardial disease, the functional murmurs disappear only with suitable recovery and treatment.

Functional murmurs associated with relative insufficiency of the atrioventricular valves also are relieved only by recovery and appropriate treatment. Such murmurs are primarily heard in poorly-trained horses that have been over-exerted.

Functional murmurs are distinguished from organic murmurs by their softer intensity and blowing quality, and by their characteristic variations in intensity during the relatively brief period of the examination.

It must be acknowledged that the causes of functional murmurs in the fit horse have not been adequately clarified. For example, it is difficult to account for the fact that 28 % of the well-trained horses that were selected for entry in the Tenth World

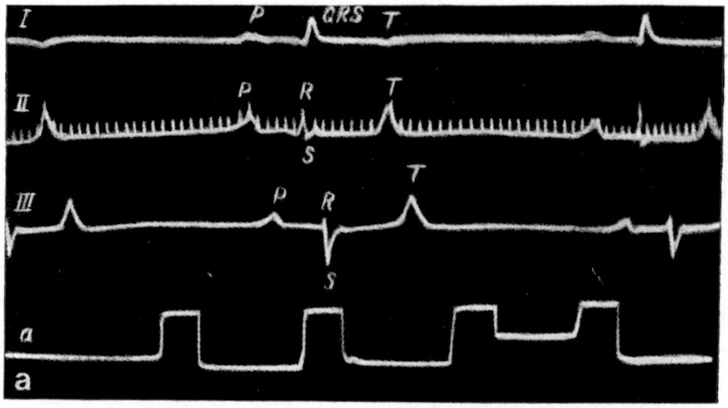

Fig. 2.1.3. — 13. EKG of a race horse: left ventricular hypertrophy; a = standardization marks.

Championships of the Modern Pentathlon were found on examination to have resting systolic murmurs. All these murmurs were audible at the pulmonary valve. The clinical, electrocardiographic, arteriotonometric and phlebotonometric studies, as well as the laboratory analysis of blood, urine and feces revealed no abnormalities. The only unusual finding was a marked increase in blood velocity, which probably was also the major cause of the murmurs. The murmurs disappeared after exercise, thus confirming their functional nature. Apparently the appearance of these murmurs is related to the rigorous training of the animals, overall fitness of the cardiovascular system, and the attendant hemodynamic changes. The veterinarian must be able to distinguish systolic functional murmurs not only from the pathological murmurs associated with valvular defects, but also from other waxing and waning murmurs. Murmurs of this type have been observed in only about 2% of the Thoroughbreds and trotters of the Central Moscow Hippodrome. Occasionally these murmurs are audible during systole, becoming more distinct during inspiration. They are blowing, weak, short and of varying intensity. They disappear completely when breathing is inhibited by compressing the nostrils. Most cardiologists believe that these murmurs result from the aspiration of air into the pulmonary region that is compressed by the heart during diastole. With the reduction of cardiac volume that occurs during systole, local compression on the lung is relieved, and air is aspirated into that region.

Electrocardiographic studies in athletic horses have demonstrated the prime importance of this technique in monitoring the response to training. Well-trained horses frequently show EKG changes that are characteristic of physiologic left ventricular hypertrophy. This 'LVH pattern' was recorded in 40% of the horses entered in the Tenth World Championships of the Modern Pentathlon. The physiologic hypertrophy varied in degree from one animal to the next.

The EKG of the stallion 'Žgučij', for example, was characterized by a negative QRS complex and a tall T wave of opposite polarity ('discordant' T wave) in limb lead III (fig. 2.1.3. — 13). The horse 'Rajgur' had a more pronounced LVH pattern in its EKG, signifying a still greater degree of left ventricular hypertrophy. Besides a negative QRS complex and discordant T wave in lead III, the EKG of this horse featured a biphasic QRS complex in limb lead II. The EKG of the horse 'Achtyrka' showed the strongest LVH pattern (fig. 2.1.3. — 14) with negative QRS complexes and discordant T waves in limb leads II and III. The left ventricular hypertrophy demonstrated for this horse by EKG was confirmed on clinical examination — percussion of the chest wall revealed a shift of the posterior percussion boundary of the heart to the 7th rib.

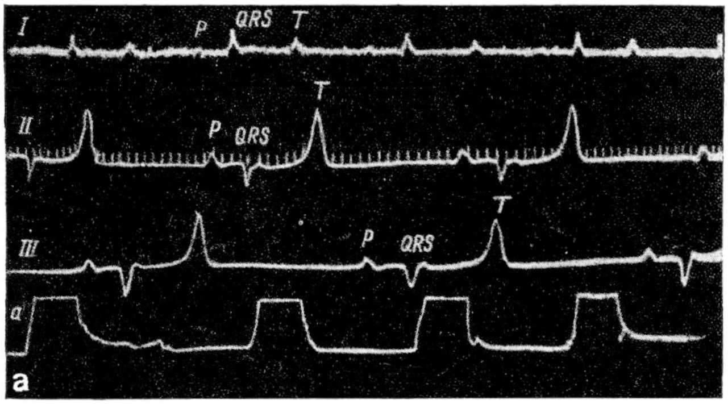

Fig. 2.1.3. — 14. EKG of a race horse: marked left ventricular hypertrophy; a = standardization marks.

Exercise accentuates the LVH pattern in the EKG, indicating a marked delay in the excitation of the hypertrophied left ventricle compared to the right ventricle.

When interpreting an LVH pattern in the EKG of a fit athletic horse, attention should be given to the duration of the QRST ventricular complex (the QT interval) and of its initial portion, the QRS complex. In physiologic left ventricular hypertrophy, the length of the QT interval is within normal limits for Standardbreds and Thoroughbreds, amounting to an average of 0.50 s with variation from 0.40 to 0.55 s. The average duration of the QRS complex in such cases is 0.10 s with variation from 0.07 to 0.15 s. The duration of the foregoing complexes is reduced after exercise.

Pathologic cardiac hypertrophy, especially of the left ventricle, secondary to dystrophic or degenerative myocardial disease, is characterized in the EKG by a considerable prolongation of the entire QRST ventricular complex, with a lengthening of the QT interval to more than 0.60 s and a widening of the QRS complex to more than 0.15 s. This is often accompanied by wide T waves and abnormally-shaped, displaced ST segments signifying inadequate blood delivery to the myocardium (especially the hypertrophied ventricular wall) and a disturbance of metabolic processes within the heart muscle. After exercise the duration of the QRST complex (QT interval) and width of the QRS complex in horses with pathologic cardiac hypertrophy do not decrease as in horses with physiologic hypertrophy. They are in fact increased.

An EKG pattern characteristic of right ventricular hypertrophy is uncommon in athletic horses.

Because physiologic and pathologic cardiac hypertrophies cannot always be clearly distinguished from each other, every horse that shows evidence of pronounced hypertrophy of either ventricle during the training period should undergo a systematic clinical and electrocardiographic examination. This makes it possible to assess exercise tolerance and estimate the necessary post-exercise recovery period; otherwise a physiologic hypertrophy can progress rapidly and insidiously to a pathologic form. If accompanied by dystrophic and degenerative myocardial changes, it can seriously hamper the working capacity of a race horse. The nature of the EKG changes that develop in the horse under the influence of exercise training depends mainly on the animal's state of training. In well-trained horses the post-exercise EKG shows high-amplitude P, R and T waves in all limb leads, a shortening of the PQ and QT intervals, and in most cases a left deviation of the electrical axis. In the EKG of the fit

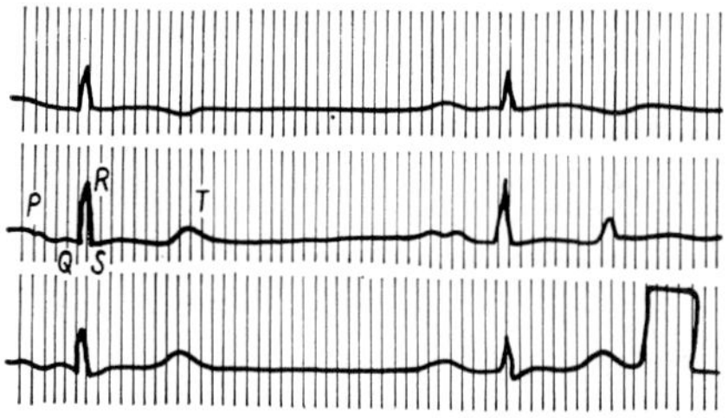

15

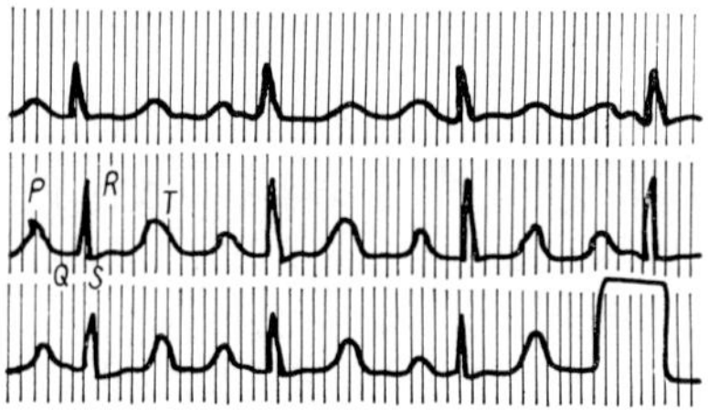

16

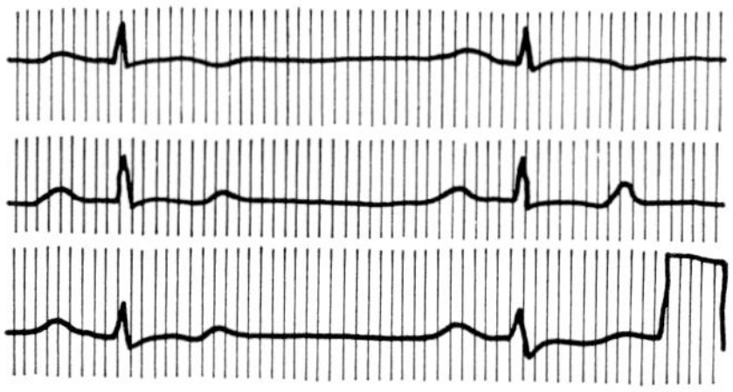

17

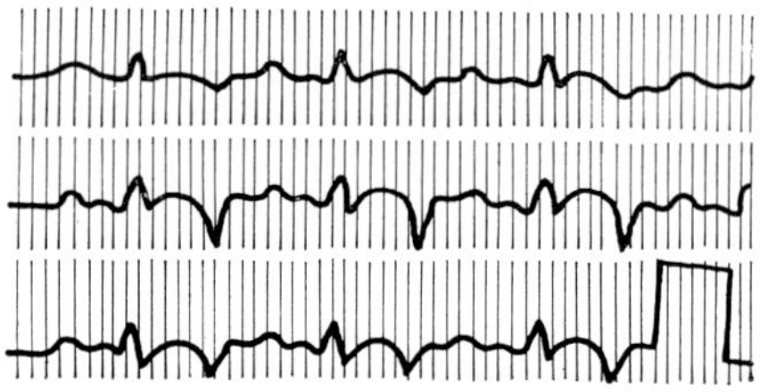

18

Fig. 2.1.3. — 15. EKG of a stallion at rest.
Fig. 2.1.3. — 16. EKG of a stallion after two fast heats.
Fig. 2.1.3. — 17. EKG at rest before the start of training.
Fig. 2.1.3. — 18. EKG of the same horse as in 2.1.3. — 17 after a fast heat.

stallion 'Kamennyj Svetok', for example, the high P, R and T waves and short PQ and QT intervals are obvious on comparison with the resting EKG (figs. 2.1.3. — 15 and — 16). These EKG changes were characteristic of a healthy myocardium. This could be confirmed by clinical examination and arterial blood pressure measurement. Analysis of the EKG records of this horse made before and after workouts revealed a number of changes. While the P waves in limb leads II and III were flat and split before exercise, as is normally the case in horses at rest, they were tall, peaked and unsplit after exercise. This indicated an acceleration of the excitation processes in the atria in response to physical exertion. The amplitudes of the R and T waves were also increased after exercise, owing to the greater coronary blood flow and increased metabolic processes in the myocardium. The T-wave changes, reflecting the repolarization in the ventricular myocardium, were highly characteristic. The biphasic T wave frequently found in limb lead II of normal horses changed to a tall positive wave after exercise. This reflected an increase of metabolic activity in the heart muscle and demonstrated a healthy myocardium.

In unfit as well as overtrained horses, different EKG changes appear after exercise. The amplitudes of the P, R and T waves are diminished, and the PQ interval and QRST complex (QT interval) are prolonged. These are signs characteristic of a poorly functioning myocardium. In addition, EKG changes appear that are characteristic of metabolic disturbances in the myocardium as well as dystrophic-degenerative lesions with associated coronary insufficiency. For example compare the pre- and post-exercise EKG records of the untrained horse 'Lazur', shown in figures 2.1.3. — 17 and — 18. The EKG after one heat shows widening and distortion of the T waves as well as abnormally shaped ST segments with upward deviation of the isoelectric line in all leads. Such changes are indicative of abnormal myocardial metabolism and pronounced coronary insufficiency. These lesions produce low-amplitude waves in all leads and a relative prolongation of the PQ and QT intervals. On clinical examination of this horse after exercise, muffled heart sounds were noted. Analogous changes

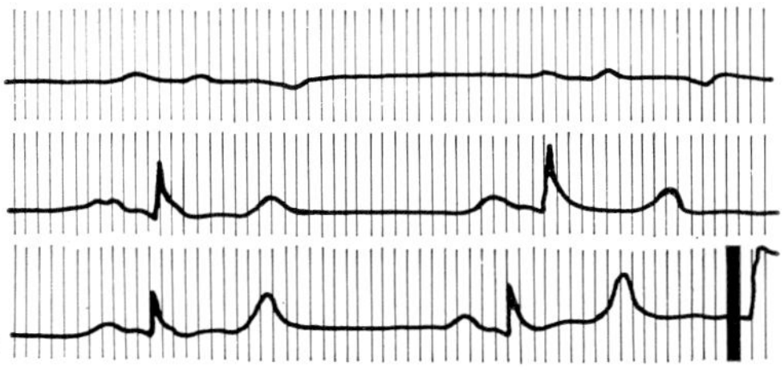
19

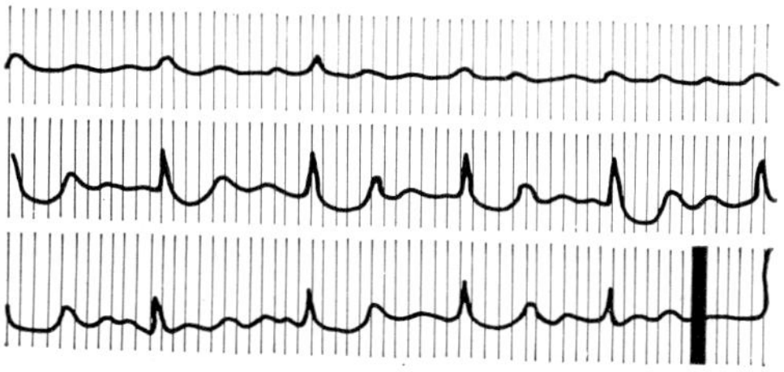
20

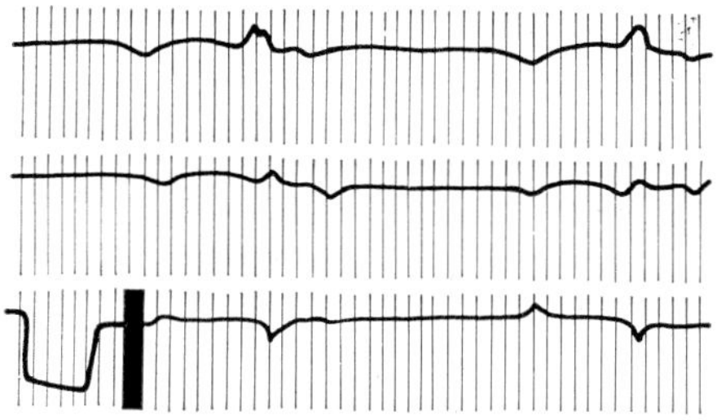
21

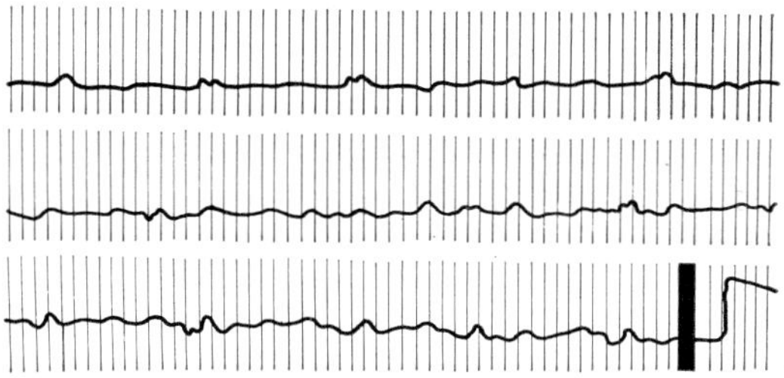
22

Fig. 2.1.3. — 19. EKG of a horse at rest.
Fig. 2.1.3. — 20. EKG of the same horse as in 2.1.3. — 19 after a fast heat.
Fig. 2.1.3. — 21. EKG of a horse at rest.
Fig. 2.1.3. — 22. EKG of the same horse as in 2.1.3. — 21 after training.

were observed in the EKG of the poorly-trained horse 'Basnja' after exercise at a fast gait (figs. 2.1.3. — 19 and — 20). This animal also exhibited dyspnea, cyanosis of the visible mucous membranes, and pronounced tachycardia after exercise.

When training is intensified, horses that have had little conditioning are especially apt to develop dystrophic-degenerative myocardial lesions and arrhythmias. In the horse 'Potschka', for example, a heart block was observed due to severe dystrophic-degenerative myocardial damage (low amplitude of all waves, broadened, slurred, notched QRS complex in all leads; figs. 2.1.3. — 21 and — 22). After exercise the voltage of all waves decreased. The P wave was widened and distorted, the QRS complex was also widened and further distorted, and the T wave was shortened. Post-exercise clinical examination of this horse revealed a muffling of the heart sounds with a prolonged first sound, dyspnea, severe tachycardia, and splitting of the second heart sound. Such horses should be immediately removed from training and placed under veterinary care. If the myocardial changes are irreparable, the animal must be retired from competition and in some cases is unsound even for breeding purposes.

During interpretation of the EKG, the systolic index is also calculated. This index represents the ratio of the duration of the QRST complex (electrical ventricular systole) to the duration of the total cardiac cycle (R-R interval) and characterizes the functional state of the myocardium. The systolic index increases after exercise, especially in unfit horses, as an expression of the elevated heart rate. In fit horses, it increases from 32 to 56 %, on the average, and from 36 to 78 % in unfit animals. Horses with little training are far more apt to develop arrhythmias than are well-trained horses. The most frequent form is the partial AV block, which we detected in 12—16 % of the horses examined. Generally this arrhythmia is observed only at rest and disappears with exercise. Nevertheless, this disturbance cannot be considered entirely benign, for it is not rare for a partial intermittent AV block to progress

23
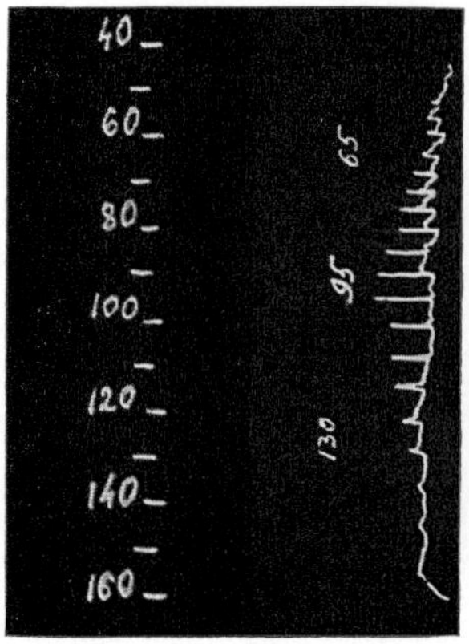

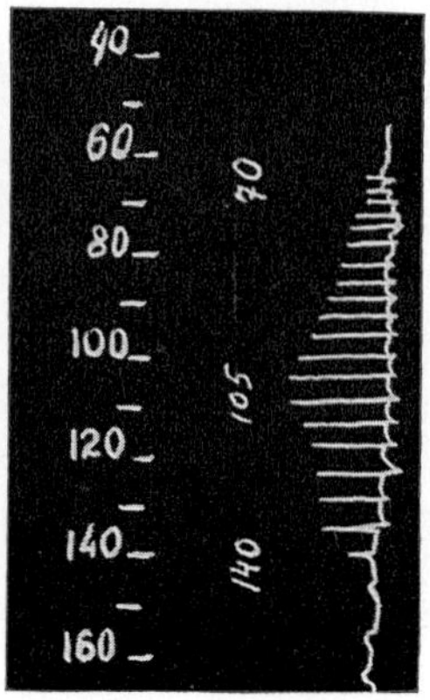

24

Fig. 2.1.3. — 23. Oscillogram of a well-trained horse at rest.
Fig. 2.1.3. — 24. Oscillogram of a well-trained horse after strenuous exercise.

to a permanent or even complete heart block. Besides AV block, athletic horses may also exhibit arrhythmias such as sinoatrial block and premature beats, especially ventricular premature beats. Our findings indicate a prevalence of 8—10 % for sinoatrial block. It is most commonly associated with long training breaks or a lack of systematic training and is indicative of excessive vagal tone. Premature beats are mainly a post-exercise phenomenon in poorly-trained horses and have a prevalence of 3—5 % according to our findings.

Clearly, electrocardiography plays an important role in the physiologic monitoring of the athletic horse. The development of the bioradiotelemetric method of EKG recording holds particular promise in this regard [Novošinov et al., 1973].

The measurement of arterial blood pressure in the race horse before and after prescribed workloads can also provide valuable information which supplements and enhances the accuracy of clinical and EKG findings. Our data indicate that the systolic arterial blood pressure of well-trained Standardbreds increases by an average of 1.3—2.0 kPa (10—15 mm Hg[1]) during the training period after exercise at a fast gait. In fit Thoroughbreds preparing for the Tenth World Championships in the Modern Pentathlon, it increased by an average of 2.0—2.7 kPa (15—20 mm Hg) after workouts comparable in intensity to competitive conditions. The post-exercise rise of systolic pressure in fit horses takes place mainly at the cost of increased cardiac work, a greater circulating blood volume, and a significant increase in arterial tone.

The diastolic arterial pressure also increases in fit horses after exercise, but to a lesser degree than the systolic. In our investigations in Standardbreds and Thoroughbreds, it increased by an average of 1.3—2.0 kPa after intensive exercise. In fit horses this increase is accomplished essentially by a rise in heart rate and an increase in peripheral arterial tone.

The fit horse also shows an increase in mean arterial pressure following exercise. This increase is small compared to the systolic and diastolic pressure changes, however. We found an average elevation of 0.7—1.3 kPa in Thoroughbreds and Standardbreds.

The pulse pressure (difference between systolic and diastolic pressures) remained unchanged or rose slightly in these horses.

1 Conversion: kPa × 7.501 = mm Hg, mm Hg × 0.1333 = kPa.

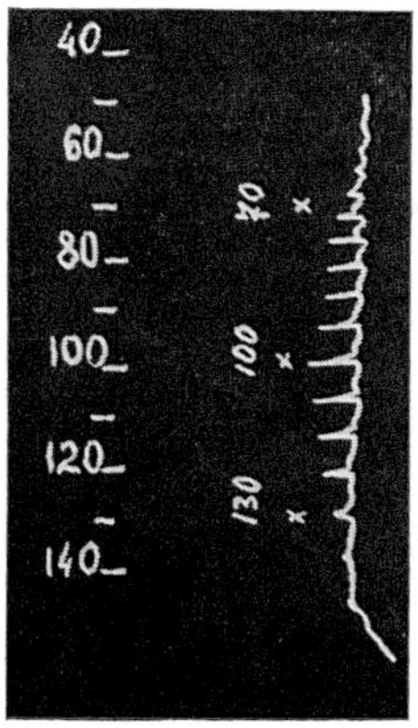

25

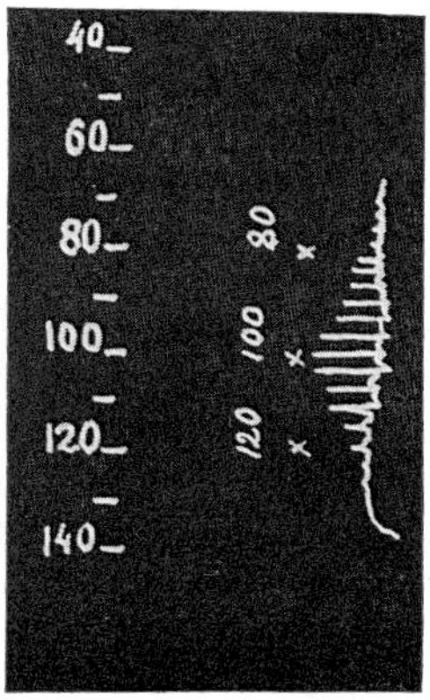

26

Fig. 2.1.3. — 25. Oscillogram of a poorly-trained horse at rest.
Fig. 2.1.3. — 26. Oscillogram of a poorly-trained horse after strenuous exercise.

The changes in the arterial blood pressure parameters of fit race horses during an intensive training period are shown in figures 2.1.3. — 23 and — 24. These parameters show different post-exercise changes in unfit and overworked horses than in fit horses. The systolic pressure in such animals does not increase and tends to actually decrease. The systolic pressure of Standardbreds with minimal training decreased an average of 0.7—1.3 kPa after strenuous exercise (2-mile sprint or 2 heats). In inadequately-trained Thoroughbreds that met the requirements of the Tenth World Championship in the Modern Pentathlon, a fall of 1.3—2.0 kPa was measured. Systolic pressure changes of this type indicate a weakness of cardiac activity (decreased myocardial contractility) and a significant decrease in arterial vascular tone due to an accumulation of toxic metabolic products (e.g. lactic acid) in the body.

The diastolic pressure of unfit horses typically increases by an average of 1.3—2.0 kPa (10—15 mm Hg) after exercise. This elevation is mainly the result of pronounced tachycardia due to a decrease in myocardial contractility, as confirmed by clinical and EKG findings. The pulse pressure in such horses falls to 5.3 kPa or lower after exercise, pointing to a considerable decline in the functional capacity of the heart and a disturbance of vascular tone.

The mean arterial blood pressure of unfit horses also usually falls after exercise — by about 0.7—1.3 kPa (5—10 mm Hg) according to our findings.

The changes in the arterial blood pressure parameters of unfit race horses after strenuous exercise are illustrated in figures 2.1.3. — 25 and — 26.

The time required for blood pressure parameters to return to initial values after exercise is also useful for assessing an animal's state of training. Based on our experience, the blood pressure parameters of fit horses return to initial values within 30—40 min. In unfit horses, this recovery takes 50—60 min.

Thus, the findings of arteriotonometry, when combined with the results of clinical and electrocardiographic examinations, provide considerable valuable information in assessing the working capacity and state of training of the equine athlete. They provide sufficiently objective criteria for regulating the intensity of the training regimen.

References

Bobylev, I. F.: Naučnye osnovy zootechničeskogo i veterinarnogo kontrolja v konnom sporte. Vet.-med. Diss., Moskva (1968).

Danilevskij, V. M.: Lečenie vnutrennich nezaraznych boleznej životnych (kratkij spravočnik), Izdat 'Kolos', Moskva (1967).

Davydovskij, I. V.: Patologičeskaja anatomija i patogenez boleznej čeloveka. Moskva (1956).

Deegen, E.: Klinische Elektrokardiographie beim Pferd unter Berücksichtigung der Muskelmassenverteilung am Herzen. Vet.-med. Habil.-Schrift, Hannover (1976).

Detweiler, D. K.; Patterson, D. F.: The cardiovascular system. In: Catcott, E. J.; Smithcors, J. F. (Ed.): Equine Medicine and Surgery, 2nd ed., p. 277. Amer. Vet. Public., Wheaton/Ill.

Domračev, G. V.: Aritmii i bolezni miokarda u lošadej, Sel'chozgiz, Moskva (1950).

Filatov, P. V.: Kliničeskaja elektrokardiografija u sel'skochozjajstvennych životnych. Vet.-med. Diss., Moskva (1956).

Filatov, P. V.: Aritmii serdca. In 'Veterinarnaja enciklopedija', *1*, Izdat. 'Sovjetskaja enciklopedija', Moskva (1968).

Filatov, P. V.; Sudakov, N. A.; Beljaev, I. M.: Praktičeskie zanjatija po kliničeskoj diagnostike s rentgenologiej. Izdat. 'Kolos', Moskva (1964).

Fogelson, L. I.: Bolezni serdca i sosudov. Atlas. Part I, Moskva (1961).

Hutyra, F.; Marek, J.; Manninger, R.; Mócsy, J.: Častnaja patologija i terapija domašnych životnych. Izdat. sel.-choz. lit. i plakatov, Moskva (1963).

Kedrov, A. A.: Bolezni myšcy serdaca. Medgiz. Leningrad (1963).

Laskov, A. A.: 'Adaptacija lošadekj chroničeskoj i ostroj gipoksii' Rossel-chozizdat., Moskva (1972).

Laskov, A. A.: Dinamika fiziologičeskich funkcij i rabotosposobnosti lošadej pod vlijaniem gipoksii. Vet.-med. Diss., Moskva (1973).

Lightowler, C. H.; Grisolia, J. O.: Parasistolia ventricular en el equino. Rev. Méd. Vet. *53:* 253 (1972).

Mozgov, I. E.: Farmakologija. 6th ed. Izdat 'Kolos', Moskva (1974).

Muylle, E.; Roose, P. de: An interventricular septal defect and a tricuspidal valva insufficiency in a trotter mare. Equine Vet. J. *6:* 174 (1974).

Nagorski, F.: Choroby ukladu krazenia zwierzat. Panstwowe Wydawnictwo Rolnicze i Leśne, Warszawa 1972.

Nedosekin, G. P.: Protivovospaltitel'nye preparaty v sportivnoj veterinarii. Konevodstvo i konnyj sport *6:* 29 (1966).

Novošinov, G. P.: Zvuki i biolektričeskie potencialy serdca u životnych v norme i pri patologičeskich processach. Vet.-med. Diss., Kasan (1969).

Novošinov, G. P.; Tuksaitov, R. Ch.; Čelyšev, A. A.: Bioradiotelemetričeskij metod kardiografii. Veterinarija *11:* 90 (1973).

Pauli, B.: Koronarsklerose beim Pferd. Schweiz. Arch. Tierheilk. *115:* 517 (1973).

Rapoport, Ja. L.: Miokardit. Patologičeskaja anatomija i patogenez. Idiopatičeskij miokardit. Med. Enciklopedija *18* (1960).

Roščevskij, M. P.: Evoljucionaja elektrokardiologija. Izdat. 'Nauka', Leningrad (1972).

Sevestre, I.; Baron, M.: Modifications de l'electrocardiogramme provoquées par une épreuve de fond chez le cheval. Rec. Méd. Vét. *149:* 911 (1973).

Skvorcov, M. A.: Osnovnye etapy v razvitii učenija o revmatizme. Sovetskaja Medicina *10* (1949).

Spörri, H.; Leemann, W.: Zur Pathophysiologie der Aortenklappeninsuffizienz des Pferdes. Berliner Münchener Tierärztl. Wschr. *85:* 441 (1972).

Sudakov, N. A.: Rezul'taty elektrokardiografičeskogo i arteriotonometričeskogo issledovanija lošadej. In: 'Metodičeskie sovety konnomu sportu'. Izdan. Moskovsk. vet. akad. (1963), p. 64.

Sudakov, N. A.: Elektrokardiografičeskie issledovanija v sisteme kliniko-fiziologiceskogo kontrolja pri treninge sportivnych lošadej. In: 'Fiziologičeskie osnovy elektrokardiografii životnych'. Izdat. 'Nauka', Moskva-Leningrad (1965), p. 38.

Sudakov, N. A.: K voprosu o differential'noj diagnostike miokardita i miokardoza u domašnich životnych. Trudy Baschkirsk. sel. choz. inst. Ufa *12* (1966), part 4.

Sudakov, N. A.: O klassifikacii i diagnostičeskom značenii šumov, vyslušivaemych v oblasti serdca u sel'skochozjajstvennych životnych. Trudy Baschkirsk. sel. choz. inst. Ufa *12* (1966), part 4.
Sudakov, N. A.: Miokardit, Veterinarnaja enciklopedija. *4*, Izdat. 'Sovestkaja enciklopedija', Moskva 1973.
Sudakov, N. A.: Miokardoz, Veterinarnaja enciklopedija. *4*, Izdat. 'Sovetskaja enciklopedija', Moskva 1973.
Sudakov, N. A.: Perikardit, Veterinarnaja enciklopedija. *4*, Izdat. 'Sovetskaja enciklopedija', Moskva 1973.
Toutain, P. L.: La physiologie de l'exercice musculaire. Rev. Méd. Vét. *125:* 1385 (1974).
Tschervjakov, D. K.; Evdokimov, P. D.; Vischker, A. S.: Izdat. 'Kolos', Moskva 1970.
Urazaev, N. A.: Fonokardiografija i ee primenenie v veterinarii. Vet.-med. Diss., Witebsk (1965).
Wirth, D.: Vorhofflimmern und -flattern beim Pferd. Wiener Tierärztl. Mschr. *29:* 241 (1942).
Zajcev, V. I.: Kliničeskaja diagnostika vnutrennich boleznej sel'skochozjajstvennych životnych. Izdat. 'Kolos', Moskva 1971.

2.1.3.2. Diseases of the Blood and Blood-Forming Organs

2.1.3.2.1. Anemias

Classification. Anemia is an abnormal reduction in the quantity of hemoglobin and erythrocytes in the blood. It is characterized by disturbances of oxidative processes in the body and the development of hypoxia in the tissues. Anemias in athletic horses may be classified according to their origin as hemorrhagic, hemolytic, hypoplastic or aplastic.

Hemorrhagic Anemia (Posthemorrhagic Anemia)
Definition. This form of anemia represents a volume deficit caused by an acute or chronic blood loss.
Symptoms. Obvious signs are weakness, fatigue, unsteady gait, and pallor and dryness of the visible mucous membranes; with severe blood loss there may also be muscular tremor and a fall of the internal body temperature. The cardiac impulse is markedly increased. The first heart sound is accentuated and may be snapping, while the second heart sound is weak. Tachycardia and dyspnea are present. The arterial blood pressure is low, and diuresis is depressed. The ESR is accelerated. There is a reduction in the number of erythrocytes and hemoglobin content per unit blood volume. Initially the anemia is normochromic but quickly becomes hypochromic. As a result of increased bone marrow activity, immature and abnormal erythrocyte forms appear in the peripheral blood — reticulocytes, normoblasts, erythroblasts, megaloblasts, anisocytes, poikilocytes and polychromatophilic cells.
Etiology. This form of anemia may result from an acute, heavy blood loss or from smaller intermittent hemorrhages. Causes include vascular trauma as well as vascular damage secondary to inflammatory changes or other lesions of the internal organs (lungs, stomach, bowel, liver, kidneys, uterus). Hemorrhagic diseases are also associated with extravasation of blood.
Pathogenesis and Lesions. The rapid loss of more than 30 % of the total blood volume leads to shock or collapse. With a blood loss of this magnitude the arterial blood pressure cannot be maintained, and there is a consequent disruption of hemodynamics and oxidative processes in the tissues. Sustained blood losses lead to degenerative changes in parenchyma of various organs. Necropsy reveals pallor of the organs and tissues and, not infrequently, signs indicative of degenerative changes.

Diagnosis. The diagnosis is based upon the characteristic symptoms, taking into account the results of the blood study and examination of the urine, feces and abdominal fluid for the presence of blood.

Treatment and Prophylaxis. The animal should be restrained, and prompt measures are taken to achieve hemostasis. For internal hemorrhage a 10% calcium chloride solution (100—150 ml) is slowly infused into the jugular vein. This should be combined with the injection of 3.0—5.0 ml epinephrine solution (1 : 1,000), 1.0—2.0 g ascorbic acid and 10% gelatin solution. For severe blood loss the administration of stabilized blood (1—3 l) by continuous drip infusion is the therapy of choice. Blood plasma and serum also have hemostatic properties and in emergencies may be infused without regard for blood group. A variety of blood substitutes may be given intravenously such as Ringer-Locke solution, dextrans or isotonic saline (infusion rate 1,000 ml in 5—10 min). For long-term treatment, the diet should be high in protein, vitamins and minerals. In particular, ample amounts of the trace elements cobalt, copper and iron should be given. Water intake is not restricted.

The prophylaxis of hemorrhagic anemia consists in the prevention of injuries in the athletic horses and in the prompt treatment of diseases that are associated with hemorrhage.

Hemolytic Anemia

Definition. This anemia results from an excessive destruction of erythrocytes. Both acute and chronic forms are known to occur.

Symptoms. Signs suggestive of hemolytic anemia are weakness, pallor and yellowness of the visible mucous membranes, tachycardia and dyspnea. Enlargement of the spleen will also occur. The erythrocyte count and hemoglobin content of the peripheral blood are altered as in hyperchromic anemia. Immature erythrocytes appear — reticulocytes, normoblasts, erythroblasts, megaloblasts and polychromatophils. Anisocytosis, poikilocytosis, basophilic stippling, Jolly bodies and Cabot rings are also observed. The indirect serum bilirubin is elevated to 219 μmol/l or higher. Increased urobilin is detected in the urine and increased stercobilin in the stool. In severe cases the blood sugar and cholesterol levels are elevated, and hemoglobinuria is present.

Etiology. Hemolytic anemia is caused by the ingestion of certain hemolytic poisons, burns, or the action of toxins on the formed elements of the blood in infectious or parasitic diseases, including equine babesiosis.

Pathogenesis and Lesions. The pathogenesis of this anemia is based on the breakdown of erythrocytes by the action of poisons or toxins and a reactive hyperplasia of the blood-forming organs with increased hemolytic activity of the reticuloendothelial tissues. This leads to the development of hemolytic jaundice and hemoglobinuria. The mucosae and serous membranes take on a yellow appearance. Blood effusions are seen on the skin, mucosae and internal organs. The spleen is congested and enlarged. Often destructive changes are seen in the liver and bone marrow, with manifestations of hemosiderosis.

Diagnosis. The diagnosis of hemolytic anemia is based upon laboratory findings in conjunction with the history and clinical signs. Differentiation from other anemias, especially Equine Infectious Anemia (EIA) and anemias due to leptospirosis or babesiosis, is necessary.

Treatment and Prophylaxis. The gastrointestinal tract should have the offending poisons or toxins removed by the administration of laxatives and diuretics. Then hypertonic solutions of sodium chlorate, calcium chlorate or glucose are administered intravenously. Other frequently used agents are liver extracts such as Kampolon or Antianemin, essential amino acids, vitamin B_{12} (1,000—2,000 μg i.m. or s.c.), and the trace elements cobalt, copper and iron, administered by addition to the feed. Stringent control of feed quality is a useful preventive measure. The specific prophylaxis of babesiosis and other infectious and parasitic diseases that are accompanied by hemolysis also contributes to the prevention of this form of anemia. Affected horses should receive prompt treatment.

Hypoplastic Anemia

Definition. Hypoplastic anemia is based upon a deficiency of blood formation, especially erythropoiesis.

Symptoms. The clinical picture is one of apathy, poor exercise tolerance, tachycardia, dyspnea, and pallor and frequent bleeding of the visible mucosae. The erythrocyte count and hemoglobin content of the peripheral blood are decreased. Anisocytosis, poikolocytosis, thrombocytopenia and leukocytopenia are frequently demonstrated. The ESR is increased. Aspirated bone marrow shows a reduced content of erythroblasts and reticulocytes.

Etiology. Hypoplastic anemia is caused by a dietary deficiency of protein, iron, copper, cobalt, folic acid and other vitamins, or by their deficient utilization by the body. It can also result from a depression of bone marrow function secondary to intoxications based upon metabolic disturbances (ketosis, osteodystrophy), diseases of the liver, digestive tract or kidneys (nephritis), radiation sickness, as well as infectious and parasitic diseases.

Pathogenesis and Lesions. The deficiency state leads to disturbances in the intermediary metabolism of iron, copper, cobalt, essential vitamins and amino acids. In nephritis the formation of erythropoetin is impaired, and in liver disease, the storage of vitamin B_{12}.

Necropsy findings include pallor of the mucosae and serous surfaces, hemorrhages and degenerative lesions of the parenchymatous organs.

Diagnosis. The diagnosis is established by clinical and hematologic findings. Differentiation from aplastic anemia, radiation sickness, leukosis, and infectious diseases and parasitisms is necessary.

Treatment and Prophylaxis. An ample supply of protein, vitamins and minerals should be provided in the ration. Treatment with blood transfusions; tissue preparations; liver extracts; arsenic compounds (potassium arsenite solution or Fowler's solution, 10—50 ml orally, arsenous acid, 0.1—0.5 g, methylarsinic acid, 1.0—4.0 g orally), trace elements such as iron, cobalt and copper; and vitamins (B_{12}, K, folic acid) is indicated. Calcium chlorate may also be administered.

The key to the prophylaxis of hypoplastic anemia is sound nutrition and the prevention of various infectious or parasitic diseases as well as metabolic disorders and diseases of the liver, kidneys and gastrointestinal tract.

Aplastic Anemia

Definition. In aplastic anemia there is a profound decrease in blood formation, especially erythropoiesis.

Symptoms. The principal signs are apathy, exercise intolerance, anorexia, pallor and bleeding of the visible mucosae, tachycardia, dyspnea, a marked fall in the erythrocyte count and hemoglobin level, and a high ESR. The content of erythroblastic cells in the bone marrow is substantially reduced.

Pathogenesis and Lesions. The first change is hypoplasia or aplasia of the bone marrow. This leads to the development of a normochromic, normocytic or microcytic anemia, accompanied by thrombocytopenia and leukopenia. The blood vessels become fragile and abnormally permeable, and a bleeding tendency results. The immune system is severely depressed.

Necropsy reveals extreme pallor of the mucosae and serous membranes with petechial and striate hemorrhages as well as passive hyperemia and necrosis in the parenchymatous organs. The bone marrow, especially of the long bones, appears pale and yellow. In addition, marked destructive changes are found in the myocardium, liver and kidneys.

Diagnosis. The clinical and hematological findings form the basis for the diagnosis. Differentiation from hypoplastic anemia, radiation sickness and leukemia/lymphosarcoma is necessary.

Treatment and Prophylaxis. Treatment is with blood transfusions; calcium chloride; ascorbic acid; the trace elements cobalt, copper and iron; liver preparations; arsenic preparations such as Fowler's solution, arsenic and methylarsinic acid (Arrhenal); and the vitamins B_{12}, K and folic acid. Prophylaxis is based on the prevention of severe acute toxicoses.

2.1.3.2.2. Hemolytic Disease of Newborn Foals

Definition. Hemolytic disease of newborn foals, or neonatal isoerythrolysis, is the term applied to a disease entity based upon a genetic immune disorder, in which there is an incompatibility between the erythrocyte antigens (blood group factors) of the foal and the antibodies (serum immunoglobulins) of the mare. The major symptoms are hemolytic anemia (neonatal anemia) and jaundice (neonatal icterus). These are accompanied by evidence of malaise and, in acute and peracute cases, by hemoglobinuria, circulatory disturbances and dyspnea.

History and Prevalence. The similarity between certain hemolytic disease symptoms on the fetus and in the newborn foal has been recognized for well over a century. But productive research on hemolysis in foals had to await the discovery of the human Rh blood factor system by WIENER [1940], the recognition of blood group incompatibilities in the ABO system, and the observation that Rh antigens are responsible for the occurrence of the dreaded fetal erythroblastosis. The first important results on hemolytic disease in newborn foals came during the period 1947—1950 from studies on Thoroughbred foals in Great Britain [COOMBS et al., 1948] and the USA (BRUNER et al., 1948, 1950; PARRY et al., 1949] and on mule foals in France [CAROLI and BESSIG, 1947]. These early results were subject to much misinterpretation due to a lack of knowledge of equine blood groups.

COOMBS et al. [1948] were the first to demonstrate hemolysins in the mare against erythrocyte antigens of the stallion and foal. While much was published subsequently on the prevalence of the disease in individual series, comprehensive epidemiologic data have been lacking. Available results would indicate that only about 1% of foals in a general population are affected [CRONIN, 1955]. However, this value is almost certainly too low if we consider that many fatalities are not recorded as 'death due to neonatal isoerythrolysis' because cases with a mild course cannot be diagnosed without laboratory tests. The prevalence appears to be higher when animals of different erythrocyte genotypes are bred (cross-breeding or the importing of sires). For example, when mares are bred to donkeys, the disease appears in 10% of the mule foals [CAROLI and BESSIG, 1947].

Clinical Symptoms and Lesions. In most cases the foal is healthy at birth and does not develop symptoms until it ingests colostrum. In typical cases the foal becomes lethargic and anorexic within 8 hours to 3 days after birth. This is followed by weakness and asthenia which become progressively more severe. There is pallor of the conjunctivae and mucous membranes, and icteric discoloration is apparent. Other clinical signs are a rapid heart and respiratory rate, an increased apex beat, pulsation of the jugular vein, hemoglobinuria, and later dyspnea. Subnormal temperatures are sometimes recorded. The hematologic picture is one of progressive hemolytic anemia. The hematocrit value, erythrocyte count and hemoglobin level are low. The symptoms are most pronounced within 2 to 4 days after birth but are still evident up to 8 days postpartum. Peracute cases die within 8 to 36 hours, acute cases within 2 to 4 days, and subacute cases within 5 to 6 days [Parry et al. 1949; Doll and Hull, 1951; Doll, 1952]. In milder cases the foals appear weak and are reluctant to nurse, but recovery is rapid.

The necropsy findings vary according to the degree and duration of the disease, i.e., the amount of antibodies ingested and the proportion of damaged cells. Anemia is the only symptom in peracute cases. In other cases anemia is accompanied by hemolytic icterus, or obstructive icterus if liver damage has already occurred. In addition there is hyperemic, noninflammatory swelling of the liver and spleen and centrilobular hypoxemic hepatic changes. In subacute cases there is nephrosis, bleeding in the serous membranes, mucosae and parenchymae, moderate transudation in the serous cavities, and hemoglobinuria. The erythrocyte count, hematocrit and Hb level are reduced by about 50% (hypochromasia). Anisocytosis and poikilocytosis are present in some cases. Regenerative cells and erythroblasts are absent in affected foals. 'Kernicterus' (deep yellow staining of the basal ganglia with associated neurotoxic symptoms) is also unknown in the horse, which is why the terms icterus gravis neonatorum and fetal erythroblastosis are not applied, as they are in human beings.

Etiology and Pathogenesis. The primary cause of neonatal isoerythrolysis in foals is a reaction between antigenic determinants on the erythrocyte membrane of the newborn and antibodies (serum immunoglobulins) of the mother. These antigens are identical to normal blood group factors. A_1 (A system) and Q (Q system) are involved according to one US study [Stormont, 1975]. Because the numerical system of the blood group nomenclature is inconsistent in the older literature, and all blood group systems probably have the same potential, there appears to be little value in interpreting older findings or emphasizing particular factors.

The antibodies (hemolysins and hemagglutins) of the mother may be iso- or heteroimmune antibodies as well as natural iso- or heteroantibodies. The transmission of maternal antibodies or immunoglobulins to the foal via the colostrum is a natural mechanism for protecting the newborn during its first weeks of life. In neonatal isoerythrolyis, however, the foal has inherited from the stallion, antigenic determinants to which the mare has antibodies, or to which she has developed such antibodies during pregnancy. When the antibodies are ingested in the colostrum and absorbed, an antigen-antibody reaction occurs in which the suckling's erythrocytes are attacked and destroyed. Some of this erythrocytolysis takes place in the circulating blood, but most occurs in the spleen and liver. If the liver cannot break down the excess bilirubin that is formed, icterus develops. If the sensitized cells are destroyed more rapidly than they can be replaced, anemia occurs, accompanied by various degrees of icterus and hemoglobinuria.

Isoimmunization of the mare can take place in a variety of ways. Transplacental immunization of the pregnant mare appears to be the most important mechanism in racing breeds. For this to occur, the fetal erythrocyte antigens must pass through the placental barrier into the maternal circulation. Given the epitheliochorial placenta of the horse, this is not readily accomplished, for the fetal and maternal circulations are separated by six tissue layers. The placenta becomes permeable to antigens and antibodies only if it is damaged (petechia-like retroplacental hemorrhages at or near foaling time) or diseased (inflammatory processes, adhesions, necrotic foci).

Because the normal antibody titer must first exceed a certain threshold, antibody formation generally occurs too late in the same pregnancy, i.e. is not intensive enough, to affect the foal. Hence the syndrome is usually observed only after several prior pregnancies [Franks, 1962; Stormont et al., 1964]. Isolated cases in first pregnancies are known, however [Brion, 1949].

Isoimmunization of the mare can also be induced by immunization with blood group antigens of the sire to which she was bred, by blood transfusion, or by use of homologous (pooled) blood vaccines or polyvalent tissue vaccines containing horse erythrocytes. Horse viral abortion vaccine prepared from homogenized lung tissue containing blood has been implicated in particular [Doll et al., 1952]. Heteroimmunizations can lead to the same result. For example, Rensmeyer [1977] demonstrated partial antigenic properties between the sheep and horse. An ovine immune serum was found to contain heterohemolysins that reacted specifically with the blood group factor C_a of the horse. Natural isoantibodies have also been suggested as a primary cause.

The serologic reaction is first manifested postnatally after the ingestion of colostrum, for normally the placenta is impermeable to unchanged antibodies, and the intestinal mucosa of the foal generally is permeable only up to 36 hours after birth [Bruner et al., 1950]. There are exceptions, however. In isolated cases the permeability to antibody has persisted for up to 2 weeks. Damage to the fetus in utero is rarely reported [Priouzeau, 1952]. In other species, prenatal isoerythrolysis is known to cause abortion, prematurity, fetal maceration, failure to thrive after birth, perinatal death, and fetal or congenital hydrops.

Diagnosis. Neonatal erythrolysis can be diagnosed only on the basis of adequate laboratory tests. The clinical, hematologic and pathomorphologic findings provide indications. The syndrome must be differentiated from hemolytic icterus or septicemia in infectious diseases that are accompanied by a low erythrocyte count, hemoglobin level and hematocrit or by anemia and jaundice. Hemolytic anemia and septicemia are distinguished by fever, lethargy and failure to nurse a short time after birth. In addition, corresponding organ findings (lungs, digestive system, brain, kidneys, liver and joints) are generally present. Noninfectious diseases include prematurity and immaturity (hepatic immaturity with deficient breakdown of bilirubin) as well as fetal and neonatal stress (asphyxia, trauma at birth, neonatal maladjustment syndrome). The latter are excluded on the basis of low birthweight, the appearance of clinical symptoms shortly after birth (cardiovascular, pulmonary) as well as behavioral abnormalities. Such abnormalities are characteristic of cerebral hemorrhage, such as inability to stand and to nurse and disinterest in the mare, and occasionally on the basis of other disturbances (motor unrest, exaggerated extensor tone, spasms, convulsions) [Schmid, 1967; Rossdale, 1972].

The diagnosis is confirmed by the technique of blood group serology that is optimum for the species involved. Because hemolytic procedures are better suited for the equine blood group systems (with the exception of the D system) than are hemagglutination techniques [Stormont, 1975; Stormont et al., 1964; Sandberg, 1973], blood type testing in horses is generally done by the hemolytic method. Preferably this is done 1—2 weeks before birth or immediately postpartum if the disease is suspected. The serum isoantibodies in the blood and colostrum or precolostrum of the mare are tested against antigens of the stallion and/or foal as well as against test antigens. The fall of the blood titer during the period of heavy colostrum production is noted. The tests are done using 1 : 4 and 1 : 6 dilutions of the mare and foal serum, and 1 : 16 and 1 : 64 dilutions of the precolostrum and colostrum. 2.5% erythrocyte suspensions serve as the antigen, and absorbed rabbit serum as the complement.

Any degree of hemolysis that definitely exceeds the negative control (reaction with erythrocytes of unsuspected foals and horses) is counted as a positive, meaning that the mare is a carrier of isoantibodies against the erythrocyte antigens of the stallion and foal. The nature of the antigens can be clarified with test sera (factor sera), and that of the antibodies with test antigens. The antibodies absorbed to the foal's erythrocytes can be recovered by elution. Another means of demonstrating isoimmunization is by use of the anti-horse globulin test of Coombs et al. [1948], but this method is no longer generally recommended [Stormont, 1975].

Treatment and Prophylaxis. Treatment is directed toward removal of the ingested antibodies, the susceptible erythrocytes and the erythrocyte breakdown products by means of an exchange transfusion (blood withdrawal and replacement transfusion). In milder cases blood withdrawal alone is sufficient. The blood of the dam is a suitable erythrocyte source, provided the blood cells are washed free of the antibody-bearing plasma. The erythrocytes are resuspended in physiologic saline or a suitable donor plasma and infused i.v. at a rate of 1 l/h. The number of repetitions depends on the progress of the foal's hemogram. Transfusions should be repeated until the erythrocyte count reaches 5,000,000/ml. A total of 2 to 7 l of blood is required. Other donor erythrocytes or blood must be tested for compatibility by cross-matching, especially if the donor is related to the dam. The donor's serum must cause no lysis or agglutination of the foal's erythrocytes. Foals tolerate well repeated transfusions with blood of their own type. Hypothermia is treated symptomatically by raising the ambient temperature, myocardial asthenia by the administration of cardiac glycosides, and hypoimmunoglobulinemia by giving compatible donor colostrum (or plasma or corresponding gamma globulin preparations). Complete rest is indicated, and a course of prophylactic antibiotics is recommended.

Neonatal isoerythrolysis can be prevented by testing the mare's serum against the sire's cells before the birth of the foal. After birth the foal's erythrocytes may also be tested. If the test is positive, the foal should be muzzled or removed from the dam for 36—48 h to prevent ingestion of maternal colostrum. It should be fed colostrum from a nonsensitized mare or diluted cow's milk and immunoglobulins should also be given. In the interim the foal is permitted to nurse the dam for 5 min at a time after first milking the dam. If serologic testing of the foal's erythrocytes against maternal colostrum or milk confirms the absence of potentially harmful antibodies, normal nursing may be resumed.

It has been suggested that isoerythrolysis can be prevented by testing all mares and stallions before breeding or by routinely screening all pregnancies, but this is hardly practical from a technical standpoint.

Prognosis. Under ordinary circumstances the mortality rate is high. The prognosis is more favorable if the foal is treated with transfusions. The outcome depends on the rapidity with which the condition is diagnosed and treated, and on the severity and course of the disease. With erythrocyte counts below 2,500,000/ml and hemoglobin levels below 5 g/dl, the prognosis is poor; with counts below 2,000,000/ml, death is certain. Foals with counts above 4,000,000 can be expected to recover.

2.1.3.2.3. Hemorrhagic Diseases

Classification. Three main groups of hemorrhagic disease, or abnormal bleeding tendency, can be distinguished according to their pathogenesis:

— diatheses due to vascular causes (vascular disease, vagogenic bleeding tendencies),
— coagulation defects,

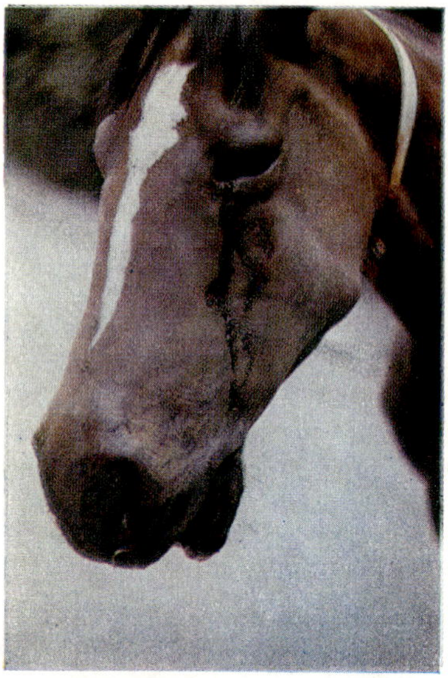
27

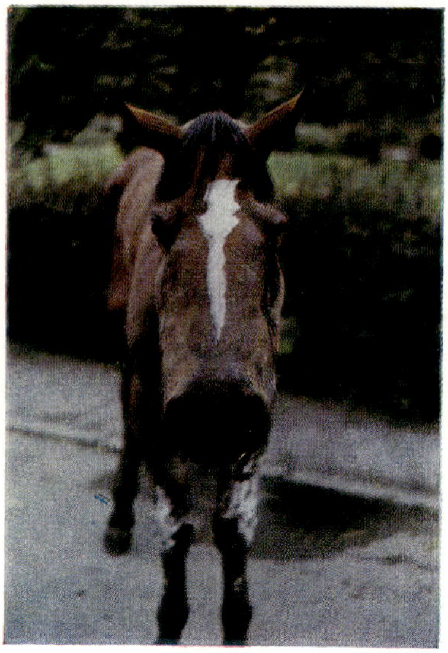
28

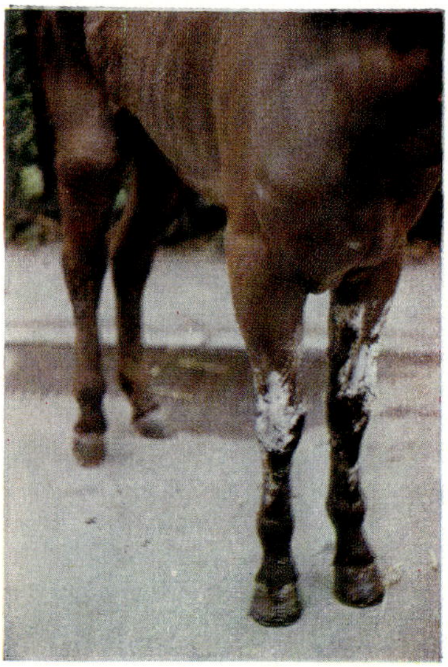
29

Fig. 2.1.3. — 27. Purpura hemorrhagica: swelling of the face and muzzle.

Fig. 2.1.3. — 28. Purpura hemorrhagica: swelling of the ventral abdomen.

Fig. 2.1.3. — 29. Purpura hemorrhagica: edema of the limbs.

— disorders of hemostasis due to platelet abnormalities: thrombocytopenia and thrombasthenia or thrombopathia.

Vascular diseases are characterized clinically by petechial hemorrhages. They are diagnosed with the aid of vascular tests such as the prick test or suction test. In the horse they may be infectious (purpura hemorrhagic), allergic or toxic (sweet clover disease) in origin. In dogs they can result from vitamin deficiency and in man from hereditary factors.

Coagulation defects, either congenital or acquired, are characterized by a deficiency of one or more factors of the normal blood coagulation system. One such deficiency is caused by an increase in physiologic inhibitors or the formation of pathologic inhibitors. This type is generally acquired. Liver diseases are particularly important in the pathogenesis of acquired coagulation disorders.

Thrombocytopenia is a deficiency of blood platelets. This hemorrhagic disease can result from depressed platelet formation due to bone marrow pathology, from an excessive breakdown or consumption of platelets, or from the excessive destruction of platelets by antibodies. *Thrombopathia* is due to a disturbance of platelet function.

Purpura Hemorrhagica

Definition. Purpura hemorrhagica is characterized by damage to the blood vessels with the development of extensive, symmetrical edematous swellings and multiple hemorrhages in the skin, subcutaneous tissue, muscles, mucosae and internal organs.

Symptoms. The first sign is bleeding from the nasal mucosa and conjunctivae, followed later by a nasal discharge. Extensive edematous swellings appear in the region of the head, thorax, ventral abdomen and limbs (figs. 2.1.3. — 27 to — 29). The severe swelling of the nostrils, lips, cheeks and dorsum of the nose greatly alters the shape of the head in the region of the visceral cranium. Initially the swellings are hot and painful, but later they are cold and nontender. The margins of the swellings are sharply delineated. The skin over the edematous areas becomes coated with a yellow, sticky, serous fluid that soon dries leaving a yellow-brown scale. In severe cases the tissue at the center of the edematous areas may undergo a gangrene with subsequent sepsis and possibly septacemia. The swellings may interfere with eating, respiration and urination. Protein, hemoglobin, cellular blood constituents, epithelial cells, casts and high urobilin levels are found in the urine. The body temperature is normal or slightly elevated. Remittent fever is seen only in severe cases. Tachycardia and premature beats may occur, and systolic murmurs are occasionally heard. Examination of the blood usually reveals eosinophilia and neutrophilia as well as changes in the red blood count resembling those in posthemorragic anemia. The indirect serum bilirubin is increased to more than 855 μmol/l[1].

Etiology. The disease usually develops as a result of a postinfectious allergic reaction. It is seen most frequently as a sequel to strangles (Streptococcus equi) or other streptococcal diseases. Cold, excessive fatigue and vitamin deficiency states may be predisposing factors.

Pathogenesis and Lesions. The toxins and inflammatory products that are formed in infections and other diseases trigger an allergic reaction. This in turn leads to vascular changes with wall damage, resulting in extravasation of plasma and blood into the tissues.

Necropsy reveals hemorrhages and gelatinous fluid in the skin, subcutaneous tissue, mucosae, muscles and parenchymatous organs. Mucosal ulcerations are frequent.

Diagnosis. The sudden appearance of extensive, symmetrical, sharply-defined edematous swellings with associated hemorrhages of the skin and mucosae and a normal or slightly elevated body temperature is significant. There may be a history of recent infection, and characteristic hematologic findings are present. The demarcated, symmetrical edematous swellings of purpura hemorrhagica serve to distinguish it from thrombopenia, lymphosarcoma, radiation sickness, anthrax, and clostridial diseases. These diseases are usually associated with high fever.

Treatment and prophylaxis. Treatment centers on the use of antiallergic agents: procaine (200 or 100 ml of a 0.5 or 1.0 % solution, i.v.), sodium salicylate (10.0—50.0 g orally), aminophenazone (30.0—50.0 g orally), calcium chlorate or calcium gluconate

1 Conversion: mg/100 ml × 17.1 = μmol/l; μmol/l × 0.0585 = mg/100 ml.

(10.0—20.0 g, given i.v. in a 5—10% solution), diphenhydramine hydrochloride (0.1—0.5 g, given s.c. in a 1% solution), ACTH, cortisone and other highly active depot glucocorticoids. Corticotropin (ACTH) is administered intramuscularly in isotonic saline in a dose of 0.08—0.13 I.U./kg BW 3—4 times daily. ACTH zinc phosphate is given only once daily or 2—3 times weekly in the same dose. Ascorbic acid, menadione sodium bisulfite, cardiovascular agents and serotherapy are also beneficial. Moskalik has obtained good results with diphenylhydramine hydrochloride and menadione sodium bisulfite administered in 2 to 4 doses. In severe cases antimicrobial agents (sulfonamides, antibiotics) are also indicated. An alkalizing diet is recommended.

Prophylaxis consists in the prevention of the inciting infectious diseases. When such diseases occur, the prompt administration of desensitizing drugs forestall complications.

Hemophilia

Definition. Hemophilia is a relatively rare hereditary disease that is characterized by a severe and persistent bleeding tendency.

Symptoms. Affected animals suffer recurrent bouts of epistaxis which vary in degree from profuse hemorrhagic episodes to the formation of small clots in the nasal cavities. Sudden death can result from the aspiration of blood into the lungs. Sometimes the hemorrhages are completely spontaneous, but often they occur only with extreme exertion. On the other hand, horses with epistaxis frequently withstand very severe exertion without developing nosebleed. The large, frequent blood losses lead to posthemorrhagic anemia.

Etiology. Hemophilia in humans, known also as 'bleeder's disease', was formerly attributed to a defect of thrombin or fibrin formation. However, the classic form, hemophilia A, is based upon an hereditary deficiency of Factor VIII (antihemophilic globulin, antihemophilic factor). This deficiency is inherited as a sex-linked recessive trait, i.e., the disease is inherited by both sexes but tends to affect males only. The second and most common hereditary form of hemophilia in man is hemophilia B or Christmas disease, based upon a deficiency of Factor IX (Christmas factor, PTC = plasma thromboplastic component).

Unlike classic hemophilia in man, hereditary epistaxis in horses is transmitted as a non-sex-linked recessive trait. It is recognized as a breed-intrinsic disease of the English Thoroughbred. The first historically known racehorse with nosebleed was 'Bartlet's Childers' ('Bleeding Childers'). All horses that died in the 19th century from epistaxis can be traced back to the stallion 'Herod', born in 1758, whose most famous descendant, 'Hermit', was one of the most successful racehorses of the 19th century.

Pathogenesis and Lesions. For a long time it was thought that the hemorrhages were due to the rupture of abnormally thin-walled blood vessels in the upper respiratory tracts. This excessive fragility and thinness of the vessel walls was thought to be the result of prolonged inbreeding of the English Thoroughbred. Extreme exertion such as would occur near the end of a race, the degree and state of the animal's training, and its feeding regime and care were considered responsible for the appearance of clinical symptoms. Only recently has the theory relating hereditary epistaxis in Thoroughbreds to coagulation disturbances gained wide support. Stolpe in 1969 and Stolpe and Wiesner in 1970 showed that the condition was based upon a defect in the formation of fibrinogen. The disturbance is probably localized in the second stage of blood coagulation, during which fibrin is formed from fibrinogen by polymerization under the action of thrombin. Population-genetic studies in Thoroughbreds and trotters confirm that the defect is inherited as a simple recessive trait.

Diagnosis. Photometric extinction measurements of the selective precipitation of fibrinogen by ammonium sulfate demonstrate a quantitative difference in fibrinogen content between normal and affected horses. The fibrinogen extinctions of 'bleeders' (0.060 s $\pm$ 0.004 ext.) are significantly lower than those of clinically healthy animals (0.109 s $\pm$ 0.011 ext.). Gravimetric fibrinogen determinations expressed in g % show similar values for normal and affected horses. However, the ratio of g/100 ml to extinction is substantially higher in horses with epistaxis (4.24 [4.00—4.64]) than in normal animals (2.66 [2.50—2.85]), indicating an alteration in the quality of the fibrinogen. Clinically healthy horses with an elevated ratio can be regarded as heterozygous for epistaxis.

Treatment and Prophylaxis. Treatment consists in the transfusion of whole blood or plasma and the administration of ACTH, ascorbic acid, menadione sodium bisulfite, and hypertonic saline and glucose solutions. Hydrogen peroxide solution and iron sesquichlorate are used locally. When anemic symptoms are present, the usual treatment for hemorrhagic anemia is instituted. The avoidance of inbreeding is a prophylactic measure that may be adopted in breeding practice. Horses with hemophilia should be excluded from breeding.

Thrombocytopenia

Definition. The disease is characterized by the occurrence of minute hemorrhages and a decreased platelet count per unit blood volume.

Symptoms. The disease is manifested by weakness, rapid fatigability, anorexia, and numerous small hemorrhages in the skin and mucosae. The latter are markedly pale. The pulse and respiratory rate are increased. The hematologic findings are typical of chronic hemorrhagic anemia. Examination of blood smears reveals erythrocytes with Jolly bodies or Cabot rings as well as poikilocytosis. The platelet count is severely depressed and may be 11×10^9/l or lower. Normal platelets are interspersed with basophilic platelets and giant cells. The retractibility of the clot is greatly reduced. The megakaryocyte content of the bone marrow is low.

Etiology. The disease is based upon an inhibition of thrombocytopoiesis or an excessive platelet destruction. Often the disturbance of thrombopoiesis is caused by 'stress' factors, but it may also be associated with lymphosarcoma or excessive radiation exposure.

Pathogenesis and Lesions. The inhibition of thrombopoiesis or increased destruction of blood platelets leads to a bleeding tendency with the development of hemorrhagic syndrome.

Necropsy reveals many small hemorrhages in a variety of organs and tissues as well as enlargement of the spleen.

Diagnosis. The diagnosis is based on the presence of hemorrhagic syndrome, a reduced platelet count in the peripheral blood, and a low megakaryocyte count in aspirated bone marrow. Thrombocytopenia must be differentiated from infectious anemia, radiation sickness and lymphosarcoma.

Treatment and Prophylaxis. Green feed should be added to the ration. Measures are taken to influence the functional capacity of the bone marrow, digestive tract and liver. Treatment is with vitamin K (menadione sodium bisulfite, 0.02 g/100 kg BW i.m.), vitamin B_{12}, calcium chloride, ascorbic acid, liver extracts, and the trace elements cobalt, iron, copper and manganese. Prophylaxis consists in the prevention of toxicoses and the elimination of 'stress' factors.

2.1.3.2.4. Leukemia

Definition. Leukemia is a systemic illness characterized by a progressive malignant disease of the blood-forming tissue, involving a distorted proliferation of leukocytes and their precursors in the blood. According to JARMAY [1954], WIRTH [1950], ČERNJAK [1960] and other authors, its occurrence in horses is rare. Leukemia was first reported in the horse by the Dresden pathologist LEISERING in 1858. Later the disease was also described by SIEDAMGROTZKY, NOCARD and others. HENSCHER refers in 1931 to the description of 100 cases of leukemia in the horse.

According to WIRTH [1950], SINEV, DEKKER and others, leukemia occurs in horses over 6 years of age. Most cases are of the lymphatic form, although recently cases of myeloid leukemia have also been reported.

Symptoms. According to the descriptions of HABERSANG, HELL, NEUMANN-KLEINPAUL, SINEV, ALMEJEW, ČERNJAK and other authors, the major signs of leukemia in the horse are apathy, weakness, anorexia, rapid weight loss or even cachexia, and pallor of the mucous membranes. In the early stage transient temperature elevations and colicky episodes can also be observed. As the disease progresses, signs of heart failure (abnormalities of rate and rhythm, dyspnea, cyanosis, edema) and hemorrhagic disease become increasingly severe. LEISERING, LANDMANN, FOMLER, MAROLT and others have observed considerable enlargement of the spleen and superficial lymph nodes due to tumor formation. Hematologic studies in horses with lymphatic leukemia reveal the presence of immature leukocytes (prolymphocytes, lymphoblasts, lymphoreticular cells; fig. 2.1.3. — 30) in large numbers. In the leukemic form, the total leukocyte count is elevated by the abundance of immature lymphocytes in the blood. As a rule the erythrocyte and platelet counts and hemoglobin levels are markedly reduced. Many microcytes are found among the red cells.

Myeloid leukemia is characterized by the presence of immature granulocytes (juveniles, myelocytes, promyelocytes, myeloblasts and hemocytoblasts) in the peripheral blood.

Etiology. The etiology of the disease is not clearly understood. Most investigators regard equine leukemia as having multiple etiologies, with viruses and genetic factors playing the major role.

Pathogenesis and Lesions. There are three stages in the development of leukemia: the incubation stage and the subclinical and clinical stages. The subclinical (latent) stage is the longest. The clinical course is relatively brief. Usually death occurs several weeks after the first clinical signs appear, though some cases prove fatal within a few days. Leukemia in horses may take a leukemic or aleukemic course. In the leukemic form the number of leukocytes in the peripheral blood is markedly increased (50,000—500,000/mm^3). This is due mainly to the presence of immature lymphocytes (prolymphocytes, lymphoblasts and lymphoreticular cells), which make up 90—95 % of the differential blood count [WIRTH, 1950; NEUMANN-KLEINPAUL].

According to reports by SEILS and others, the various forms of equine leukemia are associated with the following changes in the peripheral blood: The leukocyte count ranges from 3.6 to 30×10^9/l (60—98 % of which are lymphocytes, 8.8—25 % lymphoblasts, 10—17 % neutrophils, 0.5—4 % monocytes, 0.01—1 % eosinophils and 0.03—0.5 % basophils, with isolated myelocytes and undifferentiable reticular cells), the erythrocyte count is from 1.06—4.30×10^{12}/l, and the hemoglobin content is between 2 and 5 g/dl. The red cells show anisocytosis, poikilocytosis and polychromasia.

The organic changes of lymphatic leukemia in the horse involve mainly the lymph nodes, spleen, liver, kidneys and heart [ČERNJAK, 1960; SINOV, 1957; PALLASKE,

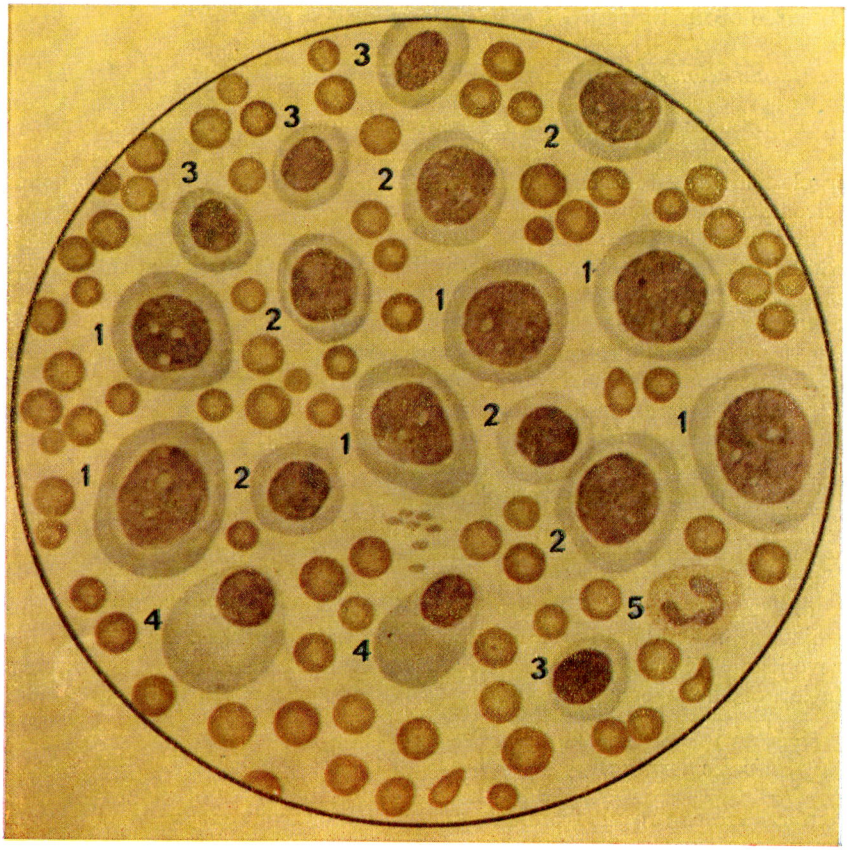

Fig. 2.1.3. — 30. Blood picture of a horse with lymphatic leukosis. *1* lymphoblasts; *2* prelymphocytes; *3* lymphocytes; *4* lymphoreticular cells; *5* segmented granulocyte.

1958; Almejew, 1963]. They consist in an enlargement of these organs, the presence of leukemic infiltrates, and in most cases tumor infiltration. Splenic enlargements up to 50—55 kg have been reported. Not infrequently the lungs and digestive tract are also involved. In addition, changes arise that are characteristic of hemorrhagic syndrome and anemia. Death usually results from severe myocardial damage.

Diagnosis. The collection and examination of blood specimens and biopsy samples from the lymph nodes, bone marrow, spleen and liver, together with the clinical picture, offers the best chance of reaching a prompt diagnosis in the living animal. In most cases a histopathologic examination is necessary to confirm the clinical and hematologic diagnosis.

Leukemia must be differentiated from radiation sickness and various diseases that are accompanied by a leukocytosis of the blood-forming tissues.

Treatment, Control. Measures for the control of leukemia in horses are prescribed by law internationally.

2.1.3.3. Diseases of the Spleen

2.1.3.3.1. Inflammation of the Spleen (Splenitis)

Symptoms. The major symptoms are weakness, anorexia or refusal to feed, and, in suppurative cases, fever, tachycardia, an extended area of splenic dullness, and splenic enlargelement and tenderness on rectal exploration. In severe cases hematopoiesis and circulation are impaired.

Mild cases may be asymptomatic.

Etiology. Splenitis usually occurs as a complication of infectious or other diseases.

Pathogenesis and Lesions. Toxins and inflammatory products that accumulate in the blood during the course of the primary disease (usually an infection) enter the spleen. There they initiate inflammatory processes which may spread to the peritoneum, causing peritonitis. The inflammation leads to enlargement of the spleen, disturbances of blood formation and circulation, as well as to functional impairment of the digestive organs and colic.

Necropsy reveals splenomegaly from inflammatory edema and, in severe cases, destructive changes of the parenchyma.

Diagnosis. It is based on the clinical findings, taking into account the hematologic examination and the animal's history. Anthrax, infectious anemia and leukemia must be excluded.

Treatment and Prophylaxis. The administration of antimicrobial drugs (sulfonamides, antibiotics) is combined with symptomatic treatment. Prophylaxis is based upon the prevention of infectious and other diseases that are frequently complicated by inflammation of the spleen.

2.1.3.3.2. Splenic Hemorrhage

Splenic hemorrhage can result from a blunt trauma or from excessive engorgement due to inflammatory or other pathologic processes in the spleen. Splenic hemorrhage leads to hematoma formation or to a uniform enlargement of the entire organ. The splenic enlargement and function impairment have effects on the functions of other organs and systems. Frequently the animal will show peculiar colicky behavior, arching the back and standing with the limbs drawn together beneath the body.

2.1.3.3.3. Rupture of the Spleen

Splenic rupture can be caused by direct, severe violence or may be secondary to anthrax, lymphosarcoma, echinococcosis infestation or splenic hemorrhage. The clinical picture is one of internal bleeding, accompanied by marked pallor of all mucosae, tachycardia, dyspnea, profuse sweating and colic. Immediate surgical treatment is indicated.

2.1.3.3.4. Tumors of the Spleen

Most splenic tumors are melanosarcomas, which mainly affect gray horses. The neoplasm is detected by rectal examination. It may reach the size of a child's head. The disease must be differentiated from echinococcosis, lymphosarcoma and hematoma. The clinical manifestations include colic, impaired hematopoiesis, and pigmentary change.

References

ALIKAEV, V. A.; ZAMARIN, L. G.; DANILEVSKIJ, V. M.: Vnutrennie nezaraznye bolezni sel'skochozjajstvennych životnych. 4th ed. Izdat. 'Kolos', Moskva 1972.

ALMEJEW, CH. S.: Lejkozy u životnych. Vestnik sel. choz. nauki *7* (1963).

BOLLINGER, O.: Über Leukämie bei den Haustieren. Virchows Arch. *59:* 344 (1874).

BRION, A.: Sur l'ictère hémolytique du poulain noveau-né. Rec. Méd. vét. *100:* 229 (1949).

BRUNER, D. W.; HULL, F. E.; DOLL, E. R.: The relation of blood factors to icterus in foals. Amer. J. vet. Res. *9:* 237 (1948).

BRUNER, D. W.; DOLL, E. R.; HULL, F. E.; KINKAID, A. S.: Further studies on hemolytic icterus in foals. Amer. J. vet. Res. *11:* 22 (1950).

CAROLI, J.; BESSIG, M.: Recherches sur la cause de l'ictère grave familial des muletons. Rev. Hématol. *2:* 207 (1947).

ČERNJAK, V. Z.: O lejkozach domašnich životnych. Sb. 'Problemy lejkozov i immunologii', Leningrad 1960.

ČERNJAK, V. Z.; SACHAROV, S. F.: Materialy po lejkozam mlekopitajuščich. Trudy mezdunarodn. konfer. patol. anat. sel. choz. živ., Woronesh 1961.

CHRUSTALEV, A. S.: Gemofilija. Veterin. enciklopedija *2:* 353 (1969). Izdat. 'Sovetskaja enciklopedija', Moskva.

COOMBS, R. R.; CROWHURST, R. C.; DAY, F. T.; HEARD, D. H.; HINDE, I. T.; HOOGSTRATEN, J.; PARRY, H. B.: Haemolytic disease of newborn foals due to isoimmunization of pregnancy. J. Hyg. *46:* 403 (1948).

CRONIN, M. T. I.: Haemolytic disease of newborn foals. Vet. Rec. *67:* 479 (1955).

DOLL, E. R.: Observations on the clinical features and pathology of hemolytic icterus of newborn foals. Amer. J. vet. Res. *13:* 504 (1952).

DOLL, E. R.; HULL, F. E.: Observations on hemolytic icterus of newborn foals. Cornell Vet. *41:* 14 (1951).

DOLL, E. R.; RICHARDS, M. G.; WALLACE, M. E.; BRYANS, J. T.: The influence of an equine fetal tissue vaccine upon hemaglutination activity of mare serums: its relation to hemolytic icterus of newborn foals. Cornell Vet. *42:* 495 (1952).

FRANKS, D.: Horse blood groups and hemolytic disease in the newborn foal. Ann. N. Y. Acad. Sci. *97:* 235 (1962).

HUTYRA, F. v.; MAREK, J.; MANNINGER, R.; MÓCSY, J.: Spezielle Pathologie und Therapie der Haustiere. 11th ed. Izdat. sel. chou. lit. žurnal. plakatov, Moskva 1963.

JARMAY, K.: Die Leukosen der Haustiere. Budapest 1954.

KUDRJAVCEV, A. A.; KUDRJAVCEVA, L. A.: Kliničeskaja gematologija životnych. Izdat. 'Kolos', Moskva 1974.

LEISERING, A. G. T.: Leukämie beim Pferd. Ber. Vet.-Wesen Kgr. Sachsen *11* (1858).

MALININ, A. I.: Anemija. Veterin. enciklopedija *1:* 247 (1968). Izdat. 'Sov. enciklopedija', Moskva.

MALININ, A. I.: Diatez. Veterin. enciklopedija *2:* 798 (1969). Izdat. 'Sov. enciklopedija', Moskva.

MOSKALIK, R. S.: O krovopjatnistom tife losadej. Veterinarija (1975), No. 2, p. 59.

NOCARD, E.: Sur la leucocythemie. Arch. vét. Alfort *5:* 625 (1880).

PALLASKE, J.: Pathologische Anatomie der Säugetierleukosen. Mh. Vet.-Med. *13:* 65 (1958).

PARRY, H. B.; DAY, F. T.; CROWHURST, R. C.: Diseases of newborn foals. I. Hemolytic disease due to iso-immunization of pregnancy. Vet. Rec. *61:* 435 (1949).

PJANIKOV, L. C.: Atlas kletok krovi kostnogo mozga lošadej. Gosizdat. sel. choz. lit., Moskva-Leningrad 1953.

PRIOUZEAU, M.: Ictère hémolytique du muleton. Rec. Méd. vét. *128:* 79 (1952).

RENSMEYER, W.: Beiträge zur vergleichenden Blutgruppenserologie bei Schaf, Rind, Schwein und Mensch unter besonderer Berücksichtigung der Lymphozyten. Vet.-med. Diss., München (1977).

ROSSDALE, P. D.: Differential diagnosis and treatment of equine neonatal disease. Vet. Rec. *91:* 581 (1972).

SANDBERG, K.: The D blood group system of the horse. Anim. Blood Groups biochem. Genet. *4:* 193 (1973).

SCHMID, D. O.: Immunogenetische Untersuchungen bei Pferden. Wiener tierärztl. Mschr. *54:* 375 (1967).

SEILS, H.: Über einen Fall lymphatischer Leukose bei einem Fohlen. Mh. Vet.-Med. *15:* 522 (1960).

SIEDAMGROTZKY, O.: Über die Leukämie bei den Haustieren. Pflügers Vortr. f. Tierärzte *10:* 395 (1878).

SINOV, A. V.; DOBIN, M. A.; JUŠKOVSKIJ, M. A.: K voprosu o lejkozach mlekopitajuščich. Sb. rabot Leningradsk. vet. inst. *16* (1957).

STOLPE, J.; WIESNER, E.: Das Fibrinogen bei nasenblutenden Galopprennpferden und Trabern. Arch. exp. Vet.-Med. *24:* 903 (1970).

STORMONT, C.: Neonatal isoerythrolysis in domestic animals. A comparative review. Acta veterin. Sci. comp. Med. *19:* 23 (1975).

STORMONT, C.; SUZUKI, Y.; RHODE, E. A.: Serology of horse blood groups. Cornell Vet. *54:* 439 (1964).

THEILEN, G. H.; FOWLER, M.: Lymphosarcoma (Lymphocytic leukemia) in the horse. J. Amer. vet. med. Assoc. *140:* 923 (1962).

VASILEV, N. T.; RUMJANCEV, N. V.: Lejkozy sel'skochzjajstvennych životnych. Izdat. 'Kolos', Moskva 1975.

WIRTH, D.: Grundlagen einer klinischen Hämatologie der Haustiere. 2. Aufl. Wien und Innsbruck 1950.

2.1.4. Diseases of the Respiratory System

2.1.4.1. Endoscopy of the Nasal Passages, Pharynx, Larynx and Bronchi

Diseases in the region of the nasopharynx and larynx generally are not accessible to direct clinical inspection. While direct examination of the pharyngeal cavity without aids can be attempted in the recumbent, anesthetized horse by holding the mouth open and depressing the base of the tongue, only a limited portion of the pharynx can be visualized in this way. Hence, this type of examination is of only minor importance in the clinical diagnosis of nasopharyngeal diseases in the horse. Because of the many diseases affecting this region, the endoscope has become an indispensible tool. In many cases it provides the only means of obtaining a definitive diagnosis.

Both rigid and flexible endoscopes are available. Illumination is provided either by an incandescent bulb at the tip of the instrument or by an external high-intensity lamp that transmits light into the endoscope through a fiberoptic bundle. Modern fiberoptic light eliminates the problem of heat generation at the instrument tip while providing a more intense illumination and thus a brighter, more detailed field of view. The optimum endoscopic barrel size is 10—12 mm. Today, wide-angle optics make it possible to survey a much larger area than was possible with traditional lens systems. In the prelaryngeal region, for example, the epiglottis, arytenoid cartilage and pharyngeal roof can be observed in the same field of view. A film or photographic record can be made through the endoscope if desired.

The special diagnosis of guttural pouch diseases requires the use of angled instruments or instruments with an angled light source, for straight instruments will miss the entrance to the guttural pouch. The endoscope should be at least 60 cm in length so that the posterior recesses of the pouch can be examined even in large horses. Flexible instruments are used for bronchoscopy.

Technique of Endoscopic Examination. The use of stocks for restraint is optional. There are horses that will resist and there are others that are quite cooperative. In either case the examination may be attempted with the animal standing. Caution is always advised, however, for freely standing horses are more apt to lunge forward or rear. A twitch should be used if possible, and two assistants should restrain the animal's head. If the horse will not tolerate a twitch, it should be sedated in the interest of its own safety and that of the examiner. A 500- to 600-kg horse is sedated with 15 ml of methadone and 10 ml of 2 % xylazine i.v. or with 20 ml of methadone and 2—3 ml of propionyl promazine i.v.

Before the endoscope is inserted, it should be immersed in water heated to 40 °C, or the objective should be treated with an anti-misting compound.

For introduction of the endoscope, the examiner stands in front and somewhat to the side of the animal. With one hand he raises the ala nasi, and with the other he slides the endoscope, held next to the eyepiece, into the ventral nasal meatus. Care must be taken that the twitch does not occlude the nasal opening, for a horse may struggle if the nasal airflow is blocked. If downward pressure is exerted on the endoscope, it will slide quickly and easily into the ventral meatus. If the endoscope encounters an obstacle before it is in the pharynx, it is retracted somewhat and then readvanced. The horse may become anxious initially as the endoscope traverses the anterior portion of the nasal passage. During the examination the instrument is secured with one hand against the medial alar fold at the nasal inlet so that it will follow any unexpected head movements. An endoscope held only at the eyepiece end could cause serious nasal injury during unexpected movements. If the animal struggles excessively, the instrument should be removed at once to avoid injury to the turbinates and ethmoids.

a) Nasal examination: The endoscope is advanced to the larynx and then slowly retracted. The objective is pointed upward to look for abnormalities in the dorsal turbinate and ethmoid labyrinth.

b) Examination of the pharynx and larynx: The endoscope is advanced as far as possible and then slowly retracted and rotated to allow a general inspection. With a wide-angle lens it is possible to visualize the arytenoid cartilage, aryepiglottic fold, epiglottis, vocal cords and laryngeal ventricles; portions of the tracheal mucosa may even be visible between the vocal cords.

c) Examination of the guttural pouches: For endoscopy of the guttural pouches, the laryngoscope is advanced to the larynx and slowly retracted. The cartilage flap which covers the opening of the eustachian tube will be seen on the lateral wall of the pharynx. When this flap is visualized, the endoscope is withdrawn about 5 cm further and then carefully readvanced while rotating it laterally about 60—90°. The instrument will enter the pouch cavity for a distance of about 10 cm without encountering any palpable resistance. If the instrument slips past the entrance to the pouch, the resistance of the vertebral pharyngeal wall is quickly felt. With disease of the guttural pouch, the cartilage flap may gape somewhat and so will facilitate insertion of the endoscope. The instrument first enters the small anterior portion of the pouch, from which it can be advanced into the medial compartment. The great cornu of the hyoid bone divides the ventral portion of the pouch into a lateral and medial compartment. If necessary, the lateral compartment can be reached with flexible instruments. If the endoscope is inserted into the guttural pouch with the objective pointed downward, it will be seen that the ventral wall of the pouch ends in a recess. This recess cannot be identified if nearby lymph nodes are swollen. The pouch mucosa is raised medially by the underlying external carotid artery and the internal maxillary artery arising from it. The glossopharyngeal nerve courses over the external carotid artery.

d) Soft palate paresis or elongation: On endoscopic examination the soft palate may appear 'elongated', as its free edge covers the laryngeal aspect of the epiglottis.

This finding must be carefully reconfirmed if corresponding clinical symptoms are present.

e) Epiglottic entrapment: The mucous membrane fold extending from the arytenoid cartilage to the epiglottis becomes displaced over the epiglottis, entrapping it. The endoscopic appearance is unmistakable.

f) Epiglottic cyst: The epiglottis is found to be displaced upward from below by a cystic-like structure.

g) Bronchoscopy: The bronchoscope is advanced as far as the tracheal bifurcation. The color and consistency of the exudate in the trachea can be determined.

Complications. Struggling of the animal during endoscopy can cause injury to the mucosa, the turbinates or the ethmoid area and results in profuse epistaxis, usually venous, that seldom persists for more than 10—30 min. If bleeding is prolonged, the nasal cavity may be packed, and epinephrine-base drugs and hemostatics are administered. Immediately after use the endoscope is cleaned with warm water and disinfected. Formaldehyde is sometimes used for sterilization. For rapid disinfection, endoscopes intended for repeated use may be cleaned with alcohol-base skin antiseptics

2.1.4.2. Diseases of the Nose, the Nasal Cavities and the Paranasal Sinuses

2.1.4.2.1. Epistaxis

Definition. Hemorrhage from the vessels of the nose or sinuses is called epistaxis (rhinorrhagia).

The bleeding may be due to *local causes*, or may be *symptomatic* in nature. The former may result from trauma, tumors or the entry of foreign bodies into the nasal passages; the symptomatic form is associated with idiopathic epistaxis (defects of fibrinogen formation), hemorrhagic disease, vascular disease, circulatory disorders, febrile infectious diseases, or hemorrhage from the guttural pouch in mycotic infections.

Epistaxis may occur as an isolated episode, or it may be recurrent and paroxysmal. The bleeding may be spontaneous or may have an obvious precipitating cause. It may issue from one or both nostrils.

Symptoms. Sudden hemorrhage occurs after injuries to the ethmoid area (nasogastric tube or endoscope), fractures as well as contusions in the region of the nasal cavities and maxillary sinuses. With injury to the ethmoid area, blood streams profusely from one or both nostrils. Nasal respiration becomes stertorous and rattling, and the animal may cough from the aspiration of blood. The bleeding becomes heavier when the head is lowered and may stop completely when the head is raised. The intensity of the hemorrhage may fluctuate with time; often the bleeding stops for several minutes, only to recur suddenly and persist for several hours. In hemorrhagic diseases, the blood flows from the nose in drops or in a thin stream. With ulcers of the nasal mucosa, polyps or tumors, the bleeding due to necrosis of the lesions is dark, serosanguinous, and occasionally contains necrotic fragments or reddish-black clots (bloody exudate). 'Epistaxis in racehorses' [Mahaffey, 1962; Stolpe and Wiesner, 1970] is a condition in which nosebleed develops suddenly after heavy exertion, and fine blood droplets are expelled from the nostrils in spray form (see 2.1.3.2.3.). The blood losses associated with the various forms of epistaxis are difficult to assess, because the animals swallow a portion of the blood or wipe it off on nearby objects (wall of stall, feed box). In bleeding of ethmoidal origin, losses may be as high as 500—1,000 ml before the hemorrhage stops spontaneously after about 15 min.

Etiology. Trauma to the head and nasal mucosa and the entry of foreign bodies into the nasal passages are the most frequent causes of epistaxis. Idiopathic epistaxis is a disease of racehorses and as such occurs without an exogenous cause; the recurrent hemorrhages are apparently unrelated to time or degree of exertion. This form of epistaxis has complex causes and may be based upon an inbred defect such as a low platelet count or a qualitative abnormality of the fibrinogen ratio (formation of defective fibrinogen) (see 2.1.3.2.3.).

Diseases accompanied by hemorrhagic tendency can also cause bleeding from nasal mucosal vessels. Hypersensitive horses fed foreign proteins (purpura anaphylactica) may react with epistaxis. Drops of blood from the nostrils may be observed in purpura hemorrhagica and toxic states, and recurrent epistaxis in guttural pouch mycosis. Not infrequently, mild epistaxis (bloody exudate) occurs from tumors of the nasal mucosae (chondromas of the nasal septum) or tumors of the nasal cavity. Paroxysmal epistaxis has been described following the rupture of an aneurysm (internal carotid artery) [Boucher et al., 1964].

Diagnosis. Often the seat of the hemorrhage is not obvious and must be determined by endoscopy [Gratzl, 1964]. When the hemorrhage originates from the lungs, the blood is bright red and frothy, and some coughing is usually present. Hematologic studies (platelet and erythrocyte counts, hematocrit, hemoglobin, clotting time) are useful in ascertaining the probable cause of the epistaxis. If trauma, foreign bodies and tumors can be excluded, the possibility of infection, myocardial damage or allergic disease should be considered.

Prognosis. In epistaxis of traumatic origin, the prospect for healing is usually good; profuse hemorrhages however can be fatal. The prognosis is doubtful in hemorrhagic diseases and it is poor if the bleeding is of neoplastic origin.

Treatment. Mild acute hemorrhages soon stop by themselves. Recumbent animals should be made to stand if possible. Any exercise must be avoided. Packing of the nasal passages is contraindicated! If bleeding is severe the animal should be transfused with 2,000—3,000 ml whole blood or infused with 1,000—2,000 ml plasma expander. Hemostatics, vitamin C + K, calcium infusion solutions, and 1 : 1,000 epinephrine may be administered s.c. or slowly i.v. as adjunctive measures.

If the site of bleeding has been located and is accessible, hemostasis can be achieved by cauterization or electrocoagulation. The application of epinephrine- or thrombin-containing sprays may be effective in controlling small hemorrhages. The spray consists of 1 % saline solution containing 1 : 1,000 epinephrine or 100 NIH units of thrombin and is applied by means of a flexible spray catheter and Janet syringe. Bleeding from the guttural pouch is controlled by ligating the maxillary artery or carotid artery [Owen and McKelvey, 1979].

2.1.4.2.2. Nasal Catarrh (Rhinitis, Coryza)

Definition. Rhinitis is the term applied to inflammation of the nasal mucosa. The condition may be described as catarrhal, purulent, or necrotic, depending on the nature of the lesions and exudate. Rhinitis may be present as a separate entity but usually occurs in conjunction with other respiratory tract diseases.

Symptoms. In uncomplicated catarrhal diseases of the nasal mucosa, there is a serous to mucoid discharge from both nostrils (figs. 2.1.4. — 1 and — 2). The nasal mucosae are reddened, and sneezing or snorting may be present. In most cases systemic effects are absent. Fever and anorexia are characteristic of the purulent, or necrotizing forms of rhinitis. With more severe swelling of the nasal mucosa and

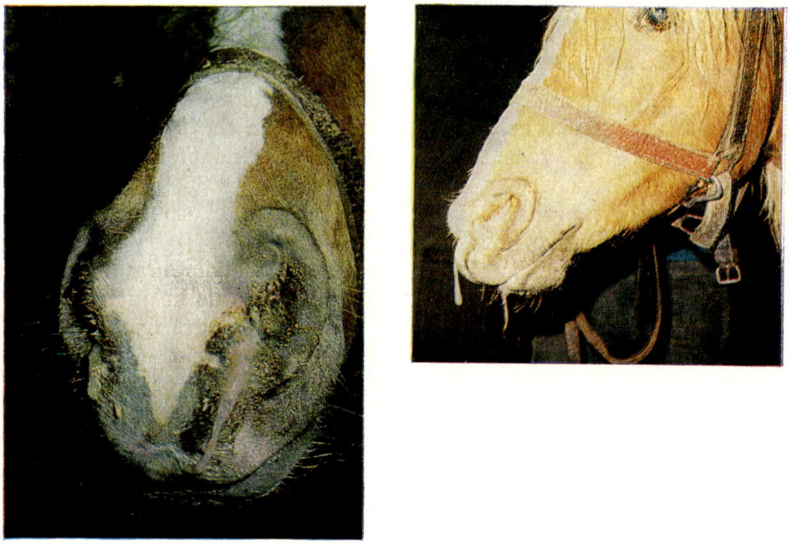

2

1

Fig. 2.1.4. — 1–2. Nasal catarrh: purulent discharge from both nostrils.

hypertrophy of the turbinates, stenotic sounds are heard during inspiration and expiration. The intermandibular lymph nodes are often unchanged; only in severe forms do they become swollen and painful. All forms of rhinitis may take an acute, subacute or chronic course. Uncomplicated forms (catarrhal rhinitis) often heal swiftly and without complications. Occasionally purulent inflammations give rise to secondary sinusitis, laryngitis, tracheitis or bronchopneumonia. Rarely does a necrotizing inflammation spread to involve cartilaginous or bony structures of the nose.

Etiology. Noninfectious diseases of the nasal mucosa can result from the inhalation of smoke or irritating gases, fumes or dust. Naturally occurring allergens (e.g., pollen from various grasses, rape or conifers) can also provoke rhinitis ('hay fever'). However, no methods are available in veterinary medicine for directly demonstrating the allergen responsible for the disease.

Inflammations of the nasal mucosae are associated with the following bacterial or viral diseases [Beer, 1980; Hutyra et al., 1954; Teufel et al., 1974; Wirth and Diernhofer, 1950]:
— equine influenza,
— rhinopneumonitis,
— upper respiratory tract infections,
— strangles (Streptococcus equi).

Diagnosis and Differential Diagnosis. The etiologic diagnosis of rhinitis is often difficult. A symptomatologic diagnosis can be quickly made by inspection of the mucous membranes, if necessary with the aid of a rhinoscope. The consistency of the nasal discharge (seromucous, purulent), its unilateral or bilateral occurrence, and exploration of the nasal cavities and guttural pouches aid in the differential diagnosis. The diseases that are accompanied by nasal discharge can, according to Deegen [1973], be divided into six main groups:

1. Infectious respiratory tract diseases:
   a) viral diseases,
   b) bacterial diseases.
2. Chronic respiratory tract diseases.
3. Allergic and toxic diseases.
4. Tumors or growths of the upper respiratory tract.
5. Specific inflammation of the respiratory tract.
6. Diseases in the upper gastrointestinal tract.

Previous research indicates that follicular changes in the region of the guttural pouches and pharynx, possibly combined with accumulations of exudate, may be attributable to certain species of virus (equine herpesvirus). If a rhinitis outbreak occurs in a given group of horses, an attempt should be made to isolate the causal agent by taking nasal swabs or washings and blood samples for bacteriologic or virologic analysis. The nasal discharge of strangles has a characteristic yellow color [Ebert, 1969; Waagenar and Schaaf, 1965].

Sinus empyema (maxillary, frontal, sphenoidal) and guttural pouch empyema must be considered in the differential diagnosis. Unilateral nasal discharge that increases when the head is lowered and is accompanied by mild nasal mucosal changes is characteristic of sinusitis.

Prognosis. Horses with acute rhinitis, may be given a favorable prognosis especially if it is sporadic in nature. Purulent and necrotic rhinitis respond poorly to therapy, and improvement is slow. Complications arise if the rhinitis spreads to the ethmoid area and maxillary sinus.

Treatment. Acute rhinitis responds to removal of the causative agent and exposure to fresh air and dust-free feeds. In more severe cases the nasal cavities should be irrigated with astringent and antiseptic solutions by means of a spray catheter. With severe swelling of the mucosae, 1 : 1,000 epinephrine should be added to the irrigating solution. Mucosal inflammation accompanied by bacterial infection of the upper respiratory tract responds well to treatment with aerosols containing antibiotics and ethereal oils [Gruner, 1956; Reuter, 1967]. Nasal sprays (OTC, chloramphenicol, Risoco) can also be beneficial. If it is suspected that the rhinitis is due to hypersensitization, antihistamines and antiallergic drugs must be administered for a period of several days. The use of antibiotics or sulfonamides should be considered if fever is present.

2.1.4.2.3. Inflammation of the Maxillary and Frontal Sinuses (Maxillary and Frontal Sinusitis)

Definition. Excessive accumulation of secretions in the maxillary sinus may be due to a congenital or acquired obstruction of the nasomaxillary opening.

Symptoms. The condition is usually unaccompanied by systemic signs. A bulge may appear over the maxillary sinus which is neither warm nor painful. The skin can be moved over the bulge. Percussion elicits a dull sounds. In rare cases there is a unilateral nasal discharge, but lacrimation is often present. In uncomplicated cases the intermandibular lymph nodes are enlarged but not painful.

Etiology. Inflammation and fluid accumulation is usually caused by the spread of inflammation from the nasal mucosae. The inflammatory processes and secretions cause a blockage of the narrow openings between the nasal passages and the maxillary sinus. Congenital occlusion of the nasomaxillary opening is rare.

Diagnosis. Radiography [Kovács et al., 1964] of the standing horse reveals densities in the region of the maxillary sinus. A horizontal fluid line may be visible within the sinus. Several films should be taken at various angles (oblique views) [Schebitz and Weber, 1963].

On endoscopy, a bulge is sometimes noted in the area of the ventral as well as dorsal meatus at the level of the maxillary sinus. Trephination confirms the clinical diagnosis. When the thin bone flap made by the trephine is raised, a hypertrophic mucosa is usually evident. If this is incised, an odorless, serous to mucoid fluid is exuded. Sinusitis must be differentiated from follicular cysts. In a follicular cyst, incision of the maxillary sinus mucosa, reveals a further mucosa within the cyst. When this is incised, a brown, turbid fluid is discharged. The inner surface of the opened cyst is rough and villous, and the wall of the cyst may show bony inclusions. Osteodystrophia fibrosa (bighead, bran disease) may produce symptoms and an external appearance similar to maxillary sinusitis.

Prognosis. The prognosis is good when prompt surgical treatment is performed.

Treatment. Following trephination of the maxillary sinus the septum between the rostral and caudal compartments of the sinus is removed [Popesko, 1961]. The accumulated fluid is aspirated, and any loose bone fragments or abnormal tissue are removed. This is followed by daily irrigation with mild antiseptic solutions. Strongly irritating solutions should be avoided; warm saline solutions are used toward the end of the healing period. To avoid secondary suppuration of the wound and sinus, care should be taken that the trephine opening does not close prematurely.

2.1.4.2.4. Maxillary and Frontal Sinus Empyema

Definition. Sinus empyema refers to an accumulation of pus in the maxillary or frontal sinus (figs. 2.1.4. — 3 and — 4).

Symptoms. Most cases are unilateral. The main presenting complaint is nasal discharge, which is typically purulent, discolored, fetid and sometimes blood-tinged. The purulent discharge may be continuous or intermittent. Typically it decreases during rest and increases when the head is lowered or when the depth and rate of respiration are increased. There is slight swelling of the intermandibular lymph nodes on the affected side, but the nodes are usually not tender. The nasal discharge may cease during certain periods when the inlets to the nasal passages seal over. A bulge often develops over the maxillary sinus. The bone may be abnormally thick or thin. Often marked tenderness is noted on digital palpation. The affected sinus is dull on percussion, in contrast to the healthy side. Fever and lethargy may be noted early in the disease. If dental disease is present, the animal will be reluctant to eat. As the disease progresses, signs of chronic inflammation result and the condition may persist for many months. Possible complications in longstanding cases are turbinate and ethmoid necrosis and rarely meningitis.

Etiology. Maxillary and frontal sinus empyema is usually secondary to inflammation of the upper respiratory tract or to strangles. Maxillary dental diseases are another major cause. Cases with purulent periodontitis can break through into the maxillary sinus, causing empyema. Traumatic empyemas due to a maxillary fracture or the entry of foreign bodies are rare [Leyland and Baker, 1975).

Diagnosis and Differential Diagnosis. Clinical findings are substantiated by inspection, palpation and percussion as well as by radiography and endoscopy. A careful examination of the teeth in the maxillary region is necessary to exclude dental disease as a possible cause of the empyema.

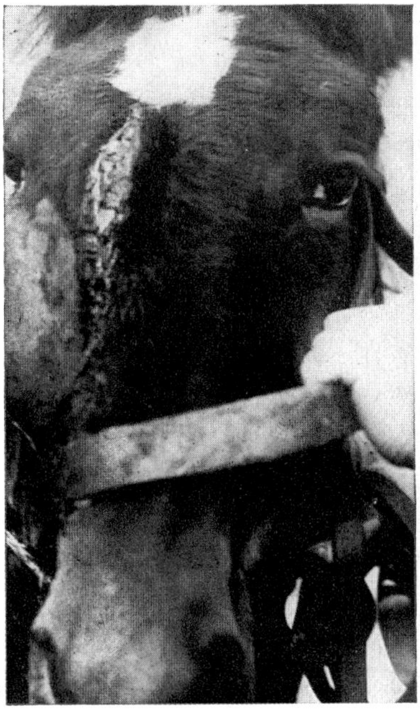
3

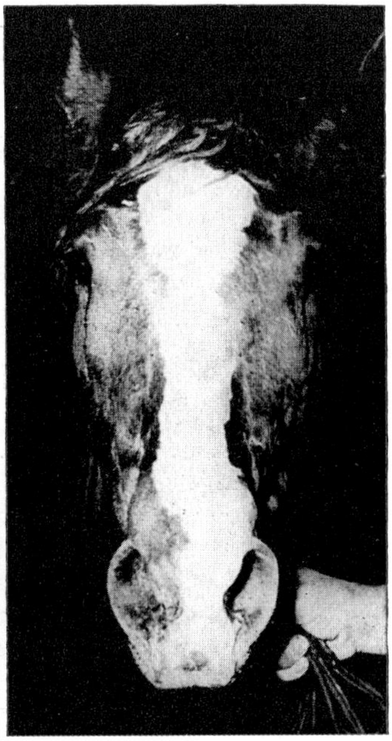
4

Fig. 2.1.4. — 3. Frontal sinus empyema.
Fig. 2.1.4. — 4. Maxillary sinus empyema.

Follicular cysts, myxofibromas, adenofibromas, chondromas, osteomas and squamous cell carcinomas must be excluded. Guttural pouch empyemas can mimic a maxillary sinus empyema, but in guttural pouch disease the nasal discharge is commonly bilateral unless one pouch is involved. In addition, the discharge of guttural pouch empyema is odorless and is increased by deglutition or feeding. With sinus tumors, the quantity of the discharge is usually small but constant, and blood and tissue fragments are sometimes present. Respiration may be impaired with tumors in this region.

Prognosis. In empyemas of non-dental origin, the prognosis with surgical treatment is good. Empyemas due to dental disease have a less favorable prognosis.

Treatment. When sinusitis is detected early, treatment by centesis of the maxillary sinus and the instillation of penicillin for several days should be attempted.

When empyema is present, trephination is indicated [Dietz et al., 1980]. The inspissated pus and necrotic tissues are removed by curettage and irrigation. The septum between the two compartments of the maxillary sinus must be penetrated during the operation. Postoperatively the horse is returned to its stall, and about 3—4 h later the sinus is copiously flushed with a warm, nonirritating antiseptic solution. This treatment is repeated at 2-day intervals. After a week or two the irrigating solution flowing from the nostrils and the operative wound should be clear; from that point on irrigation is done only with warm water or saline. The trephine opening will heal within 3 to 5 weeks. If a tooth or teeth had to be removed because of periodontitis, a fracture or caries, the trephine wound must be kept open longer. In the maxillary sinus region the channel leading from the alveolar socket to the sinus cavity usually is slow to heal and granulate closed. Treatment of the alveolar wound should always be combined with irrigation of the maxillary sinus.

2.1.4.2.5. Follicular Cysts of the Maxillary Sinus

Definition. Dental follicles which undergo cystic enlargement and fill the maxillary sinus are called follicular cysts. They can cause bulging of the maxillary bone and compression of the turbinates, giving rise to secondary obstructions and necrosis of surrounding tissues.

Symptoms. Sinus cysts develop mainly in the yearling foal during the growth of the 3rd premolar and cause a slowly progressive swelling in the maxillary region that often extends to the orbit. In most cases these swellings are neither hot nor tender to pressure. Percussion elicits a loud sound. Often there is a unilateral ocular discharge that forms tracks in the haircoat of the upper jaw (obstruction of naso-lacrimal canal). Large cysts are characterized by a unilateral nasal discharge, and sometimes by a stenosis of the nasal airway which produces an inspiratory and expiratory sound.

Etiology. Cysts can develop in the alveolar process of the maxilla from supernumerary and unerupted tooth primordia and extend in the direction of the maxillary sinus and turbinates. There is compression and displacement of surrounding structures, which gradually unites the maxillary sinuses and nasal cavity into a single (arge cavity occupied by the follicular cyst. This is accompanied by a partial occlusion of the medial meatus, which impairs respiration. Tissues adjacent to the cyst sturbinate, nasoturbinal, maxilloturbinal) undergo degenerative changes and may secrete mucous. The surrounding bony substance also may undergo enlargement similar to that seen in osteodystrophia fibrosa (bighead, bran disease).

Diagnosis and Differential Diagnosis. The diagnosis is based upon clinical symptoms and is confirmed by radiography and endoscopy. The oral cavity should be carefully examined for delays in tooth eruption, an impacted premolar or nonocclusion of the molars ('open bite'), as these signs may indicate a follicular cyst. In most cases a bulging of the maxilla on the buccal side is also palpable within the oral cavity.

Cysts must be differentiated from other types of tumor.

Prognosis. The prognosis is guarded, because both the protracted postoperative course and subsequent abnormalities of tooth eruption can cause a loss of condition due to poor feeding.

Treatment. Treatment consists of radical surgical removal. The foal is anesthetized and placed in lateral recumbency for the procedure. An infraorbital nerve block may be administered to supplement the anesthetic regime and the anterior nares is positioned lower than the neck. Three trephine openings are made and are interconnected with bone forceps. The cavity of the cyst can be displaced from the mucosa of the maxillary sinus with the finger, producing a parchment-like crackling sound. The cyst wall is up to 10 mm thick and contains a thin bony cavity. Sharp division yields a reddish-yellow, serous fluid that may have fine, rice-like particles in it. The inner lining of the cyst wall appears rough. The cyst is now removed piece by piece from the maxillary sinus cavity. Its deep portion abuts on the root of a molar, and the root is exposed during the excision. It is important that all portions of the cyst be removed. The remnants of the turbinate are removed through the nostril. The resultant heavy bleeding creates a danger of aspiration, and so at this point the operation must be terminated and the horse returned to its feet as quickly as possible. Postoperative irrigation should be done as described under the treatment of sinus empyema.

2.1.4.2.6. Turbinate Necrosis

Definition. This is a partial necrosis due to bacteria that affects the middle portions of the turbinate. It is seen in older horses.

Symptoms. A curved swelling about the width of a hand appears in the midportion of the dorsum of the nose. It extends from a line connecting the two medial canthi down to the level of the 2nd premolar. Initially the swelling is hard but later it softens and becomes painful. This is accompanied by a bilateral purulent, fetid nasal discharge.

Inspiratory and expiratory noise is present as a result of airway stenosis. The intermandibular lymph nodes are only mildly enlarged and are painless. The visible nasal mucosa appears edematous and glassy. In the terminal stage of the disease, cerebral signs may appear due to spread of the inflammatory process via the ethmoid bone. This is usually accompanied by maxillary sinus empyema.

Etiology. Inflammation of the upper respiratory tract and strangles following complicated cases are believed to be responsible for the gradual and progressive turbinate necrosis.

Diagnosis and Differential Diagnosis. The diagnosis is established by the externally visible changes, the radiographic and endoscopic examination, and clinical findings (nasal discharge). A stomach tube introduced when swelling first appears, will encounter or meet resistance. If inserted forcefully, it can easily cause epistaxis.

Endoscopically, portions of the turbinate are found to be necrotic and embedded in well-circumscribed granulation tissue. Percussion elicits a dull sound over the swelling on the nasal dorsum.

Turbinate necrosis must be differentiated from tumors. These are usually distinguished by ill-defined swellings in the region of the maxillary sinus and nasal cavities. Maxillary and frontal sinus empyemas must also be considered in the differential diagnosis. In the case of a follicular cyst or 'mucoid degeneration' of the turbinate, seen only in yearlings, the nasal discharge is serous and non-fetid.

Prognosis. If cerebral signs are present, or if secondary aspiration pneumonia has developed, the prognosis is usually hopeless. In the early stage of the disease, surgical removal of the necrotic turbinate is usually sufficient to prevent complications and enhance the prospect of recovery.

Treatment. Respiratory distress, if present, is relieved by a temporary tracheostomy. If maxillary sinus empyema is suspected, the sinus is opened by trephination, and then the dorsum of the nose is split 2 cm from the midline over the swelling. Overlying tissues are reflected until the periosteum is well exposed. Then trephine holes are made near the upper and lower ends of the wound, the bone between the openings is removed with a ronguer, and the bony edges are smoothed. The areas of turbinate necrosis are usually well demarcated and can be removed through the surgical opening. Then the head is lowered and the operative wound is irrigated and packed. In advanced and complicated cases, complete removal of the turbinates is indicated. Through the trephine opening, the dorsal turbinate is carefully detached from the dorsolateral wall of the nasal cavity and removed in pieces. The bulk of the turbinate must be extracted through the nostrils with forceps. This causes profuse bleeding, and the horse should be brought to its feet as quickly as possible following removal of the turbinates. The bleeding will stop usually spontaneously once the animal is standing. Postoperative care should include the administration of antibiotics. Irrigation should be performed at 2- to 3-day intervals.

2.1.4.2.7. 'Mucoid Degeneration of the Turbinate' (Myxomalacia Concharum, Hydropic Degeneration, Congenital Mucoid Cyst, Sand's Disease)

Definition. This disease is characterized by the formation of mucoid cysts, usually unilaterally, which fill the space between the floor and roof of the nasal passage, the maxillary bone and the nasal septum. It is seen primarily in yearlings.

Symptoms. A bulge between the dorsum of the nose, facial crest and orbit gradually appears at the level of the maxillary sinus. Wheezing or stertorous respiratory sounds develop as a result of stenosis. The animal's general condition is usually unimpaired. The clinical picture resembles that of a maxillary sinus cyst. The dorsal turbinate is compressed by the protruding cyst, and the ventral turbinate also undergoes changes due to compression. There is a local accumulation of mucus and gelatinous fluid, and a serous to mucoid nasal discharge. The intermandibular lymph nodes may be enlarged.

Etiology and Differential Diagnosis. The cause of the disease is unknown. Sand [1893] characterized the disease as a 'mucoid degeneration'. Merz rejected this theory, however. According to Bolz [1970], the disease is identical with the follicular cyst. Its clinical appearance does not correspond to that of osteodystrophia fibrosa. Rubarth and Krook [1968] suggest that the changes are the expression of a nutritional secondary hyperparathyroidism on the basis of the morphologic picture.

Prognosis. Prompt surgical treatment offers the only hope of a cure especially in acute cases.

Treatment. Removal of the turbinates is performed by the technique described for turbinate necrosis.

2.1.4.2.8. Soft Palate Elongation (Dorsal Displacement of the Soft Palate)

Definition. This was thought to be a paresis or elongation of the soft palate causing respiratory embarrassment. Current theories now feel the condition is a 'dislocation' of the larynx with respect to the soft palate.

Symptoms. Sudden dyspnea occurs when the horse is exercised at a fast gait. The animal breathes with a characteristic vibrating, rattling sound and has frequent paroxysisms of coughing. The sounds disappear when the animal is calm and rested. The airway obstruction can be localized to the pharynx by auscultation.

Etiology. The causes are not fully understood. Soft palate paresis can occur as a sequel to strangles or viral infection of the upper respiratory tract. Such cases may involve a paralysis or paresis of the palatinus muscle or levator palatini muscle, which are innervated by branches of the vagus nerve. This results in the soft palate, covering of the epiglottis. Paresis of the soft palate is sometimes combined with unilateral laryngeal hemiplegia [Cook, 1962, 1964, 1965; Gerber, 1968].

Diagnosis and Differential Diagnosis. The disease is localized by auscultation before, during and after exercise. Examination of the oral cavity is usually unrewarding. The laryngoscope reveals continuous or intermittent covering of the epiglottis by the soft palate.

If the tissues surrounding the larynx are flaccid, the larynx itself may appear small, and the epiglottis may be displaced upward. As a result, the vocal cords are difficult to visualize. Paralysis of the recurrent laryngeal nerve (left-sided laryngeal hemiplegia) is characterized by inspiratory dyspnea, and laryngoscopy shows a definite asymmetry of the vocal cords with sagging of the arytenoid cartilage. Spasm of the cricoarytenoid muscles can cause dyspnea and even respiratory arrest if the arytenoid cartilage obstructs the dorsal region of the glottis [GOULDEN et al., 1975]. Retrolingual and subepiglottic cysts are ruled out on endoscopy and physical examination. Acute pharyngeal inflammation, which may be associated with soft palate edema, is also identified by endoscopy. Chronic bronchitis and laryngitis with hypertrophy of the mucosa as well as certain heart diseases can mimic some symptoms of the soft palate (respiratory distress, stenotic sounds). Therefore a thorough clinical examination of the heart and lungs is indicated. A cleft soft palate in the foal causes difficulty in nursing. A persistent right aortic arch with compression of the esophagus can also mimic defects of the soft palate [BARTELS and VAUGHAN, 1969].

Prognosis. In severe cases surgery is indicated. The prognosis for a complete recovery is guarded.

Treatment. The surgical treatment for soft palate elongation is a partial soft palate resection by the method of Hofmayer [DIETZ et al., 1980]. A more recent technique involves a myectomy of the sternothyrohyoideus muscle [COOK]. If the soft palate is cleft, correction may be attempted following a mandibular symphysiotomy [STICKLE et al., 1973) (see 2.1.5.8.6.). Attempts at nonoperative treatment are ineffective in most cases.

2.1.4.2.9. Neoplasms of the Anterior Airways

Neoplasms of the nose and its cavities are relatively frequent in the horse. The tumors may arise primarily from the mucosa or bony wall, or they may invade the nose secondarily from the oral or pharyngeal cavity [HANSELKA et al., 1975; LEUTHOLD; LINGARD and CRAWFORT, 1970; MASON, 1975; MENSA; RAHKO et al., 1972].

Localization

- Nasal mucosa: Besides myxofibromas and adenofibromas with cystic enlargement of the mucous glands, hyperplasia of the nasal mucosa (polyps) and cutaneous papillomas are observed at the junction of the skin with the mucous membrane at the nares [NJOKU and BURWASH, 1972]. Mucosal tumors may appear as lobular or nodular growths and may have a broad site of attachment with the mucosa. Angiomas may arise from the venous plexus of the nose.
- Nasal septum: The septum is affected mainly by chondromas, which can cause it to deviate in either direction. Osteomas which arise from the nasal septum may also occur.
- Turbinate: Neoplastic changes can develop in this area as a result of amyloidosis. They often appear at the rostral end of the turbinate and are visible or palpable through the nostril as a cone-shaped growth. Occasionally metastatic tumors in older gray horses with melanomas appear as nodular thickenings of the turbinates.
- Ethmoid bone, hard palate, paranasal sinuses: Spindle-cell carcinomas, squamous-cell carcinomas, odontomas, osteofibromas, myxomas and hemangiomas have been observed in these areas. Mucosal and bone changes that are characterized by granuloma formation can arise from the frontal sinus in response to infection by yeastlike organisms *(Cryptococcus neoformans)* or *Micronema* nematodes *(M. deletrix)* [JOHNSON and JOHNSON, 1966; SCOTT et al., 1974; WATT, 1970].

Symptoms. Smaller neoplasms in the early stage cause no obvious clinical changes in the aforementioned regions. Only when tissue destruction occurs or there is compression due to tumor growth can one expect to find changes about the face and head, epistaxis, nasal discharge and respiratory impairment (fig. 2.1.4. — 5). In

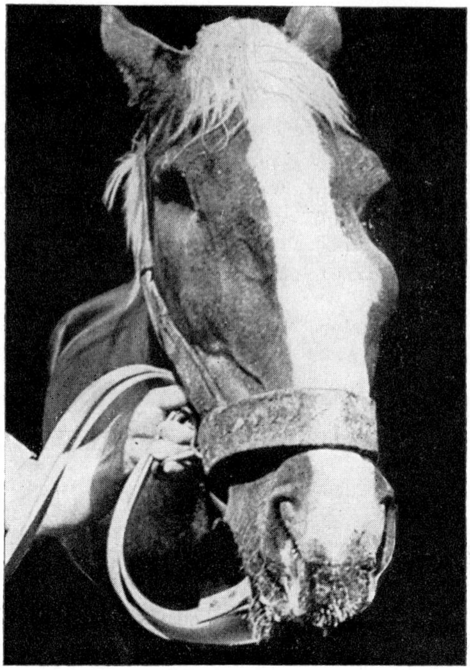

Fig. 2.1.4. — 5. Turbinate osteosarcoma with nasal discharge.

maxillary sinus carcinomas, examination of the oral cavity often reveals a defect in the hard palate beside the cheek teeth. Individual teeth are loosened, the tissue surrounding the dental lamina is fragile, and the mucosa shows dark-red discoloration.

Diagnosis. The nature of the tumor can be determined by the histologic examination of biopsy material. Carcinomas and sarcomas show a rapid infiltrative growth with swift bony tissue destruction. Space-occupying lesions within the nasal passages cause dyspnea and a multitude of abnormal inspiratory and expiratory sounds. Catheterization of the nasal meati and endoscopic inspection can in many cases disclose the size, shape and extent of the tumor. Radiographs of the head in several planes provide useful information on the localization, extent and perhaps even the nature of the neoplasm [Ammann and Fackelmann, 1971].

Prognosis. Sarcomas and carcinomas are generally incurable. Tumors in the ethmoid region that have invaded the nasal cavity from the palatine process of the maxillary bone are inaccessible to surgery and so are inoperable.

Treatment. Tumors visible in the nasal cavity can be removed through the naris. Occasionally it is necessary to split the outer ala nasi in order to gain access. The incisions must be carefully made and meticuously sutured to avoid disfigurement postoperatively. Deep-seated tumors can be removed only after the nasal cavity and paranasal sinuses have been radically opened and combined if necessary with removal of the turbinates. Ethmoid hematomas must be approached with care and may require the use of electrosurgical or cryosurgical techniques to avoid excessive hemorrhaging.

References

Anonymous: Chondrom in der Nasenscheidewand eines Pferdes. Bildbericht. Dtsch. Tierärztl. Wschr. *79:* 219 (1972).

Ammann, K.; Fackelmann, G.: Zur Röntgendiagnose geschwulstartiger Prozesse der Nasengänge und Nasennebenhöhlen beim Pferd. Wiener tierärztl. Mschr. *58:* 151 (1971).

Bartels, J. E.; Vaughan, J. T.: Persistent right aortic arch in the horse. J. Amer. vet. med. Assoc. *154:* 406 (1969).

Bayer; Fröhner, E.: Handbuch der tierärztlichen Chirurgie und Geburtshilfe (Wilhelm Braumüller, Wien und Leipzig 1910).

Beer, J.: Infektionskrankheiten der Haustiere, 2. Aufl. (VEB Gustav Fischer Verlag, Jena 1980).

Bolz, W.: Lehrbuch der Allgemeinen Chirurgie für Tierärzte, 4. Aufl. (VEB Gustav Fischer Verlag, Jena 1970).

Bolz, W.; Dietz, O.; Schleiter, H.; Teuscher, R.: Lehrbuch der speziellen Veterinärchirurgie, 2. Aufl. (VEB Gustav Fischer Verlag, Jena 1975).

Boucher, W. B.; Elliot, G. A.; Schmucker, B.: Epistaxis due to rupture of an aneurysm in a horse. J. Amer. vet. med. Assoc. *145:* 1004 (1964).

Cook, W. R.: Clinical observations on the equine soft palate. Proc. 1st. Ann. Congr. Brit. Equine Vet. Assoc. p. 5 (1962).

Cook, W. R.: The diagnosis of respiratory unsoundness in the horse. Proc. Brit. Equine Vet. Assoc., p. 18 (1964).

Cook, W. R.: The diagnosis of respiratory unsoundness in the horse. Vet. Rec. *77:* 516 (1965).

Cook, W. R.: Clinical observations on the anatomy and physiology of the equine respiratory tract. Vet. Rec. *79:* 440 (1966).

Cook, W. R.: Instrument specifications for endoscopy of the equine upper respiratory tract and Eustachian tube diverticulum. Vet. Rec. *87:* 429 (1970).

Deegen, E.: Ursache des Nasenausflusses beim Pferd. tierärztl. praxis *1:* 169 (1973).

Dietz, O.; Schleiter, H.; Schaetz, F.; Teuscher, R.: Anästhesie und Operationen bei Gross- und Kleintieren, 2. Aufl. (S. Hirzel Verlag, Leipzig 1980).

Ebert, E. F.: Some observations on equine strangles. Vet. Med. and Small Animal Clinician *64:* 71 (1969).

Gerber, H.: Zur Therapie chronischer Respirationskrankheiten des Pferdes. Schweiz. Arch. Tierheilk. *110:* 139 (1968).

Gerber, H.: Klinik und Therapie chronischer Lungenleiden des Pferdes. Dtsch. tierärztl. Wschr. *76:* 234 (1969).

Goulden, B. E.; Barnes, G. R. G.; Quinlan, T. J.: A case of equine laryngospasm. New Zealand vet. J. *23:* 148 (1975).

Gratzl, E.: Instrumentarium zur Rhinoskopie und Laryngoskopie an Pferden von Polansky und Schindelka 1888/89. Wiener tierärztl. Mschr. *51:* 203 (1964).

Gruner, J.: Zur Aerosoltherapie bei Erkrankungen des Respirationstraktes des Pferdes. Neue Ergebnisse der Aerosolforschung. Bericht über den 2. Aerosol-Kongress 1955. (Schattauer, Stuttgart 1956).

Hanselka, D. V.; Young, M. F.: Ethmoidal hematoma in the horse. Vet. Med. and Small Animal Clinician *70:* 1289 (1975).

Hutyra, F. v.; Marek, J.; Manninger, R.; Mócsy, J.: Spezielle Pathologie und Therapie der Haustiere, 10. Aufl. (VEB Gustav Fischer Verlag, Jena 1954).

Johnson, K. H.; Johnson, D. W.: Granulomas associated with Micronema deletrix in the maxillae of a horse. J. Amer. vet. med. Assoc. *149:* 155 (1966).

Kovács, Gy.; Glósz, L.; Gertner, M.: Die Röntgenanatomie der Hirnschädelknochen des Pferdes. Acta vet. Acad. Sci. Hung. *14:* 309 (1964).

Leuthold, A.: Vorkommen und Diagnose des Kieferhöhlenkarzinoms beim Pferd. Festschrift Theodor Schmidt: Fortschritte der neuzeitlichen Veterinärchirurgie (undated).

Leyland, A.; Baker, J. R.: Lesions of the nasal and paranasal sinuses of the horse causing dyspnoea. Brit. vet. J. *131:* 339 (1975).

Lingard, D. R.; Crawfort, T. B.: Congenital ameloblastic odontoma in a foal. Amer. J. vet. Res. *31:* 801 (1970).

MAHAFFAY, L. W.: Respiratory conditions in horses. Vet. Rec. *74:* 1295 (1962).
MASON, B. J. E.: Spindle-cell sarcoma of the equine para-nasal sinuses and nasal chamber. Vet. Rec. *96:* 287 (1975).
MASON, B. J. E.: Empyema of the equine paranasal sinuses. J. Amer. vet. med. Assoc. *167:* 727 (1975).
MENSA, A.: Über die odontogenen Tumoren der Kiefer. Festschrift Theodor Schmidt: Fortschritte der neuzeitlichen Veterinärchirurgie (undated).
NJOKU, CELESTINE O.; BURWASH, W. A.: Congenital cutaneous papilloma in a foal. Cornell Vet. *62:* 54 (1972).
OWEN, R.; MCKELVEY, W. A. C.: Ligation of the internal carotid artery to prevent epistaxis due to gutteral pouch mycosis. Vet. Rec. *104:* 5, 101 (1979).
POPESKO, P.: Atlas der topographischen Anatomie der Haustiere (VEB Gustav Fischer Verlag, Jena 1961).
RAHKO, T.; ALITALO, I.; PAATSAMA, S.: Myxoma in the nasal cavity of the Finnish-bred horse. A report on three cases recently observed in Finland. Acta. vet. scand. *13:* 131 (1972).
REUTER, U.: Untersuchungen über die Aerosol-Therapie einiger unter dem Symptomen-Komplex der Pferdegrippe verlaufenden Erkrankungen der Atmungsorgane. Vet.-med. Diss., München (1967).
RUBARTH, S.; KROOK, L.: Etiology and pathogenesis of so-called mucoid degeneration of the nasal conchae in the horse. Acta vet. scand. *9:* 253 (1968).
SCOTT, E. A.; DUNCAN, J. R.; MCCORMACK, J. E.: Cryptococcosis involving the postorbital area and frontal sinus in a horse. J. Amer. vet. med. Assoc. *165:* 626 (1974).
SCHEBITZ, H.; WEBER, W.: Zur Röntgenuntersuchung des Gesichtsschädels vom Pferd. Dtsch. tierärztl. Wschr. *70:* 450 (1963).
STICKLE, R. L.; GOBLE, O.; BRADEN, T. D.: Chirurgische Korrektur eines gespaltenen Gaumensegels beim Fohlen. Vet. Med. and Small Animal Clinician *68:* 159 (1973).
STOLPE, J.; WIESNER, E.: Das Fibrinogen bei nasenblutenden Galopprennpferden und Trabern. Arch. exp. Vet.-Med. *24:* 903 (1970).
TEUFEL, P.; GRUND, S.; ZELLER, R.: Experimentelle Infektion der Nasenschleimhaut eines Pferdes mit dem Rhinopneumonitis-Virus (Herpesvirus-equi-1). Berliner Münchener tierärztl. Wschr. *7:* 61 (1974).
WAGENAAR, G.; SCHAAF, A. V. D.: Druse. Tijdschr. Diergeneeskd. *90:* 315 (1965).
WATT, D. A.: A case of cryptococcal granuloma in the nasal cavity of a horse. Aust. vet. J. *46:* 493 (1970).
WIRTH, D.; DIERNHOFER, K.: Lehrbuch der inneren Krankheiten der Haustiere (Enke, Stuttgart 1950).

2.1.4.3. Diseases of the Larynx and Trachea

2.1.4.3.1. Laryngitis

Definition. Laryngitis is a collective term applied to catarrhal or purulent inflammation of the laryngeal mucosa and inflammation of the laryngeal cartilage. The various inflammatory diseases of the laryngeal mucosa are of main clinical interest because of the frequency of their occurrence. Laryngitis may take an acute or chronic course.

Etiology. Laryngeal inflammation frequently develops as a sequel to the viral upper respiratory infections which have the same general etiology as pharyngitis (q.v.). Mechanical injuries from the entry of foreign bodies into the larynx, such as feed particles or awns, are infrequent causes. The repeated inhalation of irritants (ammonia, toxic gases) can trigger inflammatory reactions in the laryngeal mucosa or promote their development.

Often laryngitis is associated with rhinitis and pharyngitis. It may also occur in chronic obstructive pulmonary disease and pneumonia. It regularly accompanies inflammation of the upper respiratory tract and so is seen in rhinopneumonitis, influenza and viral arteritis. Heat, dryness, exposure to dust and extreme temperature fluctuations predispose to the development of respiratory tract disease.

Sudden cooling may reflexly provoke vasoconstriction and ischemia. This may lower the natural resistance of the mucosa to microbial infection, enabling the microorganisms normally present on the mucosa (streptococci, staphylococci, coliforms) to invade the tissue and cause inflammation.

Laryngitis is also a feature of specific infectious diseases. It is observed in strangles, glanders, purpura hemorrhagica and epizootic lymphangitis.

Symptoms. In the early stages of acute laryngitis there is a short, harsh, dry cough which later becomes moist and in many cases is painful. Persistent coughing spells are frequent. Spontaneous coughing is especially noted when the horse is led out of its stall, during exercise, during sudden exposure to cold air, and during ingestion of dusty feeds. A bilateral, serous to mucopurulent nasal discharge develops during the course of the disease. Often the intermandibular lymph nodes are swollen, and the throat region is tender to palpation. With swelling of the laryngeal mucosa abnormal respiratory sounds will result. These have a rattling or sterterous quality and may be mistaken for roaring. Local inflammation is usually unaccompanied by fever.

In chronic cases the cough is dry, harsh and less frequent, and it does not produce the pain of the acute form.

In acute inflammation the laryngeal mucosa is reddened and edematous. The mucosa of the epiglottis is also red and swollen and is covered with mucopurulent exudate. Severe mucosal redness signifies an inflammation of the upper airways. Strangles may be accompanied by a marked swelling of the laryngeal mucosa, which may also be coated with a purulent exudate. Rhinopneumonitis may form vesicles in the mucosa which later develop into pinhead-size nodules.

Diphtheritic coatings and ulceration may be noted during the course of certain specific infectious diseases (epizootic lymphangitis, purpura hemorrhagica).

In chronic inflammation the mucosa is grayish-white in color and its surface is rough and thickened.

Treatment. Treatment aims at relieving the primary disorder. If the laryngitis is a clinical manifestation of a systemic infection, chemotherapeutic measures form the basis of treatment. Antibiotics, sulfonamides and expectorant therapy are employed. Prophylactic innoculations with commercially available or stable-specific vaccines may be given with the object of increasing the resistance to certain common infectious diseases. Inhalation of anti-inflammatory and antiseptic aerosols or of secretolytic vapors are a useful adjunct to therapy. If dyspnea is severe, a tracheotomy is occasionally indicated. Affected animals should not be worked and should receive dust-free feed (hay should be moistened with water). Where possible, limited pasturing may be allowed. In chronic cases a change of climate has proved beneficial in conjunction with the measures listed above.

2.1.4.3.2. Tumors of the Larynx

Occurrence. Laryngeal tumors are relatively uncommon in the horse. Both benign and malignant forms are known. Benign tumors frequently take the form of pedunculated polyps attached to the epiglottis and occasionally the vocal cords. These may be papillomas, fibromas, adenomas, myxomas or lipomas. Carcinomas arising in the laryngeal mucosa tend to infiltrate surrounding tissues.

Symptoms. Because the polyps are moved back and forth by the flow of respiratory air, they cause rattling or even stenotic respiratory noises, depending on their size. Constant coughing may occur. There is no systemic reaction or fever. The noises may increase with forced respiration, creating sounds resembling roaring. Carcinomas provoke frequent coughing. The superficial tissue necrosis that accompanies carcinoma produces a bilateral, reddish, serous or mucoid nasal discharge. Fast-growing carcinomas can interfere with deglutition. Metastasis to the regional lymph nodes is common.

The *diagnosis* is established by endoscopy.

Treatment. Benign tumors can generally be successfully removed via a laryngotomy. The laryngotomy may also be used as a diagnostic aid in doubtful cases.

2.1.4.3.3. Wounds of the Larynx

Wounds can occur as a result of accidents or strangulation.

Symptoms. The symptoms in acute cases depend on the extent of the injury. Hemorrhages and perilaryngeal swelling may complicate the clinical picture. Perforating wounds are recognized by the escape of air and the exudation of a foamy, blood-tinged mucus through the cutaneous wound. If the wound edges are inverted, dyspnea can arise. Non-perforating wounds can lead to perilaryngeal cellulitis due to the entry of infectious organisms; this can spread to the larynx and cause respiratory embarrassment.

Treatment. Therapy consists of the use of systemic antibiotics and local surgical wound care. A temporary tracheostomy is indicated if dyspnea is severe.

2.1.4.3.4. Edema of the Larynx (Glottic Edema)

Definition. Laryngeal or glottic edema refers to the accumulation of a serous fluid in the loose tissue of the arytenoepiglottic folds with spread to surrounding submucosal tissues.

Symptoms. Owing to its peracute course, glottic edema may lead to acute life-threatening situations from severe respiratory embarrassment. Breathing becomes difficult and is accompanied by whistling or râles. Marked venous congestion and cyanosis are also present. Because the epiglottis can no longer seal the entrance to the larynx, the animal may have coughing spells. By contrast, congestive edemas develop relatively slowly, i.e., over a period of several days, and their symptoms are not so severe.

Etiology. Glottic edema may be congestive in nature, resulting from compression of the jugular vein (throatlatch, stable halter, strangulation), or it may take the form of a dependent edema secondary to edema of the head. Glottic edema may also be inflammatory, occurring as a sequel to fractures, contusions, mucosal inflammation (e.g., after strenuous rides on dusty roads or from the inhalation of smoke or irritating fumes), or arising during the course of specific diseases (anthrax, purpura hemorrhagica, clostridial infections) as well as allergic conditions.

Diagnosis. The endoscopic picture is characterized by a marked edema of the aryepiglottic fold. This and the clinical findings establish the diagnosis.

Treatment. Because of the peracute course of the disease, rapid intervention is sometimes necessary. A temporary tracheotomy with insertion of a tracheostomy tube will help get the animal through the acute life-threatening crisis. While the edema itself may respond poorly to treatment, an attempt should be made to ascertain the cause of the disease so that a specific therapy can be instituted. In many cases the edema will regress spontaneously once the dyspnea has been relieved.

2.1.4.3.5. Chronic Ossifying Chondritis of the Larynx

Definition. This is a chronic form of laryngitis which has resulted from partial or complete ossification of the laryngeal cartilages.

Symptoms. Affected animals stand with the head noticeably extended. The narrowing of the laryngeal lumen interferes with respiration, causing stenotic inspiratory and expiratory sounds. The site of the stenosis can be determined by auscultation. The ossification leads to rigidity of the larynx. On palpation it feels hard and inelastic, and the individual cartilages can no longer be distinguished. The vocal cords and arytenoid cartilage are immobile, and so the rima glottidis can no longer be opened. Frequently the ossification is accompanied by a chondritis with multiple abscess formation, ulceration and necrosis, in which case fistulas develop at various locations in the larynx.

Etiology. The ossifying processes are caused mainly by contusions or wounds. Other causes include faulty or unsuccessful roaring operations.

Treatment. The disease is incurable and a permanent tracheostomy may be the only means of keeping the animal alive.

2.1.4.3.6. Fractures of the Laryngeal Cartilages

Despite the elasticity of the laryngeal cartilages, they are susceptible to traumatic fracture. This applies especially to the cricoid cartilage.

Diagnosis. Generally the diagnosis presents no difficulties. The relationship to prior external trauma in conjunction with local deformity and possible respiratory embarrassment enable a strong presumptive diagnosis. The diagnosis can be confirmed by radiography.

Treatment. Treatment consists in surgical reduction of the fracture and its repair with approximating sutures.

2.1.4.3.7. Laryngeal Paralysis (Laryngeal Whistling, Roaring)

Definition. Laryngeal paralysis, recurrent nerve paralysis, or laryngeal hemiplegia is a permanent disturbance of those laryngeal functions that are responsible for regulating the flow of air to the lungs. It is due to an atrophy of some or all of the intrinsic laryngeal muscles which derive their motor innervation from the recurrent laryngeal nerve. The atrophy of the laryngeal muscles leads to the sagging of one or both arytenoid cartilages into the laryngeal lumen and to the functional impairment of one or both vocal cords. Clinically there is a respiratory stenosis that produces a characteristic whistling or roaring noise.

Occurrence. Roaring is principally a disease of large horses and large breeds. Medium-size horses are rarely affected. The disease is virtually unknown in small horses and ponies.

The disease is observed most frequently in athletic horses. Its incidence is greatest in horses less than 6 years of age ($> 80\%$ of cases according to Cook), although animals may still be affected up to age 12. The occurrence after this age is unusual. There appears to be no age or sex predisposition, though an hereditary predisposition cannot be ruled out. In over 90% of patients the laryngeal paralysis is restricted to the left side (98% according to Cook, 1968). The paralysis is bilateral in a very small percentage of cases. The isolated occurrence of right-sided laryngeal hemiplegia is disputed. Marks et al. [1970] observed 5 cases, mostly due to the result of faulty injection technic in the neck region.

Etiology. The impairment of laryngeal function is due to a degeneration of the motor nerve fibers supplying the laryngeal muscles.

The cause of left laryngeal hemiplegia is a primary, incurable paralysis of the left recurrent nerve. The cause of roaring is thought to be based upon an anatomic predisposition owing to the unique topography of the left recurrent nerve, and the apparent relationship between paralysis and the size of the horse. The left recurrent nerve branches from the vagus nerve at the base of the heart and winds around the aortic arch before ascending the neck. This anatomic course makes it effectively shorter than the right recurrent nerve. Because it must span the same distance from the vagus nerve to the larynx, it comes under greater tension when the neck is turned to the right than does the right recurrent nerve when the neck is turned to the left. When a critical degree of stretch is exceeded, degenerative changes arise. Theoretically tensile forces acting on the nerve are greater in large and long-necked horses due to the correspondingly greater radii of curvature and flexion. As a result, these animals are more susceptible to left recurrent nerve paralysis. It is also thought that enlargement of lymph nodes due to lower respiratory tract infections, growth-related enlargement of the neck muscles, and training-related changes in myocardial size and position can also contribute to recurrent nerve stretch and thus predispose to degenerative change. The importance of aortic pulsation in left recurrent nerve damage remains disputed, for histopathological evidence is lacking. In rare cases, lead poisoning or the ingestion of toxic plants (lathyrism) can produce the clinical picture of recurrent nerve paralysis. Guttural pouch mycoses, which according to Cook [1968] also show a left-sided predominance, may be associated with roaring due to damage to the vagus nerve.

Degenerative changes of the vagus and left recurrent laryngeal nerve have been produced experimentally with streptococcal toxins. These observations support the theory that Streptococcus equi infections may contribute to laryngeal hemiplegia. The significance of inflammation of the upper respiratory tract (influenza, rhinopneumonitis) in roaring remains unclear. However, inflammation of the larynx and pharynx should be considered, especially when the laryngeal paralysis is bilateral.

Acute recurrent nerve paralysis may theoretically result from strain of the neck musculature (e.g., by strong extension of the head in animals positioned dorsally for surgery), ligation of the carotid artery in esophagotomies, or transection of the nerve in accidental wounds (e.g. wire cuts). The resulting paralysis is immediate. Recurrent nerve paralysis can also occur after periphlebitis in the vicinity of the jugular vein.

Symptoms. The most prominent signs of roaring are an inspiratory sound that occurs as a roar or whistle, during physical exertion. There is also impairment of performance which varies with the degree of respiratory stenosis. This is especially marked in racehorses. In the early stages of the disease a faint whistle is heard that is similar to the sound made by blowing into an open bottle. As the disease progresses, the noise becomes more intense and assumes a 'roaring' quality more like the sound of a crosscut saw. In the early stages of the condition the noise is evident only during periods of maximal exertion and subsides quickly after a short rest. In the late stages the sounds are audible even during light trotting and persist for some time after strenuous exercise. The sagging of the arytenoid cartilage into the laryngeal lumen and the medial shift of the vocal cord significantly reduce the air flow to the lungs. The animal's working capacity is diminished, and inspiratory dyspnea dominates the clinical picture if the animal is forced to exercise. Affected horses lose their normal 'voice' due to the vocal cord paralysis.

Differential Diagnosis. Abnormal respiratory noises in the horse can have numerous causes. Inspiratory noises are frequently heard when working untrained horses or horses that have been out of training for a prolonged period of time. These noises disappear once the animal has become accustomed to the training regimen. Sometimes abnormal sounds will also occur when a horse gets its tongue over the bit and the reins are tightened. These disappear when the reins are slackened, and the problem can be remedied by changing the bit. Retraction of the tongue can also partially obstruct the pharyngeal airway and produce stenotic sounds. As a rule, however, abnormal respiratory sounds are caused by changes that obstruct the airway.

An asymmetrical air flow through the nostrils signifies an intranasal obstruction. Abnormal resistance to the passage of a nasogastric tube may be considered proof of this. The causative lesions, usually unilateral, may be tumors, maxillary retention cysts or sinus empyema. A thickened septum can obstruct one or both nasal passages. The abnormal sounds disappear when the affected passage is occluded, e.g., by holding the nostril closed. Inspiratory stenosis can result from paralysis of the muscles that dilate the nose associated with facial paralysis. Stenotic sounds can also accompany inflammatory processes in the pharynx and larynx, but these lesions are very often infectious in nature and so may be accompanied by fever and swelling of the lymph nodes of the head and neck region. Often the noises are present even at rest and are equally audible during inspiration and expiration; they disappear when the primary disorder is cured. Epiglottic cysts can produce a sound very similar to laryngeal whistling. They may be excluded by laryngoscopic examination.

Dorsal displacement of the soft palate leads to spontaneous, acute dyspnea during maximal exertion. Affected horses pull up suddenly when running and appear to choke. Trainers call this 'swallowing the tongue'. The noise that is typical of this disease occurs mainly during exhalation.

Tympanites of one or both guttural pouches, characterized by swelling in the parotid region, can lead to pharyngeal obstruction and stenotic sounds.

Tracheal obstruction due to tumors, deformation of the trachea secondary to old injuries, exuberant granulation tissue in poorly healing tracheotomy or ventriculectomy wounds, are additional causes of stenotic inspiratory and expiratory sounds.

Diagnosis. The basis for surgical intervention is an accurate diagnosis. The typical sound of laryngeal hemiplegia is a whistling inspiratory sound that occurs when air is forced through the constricted larynx, causing the edge of the paralyzed vocal cord that projects into the lumen to vibrate. Hence, the noise is audible only during exertion sufficient to cause forced respiration.

The following questions should be answered when the history is taken:

- When were the symptoms first noticed?
- Have the symptoms increased since then?
- Do they affect the horse's performance?
- Is the horse in regular training (degree of fitness)?
- Is the horse's whinny or neigh altered?

The examination begins with the patient at rest. A routine clinical examination is followed by a detailed examination of the head and neck. If there is a left-sided

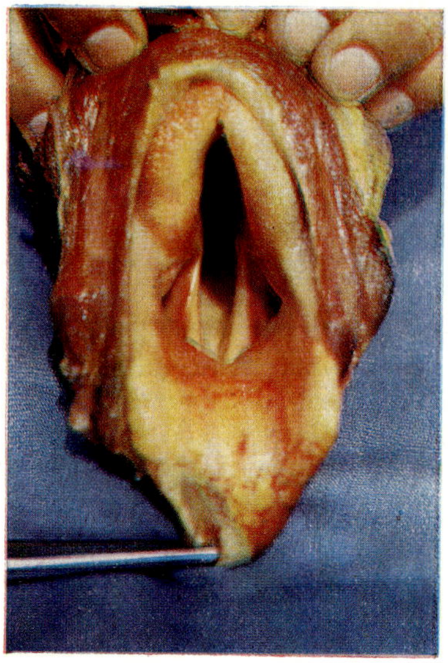

Fig. 2.1.4. — 6. Endoscopic appearance of laryngeal hemiplegia: sagging of the left arytenoid cartilage, paralysis of the left vocal cord.

atrophy of the intrinsic laryngeal muscles, the asymmetry between the right and left sides will be noted on simultaneous palpation. The muscular atrophy is recognized by a protrusion of the muscular process of the left arytenoid cartilage. The process normally lies below the cricoarytenoideus dorsalis muscle and is not palpable. If this finding is positive, the depression test may be tried. For this, the examiner stands in front of the horse with the animal's chin resting on his shoulder. With 1 or 2 fingers he presses the muscular process of the arytenoid cartilage in a cranioventromedial direction, while gently supporting the opposite side with the other hand. In left laryngeal hemiplegia an inspiratory noise can be produced with very little force. Horses may be tested by frightening them. Affected animals will emit a distinctive grunting sound (grunt to the stick test).

Next, the horse is examined during exercise. As a rule, lunging is insufficient for this purpose. The horse is ridden in a circle, and the examiner stands at the center. Affected horses will usually show abnormal respiratory sounds when galloped at an appropriate speed. It is difficult to determine when an exercising horse is inhaling and exhaling. During inhalation the nostrils are dilated.

At the canter, the respiratory excursions are synchronized with the movements of the limbs. The horse exhales when the forelimbs strike the ground and the rider drops into the saddle.

If the examination fails to yield the desired result, the horse is galloped in a tight circle in opposite directions. In left laryngeal hemiplegia the inspiratory sound will increase when the animal is ridden to the left. A healthy horse makes little or no sound during inhalation, and if a sound is present it is decidedly weaker than the expiratory sound. If the inspiratory sound is louder than the expiratory sound and is audible more than 100 m away, it is abnormal.

To correctly assess the degree of dyspnea, it is important to know whether the horse willingly maintains or increases the pace, and whether it preserves the normal gallop rhythm. In the canter the 'beat' of the limb movements determines the respiratory rhythm. The respiration rate cannot be increased independently of the limb movements. Hence, the dyspneic horse has difficulty in maintaining a normal gallop rhythm.

After the cantering test is complete, the examiner can again hold his ear to the animal's nostrils to determine whether a louder inspiratory sound is present.

Laryngoscopy. A definitive diagnosis of laryngeal hemiplegia is made by endoscopy. Frequently the laryngoscopic findings are unmistakable. The instrument should have a 60° viewing angle so that the arytenoid cartilage and vocal cords can be simultaneously inspected. The endoscopic appearance of laryngeal hemiplegia is characterized by a triad of findings: the rima glottidis is asymmetric, the vocal cord on the affected side appears shortened or set at a steep angle, and the arytenoid cartilage sags into the laryngeal lumen (fig. 2.1.4. — 6).

During inspiration the larynx is widely patent, and during expiration the rima glottidis is closed. The diagnosis of roaring relies not so much on the asymmetry of the rima glottidis (though this is typically present in well-developed cases) as on the *movement* of the arytenoid cartilage. If the left arytenoid cartilage fails to abduct normally during inspiration, laryngeal hemiplegia is present. Occasionally even healthy horses are observed to inhale and exhale through a half-open rima glottidis without moving the larynx. It may be difficult in such cases to decide whether hemiplegia is present. An attempt may be made to elicit laryngeal movements by applying a blanket strap tightly over the ribs. Often this will cause the horse to increase its respiratory effort, accompanied by movements of the larynx. If the respiratory rate at rest is 8—12 breaths/min, the rate at the canter will increase to 120—150 breaths/min. After exercise the respiratory rate is still about 50 breaths/min, and the asymmetry is much more obvious than before exercise. Left-sided hemiplegia is better recognized by endoscopy through the right nasal passage. Mild or early hemiplegia is evidenced only by a *delayed* abduction of the arytenoid cartilage' frequently associated with fluttering of the vocal cord.

Bilateral paralyses show a narrow rima glottidis which opens little or not at all when the animal inspires.

Treatment. Injuries due to stretching and contusions of the nerve itself take from several days to 4 or 5 months to heal, depending on the severity of the damage and assuming that the trauma does not recur.

The final, irreversible paralysis must be treated by surgical means. There are three main procedures available: permanent tracheostomy, ventriculectomy (as modified by Günther and Williams) and laryngoplasty [Marks, 1970].

The *permanent tracheostomy* restores the horse to temporary usefulness by establishing a patent airway. The previous loss of work capactiy is immediately relieved. The operation is done under infiltration anesthesia with the animal standing; mild sedation is also necessary in some horses. The disadvantages of this treatment are the need for changing and cleaning the tracheal tubes, granuloma formation at the tracheotomy site, and finally the fact that the surgery permanently 'brands' the horse as a roarer!

The *ventriculectomy* is an attempt to eliminate the mechanical obstruction in the larynx and thus improve respiratory stenosis. The operation is done under local anesthesia with the horse standing or with the animal anesthetized and recumbent. The operation may be facilitated by first performing a temporary tracheotomy although many surgeons prefer not to. The ventriculectomy involves removal of the mucous membrane of the left laryngeal and/or right saccule. The subsequent scar formation adheres the inner wall of the saccule, including the vocal cord to the lateral laryngeal wall. Some surgeons feel that unless a temporary tracheotomy is done, there is a danger of choking postoperatively due to aspiration of the edges of the skin wound into the larynx. Such a complication would require immediate wound retraction or an emergency tracheotomy. Problems associated with laryngeal edema, which may develop during the first postoperative days, are also theoretically prevented by an early tracheotomy. One possible complication of the ventriculectomy is ossifying chondritis of the laryngeal cartilages, causing the larynx to become hard and inelastic. A ventriculectomy in the early stage of recurrent nerve paralysis, before the onset of muscular atrophy, cannot arrest the progress of the disease and prevent sagging of the arytenoid cartilage, and so recurrences are possible some time after the operation.

Laryngoplasty. Essentially, laryngoplasty involves the fixation of the paralyzed arytenoid cartilage in an abducted position. Combined with the ventriculectomy, laryngoplasty is considered the procedure of choice. At present it is the most successful method for relieving the respiratory stenosis of laryngeal hemiplegia. The operation is performed under general anesthesia in the recumbent animal. For a complete restoration of the laryngeal lumen, the arytenoid cartilage is fixed in the maximum inspiratory (i.e., dorsolateral) position.

The inspiratory function is replaced with a prosthesis which draws the muscular process of the arytenoid cartilage caudally and laterally. The arytenoid cartilage can be stabilized with any nonabsorbable suture material, preferably used double-strength. The horse is placed in lateral recumbency with the head and neck extended. A 10-cm skin incision is made dorsal and parallel to the jugular and external maxillary veins, from the cranial border of the larynx to the level of the 2nd tracheal ring. Further exposure is achieved bluntly in order to spare the main cervical nerve branches, the thyroid gland, the esophagus, the thyrolaryngeal artery and vein, and the glossopharyngeal nerve branches supplying the laryngeal muscles. Some surgeons use a more ventral approach, incising ventral to the linguofacial vein. The omohyoideus muscle is retracted ventrally and the linguofacial vein dorsally. The caudal border of the cricoid lamina and the muscular process of the arytenoid cartilage are exposed below the fascia between the crico- and thyropharyngeus muscles. The muscular process of the arytenoid cartilage is anchored to the caudal border of the cricoid with a nonabsorbable suture. Another approach used by some surgeons is 2 separate 10-cm incisions — one cranial incision dorsal to the external maxillary vein before its bifurcation, and one caudal incision ventral to the jugular vein.

Following the laryngoplasty the ventriculectomy then is done with the horse in dorsal recumbency. A Lycra® prosthesis has been used successfully in many countries although any nonabsorbable suture is usually satisfactory. The exact inspiratory position of the arytenoid cartilage is checked intraoperatively with a laryngoscope.

Prognosis. The operation has a success rate of 80—90 %. With ventriculectomy alone, the animal must be rested 8 weeks postoperatively to allow definitive fusion of the laryngeal saccule with the side wall.

Following a laryngoplasty, the animal requires 4—6 weeks of stall rest. Follow-up endoscopic examinations are made during this period. If no pharyngitis or edema is noted, the horse may be gradually returned to training. If the prosthesis is tied too tightly, coughing may occur due to deficient glottis closure and food aspiration. Such symptoms rarely persist for more than 3 weeks postoperatively.

2.1.4.3.8. Diseases of the Guttural Pouch

The guttural pouches are air-filled, ciliary epithelium-lined diverticula of the auditory tubes which communicate between the tympanic membrane and the pharynx. They develop in the foal during the first 2 months of life. Each has a volume of

300—500 ml. The hyoid bone divides each pouch into a lateral and medial compartment. The lateral compartment is covered by a 10-mm-thick layer of parotid glandular tissue and by the outer skin. The medial compartment is closely adjacent to the wall of the nasopharynx. The regional lymph nodes are the medial retropharyngeal. In the horse the slit-like opening of the auditory tube is surrounded by tubal cartilage, which simultaneously forms a flap. The guttural pouch may suffer from inflammation transmited from the pharyngeal cavity, although purulent inflammation secondary to pharyngitis is rare in the horse because of the valve like nature of the flap.

Tympany of the Guttural Pouch

Definition. Tympany of the guttural pouch is an abnormal accumulation of air causing a balloon-like distention of the guttural pouch.

Occurrence. Guttural pouch tympany is a relatively rare disease. It can occur in horses of all age groups. Foals occasionally suffer from inflammatory guttural pouch tympanites caused by the entry of air and milk into the guttural pouches during suckling. Concretions then form through fermentation of the milk and coagulation, and a high-grade mucosal inflammation develops.

Symptoms. Tympanic distention of the guttural pouch causes a massive swelling of the parotid region. If the pouch is severely distended, the lateral pharyngeal walls bulge into the pharynx and interfere with respiration and deglutition. The dyspnea resulting from the severe pharyngeal stenosis is most pronounced during inspiration.

Etiology. A congenital malformation of the auditory tube (plication, stricture) can allow the entry of atmospheric air into the pouch. Rarely gas can form within the pouch as a result of inflammations due to gas-forming bacteria.

Diagnosis. Percussion of the swollen parotid region elicits a ringing tympanitic sound. The resonance is considered pathognomonic of guttural pouch tympany. On needle aspiration, air or gas escapes from the area of enlargement.

Treatment. As a rule, only surgical treatment yields a satisfactory result. It may be done under general anesthesia or under infiltration anesthesia with the animal standing and sedated. The tympanic pouch is opened with a 10- to 12-cm incision. The pouch is freed from any adhesions with the subcutaneous tissue. Folds in the auditory tube are excised. Another more satisfactory method to relieve tympanites is to create a fistula in the medial septum between the two pouches, allowing the 'abnormal' pouch to empty via the good pouch. After irrigation with 3 % hydrogen peroxide solution or with another antiseptic, the pouch is packed. Prophylactic antibiotics are given for 6 to 9 days. About 30 days are needed for full recovery.

Inflammation of the Guttural Pouch

Definition. Guttural pouch inflammation is an acute or chronic, insidious condition of the guttural pouch mucosa. Inflammatory products may accumulate owing to the anatomic peculiarities of the pouches. A specific form of the disease is guttural pouch empyema, in which there is an accumulation of mucopurulent material (see below).

Symptoms. The symptoms of the precipitating disease may be evident. If the guttural pouch inflammation is secondary in nature, it will take some time for obvious specific signs to develop.

A frequent sign is dysphagia. The head is held extended during deglutition, and the frequent swallowing is accompanied by a reflex cough. There may also be frequent regurgitation if swallowing is painful. Dysphagia is especially marked during drinking, and much of the water is regurgitated through the nostrils. When the head is lowered a mucoid (yellow-green) or more purulent (gray or yellow-gray) exudate drains from the nostril on the affected side. Compression of the guttural pouch during chewing, swallowing or head flexion increases the rate of discharge. If the pouch contents become inspissated, dry, condensed masses (chondroids) also appear in the discharge.

The affected guttural pouch causes the upper parotid region to bulge in the angle between the caudal border of the mandible and the cervical vertebrae. On palpation the swelling can be displaced toward the opposite side. Manual compression of the guttural pouch may intensify the discharge.

In acute cases the affected pouch is tender to pressure, and there may be swelling due to cellulitis of the surrounding area. Swelling and possible abscessation of the intermandibular lymph nodes are a sign of coexisting pharyngitis.

Etiology. Occasionally inflammation of the guttural pouch is a primary condition caused, for example, by trauma or by the irritating action of foreign bodies that have entered the pouch from the outside or from the pharynx (including food particles).

In most cases, however, guttural pouch inflammation is a secondary manifestation of a more generalized upper respiratory infection such as rhinitis, pharyngitis or strangles, with pathogenic organisms gaining entry to the guttural pouches from the pharynx. In most cases the guttural pouch infection is advanced before external signs appear, for the pharyngeal openings are situated such that exudate is discharged only if it is present in large amounts and the head is lowered.

Diagnosis. Pronounced local symptoms provide sufficient evidence for a presumptive diagnosis of guttural pouch inflammation. Endoscopy enables a definitive diagnosis to be made.

On endoscopy of the pharynx, the guttural pouch is seen to protrude caudally and obscure the arytenoid cartilages. The epiglottis is partially obscured also and there is constriction of the pharynx. Often exudate is found draining from the pharyngeal orifice. The exudation increases when the head is lowered or on manual compression of the guttural pouch. If blood appears beneath the cartilage flap, endoscopy is not advised due to the risk of a fatal hemorrhage.

In *acute cases* with low-grade mucosal inflammation, the network of blood vessels appears abnormally prominent in the edematous, translucent mucous membrane. The vessels are especially prominent on the medial guttural pouch wall. With more severe inflammation the vascular pattern becomes indistinct. The mucosa is diffusely erythematous, edematous, and has a thickened contour. Strands or pools of mucopurulent material are seen in the deepest posterior regions of the medial compartment of the pouch.

Equine rhinopneumonitis may produce typical changes in the guttural pouch mucosa which allow a relatively certain diagnosis.

In the *acute stage* pinhead-size vesicles or nodules appear in the mucosa.

As the disease progresses, mucosal thickenings develop, and the entire mucosal surface becomes nodulated. The changes are most apparent on the medial pouch wall, but in severe cases and in foals they can be demonstrated over the entire guttural pouch mucosa.

Strangles and similar streptococcal diseases lead to purulent inflammation. The regional lymph nodes (e.g., the lateral retropharyngeal) are very often involved. With swelling and abscessation, the posterior ventral recess of the medial compartment of the pouch is distorted. In some cases abscessation of the lymph node is evidenced by the appearance of red-bordered foci in the guttural pouch mucosa that exude pus. The guttural pouch fills with purulent exudate that produces an *intermittent* nasal discharge. If the pus cannot escape from the pouch due to a blockage of the pharyngeal orifice, a typical guttural pouch empyema develops. Accumulated longstanding pus may become inspissated, forming concretions that are associated with chronic mucosal inflammation (chondroids).

Radiography is useful in revealing fluid accumulations and concretions and in excluding hyoid bone fractures.

Complications of guttural pouch catarrh include laryngeal stenoses caused by displacement of the arytenoid cartilage. The occurrence of dysphagia early in the disease can lead to aspiration pneumonia. Necrosis of the guttural pouch wall can cause vascular erosions with consequent hemorrhage.

Treatment. The main therapeutic effort is directed toward the primary disorder. The drainage of exudate is promoted, and the chance for a spontaneous recovery improved, by feeding and watering the animal on the ground, depressing the head several times daily, and applying pressure to the guttural pouch region.

As long as temperature elevations and local inflammatory reactions persist, warm, moist compresses should be applied. Later the use of rubefacient ointments (e.g., camphor liniment), salicylic acid ointment, ichthammol ointment or various iodinated preparations is recommended. Irrigations of the guttural pouch will hasten the drainage of secretions. The use of antiseptic and anti-inflammatory solutions is also beneficial. A guttural pouch catheter (catheter of Gratzl) is introduced into the pouch with the aid of an endoscope passing the catheter through the ventral meatus into the pharyngeal auditory orifice. Mild non-irritating sulfonamides, antibiotics or antiseptics may be applied in spray form.

If the contents of the guttural pouch cannot be removed through the tubal orifice, surgical incision of the pouch is indicated. After removal of the pathologic material, the pouch is flushed daily with a 3% hydrogen peroxide solution or another mild antiseptic.

Prognosis. The sooner treatment is instituted, the better the prognosis. With prompt, thorough, intensive treatment, even severe cases have a good prospect for recovery.

Empyema of the Guttural Pouch

Definition. Guttural pouch empyema is an accumulation of pus within the pouch cavity. It is not synonymous with purulent guttural pouch inflammation, for in empyema there is invariably a retention and accumulation of pus in the guttural pouch. Pus may or may not be present in inflammation alone.

Symptoms. In the acute stage the symptoms are identical to those of inflammation of the guttural pouch. Even in longer-standing cases the general health is not impaired. The typical intermittent nasal discharge is not observed if there is blockage of the pharyngeal auditory orifice.

Etiology. Guttural pouch empyema has the same causes as inflammation. In addition, there may be a severe obstruction to drainage which promotes the accumulation of pus in the guttural pouch. Empyemas can also result from the breakthrough of lateral retropharyngeal node abscesses into the pouch.

Diagnosis. Local swellings in the parotid region, a recurrent purulent nasal discharge on the affected side when the head is lowered, and drainage of pus from the ipsilateral nostril on compression of the distended pouch are characteristic of empyema. On endoscopy the affected guttural pouch is seen to protrude into the pharynx. With excessive pus accumulation the larynx may be completely obscured, and sometimes only the epiglottis is visible. Occasionally the cartilage flap at its orifice is swollen and the entrance to the auditory tube is occluded, thereby preventing the escape of pus. If it is possible to pass the laryngoscope into the guttural pouch, it is immediately soiled by pus. If the scope is cleaned and reinserted, pus will be seen escaping below the cartilage flap. If the pus has become inspissated, empyema can be diagnosed only by direct endoscopy of the pouch cavity. The mucous membrane is red and swollen and partially coated with yellowish-white pus.

Treatment. Treatment follows the general guidelines for treating guttural pouch diseases. Main attention is devoted to the causal primary disorder and to cleaning the guttural pouches by flushing them with antiseptic solutions. Anti-inflammatory and antibiotic solutions can hasten recovery. If the adhesions below the cartilage flap cannot be freed, surgical treatment is recommended, including drainage through Viborg's triangle.

Chondroids of the Guttural Pouch

Definition. Occasionally pus in the guttural pouch becomes inspissated to form smooth, spherical concretions called 'chondroids' or guttural pouch stones.

Symptoms. Acute inflammatory manifestations are absent. The guttural pouch protrudes between the caudal border of the mandibular ramus and the cervical vertebrae, forming a swelling that often feels soft. The chondroids are difficult to identify by palpation. They appear as round, patchy masses on the radiograph. A nasal discharge may or may not be present.

Etiology. The chondroids form gradually from exfoliated epithelial cells, blood, inflammatory products and necrotic tissue. They are molded into their spherical shape by movements of the guttural pouch.

The liquid contents are absorbed by the mucosa, leaving mainly the dried out material behind. The pouch may then contain spherical chondroids coated with a thick mucoid film, or inspissated exudate masses that have a friable, cheesy consistency. In either case the mucosa of the guttural pouch undergoes a reactive thickening.

Diagnosis. The diagnosis is established either by endoscopy or by surgical exploration.

Treatment. If chondroids are present, surgery is indicated. An approach through Viborg's triangle is the method of choice.

After removal of the chondroids, the pouch is flushed daily with antiseptic solutions until the secretions are gone. The wound may need regular draining and packing. Thickenings of the wall and dilatation of the guttural pouch may be difficult to correct. An alternative to a protracted convalescence may be to create a permanent fistula by suturing the guttural pouch mucosa to the skin (marsupialization). The pouch can then be irrigated with astringent or mild liquids. Several weeks or even months will be needed for healing.

Tumors of the Guttural Pouch

Tumors of the guttural pouch are rare. Usually they spread to the guttural pouch from surrounding tissues. Most guttural pouch tumors are carcinomas. Melanosarcomas arising from the parotid gland or a guttural pouch lymph node can occur in gray horses. The prognosis is unfavorable, because anatomic structures generally prohibit a radical excision.

Mycosis of the Guttural Gouch

Definition. Guttural pouch mycosis is an inflammation of the guttural pouch mucosa caused by various types of fungi. The gross and microscopic lesions suggest a necrosis, which may spread to involve major blood vessels.

Occurrence. Guttural pouch mycosis is a disease of stabled horses that occurs almost exclusively during the warm months. No age dependence or breed predisposition is apparent. Both sexes are equally susceptible. The first symptoms appear in late spring and early summer. According to Cook [1968] cases are observed sporadically from April through August.

Etiology. When the history is taken there are unlikely to be common factors suggesting a cause. Various types of fungi have been demonstrated in the guttural pouches of affected horses, including *Corallium (Paecilomyces)*, *Acaulium (Scopulariopsis)*, *Penicillium* and *Aspergillus (Aspergillus fumigatus* and *Aspergillus nidulans)*. The fungi or mycelia gain entry to the guttural pouch through the pharyngeal opening of the auditory tube. With each breath small amounts of respiratory air enter the guttural pouches, and it is assumed that the fungal organisms or spores gain entry by this route. They are demonstrated relatively frequently in washings from healthy guttural pouches. The mycotic findings are apparently dependent on contamination of feeds and on stable-specific conditions. The risk of mycotic infection increases with exogenous factors. Little is known about the circumstances which promote the manifestation of a mycosis in the guttural pouches. Traumatic causes have been suggested. Both microtraumata with damage to the relatively thin mucosa at bony prominences of the tympanic bulla and exogenous influences are assumed. Cook feels that an aneurysm of the arteries in the guttural pouch may be the initiating cause.

Symptoms. The cardinal symptoms are epistaxis and pain on deglutition. However, these may coexist with other clinical signs such as parotid pain, abnormal respiratory sounds, abnormal carriage of the head, sweating and shivering, nasal catarrh, ocular defects and miosis, head-shyness, facial paralysis and colicky symptoms.

Epistaxis, most often unilateral, occurs at rest without apparent cause. All degrees of severity are observed from a slow drip to a profuse flow. The hemorrhages recur at intervals of 24 hours to several weeks. Dysphagia develops suddenly. The horse coughs when feeding and has difficulty drinking, some of the water being regurgitated through the nostrils. Emaciation may develop. Guttural pouch mycosis must be differentiated from pharyngitis and from paralysis of the pharyngeal nerves and the associated muscular atrophy.

Tenderness to pressure is noted in the area of the affected pouch. Pain is also evident on sudden turns of the head.

Affected horses stand with the head extended or lower than normal. This is also possible in pharyngitis and with local atlanto-occipital joint pain.

A unilateral mucoid or mucopurulent nasal discharge is usually present.

Left-sided guttural pouch mycoses are occasionally associated with left-sided laryngeal hemiplegia. In these cases atrophy of the cricoarytenoideus dorsalis muscle can be demonstrated.

Diffuse corneal opacities, photophobia and lacrimation, as well as colicky symptoms and sweating, are associated with sympathetic nervous system disorders (i.e. Horner's syndrome).

Differential Diagnosis. Epistaxis, dysphagia, nasal catarrh and parotid swelling are seen in a number of other diseases. For example, epistaxis, both unilateral and bilateral, occurs in pulmonary hemorrhage, in hemorrhages from the pharynx and nasal cavity due to ruptures of smaller vessels during racing or training, in turbinate necrosis, ethmoid hematoma and neoplasms of the pharynx and guttural pouch.

Dysphagia is a symptom of:

— hyoid bone fractures, marked by nasal discharge, parotid pain and painful swelling of the throat;

— abscesses of the retropharyngeal lymph nodes which penetrate the guttural pouch;
— cleft palate, which can allow soft feeds to leak from the nostrils; deglutition is accompanied by coughing.

Swellings of the parotid region are found in fractures of the great cornu of the hyoid bone, guttural pouch empyema, guttural pouch tympany, jugular vein thrombophlebitis and parotid melanomas, and intermittent epistaxis is present if there is breakthrough into the guttural pouch.

Diagnosis. It is made on the basis of clinical symptoms and endoscopic findings. If diphtheritic membranes are present, diagnosis is relatively simple. They occur as yellow-brown or mottled dry masses mainly on the roof of the medial compartment of the guttural pouch and are clearly delineated from surrounding tissues. The vascular erosions caused by the fungal colonies lead to frequent hemorrhages, which may be mixed with a purulent discharge.

If diphtheroid membranes are absent and only scars are present, diagnosis is difficult. If characteristic symptoms are present and endoscopic findings are negative, surgical exploration may offer the only means of reaching a definitive diagnosis.

Treatment. To avoid vascular damage and the often fatal hemorrhages that follow, treatment should be instituted without delay. Treatment consists in a course of systemic antifungal drugs and irrigation of the infected pouch. If results are unsatisfactory, surgical exposure and local treatment with antimycotic agents is indicated. Arterial ligatures are often neccessary in such cases. Owen and McKelvey [1975] recommend ligation of the internal carotid artery.

References

Bolz, W.; Dietz, O.; Schleiter, H.; Teuscher, R.: Lehrbuch der speziellen Veterinärchirurgie. Bd. I (VEB Gustav Fischer Verlag, Jena 1975).

Cook, W. R.: Diagnosis of respiratory unsoundness in the horse. Vet. Rec. *77:* 516 (1965).

Cook, W. R.: The clinical features of guttural pouch mycosis in the horse. Vet. Rec. *83:* 336 (1968).

Cook, W. R.: The pathology and aetiology of guttural pouch mycosis in the horse. Vet. Rec. *83:* 422 (1968).

Cook, W. R.: Procedure and technique for endoscopy of the equine respiratory tract and Eustachian tube diverticulum. Equine vet. J. *2:* 4, 137 (1970).

Damonte, F. F.: Combination of steroids, antibiotics and proteolytic enzymes in the treatment of laryngitis in the race-horses. Gac. vet. (Buenos Aires) *31:* 316 (1969).

Dietz, O.; Schaetz, F.; Schleiter, H.; Teuscher, R.: Operationen bei Gross- und Kleintieren, 2. Aufl. (S. Hirzel-Verlag, Leipzig 1980).

Dornblaser, J. H.: Some observations on roaring in horses. Vet. Med. and Small Animal Clinician *62:* 629 (1967).

Eickmeier, H.: Chronische follikuläre Laryngitis und Hauptmangel Kehlkopfpfeifen. Berliner Münchener tierärztl. Wschr. *89:* 174 (1976).

Garuffi, R.: Asportazione delle corde vocali negli equini. Nuova Vet. *44:* 39 (1968).

Huskamp, B., Böckenhoff, G.: Ergebnisse der Kehlkopfpfeiferoperation nach Marks. Prakt. Tierarzt *59:* 302 (1978).

Johnson, J. H.: Laryngoplasty for advanced laryngeal hemiplegia. Vet. Med. and Small Animal Clinician *65:* 347 (1970).

Johnson, J. H.; Johnson, D. W.: Granulomas associated with Micronema deletrix in the maxilla of a horse. J. Amer. vet. med. Assoc. *149:* 155 (1966).

Lemonier, J.-P.: La rhino-laryngoscopy chez le cheval de sport. Techn. photograph. (1973). Impr. Chastrusse.

Mackay-Smith, M. P.; Johnson, J. H.; Baker, R. H.: Laryngoplasty — A progress report. Proc. 29th Annu. Conv. Amer. Assoc. Equine Pract., p. 133 (1973).

Mahaffey, L.: Respiratory conditions in horses. Vet. Rec. *74:* 1295 (1962).

Marks, D.; Mackay-Smith, M. P.; Cushing, L. S.; Leslie, J. A.: Use of a prosthetic device for surgical correction of laryngeal hemiplegia in horses. J. Amer. vet. med. Assoc. *157:* 157 (1970).

Marks, D.; Mackay-Smith, M. P.; Cushing, L. S.; Leslie, J. A.: Observations on laryngeal hemiplegia in the horse and treatment by abductor muscle prothesis. Equine vet. J. *2:* 159 (1970).

Marks, D.; Mackay-Smith, M. P.; Cushing, L. S.; Leslie, J. A.: Etiology and diagnosis of laryngeal hemiplegia in horses. J. Amer. vet. med. Assoc. *157:* 429 (1970).

Mason, B. J. E.: Laryngeal hemiplegia. A further look at Haslam's anomaly of the left recurrent nerve. Equine vet. J. *5:* 150 (1973).

Merriam, J. G.: Laryngoplasty — An evaluation of three abductor muscle prothetics. Proc. 19th Annu. Conv. Amer. Assoc. Equine Pract., p. 123 (1973).

Monradi, R. J.: Practise tips pauel (Laryngeal ventriculectomy). 11th Annu. Proc. Amer. Assoc. Equine Pract. Conv. (1965). Miami Beach, Florida/USA.

Naumann, J.: Literaturübersicht und eigene Untersuchung zum Kehlkopfpfeifen und seine operative Behandlung. Vet.-med. Dipl.-Arb. Berlin (1973).

Nicke, K.: Zur Kehlkopfpfeiferoperation am Pferd unter Praxisbedingungen. Prakt. Tierarzt *52:* 370 (1972).

Orditge, R. M.: Epiglottic entrapment in the horse. Vet. Rec. *100:* 365 (1977).

Owen, R.; McKelvey, W. A. C.: Ligation of the internal carotid artery to prevent epistaxis due to gutteral pouch mycosis. Vet. Rec. *104:* 5, 100 (1979).

Pouret, E.: Laryngeal ventriculectomy with sticking of the laryngeal sacacles. Proc. 12th Annu. Conv. Amer. Assoc. Equine Pract., p. 207 (1960).

Quinlan, J.; Morton, D. D.: Paralysis of the branches in the N. vagus, N. recurrens, N. pharyngeus, and N. laryngeus cranialis (Palatinum molle) as an aetiological factor in 'whistling' and 'roaring' in horses. J. South African vet. med. Assoc. *28:* 63 (1957).

Quinlan, J.; Reusberg, S. W. J. van; Starke, N. C.: The soft palate (Palatinum molle) as a cause of dyspnoea in the race-horses. J. South. African vet. med. Assoc. *20:* 125 (1949).

Raker, C. W.: Neuste Erkenntnisse in der Behandlung von Erkrankungen der oberen Luftwege. Equitania (1979).

Rauf, G.: Literaturstudie über Ursache, Diagnostik und Behandlung des Kehlkopfpfeifens der Pferde. Vet.-med. Diss., Hannover (1964).

Rooney, J. R.: Laryngeal hemiplegia. Proc. 12th Annu. Conv. Amer. Assoc. Equine Pract. Mod. Vet. Pract. *51:* 1 (1970).

Rooney, J. R.; Delany, F. M.: A hypothesis of the causation of laryngeal hemiplegia in the horse. Equine Vet. J. *2:* 35 (1970).

Salerno, G.: Laryngeal and nasal paralysis in the sporting horse. Atti Soc. Ital. Scienze Vet. *25:* 13 (1971).

Schebitz, H.: Zur Hemiplegia laryngis (Kehlkopfpfeifen) beim Pferd, Untersuchung und Operationsergebnis. Dtsch. tierärztl. Wschr. *72:* 23, 548 (1965).

Speirs, V. C.: Abductor muscle prostheses in the treatment of laryngeal hemiplegia in the horse. Austral. Vet. J. *48:* 251 (1972).

Watt, D. A.: A case of cryptococcal granuloma in the nasal cavity of a horse. Aust. Vet. J. *46:* 493 (1970).

Wheat, J. D.: Tympanitis of the guttural pouch of the horse. J. Amer. vet. med. Assoc. *140:* 453 (1962).

Zeller, R.: Rhino-laryngoskopische Untersuchungen beim Pferd. In: Handlexikon der Tierärztl. Praxis, p. 712c (Medical Book Company, Kopenhagen).

2.1.4.4. Noncontagious Diseases of the Lungs and Pleura

2.1.4.4.1. Pulmonary Emphysema, Chronic Obstructive Bronchitis (COB), Chronic Obstructive Pulmonary Disease (COPD)

Definition. In chronic obstructive pulmonary disease (COPD) the alveoli become overinflated with air, and after expiration the residual air volume is abnormally increased.

Symptoms. A distinction is made between acute and chronic pulmonary emphysema.

Acute emphysema: As a result of acute bronchitis, the expiratory effort is markedly increased and abdominal breathing is accentuated. A weak cough is usually present. The nasal discharge is mucoid to mucopurulent. Auscultation reveals marked crepitation together with moist and dry râles, especially in the apical lobe region. The alveolar lung sound may be accentuated or diminished. On percussion, the edge of the lung field is found to be expanded caudally. The percussion sound is tympanitic. Acute emphysema can develop in a matter of days, particularly if the animal is exercised, despite the presence of a cough.

Chronic bronchitis: Chronic bronchitis develops as a late result of chronic obstructive bronchitis and bronchiolitis. The most obvious clinical sign is a frequent cough, which usually occurs in the morning or when the animal is first exercised. The cough may be exacerbated by a dusty environment or if dusty feed is offered. The nasal discharge is intermittent.

The cough may remain harsh and forceful for some time, but as the disease progresses it becomes softer and in extreme cases is weak. The respiratory rate is slightly elevated even at rest (18—24/min), and there is an increased abdominal effort with an expiratory lift of the abdominal wall. In severe cases the nostrils are widely flared during inspiration, and the rectum protrudes during expiration. At this stage coughing is often accompanied by flatus. The dyspnea can show considerable variation. The animal may suffer severe dyspneic episodes that last for several days and then gradually subside. The auscultatory findings are highly variable. Abnormal sounds, usually in the form of crepitation or dry râles, are heard most frequently over the apical lobes. Often they are detectable over the diaphragmatic lobes during forced respiration. Vesicular sounds may be diminished despite the greater respiratory effort. The abnormal sounds may disappear after repeated coughing; this is not unusual in animals that are examined after being transported. Forced respiration should always be induced during the examination. If auscultatory findings are negative at rest, abnormal sounds may appear following exercise (10-min trot).

Because respiration tends to be rapid but shallow after exercise, and the horse is apt to be anxious, auscultatory findings are often unsatisfactory. A more reliable method is to administer 1 % lobeline by rapid i.v. injection in a dose of 5 to 10 ml depending on the size of the patient. This induces a very deep respiration within $1^1/_2$ to 2 min that lasts for about 2 minutes. Even very mild cases of bronchitis can be reliably detected by this method [Minder, 1977]. The heart rate in emphysema is, at most, slightly elevated, but in well-developed cases the second heart sound is clearly accentuated. Show horses may still be able to jump and do dressage work for 1 to 3 years after contracting the disease. In severe cases, however, the patient is incapable of doing even light work. The animal's nutritional status will show steady deterioration.

Additional Tests. A definitive diagnosis is not difficult in well-developed cases. In other cases, especially if pulmonary distention is not yet marked, it is often difficult to make a diagnosis from the clinical examination alone, and additional tests may be warranted. The red blood cell count may be determined before and after exercise, but an observed increase can have numerous causes [GERBER, 1969]. Another method is the measurement of intrapleural pressure (normal insp. pressure 1.34 kPa[1], normal exp. pressure 0.33 kPa). With reduced elasticity or obstruction of the airways, the expiratory pressure may rise to 1.47 kPa [SASSE]. Pulmonary function can also be tested by helium washout and wash-in studies [SPÖRRI; SASSE]. These are techniques suitable only for especially equipped clinics. Finally, the pCO_2 and pO_2 of whole arterial blood can be measured. Based on our experience, we believe this method to be the most suitable. Arterial blood is easily collected from the temporal artery (normal resting value 12.7—13.3 kPa, post-exercise value 11.3 kPa; SASSE). Resting values below 12.0 kPa denote a deficiency of gaseous exchange. Bronchoscopy can be used to assess the nature and quantity of the mucus.

Pathogenesis. Pulmonary emphysema is an alveolar defect that results from chronic bronchitis and/or bronchiolitis. The accumulation of exudates in the bronchioles and inflammatory swelling of the bronchial mucosa lead to narrowing of the bronchial passages. During active inspiration the bronchi are dilated and so air can still enter the alveoli. During expiration the bronchi are constricted, and evacuation of the alveoli is hindered (COB; SASSE). The residual volume in the alveoli increases, and the alveoli become progressively overdistended. This is accompanied by a stretching and consequent narrowing of the pulmonary capillaries. The attendant rise of resistance in the pulmonary capillary space is compensated by an increase in the work of the right ventricle (accentuated 2nd heart sound). As alveolar distention increases, the alveolar septae may rupture, thereby reducing the area available for gaseous exchange. At the same time, degenerative changes develop in the overstretched elastic fibers. The obstruction to air outflow caused by the exudate, combined with the failure of passive contraction due to the loss of alveolar elasticity, makes air removal difficult from the emphysematous lung. To compensate, the animal must breathe with an increased abdominal effort, and a characteristic 'heave line' appears. It has been speculated that plant and fungal allergens may cause spasm of the bronchioles, but their etiologic significance remains unclear. The favorable response to β-receptor stimulators (epinephrine, isoprenaline) or vagal nerve blockers (atropine) points to increased spasm of the bronchi, and an allergic etiology. The response to adrenocortical prepations (prednisolone), which exert both an anti-inflammatory and anti-allergic action, suggests that an allergic component is present. Because the exudate in the bronchioles consists mostly of viscous mucus, it is difficult or impossible to expel. A vicious cycle develops which finally turns the patient into a respiratory cripple. If anatomic changes are already present in the alveoli (septal tears), a complete recovery is no longer possible.

Prognosis. The prognosis is usually unfavorable in well-developed cases. Symptomatic relief can be achieved with suitable measures, but full recovery cannot be expected.

Differential Diagnosis. Laryngitis and tracheitis occur mainly following viral infections (e.g. Herpes virus). Coughing is easily elicited by squeezing the larynx. Auscultation reveals no abnormal lung sounds, even during forced respiration. The laryngoscope shows lymphoid follicle formation in the pharynx, on arytenoid cartilages and occasionally the epiglottis.

In chronic bronchitis there are no crepitant lung sounds on auscultation, and the blood gas analysis indicates a normal pO_2.

Lesions. The lungs are pale and distended in all regions. They remain distended even when extracted. A crackling sound is heard when the altered lung regions are

1 Conversion: 1 mm H_2O = 9.81 (Pascal); 1 mm Hg = 0.133 kPa.

incised or pressure is applied to the lung. Small amounts of viscous mucus can be expressed from the finer bronchi.

On histologic examination a bronchiolitis is present in most cases. The alveoli are strongly dilated and many alveolar cells are ruptured. A thickened mucosa and exudate are found in the bronchioles. The pulmonary capillaries show marked thinning.

Treatment. Response to glucocorticoids is good in acute cases. However, use should be limited to 3 injections given at 3- to 4-day intervals. Enzyme preparations such as streptokinase may be administered intratracheally in an attempt to liquefy the tenacious exudate. Expectorants can also be beneficial. Antitussive agents (codeine preparations) are indicated only if coughing is persistent. Bronchodilator inhalations (Clenbuterol hydrochloride) also promote expectoration. Overall hygiene is important. Saw dust or shavings should be used for bedding instead of straw. Hay is best replaced with a pelleted ration. Exposure to dust should be minimized. Prolonged pasturing is advantageous in some cases. While these measures cannot reverse the anatomic changes, they can extend the animal's usefulness by 1 to 2 years. Horses with COPD should never be used for heavy work [Larson, 1972]. The treatment recommended by Deegen et al. [1980], consisting of the i.v. infusion of approx. 30 l of isotonic NaCl per 500 kg BW per day at a rate of 10 l/hr/day, appears promising.

Prophylaxis. The best preventive measure is rest.

References

Deegen, E.; Lieske, R.; Fischer, J.: Eine neue Methode der sekrolytischen Therapie bei Pferden mit chronisch obstruktiver Bronchitis. Proc. Dtsch. Vet.-med. Ges., 7. Tag. (1980), 63.

Fellenberg, M.; Minder, H. P.; Wegmann, Ch.; Frei, F.: Lungen-, Sekret- und Blutproteasen-inhibitoren von Pferd und Rind. Eine vergleichende Studie über endogene, prädisponierende Faktoren für chronisch-obstruktive Lungenerkrankungen. Schweiz. Arch. Tierheilk. *121:* 355 (1979).

Gerber, H.: Klinik und Therapie chronischer Lungenleiden beim Pferd. Dtsch. tierärztl. Wschr. *76:* 234 (1969).

Minder, H. P.: Diagnose und Prognostik chronischer Respirationsleiden beim Pferd. Schweiz. Arch. Tierheilk. *119:* 341 (1977).

Larson, V. L.; Sorenden, D. K.: The respiratory system. Equine medicine and surgery, 2nd ed. (Amer. Vet. Public., Wheaton/Ill. 1972).

Spörri, H.; Denac, M.: Lungenfunktionsprüfungen bei Grosstieren. Schweiz. Arch. Tierheilk. *109:* 252 (1967).

Spörri, H.; Leemann, W.: Zur Untersuchung der Lungenmechanik bei Grosstieren. Schweiz. Arch. Tierheilk *106:* 699 (1964).

2.1.4.4.2. Bronchitis

Definition. The disease is based upon inflammatory changes in the bronchial tree. Bronchitis refers to inflammation of the larger bronchi, and bronchiolitis to inflammation of the finer bronchial branches. The disease may take an acute or chronic course.

Symptoms. Acute bronchitis may begin with a dry, painful cough, initially unaccompanied by a nasal discharge. Within a few days the painfulness subsides, the cough becomes moist, and a serous to mucopurulent nasal discharge appears. The temperature may rise as high as 39.8 °C for 3 to 4 days, during which time the patient is lethargic. When the fever passes, the general health and appetite return to normal. The respiratory rate is slightly increased to 18—20/min. Initially dry rales, and later dry and moist rales, are heard over the entire lung. Percussion shows no expansion of the lung field. Acute bronchiolitis should be suspected if the cough and fever are accompanied by a markedly increased inspiratory and expiratory effort. The more extensive the bronchiolitis, the more labored and frequent the breathing, often combined with flaring of the nostrils. The cough is weak and dry, and nasal discharge is scant or absent. Dry rales and crepitation are heard on auscultation; the intensity of vesicular sounds may be increased or diminished. Percussion elicits a tympanitic sound and demonstrates an expanded lung field.

Chronic bronchitis and bronchiolitis may develop from an acute infection that never fully resolved. A cough suddenly recurs in a patient who has apparently recovered from the primary disorder. The coughing may be periodic, occurring only in the morning or when the horse is first exercised, or it may be more or less constant. The nasal discharge may similarly vary from occasional and mucoid to persistent and purulent. The ESR is markedly increased. The blood gases are unchanged in bronchitis, but in moderate to severe bronchiolitis the pO_2 falls below 85 %. Bacteriologic examination of the nasal discharge is generally unproductive, for the specimen is apt to be contaminated with ubiquitous organisms. However, if a specific organism such as *S. zooepidemicus*, *S. equi*, *E. coli*, *Staphylococcus* spp. and *Pseudomonas* is demonstrated, this is interpreted as a positive finding.

Etiology. Initial acute bronchitis or bronchiolitis is most frequently due to infection with A-equi-1 or A-equi-2 type influenza or equid herpesvirus I. Exposure to dust and smoke is of considerably less significance, although such factors cannot be entirely excluded. Cold is of minor importance as a primary cause, though chilling can lower the resistance to infection by non-specific organisms. The long-term inhalation of air contaminated with molds has also been incriminated.

Pathogenesis. Under normal circumstances pathogenic organisms are caught by the bronchial mucosa and destroyed. If defense mechanisms are inadequate, the ciliated epithelium becomes damaged, and the organism penetrates the submucosa and replicates there, causing a submucosal inflammation.

The sensory fibers are stimulated by the inflammation, resulting in a dry, painful cough. As the disease progresses, the inflammation leads to an increased production of bronchial mucus, which is transported cranially both by coughing and by ciliary action, and a nasal discharge results. If the pathogenic organisms succeed in invading the bronchi, the discharge becomes purulent.

If the disease spreads to the bronchioles, these passages become narrowed by secretions and by swelling of the mucosa. This interferes with air flow during both inspiration and expiration, and obstructive bronchitis results (see p. 114). Because the bronchioles are narrower during expiration than inspiration, the residual volume in the lung is increased, and the lung boundary is expanded.

Unless the disease resolves completely, a chronic bronchitis and/or bronchiolitis will develop, often leading to an incurable alveolar emphysema. The role played by allergic reactions in chronic cases is not clearly understood. Molds and plant pollens are potential allergens. Mechanical irritation of the mucosa by dust and an excessive ammonia content of the stable air can also serve to perpetuate a chronic bronchitis.

Differential Diagnosis. Pulmonary edema is rare in the horse. It is most often seen in animals that have been near a fire and have inhaled hot gases. Burns of the haircoat are usually evident. The patients are depressed, and breathing is very labored. Auscultation reveals moist râles over the entire lung, and a frothy, blood-tinged nasal discharge may be present. Occasionally pulmonary edema is observed in acute heart failure following endurance rides. The respiratory rate and effort are greatly increased, moist rales are heard over the lungs, and the pulse is weak and very rapid. In some cases bronchopneumonia is difficult to distinguish from bronchitis if the pneumonic foci are small. Generally, however, affected horses have intermittent fever and general health impairment. Blood studies invariably show a neutrophilia, and anemia may be present.

Prognosis. Bronchitis carries a favorable prognosis, given adequate care and treatment, but the prognosis for bronchiolitis is guarded due to the potential for developing chronic alveolar emphysema, chronic obstructive bronchitis or chronic obstructive pulmonary disease.

Lesions. In acute cases of bronchitis the lung is collapsed, while in bronchiolitis either the entire lung or the apical lobes or margins of the diaphragmatic lobes remain inflated. In addition to the emphysematous regions, circumscribed areas of atelectasis may be present and may be mistaken for pneumonic lesions. The bronchi show red maculae, and the mucous glands are markedly enlarged in places. Increased amount of mucoid or mucopurulent exudate are found in the bronchi. In bronchitis a viscous mucus can be expressed from the bronchioles. In chronic bronchitis there is increased mucus, the bronchial mucosa is thickened by villus-like projections, and mucus-filled areas of bronchiectasis may be noted.

Treatment. The patient is confined, in a dustfree environment (stable hygiene). A racking cough is relieved with codeine preparations or the inhalation of camomile vapors. Secondary infection is treated by the administration of antibiotics or sulfonamides.

In highly purulent bronchitis penicillin and enzyme preparations such as streptokinase are given by intratracheal injection. In chronic cases as well as in acute cases with definite pathologic findings and no nasal discharge, treatment with a combination of expectorants and antitussive agents is recommended.

2.1.4.4.3. Pneumonia

Definition. Pneumonia is an acute or chronic inflammation of the lungs. It may be classified according to cause as bronchopneumonia, interstitial, parasitic or necrotizing pneumonia.

Symptoms. Often pneumonia is preceded by another respiratory disease such as bronchitis or bronchiolitis, but it may also arise during the course of another infection such as strangles or navel infection in foals. In well-developed cases the symptoms are unmistakable. Acutely ill horses appear depressed and show little or no interest in food. Respiration is markedly labored, and there is a weak, moist, painful cough. The temperature is always elevated, often above 40 °C, and the pulse rate is about 50/min. Nasal discharge may or may not be present. Auscultation early in pneumonia reveals moist rales over the ventral third of the thorax, which later change to dry rales. If the pneumona is extensive, bronchial tones are also audible, and a pleural friction rub may be heard in later stages. If the respiratory and heart sounds are muffled, exudative pleuritis should be suspected. Percussion may reveal dullness in the area of the lower thorax after a period of 1 to 2 days. If adequate treatment is instituted within 24 hours after the first symptoms appear, the clinical signs may largely subside in 1 to 4 days. In cases of aspiration pneumonia, on the other hand, improvement is unlikely. There is a noticeable deterioration of condition in such cases. A grayish, sweet-smelling nasal discharge, which may be blood-tinged, appears in 3 to 4 days.

Laboratory Findings. There is always a marked leukocytosis with a left shift, and the ESR is increased.

Etiology. Pneumonia can arise during the course of infections with equi-1 and -2 influenza virus, herpes I, adeno-, rhino- or parainfluenza-3, as well as viral arteritis infections. It is uncertain whether bacterial pneumonias are primary infections or whether they occur secondarily to viral infections. However, it is clear that pulmonary metastases can occur in foals with navel infection; this also applies to *Streptococcus equi*. It is known, that severe pneumonias can develop during the course of severe *E. coli* and Salmonella enteritis, and that the pulmonary infection is caused by the same organisms. *Actinobacillus equi* causes mainly joint and intestinal disease in foals but can also produce severe pneumonia. A massive infestation with ascarid larvae can cause a transitory eosinophilic infiltration of the lung, and purulent pneumonia can result in such cases from secondary bacterial invasion. Aspiration pneumonia can arise duiing a severe tetanus infection or pharyngeal obstruction or may result from the passage of a nasogastric tube into the trachea. The inhalation of hot or highly caustic gases during fires is also a cause of pneumonia in horses. Factors such as preexisting disease, malnutrition and exhaustion can predispose the horse to pneumonia or increase the severity of the infection.

Pathogenesis. Pneumonia is described as lobular if it affects only individual broncho-pulmonary segments, or as lobar if one or more lobes are involved. The extent of the infection apparently depends on the virulence of the causal organism. It is assumed that the infections are introduced chiefly by inhalation and cause a primary bronchiolitis which spreads to involve adjacent lung parenchyma. In pneumonias of metastatic origin, the infection arises by the hematogenous route. In this case, however, pulmonary abscesses are more likely to develop.

The pathogenic organism produces severe inflammation with edema, and the alveoli become filled with exudate. Gaseous exchange is hampered in varying degrees, depending on the extent of the inflammation. The loss of alveoli leads to an increased ventilation of remaining healthy lung areas, and emphysema may develop. Moist râles appear due to inflammatory exudate accumulating in the bronchial tree. If large parts of the lung are involved but the bonchi are still patent, bronchial tones are detected on auscultation. The absence of any sounds over the affected lung regions indicates that the bronchi are completely filled with fibrinous material. This 'fibrinous pneumonia' is usually of the lobar type and often spreads to the pleura, giving rise to an exudative pleuritis. Infection with *Sphaerophorus necrophorus* generally leads to liquefaction of the lung tissue and cavitation. Interstitial pneumonia can arise from any other form, as well as from severe bronchiolitis. Viral pneumonia often begins with peribronchitis. Because of aggregation of histiocytes and plasmocytes, and later fibroblasts and fibrocytes, an induration takes place which results in the loss of functional lung tissue.

Because it is rare for an entire lung half to be involved, shortness of breath is seldom severe at rest. On the other hand, the pulmonary circulation is impaired by the displacement or thrombosis of pulmonary capillaries, a greater load is placed on the heart, tachycardia develops, and the second heart sound is accentuated.

Lesions. The most severe changes are found in the anterior and dependent parts of the lung. Affected lung projects above healthy tissue and may show a reddish-brown or grayish-red to yellow discoloration, depending on the duration of the illness. Dark areas of atelectatic lung devoid of air are also found. The tissue which surrounds the pneumonic areas and still contains air is usually somewhat distended (emphysema). Septic lesions ranging from small suppurative foci to cherry-size abscesses or cavities filled with a caseous material are found, depending on the causal organism. Mucopurulent material is typically found in the smaller bronchi. There is marked interstitial edema, and in chronic cases marked induration due to fibrous tissue is present.

Differential Diagnosis. In bronchiolitis a high fever is present for only 1 to 2 days. Systemic effects are mild, and the cough is initially painful. In dry pleuritis abdominal respiration is predominent, and friction sounds are present. Exudative pleuritis is characterized by a horizontally-limited area of dullness.

Prognosis. If pneumonia is treated within 24 h after initial symptoms appear, a complete recovery is possible. If treatment is delayed the prognosis is doubtful. Aspiration pneumonias always have a very guarded to unfavorable prognosis. In chronic pneumonia the prognosis is equally guarded. Even if the animal recovers, a restoration of full work performance is unlikely.

Treatment. Affected horses should be placed in quarters that are as dust- and draft-free as possible. They should not be exposed to direct sunlight. Antibiotic or sulfonamide therapy is instituted without delay. Penicillin may be given intramuscularly in doses of 10—20 million I.U. Very acute cases respond well to a combination of penicillin and streptomycin, the latter given intramuscularly in a daily dose of 10 mg/kg BW. Tetracyclines are administered in a dose of 4—10 mg/kg BW i.v.

A combination of irimetoprim and sulfadoxine (Duoprim) is also used. It is given in an initial dose of 50 ml i.v. followed by maintenance doses of 20—30 ml i.v., depending on the size of the patient. The intratracheal injection of 1—2 million I.U. penicillin combined with streptokinase in an aqueous solution has also proved effective during the first 4 days. Expectorants may be given to promote the expulsion of exudates. Therapy should be maintained for 2 days after the fever has subsided. Fresh water and palatable feeds should be offered. Fresh, good-quality grass is preferred, and if hay is offered it should be well shaken and free of dust.

References

Catcott, E. Y.; Smithcors, J. F.: Equine medicine and surgery, 2nd ed. (Amer. Vet. Public., Wheaton 1972).

Eikmeier, H.: In: Handlexikon der Tierärztl. Praxis, p. 535e (Medical Book Company, Kopenhagen).

Jubb, K. V. F.; Kenedey, P. C.: Pathology of domestic animals, vol. 1 (Academic Press, New York 1963).

Marek, J.; Manninger, R.; Mócsy, J.: Spezielle Pathologie und Therapie der Haustiere (Gustav Fischer Verlag, Jena 1945).

Potel, K.: Lehrbuch der Pathologischen Physiologie der Haustiere (VEB Gustav Fischer Verlag, Jena 1969).

2.1.4.4.4. Diseases of the Pleural Cavity

Pleuritis (Pleurisy)

Definition. This disease, which is infrequent in the horse, is based on an inflammation of the visceral and/or parietal pleura. Generally both pleural layers are involved.

Symptoms. Pleuritis is suspected if fever, depression and anorexia arise during the course of a pulmonary disorder. The respiratory rate is increased to 40/min. Thoracic breathing is shallow and is restricted in favor of increased abdominal respiration. There is a short, painful cough, the palpebral conjunctivae are markedly congested, and the pulse rate is elevated. On auscultation friction sounds can be heard in the dry form (dry pleuritis). They are most audible during maximal inspiration and at the start of expiration. In the wet form (exudative pleuritis) vesicular sounds are weak or absent in the distal parts of the lung and are accentuated in the dorsal regions. Findings on percussion depend on the type of inflammation present. In dry pleuritis the findings are negative, though tapping of the chest wall is obviously painful and may elicit a cough. With massive fibrinous exudation, circumscribed dull areas may also be present. Fluid accumulation in the pleural space is common in such cases and is evidenced by a dull area with a horizontal border, dorsally.

In exudative pleuritis there is significant impairment of general health, and the border of the dull area rises appreciably within a matter of days. In severe cases there may be increasing distention of the jugular vein, and the heart sounds become faint. Horses with extensive pleuritis are reluctant to lie down. Edema of the ventral thorax and forelimbs may be observed. Suspected exudative pleuritis may be confirmed by thoracocentesis.

Laboratory Findings. There is usually a marked leukocytosis with neutrophilia and a left shift. In acute and massive exudative pleuritis the erythrocyte counts are usually elevated, while in chronic pleuritides a normochronic anemia is observed. The tapped fluid has a total protein content in excess of 3 % and a density greater than 1.016. Neutrophilic leukocytes are found in the sediment. Various organisms may be recovered from the fluid: streptococci, staphylococci, *E. coli* and in foals *Actinobacillus equi*.

Course. A circumscribed dry pleuritis generally resolves completely within 1 to 2 weeks. In exudative pleuritis recovery is possible if severe bacterial infection is not present. Not infrequently, horses with massive exudation die from circulatory failure within 2 to 3 weeks. Chronic pleuritis leads to increasing emaciation and also is fatal within a few weeks.

Etiology. Inflammation of the visceral pleura can develop during the course of a viral or bacterial pneumonia. Pleuritis can also be caused by trauma resulting in rib fractures or chest wall perforations, and by thoracocentesis performed with poor aseptic technique. A massive invasion by ascarid larvae in the young horse also can irritate the visceral pleura and cause a circumscribed dry pleuritis.

Pathogenesis. The pleura consists of a single layer of squamous epithelial cells, the lymphatic vessels forming a dense capillary network near the epithelium. Blood capillaries and nerve fibers are also present. If a pulmonary inflammation develops, it leads to dilatation of the subserous vessels with edema formation and the entry of fluid into the pleural space. Initially the exudate is resorbed, but fibrin remains adherent to the pleural surface, giving rise do 'dry' pleuritis with associated friction sounds. If exudation exceeds resorption, the fluid accumulates in the thoracic cavity and an exudative pleuritis develops. The inflammation irritates the sensory nerve fibers, and movements of the chest wall are painful, causing respiration to become shallow. Depending on the causal agent and the severity of the process, the exudate may be serous (serous pleuritis), serofibrinous or purulent (suppurative pleuritis). The effusions and sometimes massive fibrinous deposits lead to compression of adjacent lung tissue, resulting in atelectases and an impairment of gaseous exchange. The shallow respiration combined with the reduction of ventilated lung can produce marked cyanosis of the mucosae. With a high degree of fibrinous exudation, adhesions form between the two pleural layers. In chronic cases these become converted to connective tissue proliferating into thick fibrous adhesions in which multiple abscesses may be found.

Differential Diagnosis. The crepitation sounds of bronchiolitis can mimic the friction sounds of pleuritis. However, crepitation sounds are restricted mainly to the apical lobes, whereas pleuritic friction sounds are heard mainly over the diaphragmatic lobes. Also, bronchiolitis is distinguished by an absence of pain on percussion and a tympanitic percussion sound.

Prognosis. The prognosis of dry pleuritis is favorable, and that of serous pleuritis is fair if the primary cause can be removed.

Suppurative and chronic pleuritis have an unfavorable prognosis, because complete recovery is impossible.

Lesions. In healed dry pleuritis, circumscribed thickenings of the visceral pleura are found mainly in the region of the diaphragmatic lobes. In suppurative pleuritis there are indurated deposits and adhesions of the pleural layers, and the process usually extends to the pericardium. Fibrous adhesions are present in chronic cases.

Treatment. Antibiotics or sulfonamides are administered parenterally. Excessive fluid accumulations are removed by thoracocentesis, followed by the placement of an antibiotic into the pleural cavity. Adhesion formation between the pleural layers may be prevented by combining the antibiotic with an enzyme preparation such as streptokinase. Fluid removal can be assisted, and reaccumulation delayed, by giving a diuretic or mannitol. In chronic pleuritis treatment is generally useless.

References

LARSON, V. L.; SORENSEN, D. K.: The respiratory system. In: Equine medicine and surgery, 2nd ed. (Amer. Vet. Public. Inc., Wheaton/Ill. 1972).

MAREK, J.; MANNINGER, R.; MÓCSY, J.: Spezielle Pathologie und Therapie der Haustiere (Verlag Gustav Fischer, Jena 1945).

POTEL, K.: Lehrbuch der Pathologischen Physiologie der Haustiere (VEB Gustav Fischer Verlag, Jena 1969).

Pneumothorax

Definition. Pneumothorax is a condition in which air has entered the pleural sac through an open chest wound or from the rupture of a major bronchus.

Symptoms. The most prominent sign is the sudden development of inspiratory dyspnea, whose severity increases with the magnitude of the injury. Affected horses are reluctant to lie down, the nostrils are widely flared, the inspiratory phase of each respiratory cycle is markedly prolonged, and movements of the chest wall are increased. If the parietal pleura is injured, air can also enter the subcutaneous tissue producing a cutaneous emphysema. In severe cases there is increasing cyanosis of the mucosae, and fatal anoxia can develop within 1 to 2 h. Thoracic percussion elicits a metallic tympanitic sound that is demonstrable on both sides. Pleuritis is a common sequel to traumatic pneumothorax.

Etiology. The main cause is accidental puncture of the thoracic wall with perforation of the pleural cavity. Air can also enter the pleural cavity through the puncture of a lung by a broken rib. In rare cases a necrotizing pneumonia with cavitation can break through into the pleural cavity and cause pneumothorax. Finally, thoracocentesis performed with a too-short needle can cause air to be aspirated into the pleural cavity during inhalation. In this case the amount of air entering the pleural sac is too small to produce dyspneic symptoms.

Pathogenesis. In the event of a major chest wall injury, the breaching of a large cavity communicating with a bronchus, or a lung injury with the rupture of a bronchus, the pressure in the pleural cavity becomes equal to atmospheric, and 'open pneumothorax' is said to be present. If the opening is small it may close during expiration, and air can enter the pleural space only during inspiration; then a 'valvular pneumothorax' is present. A 'closed pneumothorax' is one in which the wound is closed and further air entry is prevented. The entry of air into the pleural cavity alters the negative interpleural pressure, and this allows the elastic lung to contract or even collapse completely in severe cases. Because the mediastinum of the horse is patent, a pneumothorax quickly becomes bilateral, even after a unilateral injury. The collapse of the lung impairs gaseous exchange and embarrasses the venous return to the heart. There may be marked cyanosis of the mucosae, depending on the severity of the pneumothorax. Fatal anoxia can occur in extreme cases. If the lung is only partially collapsed and the point of entry of air is closed, the air will be resorbed in 2 to 3 weeks, and a full recovery may be expected.

Differential Diagnosis. Exudative pleuritis does not have a sudden onset, marked dullness is noted in the ventral thoracic region, and fluid is aspirated from the pleural sac. Hemothorax may occur in conjunction with pneumothorax after an injury but can also occur independently. Besides labored breathing, a dull area with a fluid line and pale mucous membranes due to anemia are the most prominent signs. Thoracocentesis is usually diagnostic.

Prognosis. Pneumothorax due to a chest wall rupture has a very poor prognosis. If further entry of air into the pleural cavity can be prevented, recovery is possible.

Lesions. In horses that die with acute pneumothorax, both lungs are collapsed. Necropsy is performed in chronic cases only if secondary pleuritis has developed. Besides the lesions of suppurative pleuritis, which are almost always present, circumscribed atelectases of the apical lobe are found.

Treatment. Traumatic wounds of the chest wall are closed quickly to prevent the further aspiration of air. In severe cases the horse must be intubated and placed on a respirator. Positive pressure is applied to reinflate the lungs and expel the air from the pleural sac. This is followed by definitive closure of the wound. To prevent secondary pleuritis, the patient should be kept on antibiotics or sulfonamides until wound healing is complete.

References

HOFF, F.: Klinische Physiologie und Pathologie, 5. Aufl. (Thieme, Stuttgart 1956).

POTEL, K.: Lehrbuch der Pathologischen Physiologie der Haustiere (VEB Gustav Fischer Verlag, Jena 1969).

SIEGENTHALER, W.: Klinische Pathophysiologie (Thieme, Stuttgart 1970).

Hydrothorax and Hemothorax

Definition. Hydrothorax and hemothorax result from the accumulation of non-inflammatory transudate or blood, respectively, in the pleural cavity. Both conditions are rare in the horse.

Symptoms. The most prominent feature is the increasing dyspnea, which can develop gradually in hydrothorax and within a few hours in hemothorax. Neither condition is accompanied by fever. Hydrothorax generally leads to edema of the ventral abdomen and limbs, while in hemothorax there is no peripheral edema but the visible mucosae are pale.

Auscultation reveals weak vesicular sounds in the lower portions of the lung and faint heart sounds. A dull area with a horizontal fluid line is percussed over the ventral thorax. Thoracocentesis will disclose the nature of the accumulated fluid.

In hydrothorax the aspirated fluid is generally clear or slightly yellowish, its density is below 1.016, and its protein content is less than 3.0 g/l. The sediment contains isolated endothelial cells with vacuoles. In hemothorax, of course, blood is obtained on aspiration.

Etiology. A longstanding right-sided heart failure can lead to venous pooling in the cranial region of the vena cava and thus to the escape of noninflammatory fluid (transudate) into the pleural cavity.

Hydrothorax can also result from a significant reduction in the total protein content of the plasma. This hypoproteinemia can have various causes: cirrhosis of the liver, a severe mycotoxicosis or, in rare cases, a massive nephrosis with sizable protein losses through the kidney.

Hemothorax is practically always due to a traumatic injury of the chest wall.

Pathogenesis. When venous congestion occurs, the flow velocity of the blood in the vena cava is reduced. This leads to a pressure elevation in the vena cava, and the oxygen supply is reduced. Both circumstances heighten the permeability of the venous wall, leading initially to the extravasation of plasma and, if the pressure elevation persists, the leakage of cellular elements may occur as well.

With hypoproteinemia there is a fall of the colloidal osmotic pressure in the vessels, the reabsorption of fluid from the tissues is decreased, and hydrothorax develops.

Hemothorax is based on vascular injuries of the lung and the extravasation of blood into the pleural cavity.

Differential Diagnosis. Pleuritis takes a febrile course, and an inflammatory exudate is obtained on thoracocentesis.

Pneumothorax has a sudden onset, and the percussion sound is tympanitic.

Prognosis. In hydrothorax the prognosis is grave to poor, because generally speaking, the primary disorder is rarely curable.

The prognosis of hemothorax depends on the severity of the hemorrhage.

Treatment. Hydrothorax is managed by treating the primary condition. In hemothorax efforts are directed toward arresting blood loss. Severe dyspnea can be relieved by the aspiration of fluid from the pleural cavity.

2.1.5. Diseases of the Digestive System and Peritoneum

2.1.5.1. Diseases of the Oral Cavity

2.1.5.1.1. Stomatitis (Inflammation of the Oral Mucosa)

Definition and Forms. The oral cavity of the horse is lined with a cutaneous, pink but well-perfused mucous membrane. The principal parts of the oral mucosa are the gingivae, palate, and the buccal and lingual mucosae.

Stomatitis refers to inflammation of the oral mucosa or large portions of it. Terms applied to more localized inflammations are cheilitis (inflammation of the lips), gingivitis (inflammation of the gums), glossitis (inflammation of the tongue).

Both superficial and deep inflammation can occur as primary, independent entities or may arise secondarily as complications of other diseases.

Besides physical agents of traumatic or thermal origin, stomatitis may also be caused by chemical and infectious agents. The latter group includes bacterial, viral and mycotic forms.

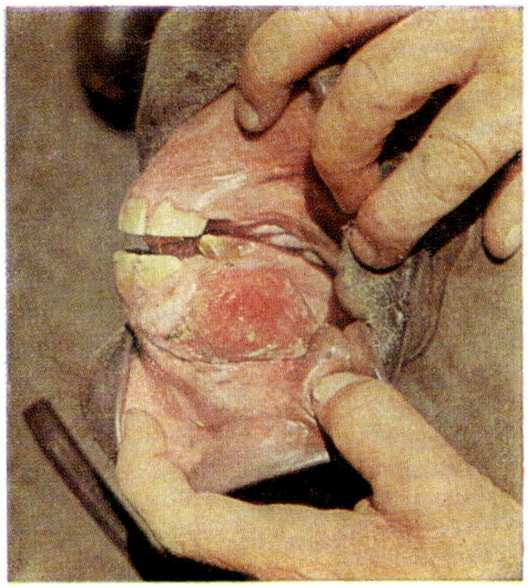

1

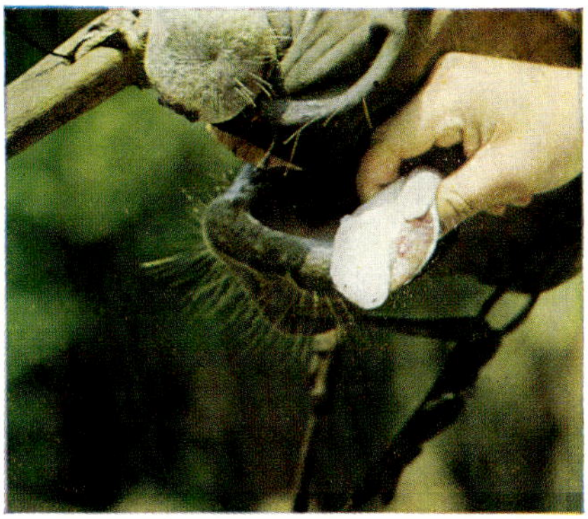

2

Fig. 2.1.5. — 1. Pseudomembranous stomatitis in the incisor area of a foal.
Fig. 2.1.5. — 2. Lingual wound.

Symptoms. All forms of stomatitis are marked by excessive salivation and difficulties in feeding. Stomatitis can also cause a horse to resist the placement of a bit and may be a cause of sudden refractoriness in the horse's nature.

The clinical picture of acute, catarrhal stomatitis is characterized by a patchy or diffuse reddening of the swollen mucosa. The swelling due to serous infiltration of the mucosa and submucosa may be so severe in the area of the hard palate that it is mistaken for a neoplasm. Sloughed epithelial cells mix with the secretions of the mucous glands and saliva and form a grayish-white or dirty-gray coating which decomposes and produces a fetid breath odor.

Pea-size vesicles are characteristic of *vesicular stomatitis.* The vesicles rupture leaving shallow erosions which heal in a few days in the absence of secondary infection.

If pathogenic organisms gain entry to the vesicular contents a secondary *pustular stomatitis* develops. The nodules undergo purulent liquefaction and form larger pustules surrounded by a hyperemic zone, which in turn are converted into deep ulcers that extend into the submucosa before they finally heal with scarring.

Ulcerative stomatitis may be caused by chemical agents and is characterized by the formation of defects covered by various types of scab. *Pseudomembranous stomatitis* is characterized by profuse salivation, redness of the mucosa, and the presence of grayish-white coatings and crusts (fig. 2.1.5. — 1). The swellings may spread to the lips and angle of the mouth. Invasion by certain bacteria causes perforating labial tissue losses and necrosis.

Etiology. Acute catarrhal stomatitis may be a primary entity caused by physical, chemical or infectious agents, but frequently it occurs as a clinical manifestation of infectious diseases.

Vesicular stomatitis is caused by a different etiological agent than that which causes viral vesicular stomatitis. This disease has been known since the turn of the century. It caused great losses, especially among military horses in the USA. The disease has been recognized in Europe for over 50 years.

In animals with horse pox, pustular stomatitis develops in 3 to 7 days following inoculation with the virus.

Ulcerative stomatitis may be caused by trauma from sharp awns in unthreshed wheat as well as by chemical injuries, either from agents applied to the mucosa externally or from toxic substances such as mercury, lead, silver or copper that are excreted in the saliva.

Spoiled feeds, such as moldy or rotten hay, can lead to pseudomembranous stomatitis within a few days.

Diagnosis. The diagnosis is based upon the clinical examination and especially upon local or diffuse macroscopic lesions that are noted during inspection of the oral cavity. The clinical picture may change daily, depending on the cause and duration of the disease.

Treatment. The cause of the stomatitis should be ascertained and if possible removed. The animal should then be placed on a diet of soft feed or perhaps green feeds and soft hay. If the patient cannot drink from the automatic waterer on account of pain, fresh water must be offered several times daily. Fresh water or water slightly acidified with vinegar can be given by slow, careful drenching with the aid of an irrigator. A 0.1 % $KMnO_4$ solution or 1 % H_2O_2 solution may also be added to the water. Ulcers should be cauterized once or twice daily, the oral cavity flushed with 1 % saline solution. Local therapy is supplemented by the parenteral administration of antibiotics.

2.1.5.1.2. Pharyngeal Cysts

See Sec. 2.1.5.8.5.

2.1.5.1.3. Glossitis (Inflammation of the Tongue)

Definition. The term glossitis is applied both to inflammation of the lingual mucosa and to inflamation of the muscles of the tongue.

Forms. The lingual mucosa is involved in almost all cases of stomatitis, and glossitis is a feature of various infectious diseases (anthrax, malignant edema). For the most part, however, inflammations of the lingual mucosa and musculature occur following superficial or deep mechanical, chemical or thermal injuries.

The tongue is subject to incised, lacerated, puncture, contused, caustic or burn wounds. These may extend longitudinally or parallel to the midline or extend transversely across the tongue and may involve the dorsum of the tongue (fig. 2.1.5. — 2).

Symptoms. The main symptom is a difficulty or inability to drink or masticate. The pain from inflammation restricts the active mobility of the tongue, so that during mastication the food cannot be adequately shifted to the side of the mouth or swallowed by pressure against the palate. As a result, food material is discharged from the mouth, accompanied by profuse salivation. The pain associated with the inflammation or injury causes the animal to resent being bitted.

With extensive transverse wounds of the muscle of the tongue the tip sometimes protrudes between the incisors. If a cellulitis or phlegmon of the tongue has developed as a result of wound infection, then in severe cases the tongue will protrude well out of the open mouth. The tongue will show visible lesions such as wounds, ulcers or areas of pressure necrosis from the cheek teeth and incisors.

In these cases respiration is impaired and a sterterous breathing may be present. A gangrenous aspiration pneumonia may result from regurgitation and dysphagia.

Withdrawing the tongue from the passively-opened mouth is painful and should be done with care. Once the tongue is withdrawn, the various wounds can be recognized.

Wounds in the aboral or basal portion of the tongue are difficult to locate. The tongue can be raised to disclose wounds on the inferior and lateral lingual surfaces.

Palpation will reveal any foreign bodies that have been driven superficially into the tongue.

Etiology. Acute glossitis occurs in conjunction with stomatitides of various causes, infectious diseases, purpura hemorrhagica and injuries.

Smaller stab wounds are caused by foreign bodies that may penetrate into the lingual musculature and migrate to a new location.

Slit wounds of the tongue can be caused by the licking of feed boxes, opened cans, etc. The tongue may even be split in two if it becomes caught on a sharp object.

If the tongue comes between the incisors during a fall, it will be bitten through, and the amputated tip sometimes remains attached by only a shread of mucosa. Tongue injuries are also caused by pointed, sharp-edged teeth, abnormally elongated teeth, shear mouth, projections from broken teeth, or by deviated, rotated or dislocated teeth. Even normal teeth can inflict tongue injuries in cases of lingual paralysis or during impairments of consciousness due to such diseases as meningitis.

Other causes of injury include the use of damaged bits. Jointed bits can cause deep lingual wounds if the hinge-like ring connection becomes excessively worn.

Rough and inhumane handling, such as tying a refractory horse by the tongue, can cause the tongue to be avulsed from the hyoid bone.

The improper use of dental instruments and the administration of pills or capsules with a balling gun are other common causes of lingual injuries.

Finally, the tongue may be injured or burned when the horse licks irritant drugs from the skin (e.g., rubefacients) or the tongue comes in contact with boiling water or hot objects.

Diagnosis and Differential Diagnosis. By a thorough physical examination and careful inspection of the oral cavity under good illumination, it is usually possible to identify the nature of the injury and in many cases ascertain its cause.

If the results of the lingual examination are inconsistent with clinical findings, a radiographic examination is recommended.

Treatment. Specific immune serum or polyvalent immune serum may be given in certain clostridial diseases. High doses of broad-spectrum antibiotics may be given for other bacterial diseases. Wounds in the oral cavity heal well owing to the bacteriostatic action of the saliva as well as the good blood supply. Even severe lingual injuries usually go on to complete, uneventful healing.

While superficial mucosal wounds generally require no special treatment, longitudinal incised wounds of the lingual musculature should be carefully sutured. A longitudinal split in the tongue can also be repaired in this way, with interrupted sutures placed on both the superior and inferior lingual surfaces.

With deep transverse wounds or necrosis of the tongue, up to 10 cm of the apex may be surgically amputated without causing feeding disturbances. If the lingual arteries or their dorsal branches have been divided, they must be carefully ligated. Following appropriate wound care, the mucosa is sutured over the amputation stump. The lingual stump apparently elongates to some degree in time.

An extensive loss of lingual tissue need not be life-threatening. The animal learns to ingest food even with a relatively short stump. Wound infections and cellulitis are initially treated by irrigating the oral cavity with antiseptic agents. The pointing of abscesses in the intermandibular area can be hastened by the application of 20 % Icthammol® ointment. Abscesses which lie in or below the tongue or in the intermandibular area are lanced.

If suffocation is a danger, a temporary tracheostomy is indicated. Fluid may be administered parenterally for several days. A liquid diet should be maintained until the wounds are completely healed. Analgesics may be indicated for the first few days.

When irritant topical medications are used, the animal should be kept from licking them by placing a permanent protective dressing over the area treated, by placing a collar about the neck to restrict movements, or by cross-tying the head for a short time.

The horse should be watched carefully during the inhalation of hot vapors and guarded against burns or scalding.

The mouthpieces of snaffle or curb bits should be checked before use. A rubber snaffle is preferred for the young, sensitive mouth. If a curb-type bit is used, a Pelham (curb bit with a movable snaffle mouthpiece) is recommended.

2.1.5.1.4. Lingual Paralysis

Definition. Neurogenic paralysis of the tongue can result from a uni- or bilateral paresis or paralysis of the hypoglossal nerve (see Sec. 2.1.14.2.3).

Symptoms. With bilateral paralysis of the hypoglossal nerve, the tongue hangs from the mouth at the center of the lips. With unilateral paralysis the tongue deviates toward the affected side when extended and toward the unaffected side when retracted. Salivation is excessive. Initially the tongue is unchanged but may develop secondary mucosal injuries, either self-inflicted or from external trauma. It may be difficult or impossible for the animal to masticate and swallow food.

Etiology. The hypoglossal nerve can be contused, strained or torn in the intermandibular area by strangulation, mandibular fracture, struggling to free the entrapped head, or by forcible withdrawal of the tongue. In many places farriers still tie refractory horses by their tongue for shoeing! This can also lead to myogenic peripheral paralyses from muscular contusions. Lingual paralysis of central origin usually occurs as a symptom of encephalomyelitis, rabies, brain tumors and severe intoxications.

Diagnosis and Differential Diagnosis. In the vice of 'tongue-lolling', there is no demonstrable impairment of lingual muscular activity. Fracture of the hyoid bone, facial paralysis and dislocation of the mandible must be excluded. Wounds and cellulitis of the tongue are painful.

Treatment. The prolapsed parts of the tongue should be protected from injury if at all possible. Pareses usually disappear in about a week even without treatment. Vitamin B complex preparations may be administered. Attention should be given to appropriate nutrition and to removal of the causative factor.

In paralysis of central origin, the course of the primary disease will decide the outcome.

Chronic lingual paralysis leads to gradual atrophy of the tongue and makes it extremely difficult for the horse to feed itself. Paralyses that do not improve after 14 days have a poor prognosis.

2.1.5.1.5. Diseases of the Teeth

Dental Calculus

Definition. Dental calculus, or tartar, is a salivary concretion that forms on dental surfaces.

Occurrence. According to Beier [1915], dental calculus occurs in 83.33 % of all horses. Teeth located close to the excretory ducts of the salivary glands are mainly affected.

Symptoms. Affected teeth exhibit a grayish-white to dark-gray or sometimes yellow-green coating of a friable consistency. The deposits taper from the base of the extra-alveolar part of the tooth toward the occlusal surface and extend up to about the middle of the visible portion of the tooth. The occlusal surface itself is unaffected. The calculus forms most frequently on the maxillary premolars situated near the excretory ducts of the salivary glands, in the region of the two furrow-shaped depressions in the buccal surfaces, and on the mandibular canine teeth.

In abnormalities of dentition, such as overgrowth, shear mouth or step mouth, the calculus forms preferentially on the buccal surfaces of abnormally elongated teeth. On the incisors it fills the space between the proximal surfaces and completely encircles the neck of the tooth.

As a rule, dental calculus produces no clinical signs. In severe cases there may be a pronounced hyperemia or inflammation of the gum (gingivitis). If the deposits encroach upon the gum, ulcerative changes develop below the calculus, and a fetid breath odor results.

Etiology. According to Becker [1970], the soluble calcium bicarbonate in the saliva is converted to insoluble calcium carbonate with the release of CO_2 and is deposited upon the teeth. This calculus is composed mainly of porous, pumice like calcium carbonate mixed with epithelial cells from the oral mucosa, food debris and oral bacteria.

The diet is an important factor in the formation of dental calculus, for it influences the composition of the saliva. A calcium-rich diet may predispose to calculus formation.

According to Wittmann [1908] dental calculus in the horse has the following composition:

	%
Water	1.21
Water-soluble substances KCl, K_2SO_4	0.24
Organic constituents (mucus and food residue)	11.35
Calcium phosphate	2.76
Calcium carbonate	83.45
Sulfur (determined as H_2S)	0.17

Treatment. Dental calculus is removed mechanically with a small curette. Large calculi can be dislodged by inserting a suitable dental instrument between the tooth and calculus and exerting a gentle prying action.

Calculus can be removed gently and painlessly by means of suitable ultrasonic devices.

Following calculus removal the gingival pockets and necks of the teeth are swabbed with tincture of iodine, or glycerine/iodine combination.

Periodontitis (Alveolar Periostitis)

Definition. Periodontitis refers to a pyogenic inflammation of the dental supporting tissues, which may extend to the tooth and alveolar wall. The lower arcade is most frequently involved.

Forms. In *marginal periodontitis* the infection originates at the edge of the alveolus. An infection of the pulp may spread to the periodontium from the root apex, leading to *apical periodontitis.* In *total periodontitis* the entire alveolar dental membrane is involved. The inflammatory process often results from the extension of a gingival inflammation. If the gum margin is involved, the condition is called paradontitis or paradentitis. Conversely, gingivitis can also develop secondarily to periodontitis.

Symptoms. Affected horses eat slowly and consume little food. The haircoat appears dull. Seasonal shedding is delayed or incomplete. The animal's nutritional status deteriorates, it has a dull and lethargic appearance and sweats inadequately during exercise. Gastrointestinal disorders arise in the form of colic or enteritis. Poorly masticated grains may be found in the feces.

There may be excessive salivation and a fetid breath odor. Although the affected area is initially tender to pressure, the animal is reluctant to drink cold water.

Inspection of the oral cavity discloses hyperemia, bleeding and swelling of the gum surrounding the tooth (marginal periodontitis). The affected tooth, which appears elongated, is mobile and may show buccal or lingual deviation (total periodontitis).

Radiography shows marked alteration of the alveolar region with a characteristic atrophy of the lamina at the margin of the affected alveolus.

The pus that accumulates in the alveolus may rise toward the oral cavity or find drainage through the bone. Fistulae of this type may develop at the mandibular border in the region of the premolars.

From the affected alveoli of the maxillary premolars, the pus may either travel medially into the nasal cavity or erupt laterally through the maxillary cortical bone and outer skin.

Maxillary sinusitis develops if pus breaks through the alveoli of the upper molars. A unilateral, purulent, intermittent nasal discharge that increases when the head is lowered is characteristic of this complication.

Etiology. Periodontitis is generally caused by bacterial infection. The rare aseptic periodontitis may occur as a sequel to direct trauma, and is characterized by the resorption of blood and regenerative processes in the periodontium. This form includes the aseptic inflammation that occurs in the region of the root apices of the replacement premolars when their eruption is excessively delayed by retention of the deciduous premolars. The periodontium of the milk teeth also becomes inflamed during eruption of the permanent teeth, but these inflammations subside as the milk teeth are shed and so do not spread to involve the periodontium of the replacement teeth. Pyogenic periodontitis, on the other hand, usually results from food entrapment between the tooth and gum (marginal periodontitis). Often awns become lodged between the third premolar and first molar from the buccal or lingual side; a soft diet and the feeding of molasses encourage the decomposition processes between the teeth and predispose to infection by the introduction of bacterial pathogens.

This process is further predisposed by gap between the cheek teeth, by the loosening of teeth from other causes, through displacements by supernumerary teeth, and by fissures or fractures of the teeth.

A pulpitis can spread to the periodontium via the root canals (apical periodontitis). Again, food entrapment plays a role, for if the pulp cavity is exposed due to a failure of secondary dentine formation, food matter can enter the cavity and initiate the inflammation.

Periodontitis of mandibular first and second molars is usually chronic and often leads to secondary ossifying periostitis, characterized by marked mandibular enlargement.

Treatment. Initially trapped food material between the teeth is removed. Then, in the early stage of a marginal periodontitis, a partial resection of the extra-alveolar portion of the tooth is undertaken if the patient is young and the dental root is still long enough to allow good occlusion of the tooth later on (radiography!).

In all other cases the affected tooth must be extracted. Often it is found at operation that the interalveolar bony septum is already necrotic, so that the contact surface of one or both adjacent teeth is deeply exposed. These teeth, too, will have to be extracted sooner or later. As a rule, however, only one tooth may be pulled on each side without causing permanent abnormalities of mastication.

In cases of extensive secondary ossifying periostitis, extraction may prove extremely difficult, requiring that the tooth be repelled with a dental punch following trephination to gain access to its base. After the removal of the tooth, the alveolus is irrigated with an antiseptic solution and filled with packing. This also applies to the trephine wound.

If maxillary sinusitis is present, the sinus is opened by trephination and also treated with antiseptic solutions. Food material is carefully flushed from the cavity. It is essential that the alveolus be packed to prevent contamination with food material.

Pulpitis

Definition. Pulpitis refers generally to a pyogenic inflammation of the dental pulp, the richly vascularized and innervated connective tissue contained in the pulp cavity of the tooth.

Occurrence. Purulent pulpitis can occur in the incisors and cheek teeth of horses of all ages.

Symptoms. Pulpitis, which begins with hyperemia and inflammatory edema of the dental pulp, leads to compression of the sensory pulpal nerves with subsequent pain. In the confines of the pulp cavity the diseased pulp undergoes a rapid necrosis in acute cases due to the action of bacterial invaders. When this process has run its course, the tooth is 'dead', and the pulp is no longer sensitive to stimuli. The pain during this time causes feeding disturbances and is especially severe when cold water is consumed. If the gangrenous pulp communicates with the outer tooth surface as a result of caries, fracture or erosion, the breath takes on a fetid odor.

Chronic pulpitis causes the horse to favor the affected tooth or the entire row of teeth for a prolonged period of time, possibly leading to abnormalities of dentition (sharp edge formation, shear mouth).

The absence of secondary dentine formation in the affected tooth eventually leads to exposure of the pulp cavity on the occlusal surface. Openings appear which communicate directly with the pulp cavity and represent cross-sections of the opened division of the pulp cavity ('porodontia'). The defect is filled with food debris, which when removed exposes the pulp cavity. The dentine surrounding the opening is neither softened nor discolored. The inner wall of the cavity is brown and smooth. The pulp itself is no longer present.

In acute pulpitis the regional lymph node is enlarged and tender. Percussion of the affected tooth is painful.

A lateral radiograph made with dental film will clearly demonstrate secondary changes at the root apex.

Etiology. The bacteria responsible for the pyogenic infection may gain entry to the pulp by the hematogenous route, directly from the crown of the tooth, or indirectly from the diseased periodontium.

Dental caries is of minor importance in the occurrence of a *direct* infection, for the folded enamel of the equine tooth generally prevents decay from extending very deep into the tooth. Moreover, caries in the horse is almost always a 'dry' form, which is less apt to cause complete dissolution of the teeth.

Fissures and fractures in the crown of the tooth can expose the pulp cavity to bacterial invasion and thus lead to pulpitis.

The senile or presenile erosion of one or more cheek teeth is associated with such rapid wear of the crown that continuous secondary dentine formation can no longer prevent a communication of the pulp cavity from the occlusal surface. Pulpitis also occurs in cheek teeth or incisors subjected to abnormal wear by other mechanisms (cribbing, etc.).

Partial pulpitis occurs after the completion of dental growth when only *one* division of the pulp cavity is exposed and the resultant inflammation does not spread to the other cavity divisions.

Indirect infection of the dental pulp can occur through the diseased periodontium. This is most frequently caused by the trapping of food between the proximal surfaces of diastemic cheek teeth, and the subsequent entry of the infectious organisms into the pulp via the root canals following partial destruction of the periodontium. The formation of secondary dentine is arrested as a result of pulpal necrosis or necrobiosis, and the pulp cavity is spontaneously opened by porodontia. The disease may be restricted to one division of the pulp cavity if it originated with a periodontitis of only one root branch, and the remaining divisions of the pulp cavity are sealed off from the infection.

While a serous pulpitis may regress in favorable cases, a pyogenic or necrotizing inflammation invariably leads to the destruction of the pulp.

In acute cases the apical periodontitis that is almost always present in pulpitis leads to an ascending periodontitis of the lateral surfaces with loosening of the tooth, sometimes accompanied by dental abscesses and dental fistulas on the outer jaw surface and occasionally by invasion of the maxillary sinus with consequent sinus empyema. In chronic cases of pulpitis, areas of hypercementosis form on the root which seal off the apical foramen and present as rough, plaster-like, spherical structures in the apical area. Often they are an impediment to extraction and can be removed only after trephination.

Treatment. According to EISENMENGER [1959] the dental roots can be exposed from the side in young horses and resected after removal of the granuloma. A tooth already loosened as a result of periodontitis should be extracted. Soft granulation tissue at the root apex and areas of hypercementosis remaining in the alveolus are removed with a curette.

References

EISENMENGER, E.: Über die Zahnfacherkrankungen des Jungpferdes, ihre Ursachen und operative Behandlung unter Erhaltung des vollständigen Gebisses. Wiener Tierärztl. Msch. *46:* 51 (1959).

ZETNER, K.; EISENMENGER, E.: Wurzelspitzenresektion zur Behandlung der Zahnfistel des Pferdes. XIII. Congr. Europ. Soc. Vet. Surg., Budapest 1980.

Dental Fractures

Definition. A dental fracture is the fragmentation of a tooth from traumatic causes.

Forms. The dental accident may take the form of a simple chip fracture, a longitudinal or transverse fracture, or a fissure.

Symptoms. With the lips rolled back, fractures of the *incisors* are recognizable by an absence of portions of the crown or by an apparent labial or (in rare cases) lingual deviation of the tooth. In reality only the broken portion is deviated. It may cause injury to the oral mucosa, lip or tongue, accompanied by transitory bleeding. After careful opening of the oral fissure, fractures on the lingual side of the incisors may also be seen. Fractures of several adjacent incisors are not uncommon and may be accompanied by tearing of the gum. In transverse fractures the entire coronal portion of the tooth may be lost in some instances, and only the alveolar portion (root) remains attached.

Longitudinal fractures are most frequently observed in the *cheek teeth* and may also be evidenced by buccal or lingual deviation of the fragments, assuming they are retained in the mouth. Larger fractures and any associated mucosal injuries can be well diagnosed by palpation and inspection with the aid of a mouth speculum and good illumination.

Food residue becomes lodged between the tooth fragments that are still attached to the alveolus or held in place by the gum, and if pressed into the alveolus this residue can lead to alveolar periostitis with marked pain symptoms.

Fissures are easily overlooked.

Difficulties in eating and drinking arise only if the fracture is associated with an injury to the oral mucosa, tongue, alveolus or jaw, or if the pulp cavity has become exposed. Pain is especially severe when cold water is consumed. However, feeding difficulties seldom persist for more than a few days after the occurrence of the fracture. Evidence of slow and careful mastication is mainly observed in fractures of the cheek teeth with secondary pulpitis or alveolar periostitis. Often deviations cause 'quidding' in the horse, and the expelled material may be found on the feeding table and stall floor.

Chip fractures that do not expose the pulp frequently show no clinical signs. Fracture sites predispose to caries, and a longstanding fracture of a molar or premolar can lead to abnormal elongation of the opposing tooth.

Etiology. Dental fractures, especially of the upper and lower incisors, can occur during falls, during violent rolling from colic, in collisions with obstacles, or when the animal is being cast for anesthesia.

Fractures of the cheek teeth, especially the maxillary premolars, can occur when the upper and lower arcades snap together violently during a fall, or when the animal bites down on a rock or other hard object that is present in the feed.

Transverse fractures that extend obliquely backward through the tooth sometimes occur during the rasping of protruding cheek teeth.

In the presenile and senile mouth, the teeth lose their original strength, and even the normal stresses of mastication can lead to a dental fissure or fracture.

Teeth that are weakened by structural abnormalities or dental disease are susceptible to secondary fractures during normal loading by the opposing tooth.

The 1st molar often shows hypoplasia of the enamel invaginations with resultant presenile erosion and abnormalities of dentine formation, making it especially prone to fracture.

Porodontia and caries are further potential causes of spontaneous dental fractures.

Prognosis. In chip fractures the tooth can be saved provided the pulp cavity has not been exposed and there is no pulpal infection. Such fractures seldom cause clinical signs and in most cases their detection is fortuitous. If only portions of the crown or enamel invaginations are broken from the lingual aspect of the tooth, then the defect will eventually disappear through normal wear.

In exceptional cases a fissure in a juvenile tooth that extends to the pulp will heal by secondary dentine formation in the absence of pulpal infection. This is possible only in young animals.

Treatment. Any sharp edges or points left by the fracture are filed smoothed. Large splinters that remain attached by the gum and fracture fragments that have a wedge- or spike-shaped termination in the alveolus are removed. As a rule, teeth with a primary or secondary longitudinal fracture should be extracted, for generally a periodontitis, fragment deviation or caries develops that makes preservation impossible. Following the extraction of a cheek tooth, the dentition should be checked regularly so that excessive elongation of the opposing tooth can be promptly recognized and corrected.

Dental Caries

Definition. Dental caries is a circumscribed decay of the calcified tissues of the tooth (enamel, dentine, cement) which generally progresses from the outside of the tooth inward.

Forms. Caries is described according to the type of tissue affected (enamel, dentinal, cemental) or according to its localization (occlusal surface, proximal surface, buccal or lingual surface, neck, root).

Caries in horses is mainly of the dry form (caries sicca); the moist form (caries humida) is extremely rare.

Occurrence. Dental caries is relatively uncommon in the horse. BECKER [1945] found a prevalence of only 1.05% in a population of 30,000 military horses. Nearly half of all affected horses were between 16 and 19 years of age.

Caries affects mainly the cheek teeth, especially the maxillary first molar. It is rarely observed in the incisors and canines.

Symptoms. Pain and consequently difficulties in mastication will be present. This will occur especially if the caries has invaded the enamel and dentine and has created large tubular defects that extend to the pulp and root apex causing secondary pulpitis, periodontitis, dental fracture or loosening and deviation of the tooth. Such defects are recognized by their brownish discoloration and by the dryness of the decaying tissue. The cement appears fissured and eroded at its free border, but pits with foul-smelling carious material are not observed.

Cemental caries (cement necrosis) develops within the infundibulum, but usually its progress is halted once the enamel is reached. Pulpitis occurs only if the caries erodes from the cement covering the enamel folds to the periodontium, whence it invades the body of the tooth from the side.

In rare cases, caries develops from the interior of the tooth outward as a result of secondary root caries. This is caused by a spread of the lesion from the cement of the enamel cylinders to the pulp. Given the size of the apical foramen, this form is invariably associated with apical periodontitis.

Thus, caries of the occlusal surfaces arises from the enamel cylinders and enamel folds of the molars and less frequently from the dentinal islets. Caries of the lateral surfaces arises from the contact surfaces of adjacent teeth (interstitial caries), usually maxillary first and second molars, while root involvement is secondary to other forms of dental decay.

Etiology. Dental caries is observed far less frequently in the folded-enamel teeth of equidae than in the cusped-enamel teeth of the carnivore. Moreover, equine teeth undergo a constant erosion, with the continual appearance of new dental tissue on the occlusal surface.

Despite varying opinions as to the causes of dental caries in horses, it is clear that the action of certain chemical and bacterial agents is important in the etiology of the disease.

Treatment. Caries of the occlusal surface is only treatable in exceptional cases. The necrotic tissue is removed from the defect with a burr, and the prepared cavity is disinfected and filled with a suitable filling material. According to BECKER [1938] an amalgam filling is satisfactory for smaller defects, while a cast filling is required for larger defects.

In cases of interstitial and root caries, or when additional complications arise in the form of periodontitis or pulpitis, the tooth cannot be saved and must be extracted especially if significant masticatory difficulties exist.

The bridging of adjacent teeth is practiced in horses but is a procedure reserved for specialists.

2.1.5.1.6. Abnormalities of Dentition

Inferior and Superior Brachygnathia (Parrot and Sow Mouth)

Definition. Congenital shortness of one jaw with normal development of the remaining jaw is called brachygnathia. An apparent brachygnathia may be present if there is abnormal protrusion (prognathia) of one jaw. Comparative cranial measurements will make it possible to differentiate a prognathic from a brachygnathic deformity.

In 'parrot mouth', or inferior brachygnathia (cf. Sec. 2.8.2.1.), the lower jaw is shorter than the upper jaw; in 'sow mouth', or superior brachygnathia, the lower jaw is longer.

Symptoms. The changes affect mainly the incisors, which are in abnormal apposition to one another. This can cause the development of hooks on the labial borders of the upper incisors (inferior brachygnathia) or lower incisors (superior brachygnathia).

If the condition is severe there may be no contact at all between the occlusal surfaces of the incisors, resulting in the elongation of all incisors due to an absence of erosion. This can cause wounds or ulceration of the exposed gingiva behind the upper incisor arcade in inferior brachygnathia, and injuries to the gingiva, periosteum and bone of the lower bar region in superior brachygnathia. In addition, these deformities prevent food prehension with the teeth, and so affected animals may exhibit gastrointestinal disturbances and general emaciation. Often the deformity results in a longitudinal displacement of the cheek teeth relative to one another, creating an altered alignment between the maxillary and mandibular arcades. In inferior brachygnathia, for example, maxillary P2 and mandibular M3 lack an opposing tooth and consequently elongate or develop long points (exsuperantia dentium) that can cause severe injuries to the opposing jaw. In superior brachygnathia such points form on mandibular P2 and maxillary M3.

Therefore, in both inferior and superior brachygnathia as well as in prognathia, the cheek teeth should be carefully examined for the presence of abnormal projections and any associated gingival lacerations or bone damage.

Treatment. The sharp hooks on the mandibular incisors (superior b.) or maxillary incisors (inferior b.) should be removed with a rasp at intervals of 6—9 months. In severe cases the extraction of the upper or lower incisors may improve the animal's condition. Points on P2 or M3 are carefully removed by rasping. Wounds of the gum or bone are treated by daily irrigation with antiseptic and astringent solutions.

Polyodontia (Supernumerary Teeth)

Definition. Polydontia refers to the presence of extra or supernumerary teeth in addition to the normal number (figs. 2.1.5. — 3 and — 4).

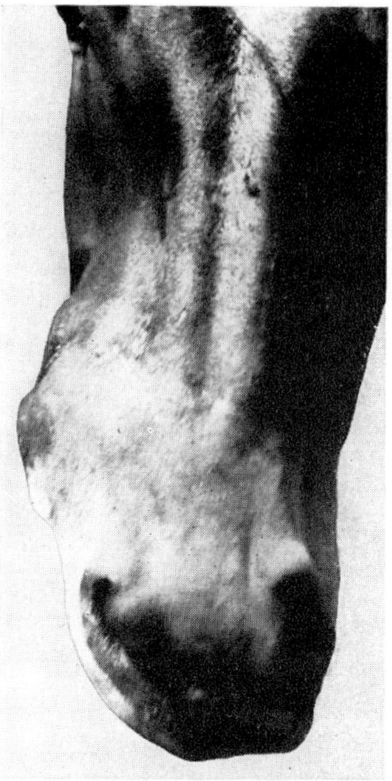

3

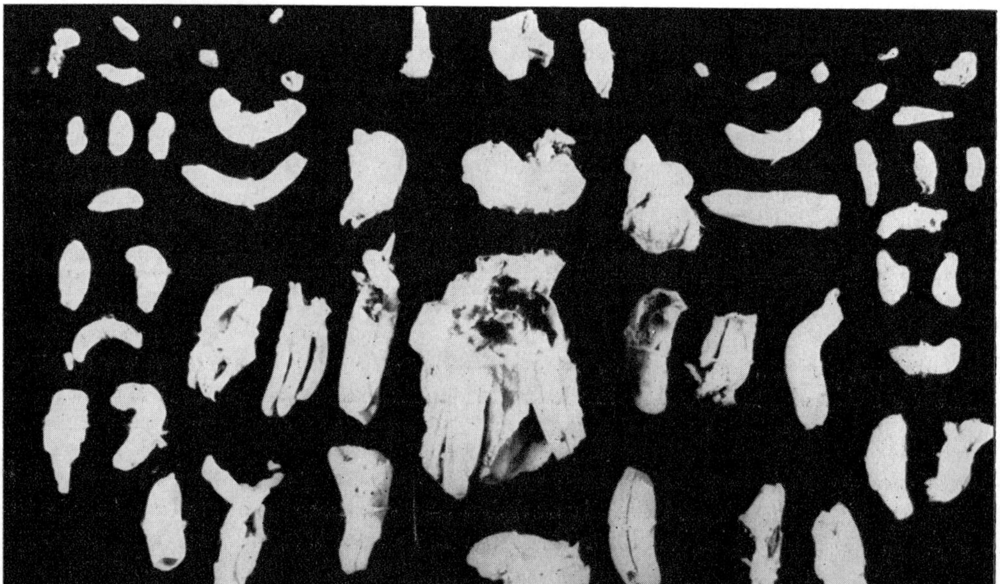

4

Fig. 2.1.5. — 3. Supernumerary teeth in the premolar area.
Fig. 2.1.5. — 4. Extracted supernumerary teeth (archive photo of Chirurgische Tierklinik of Humboldt University, Berlin).

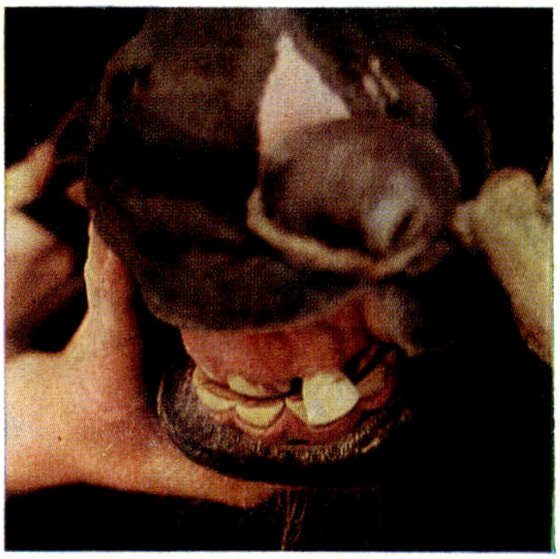
5

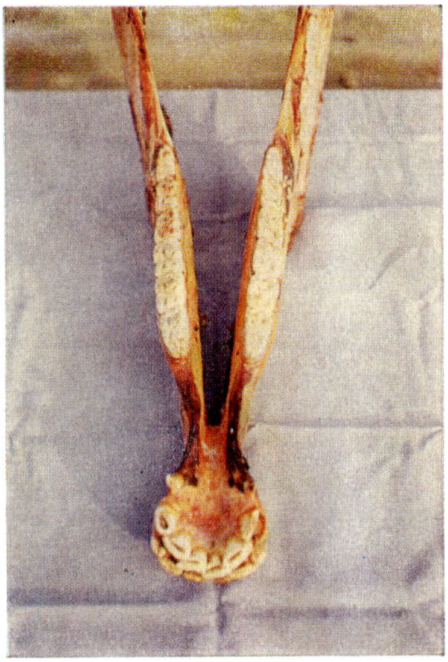
6

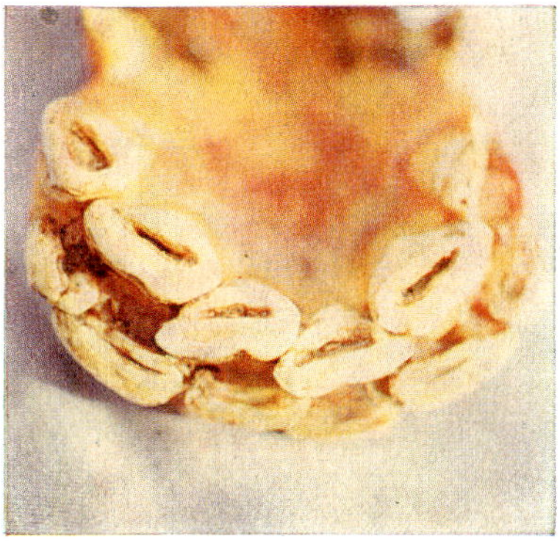
7

Fig. 2.1.5. — 5. Retention of a deciduous upper incisor.

Fig. 2.1.5. — 6–7. Retention of all deciduous lower incisors.

Symptoms and Etiology. BECKER and EWERT [1945] found supernumerary teeth in 0.46 % of a population of 30,000 horses of varying age and gender. According to Becker the condition may be one of three types:

1. Pseudopolyodontia. Polyodontia may appear to be present if teeth of different kinds come abnormally close together as a result of transposition, such as a canine occurring directly adjacent to a 3rd incisor. The retention of some or all deciduous teeth similarly leads to an apparent polyodontia in which deciduous and permanent teeth are juxtaposed or, in the case of the incisors, form a double row.

2. Typical polyodontia. This is a phenomenon marked by the presence of supernumerary teeth that arise as a result of an increased number of tooth germs. A typical pattern in horses is the presence of a 4th incisor together with a 1st premolar (wolf tooth). The latter in particular occurs so frequently that it cannot be strictly regarded as pathological.

These teeth often possess the characteristics of retained deciduous teeth (figs. 2.1.5. — 5 to — 7) or they may have a primitive conical or peg shape that is similar to the dentition of early mammalian ancestors.

3. Atypical polyodontia. This is a true malformation or variation in the number of teeth that generally bears no relation to the phylogenetic development of the dentition. This form of polyodontia is based either on an increased number of tooth germs, a division of tooth germs, or a displacement or fragmentation of parts of the dental lamina or odontogenic tissue of the rudimentary jaw. Such teeth seldom exhibit simple conical shapes, but possess either deciduous or permanent tooth

characteristics with a complicated or malformed structure; they are not shed as a rule.

Supernumerary teeth may be located within the normal dental arcade or just outside it.

Oligodontia (Absence of Teeth) (cf. Sec. 2.8.4.1.)

Definition and Occurrence. Oligodontia is a congenital failure of tooth development. It may result from retention and impaction of one or more teeth in the jaw, in which case pseudo-oligodontia is present. But the true forms are due either to an absence of the tooth bud (reductive o.) or to the destruction or suppression of the tooth bud during embryonic life (sporadic o.).

1. Pseudo-oligodontia occurs most frequently in the mare in the form of retention and impaction of the canines. This form is rarer in stallions and geldings. Pseudo-oligodontia is often indistinguishable clinically from true oligodontia, and radiographic examination may be necessary for a definitive diagnosis.

2. True oligodontia may be based upon a phylogenetic reduction of the dentition (reductive o.), but this form is rare in horses. Much more common is sporadic oligodontia, which results from the formation of a deficient number of tooth germs during differentiation of the dental enamel or from a suppression of the tooth germs during their embryonic or postembryonic development. In other cases the development of the tooth germs is inhibited such that the formation of the corresponding teeth is prevented.

True oligodontia usually involves individual teeth, but occasionally an entire arcade or a particular kind of tooth is affected. The absence of canines in mares (see above) is the most frequent; in 70—75 % of cases this deficit is based upon a true oligodontia. The incisors may also be affected.

Losses of teeth due to dental or periodontal disease, trauma or old age are acquired rather than congenital, and so we do not classifiy them as forms of oligodontia.

Treatment. Only the sequelae are treated. Thus, opposing teeth that show abnormal elongation should be regularly shortened or floated to prevent damage to the mouth.

Abnormal Wear of the Incisors (cf. Sec. 2.8.4.1.)

Definition and Forms. Certain stable vices of the horse such as cribbing or whetting can lead to extreme abnormal wear of the incisors. This can be a cause of digestive problems on the one hand, while providing presumptive evidence for the presence of the vice on the other.

Symptoms and Etiology. Cribmouth is characterized by severe erosion of the labial borders of maxillary first and second incisors. These changes occur when the horse places the upper incisors over the edge of the feeder or some other hard object and then arches the neck, thereby pressing the teeth forcibly against the object. The wear spot may be rounded, flat or indented, depending on the shape of the object grasped. Usually air is swallowed when the neck is arched ('wind sucking'), but the horse may swallow air without cribbing, in which case the incisor wear will be absent ('pure wind sucking') (cf. Sec. 2.9.1.).

Years of cribbing can lead to extreme wear, and the entire tooth may be shortened. Constant replenishment of the incisors and normal occlusal wear keep the changes within normal limits, and rarely is the tooth worn down to the enamel cylinders or pulp cavity. Disturbances of eating and drinking are generally noticed in such cases.

Treatment. In many cases the vice can be cured by a change of environment, or crib-biting can be made difficult or impossible by a myectomy of the sternohyoid, sternothyroid or omohyoid muscles including resection of the ventral branch of the spinal accessory nerve. Removal of the sternocephalicus muscle can be performed as an alternative to resection of the nerve (Forssell's procedure). Horses that are stalled next to cribbers have been known to pick up the habit in a short time.

Whetmouth develops in horses that constantly move their head back and forth or shift their weight from one foreleg to the other, simultaneously rubbing the incisors against the edge of the crib or rail. This erodes the labial surfaces of the maxillary incisors and in many cases the mandibular incisors until the enamel invaginations are exposed, the pulp cavity is opened, and the occlusal surfaces acquire a chisel shape. In extreme cases bleeding wounds and ulcers form at the gingival margin, and blood is found in the feed trough or on the lips. Food prehension may become difficult.

Treatment. Despite pain, affected horses cannot be broken from the habit. Therefore, they must be tied in such a way that they can no longer whet the teeth, or the trough must be removed after feeding. Performance of the swaying movement without rubbing the teeth against objects is called 'weaving'.

2.1.5.2. Facial Nerve Paralysis

See Sec. 2.1.14.2.1.

2.1.5.3. Diseases of the Masticatory Muscles

2.1.5.3.1. Contusions of the Masseter Muscle

Definition. These involve tears or hematomas of the masseter muscle.

Symptoms. The affected buccal region is swollen, tender and slightly warm. The horse chews slowly and cautiously. No external wounds are apparent. Sometimes a defect may be felt in the muscle on palpation.

Etiology. Contusions of the masseter muscle are caused by the action of blunt trauma. Masseter contusions sometimes occur when the animal's head strikes against the table or floor during casting or anesthetic induction.

Prognosis and Treatment. The functional prognosis is good. Acetate solutions, short-wave radiation or dry heat may be administered locally for gradual relief of clinical symptoms.

2.1.5.3.2. Cellulitis (Phlegmon) and Abscess of the Masseter Muscle

Definition. A cellulitis (phlegmon) of the masseter muscle following a pyogenic wound infection will undergo abscessation if resorption does not occur.

Symptoms. The buccal region is swollen. Usually the skin can still be shifted about over the swelling. Tenderness and increased warmth are noted on palpation. The animal has obvious difficulty in eating and drinking. Fever may be present. Evidence of a small wound may be visible on the skin or within the oral cavity. If the cellulitis becomes abscessed, a circumscribed fluctuation will be found at the lower border of the masseter muscle. There is a continuous rise of body temperature up to this point.

Etiology. Cellulitis and abscesses of the masseter muscle are always caused by pyogenic organims, usually streptococci, that gain access to the buccal muscles through wounds in the oral cavity or small cutaneous wounds.

Prognosis and Treatment. With resorption and resolution, the prognosis is good, even if abscessation has taken place. Treatment is like that for cellulitis of other body areas. A course of systemic antibiotics is always indicated and should be started promptly with the earliest signs of abscessation. The abscess should be lanced from the top downward to reduce the risk of severing the facial nerve, followed by treatment of the open wound in the usual fashion.

Sequellae. Chronic interstitial myositis sometimes occurs as a sequel to masseter cellulitis and abscessation.

2.1.5.3.3. Masseter Paralysis

See Sec. 2.1.14.2.2.

2.1.5.3.4. Trismus (Spasm of the Masseter Muscle)

Definition. Spasm of the masseter muscle is not a separate disease entity. It is a secondary condition whose primary cause lies mostly in metabolic infectious or toxic diseases of the central nervous system.

Symptoms. Typically there is a paroxysmal, bilateral spasm of the masseter muscles, which feel hard and board-like on palpation. The muscles are not swollen and may even be indrawn somewhat. The jaw appears 'locked' and the mouth can open by no more than 1—2 cm. Usually the horse has an anxious expression during the attacks, which may be of long or short duration before subsiding. Systemic effects are always present. The animal salivates excessively and is unable to eat or drink or does so with great difficulty; gradual emaciation develops.

Etiology. Trismus occurs as a result of central nervous disorders and is a characteristic early symptom of tetanus. Because the symptoms appear about the head, trismus is usually recognized early and tends to appear in response to sudden acoustic or visual stimuli. Sedatives can prevent the occurrence of attacks for a period of hours or days. Trismus may also occur as a sequel to other central nervous disorders and hypocalcemia.

Prognosis and Treatment. The prognosis depends mainly upon successful control of the primary infectious disease. The injection of local anesthetic into the masseter muscles is contraindicated, for this tends to cause additional lesions, provoke further spasms and could be a source of infection. Spasmolytic agents, especially neuroleptics, as well as central-acting muscle relaxants should be given for the control of spasm. Hypocalcemia should be treated appropriately.

2.1.5.3.5. Chronic Interstitial Myositis of the Masseter Muscle

Definition. This is a chronic muscle inflammation in which there is wasting of the muscle fibers that results in atrophy or even dystrophy of the masseter muscle, followed by the proliferation of interstitial connective tissue. The entire process leads to severe loss of function in the affected muscle.

Symptoms. Initially the masseter muscle feels abnormally hard and tense on the affected side. The first visible sign is a swelling, usually not tender, in the area between the facial crest, zygomatic arch and lower mandibular border; later marked atrophy is apparent in this area. The proliferation of interstitial connective tissue at the expense of muscle fibers leads to a decrease in the elasticity and contractility of the masseter muscle. The mouth cannot be completely closed, nor can it be opened sufficiently. The animal has difficulty in chewing, and if the disease is unilateral, chewing on one side leads to a marked angulation of the table surfaces of the cheek teeth and thus to a unilateral 'shear mouth'. Initially there is no impairment of general condition, but eventually gradual emaciation ensues.

Etiology. Chronic interstitial myositis develops gradually following wounds that have undergone irregular secondary healing. It is especially common after cellulitis and abscesses of the masseter muscle and its fascial planes. The disease may also be caused by long-standing dental and mandibular fistulae which communicate with the exterior through the masticatory muscles.

Differential Diagnosis. Similar phenomena are seen in long-standing inflammation of the temporomandibular joint, especially chronic degenerative joint disease of that joint. Mandibular fractures also can lead to chronic interstitial myositis.

Prognosis. A complete recovery cannot be anticipated.

Treatment. While the damage cannot be reversed, an attempt may be made to arrest the progress of the fibrosis by massage or by short-wave or microwave therapy. If the muscles are repeatedly and forcibly stretched with increasing trismus, there will be further tearing and additional shortening of the affected muscle, which has lost its contractile power.

Reference

Bolz, W.; Dietz, O.; Schleiter, H.; Teuscher, R.: Lehrbuch der Speziellen Veterinärchirurgie, Teil I (VEB Gustav Fischer Verlag, Jena 1975).

2.1.5.4. Diseases of the Mandible

See Sec. 2.1.17.1.3.

2.1.5.5. Diseases of the Temporomandibular Joint

2.1.5.5.1. Wounds of the Temporomandibular Joint

Definition. The temporomandibular joint is subject to puncture wounds and contusion.

Symptoms. A puncture wound of the temporomandibular joint causes no impairment of food prehension or mastication during the first few hours after the injury. If functional disturbances are observed initially, an associated chip fracture may be present at the joint margin. Clear, amber-colored synovial fluid flows from the wound when the horse moves its lower jaw. Sometimes air is aspirated into the joint during masticatory movements, and becomes mixed with the synovial fluid, forming a foam-like plug that exudes from the wound and dries.

Etiology. Puncture wounds of the temporomandibular joint in the horse are caused by the entry of pointed foreign objects, such as nails. Open contused wounds can occur during casting and may also be accompanied by the chip fractures at the joint margin.

Diagnosis. The diagnosis is based upon the symptoms described. The wound is considered 'fresh' only as long as clear, amber-colored synovial fluid is discharged.

Prognosis. The prognosis is good if the puncture wound is treated within 24 h after its occurrence. The prognosis is worse if associated chip fractures are present. If a puncture wound of the temporomandibular joint is not treated within 24 h, the disease progresses to an infectious arthritis with a poor prognosis.

Treatment. A puncture wound of the temporomandibular joint should be treated surgically within a few hours of its occurrence. Ideally, temporary immobilization of the wound and the joint is necessary if optimum healing is to occur. This is not practical in the horse, however. The temporomandibular joint is flushed with an antibiotic solution, and then 1 to 2 million I.U. of a crystalline penicillin solution are instilled. One should avoid entering the joint through the puncture wound if at all possible. It is better to pass a cannula into the synovial space through the joint capsule as far from the puncture wound as possible and inject the antibiotic into the joint until it appears in the wound. Very small puncture wounds are closed by applying a 10 % iodine ointment. This will produce a periarticular swelling that will close the wound. Larger wounds should be closed in two layers if possible, with the capsule sutured before the skin; a liquid sealant is then applied for extra protection. The joint can be rested temporarily by withholding food for about 24 h. Systemic antibiotics are administered for 4 to 5 days. No further local treatment is necessary. The skin sutures are removed when they begin to loosen.

Sequellae. Puncture wounds of the temporomandibular joint require careful treatment during the first 24 h to prevent the development of an infectious arthritis.

2.1.5.5.2. Temporomandibular Arthritis

Definition and Occurrence. There are three types of inflammation of the temporomandibular joint in the horse:
— acute serous temporomandibular arthritis,
— infectious (pyogenic) temporomandibular arthritis,
— chronic degenerative joint disease.

Symptoms. Acute serous temporomandibular arthritis is associated with disturbances of mastication. The affected joint is visibly swollen. On palpation the joint capsule protrudes above the groove of the joint margin. This is most obvious when the examination is done during mastication. Pain is elicited by pressure on the joint.

Infectious temporomandibular arthritis (figs. 2.1.5. — 8 and — 9) is usually secondary to a penetrating wound and is characterized by a worsening of the clinical signs 2 to 3 days after the injury has occurred. If the joint wound is still open, a turbid, yellowish synovial fluid is discharged which dries forming a crust below the joint. If one temporomandibular joint is sound, the horse chews rough feeds on the healthy side, with the result that mastication is less effective than normal. By the 4th or 5th day after the injury the area surrounding the temporomandibular joint is swollen, hot and very tender to pressure. The horse will resist violently if an attempt is made to open its mouth. The rectal temperature is mildly elevated starting on the 4th or 5th day after the onset of the disease and may be significantly elevated in advanced cases. Often the wound is sealed off by a plug of yellow, coagulated, synovial fluid by the 5th or 6th day. The entire cheek may be caked with dried synovial fluid.

If the joint disease progresses unchecked, the infectious arthritis leads to a capsular cellulitis and finally to a suppurative panarthritis. The meniscus of the temporomandibular joint undergoes degeneration. Severe emaciation develops, despite the

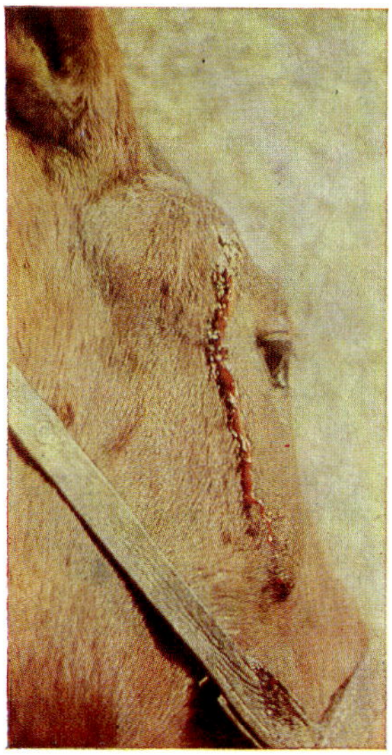

8

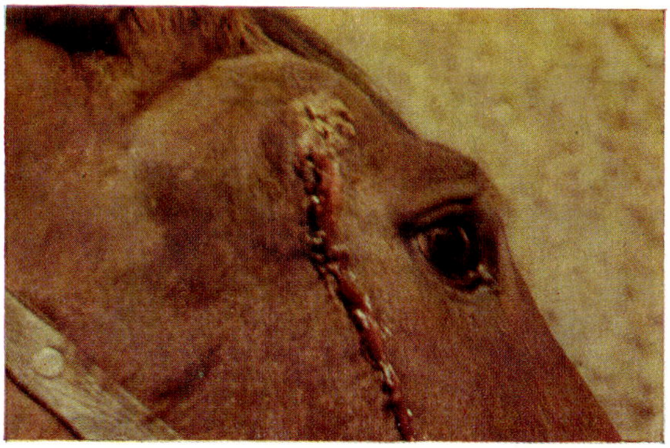

9

Fig. 2.1.5. — *8–9.* Suppurative arthritis of the temporomandibular joint.

fact that the horse is usually hungry and makes constant attempts to eat. Septicemia is not uncommon in horses with suppurative temporomandibular panarthritis.

In chronic degenerative joint disease, the transverse groove of the healthy joint is no longer palpable due to thickening of the joint margins. Only a relatively nontender bulge is felt directly at the temporomandibular joint. Opening of the mouth is extremely difficult and causes obvious pain. Frequently the mandible deviates toward the healthy side, so that when the lips are rolled back the upper and lower incisors are not in apposition. If the arthritis has been present for several weeks or even months, the occlusal surfaces of the incisors slant downward toward the healthy side when viewed from the front. Radiographs reveal periarticular changes about 8—10 weeks after the onset of the joint disease. Horses with chronic degenerative joint disease make slow, tentative chewing movements. Also typical are a shear-mouth erosion of the cheek teeth and a marked disuse atrophy of the masticatory muscles on the affected side. Gradual, severe emaciation develops.

Etiology. Acute serous temporomandibular arthritis may be caused by excessive joint strain due to the chewing or biting of hard objects. This is a relatively infrequent cause in the horse. It can also result from blunt trauma to the temporomandibular joint, such as may occur when the horse lays its head on a hard floor or strikes it repeatedly against a hard surface.

Septic temporomandibular arthritis almost always occurs as a sequel to neglected puncture wounds of that joint. The invading infectious organisms cause necrosis of the articular cartilage and meniscus.

Chronic degenerative joint disease occurs as a result of chronic excessive joint strain. Rarely does it arise from an acute serous arthritis. Other frequent causes are unilateral mastication as a result of dental disease, irreversible facial or trigeminal paralysis of the contralateral side, and chip fractures of the joint margins.

Diagnosis. Acute serous temporomandibular arthritis is diagnosed on the basis of clinical signs. In septic arthritis, an old puncture wound can usually be demonstrated, and characteristic clinical symptoms are present.

In chronic degenerative joint disease, radiographs taken 8—10 weeks after the onset of the disease will demonstrate the extent of the process.

Differential Diagnosis. Chronic degenerative joint disease may be confused with chronic interstitial myositis. In the latter, as in all muscular atrophies, the affected joint is abnormally prominent.

Prognosis. Prognosis is favorable for the acute, serous form and guarded to poor for infectious arthritis. Even after the inflammation has subsided, there is always a chance that degenerative joint disease will develop, resulting in chronic life-long feeding trouble. In degenerative joint disease the prognosis is always guarded to poor.

Treatment. During the first hours of an acute serous temporomandibular arthritis, anti-inflammatory treatment is administered. The cause of the inflammation should be identified and corrected.

On the 2nd to 3rd day of an infectious temporomandibular arthritis, one should try to instill crystalline antibiotic solutions into the joint at least twice daily. Meanwhile, hot packs or rubefacient solutions should be applied to the joint. If treatment is not initiated until the disease has reached the capsular cellulitis or panarthritic stage, partial resection or opening of the joint is indicated. In this procedure the joint capsule is opened parallel to the joint margin. Then the joint cavity is pried open, and an attempt is made to excise as much of the meniscus as possible, also removing the cartilage from both articular surfaces. The joint cavity is then packed with gauze soaked in an antibiotic solution. The skin is then sutured. The gauze packing is left in place for several days. A regimen of open wound treatment is followed until granulation healing occurs. The aim is to construct a pseudarthrosis to replace the diseased joint. Infectious arthritis is frequently followed by chronic degenerative joint disease.

In chronic degenerative joint disease, local treatment with rubefacient ointments (iodine, camphor, bi-iodate and cantharidin) may be tried for symptomatic relief. Intra-articular injections of glucocorticoids may also be of temporary benefit. Forcible opening of the mouth in an attempt to mobilize the joint usually brings only temporary improvement, and afterward the condition may worsen. A joint resection may be attempted as a last resort.

Sequellae. The foregoing guidelines should be followed in all types of temporomandibular joint disease, for they offer the only means of preserving the athletic as well as breeding potential of the affected horse.

2.1.5.6. Diseases of the Salivary Glands and Salivary Ducts

2.1.5.6.1. Wounds of the Salivary Glands and their Excretory Ducts

Occurrence. These wounds occur in the region of the parotid and mandibular glands. Wounds of the salivary ducts affect mainly the 'Stensen's duct', which extends from the parotid gland to the salivary papilla in the buccal vestibule within the oral cavity. These wounds usually occur in the area of the ramus of the mandible.

Symptoms. Puncture wounds in the region of the salivary glands produce few obvious clinical signs. Sometimes the surrounding area shows circumscribed swelling and is tender for several days after the injury. Bleeding is not characteristic. If the puncture wound becomes infected, cellulitis and salivary gland abscesses may develop, producing a clinical picture of parotitis. The entire region of the salivary glands extending down below the mandible is diffusely swollen and tender. Head movements are painful, and affected horses usually stand with the head extended. The increasing parotid swelling may exert pressure on the pharynx, causing dysphagia. If abscesses develop from the inflammation, the swelling becomes fluctuant. In the case of larger incised wounds, the glandular tissue may be visible. There may be a salivary discharge from the wound that increases during feeding. In contused wounds with glandular tissue necrosis, the salivary discharge may account for the major portion of the wound exudate.

If the salivary duct has been completely severed, a large amount of saliva will dribble from the wound. During feeding the saliva may even spurt from the wound in a stream. Wounds of Stensen's duct usually occur at the point where the duct curves from the inner to outer aspect of the mandible.

Diagnosis and Differential Diagnosis. Clinical symptoms should provide an adequate basis for diagnosis. It is difficult to differentiate an injury of the parotid gland from one of the mandibular gland.

Prognosis and Treatment. The prognosis is always good. Initially the horse should be fasted for a time. Because the secretion of saliva is reflexly activated when nearby animals are fed, the animal should be temporarily housed in separate quarters. Small puncture wounds in the region of a salivary gland do not require treatment initially. For animals that are not actively immunized, tetanus prophylaxis is indicated. The puncture track and its opening are painted liberally with iodine. If cellulitis is already present in the region of the parotid or mandibular salivary gland, the application of camphor or iodine ointments is indicated. In addition, large doses of penicillin are given for 4 to 5 days. This is usually sufficient to prevent the necrosis of glandular tissue and abscessation. If abscessation is unavoidable, the absesses are not incised until the 'point' of the abscess is thin.

Fresh incised wounds in the region of the salivary gland or salivary duct are sutured to ensure primary healing. We do not recommend excision of the wound edges with subsequent packing or drainage. Systemic antibiotic protection is maintained for several days. The salivary duct may occasionally be repaired with fine silk sutures.

2.1.5.6.2. Salivary Fistula

Definition. The salivary fistula is marked by a funnel-shaped wound from which there is a continuous salivary discharge. Discharge occurs especially during feeding. The fistulous tract can be reached by inserting a probe into the wound opening. The base of the fistula is formed either by salivary gland tissue or by the excretory duct of a salivary gland.

Symptoms. The track of an old salivary-gland or -duct wound undergoes epithelialization instead of healing. The result is a salivary fistula with a small opening from which saliva drips or even spurts. The subcutaneous tissue surrounding the fistulous opening undergoes a fibrous thickening. If this tissue can be raised between the fingers, a scar-tissue cord about the thickness of a pencil will be felt extending into the glandular parenchyma. In some cases this cord is quite short, and if located at the mandibular border it may extend into the excretory duct of the salivary gland. Systemic signs do not occur.

The *diagnosis* is based on symptoms and generally presents no difficulties.

Prognosis. It is favorable. The lesion cannot heal however without operative treatment.

Treatment. The affected horse is housed away from other animals. One or two doses of a drug are administered to inhibit salivary secretion. If the fistula extends into the glandular tissue, one may first roughen it with caustic agents in an attempt to promote the formation of adhesions. If the salivary discharge is scant, this method alone may work. A rubefacient ointment may be rubbed into the area surrounding the fistulous tract with the object of inducing an inflammation that will occlude it. Alternatively, the area may be infiltrated with agents that promote connective tissue proliferation, such as tincture of iodine or Lugol's solution. Sometimes this will also cause the fistula to close by swelling.

In fistulae of the salivary duct, the edges of the channel can be excised down to the duct to enable a suture repair of the duct system. If this is unsuccessful, ligation of the salivary duct may prove necessary. The resulting accumulation of secretions leads to a temporary distension of the gland and ultimately to pressure atrophy. Another method is to obliterate the gland by injecting tincture of iodine into the salivary duct through the wound. This is best done with sterile 60 % glucose solutions, 20 % saline or 30 % alcohol. These injections are repeated if necessary at one-week intervals. An attempt may be made to transpose the fistulous tract or fistulous opening into the oral cavity to form a new salivary duct orifice. If carefully done, this operation is almost always successful.

2.1.5.6.3. Ectasia of the Salivary Duct

Definition and Occurrence. Salivary duct ectasia refers to an overall dilatation of the excretory duct of the parotid gland (Stensen's duct).

Symptoms. The parotid duct is dilatated, in some cases to thumb size, over its entire course or only in its anterior portion. On palpation it slides back and forth on the anterior border of the masseter muscle. It is soft, having somewhat the consistency of an engorged vein, and the saliva within it is displaced when pressure is applied. No systemic signs occur.

Etiology. Salivary duct ectasia is caused by an obstruction of the salivary flow. Inflammation of the oral mucosa, chemical injuries and wounds can cause a stenosis due to scarring of the salivary duct orifice in the region of the papilla. This interferes with the excretion of saliva. Sometimes oat grains or chaff can become lodged in the papilla, leading to inflammation and subsequent obstructive stenosis. In very rare cases the salivary duct orifice may become obstructed by salivary calculi.

Treatment. An attempt is made to probe the orifice with the animal standing and sedated or recumbent. A narrowed orifice is incised with a probe-ended scalpel. The salivary papilla is found behind the buccal pouch at the level of the 2nd to 5th maxillary cheek tooth. The bulging duct may also be located within the oral cavity and incised at a favorable site. The incision should be at least 1 to $1^1/_2$ cm long. This artificially created internal fistula will provide an outlet for continuous salivary drainage. The constant secretions prevent wound closure, and so no sutures need be placed between the salivary duct wall and oral mucosa.

2.1.5.6.4. Sialoliths (Salivary Calculi)

Definition. Salivary calculi are formed in the parotid duct by the precipitation of calcium carbonate. They cause an obstructive stenosis and ectasia of the salivary duct.

Symptoms. The calculi may occur singly or in groups. Individual calculi may act as a valve in the distended duct, shutting off the flow of saliva to the oral cavity. But several smaller calculi arranged like string-of-beads are more commonly found in the horse. A thumb-size cord may be found running obliquely forward and upward, terminating approximately at the salivary papilla. With digital palpation this duct can be followed a short distance caudally on the inner aspect of the mandible. It often feels hard and is nontender. On examination of the oral cavity, ulcers and scars are seen in the region of the salivary papilla. The papilla itself is sometimes enlarged, and a stonelike object may be detected on probing. Frequently, pathogenic organisms migrate from the oral cavity into the engorged salivary duct, and an inflammation develops. If external pressure is applied to the congested duct, a yellowish, turbid fluid is exuded from the papilla. In extreme cases, abscessation can occur. The calculi vary in size from a cherry stone to a fist. It is not uncommon to find a foreign body at the center of the calculus, which served as a nidus. Adjacent calculi within a salivary duct show facet-like erosions at points of mutual contact. Most are white or yellowish in color, have a plaster-like consistency or are stony hard. Atrophy of the parotid gland may be seen in long-standing cases.

Etiology. Most salivary calculi are caused by the entry of oat grains, chaff, awns, spicules, wood splinters or other small foreign bodies into the salivary duct through the papilla. There they act as a nidus for the precipitation of calcium salts that are contained in the saliva. It takes months for the salivary calculi to reach a corresponding size. Sometimes sloughed epithelial cells from the salivary duct can act as a nidus.

Treatment. The horse is cast onto the healthy side. If multiple small, 'string-of-beads' calculi are present and are palpable externally, an attempt is made to remove them first by massaging the duct in the direction of the papilla. If the papilla is too narrow for this, it is expanded by making an incision from within the oral cavity. The duct should be opened only as far as necessary to allow delivery of the calculi. If the calculi are found to be lodged firmly in the duct, then a needle is inserted into the engorged duct from the outside, and mineral oil is injected as a lubricant to facilitate the removal, Once the calculi have been removed, the injection needle is again used to irrigate the patent duct. In most cases, very large solitary calculi cannot be removed in this way, and it becomes necessary to open the salivary duct by an incision from the outside. After the calculus is removed, the duct is probed in the direction of the papilla to restore patency. The final step is closure of the salivary duct with closely-spaced sutures, taking care to invaginate the wound edges during the repair. The skin is also closed with closely-spaced interrupted sutures. With careful technique, this procedure will usually assure primary healing.

Reference

Bolz, W.; Dietz, O.; Schleiter, H.; Teuscher, R.: Lehrbuch der Speziellen Veterinärchirurgie, 2. Aufl. (VEB Gustav Fischer Verlag, Jena 1975).

2.1.5.7. Diseases of the Hyoid Bone

2.1.5.7.1. Fractures of the Hyoid Bone

Definition. These mainly involve simple or multiple, closed or open fractures of the basihyoid, its lingual process and the thyrohyoid. Fractures of the kerato-, epi- or stylohyoid may also occur if there is an associated comminuted fracture of the mandible. Fractures of the hyoid are uncommon, situated as it is between the mandibular rami, and it is somewhat protected.

Symptoms. The tongue hangs flaccidly from the mouth, accompanied by the drooling of saliva. This is especially typical in fractures of the basihyoid and lingual process. When the tip of the tongue is pulled, the horse is unable to draw it completely back into the mouth. All lingual movements cause obvious pain. The fracture hematoma and associated inflammation cause swelling of the intermandibular area. The horse is unable to eat or drink or does so with great difficulty. If a bolus of food is pushed into the mouth over the dorsum of the tongue, deglutition also appears to be very painful. Bony fragments may perforate the floor of the mouth or lateral pharyngeal wall, which in acute cases causes hemorrhage from the oral cavity or a discharge of frothy, blood-tinged saliva. If portions of the fractured hyoid bone protrude into the guttural pouch or larynx, a uni- or bilateral epistaxis may be present. Opening the mouth for examination is resisted, and compression of the hyoid bone or posterior intermandibular area from the exterior causes obvious pain. Crepitation is seldom detected. Guttural pouch empyema with a unilateral purulent nasal discharge can occur as a late symptom of hyoid bone fractures. Trismus and a fetid breath odor are usually present in such cases. The tongue shows a marked unilateral atrophy with an ipsilateral disturbance of sensation [Hertsch and Wissdorf, 1975]. The atrophy is usually accompanied by folding of the lingual mucosa.

Etiology. Hyoid fractures usually have a traumatic etiology and generally result from direct violence to the intermandibular area. They may be associated with mandibular fractures. Inhumane measures to subdue a fractious horse by forcibly withdrawing or even tying the tongue can provoke hyoid fractures. In rare cases kicks from other horses or the use of poor technique in the repulsion of lower cheek teeth are responsible.

Differential Diagnosis. Hyoid fractures must be differentiated from tears of the lingual muscles and lingual paralysis from neurogenic causes — the former by inspection and palpation, the latter by an absence of swelling, loss of mobility and absence of pain.

Diagnosis. The history and clinical picture are diagnostic. The horse may be cast and the mouth radiographed to demonstrate the fracture.

Prognosis. The prognosis is poor for bilateral fractures of the basihyoid, because food intake and deglutition prevent immobilization of the fragments. Death from starvation is common. Unilateral subcutaneous or submucosal fractures heal in 4 to 8 weeks after fibrous union has occurred. Open, infected fractures carry a poor prognosis, for they tend to cause cellulitis or hyoid bone necrosis with subsequent fistulization.

Treatment. In open fractures the wound is examined, and foreign bodies including loose bone fragments are removed. The fracture is reduced, and internal fixation with cerclage wire may be attempted. Antibiotics are administered for 6 to 8 days. In unilateral closed fractures the animal is fed by stomach tube on the 1st day, and later, liquid feeds and mash are give. After 3 to 4 weeks the horse should again be able to feed normally. Fixation wires are removed after about 8 weeks, if indicated (e.g. drainage and fistulation).

Sequellae. In complicated and multiple hyoid bone fractures, destruction of the animal should be considered if there has been no improvement in local or general condition after 3 to 4 weeks.

2.1.5.7.2. Hyoid Bone Necrosis and Hyoid Bone Fistula

Definition. Here a bony or cartilaginous necrosis occurs, usually as a secondary condition. It leads to the formation of fistulae in the intermandibular area.

Symptoms. The first sign is a circumscribed, hard swelling in the intermandibular area that goes on to abscessation. The abscess cavity does not fully heal by granulation, and a fistulous tract remains. This tract may be followed through indurated scar tissue to the base of the fistula, formed by necrotic hyoid bone or hyoid cartilage. The fistulous opening is located in the mid-intermandibular area approximately at the level of the 2nd molar. The pus has a carious odor, is yellowish-gray in color and has a watery consistency. Abnormalities of mastication or deglutition are seldom present. A probe encounters the necrotic portion of the hyoid bone at a depth of 5—15 cm. The base of the fistula is rough and hard or cartilaginous. Sometimes the necrotic focus can be localized by simultaneous examination of the oral cavity.

Etiology. Local hyoid bone necrosis or a subsequent fistula may be the result of a complicated fracture. But the disease may also occur following intermandibular cellulitis or abscessation of the mandibular lymph nodes.

Differential Diagnosis. Mandibular and dental fistulae and intermandibular staphylococcal infections must be excluded.

Diagnosis. If probing does not yield a definitive result, a fistulogram is recommended.

Prognosis. The prognosis is good if the necrosis is limited to the lingual process of the basihyoid, or if the continuity of the hyoid apparatus is preserved.

Treatment. The fistulous tract is incised in the middle of the intermandibular area, obtaining exposure sufficient for digital palpation or, preferably, direct visual inspection of the base of the fistula. Necrotic cartilage is excised with a blunt-ended knife, and necrotic bone tissue removed with a gouge or curette. In some cases it is best to initially extirpate the mandibular lymph nodes, as this will improve exposure of the operative area as well as facilitate the control of hemorrage. Hemorrhage can be profuse at times. The wound is packed, sutured, and antibiotics are administered postoperatively for 5 to 6 days.

Sequellae. Careful operative treatment with the liberal excision of necrotic tissues usually ensures a complete recovery.

Reference

Hertsch, B.; Wissdorf, H.: Beitrag zur Behandlung von Frakturen am Kopf des Pferdes. II. Zungenbeinfrakturen. Dtsch. Tierärztl. Wschr. *82:* 473 (1975).

2.1.5.8. Diseases of the Pharynx

2.1.5.8.1. Pharyngitis

Definition. Pharyngitis is a catarrhal, purulent, diphtheroid or necrotizing inflammation of the pharyngeal mucosa. It may be superficial or may involve the submucosa. It may affect the oral portion of the soft palate as well as the lymphatic tissue of the dorsal pharyngeal recess.

Symptoms and Diagnosis. The horse stands with the head extended. It eats slowly and cautiously and may interrupt its feeding at frequent intervals. During swallowing the head is extended even further or is moved in a nodding or shaking fashion. Affected horses often move about restlessly and paw the ground with their forelegs. In severe cases food is dropped from the mouth or regurgitated through the nostrils, the animal makes frequent, tentative jaw movements and may refuse to eat or drink altogether. There is a bilateral mucoid or purulent nasal discharge that may contain particles of feed. The throat feels warm on palpation, and compression of the throat with both hands elicits moderate to severe pain. The mandibular lymph nodes are swollen, and the intermandibular space is obliterated. Unilateral swellings or deeper masses may indicate the presence of foreign bodies, neoplasms or abscesses. The horse usually resists the insertion of a laryngoscope. This permits only a fleeting view in the standing animal. It may be necessary to anesthetize the horse for laryngoscopic examination. The inspection and subsequent palpation of the pharynx with the aid of a mouth speculum (if necessary under xylazine-promazine sedation) provides more immediate information. Severe redness, swelling, mucus, pus, and a diphtheroid coating may be evident. There may be swelling of the soft palate and epiglottis. The epiglottis may appear abnormally upright. Foul-smelling, decomposing food particles may also be found.

A painful cough is not uncommon. The body temperature is initially normal, but fever and depression may appear later if the pharyngitis becomes severe. Abscessation of the regional lymph nodes is rare.

Etiology. Pharyngitis seldom occurs in the horse as a primary entity. It may result from injury during the swallowing of sharp objects. At one time, primary pharyngitis was commonly caused by the use of balling guns. In rare cases gasterophilus larvae are found on the lateral or dorsal pharyngeal wall. Horses rarely ingest materials sufficiently irritating or caustic to inflame the pharynx. A fibrinous, diphtheroid pharyngitis has been observed following stable fires. Pharyngitis mainly occurs in combination with infectious diseases of the upper respiratory tract such as influenza, viral arteritis, herpesvirus infection, strangles and bacterial inflammation.

Differential Diagnosis. Tumors of the pharynx are distinguished by an absence of pain. In pharyngeal paralysis there is a loss of the swallowing reflex normally present when a foreign object is inserted into the pharyngeal area, pain and redness are absent, and the head is not held extended.

An esophageal obstruction can be excluded by passing a nasogastric tube. Diseases of the guttural pouch are excluded by endoscopy, localization, tenderness, and by the absence of nasal discharge when the head is lowered.

Pharyngeal and sub-epiglottic cysts are most commonly seen in foals between the age of 6 months and 1 year.

Soft palate defects, including cleft palate, should be considered in foals and ponies. They can be excluded by manual or digital palpation of the oral cavity, taking into account the animal's history.

A roughened mucosa covered with multiple small nodules is characteristic of pharyngitis.

Treatment. Soft or liquid feeds should be offered. In severe cases the horse must be fasted or force fed for 1 to 2 days. The water and energy balance can be regulated with intravenous electrolyte and glucose solutions. Usually the passage of a nasogastric tube is painful. With the head lowered, the pharynx may be flushed with boric-acid solution, potassium permanganate or H_2O_2 solutions (3 %). In purulent cases, the pharynx is also sprayed with solutions containing chloramphenicol and prednisolone. This may be repeated 2 or 3 times daily. If fever or other systemic signs are present, high doses of antibiotics are administered until the fever subsides. Topical agents applied externally are not much favored today due to hair loss associated with their use.

Flushing the pharynx with Lugol's solution has also proved beneficial, in certain cases.

Prognosis. Acute primary pharyngitis runs a course of 8 to 14 days. Purulent pharyngitis may go on to abscessation before resolving. Secondary pharyngitis will subside once the primary disorder has been cured.

Sequellae. If secondary pharyngitis of viral origin is suspected, the affected horse should be isolated from other animals until the cause has been ascertained.

2.1.5.8.2. Foreign Bodies in the Pharynx

Definition. Large, hard root crops (sugar beets), corn cobs and foreign bodies that are too big to swallow can cause obstruction of the pharynx. While horses are disinclined to ingest sharp foreign bodies, such objects are capable of lodging in the pharyngeal wall, soft palate or root of the tongue, where they cause the formation of foreign-body abscesses.

Symptoms. While attempting to eat a large vegetable or piece of fruit, the animal suddenly coughs, shakes its head and may drool saliva. The breathing becomes stertorous in some cases.

Pointed foreign bodies such as nails, wood splinters or pieces of wire cause wounds when ingested. The foreign bodies migrate rapidly into surrounding tissues. The clinical manifestations are those of pharyngitis with subsequent cellulitis and abscessation in the pharyngeal space.

Diagnosis and Treatment. The diagnosis is based upon a manual examination of the oral cavity. A large bolus or foreign body lodged in the pharynx is removed at once.

If it is suspected that pointed foreign bodies have entered the mucosa (localized pain and swelling, internal abscessation), radiographs should be taken in at least two planes. Such objects are frequently radiopaque.

The object is removed through an incision made from within the oral cavity or from the exterior, depending on its localization.

Differential Diagnosis. See Sec. 2.1.5.8.1. and 2.1.5.8.3.

Prognosis and Sequellae. Recovery is rapid and complete.

2.1.5.8.3. Wounds, Phlegmons and Abscesses of the Pharynx

Definition. Perforating wounds in particular lead to cellulitis and abscesses of the pharynx.

Symptoms. With larger wounds of the pharynx, there may be transitory bleeding from the nose, or the saliva may be frothy and blood-tinged. Difficult swallowing is apparent. Wounds that perforate the pharyngeal mucosa lead to pharyngeal cellulitis. If the inner fascial planes of the pharynx are perforated, intermuscular cellulitis develops, causing severe dysphagia. If the perforation extends to the outer pharyngeal fascia, a diffuse peripharyngeal cellulitis develops which spreads to the respiratory portion of the pharynx leading to dyspnea and asphyxia.

The pharyngeal region is swollen, and the animal stands with the neck low and the head extended. Radiographs may disclose metallic foreign bodies and abscesses accompanied by gas formation. Radiographs will not reveal wood splinters, plastic objects, awns or light metals. Retropharyngeal abscesses develop within 8 to 10 days, or somewhat sooner if local hyperemia is artificially induced. A fluctuating bulge appears in the middle of the parotid area, or a swelling appears in the submaxillary region. Abscessation of the mandibular lymph nodes is not uncommon.

Etiology. Cellulitis of the pharynx can occur following wound infections from the inhumane use of sticks and whips, the faulty use of dental rasps or chisels, and accidental abrasions during the use of certain dental grinders. Injuries from perforating foreign bodies may also be responsible in rare cases.

Differential Diagnosis. All degrees of pharyngitis must be excluded.

Treatment. Hemorrhages usually stop spontaneously in a matter of minutes. Cellulitis and abscesses are managed according to general principles of wound management. The spread of wound infection may be prevented with systemic antibiotics.

The *prognosis* is good following the removal of foreign bodies and abscessation.

Reference

HAMILTON, D.: Pharyngeal rupture in a horse. J. Amer. vet. med. Assoc. *162:* 466 (1973).

2.1.5.8.4. Chronic Follicular (Lymphoid) Pharyngitis

Definition. This is a chronic follicular or papillary inflammation of the pharyngeal mucosa that may lead to constriction of the upper airways. The disease is most common in 2- to 3-year-olds, although any older, fit, athletic horse is susceptible.

Symptoms. The first clinical signs are harsh inspiratory and expiratory noises that increase with exercise. Affected horses may suffer severe coughing fits at the start of and following physical exertion. The respiratory rate is generally increased and takes some time to return to normal. Sometimes there is only a serous or mucoid nasal discharge that disappears for a time, only to recur after coughing.

Usually the animals are afebrile and do not appear clinically ill while in their stall. There is slight swelling of the mandibular nodes. Coughing can be stimulated by compression of the larynx. No abnormal lung sounds are heard.

Etiology. Chronic follicular lymphoid hyperplasia of the pharynx occurs as a sequel to acute viral or bacterial infections of the upper airways. The disease is frequently seen weeks or months after the animal has recovered from an attack of influenza or equine rhinopneumonitis. The nasopharynx of the horse is lined with lymphoid tissue. Any irritation of this tissue by various noxious stimuli can lead to follicular lymphoid hyperplasia, combined in some cases with connective tissue proliferation and the development of polyps. Polyps may appear on the pharyngeal wall and in the dorsal pharyngeal recess.

Diagnosis. The diagnosis is made from the history and laryngoscopic examination. The laryngoscope reveals either edematous, hyperemic or ulcerated areas with swollen lymph follicles, or fibrotic changes. The affected mucosal areas have a grayish-yellow color. On digital palpation the mucosa feels rough, dotted, with tiny nodules.

Differential Diagnosis. Endoscopy is useful for excluding laryngeal hemiplegia, soft palate paresis, epiglottic entrapment, and acute inflammation of the pharynx and guttural pouch regions. In most cases streptococcal organisms can be isolated from the lesions. Individual follicles surrounded by unchanged mucosa may also occur in the normal equine pharynx, but the clinical changes become more intense as the follicles or polyps increase in number.

Prognosis and Treatment. The prognosis is somewhat guarded, for it is difficult to predict which treatment will be most effective. Sometimes regression will occur with $1^1/_2$ to 2 months of rest. The nasopharynx may be sprayed with organic iodine solutions. This treatment appears to be successful only in the early stage of the disease, however. RAKER [1976] has evaluated a spray containing dimethyl sulfoxide (DMSO), prednisolone and Furacin® (nitrofurazone) and found it to be effective. RAKER also notes that electrocauterization yields excellent results, the object being to induce a severe inflammation and consequent necrosis that will lead to resolution of the hyperplastic follicles. General anesthesia and a laryngotomy are required for this treatment. Other authors, such as MCALLISTER and BLAKESLEE [1977], report good results with 50 % trichloroacetic acid applied topically through a tube passed into the ventral meatus with the horse standing and sedated. Care must be taken to prevent the highly caustic acid from coming in contact with the laryngeal cartilage. The treatment is repeated after 3 to 5 days until necrosis of the affected mucosal areas has been achieved. Four to six weeks' stable rest is necessary following treatment.

References

BLAKESLEE, J. R.; OLSEN, R. G.; MCALLISTER, E. S.; FASSBENDER, J.; DENNIS, R.: Evidence of respiratory tract infection induced by equine herepesvirus, type 2, in the horse. Canad. J. Microbiol. *21:* 1940 (1975).

FLOER, V. W.; SCHMIDT, R.; PETZOLDT, K.: Mikrobiologische Untersuchungen zur Frage von Herpesvirusinfektionen des oberen Respirationstraktes des Pferdes. Dtsch. Tierärztl. Wschr. *80:* 49 (1973).

HARVEY, C. E.; RAKER, C. W.; O'BRIEN, J. A.: Pharyngeal and laryngeal diseases causing airway obstruction in the dog and horse. Arch. Amer. Coll. Vet. Surg. *2:* 15 (1973).

LARSON, V. L.; SORENSON, D. K.: The respiratory system. In: Equine medicine and surgery, 2nd ed. (Amer. Vet. Public. Inc., Wheaton/Ill. 1972).

MCALLISTER, E. S.; BLAKESLEE, J. R.: Clinical observations of pharyngitis in the horse. J. Amer. vet. med. Assoc. *7:* 739 (1977).

MCGUIRE, T. C.; CRAWFORD, T. B.; HENSON, J. B.: Prevalence of antibodies to herpesvirus Types 1 and 2, arteritis and infectious anemia viral antigens in equine serum. Amer. J. Vet. Res. *35:* 181 (1974).

RAKER, C. W.: Diseases of the pharynx. Mod. Vet. Pract. *57:* 396 (1976).

ROEDER, P. L.; SCOTT, G. R.: The prevalence of equine herpesvirus 2 infections. Vet. Rec. *96:* 404 (1975).

STUDDERT, M. J.: Comperative aspects of equine herpesviruses. Cornell Vet. *64:* 94 (1974).

TURNER, A. J.; STUDDERT, M. J.; PETERSON, J. E.: Persistence of equine herpesvirus in experimentally infected horses and the experimental induction of abortion. Austral. Vet. J. *46:* 90 (1970).

2.1.5.8.5. Pharyngeal Cysts, Epiglottic Cysts

Definition. Pharyngeal cysts are rounded, fluid-filled structures that form in the retrolingual region at the entrance to the pharynx. Epiglottic cysts occur as solitary structures and may be located in the glossoepiglottic fold extending from the base of the epiglottis to the root of the tongue, on the free border of the epiglottis, or in rare cases on the isthmus faucium extending from the last cheek teeth to the base of the epiglottis.

Symptoms. The symptoms have a gradual onset and usually appear in young, growing horses. The first signs are dysphagia and dyspneic episodes that may accompany forced respiration. Episodes may occur without apparent cause. The cysts gradually become pedunculated as a result of the tension exerted on them during deglutition. The mucous membrane over the cyst is altered by thickening and erosion. Symptoms become more severe as the pedicle elongates. During deglutition the cyst is drawn into the oropharynx, causing a partial or complete obstruction with associated food regurgitation. Cysts with very long pedicles may even be swallowed, and on entering the pharynx they act, with the epiglottis, to obstruct the larynx. This causes immediate choking and spasmodic coughing in an effort to expel the cyst and clear the airway. Finally, the cyst can enter the larynx during inspiration and likewise precipitate a choking fit.

The prolonged presence of smaller cysts that partially obstruct the airway causes chronic interference with swallowing and eventually leads to aspiration pneumonia.

Diagnosis. With the mouth widely opened and the tongue withdrawn, larger cysts can be seen as rounded, grayish-white or reddish structures. Cysts near the epiglottis can be clearly identified with the laryngoscope. All cysts, regardless of their location, are easily palpated in the anesthetized horse by inserting the hand, with fingers together, into the pharyngeal cavity. Even in the 6-month-old foal, the cysts may reach the size of an egg. Many are loculated. Their contents are mucoid and gray to yellow in color.

Etiology. The growths represent retention cysts of the mucosal glands, epithelial mucosal cysts, or remnants of the thyroglossal duct.

Treatment. Incising or crushing the cysts will lead to a recurrence. They must be resected at the base of the pedicle. The simplest and safest way of doing this is by means of a snare introduced through the mouth.

In rare cases the cyst must be approached through a laryngotomy. The *prognosis* is good.

Reference

ÜBERREITER, O.: Zungengrundzysten, ausgehend von Resten des Ductus thyreoglossus beim Pferd. Wien. tierärztl. Mschr. *55:* 175 (1968).

2.1.5.8.6. Defects of the Soft Palate

Definition and Occurrence. Cleft palate or palatoschisis is the term applied to a failure of closure of the embryonic palatine fissure due to deficient development of the palatine process of the maxillary bone. This anomaly is rare in the horse (fig. 2.1.5. — 10).

More frequent are congenital defects or a cleft involving the soft palate.

Symptoms. The defects are usually apparent a few days after birth. Milk escapes through the foal's nose when it attempts to nurse. The foal chokes, snorts, sneezes and coughs. Its nutritional status progressively deteriorates. Dehydration also becomes apparent. The animal's condition may become critical when it starts to take solid foods. Food is regurgitated through the nostrils, and any water that is taken is ejected from both nostrils in a stream. This leads to a bilateral, chronic rhinitis with a mucopurulent discharge. Symptoms of aspiration pneumonia may also appear.

Diagnosis. The extent of the soft palate defect is easily assessed with the aid of a mouth speculum, tongue depressor and illuminator. The defect or cleft always starts at the free margin of the soft palate. Sometimes they are unilateral and sometimes they are located on the midline. The margins of the soft palate are usually thickened. When a nasogastric tube is passed, mucus or ingesta is pushed back into the pharyngeal cavity.

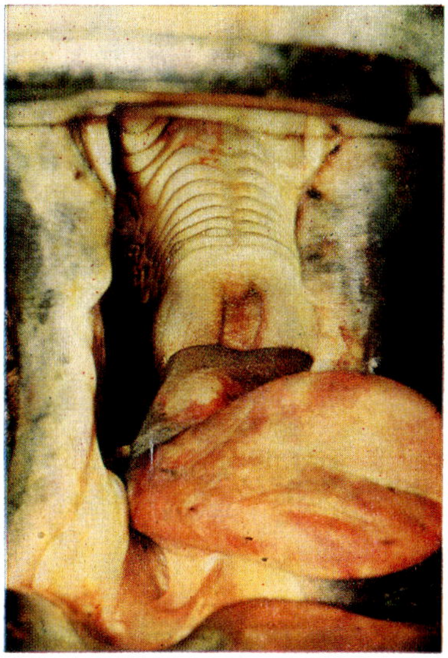

Fig. 2.1.5. — 10. Cleft palate.

Differential Diagnosis. Pharyngitis must be excluded. Esophageal spasm must also be considered, although this tends to affect only adult animals. Cardiospasm is rare in horses.

Treatment. Access to the soft palate is gained by means of a mandibular symphysiotomy. The operation is performed under general anesthesia with the animal in dorsal recumbency. An incision is made down to the mandibular symphysis, taking care not to split the lower lip, and from there the skin incision is carried inward along the left or right ramus into the rear portion of the intermandibular area. From there the retrolingual area is exposed on either the right or left side, and the mandibular symphysis is divided with a saw to obtain broad access to the pharynx and soft palate. The edges of the cleft soft palate are freshened, and the two mucosal layers are separated. Then the cleft is closed in two layers with silk sutures. The oral cavity is closed in layers. The divided symphysis is reapproximated and fixed with Kirschner wires, compression screws or cerclage wire passed around the incisors and through drill holes in the bone. Wound healing is generally complete in 10 to 14 days, during which time a course of systemic antibiotics is given.

Prognosis. It is guarded, although suture dehiscence is sometimes unavoidable and may necessitate reoperation.

Sequellae. Soft palate defects and clefts are usually inherited, and so animals with repaired defects should not be used for breeding.

References

Stickle, R. L.; Goble, D. O.; Braden, T.: Chirurgische Korrektur eines gespaltenen Gaumensegels beim Fohlen. Vet. Med. and Small Animal Clinician *68:* 159 (1973).

Hofmeyer, C. F. B.: Eine Technik zur Wiederherstellung des gespaltenen Gaumens. J. South African vet. med. Assoc. *30:* 149 (1959).

2.1.5.8.7. Tumors of the Pharynx and Tonsils

Carcinomas of the tonsils are very rare in the horse. Older horses are affected. Foci soon become palpable in the lymph nodes of the neck and throat region as a result of rapid metastasis.

Clinical signs include anorexia, cachexia, dysphagia, coughing and dyspnea. The diagnosis can be verified by the histologic examination of biopsy material. The prognosis is poor.

2.1.5.8.8. Epiglottic Entrapment

Definition. Epiglottic entrapment is an entrapping of the epiglottis as a result of displacement of the arytenoepiglottic fold. In the normal horse this structure is a broad, movable fold which is located ventral to the epiglottis and attaches to its lateral margins.

Symptoms. The horse exhibits sudden symptoms of upper airway obstruction, including coughing and head-shaking. If eating or drinking is attempted, the coughing fits become more severe.

Etiology. The cause of epiglottic entrapment is unknown. It is thought that hypoplasia of the epiglottis may be involved.

Differential Diagnosis and *Diagnosis.* Laryngoscopic examination is necessary for a definitive diagnosis. The epiglottis appears to be displaced downward, and its margins and apex cannot be seen. This also applies to the epiglottic vasculature, which normally is distinct. Soft palate elongation and roaring can be excluded on the basis of laryngoscopic findings. In intermittent dorsal displacement of the soft palate the pharynx and larynx have a normal endoscopic appearance; this symptom ordinarily occurs only in race horses or gaited breeds.

Treatment and Prognosis. The diagnosis can be confirmed by examination through the oral cavity with the horse standing and sedated. In the anesthetized horse the entrapped epiglottis can occasionally be freed by digital manipulation. Surgical correction is carried out through a laryngotomy in the dorsally recumbent horse. The arytenoepiglottic fold is grasped after first rotating the epiglottis 90° and is resected from the arytenoid cartilage to the median plane. Resection is necessary on both sides of the epiglottis. Bleeding is controlled by electrocautery. The horse should not be ridden or driven for 8 to 10 weeks postoperatively.

References

Boles, C. L.; Raker, C. W.; Wheat, J. D.: Epiglottic entrapment by aryteno-epiglottic folds in the horse. J. Amer. vet. med. Assoc. *172:* 338 (1978).

Ordridge, R. M.: Epiglottic entrapement in the horse. Vet. Rec. *100:* 365 (1977).

2.1.5.9. Diseases of the Esophagus

General. All diseases of the esophagus are accompanied by some degree of dysphagia. Normally the act of swallowing is initiated by the pharyngeal muscles. This is followed by a second, involuntary stage that is reflexly controlled and is initiated when the bolus comes in contact with sensitive areas of the pharynx. The bolus is transported further by successive contractions of the esophageal muscles. Even during drinking, this stage of deglutition is clearly visible on the left side of the neck. The peristaltic wave begins at the top of the esophagus and propels the bolus toward the stomach, preceded by a wave of relaxation. The food is delivered to the stomach in portions by the cardiac sphincter.

Under normal circumstances esophageal peristalsis is reflexly initiated only when the bolus or liquid has traversed the pharynx. On the other hand, a partial or complete peristaltic wave can be reflexly triggered by stretching (foreign body) and by local irritants such as inflammation, ulcers, parasites and wounds.

2.1.5.9.1. Esophageal Wounds

a) *Mucosal wounds* are inflicted on the luminal surface of the esophagus. They may be caused by foreign bodies or careless intubation.

Symptoms. Affected animals drink only liquids, and this is done carefully and deliberately. Some water may be partially regurgitated. A mucosal wound of the cervical esophagus can be demonstrated by contrast radiography (barium swallow).

Treatment. Soft feeds are offered, and systemic antibiotics are administered for 8 to 10 days.

If swelling due to cellulitis is present in the left jugular furrow, poultices may be applied locally to promote abscessation. The abscesses are then incised. This is done carefully to avoid injuring the cervical vessels. If foreign bodies are present in the mucosal wounds, primary treatment is surgery and involves exposing and opening the affected esophageal segment.

The *prognosis* is good.

b) *Mucosal ulcers* are caused by pressure necrosis from enlodged foreign bodies, corrosive lesions, and by gastrophilus larvae attached to the esophageal mucosa; the latter cause may be the most frequent [Wejda, 1961; Alexander, 1967].

Symptoms. Ulcers can lead to chronic esophageal spasm, stricture, and dilatation anterior to the stricture. The events initiated by these changes can be observed on the left side of the neck. The ulcer itself can be detected radiographically. Ingestion of a positive contrast mixture will demonstrate a defect of the mucosal contour in the esophageal lumen.

Treatment. The cause should be removed and soft feeds given for 8 to 14 days, supplemented by hyperalimentation with glucose and essential amino acids.

The *prognosis* is poor.

c) *Perforating esophageal wounds*

Etiology. Such wounds may result from direct trauma to the jugular furrow, but this mechanism is rare and occurs mainly in horses that run into a pointed object. Gunshot wounds are another cause.

A more important cause of esophageal wounds is iatrogenic perforation, especially when a whip handle, metal coil or metal cattle probang is inserted to relieve an obstruction. The tip is apt to slip off the mucus-covered foreign body, perforating the esophageal wall from the inside.

Symptoms. A perforation *from the outside* is recognized by the appearance of saliva, blood and food particles in the wound. Water leaks from the perforation site during drinking. A blunt-ended metal probe can be inserted into the esophageal lumen from the exterior. Swallowed contrast medium will also appear in the wound.

A perforation *from the inside* creates a tear through which saliva, food residue, and even the foreign body itself can enter the surrounding connective tissue. A doughy, painful swelling that continuously enlarges and often is crepitant, appears in the neck region. Dependent edema develops at the thoracic inlet. A perforation of the thoracic esophagus is recognized by the presence of marked systemic signs (fever, refusal of food and water). Severe dyspnea eventually occurs as a result of mediastinitis.

On radiography, contrast medium can be demonstrated in the mediastinal space.

Treatment. External puncture wounds of the esophagus will heal well with conservative treatment, which is the same as that for smaller incised wounds.

With larger perforating wounds, the wound edges are excised and the defect is closed in layers. The mucosa is repaired with continuous or interrupted silk sutures. The muscular layer is repaired with absorbable suture material. Postoperative healing is frequently attended by complications such as suture dehiscence, esophageal stricture and proximal dilatation. Sometimes a 2nd or 3rd operation is necessary.

Interior perforating wounds of the cervical esophagus require immediate treatment if there is to be any chance of recovery. The skin is incised parallel to the great vessels, and the torn esophagus is exposed by dissection. The perforation is sutured in layers, drains are placed in the infected surrounding tissue, and the upper part of the skin wound is closed, the bottom portion being left open. For 8 to 10 days the horse is offered only water and soft feeds, during which time systemic antibiotics are administered.

Prognosis. The prognosis is good for external perforating wounds but poor for internal wounds more than 24 h old. Treatment is useless if the perforation is in the thoracic esophagus.

Sequellae. An esophageal wound requires prompt diagnosis. The chance of recovery is greatly enhanced by early surgery.

2.1.5.9.2. Esophageal Fistula

Definition. In esophageal fistula there is a fistulous opening to the esophageal lumen that usually emerges on the left side of the neck, the fistulous tract passing through the skin, subcutaneous tissue, cervical fascia and esophageal wall.

Symptoms. When the animal eats and drinks, varying amounts of water, food and saliva are discharged through the skin, depending on the size of the fistulous opening and diameter of the tract. Ingested dye solutions will appear in the fistulous opening. The fistulous tract itself can be demonstrated by contrast radiographs or by passing a blunt-ended probe through the tract and into the esophageal lumen. Long-standing esophageal fistulas cause emaciation and dehydration.

Etiology. Esophageal fistulas occur as a result of perforating esophageal wounds or suture dehiscence following an esophagotomy.

Treatment. The most successful treatment is to explore the fistulous tract to its base, dissect free the esophageal mucosa and repair it with sutures, then suture the muscularis layer and skin.

Conservative treatment with poultices, agents that promote connective tissue proliferation, and cauterization or curettage of the fistulous tract are effective only if the tract is small.

Prognosis. The prognosis is good, even with multiple operations, because the fistulous tract usually becomes smaller with each operation and eventually closes.

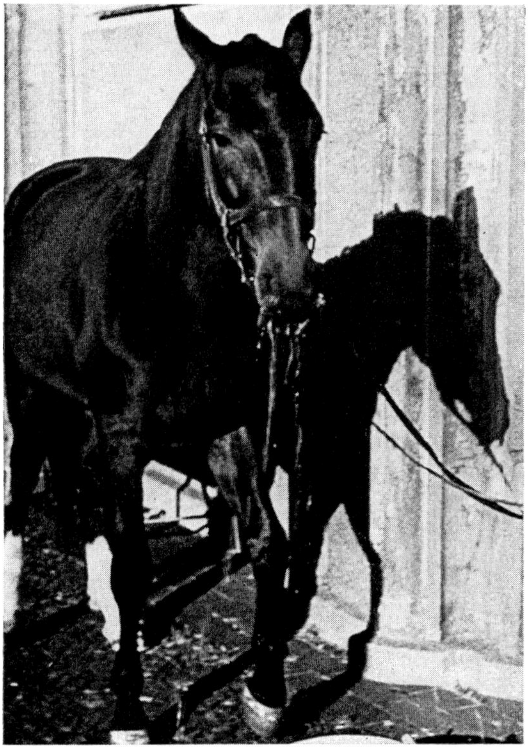

Fig. 2.1.5. — 11. Esophageal spasm: regurgitation.

2.1.5.9.3. Esophageal Spasm (Esophagism)

Definition. Esophageal spasm is a functional stenosis of the esophagus involving a painful, reflex, ring-shaped constriction of the esophageal muscles. This leads to the retention of foreign bodies and to an accumulation of ingesta anterior to the constriction. Frequently the food is shunted back and forth in the esophagus by peristaltic and antiperistaltic waves initiated by the spasm.

Symptoms. Local damage to the esophageal mucosa can result from the passage of a stomach tube or food bolus that is too large. A ring-shaped spastic constriction develops at this site which may be visible on the left side of the neck. This leads to a pooling of fluids and ingesta above the constriction. Sometimes the spasm gradually relaxes and the esophageal contents pass on to the stomach, or the ingested material may be regurgitated and expelled. In some cases the entire cervical esophagus is contracted and feels like a hard cord on palpation. This type of spasm also relaxes gradually, sometimes taking hours to subside.

The annular constriction of esophageal spasm is accompanied by an antiperistaltic wave. Initially the swallowed food and liquids move toward the stomach, but they abruptly reverse direction and are propelled cranially accompanied by stretching of the esophagus. A portion is regurgitated, and water is ejected from both nostrils when drinking is attempted (fig. 2.1.5. — 11).

The horse with esophageal spasm appears restless and stands with the neck and head extended and the neck muscles strongly tensed. After a while the animal becomes quiet again owing to partial esophageal clearing. The entire process is readily observed on the left side of the neck in the area of the jugular furrow. The last wave of the spasmodic episode disappears at the thoracic aperture.

Etiology. Esophageal spasm can result from the ingestion of poisonous plants or substances to which the animal is allergic. It can be triggered by the swallowing of an oversize bolus or pieces of food that cause mucosal wounds, inflammation or corrosive lesions. Spasm occurs the next time food is ingested. Mucosal wounds caused by hard rubber or metal probes occur in the upper esophagus or at the thoracic inlet.

Treatment. The cause must be eliminated. Soft or liquid feeds are offered. An attempt is made to temporarily relieve the esophageal spasm by giving 3 to 4 ml of 1 % atropine sulfate s.c., combined if desired with 3—5 ml promazine hydrochloride. The combination of a spasmolytic (i.v.) such as sodium noramidpyrine methane sulfonate (e.g., Metapyrin, 40—60 ml, Novalgin) with a neuroleptic (s.c.) has also proved effective. Devulder and Lefèvre [1974] supplement treatment with doses of vitamin B_1, B_{12} and iodine. Fretz [1972] reports less-than-satisfactory results with surgical myotomy.

Sequellae. The relief of esophageal spasm in the horse depends upon the elimination of the primary disorder. The repeated passage of a stomach tube should be avoided.

2.1.5.9.4. Cardiospasm, Achalasia

Definition. Cardiospasm refers to a spastic occlusion of the terminal portion of the esophagus, or cardia, which leads to the stasis of ingesta and to dilatation of the thoracic and cervical parts of the esophagus. The condition, which affects foals, is also termed megaesophagus, dysphagia paradoxica, and cardiotonic or idiopathic esophageal dilatation.

Symptoms. When a liquid is swallowed, a pouch-like bulge appears in the left jugular furrow which splashes on palpation due to the presence of air. If esophageal dilatation is severe, this bulge can extend up to the border of the mandible. Esophageal emptying is gradual. If the head of an affected foal is lowered near the ground, ingested food, saliva or liquid is discharged through the nose. A small tube can be freely passed through the dilated esophagus and even rotated there, but passage is impeded when the cardia is reached. The dilated esophagus is clearly demonstrated by contrast radiography. Often two separate areas of dilatation are seen: a thoracic dilation located caudal to the heart, and a sack-like cervical dilation with a dependent bulge.

Affected foals are emaciated and appear dehydrated. The disease may be complicated by inhalation pneumonia with severe systemic signs.

Etiology. The disease involves a disorder of esophageal function with discoordinated opening of the cardia during the act of swallowing. The cardia is that portion of the esophagus which reflexly contracts and subsequently relaxes in response to vagal stimulation initiated from within the oral cavity. The failure of this sphincter to relax on deglutition may be congenital in the nursing foal. It may also develop as a result of unknown factors and so may not appear until several days or weeks after birth.

Idiopathic cases may theoretically arise when the intrinsic intramural ganglia of the esophagus have become damaged as a result of repeated intubation.

Diagnosis. The diagnosis is based on the history, clinical signs and, if necessary, radiographic findings.

When a stomach tube is passed, a slight resistance must be overcome at the diaphragm.

Prognosis. The prognosis in foals with congenital cardiospasm is poor.

Treatment. Cardiospasm may initially be treated medically, like esophageal spasm. In addition, measures must be taken to restore hydration.

If medical therapy proves inadequate, surgical treatment may be attempted (Ramsted's operation).

Sequellae. Congenital cardiostenosis should not be treated.

2.1.5.9.5. Esophageal Obstruction

Definition. This refers to a partial or complete obstruction of the esophageal lumen.

Symptoms. The disorder is most common in greedy eaters. These horses eat ravenously and swallow large food boluses without proper mastication by the cheek teeth. As a result, the bolus becomes lodged in the upper part of the esophagus. The animal suddenly stops eating, shakes its head, coughs and steps back from the feed trough with the head somewhat extended. Many horses stamp the ground with their forelegs. The esophagus above the obstruction fills with saliva, which is later discharged through the partially-open mouth and nostrils. Rarely will the bolus slip down to the thoracic inlet unless pushed to that point with a stomach tube or probang. The head and neck are held low. If the obstruction is in the cervical esophagus, the foreign body can be detected by palpation over the larynx or in the left jugular furrow.

A second type of esophageal obstruction is more common in horses. Large portions of the esophagus, starting from the cardia and progressing cranially to the thoracic and cervical portions, become engorged with swollen things such as beet slices. A sausage-shaped obstruction may extend to the pharynx. It is evidenced by a cordlike swelling about the diameter of a broomstick located in the visible and palpable region of the esophagus in the jugular furrow. When the animal coughs, saliva mixed with bits of ingesta is expelled from the nostrils.

Etiology. Esophageal obstructions in the horse may be initiated by a transitory narrowing of the pharynx. The equine esophagus is a very long and narrow tube. The narrowest points occur in the lower cervical part and above the cardia, where the esophageal diameter is 1 cm less than in the remaining segments. The widest points are in the pharyngeal and upper thoracic part of the esophagus. Each bolus takes about 7 to 12 s to reach the stomach. Compacted foreign bodies become lodged in the esophagus just below the pharynx, at the entrance to the thorax, or above the diaphragm. Muscular tone increases at the site of the narrowing.

One of the most frequent causes of obstruction is the ingestion of chopped beets or feeds mixed with chaff. The dry, poorly-insalivated food boluses lodge in the thoracic part of the esophagus. Following lodgment, the local spasm serves to fix the obstruction, whereupon the food begins to build up. The animal continues to eat until the entire esophagus is impacted and dilated with food. For this reason dry chopped feeds should be soaked in water for 6—12 h before feeding.

Compact foreign bodies usually consist of poorly-masticated pieces of beet, carrot, potato or fruit.

Differential Diagnosis. Esophageal diverticula, scarring, functional and compressive stenoses and mucosal tumors can be excluded, if necessary by contrast radiography.

Horses sometimes regurgitate as a result of strangles, follicular pharyngitis and laryngitis, and abscessation of the retropharyngeal lymph nodes. Similar signs are associated with mucosal necrosis, mucosal ulceration and esophageal spasm.

Diagnosis. In cases where a foreign body is lodged in the cervical esophagus or the esophagus is impacted up to the pharynx with chopped or mixed feeds, palpation will enable a diagnosis of esophageal obstruction. Compacted foreign bodies lodged at the thoracic inlet or above the esophageal hiatus are localized by stomach tube intubation. Many compact foreign bodies slip spontaneously into the stomach, especially if spasmolytics, or analgesics have been previously administered. Esophageal obstruction is absent or has been relieved if the horse is able to drink a full bucket of water in long draughts without incident. Drinking in small gulps is not proof of recovery.

Prognosis. When esophageal obstruction has persisted for 24 h, the first signs of complications appear. The most serious is aspiration pneumonia. A gangrenous pneumonia can result from the aspiration of saliva and food particles. Less common are localized necrotic areas of the esophageal mucosa at the site of the foreign body with subsequent stricture formation. These complications are prevented by taking prompt, aggressive measures to relieve the obstruction. Aspiration pneumonia is sometimes fatal or may lead to chronic irreversible lung damage.

Treatment. Smooth, compacted foreign bodies in the upper esophagus are removed through the mouth by means of massage in a cranial direction either with the horse standing or anesthetized onto its right lateral recumbency. A previously administered spasmolytic is indicated. A mouth speculum is employed for the procedure. If the obstruction cannot be extricated in this way, the animal is prepared for the so-called 'operative-conservative' procedure of Podgersky [1949] and Dietz-Wintzer [1955]: Under general anesthesia the esophagus is surgically exposed in the area of the foreign body through an incision made in the left jugular furrow. Then, without opening the esophagus, the object is massaged into the pharynx where it is removed by an assistant. Sometimes the object slips past the soft palate and temporarily enters the nasal passages.

If a compacted foreign body is lodged in the area of the thoracic inlet or anterior to the diaphragm, one may first attempt to push the object onward with a stomach tube. Spasmolytics are first administered systemically, and if necessary a concentrated local anesthetic is deposited in the area of the foreign body. The stomach tube must be introduced slowly and carefully, with constant pressure exerted against the foreign body. If the mass cannot be moved into the stomach, an esophagotomy must be performed at the thoracic inlet. The foreign body is then extracted in pieces with forceps. We do not believe that an intrathoracic esophagotomy is called for in the horse.

In obstructions due to accumulations of chopped or mixed feed, removal by irrigation or air insufflation may be attempted. *Esophageal irrigation* may be done in calm or sedated horses with the animal standing but restrained, the head lowered and the hindquarters elevated. The procedure is safer if done in the recumbent horse, with the head hanging over the edge of the operating table. A nasogastric tube is passed to the point of the obstruction, the tube is connected to a pump, and water is forced against the mass in bursts of varying pressure. As pieces of food are dislodged, they pass into a second inserted tube or are flushed out past the irrigating tube. After 2 to 3 l of water have been pumped, irrigation is stopped momentarily to allow the water and dissolved food particles to drain. The tube is advanced as the esophagus is cleared. The procedure may take a few minutes or as much as several hours if the esophagus is impacted from the cardia to the hypopharynx.

In *esophageal insufflation,* a stomach tube is used to apply bursts of compressed air which dilate the entire esophagus anterior to the tip of the tube. Food shavings or particles are loosened and are discharged with the saliva, mainly through the nose. The tube is slowly advanced toward the stomach during the insufflation. In the terminal portion of the esophagus the obstruction should no longer be moved cranially but pass through the dilated esophagus into the stomach. The tip of the tube will have reached the stomach when gastric gases are detected. Esophageal ruptures are extremely rare during this procedure, for excess air between the tube and esophagus can escape to the outside.

Aftercare. Large doses of antibiotics are given systemically and even intratracheally for 5 to 6 days. If the esophagus has not been surgically opened, only water or soft feeds are offered for 1 or 2 days. After an esophagotomy the animal is fasted for 6 to 7 days or is only allowed liquids.

Esophageal obstructions in the horse should be relieved within 24 h.

2.1.5.9.6. Esophageal Stricture and Cicatricial Stenosis

Definition. Strictures are ring-shaped narrowings of the esophageal lumen. Cicatricial stenoses may involve large portions of the esophagus and reduce its lumen to pencil-size. Strictures and cicatricial stenoses are caused by excessive stretching and consequent tearing of the muscularis layer with subsequent scar formation and contraction.

Symptoms. An affected horse starts to feed normally, but within a short time it begins to nod or shake its head. The swallowed boluses are not carried completely through the esophagus, and soon the esophagus feels like a hard cord on the left side of the neck. A reduction in diameter occurs at the site of the stricture or cicatricial stenosis. The stenosis feels rubbery on palpation. Strictures of the cervical or thoracic esophagus and the proximal dilatation that is often present can be easily recognized by inspection and palpation.

Etiology. Esophageal strictures and cicatricial stenoses in the horse are most frequently caused by the passage of metal tubes or may occur as true cicatricial strictures following esophagotomies. The attachment of isolated gastrophilus larvae to the esophagus may also lead to strictures [Wejda, 1961].

Diagnosis. Swallowed liquids usually reach the stomach without difficulty. Accumulations of ingested food generally occur only after feeding with things such as oats, hay or pellets. The passage of a rubber tube is impeded at the constriction. It can be well visualized by air insufflation. A cervical or thoracic stenosis is clearly demonstrated by contrast radiography with barium.

Differential Diagnosis. Obstructions and functional stenoses of the esophagus must be excluded.

Treatment and Prognosis. Careful dilation (bougienage) of the stricture or cicatricial stenosis usually gives only temporary relief. Scarring and contracture soon recurs. An attempt may be made to treat the disease surgically by exposing the lesion and making several longitudinal, centimeter-long incisions in the muscularis layer parallel to the direction of the esophagus, taking care not to injure the mucosa. A normal diet should be offered immediately after the operation.

Epicrisis. A large percentage of horses with cicatricial stenoses and strictures of the esophagus can be kept alive only with a liquid or soft diet, so their usefulness is limited.

2.1.5.9.7. Esophageal Diverticulum

Definition. An esophageal diverticulum is a sacculation of the mucous membrane through a defect in the esophageal musculature. Diverticula occur most frequently in the cervical esophagus, at the thoracic aperture, in the thoracic esophagus or in the area near the diaphragm. They vary markedly in size.

Symptoms. Symptoms appear after eating or drinking. The horse backs away from the feed trough, becomes restless and exhibits the clinical signs of esophageal spasm, sometimes accompanied by regurgitation. In other cases prolonged esophageal peristalsis may gradually empty the contents of the sac until the next feeding. Many horses cough violently and show signs of choke. The respiratory rate is increased during such episodes, but the pulse may be slowed as a result of a vagal bradycardia.

Very small diverticula cause only a transient interruption of feeding. Filled diverticula in the cervical esophagus are easily recognized by the appearance of a bulge on the left side of the neck. The diverticula are not painful and sometimes can be emptied by massage. A stomach tube has a tendency to enter the diverticulum when first passed, but it can easily be withdrawn and routed back into the esophageal lumen. Barium radiographs are required for the visualization and accurate localization of thoracic diverticula.

Etiology. Causes are frequent intubation, foreign bodies, obstruction and rapid swelling of ingesta. Congenital diverticula are rare.

Treatment. Spasmolytics are administered. Initially then an effort is made to empty the diverticulum by introducing a nasogastric tube and carefully irrigating the sac with a very low-pressure jet of water. The head must be held low when the irrigating liquid is regurgitated. Cervical as well as thoracic diverticula caused by a rent in the muscularis are amenable either to resection or invagination. In any case it is necessary to repair the tear in the muscularis with closely-spaced interrupted sutures. If the herniated mucosa is resected, the mucosal wound is repaired with securely-placed silk sutures before the muscularis is sutured. An intrathoracic diverticulectomy or invagination always requires positive-pressure ventilation during anesthesia with a thoracotomy and partial rib resection.

Prognosis. The outcome depends on the size and location of the diverticulum. Usually the prognosis is good for cervical diverticula. Thoracic and especially epiphrenic diverticula are not that accessible, and so their prognosis is poor.

Foals with congenital diverticula should be destroyed.

References

Devulder, E.; Lefèvre, P.: Sur un cas d'oesophagite chez le cheval. Bull. mens. Soc. vét. prat. *58:* 115 (1974).

Fretz, P. B.: Repair of esophageal stricture in a horse. Mod. vet. Pract. *53:* 31 (1972).

Schebitz, H.; Schulze, D.: Zur Obstipatio oesophagi beim Pferd. Dtsch. tierärztl. Wschr. *71:* 538 (1964).

Tredten, H. W.; Keahey, K. K.: Esophagotracheal fistulation after esophageal stenosis in a horse. Vet. Med. and Small Animal Clinician *69:* 868 (1974).

Wejda, E.: Dilatatio et Stenosis Oesophagi bei einem Fohlen, hervorgerufen durch wandernde Gastrophiluslarven. Mh. Vet.-Med. *16:* 317 (1961).

2.1.5.10. Diseases of the Stomach and Intestine

2.1.5.10.1. Gastritis (Gastric Catarrh)

Definition and Pathology. Gastritis is a disease of the gastric mucosa of which various stages are known. *Acute gastritis* is associated with hyperemia and edema of the mucosa, a reduced secretion of gastric juice and increased secretion of mucus. Deeper inflammation leads to hemorrhagic changes with serosanguinous effusion (e.g., purpura hemorrhagica). The normally acid gastric juice may become alkaline, as in diseases such as grass sickness (see p. 229).

Chronic gastritis is a result of continual irritation with ulceration and scarring. Parasitism (e.g., bot infections, see Sec. 2.2.3.8.) is a frequent cause. The lesions are usually located in the cutaneous mucosa of the proximal, cardiac portion of the stomach and are associated with hypertrophy of the mucous membrane.

Symptoms and Diagnosis. In acute gastritis the appetite is always reduced or absent. Affected horses yawn frequently, bare the upper teeth and appear to like licking cool objects. A rancid smell is noted on examination of the oral cavity. Gastric juice obtained by nasogastric tube has the same smell, has a high mucus content, and may contain blood. In chronic gastritis the symptoms are similar but more protracted, and the gastric contents contain viscid mucus and blood. Examination of the gastric juice with indicator paper will indicate its degree of acidity (pH 2—3 is normal).

Etiology. Primary acute gastritis is rare in horses. Corrosive lesions of the gastric mucosa do not occur under ordinary circumstances, owing to the horse's natural aversion to caustic substances. But primary gastritis still occurs as a result of administering irritating or hot medications by mouth or due to feeding errors (e.g., dry chopped vegetables, moldy feeds). Poor dentition, leading to incomplete mastication, is a potential cause of mild gastritis. Periodic anorexia may be observed in young or nervous horses that have been overexerted.

The most frequent cause of chronic gastritis is infestation with *Gastrophilus* spp. larvae. Other parasitic lesions, like those caused by *Habronema megastoma* and *Trichostrongylus axei*, are rarely observed. Secondary disorders of the gastric mucosa may arise during the course of systemic diseases (viral infections, strangles, purpura hemorrhagica) or as a sequel to stress in the form of gastric ulcers (foals).

Differential Diagnosis. Gastritis must be differentiated from diseases of the bowel. Abnormalities of mastication or a refusal to feed may be the result of bad teeth. Metabolic diseases are excluded on the basis of laboratory tests (hyperbilirubinemia, hyperlipemia and hypocalcemia in ponies).

Prognosis. The prognosis for simple gastritis is generally favorable, and symptoms should pass in 1 to 2 days with proper care. For secondary forms the prognosis is determined by the primary disorder.

Treatment. Food is withheld for at least 24 h to empty the stomach. Gastric emptying with the normalization of gastric secretion can be promoted by giving small amounts of neutral salts (50—80 g sodium sulfate) in a linseed gruel. Chlorine-ion losses due to heavy sweating or repeated gastric emptying are replaced by giving hydrochloric acid (10—20 g HCl in 1 bucket of gruel). Then easily-digested concentrate and green feed or good hay are offered. Small amounts of feed should be given at frequent intervals, and pasturing should be limited to periods of about an hour.

2.1.5.10.2. Gastric Dilation

Enlargement of the stomach to nearly the size of a bovine rumen have been described in the horse. The dilation is always associated with gastric overload; neurogenic dilation is unknown. Three etiologic forms are recognized: acute primary and secondary dilation; chronic dilatation may develop from the acute form.

Acute Primary Gastric Dilation

Symptoms. An affected horse suddenly exhibits signs of unrest, stops eating, and may drool saliva. It displays signs of abdominal pain and makes retching movements with the back arched and the neck extremely tense and arched downward. Vomiting may occur if the gastric contents are fluid, but owing to the peculiar anatomy of the equine pharynx the vomitus is expelled from the nostrils not the mouth. Despite severe colic, the animal moves but very slowly and cautiously. The dilated stomach exerts considerable pressure on the diaphgram. To ease this pressure, affected horses often assume a 'dog-sitting' posture, and yawning and teeth-bearing may be observed. The elevated diaphragm has a marked effect on respiration and circulation, leading to dyspnea, tachycardia and shock symptoms due to the fall of blood pressure.

Diagnosis. The primary diagnostic technique to perform when gastric dilation is suspected is the passage of a nasogastric tube. Fermenting or liquid contents will escape from the tube. Rectal examination is usually unrewarding. In small horses, or if dilation is extreme, the stomach can sometimes be felt with the fingertips per rectum as a smooth-walled, bloated sack that moves synchronously with respiration. Caudal displacement of the spleen is not a very reliable sign in larger horses. Rectal examination is necessary in any case in order to exclude diseases of the bowel and thus differentiate between a primary and secondary gastric dilation.

Etiology. The most common cause of primary gastric dilation is the ingestion of large amounts of feed (e.g., overeating of grain by a horse that has escaped its stall) or the bolting of swelling or fermenting feeds (chopped beets, fruit, large amounts of pelleted feed). The rapid consumption of large amounts of water has also been incriminated.

Differential Diagnosis. Similar signs are observed in esophageal obstruction, and so the esophagus should always be checked for patency (this can be assessed by passing a tube with length markings). The presence of solid ingesta in the stomach may be confused with an obstruction in the area of the cardia. A thorough rectal examination is necessary to exclude intestinal disease.

Prognosis. The prognosis of primary gastric dilation depends on the nature of the stomach contents. It is relatively favorable in the case of liquid or fermentable contents, which can be flushed from the stomach rapidly and completely. If the gastric contents are doughy and 'dry', rapid removal is often impossible. Atony and necrosis of the stomach wall may develop. The danger of gastric rupture is always present.

A possible *complication* of gastric dilation is dietary-induced laminitis. Therefore, after the dilation is treated, the pulsation of the digital arteries and animal's gait should be closely assessed for two days.

Treatment. First a spasmolytic is administered i.v., and if the ingesta is fluid, it is siphoned from the stomach. Mineral oil doses can be helpful in hastening the emptying of fermentable ingesta (fruit, pellets) into the intestine. Careful gastric lavage with the stomach tube following the administration of noramidopyrine methane sulfonate sodium (Novalgin) is effective if the gastric content is finely divided (Gratzl's technique of gastric lavage). In the presence of coarse-stemmed or fibery ingesta, the introduction of further material into the stomach is hazardous, and attempted lavage can cause a lethal rupture. In this case measures are limited to administering spasmolytics and repeated siphoning until natural gastric emptying can occur. The use of peristalsis-stimulating drugs such as neostigmine (Prostigmin) or carbachol (Lentin) is contraindicated, for the resultant increase in muscle tone will aggravate the risk of gastric rupture.

Acute Secondary Gastric Dilation

Symptoms and Diagnosis. The symptoms of secondary gastric dilation are similar to those of primary dilation but may be masked by colicky signs associated with a primary intestinal obstruction. Because every intestinal obstruction may potentially lead to reflux gastric filling, the passage of a stomach tube is indicated whenever colic is present. In severe cases a large amount of yellow-green to brown, watery material is passed via the tube. Solid ingesta may also be present in the stomach, in which case a portion of the content is removed by careful, gastric lavage in order to decompress the stomach and forestall rupture. Of primary importance, however, is the continual removal of accumulated fluid.

Etiology. An intestinal obstruction can lead directly or indirectly to a stagnation of small intestinal contents that prevents gastric emptying. In later stages intestinal contents are refluxed into the stomach. The higher the obstruction, the more rapid the onset of gastric dilation. A duodenal obstruction can produce a retrograde gastric overload within 2 h. However, the dilation may also be the consequence of paralytic ileus. Gastric filling is not observed as often in obstruction of the large intestine. Nevertheless, it frequently occurs via the reflex pathway (pylorospasm) or as a result of compression of the duodenum by displacement of the colon, such as occurs in herniation into the nephrosplenic space (left dorsal displacement).

Prognosis. The prognosis depends on the success in treating the primary obstruction. A secondary gastric dilation can almost always be relieved temporarily by siphoning of the stomach contents. This must be done repeatedly until the initiating intestinal obstruction is relieved.

Treatment. A stomach tube is passed. The failure of gastric contents to escape spontaneously through the tube does not necessarily mean that the stomach is not dilated. In many cases the gastric contents can be removed only by suction on the end of the tube and frequent siphoning.

2.1.5.10.3. Gastric Rupture

Etiology and Pathogenesis. Gastric rupture can occur as a consequence of any severe stomach disorder. Usually it is a result of secondary gastric dilation, and less frequently of a primary dilation. Perforations caused by ulcers and tumors are extremely rare. Gastric rupture due to a heavy infestation of *Gastrophilus* spp. larvae is conceivable but is seldom observed in practice. Besides spontaneous rupture, the overstretching of the stomach wall that accompanies gastric dilation can also lead to ischemic necrosis with secondary perforation. Most ruptures occur in the area of the greater curvature. Incomplete ruptures of the muscular coat have also been observed and may lead to fatal hemorrhage.

Symptoms and Diagnosis. When the stomach ruptures, a horse that has previously exhibited colicky symptoms suddenly becomes calm. All symptoms referable to choke or abdominal pain abruptly disappear. However, signs of shock soon appear along with a heavy cold sweat. Food particles can now be recovered by abdominal paracentesis. If the rupture is small, allowing little material to escape, or if the omentum temporarily prevents the gastric contents from entering the abdominal cavity, food particles may not be recovered. The animal becomes dull, depressed, and sweats profusely. The nostrils are flared, the respiration is shallow and increased in rate, the pulse becomes rapid and thready. Everything about the horse's appearanc suggests that death is imminent. This is described as the 'stage of painlessness'. In most cases death occurs within 2 h after the rupture.

Differential Diagnosis. The same signs can be produced by an intestinal rupture. Peritonitis can cause severe signs of shock with abscence of pain. It is distinguished by a bloody abdominal fluid with a high leukocyte content and an absence of food particles.

Treatment. Treatment is useless. Immediate slaughter or euthanasia is indicated.

2.1.5.10.4. Catarrhal and Inflammatory Diseases of the Intestine

Definition and Pathology. The complex of catarrhal and inflammatory diseases of the bowel is difficult to categorize in terms of specific disease entities. The causes are manifold and the boundaries indistinct. Primary inflammatory processes are uncommon in the equine digestive tract. Almost all conditions occur secondarily to other diseases or to stress.

The simplest form is *acute catarrhal enteritis,* which occurs during the course of systemic diseases or parasitism. It is associated with hyperemia and mucous secretions of the intestinal mucosa with a transitory impairment of absorption. This may progress to a *chronic catarrhal enteritis* with degenerative or proliferative-hyperplastic changes in the mucosal surface of the intestine. Of special importance are the thrombosis and intestinal wall damage caused by migrating strongyle larvae. If larger portions of the intestine are affected, malabsorption symptoms such as hypoproteinemia and cachexia may develop.

If the intestinal mucosa is damaged or the intestinal flora is disturbed (e.g., following antibiotic usage), facultative pathogens may become virulent and cause an acute enteritis. For example, if the intestinal flora is altered, certain coliform bacteria can ascend from the colon into the small intestine and produce inflammation. A special form of enteritis is *colitis x* (hemorrhagic-edematous colitis).

All forms of enteritis are marked by severe damage to the intestinal wall with epithelial necrosis, hemorrhage and excessive mucous secretion.

Symptoms and Diagnosis. The outstanding symptom of almost all catarrhal and inflammatory intestinal diseases is diarrhea. The spastic intestinal contractions cause mild to severe colicky pains. In simple enteritis, which may regress spontaneously in 1 to 2 days, these are often the only symptoms noted. Rigid bowel segments in a state of spastic contraction are palpable on rectal examination. Increased peristalsis may be apparent even at a distance (hyperperistalsis). Long-standing inflammation is associated with mild to moderate dehydration, hypokalemia and hyponatremia. Thirst may be excessive. Straining (tenesmus) will be present if the colon and rectum are involved. In chronic enteritis these signs are accompanied by a dull haircoat, emaciation, electrolyte losses and persistent diarrhea of a watery or pasty consistency.

E. coli and Cl. perfringens infections in foals and salmonellosis take a peracute to acute course and are associated with severe signs of intoxication and metabolic disturbances. An initially high fever is followed by profuse diarrhea with substantial water and electrolyte losses. Shock and acidosis may develop within a short time. Colitis x is associated with similar signs. The hematocrit may rise in a short time to 65 to 70 (65—70 % increase), while the pH of the blood falls from a normal 7.36—7.42 to around 7.0.

Changes similar to those of colitis x are occasionally observed in the duodenum and initial portion of the jejunum. The clinical signs are also like those of colitis x, and acute gastric dilation soon develops additionally as a result of paralytic ileus. If the enteritis is of bacterial origin, the causal organisms may be demonstrated in culture.

The following criteria enable a diagnosis of acute salmonellosis to be made in the horse:

Stress (transportation, surgery), leukopenia, high fever and profuse diarrhea.

The diagnosis is confirmed by a bacteriologic examination of the feces. The most frequent causal organism in the horse is *S. typhimurium* (see Sec. 2.2.4.1.).

Etiology. The most common causes of acute enteritides in the horse are feeding errors, stress (overexertion of young horses, colic, transportation), systemic infections and parasitism (diarrhea in young foals due to strongyle infection), including the migration of strongyle larvae.

Salmonellosis is most frequently observed after colic, long transport, severe systemic diseases (e.g., respiratory tract infections) and extreme surgical stress.

Colitis x reportedly is precipitated by prolonged antibiotic usage and by the premature resumption of training after respiratory tract infections.

Differential Diagnosis. Diarrhea and fever are also characteristic of peritonitis and necrosis of the colon and cecum. These are differentiated from enteritis by abdominal paracentesis. Hyperlipemia and grass sickness may also be accompanied by diarrhea, and pasty feces may be observed in chronic, recurrent obstructions of the cecum. The ingestion of poisonous plants also must be considered whenever signs of acute gastrointestinal distress appear.

Course and Prognosis. Acute enteritis takes a mild course and generally subsides in 1 to 2 days when food is withheld. Chronic enteritis can cause irreversible damage to the gut wall resulting in chronic malabsorption and diarrhea that often respond poorly to treatment. Acute enteritis usually takes a favorable course, and affected horses should recover within a few days with proper treatment. *E. coli* and *Cl. perfringes* infections in foals as well as salmonellosis often take a peracute course and are fatal within 12 to 24 h. The same applies to colitis x and the similar disease that affects the duodenum. In many cases prompt replacement of the fluid and electrolyte losses and correction of acidosis by intravenous therapy may effect a cure.

Treatment. The first priority in simple enteritis is to remove the offending substances. Withholding food for 1 to 2 days and administering mineral oil has proven useful for this purpose. Severe diarrhea can be relieved by giving activated charcoal. Secondary bacterial infection is prevented by administering antibiotics and sulfonamides that are active against the offending bacteria (e.g., tetracycline, streptomycin, sulfaguanidine, trimethoprim sulfadiazine). In all enteritides that are associated with dehydration, intravenous therapy infusions are indicated to correct the water and electrolyte losses. Acidosis can be corrected with sodium bicarbonate infusions in 5 % solution. Specific antibiotics should be administered if time permits the organisms to be cultured and their sensitivity determined. For all enteritides of parasitic origin, a specific antiparasitic therapy is necessary.

If food is totally refused, the force-feeding (by nasogastric tube) of commercial feeds dissolved in water starting on the 2nd day of the illness has proven beneficial. This mash, to which various nutrients may be added, coats the mucous membranes and has some effect on peristalsis and the activity of the gastric and intestinal glands.

2.1.5.10.5. Colic

General. 'Colic' is a term coined centuries ago for gastrointestinal disease. It is derived from the word 'colon', the presumed seat of the disorder. Gradually laymen, veterinarians and veterinary researchers have come to apply the term to all pathologic states in which the animal exhibits behavior strongly indicative of pain or discomfort, arising from the abdomen.

With advances in diagnostic methods and the recognition of specific diseases underlying colicky symptoms, there have been numerous attempts to eliminate the term 'colic' from the veterinary nomenclature [Marek, 1956]. Today there should be no hesitation in using the word 'colic' to facilitate communication between the veterinarian and layman. It must be remembered, however, that for the veterinarian, colic is only a symptom:

Colic is not a disease but a symptom and represents a challenge of differential diagnosis.

There is no need to classify colics into 'true' forms with pain localized to the gastrointestinal tract and 'false' forms in which the pain emanates from other organs. A healthy horse does not have colic. Colic is always the product of a genuine disease or discomfort, may it be an intestinal or uterine torsion or dehydration (malfunction of automatic waterer).

Colic may be a feature of the following disease groups:

— Stomach and intestinal diseases,
— Liver and biliary diseases,
— Diseases of the urogenital organs,
— Diseases of the thorax and esophagus,
— Infectious diseases (tetanus, rabies, salmonellosis, anthrax),
— Skin diseases,
— Diseases of the locomotor system (back pain, laminitis),
— Starvation or thirst.

Causes and Development of Gastrointestinal Colics. There is no question that the *anatomic peculiarities* of the equine digestive tract play an essential role in the development of the foregoing diseases in the horse: The horse's relative inability to vomit makes gastric emptying more difficult if the stomach becomes distended. Gastric rupture may result. The very long mesentery of the horse allows the small intestine, which is 19 to 30 m in length, wide excursions into all parts of the abdominal cavity, with an associated risk of incarceration in preexisting apertures (e.g., epiploic foramen, vaginal ring). The double-horseshoe-shaped large colon, which is about 3 to 4 m long and has a capacity of 60 to 130 l, is freely mobile except where it is fixed in the region of the anterior mesenteric root. The large colon for example, may be trapped over the nephrosplenic ligament. The nephrosplenic ligament together with the dorsal edge of the spleen and left dorsal abdominal wall forms a ready-made place to trap loops of left colon that are displaced laterally and dorsally.

Strangulation through abnormal openings can also occur: pseudoligaments (cords or bands of fibrous tissue) usually lead to strangulation of the small intestine. Pedunculated lipoma, Meckel's diverticula, and congenital or acquired defects in the mesentery are additional causes of intestinal obstruction that occur with frequency only in the horse.

The junction between narrow and broad intestinal segments of the large colon such as the pelvic flexure is a predilection site for the accumulation of ingesta and the consequent formation of an impaction (fig. 2.1.5. — 12).

Colic due to *internal parasitism* is commonly the result of verminous endarteritis caused by 4th-stage larvae of *Strongylus vulgaris* in the region of the anterior mesenteric artery. Gasterophilus infestation of the stomach is an infrequent cause. Inflammatory *vascular changes* (aneurysm, thrombosis, stenosis) can chronically impair the blood supply to various parts of the intestine and predispose to bowel dysfunction. Arterial and venous thromboses can be a cause of acute blood flow disturbances (infarction and necrosis).

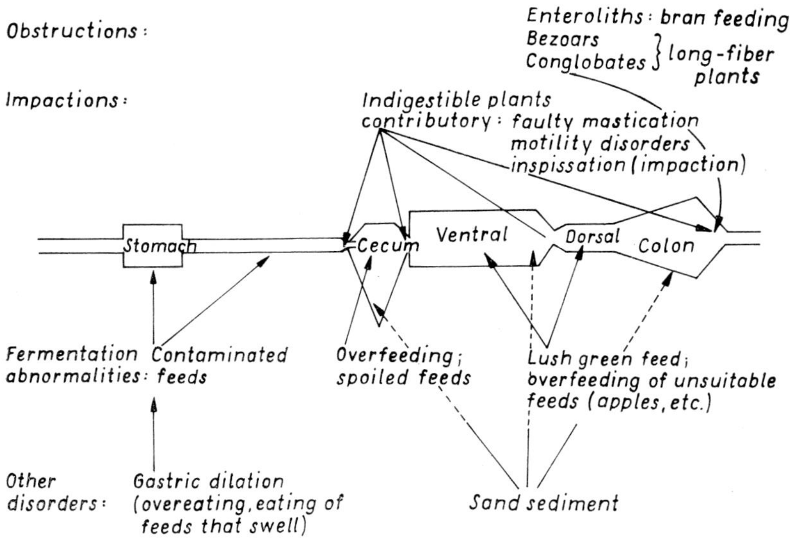

Fig. 2.1.5. — 12. Alimentary-tract related causes of colic in the horse. Classification and localization of major disorders (after Meyer, 1979).

Gratzl has theorized that the sensitivity of the equine gastrointestinal tract to autonomic control offers a pathophysiologic explanation for the susceptibility of this species to gastrointestinal colic. To this day his fundamental discussions on vagotonia in the horse remain unrefuted.

Specifically, the causes may lie in meteorological influences (weather changes, thunderstorms), feeding errors (feeding technique, feed quality and quantity) and improper care and management (cold, overexertion) (figs. 2.1.5. — 13 and — 14).

Gratzl showed that the typical pain of colic is caused by spasm in the intestinal wall and distinguished three conditions:
— spastic peristalsis,
— tonic intestinal spasm, and
— intestinal pain from mesenteric and intestinal strangulation.

Spastic peristalsis refers to an abnormal increase in muscular tone with a markedly accelerated peristaltic rhythm. Intestinal movements assume a violent character, resulting in loud, splashing and gurgling sounds accompanied by intense abdominal pain.

Tonic intestinal spasm is a sustained, localized increase in intestinal muscle tone that can cause a complete spastic occlusion of the intestinal lumen. The intestinal pain caused by *mechanical insults* is continuous and is the result of abnormal stretching compression or traction of the intestinal wall and mesentery. It can be increased on rectal examination by exerting traction on the affected part of the intestine.

Restriction in blood flow can also cause severe pain from hypoxia before necrosis occurs.

The severe intestinal pain caused by intermittent spastic peristalsis leads to the intense, intermittent attacks that are characteristic of *spasmodic colic.* The ingesta are propelled through the intestine at an accelerated rate, resulting in inadequate

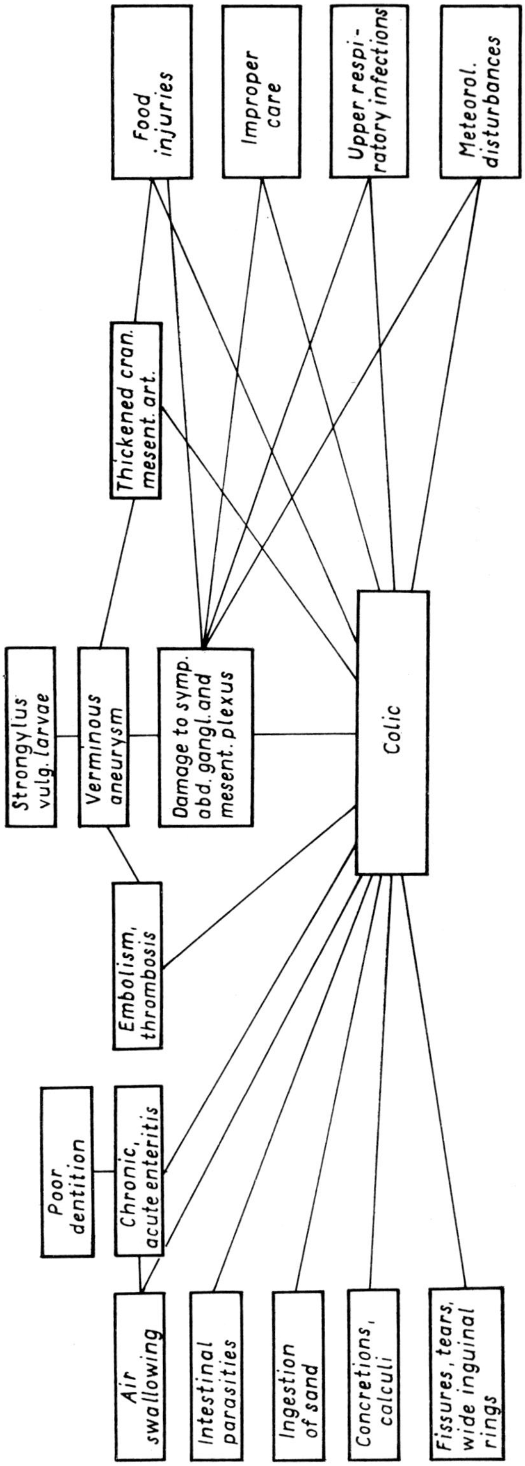

Fig. 2.1.5. — 13. Etiology of equine colic (after GRATZL, 1942).

water absorbtion. Untreated, spastic peristalsis can lead to volvulus, torsion, intussusception or incarceration, although such complications are infrequent.

The continuous pain caused by tonic intestinal spasm is manifested clinically by a general depression of the horse's behavior.

In cases of intestinal and mesenteric pain and the ischemic pain in the early stage of thromboembolism, the animal is restless and gets up and lies down frequently.

Signs of Colic. Depending on the intensity of the pain, affected horses may lie down at unusual times, stand quietly with the head and neck extended, move about restlessly, stamp and paw the ground, turn its head repeatedly toward the flank as well as stand up and lie down frequently. Severe cases may be marked by rolling, periods of calm behavior or the temporary assumption of an unusual posture, such as lying on the back. In extreme cases the animal will throw itself to the ground and roll, doing injury to itself and as well to persons standing nearby. Especially in impactions of the large intestine, the horse passes small amounts of urine at frequent intervals or is anuric for long periods of time. The severity of the colicky signs does not necessarily correspond to that of the disorder. For example, the relatively innocent intestinal spasm may be associated with severe colic symptoms, while extensive ischemic necrosis of the colon may produce only mild signs. In impactions of the large intestine the pain is almost always mild and intermittent, and the animal appears comfortable and takes food between attacks. The most dramatic symptoms are produced by torsion of the entire large colon of 360° or more. The resulting pains are so intense that examination becomes impossible. Horses with colic assume various unusual postures in an effort to alleviate the pain and tension:

- dog-sitting posture in gastric dilation and diaphragmatic elevation as a result of the tympany,
- dorsal recumbency in intestinal torsion, and
- saw-horse or kneeling posture in impactions.

Another major symptom of colic is *sweating*. It usually starts on the neck (root of mane) and shoulder area, its extent and intensity varying as a rule with the severity of the attack. The haircoat dries as soon as the pain subsides. After a severe colic attack the animal often will drip with sweat and give off steam. *Cold* sweat, with an apparent relief of pain, is characteristic of gastric or intestinal rupture.

Systematic Examination (cf. Sec. 1.1.1.4.).

Examination of the colicky horse includes the following:

- History
- Clinical examination
  External inspection and palpation (scrotum in stallions)
  Heart and circulation
  Lungs and respiration
  Body temperature
  Auscultation of abdominal cavity
  Passage of stomach tube
  Rectal examination
  Abdominal paracentesis
  Laboratory tests
  Diagnostic-therapeutic medication
  Enterocentesis (if necessary)
- Documentation of findings.

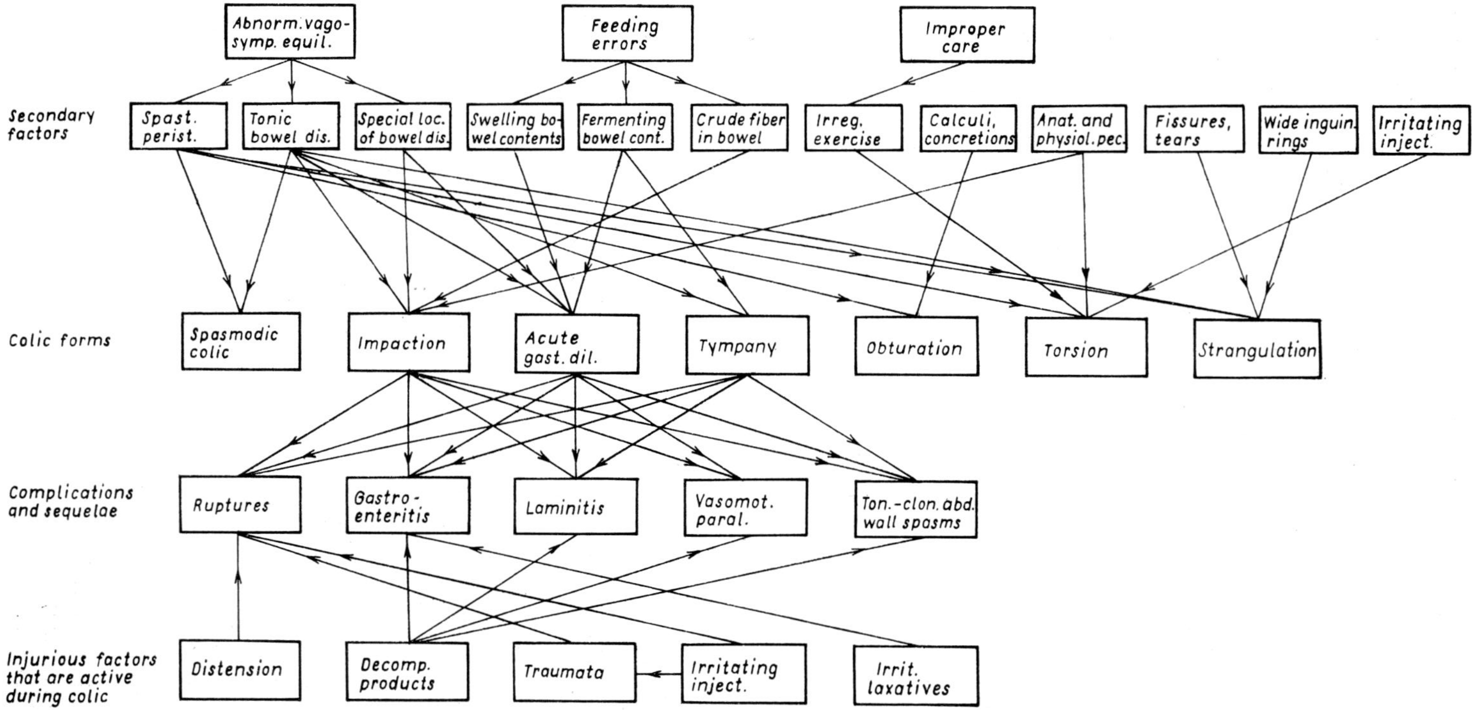

Fig. 2.1.5. — 14. Pathogenesis of equine colics caused by disturbances of vagosympathetic equilibrium (after GRATZL, 1942).

Essentially a systematic examination means the application of a designated sequence of examination procedures that are adapted to the status of the patient, followed by an accurate interpretation of the results.

The ideal goal of the examination is an etiologic diagnosis.

Given the complex nature of the examination, an unsystematic approach will most likely lead to a misdiagnosis. The fact that incipient colic may show a good and rapid response to treatment or may just as easily progress to a severe, fatal illness makes it essential that the examining veterinarian adopt a watchful, skeptical attitude. All diagnostic and therapeutic measures that are deemed appropriate should be systematically applied. For economic and practical reasons, of course, the veterinarian cannot always carry out the full range of diagnostic procedures during the initial visit. Nor would this be prudent on pathophysiologic grounds. Colic is not a static condition. The primary disorder may give rise to complications which require that modifications be made in terms of diagosis and management.

Often the diagnosis becomes easier during the course of the disease, while treatment becomes increasingly more difficult. An accurate and thorough appreciation of the nature of the disorder (impaction, tympany, displacement) is essential. The potential pathophysiologic consequences on both a local (necrosis, rupture) and systemic scale (dehydration, circulatory insufficiency, intoxication, shock, etc.) should be appreciated if the correct treatment is to be given.

The ideal management of the colicky horse involves uninterrupted diagnostic and therapeutic care, following the principles of modern intensive medicine. We employ and recommend the following diagnostic-therapeutic routine:

Stage I: 1 to 3 h after onset of disease

A. History
B. Clinical examination
C. Special examinations
   a) Stomach tube
   b) Rectal examination
   c) Diagnostic-therapeutic medication (intestinal puncture in cases of gas accumulation)
D. Documentation of findings

Stage II: 3 to 5 h after onset

B. Clininal examination
C. Special examinations
   a), b), c) and
   d) Laboratory examinations
D. Documentation and interpretation of findings

Stage III: 5 + h after onset

If a diagnosis cannot be made right away and no definite improvement is noted, the examination is repeated at 2-hour intervals according to the scheme in Stage II. If there is marked deterioration, immediate hospitalization is indicated.

Even if the veterinarian is not summoned until a later stage of the disease, he should start the entire examination routine from the beginning. (He should not rely on the findings of other veterinarians.)

History. Of special note is the time at which symptoms first appeared, the time at which the last food and water were ingested, and whether there have been recent quantitative or qualitative changes in the diet: Fermentable feed can produce tympany, spoiled corn silage can cause enteritis, and feeds that are high in coarse or crude fiber promote impactions, especially of the small colon. Torsion of the large colon occurs mainly in nursing mares, especially when they are fed on grass that is low in crude fiber. In foals with heavy ascarid infestations, anthelmintic therapy can lead to obstruction of the small intestine by the dead worms.

The nature of previous illnesses can also be helpful. In a horse with chronic colic, for example, a previous strangles infection may suggest abscessed abdominal lymph nodes. Abdominal operations for cryptorchidism or colic may show evidence of intestinal stenoses or displacements due to fibrous adhesions. In mares that have foaled, it should be determined whether any postpartum irregularities have been noted in the estrous cycle (uterine torsion). Excessive doses of prostaglandins may produce colic. 'Internal' hernias or adhesions can be caused by contusion of the bowel as a result of dystocia.

Finally, it should be determined whether the animal has undergone any previous examinations or treatments by third parties (rectal tears).

Clinical Examination

External Inspection. First the colicky horse is inspected in its stall and its behavior is observed. The examiner records the nature and degree (mild, moderate, severe) of the colicky signs, notes or inquires if the horse has adopted any unusual postures, and ascertains the amount of quality of the feces. Any distension of the flanks, localized sweating, and skin injuries about the head and tuber coxae are noted. In stallions the scrotum is palpated for inguinal hernia. If signs are severe a stomach tube should be passed, and trocarization is advised if bloating is present. If the colic is so severe that an orderly examination is impossible, heavy sedation and analgesic therapy are indicated. Noramidopyrine methane sulfonate sodium (Novalgin, Metapyrine), 50 ml i.v., and methadone (Polamivet), 25 ml i.v., are satisfactory for this purpose.

Phenothiazine derivatives are to be avoided due to their strong hypotensive action. In addition, the pooling of erythrocytes in the spleen further impairs oxygen transport in shock and makes it difficult to assess the hematocrit. In male horse, this medication may cause prolapse of the penis with injury during colicky episodes.

Examination of the Heart and Circulation. Many gastrointestinal diseases, especially intestinal obstruction, are accompanied by shock. This is manifested clinically by an increase in the heart and pulse rate, coldness of the extremities, cyanosis of the visible mucosae, increased capillary refill times, oliguria or even anuria (for details see Sec. 1.6.2.). All these are symptoms of the body's attempt to maintain a blood supply to vital centers despite hypovolemia by a redistribution of blood flow (selective vasoconstriction). In particular, the rate and quality of the pulse should be noted. As the degree of shock becomes more severe, there is an increase in the pulse rate in the facial artery, and the pulse wave becomes harder, thinner, bounding and finally impalpable, so that the heart rate must be determined by auscultation. The capillary refill time is tested on the gingiva of the incisor teeth by creating a blanched area with the fingertip and measuring the time required for the white spot to disappear. The normal refill time is 2 s or less. When inspecting the conjunctivae, it must be considered that conjunctivitis often occurs as a result of rolling or of striking the head and so is undependable for circulatory assessment (asymmetrical reddening). Its normal pink color often becomes pale pink at the onset of colic, later becoming red, then dark red and finally a muddy red when endotoxemia occurs later. The venous blood pressure is also important for circulatory assessment. If the jugular vein is poorly filled as a result of a diminished blood supply, the central venous pressure will be low or even negative. If the jugular vein appears distended even when it is not compressed, a presumptive diagnosis of congestive heart failure may be made.

The *respiratory rate* is slightly increased in most forms of colic. It is very rapid and shallow in gaseous distention, gastric dilation and peritonitis. A dyspnea with costal respiration is present in such cases. Metabolic acidosis is also associated with an increased respiratory rate. Transportation, excitement and rolling likewise increase the pulse and respiratory rate, but the rise is transitory. The animal should be given time to calm down before these rates are measured.

The internal body temperature is usually normal but may be subnormal if the horse is in shock (hypothermia). Fever signifies intestinal necrosis and peritonitis. It is also a sign of aspiration pneumonia (vomiting, intubation).

Auscultation of the Abdomen. Auscultation should be carried out on the left and right flanks. The gurgling sounds of the small intestine are heard well on the left side and may be increased, decreased or absent, have a dry or splashing character, or may start softly, rise quickly in intensity and then fade or stop abruptly (spastic inhibition).

Auscultation over the right costal arch at the level of the base of the cecum will reveal a periodic squirt of fluid through the ileocecal orifice. In the healthy horse this sound is heard from 1 to 3 times per minute, depending on food and water intake. If the cecum is filled mostly with gas, the sounds will have a hissing, tympanitic quality. If it is filled with fluid and gas, splashing sounds predominate. In the presence of a small bowel obstruction, peristalsis may be increased initially (to work against the obstruction), but later it is inhibited and finally suppressed altogether. In paralytic ileus the abdomen is silent.

The normal ileocecal valve sound is absent if the ileum is impacted and eventually disappears during the course of any small intestinal ileus. In impactions of the cecum the sound is suppressed.

The sounds of the large intestine are duller and deeper in intensity. They are not as undulating as the small intestinal sounds. In small intestinal ileus they often remain audible long after small bowel peristalsis has ceased.

Ausculation should not be done hurriedly. A minimum of 5 minutes per side is necessary in order to detect sounds recurring at longer intervals. The results of the auscultation should be interpreted very carefully. Their primary importance is for monitoring the progress of the disease, rather than arriving at a diagnosis.

Special Examinations

Passage of a Stomach Tube. Besides its diagnostic value, the passage of a stomach tube is also helpful in reducing the danger of gastric distention and rupture that is associated with many forms of colic. We use a transparent plastic tube that carries two markings: The first indicates the distance from the nose and esophageal inlet (so that the tube can be accurately directed into the pharynx), and the second shows when the end of the tube is in the stomach. In many cases the cardia can be passed only after air has first been insufflated under pressure. Once the tube has reached the stomach, any gas that is present is evacuated. Then the tube is passed somewhat deeper, and suction is carefully applied. With some practice it will be apparent at once whether gastric mucosa or gastric fluid is being aspirated. If the tube opening is blocked by a fold of gastric mucosa, the tube is advanced farther under suction to locate the gastric fluid level. The aspiration should be repeated several times even if no fluid is obtained initially because only in this way, can one be certain that the stomach is indeed empty. Aspirated fluid volumes in excess of 3 to 5 l signify an acute gastric dilation. The fluid consists of saliva and gastric juice that can no longer drain

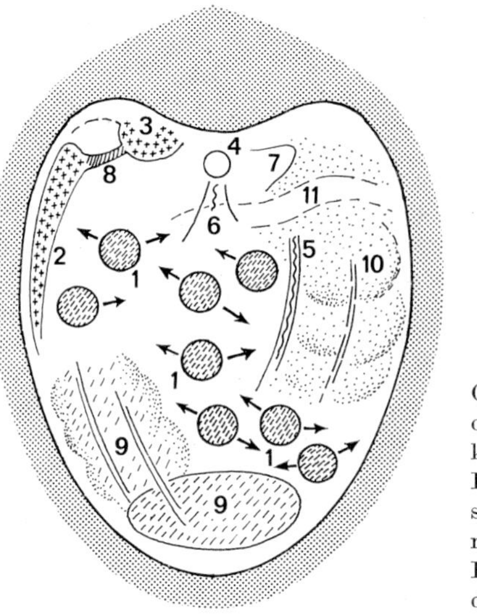

Fig. 2.1.5. — 15. Rectal findings in the normal horse. Generally palpable: *1* freely movable fecal balls in small colon; *2* caudal edge of spleen; *3* caudal pole of left kidney; *4* abdominal aorta; *5* medial band of cecum; Frequently palpable: *6* cranial root of mesentery; *7* dorsal attachment of base of cecum; *8* nephrosplenic ligament; *9* pelvic flexure and parts of left ventral colon; Rarely palpable: *10* body and base of cecum; *11* duodenum (if cecum is distended).

into the small intestine. In advanced small intestinal obstructions, brownish-yellow fluid refluxes from the small intestine into the stomach. If solid food particles are found in the stomach, a gastric lavage should be performed. This is done by introducing 3 to 5 l of cold water through the nasogastric tube and then siphoning it back off from the stomach. In primary gastric dilation this procedure must be repeated until the bulk of the stomach contents has been removed. This is done more easily and rapidly by passing a thick stomach tube through the mouth using a mouth gag. The passage of a stomach tube is so important in reducing the danger of gastric rupture that negligence in this area constitutes malpractice.

Rectal Examination. The rectal examination (fig. 2.1.5. — 15) is one of the most rewarding special examinations in the colicky horse. It is comparable in importance to the intestinal radiograph in man and small animals. It should be performed during the initial examination. Repeated rectal examinations in the same animal make it possible to clarify the initial findings. These often are ambiguous. It is also useful to monitor the response to treatment.

The rectal examination is not without risks for the patient or examiner. The veterinarian must think of his own safety; to be careless is to invite an accident. The horse also must be protected from injury (rectal perforation). In horses that strain heavily, are unusually restless or have a very small rectum, sedation, epidural anesthesia and a warm enema will generally enable a rectal examination to be carried out at minimal risk. A rectal examination should never be done forcefully. If force is necessary it is better that the examination not be done at all. Most rectal perforations occur in racehorses that have a very narrow rectal lumen. The examiner should never forcibly oppose a straining force or a peristaltic wave, but should allow the hand to relax and retract with it. If there is a ballooning of the intestine that makes exploration difficult, the examiner should await relaxation or induce it by means of an enema. The arm should be bare up to the shoulder and gloved in a thin, disposable glove that is well lubricated. First all feces are removed from the rectal ampulla. The examiner should proceed systematically so that nothing is overlooked.

Normally the fecal balls in the small colon, the caudal edge of the spleen, the caudal part of the left kidney and the abdominal aorta can be felt; the cranial mesenteric root is palpable if the examiner has a sufficiently long reach. The tense, sickle-shaped ventral band of the cecum is always easily discerned to the right of the midline. The dorsal attachment of the base of the cecum is reached by feeling along the right dorsal abdominal wall. The renosplenic or nephrosplenic ligament is palpable only in medium-size horses if the dorsal edge of the spleen and left kidney are not too close together. The pelvic flexure and several bands of the left ventral colon are usually palpable but may not be obvious. In male horses the inguinal rings can be felt about a hand's width anterior to the pelvic inlet. Abnormally palpable segments of bowel are assessed in terms of their position, size and content. They are identifiable by their anatomic structures (bands, sacculations). The examiner should note their position relative to other abdominal organs (e.g., the pelvic flexure in the pelvic cavity), their content (gas, liquid, semiliquid, pasty or firm ingesta), their size, which is conveniently referred to parts of the human extremities (e.g., arm-size loops of small intestine), their mobility (e.g., loop of small intestine abnormally anchored at the left inguinal ring), their tension (lax or tight) and their consistency (normal or thickened and fleshy). The fecal balls should be moist and of normal size. They are dry, hard and small if the intestinal transit time is prolonged leading to a greater fluid absorption. If the transit time is decreased, the fecal consistency will be pasty to watery. The rectal wall should be loose and distensible. Its lumen may be dilated cranially or obstructed by lesions external to the bowel wall. The mucosa can be shifted about and unfolded, and its surface is slippery; a velvety or sandpapery texture is abnormal. Superficial lesions are most easily felt without a glove; a bare-handed exploration is especially important if a rectal perforation is suspected (clotted blood in the ampulla). The feces may contain whitish mucous strands, oxyurids, gastrophilus larvae or blood, which is red and clotted when emanating from the terminal part of the intestine or dark when emanating from the anterior bowel (melena).

In ileus of more cranial portions of the intestinal tract the rectum may be empty and contain small amounts of sticky mucus.

From the pelvic brim, the first structures to be examined are the urinary bladder, the urethra, and in mares the uterus, ovaries and uterine ligaments. Suspected uterine torsion should be excluded in mares that are close to foaling. The inguinal (vaginal) rings are examined in stallions. Normally the tips of 1 or 2 fingers can be inserted painlessly from a dorsolateral direction. The examiner should note the presence of finger-thick, fleshy cords entering the ring that are tender to traction (inguinal hernia). Next the spleen is located. Its caudal edge touches the left abdominal wall at about the level of the last rib but often lies a hand's width caudal to it; normally the edge is sharp and distinct. In gastric dilation, after injections of phenothiazine derivatives, or often for undisclosed reasons the spleen may be displaced far caudally. In such situations it may present a blunt edge, and not be in contact with the abdominal wall.

When the large colon herniates into the nephrosplenic space, the spleen is often displaced medially. The nephrosplenic ligament can be reached from the dorsal edge of the spleen only if the ligament is free. If colon is draped over the ligament, the latter must be palpated from the direction of the left kidney. Because of stretching by the herniated bowel, the ligament will be abnormally tender to pressure. In rare cases a dilated stomach can be reached by passing the fingertips below the left kidney and far anteriorally until the smooth gastric wall is felt. The anterior mesenteric root is palpable only in medium-size or smaller horses, in which the caudal half of the left kidney is also accessible. Normally the abdominal aorta is palpable all the way to the anterior mesenteric root, and its pulsations can be felt. The mesenteric root also should pulsate and should not be thickened, obscured or tender. If the pulse is absent or a fremitus is felt, endarteritis and/or aneurysm of the cranial mesenteric artery should be suspected. The small intestine is not palpable under normal circumstances. In small intestinal obstruction with a damming-back of ingesta to the stomach, the caudal duodenal flexure can be recognized as a short, horizontal, almost immovable tube located to the right of and caudal to the mesenteric root in the area of the base of the cecum.

Palpable loops of small intestine in spasmodic colic are soft and gas-filled or constricted in certain areas. Isolated or multiple, parallel loops of small intestine that are tightly distended with gas and difficult to move are characteristic of small intestinal obstruction. An impacted ileum is sausage-shaped and about the thickness of an arm. It feels doughy and extends from the lower middle to right upper abdomen. An ileal impaction is palpable only in its early stage, for later the distended loops of small intestine proximal to the obstruction, displace the ileum anteriorally.

Dilated loops of small intestine are always an alarming sign and should prompt a search for additional signs of obstruction until a definitive diagnosis can be made.

Like the small intestine, the cecum is normally impalpable; only its ventral band can be located by exploring downward toward the right flank from a craniomedial direction. This band often is tightly stretched, extending *medially downward and cranially* from the right upper abdomen and is frequently mistaken for a displaced section of bowel. Cords of this type are very often felt in cecal tympany, and it is a good rule to devote extra time to their palpation and identification. One should determine whether their position and tension are altered by peristaltic waves, in which case the changes are functional and benign, or whether their position and tension are constant, indicating that the bands are abnormally immobilized as a result of pathologic intestinal displacement. Dilated small intestinal loops of a fleshy consistency that are tender and seem to be abnormally fixed are characteristic of an incarceration or strangulation. A twisted, tense cord arising from the mesenteric root is a probable sign of mesenteric volvulus.

Impactions of the large intestine accentuate the normal contour of the affected bowel segments. If the body of the cecum is impacted, it is easily recognized in the right half of the abdominal cavity by its longidutinal bands, which curve from the right upper abdomen downward to the left and cranially, and by its large haustra. The base of the cecum and its overhanging extremity can be set into pendular motion with the hand in cases of isolated impaction. Occasionally the cecal base is displaced quite far caudally to the anterior pelvic brim.

Impactions of the stomach-like dilation of the right dorsal colon can be palpated only by passing the hand far forward past the right side of the mesenteric root. The caudal part of the impaction feels doughy and is easily indented with the fingers. If an enterolith is lodged anterior to the transverse colon, a smooth, stony-hard hemispherical surface is felt. The intestinal wall will mold to the shape of the calculus. Abscesses in the area of the anterior mesenteric root are recognizable by their knobby surface.

The left dorsal and left ventral colon are located below and medial to the spleen on the left side. Normally they are impossible to identify owing to their semiliquid content. Impaction of the ventral colon is recognized by its longitudinal bands and haustra and can be followed caudally to the pelvic flexure, which is smooth and about the thickness of a human thigh.

Even when the cecum and large colon are distended, their sacculations are usually palpable, and their bands are tightly stretched and lie in longitudinal furrows between the rows of haustra. Tympany of the large intestine indicates that progression is obstructed in a more distal segment of bowel. In mild torsion, strangulation or kinking of the large intestine, the extent of the tympany is variable. Severe gaseous distension of the large colon that is not relieved even by trocarization of the cecum is a sign of colonic torsion. Edema due to infarction in the large bowel is evidenced by a fleshy felt thickening of the gut wall. This is demonstrated by pressing the affected segment against something firmer and allowing it to spring back. Sometimes gelatinous edematous portions of the mesentery are also palpated. When impacted or distended, the small colon is about the thickness of an arm and forms several tight coils within and anterior to the pelvic cavity. It is identified by its characteristic tenia on its antimesenteric surface which projects slightly above the intestinal surface.

The peritoneum should be smooth and nontender. Roughness or grittiness is usually caused by food particles. Fibrinous adhesions can be separated from their undersurface. A subperitoneal emphysema may be felt in some cases of intestinal rupture.

The most common mistake in rectal examinations is to conclude the examination as soon an abnormality is found, without exploring the rest of the abdominal cavity. For example in high small intestinal obstruction the examiner may palpate a secondary inspissation of feces, interpret this as an impaction of the large colon, and, satisfied with this diagnosis, overlook the grossly distended caudal duodenal flexure that could provide evidence of high obstruction.

The results of the rectal examination of colicky horses can be classified into three groups according to their diagnostic reliability:

a) *Definite rectal findings:* These are findings which leave no doubt as to the nature and site of the obstruction. The obstruction is accessible to direct palpation and is so readily identifiable that the finding may be considered 'pathognomonic' of the particular disorder (e.g., herniation into renosplenic space, incarcerated inguinal hernia).

b) *Characteristic rectal findings:* The obstruction is palpable, but a correct interpretation can be made only in the light of other rectal findings. These findings enable a special diagnosis to be made with some degree of certainty. Most findings fall into this category (e.g., strangulation of the small colon, cecal impaction).

c) *Ambiguous rectal findings:* The obstruction is impalpable or inaccessible, and its location (small intestine, large intestine) and nature (strangulation, impaction) can be deduced only from other signs (e.g., colonic torsion, strangulation of small intestine) (fig. 2.1.5. — 16; see enclosure).

Abdominal Paracentesis. The abdominal paracentesis technique of Gratzl is safe but, we believe, unnecessarily involved. He uses a trocar with a 2-mm-wide sleeve and 2 stylets. The sharp-pointed stylet is used to perforate the skin and abdominal wall, while the blunt stylet is used to penetrate the fat and peritoneum, thus eliminating the danger of inadvertant intestinal perforation. We have obtained equally safe results with a No. 2 Braunuele® cannula. First the cannula is inserted through the skin and abdominal wall, then the cannula-like stylet is withdrawn a few millimeters and the peritoneum is penetrated with the blunt plastic cannula. The simplest but most hazardous technique employs a short-bevel needle of the type used for intravenous injections in large animals.

The skin is punctured on the linea alba about midway between the sternum and umbilicus. While one assistant controls the animal's head, a second assistant picks up the foreleg on the side on which the veterinarian is standing. It is best to stand by the animal's shoulder facing the rear, rather than by the hindquarters. Thus, a right-handed operator stands on the animal's left side, and a left-handed operator on the right side.

The cannula is grasped by the hub and with a short thrust is pushed through the skin and linea alba only. Little resistance is felt after the initial thrust. The cannula tip is moved about gently to determine whether it has already entered the abdominal cavity; this is quite possible in light and thin animals and is recognized by the escape of peritoneal fluid. If the needle remains dry, the cannula is carefully advanced farther until it penetrates the peritoneum. Blood escaping from the needle may originate from an inadvertantly punctured blood vessel or from the spleen. In either case the cannula is withdrawn and reinserted at another site. If peritoneal fluid is not obtained right away, some air can be injected to clear any blockage of the cannula. The inadvertant puncture of a loop of bowel is easily recognized by the escape of a dark, grayish-green fluid. The needle is removed at once and reinserted at a new site. The puncture of bowel loops that are not abnormally distended is seldom dangerous, for the holes are rapidly sealed. However, in colics with distended loops of small intestine with a lack of peristalsis, the leakage of intestinal contents is a danger. Therefore, if rectal examination reveals small bowel dilatation, paracentesis should be done with extreme caution, if at all. Another contraindication for abdominal paracentesis is late pregnancy in the mare, due to the risk of uterine puncture.

The amount of fluid collected is highly variable. In the healthy horse a few drops of clear, pale yellow fluid will drip from the needle with each respiratory excursion (a total of about 2 to 3 ml in 1 to 2 min). With a large fluid accumulation (e.g., in ascites), a full, continuous stream is obtained. With minimal fluid accumulation a small jet appears initially and is interrupted with each respiration. About 5—10 ml can usually be obtained in such cases. The collected fluid is grossly examined in test tubes and if necessary its cellular content is determined. This is best done by centrifuging the specimen and analyzing the sediment. The sediment will show several distinct layers, with grayish-green food particles (if present) at the bottom and erythrocytes and leukocytes at the top.

Analysis of the peritoneal fluid is conducted according to certain criteria:

a) *Functional intestinal disorders unaccompanied by pathoanatomic lesions of the bowel* (e.g., spasmodic colic, mild to moderate large intestinal impactions and mild tympany): Paracentesis yields only a small amount of fluid that is yellow, transparent and free of visible contaminants.

b) *Venous congestion without intestinal necrosis* (e.g., impaction of the ileum, kinking or flexion of the colon, dorsal displacement of the large colon into nephrosplenic space): In acute cases the peritoneal fluid is mildly increased in volume and light yellow in color, later becoming darker and slightly turbid; few erythrocytes are obtained on centrifugation.

c) *Venous congestion with significant infarction and incipient intestinal necrosis* (e.g., volvulus of the jejunum, internal hernias with incarceration, torsion of the colon): A marked erythrocyte and leukocyte layer is present in the sediment. Red cells are found almost exclusively at the onset of the infarction, but white cells become more abundant as the necrosis progresses.

d) *Extensive venous congestion and intestinal necrosis with peritonitis* (e.g., volvulus of the jejunum, complete torsion of the colon): Paracentesis yields a large volume of bright-red to muddy-red fluid. Leukocytes are predominant in the sediment, although a thick erythrocyte layer is also present. If the necrotic bowel is already permeable to bacteria, a grayish-brown sediment is obtained.

e) *Intestinal necrosis due to thromboembolism, intestinal necrosis secondary to mesenteric tears, local purulent fibrinous peritonitis* (e.g., necrosis of the cecum or colon):

The fluid is muddy yellow-red to green, turbid and has a creamy consistency. Its quantity is variable and often small. Centrifugation yields a thick leukocyte layer with relatively few erythrocytes.

f) *Gastric or intestinal rupture, diffuse peritonitis:* A large quantity of muddy-red or gray-green, highly turbid fluid is obtained. An odor of intestinal contents is sometimes noted. The sediment contains grayish-green food constituents (microscopy!), numerous leukocytes and erythrocytes.

The fluid over the sediment may be brownish-red as a result of hemolysis.

g) *Intraperitoneal hemorrhage:* In acute hemorrhage, abdominal paracentesis yields whole blood. It contains mainly red cells whose proportion in the centrifugation tube corresponds approximately to the hematocrit.

h) *Abdominal abscesses and tumors (chronic recurrent colics):* In chronic colic the peritoneal fluid may be turbid, yellow-green, and have a high density (over 1.030) and high cellular content. Erythrocytes, lymphocytes, neutrophils and eosinophils and mesothelial cells are found. Microscopic differentiation can provide evidence of strangles abscesses, lymphosarcoma and other intraabdominal neoplasms.

i) *Ascites:* Paracentesis yields large amounts of fluid that is clear and straw-colored, contains no visible impurities and has a low density (1.005 to 1.015).

j) *Rupture of the urinary bladder:* The pale-yellow, clear or very slightly turbid peritoneal fluid is collected in large amounts and consists of urine. In doubtful cases the nature of the fluid is easily demonstrated with a reagent strip (urea values of 16.7 mmol/l[1] or more).

Diagnostic-Therapeutic Medication. The use of spasmolytics and/or analgesics and in some cases parasympathomimetics can often aid in the diagnosis.

In spasmodic colic, spasmoanalgesics such as noramidopyrine methane sulfonate sodium (e.g., Novalgin) or scopolamine butylbromide (e.g., Buscopan) provide almost immediate relief of colicky symptoms, and in impactions they can calm the animal for long periods of time. In cases of mechanical obstruction and peritonitis, on the other hand, they will produce no significant improvement.

The calm produced by such medications should not be confused with the 'stage of indolence' mentioned earlier. Deep shock developing as a result of intestinal necrosis causes the patient to enter this stage and exhibit a complete calmness of behavior. This is interpreted as a good sign only if circulation and peristalsis are normal. Today, spasmolytic therapy is widely employed in veterinary medicine. Its value is undisputed and in many cases is so highly rated that it can actually represent a danger to animals with mechanical obstruction. Many equine practitioners have cultivated such faith in the prompt efficacy of spasmolytic drugs that they dispense with special examinations and rely entirely on Novalgin therapy. But the failure of spasmoanalgesics in a horse with colic is an important diagnostic sign. It indicates the presence of a serious underlying disorder, such as mechanical obstruction. Consequently, it is unwise to administer these drugs at frequent intervals or attempt to force sedation by giving extreme overdoses in combination with analgesics such as methadone (e.g., Polamivet) or tranquilizers such as xylazine (e.g. Rompun). This should only be done for the purpose of facilitating examination. The side-effects of such therapy are the masking of symptoms and a worsening of the circulatory status, making diagnosis and further treatment more difficult.

Neostigmine (e.g., Prostigmin) is suitable for use in general tympany. Rectal examination in this type of colic reveals gas-filled loops of small intestine as well as gaseous distension of portions of the large intestine, especially the cecum and

1 Conversion: mg/100 ml × 0.1665 = mmol/l; mmol/l × 6.01 = mg/100 ml.

loops of left colon. Following trocarization of the cecum and evacuation of the stomach, the use of neostigmine may be of therapeutic and diagnostic value. General tympany, if present, is controlled rapidly. If the tympany is secondary to a mechanical ileus, the therapy is not only ineffective but will exacerbate symptoms. Carbachol (e.g., Lentin) is contraindicated in the colicky horse due to its strong secretory action. If the colic symptoms increase after neostigmine, accompanied by a corresponding worsening of clinical data, conservative therapy should be discontinued and surgical treatment instituted.

Time and again we have treated cases in which the first attending veterinarian administered a saline laxative without first establishing a diagnosis. Such a therapy is contraindicated because in small intestinal obstruction it increases fermentation and stagnation of intestinal contents cranial to the obstruction and at the same time promotes secondary gastric dilation and dehydration. The use of mineral oil is less hazardous, for it does not alter the water balance. Schebitz [1961] calls the use of saline laxatives in poorly diagnosed cases 'cosmetic therapy', but 'malpractice' is an equally descriptive term.

Enterocentesis. If the cecum is found to be severely distended with gas on rectal examination, it should be tapped by trocarization from the right flank. The release of the gas will bring the patient immediate relief, will greatly facilitate rectal examination and will allow gas and ingesta again to enter the cecum from the ileum. When combined with gas- and fluid-filled loops of small intestine, a tympanitic cecum is indicative of general tympany rather than small intestinal obstruction. Treatment in such cases consists of repeated puncture of the cecum and the administration of cholinergics (Prostigmin).

A gas-filled cecum in the absence of palpable small intestinal loops indicates that the intestinal lumen is constricted or obstructed (impaction, incarceration or torsion) in the region of the large colon, or that there is an isolated distension of the cecum. While trocarization of the cecum is frequently indicated, one should be hesitant to puncture the large colon. In the rare cases where it is necessary, it is done per rectum using the narrowest-gauge cannula possible. Puncture must be limited strictly to gas-filled intestinal loops; fluid-filled loops should never be punctured. We make it a rule never to puncture small intestinal loops, first because the procedure is unrewarding, second because the puncture site often remains open, predisposing to peritonitis.

Laboratory Tests. A fully-equipped laboratory is not always available to the equine practitioner. However, measurement of the hematocrit by the microtechnique has been perfected in recent years to the point that it can now be performed simply and at small cost even 'in the field'. The veterinarian should by all means take advantage of this. Rising hematocrit values in the colicky horse signal fluid losses from extravasation much earlier and more accurately than is possible to tell by skin elasticity. In the colicky horse fluid is lost to the extracellular space of the strangulated bowel (lumen of the incarcerated and prestenotic segment) as well as to the abdominal cavity. The consequences of this are hypovolemia, dehydration and shock. The normal hematocrit values in the horse are between 32 and 36[1]. In excited horses the hematocrit may rise temporarily to 45 to 48 due to the mobilization of erythrocytes from the spleen. On the other hand, the hematocrit may be lowered by the administration of phenothiazine tranquillizers and drugs with similar actions due to the sequestration of red cells in certain organs.

1 Conversion: vol.% $\times$ 0.01 = decimal value.

The hematocrit measurement offers an important clue to the degree of systemic insult caused by the colicky disease. It enables intravenous therapy to be administered and is excellent for monitoring response. In serious diseases it enables specific fluid replacement to be started even *before* the diagnosis is established, thus gaining time for diagnosis and transportation to a hospital.

Further laboratory tests (leukocyte determination, differential blood count, sodium, potassium and calcium determinations, lactate determination, blood glucose, ESR, pH) are done at the hospital as needed and are not recommended on the initial examination. Their results should be interpreted only by experienced personnel.

Documentation. The results of the systematic examination should be carefully documented. By comparing findings recorded at different times, the veterinarian is able to discern important *trends* in the course of the illness. The sheet that we use for examining the colicky horse is drawn up such that physiologic findings are on the left, and to the right are the major pathologic findings. These are arranged in order of prognostic importance such that the most prognostically unfavorable findings are on the far right (fig. 2.1.5. — 17; see enclosure). Individual values that can be expressed numerically (e.g., pulse rate) are entered in a separate column. When results are marked on the sheet, a pattern of findings emerges that will clearly reveal significant trends. On the one hand, this procedure forces the veterinarian to adopt an exacting and systematic examination routine. On the other it gives him an opportunity for analysis and reflection which is denied under the traumatic conditions of the examination itself. A study of figures 2.1.5. — 16 and — 17 should convince the equine practitioner that he has more diagnostic capabilities at his disposal than he might suppose.

2.1.5.10.6. Special Forms of Colic

Spasmodic Colic

Definition and Occurrence. Spasmodic colic, called also catarrhal intestinal colic, rheumatic colic, irritative and cold colic, is a functional intestinal disorder that is rarely associated with histologic changes of the mucosa. It is attributed to an increase in vagal tone causing peristalsis and propensity to spasm. Spasmodic colic is by far the most common form of colic in horses and accounts for some 40% of all cases.

Symptoms and Diagnosis. The disease is characterized by severe, paroxysmal attacks of colic lasting from 5 to 10 min and separated by pain-free intervals. Initially systemic effects are mild. The respiratory and pulse rate increase little during the bouts of pain. Often the hyperperistaltic activity is audible at some distance from the horse and usually has a metallic sound. Feces are passed frequently and in small amounts and usually have a soft to semiliquid consistency.

Rectal findings are seldom remarkable. A spastically constricted loop of bowel may be palpable in some instances. In other cases small amounts of gas are found in the small intestine and cecum. Barring further complications, the colicky symptoms will pass in 4 to 6 h. Possible complications are volvulus and intussusception. In most cases the administration of a spasmoanalgesic will quickly relieve the colic attacks (diagnostic-therapeutic medication).

Etiology and Pathogenesis. Attacks can be precipitated by weather changes, overexertion, chilling and feeding errors (moldy feed or straw bedding, change from stable feeding to pasturing). The irritant substances ingested with spoiled feed are propelled into the large intestine by the violent peristalsis. An individual predisposition to this colic is not uncommon.

Differential Diagnosis. Attacks of small intestinal ileus also start with loud hyperperistalsis ('resistance' peristalsis), but a prompt response to spasmoanalgesics and unremarkable rectal findings are sufficient to exclude this disease.

Reductions of blood flow due to thromboembolic lesions of the mesenteric arteries are associated with similar symptoms. If only one artery is affected in the terminal flow region, a diagnosis is virtually impossible. But if several arteries are involved, there will be a disturbance in progression that is evidenced rectally by increased filling of intestinal loops with gas and ingesta.

Prognosis. The prognosis in spasmodic colic is favorable.

Treatment. Normally a single intravenous injection of 20—60 ml noramidopyrine methane sulfonate sodium (Novalgin) or 20—30 ml scopolamine butylbromide (Buscupan) is sufficient. The treatment may be repeated after several hours if necessary.

Gas Colic, Flatulent Colic, Intestinal Tympany

Definition and Occurrence. Intestinal tympany involves a gaseous distension of the small and/or large intestine that may lead to overstretching of the bowel and eventually to intestinal paralysis or so-called paralytic ileus. Gas production may be so severe that intestinal rupture results. Intestinal tympany may be primary or secondary. *Primary* cases are caused by the ingestion of wilted or heated green feed, lush grass that is low in crude fiber, clover, fresh bread, fruit and fresh grain. *Secondary* tympany is caused by obstruction of the small or large intestine, by impaction, or by paralytic ileus in peritonitis.

Symptoms and Diagnosis. Mild distension, especially of the large intestine (often only the cecum is affected), produce mild colicky symptoms. Systemic signs are absent. Intestinal sounds are brisk and markedly increased. In the absence of obstruction, large amounts of gas and scant feces are passed. In these cases the cecum and sometimes the large colon are found to be filled with gas on rectal examination. If both the small and large intestine are affected, *general tympany* is present, and pain is intense. Severe tympany causes respiratory embarrassment due to pressure on the diaphragm. Venous return is also embarrassed by the increased intra-abdominal pressure. Because of this, shock can develop rapidly. In severe cases, death from asphyxia occurs in 3 to 5 h.

On rectal examination, dilated loops of small intestine appear to fill the abdominal cavity. The cecum is recognized at once by its medial band, which is tightly stretched and curves medially and anteriorally from the right upper to left lower abdomen. In early flatulent colic, peristalsis is initially increased but becomes more sluggish with distension of the bowel and finally ceases altogether. Marked systemic signs appear at this time. The pulse rate rises above 80 and the respiratory rate above 30. The hematocrit may be only mildly elevated initially. In *primary tympany* there is often history of a qualitative change in the diet. In addition, primary tympany is *general* in most cases, whereas *secondary tympany* is often *local*, being confined to individual bowel segments proximal to the obstruction. In torsion of the large colon, for example, there is a stagnation of gas in the cecum; a similar stasis can be caused by impactions.

Etiology and Pathogenesis. Primary tympany is caused by the ingestion of wilted or heated green feed, lush grass that is low in crude fiber, fresh bread, fruit, fresh grain and pelleted complete feeds. *Secondary tympany* is caused by an obstruction and occurs in the intestinal segment proximal to this obstruction. The stretching of the intestinal tube leads to circulatory disturbances in the gut wall resulting in a reduced oxygen supply to the intestinal musculature. The oxygen deficit hampers intestinal peristalsis, and a vicious cycle develops that can be broken only by evacuation of the bowel.

Prognosis. The prognosis in primary tympany is very good with prompt, correct treatment. In secondary cases, it depends on the prognosis of the primary disorder.

Treatment. The main therapeutic goal is to evacuate the stomach with the aid of a stomach tube and to release the intestinal gases through surgical trocarization.

In primary tympany the cecum is always tightly distended with gas, cecal trocarization is the first step in such cases. This is best done from the flank. In severe cases the puncture may be repeated or an indwelling trocar may be used. Cecal decompression will again enable gas to enter the cecum from the small intestine as well as from the colon (reflux).

Gas removal from the small intestine can be hastened by administering neostigmine (Prostigmin) following evacuation of the cecum. Puncture of the large colon and cecum per rectum is indicated only in exceptional cases. Pain will subside quickly once the cecal gas is expelled. If it persists, however, Novalgin or Metapyrin should be given. Atropine and papaverine-containing drugs such as scopolamine butylbromide (Buscupan) are contraindicated due to their paralytic effect on the bowel.

Trocarization of the intestine is followed by a 3-day course of systemic antibiotics.

Antitympanitics and antiseptics are ineffective and so should not be used. If rectal examination reveals an impaction of the large intestine, mineral oil and sodium sulfate may be beneficial. Tympany may be accompanied by secondary gastric dilation, and so the foregoing drugs should be administered only if the stomach is empty.

Most horses recover surprisingly quickly after the gas in removed. Intravenous fluids should be instituted if early signs of shock appear, in which cases sodium sulfate solutions are contraindicated, initially.

In many cases of cecal tympany, the cecum is so grossly distended that its overhanging end blocks the cecocolic orifice. This type of obstruction was first described by GRATZL. It is relieved immediately by cecal trocarization.

Intestinal Impactions

Definition, Pathogenesis and Etiology. Impactions are the most common causes of colic in the horse. They result from the sedimentation, accumulation and drying out (inspissation) of food and fecal material. Certain sites in the intestine are anatomically or pathologically predisposed to impactions. Complete obstruction almost always accompanies impactions of the small intestine but is rare in impaction of the large intestine.

The normal content of the small intestine in the horse is about 95% water, in which food particles, ranging in size from less than 1.5 mm to 5 mm in diameter, are suspended. The dilution is similar in the cecum. Significant water absorption first occurs in the large colon, especially in the large saccular like regions. It is in this region that the inspissation of intestinal contents takes place. Impactions of the small intestine start with the sedimentation and accumulation of food particles anterior to an obstacle, from which the water is extruded by spastic contractions ('sieve effect') until finally the impaction is bound fast by a sustained spasm of the gut wall. In the large intestine, on the other hand, the mechanism of impaction is inspissation. As a result, small intestinal impactions develop rapidly and often cause excruciating pain, whereas large intestinal impactions develop gradually over several feedings and produce mild symptoms of colic.

Stenoses of the small intestine may exist for some time without noticeable symptoms. If the intestinal lumen is narrowed by only a few millimeters, then under certain

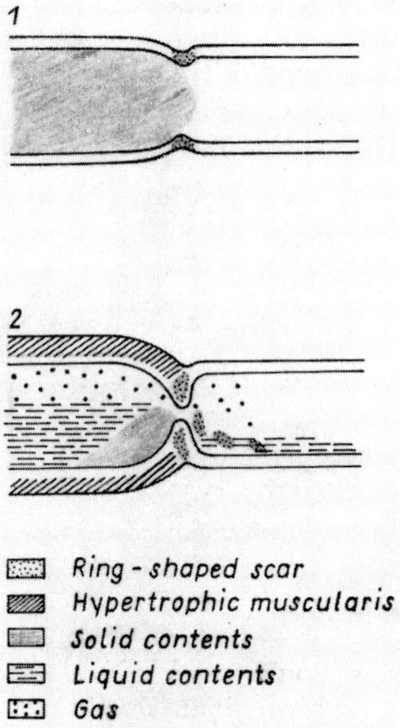

Fig. 2.1.5. — 18. Stenoses of the small intestine.
1 Ring-shaped scar *without* major luminal constriction. Obstruction caused by impaction anterior to stricture due to inadequate ability of intestinal lumen to dilate.
2 Ring-shaped scar *with* major luminal constriction. Chronic partial obstruction with compensatory hypertrophy of muscularis layer and dilation of prestenotic bowel segment.

circumstances (spasmodic colic) an obstruction can develop as a result of sedimentation of ingesta proximal to the stenosis. With more severe narrowing of the lumen, the increased resistance will eventually induce a compensatory *hypertrophy* of the intestinal wall anterior to the stenosis. This condition, called megajejunum, or muscular hypertrophy, is characterized by chronic, recurrent colicky pains following the ingestion of food. Remarkably, a hypertrophy of this type can be demonstrated over a distance of many meters proximal to the stenosis. These changes are also seen in the presence of a Meckel's diverticulum and in functional stenosis of the ileocecal orifice (ileal hypertrophy or megaileum; fig. 2.1.5. — 18).

In the large intestine, functional stenosis of the cecocolic orifice similarly leads to hypertrophy of the cecal musculature, especially in the area of the base but also in its other parts. Similar conditions are observed in the region of the right dorsal colon. In the small colon, chronic stenoses can cause hypertrophy (megacolon) at the junction of the rectum and colon.

The aboral progression of ingesta can be impeded by:
— reduced bowel motility,
— oversize food particles,
— stenosis,
— reduced water content of the ingesta.

Abnormalities of peristalsis can have various causes. Among the most frequent are:
— lack of exercise,
— overexertion,
— enteritis,
— parasitism,
— autonomic dystonias.

Mechanical causes include poor mastication as a result of dental defects or ravenous eating. Woody grain or leguminous fibers, old hay, finely-chopped roughage, spoiled corn silage and finely-chopped grass (lawn clippings) predispose to intestinal impaction, especially if microbial decomposition in the large intestine is delayed and water intake is deficient.

Heavy sweating in the summer can create an overall water deficit that leads to increased water absorption in the large intestine and thus to an abnormal degree of fecal inspissation or drying out. Small intestinal obstruction also leads to a *secondary* inspissation of ingesta in the large colon, as water reserves in the large intestine are mobilized to compensate for the hypovolemia.

Anatomic constrictions of the bowel are predilection sites for the development of impactions, although sedimentation and inspissation can occur at other locations as well (see also fig. 2.1.5. — 12). These are listed below in the order of the frequency of their involvement in impactions:

— the pelvic flexure,
— the junction of the cecum and large colon,
— the junction of the ileum and cecum,
— the small colon,
— the jejunum,
— the duodenum.

Impaction of the Small Intestine

Symptoms and Diagnosis. Symptoms of small bowel impaction usually appear soon after eating in the form of a sudden, relatively severe attack of colic. The pains are caused by overdistension of the intestinal tract and tonic spasm of the gut wall at the site of the impaction. Systemic effects are mild initially; the temperature, pulse rate and respirations show little if any change in the first hours, and the hematocrit remains normal for some time. Symptoms of shock first appear after 6 to 10 hours in most cases. A this time the pain generally subsides, only to recur when secondary gastric dilation becomes severe. The majority of small intestinal impactions occur in the terminal ileum just anterior to the ileal orifice. Often the impacted ileum can be felt on deep rectal exploration, especially in the early stage of the disease. It presents as a smooth, sausage-shaped, forearm-thick tube extending from the left of the midline obliquely upward to the base of the cecum. Often the ileum feels as if it terminates blindly in the abdominal cavity. Because the cecum is empty, the cone-shaped end of the impaction is easily palpated. In rare cases the ileocecal fold can be discerned. An impacted loop of jejunum can similarly be discerned by its circumferences and consistency, but unlike the terminal ileum it is not attached to the cecal base and so is freely mobile (fig. 2.1.5. — 19).

As the disease progresses the prestenotic stagnation becomes more extensive, and more and more distended loops of small intestine can be palpated rectally and often displace the impacted segment anteriorally until it is inaccessible per rectum. The apparently favorable effect of spasmoanalgesics in many cases does not alter the fact that impactions of the small intestine are dangerous. A high impaction of the small intestine leads very quickly to reflux filling of the stomach with the characteristic symptoms of gastric dilation. In these cases rectal examination reveals extreme filling of the duodenum, which is felt curving from right to left behind the cranial mesenteric root and forming a loop in the area of the cecal base. Definite rectal findings (impacted, sausage-shaped ileum) confirm the diagnosis of ileal impaction.

If rectal findings are indefinite, a presumptive diagnosis can be made during the course of the disease in the light of other findings.

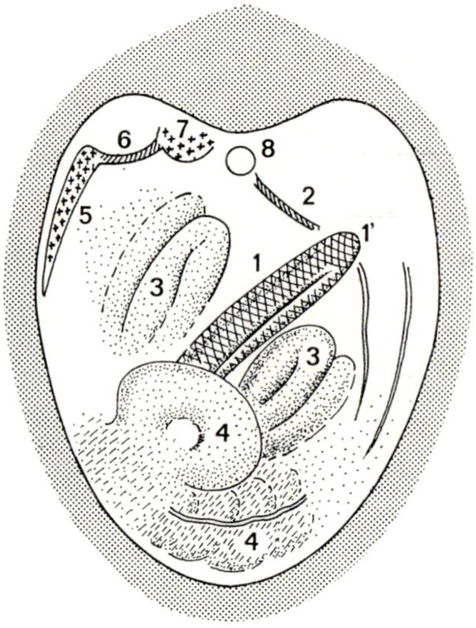

Fig. 2.1.5. — 19. Impaction of the ileum (early stage).
1 impacted ileum with cone-shaped end (ileal orifice = *1'*) due to empty cecum; *2* tense mesoileum; *3* tympanitic small intestine; *4* left ventral colon (fecal inspissation) and pelvic flexure; *5* spleen; *6* nephrosplenic ligament; *7* left kidney; *8* aorta; Findings on arm-deep rectal exploration.

A special form of small intestinal impaction in foals is caused by the accumulation of ascarids (round worms). Because a rectal examination is impossible in small patients, and shock is slow to appear, the diagnosis is presumptive.

Meckel's diverticula and chronic ileal hypertrophy can often be detected rectally. The ileum may be enlarged to the diameter of the upper arm, is firm and slightly elastic.

Differential Diagnosis. Impactions must be differentiated from small intestinal obstructions due to strangulation or incarceration. In the latter conditions spasmo-analgesics are ineffectual. Marked systemic signs develop within hours. The course in general, is more rapid and severe. In impactions the peritoneal fluid remains unchanged for some time, while in obstruction due to strangulation, it shows color changes after only 4—6 h (diapedesis).

Prognosis. The prognosis is guarded in impactions of the small intestine, and often progression to complete obstruction is unavoidable even with rational, early treatment.

Treatment. The veterinary school in Vienna recommends two doses of Novalgin given 30 min apart. Castor oil or mineral oil may additionally be given in the early stage of the disease. If this is unsuccessful, surgery is indicated. Conservative treatment in cases of secondary gastric dilation is justified only if the rectal examination shows conclusively that the ileal impaction is soft and not very large. If conservative treatment fails, the chance of recovery with surgical treatment is good. Through a midline laparotomy, the impacted mass is 'milked' into the cecum. In cases where proximal to distal massage is not possible, the fecal plug is kneaded in a proximal direction utilizing the hydraulic action of the prestenotic fluid, without doing an enterotomy. Opening of the intestine to flush out the impaction is justified only in exceptional cases, due to the danger of postoperative adhesions.

If impaction of the small intestine with ascarids is suspected in the foal, conservative treatment with an antihelmintic such as piperazine and appropriate intravenous fluid therapy is tried first. We recommend following the piperazine with Prostigmin to stimulate small bowel peristalsis. If it is suspected that the small

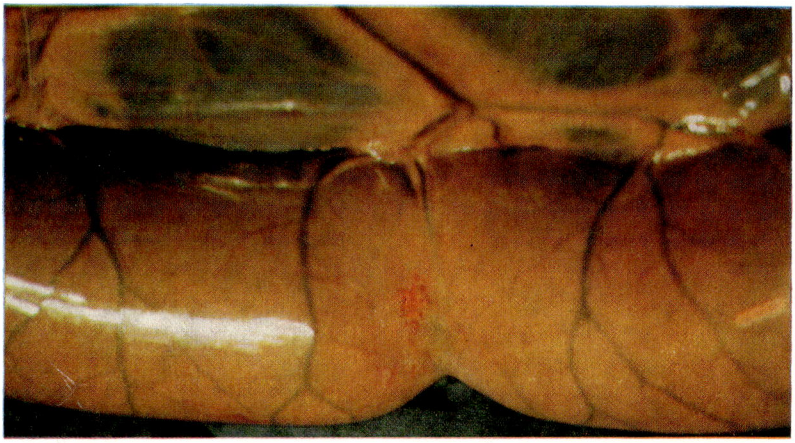

20

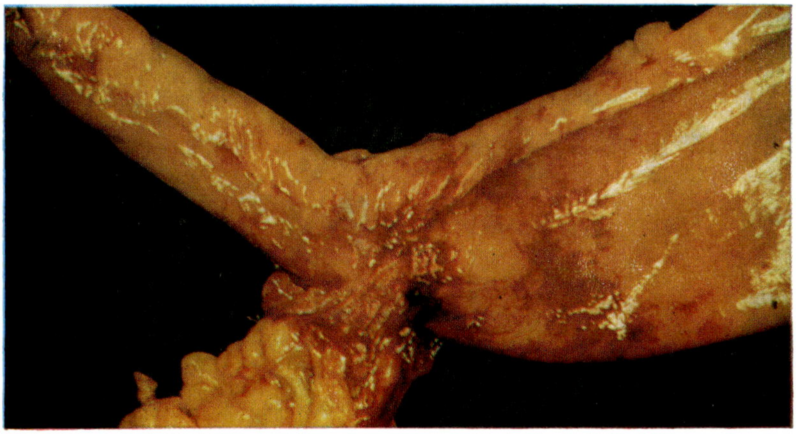

21

Fig. 2.1.5. — 20. Circular stenosis of the jejunum.

Fig. 2.1.5. — 21. A resected segment of chronically stenosed jejunum. The hypertrophied prestenotic bowel segment is on the right, the poststenotic segment on the left. The cordlike adhesion at lower left is composed of omental tissue.

intestine is obstructed by dead worms following antihelmintic therapy, Prostigmin is administered to promote elimination. The rule still holds that if secondary gastric dilation is present, surgical intervention is necessary.

In ileal hypertrophy, Meckel's diverticula or small intestinal stenoses, the chronically altered segments of bowel must be resected. The subsequent anastomosis is performed as a jejunojejunostomy or jejunocecostomy (figs. 2.1.5. — 75 to — 76).

Impaction of the Large Intestine

Impaction of the large intestine usually has an insidious onset and protracted course. Often colicky pains are absent until a considerable mass has accumulated. The first signs are constipation with the passage of small, dry feces in small amounts, a capricious appetite or anorexia, a reduced water intake, and frequent recumbency.

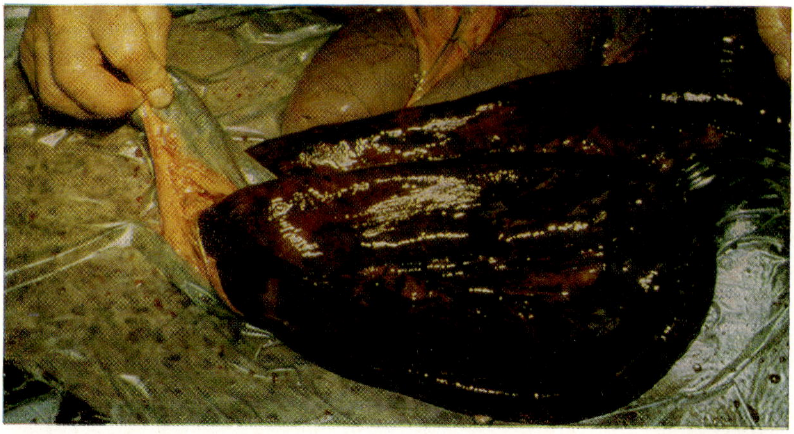

22

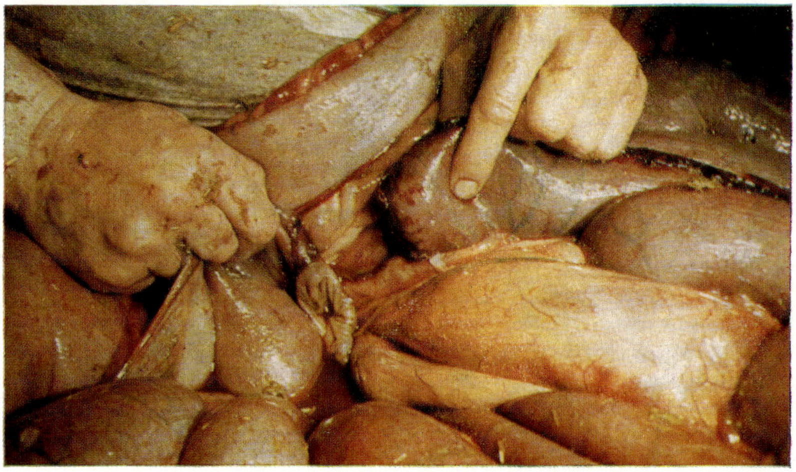

23

Fig. 2.1.5. — 22. Herniation of small intestine through a tear in the gastrosplenic ligament. The surgeon is holding the spleen. To the right are the necrotic loops of bowel.

Fig. 2.1.5. — 23. Transverse rupture of the small intestine. The surgeon is holding the two stumps. Intestinal contents contaminate the entire abdominal cavity.

The horse sweats excessively during exercise, paws the floor of the stall, stands in a straddling posture, and turns its head toward the flank. The colicky episodes are usually mild and are separated by long intervals of apparent comfort, during which the animal eats normally.

Sometimes a full urinary bladder is detected on rectal examination, which, combined with the frequent adoption of a straddling posture, can cause large bowel impaction to be misdiagnosed as 'water colic'. The cause in most cases is a reflex spasm of the bladder neck (vagotonia).

Peristalsis is usually markedly reduced. Systemic effects are mild, and the temperature, pulse rate and respiration are initially normal. In general the diagnosis is established by rectal findings.

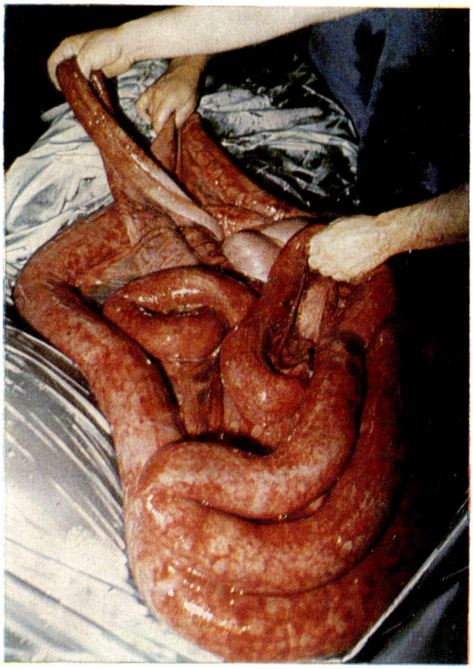

24

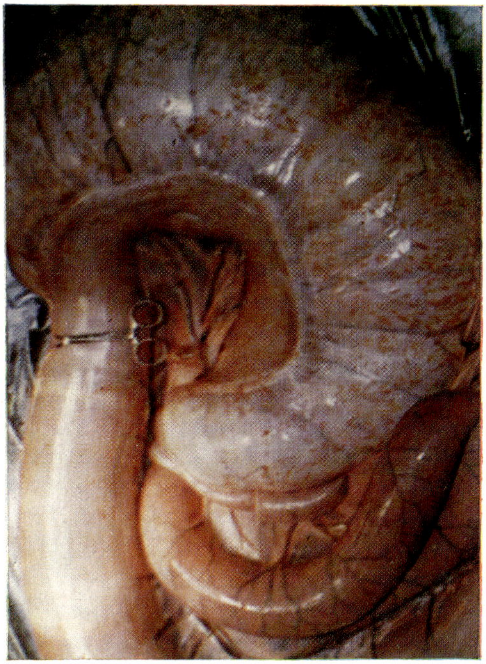

25

Fig. 2.1.5. — 24. 'Colitis x'.

Fig. 2.1.5. — 25. Meckel's diverticulum with ileal hypertrophy. The towel clamp rests upon the hypertrophic ileum. The diverticulum, shaped like a uterine horn, tapers toward the terminal ileum.

Impaction of the Cecum

Most cecal impactions occur in the base, which is then palpable as a smooth, impacted structure of limited mobility in the region of the right costal arch. It is easily indented with the fingers. The overhanging part of the base sags ventrally when it alone is impacted and forms a pendulous, head-size sac. The impacted body of the cecum is enlarged to the size of a thigh, and the contours of its bands and haustra are exaggerated.

Impaction of the Large Colon

Impactions of the pelvic flexure are the easiest to identify on rectal examination. The flexure is palpable as a horizontal U-shaped loop that usually is anterior to the pelvic cavity. It has a smooth surface and is about the diameter of a shank. Its junction with the left ventral colon can be identified by the bands of the latter. No band is felt on the left dorsal colon, but this part of the colon is usually empty and difficult to palpate in any case.

Impactions of the left ventral colon are about the thickness of a thigh. The two dorsal bands can usually be felt as smooth furrows running longitudinally between the more or less prominent rows of haustra. These bands diverge at a 90° angle owing to the dilation of the intestine and fade out at the pelvic flexure. Massive impactions may almost completely fill the left half of the abdominal cavity, making it difficult

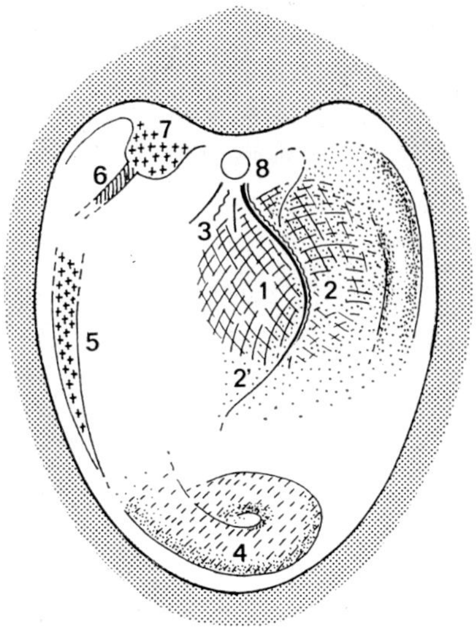

Fig. 2.1.5. — 26. Impaction of the stomach-like dilation of the right dorsal colon.
1 impacted colic ampulla; *2* tympanitic cecum with medial band (*2'*) and; *3* cranial mesenteric root are located caudal to *1*; *4* pelvic flexure (with soft impaction); *5* spleen; *6* nephrosplenic ligament; *7* left kidney; *8* aorta.

to locate the spleen. Repeated rectal examinations may disclose changes in the consistency of the left ventral colon, reflecting variations in the tone of the intestinal wall.

The somewhat rare impaction of the stomach-like dilation of the right dorsal colon is the most difficult to detect rectally. The arm must be inserted up to the shoulder in order to reach the caudal part of this dilation in the right upper abdomen anterior to the cranial mesenteric root (fig. 2.1.5. — 26).

Impaction of the Small Colon

Among the intestinal impactions, those of the small colon are the easiest to recognize on rectal examination. The arm-thick impaction of the relatively smooth intestinal tract can easily be assigned to the small colon on the basis of the prominent, 2-cm-wide longitudinal band that arches slightly forward on the antimesenteric side. The impacted intestinal loops form wheel-like coils located anterior to the pelvic inlet and within the pelvic cavity.

Differential Diagnosis. Obstruction of the small intestine can cause a secondary drying out or inspissation of the large intestinal contents that may be mistaken for an impaction of the small colon. The history offers the best means of differentiation. Whereas small intestinal obstruction develops suddenly and causes a rapid deterioration of general condition, impactions of the small intestine are characterized by symptoms of gradual onset and mild degree. Dilated loops of small intestine typical of a small intestinal obstruction are frequently missed by the examiner. A hard fecal mass is encountered in the large intestine which encourages the examiner to dispense with exploration beyond that point.

Displacements of the large colon to the left into the nephrosplenic space or to the right between the base of the cecum and right abdominal wall produce typical rectal findings that enable a differential diagnosis to be made (q.v.).

Prognosis. With prompt, specific treatment, the prognosis is good for all simple impactions. In chronic impaction of the cecum, characterized by hypertrophy or atony of the cecal musculature following degeneration of the intramural ganglia, the prognosis is poor. A large percentage of horses are rendered useless by recurrent bouts of colic or die from cecal rupture.

Treatment

Cecum: Most cecal impactions occur in the base, specifically in its overhanging blind end. In advanced cases the entire body of the cecum may be involved. Treatment is aimed at promoting the progression of the impacted mass without provoking a rupture by overloading the base of the cecum with too much fluid.

If only the base is impacted, it is sufficient to give several doses of 200—300 g sodium sulfate as a 5 % aqueous solution with 2 l of mineral oil at intervals of 8—24 h. Additionally, spasmoanalgesics are given every 8 h or 20—30 mg of atropine sulfate is given once a day. We prefer spasmoanalgesics, because their action is easier to observe and they cause minimal reduction in peristalsis. If the horse refuses to take water voluntarily, 5 l of water are given by nasogastric tube twice daily between treatments.

If the hematocrit exceeds 38, isotonic electrolyte solutions are given intravenously until approximately that value is achieved. Periodic rectal examinations are done to monitor the response and adjust the treatment as needed.

Large colon: In milder cases involving impaction of the pelvic flexure, a single administration of 300—500 g sodium sulfate as a 5 % aqueous solution and 2 l of mineral oil is often sufficient. Again, a spasmoanalgesic should be given to relieve pain and prevent intestinal spasm in the area of the impaction. If there is no improvement after 24 h (rectal examination), the treatment is repeated until the impaction is cleared.

If there is evidence of dehydration (reduced skin elasticity, increased hematocrit), it is corrected by appropriate fluid therapy. Parenteral fluid replacement not only improves the circulatory status but also indirectly softens the feces, because less water is extracted from the intestinal content when it is administered intravenously.

The administration of excessive amounts of sodium sulfate solution can seriously disrupt the fluid and electrolyte balance in the horse. If an intestinal obstruction has been misdiagnosed as an impaction, the horse's condition will deteriorate drastically following the administration of sodium sulfate solution. Thus the relatively harmless mineral oil is the laxative of choice as it does not alter the fluid and electrolyte balance.

In impactions formed by sand accumulation (sand colic), we intervene surgically only in advanced cases. With prompt treatment, the sand can be removed by a 3- to 5-day program of intensive laxative therapy. With a normal food and water intake, 300 g sodium sulfate and mineral oil twice daily should be sufficient. If severe diarrhea develops, intravenous fluid therapy is necessary to prevent dehydration.

Small colon: Impactions of the small colon can be relieved by enemas. The small colon is best flushed clear under epidural anesthesia. This requires patience and a large amount of water. The intestine may rupture if a large volume of fluid is forced into it rapidly under high pressure.

Enemas are usually unsuccessful in treatment of impactions caused by enteroliths, and surgical treatment is required.

Intestinal Obturation (Foreign-body Obstruction)

Definition and Occurrence. Obturation is the term applied to all states in which the intestinal lumen is obstructed by a foreign-body-like object that has become lodged there.

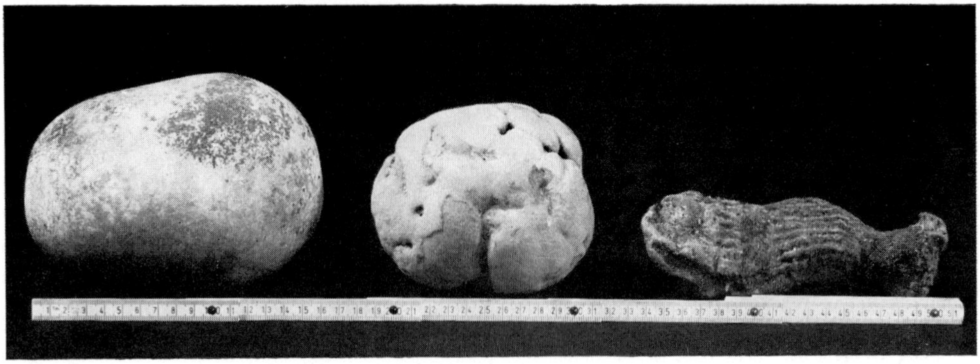

Fig. 2.1.5. — 27. Foreign bodies from the intestinal lumen. From left to right: enterolith, pyotobezoar, incrusted woolen sock.

Etiology and Pathogenesis. This form of colic is rare today, and is caused mainly by foreign bodies (textiles, plastic films), and very rarely by concretions (enteroliths). After lodging, the object becomes encrusted with mineral salts to form a pseudoconcretion (fig. 2.1.5. — 27).

Intestinal calculi may take the form of true calculi, called *enteroliths*, or *bezoars* (phytobezoars, phytotrichobezoars).

True calculi are stony hard, of high density and have a smooth surface. Ammoniomagnesium phosphate (triple phosphate) accounts for about 90% of these calculi. The stones form concentrically about a foreign-body nucleus over a period of several years and may reach a considerable size. In the past they were particularly common in mill and bakery horses fed large amounts of bran.

Phytobezoars, also called 'oat stones', contain 50% organic components (oat 'hairs') and 50% inorganic matter, mainly triple phosphate. The oat 'hairs', matted into balls, are permeated by the triple phosphate crystals to form intestinal calculi that are relatively light and have an uneven, furrowed, sandpapery surface. They can form within a matter of months.

Conglobates consist of inadequately chewed and digested, matted plant residues. Clover and other legumes can lead to the formation of round or short cylindrical masses that may reach the size of a child's head and completely obstruct the intestinal lumen. Horses with poor dentition (foals, old horses) are predisposed.

Foreign bodies and intestinal calculi can reside in the large colon for a long time without causing damage, and may go undetected until necropsy or slaughter. They cause obstruction only if they find their way into the narrower parts of the bowel. Intestinal calculi may block the funnel-shaped junction between the large and small colon, and rarely they may obstruct the pelvic flexure. Resistance peristalsis is stimulated proximal to the stenosis, thereby wedging the calculus farther into the isthmus. The gut wall surrounding the calculus itself develops a heightened sustained tone, which can lead to ischemic necrosis first of the musosa and then of the muscularis and serosa. The ischemic necrosis, in turn, can lead to intestinal rupture. Proximal to the stenosis there is massive impaction of the entire large intestine complicated by secondary tympany. Secondary gastric dilation may develop but is uncommon.

Symptoms and Diagnosis. There may be a gradual or sudden onset of mild to severe colicky pains. At first the clinical picture resembles that of large intestinal impaction, but the elimination of feces ceases. As the condition progresses the

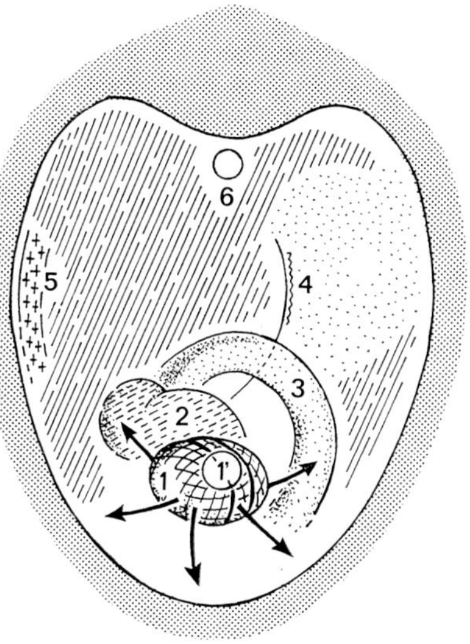

Fig. 2.1.5. — 28. Obturation of the small colon by a conglobate.
1 conglobate in small colon (movable in all directions); *1'* free band of small colon (tender to pressure); *2* prestenotic impaction; *3* prestenotic tympanitic loop of small colon; *4* cecum; *5* spleen; *6* aorta; Shaded area not explorable due to limited excursions.

horse may adopt a dog-sitting or kneeling posture. The colicky pains are temporarily relieved by spasmoanalgesics, but the animal continues to have a dull, depressed appearance. Systemic effects are very minor initially. Because water absorption continues in the large colon and there is no pronounced extravasation, the hematocrit remains unchanged for many days or is only slightly elevated. Rectal examination, even in large horses, may reveal an intestinal calculus at the junction of the large and small colon. It presents as a solid, hard, usually smooth but in some cases knobby, rounded object in the area of the anterior mesenteric root. The small colon is empty.

Foreign bodies and plant conglobates usually obstruct the small colon. The obstruction is preceded by an impaction that usually spans several loops of small colon and extends into the large colon, producing characteristic rectal findings: The arm-size, movable, impacted intestinal loops are easily identified by their antimesenteric longitudinal bands. In horses with intestinal calculi that have been previously treated with laxatives or purgatives, a temporary relief of the obstruction may be observed in some cases. If a phytobezoar is present, a small amount of thin intestinal contents can get by its knobby surface and enter the small colon. The diagnosis is based on the discovery of a calculus on rectal examination, absent defecation and, in small colonic obstruction, on the presence of a prestenotic impaction (fig. 2.1.5. — 28). Occasionally the history may suggest a diagnosis if the animal has been seen ingesting plastic materials, textiles or large amounts of clover.

Obturation of the cecum is uncommon but by no means unknown. Its clinical course is like that of small intestinal ileus (q.v.).

Differential Diagnosis. Tumors in the area of the anterior mesenteric root have very similar rectal findings. The course is chronic and defecation is scanty but present. Tumors feel firm and slightly elastic on rectal palpation. Impactions of the small colon present the same rectal picture but respond to enemas. This treatment is rarely beneficial in the case of conglobates and foreign bodies. In primary impactions of the stomach-like dilation of the large colon, the rectal findings are similar, but the impaction pits on pressure. If the impaction is composed of sand, the examiner has the feeling of palpating a sand bag.

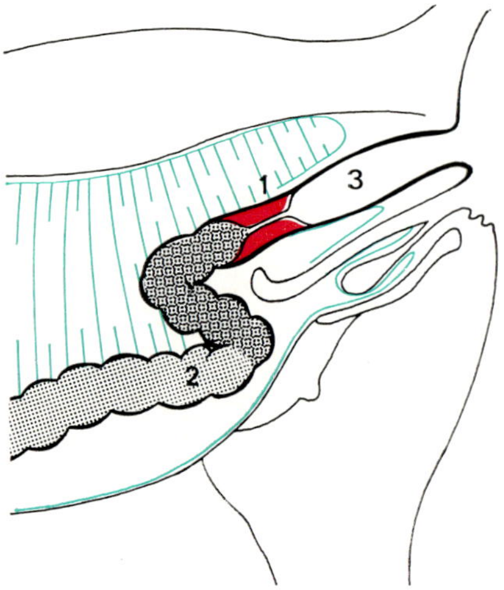

Fig. 2.1.5. — 29. Edema of the terminal small colon. *1* edema; *2* prestenotic impaction; *3* rectal ampulla.

Treatment. Apart from sand colic, which often can be successfully managed with primary conservative treatment, the other impaction colics are best treated surgically. The removal of an intestinal calculus at the junction of the large and small colon is most easily accomplished through a preumbilical, midline laparotomy. Starting at the pelvic flexure, the large colon is exteriorized as far as possible without traumatizing the prestenotic, impacted area. The dorsal colon is opened at the junction of the left colon and diaphragmatic flexure, and the intestinal contents are flushed by irrigation. Then the calculus is removed.

Operations on the small colon are done through a left-flank laparotomy or postumbilical midline laparotomy. Owing to its long mesentery, the intestine can be exteriorized without much difficulty. However, the intestinal tract is sensitive to stresses in the area of the obturation and impaction, and it should be exteriorized with extreme care to avoid rupture. Over the foreign body an enterotomy is made that is about 1 to $1^1/_2$ times the length of the bowel diameter, the incision being placed in the middle of the longitudinal band. The conglobate can then be removed without difficulty. The prestenotic impaction is removed by irrigation. The intestine is closed in two layers.

Prognosis. Obturations carry a favorable prognosis, for their gradual course allows ample time to reach a diagnosis, and their operative treatment is not especially difficult.

Edema of the Terminal Small Colon

Definition and Occurrence. A submucosal edema can develop at the junction of the small colon and rectum, producing a luminal obstruction over a distance of 10 to 20 cm preceded by an impaction. This fecal accumulation can lead, secondarily, to a kinking of the small colon anterior to the retroperitoneal region, thereby completing the obstruction (fig. 2.1.5. — 29).

Symptoms and Diagnosis. Mild colic and a protracted course are characteristic. Defecation is absent. The large colon and cecum become tympanitic in long-standing cases. The caudal part of the edema can be reached with the fingertips by inserting the hand into the empty rectal ampulla. A grossly swollen mucosa is felt. This will have lost its slippery, mucous quality as well as the normal plication and instead,

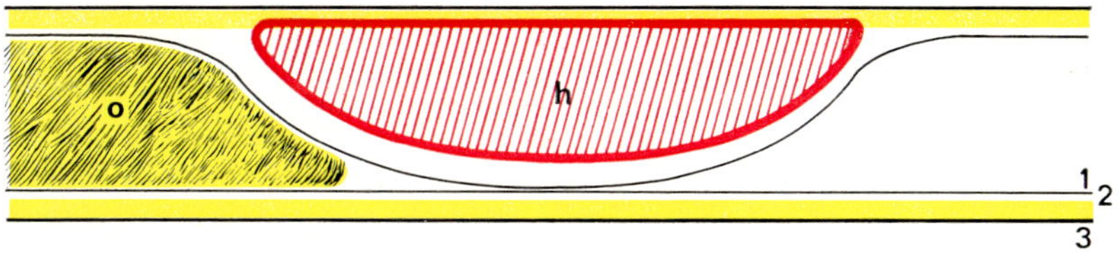

Fig. 2.1.5. — 30. Intramural hematoma. *1* mucosa; *2* muscularis; *3* serosa; *h* hematoma; *o* impaction anterior to hematoma.

presents a dry, sandpapery surface. If the edematous segment is short, the fecal plug can be reached through it, and the boundary between altered and normal mucosa can be felt. Greasy-brown traces of blood from the surface of the diseased mucosa are visible on the examiner's fingers.

Additional loops of impacted small colon can be palpated. This rectal finding is typical.

Etiology and Pathogenesis. The cause of primary edema of the terminal small colon is as yet unknown. It may conceivably be due to an interference with venous drainage in the junction between the portal vein and caudal vena cava. This itself may be caused by kinking of the bowel at the junction of the long descending mesocolon and short mesorectum. The stagnation of feces anterior to the edema further embarrasses the venous return. A thromboembolic etiology is also conceivable.

Differential Diagnosis. Findings are similar in early necrosis of the terminal segment of the small colon resulting from a mesenteric rupture following rectal prolapse or bowel contusions due to dystocia. The kinking in such cases is a result of defective intestinal mesentery in the area of the necrosis. Impaction is due to a loss of peristalsis. The submucosal edema that develops in these disorders is secondary in nature.

Prognosis. The prognosis is favorable.

Treatment. Conservative treatment is successful in most cases. Enemas are given carefully. Bougienage or pressure enemas should be avoided. Enemas are used in an attempt to gradually break up the prestenotic impaction. Sodium-sulfate and mineral-oil therapy are indicated for several days. Treatment is continued until rectal examination shows a reduction of mucosal swelling, and spontaneous defecation is reestablished. In neglected cases it may be necessary to do a laparotomy and empty the small colon through an enterotomy, followed by the correction of secondary 'kinks'.

Intramural Hematoma

A similar internal obstruction may be caused by intramural (usually submucosal) hematomas of the small or large intestine. These hematomas range from a few centimeters to several meters in length and can lead to ileus or in rare cases to death from blood loss. Resection of the affected bowel segment is almost always necessary (fig. 2.1.5. — 30).

Internal Hernias (Intra-abdominal Hernias)

These hernias are not visible externally, the hernial ring, contents and sac (if present) being located entirely within the abdominal or thoracic cavity. Most of these hernias involve the incarceration of parts of the small intestine, although colonic incarcerations are not uncommon. The internal ring may be congenital or acquired. Two typical, frequently-occurring internal hernias that involve the equine bowel are incarceration of the small intestine in the epiploic foramen and herniation of the large colon into the nephrosplenic space (left dorsal displacement).

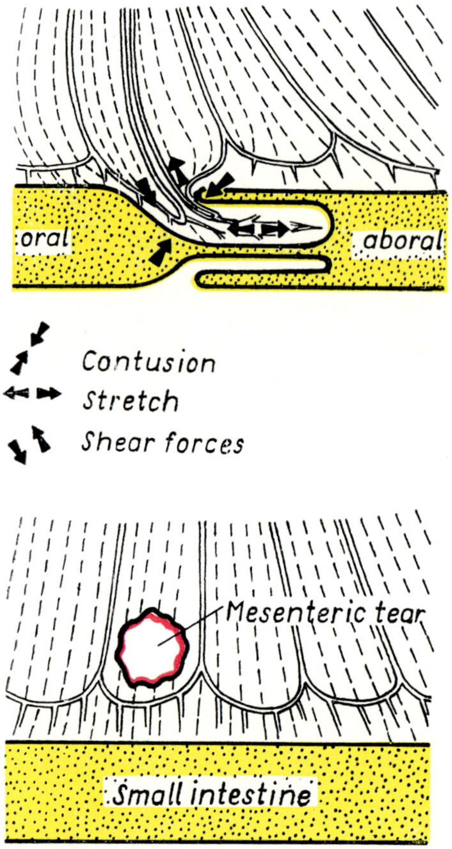

Fig. 2.1.5. — 31. Spontaneous development of mesenteric tears, shown here for an intussusception (after Kopf).

Acquired hernial rings are the result of internal injuries.

According to Kopf, spontaneous tears of the mesentery are associated with physiologic invaginations due to hyperperistalsis, during which the mesentery of the intususceptum becomes stretched and possibly torn at the edge of the intussuscipiens. Following reduction of the invagination, a defect remains in the mesentery a short distance from the bowel (see fig. 2.1.5. — 31).

A typical example is a tear in the descending mesocolon caused by rectal prolapse with intussusception of the small colon. The junctions between short and longer segments of mesentery form predilection sites for mesenteric tears. The shorter mesentery tears because it cannot follow the excursions associated with physiologic intussusceptions.

Defects in the area of attachment of the greater omentum, the mesoduodenum and the ascending mesocolon in the region of the pelvic flexure can also occur when the normally mobile serosal layers are stretched tight as a result of distension. They can also be caused by resisting the violent movements of other parts of the intestine.

Such lesions become clinically apparent only when accompanied by an incarceration of the bowel. The signs are those of a small or large intestinal ileus, depending

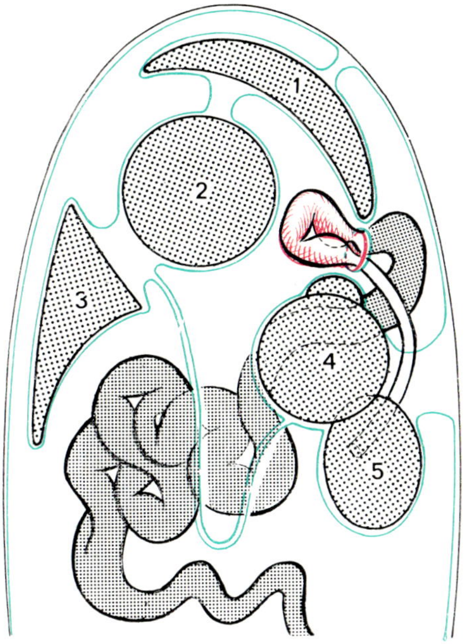

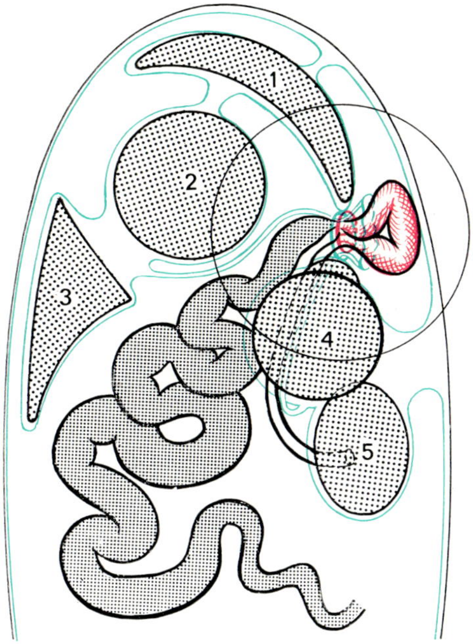

Fig. 2.1.5. — 32. Herniation through the epiploic foramen from the lateral side. The omental bursa is not displaced. *1* liver; *2* stomach; *3* spleen; *4* large colon; *5* cecum.

Fig. 2.1.5. — 33. Herniation through the epiploic foramen from the medial side. The omental bursa is involved in the herniation and is torn (omental hernia). *1* liver; *2* stomach; *3* spleen; *4* large colon; *5* cecum.

on whether the small or large intestine is incarcerated. The course is determined by the extent and degree of the strangulation.

The major internal hernias are presented below in the order of their frequency in the horse:

Frequent:
Herniation through epiploic foramen
Herniation into nephrosplenic space (left dorsal displacement)
Common:
Pseudoligamentous hernia (herniation through anomalous mesodiverticular band)
Omental hernia
Mesojejunal hernia
Descending mesocolic hernia
Mesoduodenojejunal hernia
Uncommon:
Diaphragmatic hernia
Mesoileal hernia
Ascending mesocolic hernia
Herniation through gastrosplenic ligament
Herniation through hepatogastric ligament
Herniation through hepatoduodenal ligament

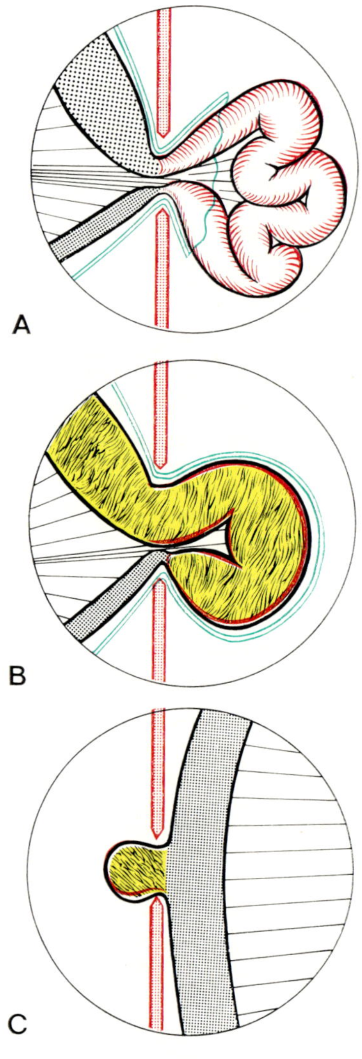

Fig. 2.1.5. — 34. Various types of medial incarceration of the small intestine in the epiploic foramen. *A:* incarceration of a large segment of small bowel; *B:* incarceration of feces-filled bowel; *C:* protrusion of bowel wall (Littre's hernia) from the lateral side.

Herniation through the Epiploic Foramen

Definition and Occurrence. The incarceration of loops of small intestine in the epiploic foramen is especially common in older horses. In the older horse the foramen is abnormally enlarged as a result of pressure atrophy of the right hepatic lobe. The intestine may enter the omental bursa (the space delimited by the omentum) from right to left (i.e., from the lateral side), or it may slip through the foramen from left to right (i.e., from the medial side). In this latter situation the intestine may push the omentum before it or may protrude through a tear (figs. 2.1.5. — 32 and — 33).

The differentiation between a lateral and medial incarceration is important from the standpoint of surgical correction.

In 38 of our own cases the average age was 7 years, though 5 horses were only 3 years old.

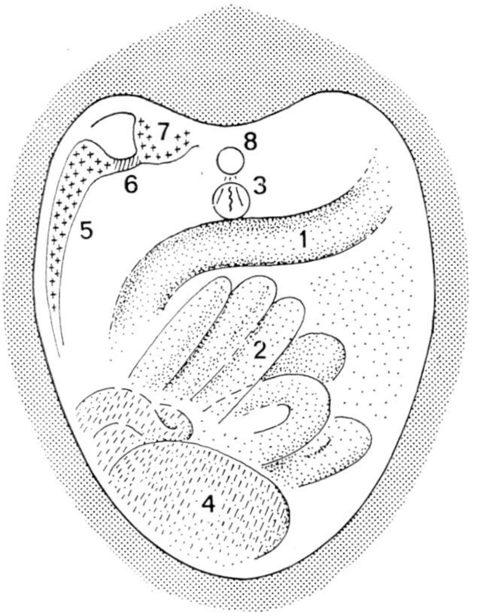

Fig. 2.1.5. — 35. High small intestinal ileus (e.g., hernia through epiploic foramen).
1 tympanitic duodenum; *2* row of gas-filled small intestinal loops; *3* tense, painful mesenteric root; *4* parts of large colon in correct location with inspissated ingesta; *5* spleen; *6* renosplenic ligament; *7* left kidney; *8* aorta; Findings on arm-deep rectal exploration.

Most incarcerations are from the medial side, the hernial contents consisting of 3 to 10 m of small intestine. Shorter lengths are rare, and even rarer are cases in which only a few centimeters of feces-filled bowel are incarcerated. We found a Littre's hernia in 4 cases (see fig. 2.1.5. — 34).

Symptoms and Diagnosis. The symptoms are those of a small intestinal ileus and vary with the nature and severity of the damage to the incarcerated bowel.

In most cases rectal exploration in the upper right quadrant shows evidence of the herniation in the form of abnormally fixed, edematous loops of small intestine whose mesentery extends toward the epiploic foramen (fig. 2.1.5. — 35).

In herniations from the lateral side, the peritoneal fluid may retain a normal color for some time, because the transudate enters the undamaged omental bursa and is not collected on paracentesis. In other cases a reddish fluid mixed with erythrocytes can be obtained 4—6 h after the onset of the disease.

The preoperative diagnosis is usually limited to the determination of a small intestinal obstruction.

Prognosis. The prognosis depends on the promptness of surgical correction and the severity of intestinal lesions. It is reasonably good for incarcerations of small segments of bowel but poor beyond 12 hours in cases of extensive intestinal necrosis.

Treatment. Conservative treatment is useless, and surgery should be performed at the earliest opportunity (q.v.).

Herniation into the Nephrosplenic (Renosplenic) Space. Left Dorsal Displacement of the (Large) Colon

Definition and Occurrence. This involves the displacement of the large colon into the nephrosplenic space, usually from a cranial direction. The loop of colon becomes incarcerated in a dorsally-open ring formed by the left kidney, the nephrosplenic ligament, the dorsal edge of the spleen and the dorsal abdominal wall. The incarceration may be complete or partial, depending on whether the edge of the spleen is laterodorsal (complete) or ventral (partial) to the displaced bowel. As a rule the spleen is engorged. The loop of colon draped over the tightly-stretched nephro-

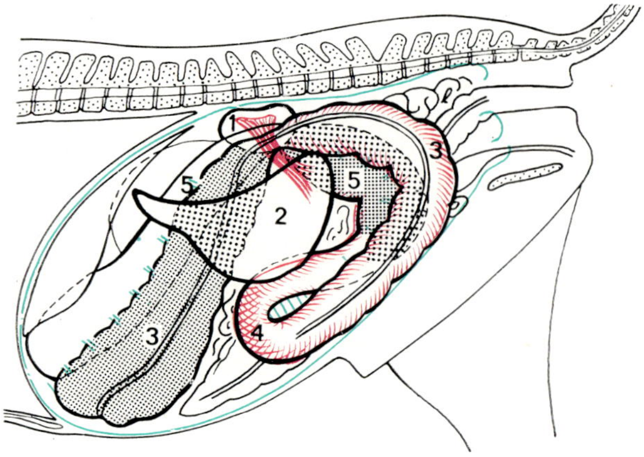

Fig. 2.1.5. — 36. Herniation into the nephrosplenic (renosplenic) space. Pathologic relationships as viewed from the right side.
1 kidney; *2* spleen; *3* ventral colon; *4* pelvic flexure; *5* dorsal colon. Red band: nephrosplenic ligament; red shading: strangulated portion of large colon; stippled areas: prestenotic fecal impaction in ventral and dorsal colon.

splenic ligament is almost always *twisted 180°* about its long axis, so that the ventral colon overlies the dorsal colon on the ligament. The large colon may herniate into the nephrosplenic space as far as the middle of the right dorsal and ventral colon. The disorder is seen mainly in mature horses, especially in large geldings; mares, small horses and foals are seldom affected. There is no breed predilection. The disease was first described by MAREK [1902]; MILNE [1977] suggested the term 'left dorsal displacement of the colon' (fig. 2.1.5. — 36).

Symptoms and Diagnosis. The disease generally takes a protracted course and produces mild colicky symptoms. In rare cases it is associated with severe colic and takes a peracute course, with shock developing within 3—6 h. It is possible to confuse torsion of the colon with such cases. In the mild form there is little or no increase in the pulse rate, temperature and respiration, and systemic signs are initially absent. The colic responds poorly to spasmoanalgesic therapy, however, and this provides a diagnostic clue. Transitory sweating may occur. The abdomen usually appears slightly bloated about the flanks. Peristaltic sounds have a ringing, truncated quality; peristalsis is spastically inhibited and in rare cases is abolished.

In mild cases the hematocrit is within normal limits or moderately increased (40—50). In long-standing or peracute cases it may rise to over 50. The pH of the blood is usually normal (7.38—7.42).

On passage of a *stomach tube*, foul-smelling gases are frequently emitted. Acute gastric dilation develops in about 30 % of cases.

Abdominal paracentesis usually yields a small volume of clear fluid with a color similar to white wine. If marked strangulation has occurred, the fluid appears blood-tinged and is increased in volume.

The *rectal examination* may be diagnostic during the initial examination. Because the rectal findings are almost pathognomomic, they represent the most outstanding diagnostic signs of the disorder: The rectal ampulla is empty and sticky or contains small amounts of dry feces. The small colon is empty and so cannot be located. Most

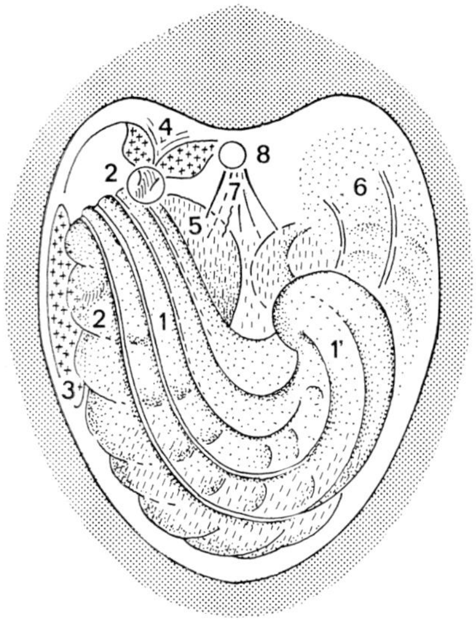

Fig. 2.1.5. — 37. Displacement of the large colon over the nephrosplenic ligament.
1 displaced loop of colon with tense longitudinal bands ('clothesline bands'); *1'* tympanitic pelvic flexure displaced to the right and cranially; *2* nephrosplenic ligament (tightly stretched and painful); *3* spleen (difficult or impossible to reach); *4* left kidney (pulled away from abdominal wall); *5* distended stomach (very rare finding); *6* tympanitic cecum; *7* cranial mesenteric root; *8* aorta.

striking is the presence of a succession of cords that extend transversely through the abdominal cavity, are immovable and converge upward, forward and to the left, where they are abnormally anchored. The partially tympanitic and partially feces-filled sacculations identify these cords as being colonic bands. The extended arm cannot be swept freely from the aorta to the ventral abdominal wall as it normally can. From the caudal edge of the left kidney, the tightly-stretched nephrosplenic ligament extends downward and to the left beneath the tense colonic bands and cannot be followed to the spleen. The spleen is usually difficult to reach and is located by exploring up and down along the left abdominal wall. Frequently the spleen lies farther ventrally and caudally than normal but may retain contact with the abdominal wall (fig. 2.1.5. — 37).

An impaction usually forms anterior to the strangulation in the dorsal colon, while the ventral colon contains gas.

If only the pelvic flexure is incarcerated, its greater curature is directed caudally and can be palpated close to the pelvic inlet. If a longer segment of the left or even right colon is incarcerated, then the pelvic flexure is displaced cranially and cannot be reached through the rectum.

In these cases the colonic bands passing from the upper left abdomen curve to the right, downward and forward in front of the pelvic inlet. In the somewhat rare cases with extravasation sufficient to cause shock, edema of the bowel wall can be detected rectally by the thickening and fleshy consistency of the sacculations.

Etiology and Pathogenesis. The true cause of this displacement is unknown. Presumably the left loops of colon ride up along the lateral abdominal wall, becoming engaged onto the nephrosplenic ligament. It is believed that gastric fullness with caudal and medial displacement of the spleen is a predisposing factor.

Differential Diagnosis. Impactions, torsions, displacements and tympany of the large colon are distinguished rectally by a free nephrosplenic ligament that is dorsal to the colon and can be followed from the kidney to the spleen.

Prognosis. If the disease is recognized during the first 3 days in mild cases or within 12 h in peracute cases, the prognosis is good with surgical treatment. Recurrences are known, however.

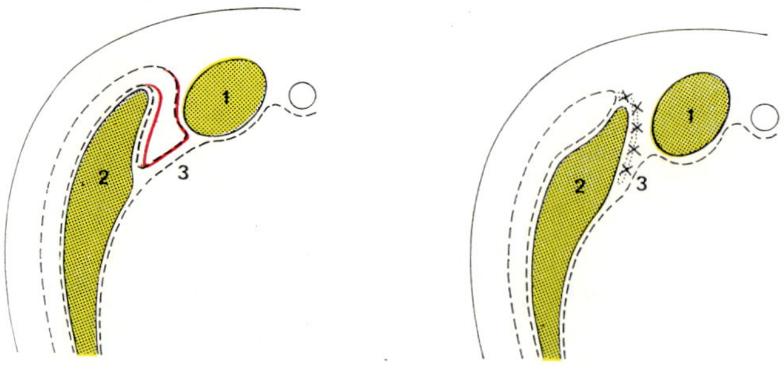

Fig. 2.1.5. — 38. Surgical closure of the nephrosplenic space, transverse section. *1* kidney; *2* spleen; *3* nephrosplenic ligament.
Left: normal situation, nephrosplenic space outlined in red; right: operative result.

Treatment. Conservative treatment is uncertain and dangerous (intestinal rupture!). If nonoperative treatment is desired in exceptional cases — it can succeed only if the incarcerated bowel contains little ingesta — its goal is to empty the affected segment. Fractionated doses of sodium sulfate solutions and mineral oil may be given in an attempt to soften the impacted ingesta in the incarceated loop. The administration of spasmoanalgesics and intravenous therapy with large amounts of isotonic solutions support the laxative therapy. Severe distension of the cecum is relieved by trocarization. If evacuation of the incarcerated loop is confirmed rectally, small doses of parasympathomimetic drugs (Prostigmin) may assist spontaneous reduction by stimulating peristalsis. Alternately, reduction may be attempted in the anesthetized horse per rectum or by rolling once the intestine has been emptied.

Operative reduction is done through a midline or left lateral laparotomy (q.v.). After a midline laparotomy the colon is repositioned with one hand if the incision is short (15—20 cm) or with both hands if the incision is long (20—40 cm). The surgeon's left hand grasps the segment of colon directly covering the nephrosplenic ligament, at which site the colon is bunched into an arm-size cord, and pushes it in a dorsolateral and cranial direction, while the right hand grasps the dorsal edge of the spleen and lifts it ventromedially over the colon. These manipulations are not easy if the colon is considerably distended and impacted. In such cases the pelvic flexure must first be carefully exteriorized and opened to permit drainage of the herniated loop. Following closure of the enterotomy and replacement of the pelvic flexure in the abdominal cavity, the reduction should present no difficulties. Usually the reduction is carried out in stages with one hand. Having freed and repositioned the colon, the surgeon checks to see whether the spleen has been restored to its normal position on the left abdominal wall, and examines the mesocolon to verify that the colon is free of twists. Only then may the abdominal cavity be closed. Recurrence can be prevented by resecting the left loops of colon (q.v.) or by closing the nephrosplenic space. The latter is done through a left lateral laparotomy: After reduction of the hernia the splenic capsule is sutured to the nephrosplenic ligament, and then the peritoneum of the dorsal abdominal wall is sutured to the nephrosplenic ligament and dorsal edge of the spleen; polyglycolic acid sutures (2 Dexon) or similar synthetic absorbable sutures are used. The slight splenic bleeding is of no consequence. The abdomen is closed, and suction drainage of the flank incision is maintained for several days (fig. 2.1.5. — 38).

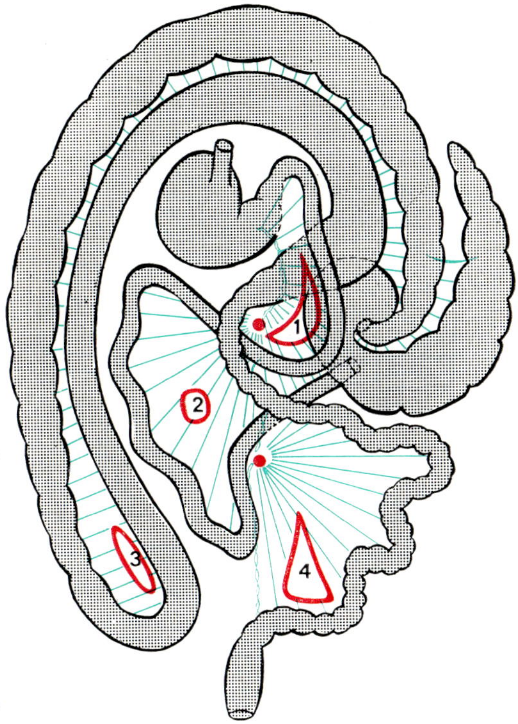

39

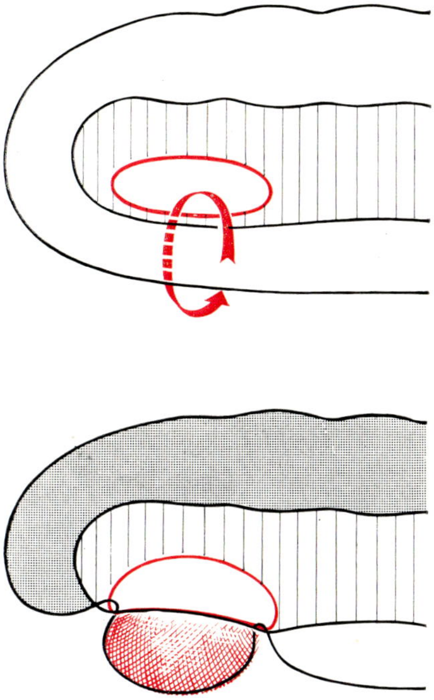

42

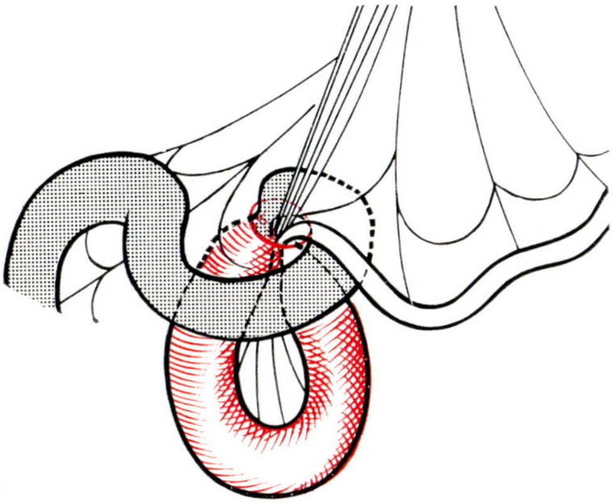

40

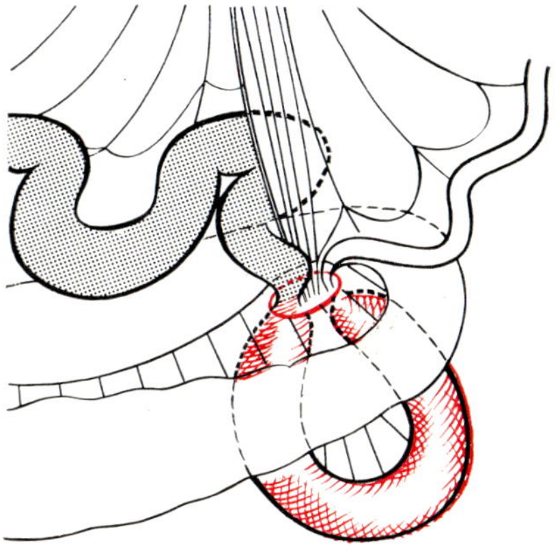

41

Fig. 2.1.5. — 39. Frequent localization of defects in the mesentery.
1 mesoduodenum; *2* mesojejunum and mesoileum; *3* ascending mesocolon near pelvic flexure; *4* descending mesocolon and mesorectum.

Fig. 2.1.5. — 40. Mesojejunal hernia.

Fig. 2.1.5. — 41. Mesocolic hernia of the jejunum.

Fig. 2.1.5. — 42. Mesocolic hernia of the colon.

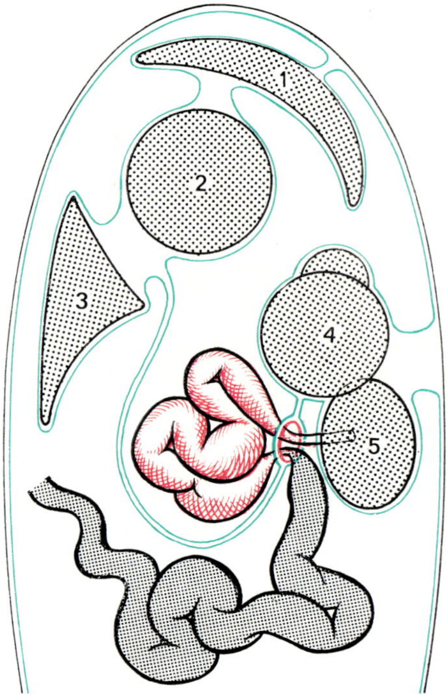

43

Fig. 2.1.5. — 43. Omental hernia.
1 liver; *2* stomach; *3* spleen; *4* large colon; *5* cecum. The small bowel incarceration is caused by a defect in the omental bursa.

Fig. 2.1.5. — 44. Herniation through the hepatogastric ligament.
1 liver; *2* stomach; *3* spleen; *4* stomach-like dilation of right dorsal colon with pancreas; *5* base of cecum.
Dark shading: prestenotic bowel segment; red shading: incarcerated bowel segment; red ring: hernial ring; green lines: peritoneal structures.

Fig. 2.1.5. — 45. Herniation through the gastrosplenic ligament.
1 liver; *2* stomach; *3* spleen; *4* large colon; *5* cecum.

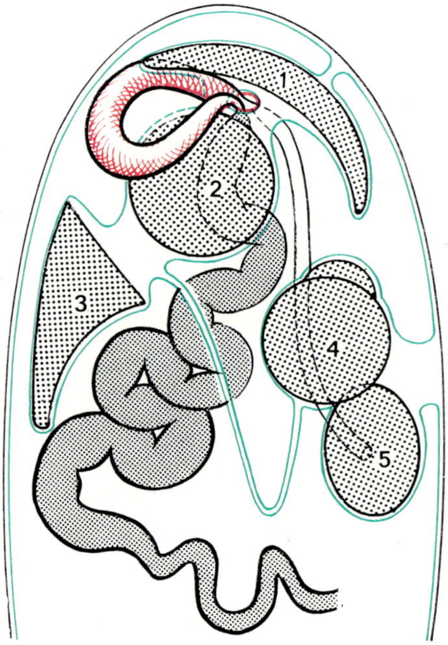

44

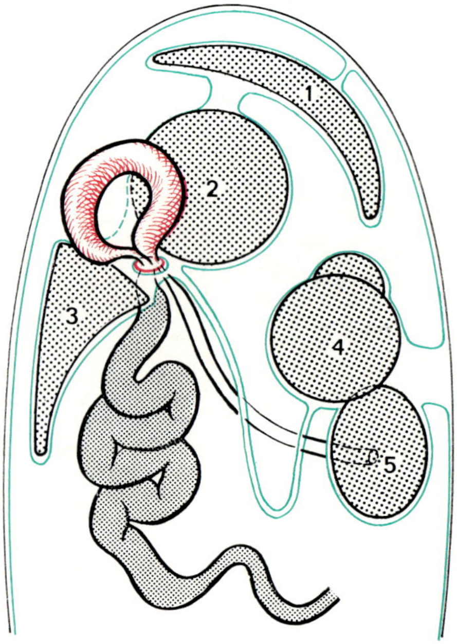

45

Mesenteric Hernia

In most cases, herniation is through the mesentery of the small intestine; hernias through the mesocolon are less frequent. Predilection sites occur where firmly-anchored bowel segments join with highly mobile segments, such as the junction of the duodenum and jejunum (figs. 2.1.5. — 39 to — 42).

Omental Hernia

Tears in the greater omentum are usually extensive. Omental trabeculae are pushed together at the tear to form a thickened, cordlike ring through which parts of the intestine can herniate (fig. 2.1.5. — 43).

Ligamentous Hernia

These hernias include those through tears in the lesser omentum (hepatogastric and hepatoduodenal ligament; fig. 2.1.5. — 44). Most such tears are slit-shaped. Herniation may also occur through defects in any of the following ligaments:
— the gastrosplenic ligament (fig. 2.1.5. — 45),
— the broad ligament of the uterus, and in rare cases,
— the fold of the ductus deferens (fig. 2.1.5. — 46).

Pseudoligamentous Hernia

This hernia corresponds to the condition called 'adhesive obstruction' in human medicine and is caused by the presence of abnormal peritoneal cords (adhesions, pseudoligaments, mesodiverticular bands). It is relatively common in the horse. The cord or band of scar tissue may be attached to the abdominal wall or some other abdominal organ, forming a portal through which parts of the intestine can herniate and become strangulated (fig. 2.1.5. — 47).

The pedicle of pedunculated tumors (e.g., lipoma) may also become knotted around a loop of bowel and cause an incarceration (fig. 2.1.5. — 48).

Diaphragmatic Hernia

See Sec. 2.1.7.1.

Twisting of the Mesentery (Mesenteric Volvulus or Torsion)

Definition and Occurrence. Mesenteric volvulus occurs when a loop of small intestine rotates about its own mesentery. While it is the intestinal lumen that actually rotates, the site of the resultant constriction is located in the mesentery. *The more times the intestine is twisted, the higher up in the mesentery the constriction occurs.* As more intestine becomes included in the volvulus, the affected loops exert an increasingly strangulating effect on one another. Ultimately the constriction reaches the mesenteric root, at which point the mesentery is twisted into a cordlike structure. The torsion may be to the left or the right.

A special form of this torsion is torsion of the jejunal and ileal mesentery, in which the entire convolution of the small intestine rotates about the mesenteric root. The torsion may amount to 360° or more (fig. 2.1.5. — 49).

Etiology and Pathogenesis. The rapid filling of a segment of small intestine exerts localized tension on the mesentery. This creates an axis about which the intestine can easily rotate during intense peristalsis (fixation by adhesions, by mesodiverticular bands, etc., has a similar effect), and a primary twist is formed. With increased peristalsis and gas formation, more and more loops of small intestine become twisted about the mesenteric axis. The very long mesentery of the horse predisposes to this process. Volvulus is arrested in the ileum and proximal jejunum due to the short

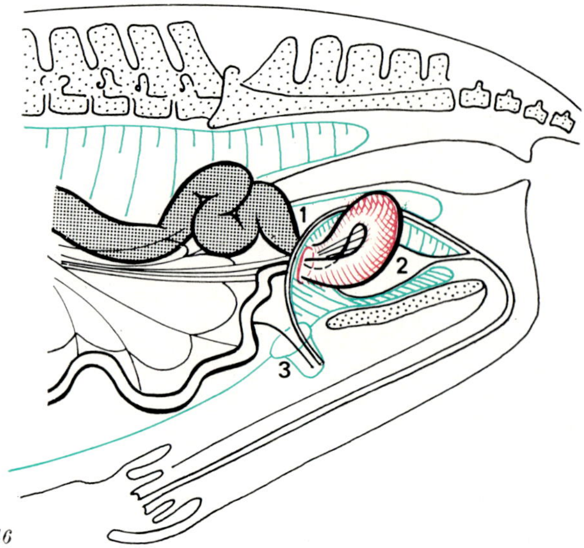

46

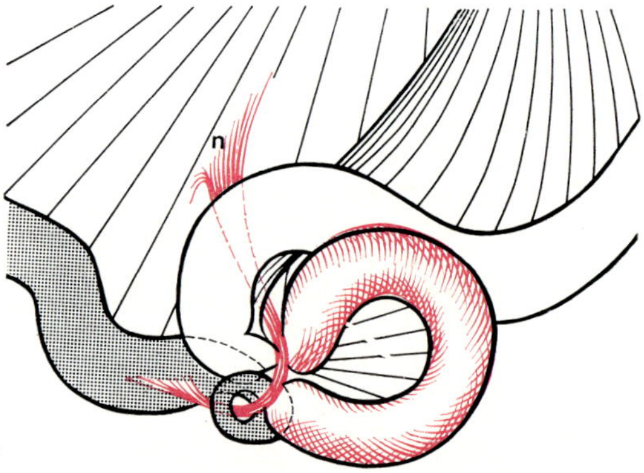

47

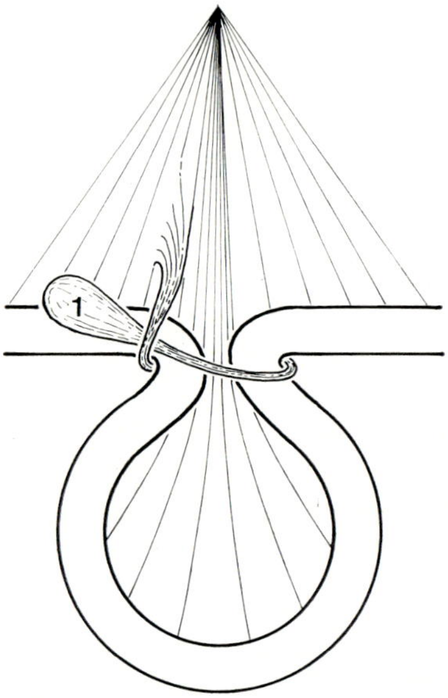

48

Fig. 2.1.5. — 46. Herniation through the fold of the ductus deferens.
1 ductus deferens; *2* urinary bladder; *3* spermatic cord stump after castration.
Fig. 2.1.5. — 47. Pseudoligamentous hernia (anomalous mesenteric band). *n* = cord of scar tissue.
Fig. 2.1.5. — 48. Incarceration of the small intestine by a pedunculated lipoma (*1*).

mesentery at these locations. The end-result of the process is a strangulating obstruction of the small intestine with all its pathophysiologic consequences (q.v.).

Symptoms and Diagnosis. The main symptom is an intense colic that usually arises suddenly. It may have been preceded by an apparently innocent episode of spasmodic colic. Spasmoanalgesics bring no relief. Marked systemic symptoms develop within a short time and severe signs appear after about 6 h, with secondary gastric dilation, severe abdominal distention and symptoms of shock. Rectal examination reveals gas- and fluid-filled loops of small intestine that are tense, cordlike and sometimes edematous. Traction on individual loops intensifies the pain. Rarely can the twisted mesentery be palpated. The peritoneal fluid shows varying degrees of hemorrhagic discoloration depending on the duration of the disease and degree of the strangulation.

Differential Diagnosis. Flatulent colic can generally be recognized on the basis of rectal findings, abdominal paracentesis and its milder clinical course. So-called volvulus nodosus (see below) and incarcerations of the small intestine present a similar clinical picture. The nature of the obstruction can be ascertained only by laparotomy.

Treatment. Treatment is surgical (see Operative Technique), otherwise the animal must be euthanatized at the earliest opportunity.

Knotting of the Small Intestine (Volvulus of the Jejunum and Ileum, so-called 'Volvulus Nodosus')

Definition and Occurrence. 'Volvulus nodosus' mainly affects the caudal segments of the small bowel. The cecum or parts of the small colon are involved in exceptional cases. The 'knot' that forms is progressively tightened by peristalsis and gas accumulation in the stenostenotic part and vessels are strangulated. Sometimes the mesentery of the affected loops becomes torn, making it difficult intraoperatively to distinguish the volvulus from a mesenteric hernia. The simple form of this type of volvulus occurs most frequently in the foal; usually only 30—150 cm of small intestine are affected at the junction of the jejunum and ileum (fig. 2.1.5. — 50).

This type of volvulus is extremely rare in mature horses.

Symptoms, Diagnosis and Treatment. They are the same as described for Mesenteric Volvulus.

Torsion of the Cecum

Definition and Occurrence. Cecal torsion involves a twisting of the cecum about its long axis. The constriction site is usually in the area of the base, and the ileum may also be involved. This extremely rare disorder leads to obstruction and necrosis of the twisted segment.

Symptoms and Diagnosis. The symptoms are those of a small intestinal obstruction. The diagnosis is established by rectal examination: Prominent cecal edema and tympany in conjunction with prestenotic dilatation of small intestinal loops typify strangulation of the cecum.

Kinking of the cecum in a caudal direction is the only condition to be differentiated.

Treatment. A midline laparotomy is performed, the direction of the twist is determined, and reduction is effected by counter-rotation of the previously emptied cecum. If cecal necrosis has developed in advanced cases, the only recourse is a cecectomy (typhylectomy).

Kinking of the Cecum

Definition and Occurrence. Caudad kinking of the cecum can occur even under *physiologic* circumstances. When this occurs the body of the cecum is displaced in a lateral and caudal direction, so that the apex points caudally. A kink forms in the area of the base. Advanced cases with marked filling of the body of the cecum can result in a strangulation obstruction with all its consequences. However, strangulation obstruction is a very rare complication of this displacement.

Diagnosis and Symptoms. The disease starts with mild colic and mild systemic signs. If there is much gas formation, the accumulation of gas and ingesta may be sufficient to interfere with circulation, resulting in marked systemic signs. Rectal examination

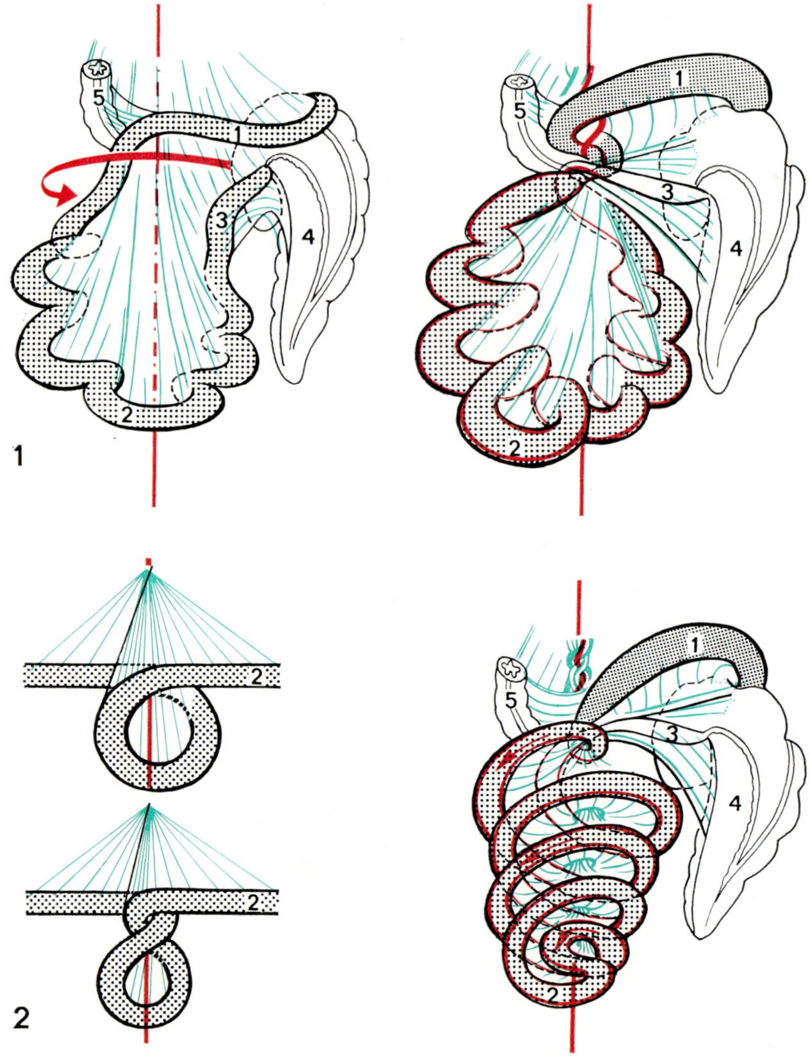

Fig. 2.1.5. — 49. Volvulus of the jejunal and ileal mesentery.
Form 1: The small intestinal convolution rotates *as a whole* about the mesenteric axis.
1 left: Normal relationships viewed from a caudal direction.
1 right: 360° rotation.
Form 2: A loop of small intestine twists several times about an axis perpendicular to the intestinal lumen, ultimately leading to a *spiraling* of the entire small intestine.
2 left: Initial twisting of the small intestine (modified from WALL); top: half twist; bottom: complete twist.
2 right: Spiraling of the entire small intestine; arrows: direction of rotation (3 × 360°).
1 duodenum; *2* jejunum; *3* ileum; *4* cecum; *5* small colon.

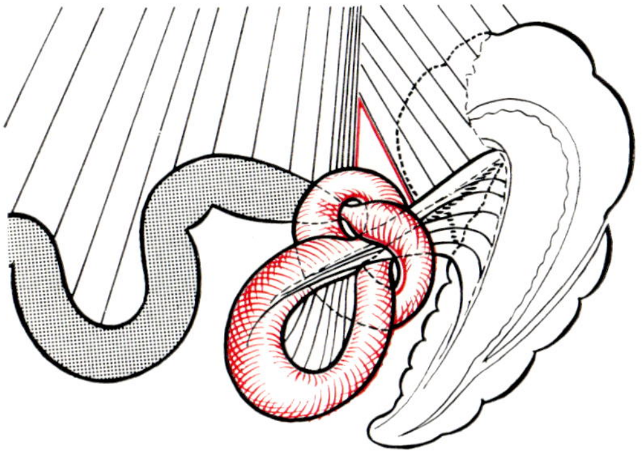

Fig. 2.1.5. — 50. So called 'Volvulus nodosus' of the jejunum and ileum with rupture of the mesentery.

shows distension of the cecum, whose caudally-directed apex is palpable or whose bands run opposite to the normal direction. Palpable edema is an indication for surgical intervention.

Treatment. In the absence of edema, careful evacuation of the gas by trocarization from the right flank is sufficient to achieve a spontaneous reduction. Surgical treatment is similar to that for torsion of the cecum.

Torsion of the Large Colon

Definition and Occurrence. Torsion of the large colon occurs when the dorsal and ventral loops of colon rotate about a common axis. The torsion may occur in a medial or lateral direction. The degree of torsion is variable: Up to 90° it is within physiologic limits; from 90 to 180° the torsion may reduce spontaneously; beyond 180° surgical reduction is required. Rotations up to 540° have been observed, but the most frequent degree of torsion is 360° (fig. 2.1.5. — 51). The length of the strangulated segment is variable. The twist, or constriction site, may occur where the loops of left colon merge with the diaphragmatic and sternal flexures, in the area of the flexures, or where the flexures merge with the loops of right colon. In these cases the torsion is said to be 'partial' (fig. 2.1.5. — 52).

In severe cases the twist moves caudad beyond the stomach-like dilation of the right dorsal colon, producing a 'complete' torsion that involves the entire large colon.

At the constriction site the loops of colon are intertwined in spiral fashion. A torsion of 180° causes a narrowing of the intestinal lumen, while greater degrees of torsion obstruct the lumen completely.

The degree of circulatory impairment depends not only on the degree of torsion that has occurred, but also on the filling of the pre- and poststenotic bowel segments (tympany) and the constriction site. Here the blood vessels are strangulated in varying degrees by the longitudinal bands.

Partial colonic torsion may occur in horses of all breeds, though small horses and ponies are infrequently affected.

Complete colonic torsion is mainly a disease of broodmares.

Colonic torsions rank first among the surgical colics of the large intestine and account for nearly 40 % of all cases.

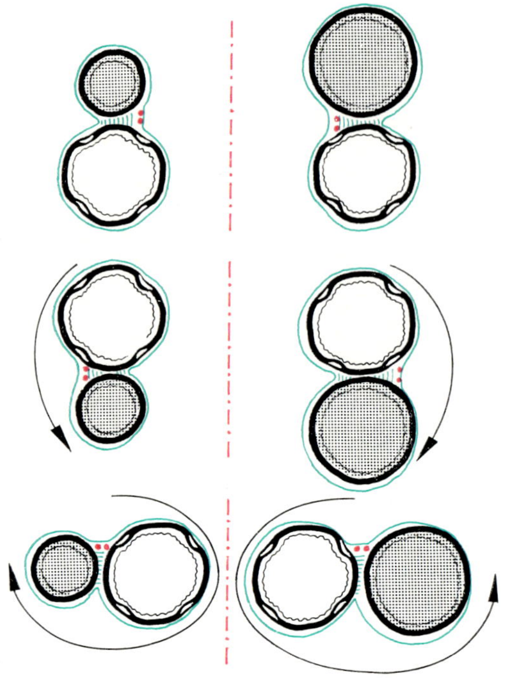

51

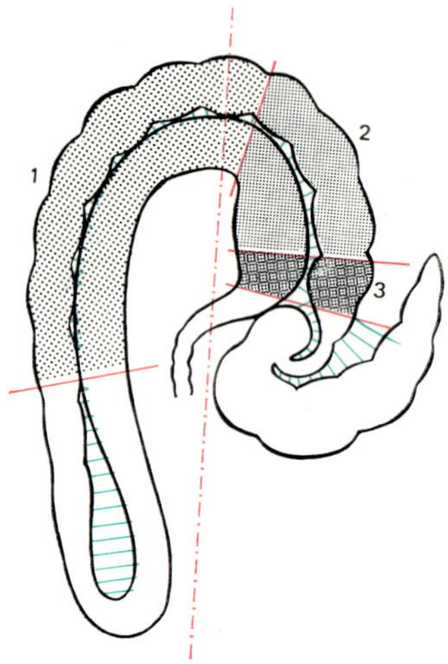

52

Fig. 2.1.5. — 51. Torsion of the large colon. Direction and degrees of torsion:
Top: normal position; Center: *180°* torsion in a *lateral* direction; Bottom: *270°* torsion in a *medial* direction.
(Transverse sections: red broken line = median plane; dorsal colon is shaded; position of vessels in ascending mesocolon indicated by red dots.)

Fig. 2.1.5. — 52. Torsion of the large colon. Location of constriction sites and their clinical significance:
1 region of left colon or diaphragmatic and sternal flexures: treatment by counter-rotation or resection; *2* region of right colon: treatment by counter-rotation or slaughter; *3* region of colic ampulla or area of attachment: untreatable except in very early cases.
Dorsal view.

Etiology and Pathogenesis. When the pelvic flexure or dorsal colon becomes impacted, gas may form in the bowel segment proximal to the impaction. The heavier dorsal colon sinks toward the floor of the abdominal cavity, while the lighter, gas-filled ventral colon 'floats' upward. The resulting torsion of 180° or less does not obstruct the intestinal lumen and reduces spontaneously once the impaction is cleared. There are exceptions, however. Sometimes during the conservative treatment of an impaction a marked exacerbation of systemic signs is noted as soon as the laxative takes effect. This occurs because the gas bubble in the ventral colon pushes the constriction site in an aboral direction, thereby increasing the degree of torsion as well as the tension at the constriction site. Some horses with partial colonic torsion present with a history that is typical of this process: A sudden exacerbation of systemic signs following prolonged treatment for impaction, with rectal signs suggestive of colonic torsion.

The situation is different in broodmares. These animals are most susceptible to colonic torsion during the change from stall feeding to grazing at pasture, when the proportion of hay and straw in the diet is greatly reduced in favor of lush grass. This can cause undesired fermentation processes to take place in the large colon, accompanied by intensive gas formation. The colonic contents in such cases have a semi-liquid, finely-frothed consistency. If a torsion occurs the contents can offer little resistance to aboral shifting of the constriction site as gaseous pressure rises. The progression to complete colonic torsion is rapid. Broodmares that are given very large volumes of feed during the winter are predisposed, for these animals possess a relatively large colon and have much 'room' left in their abdomen following pregnancy. Presumably the disease is also based upon an abnormal peristalsis that retards aboral progression of the fermenting, frothy ingesta.

If the intestinal lumen is obstructed, the disease takes a fatal course: Occlusion of the veins at the constriction site with a sustained arterial supply leads to severe congestive hyperemia and extravasation, producing extreme edema of the bowel wall and mesocolon. There is hemorrhagic infarction of the intestinal mucosa and a submucosal edema up to 10 mm thick with leakage of hemorrhagic transudate into the intestinal lumen and abdominal cavity. After only a few hours the mucosa starts to become necrotic, initially on the antimesenteric side. As much as 40 l of transudate may be present *in the intestinal wall* itself. Adding to this the transudate in the abdominal cavity and intestinal lumen, we may estimate a total loss of 60—80 l to the extracellular space — an incredibly large volume to be lost within a period of 4—6 h. This is accompanied by an endotoxemia caused by decomposition of the bowel contents, intestinal bacteria and incipient tissue necrosis. The endotoxemia leads to hemolysis and parenchymal degeneration in the heart, liver and kidneys. Tympany of the bowel — pre- and poststenotic — also has consequences. The elevated diaphragm interferes with respiration, producing a dyspnea that may be fatal. Pressure on the great vessels places an extra burden on the heart and circulation. Intestinal rupture is also possible. Death ensues in 6—12 h.

Symptoms and Diagnosis. Complete torsion of the large colon generally is marked by a severe colic of sudden onset. The symptoms are dramatic: The mare throws herself violently to the ground, rolls back and forth, jumps back to her feet, and then immediately goes down again. The animal's behavior is so frantic and unpredictable that an adequate examination is often impossible. Soon the animal is drenched with sweat, the pulse and respiratory rate are rapid, the flanks are distended, and the mucous membranes are dark red. It is not unusual for the hematocrit to rise above 60 in only 2—3 h.

Rectal examination shows severe tympanitic distension of the large colon. The wall is thickened and fleshy (fig. 2.1.5. — 53).

In the rare cases of torsion unaccompanied by significant gas formation, the colon may be displaced so far anteriorally that in large mares it can no longer be reached per rectum.

The diagnosis is easily made due to the peracute course. The animal's condition deteriorates so rapidly that often it is apparent that slaughter or at least hospitalization is indicated after only an hour.

Abdominal paracentesis, which cannot always be performed, yields a large volume of dark-red fluid which is found to contain many erythrocytes when centrifuged. Leukocytes are also obtained in later stages of the condition.

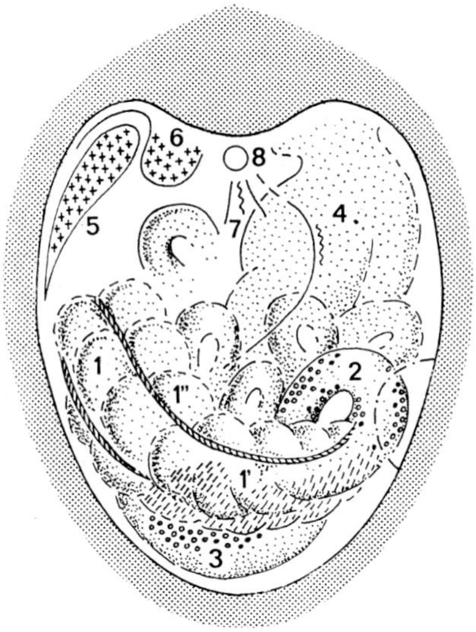

Fig. 2.1.5. — 53. Torsion of the large colon.
1 tense, tympanitic ventral colon; *1'* tightly stretched longitudinal bands; *1''* haustra; *2* distended pelvic flexure with markedly thickened, friable wall (shaded area); *3* tympanitic dorsal colon; *4* tympanitic cecum; *5* spleen; *6* left kidney; *7* cranial root of mesentery; *8* aorta.

The characteristic tympany, peracute course, rectal findings and violent behavior enable a prompt diagnosis of colonic torsion to be made.

In exceptional cases the course is more gradual, extending over several days. These are cases that are uncomplicated by tympany and involve only a partial obstruction, i.e., gas can still pass through the twisted bowel. The gut wall and mesentery are markedly edematous, but the mucosa is not infarcted, and necrosis is initially absent. Affected horses are anorexic, drink small amounts of water and suffer mild bouts of colic.

The rectal findings of an edematous colon, together with the clinical signs, establish the diagnosis.

Partial torsion of the large colon is marked by similar symptoms. The course depends on the degree of strangulation that occurs, ranging from the dramatic form with hemorrhagic infarction to the milder form.

Rectal examination almost always reveals edema of the colon and mesentery in the area of the left colon loops. This is manifested by a typical fleshy consistency.

Differential Diagnosis. A kinking of the colon (flexion or retroflexion) and right dorsal displacement of the colon present similar rectal findings with a markedly milder course. There is tympany of the ventral or dorsal colon, but the cause cannot be specified as a kink, torsion or displacement. Hence, surgery is indicated whenever *edema of the bowel wall* is detected on rectal examination. If the colon is entrapped over the nephrosplenic ligament, the palpation of ligament ventral to the colon will differentiate that condition from colonic torsion.

The relatively innocent torsions of the left dorsal and ventral colon by 180° like those occurring in impactions or tympany are not accompanied by edema formation ('physiologic' torsion).

Prognosis. Assuming the surgeon has mastered the surgical technique (which is quite difficult), the prognosis is favorable if it is not complicated by necrosis. Postoperative recovery is remarkably rapid. Colonic resection also carries a favorable prognosis if no more than two-thirds of the colon are excised. If the entire colon is

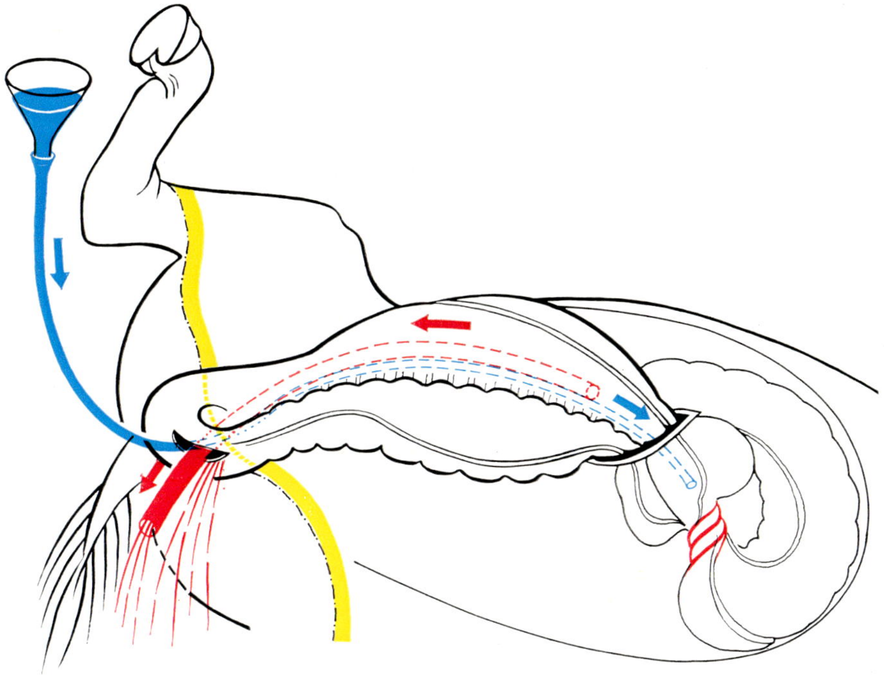

Fig. 2.1.5. — 54. Emptying the stenostenotic loop of colon by irrigation in colonic torsion.

involved in necrosis, the prognosis is grave. Unfortunately, this stage is already reached in most cases by the time the animal is hospitalized.

Treatment. In mild cases (180°) a conservative, wait-and-see approach may be adopted. These torsions are usually secondary in nature and disappear when the causal obstruction is relieved.

In torsions exceeding 180° that are accompanied by much gas formation in the poststenotic segment, deflation of the gas bubble by trocarization is sometimes sufficient to effect a reduction.

If parts of the colon are found to be edematous on rectal exploration, surgery is always indicated.

The operation is done through a preumbilical midline laparotomy. After the abdominal cavity is opened, the direction, degree and seat of the torsion are ascertained. Then the pelvic flexure is exteriorized and laid between the patient's hind legs. An incision is made in the dorsal loop and the ingesta are removed. Ingesta are removed particularly from the dorsal colon proximal to the constriction site. This is best done by means of irrigation with two tubes (fig. 2.1.5. — 54).

Only when the entire bowel segment has been emptied is the enterotomy closed and the untwisting process begun. The infusion of several liters of physiologic saline into the abdominal cavity will facilitate this maneuver, as this will 'float' the intestine and reduce adhesive forces.

If portions of the mucosa are black in the poststenotic segment, indicating necrosis, then a colonic resection is indicated especially if at least one-third of the large colon can be saved (q.v.; figs. 2.1.5. — 55 to — 58).

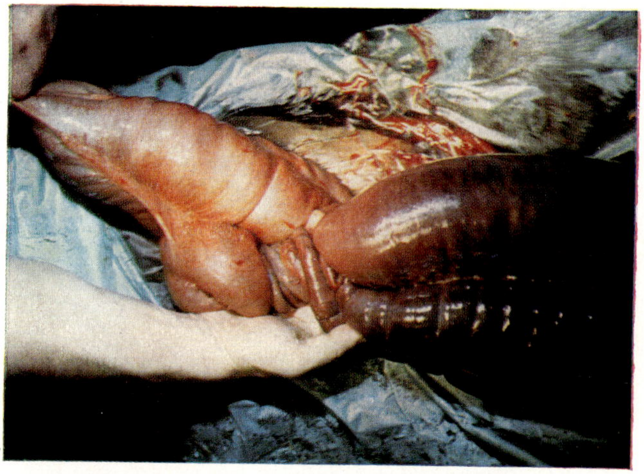
55

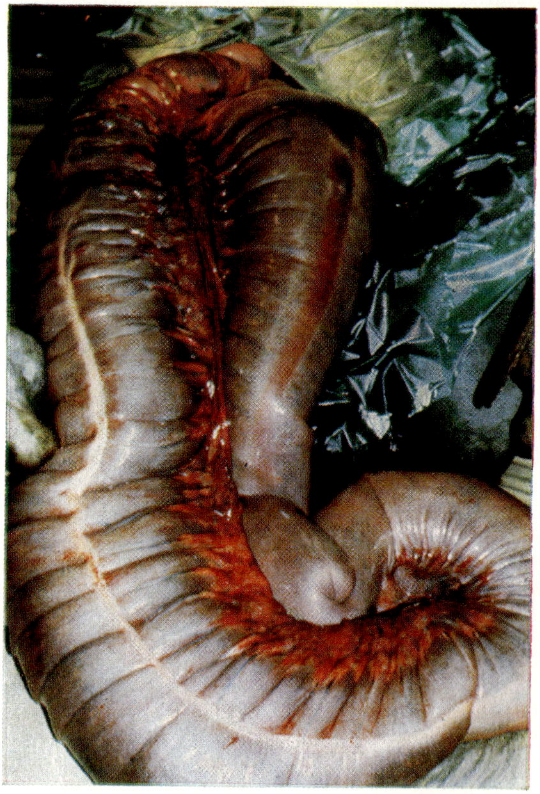
56

Fig. 2.1.5. — 55. Complete torsion of the large colon in a foal. At left is the cecum, at center is the torsion site (360°) above the surgeon's hand, and at right is the necrotic loop of colon.

Fig. 2.1.5. — 56. Complete torsion of the large colon in a broodmare. The loop of colon has been exteriorized up to and including the diaphragmatic and sternal flexures. The case shown is a 360° torsion of the sero-edematous form.

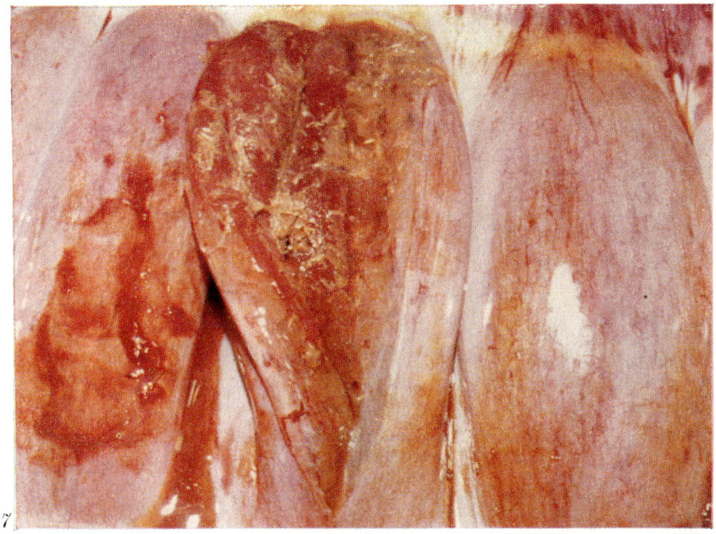

57

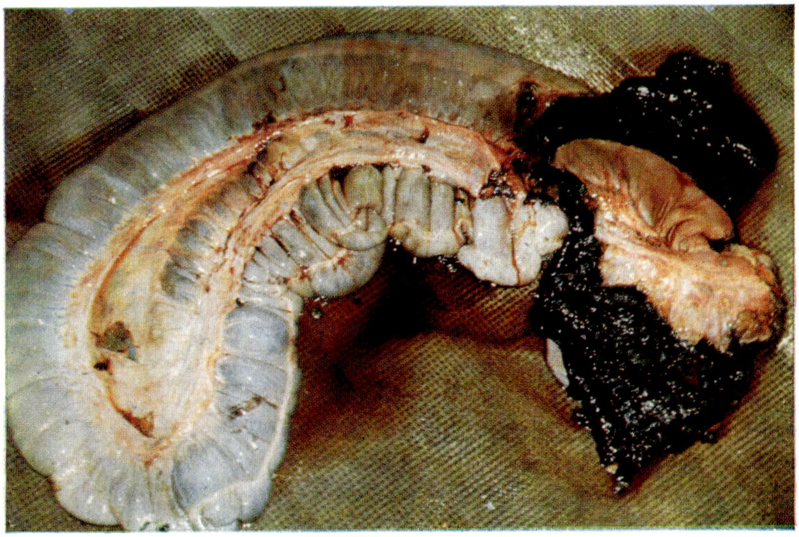

58

Fig. 2.1.5. — 57. Incision of a colonic haustra revealing submucosal edema approximately 10 mm thick. The mucosa is medium red and shows no signs of incipient necrosis.

Fig. 2.1.5. — 58. Resected loop of colon representing about two-thirds of the entire colon. The black mucosa is necrotic.

Kinking (Flexion, Retroflexion) of the Large Colon

Definition and Occurrence. Craniad displacements of the pelvic flexure lead to a kinking, or flexion, of the dorsal and ventral colon with a narrowing of the intestinal lumen (partial obstruction). The disorder is not uncommon and usually develops secondary to a tympany or impaction of the large colon. The pelvic flexure may be displaced in a lateral, medial, dorsal or ventral direction; the latter condition is also known as 'retroflexion' (fig. 2.1.5. — 59).

Symptoms and Diagnosis. Initially the symptoms are mild, for the luminal reduction is minimal and venous congestion is slight. Rectal examination shows a gas-filled colon whose dorsal and ventral parts can usually be identified from their longitudinal bands. However, the pelvic flexure is displaced craniad and consequently is out of reach.

Treatment. If tympany is pronounced and systemic signs are mild or absent, initial treatment consists of cecal trocharization. Prostigmin is administered after the gas is released. If conservative treatment fails or a marked exacerbation points to surgical intervention, a midline laparotomy is performed, and the large colon is evacuated and repositioned.

Prognosis. Conservative treatment is not always successful. Vigorous laxative therapy carries a risk of intestinal rupture.

The chance of recovery with surgical treatment is good.

A special form of displacement and kinking of the large colon is termed *right dorsal displacement of the large colon.*

Definition and Occurrence. In this condition part or all of the large colon is displaced to the right and caudally, then winds back medially and cranially around the fixed point formed by the cecum. A kink develops immediately aboral to the cecum in the initial and terminal parts of the large colon. This displacement is roughly analogous to nephrosplenic herniation on the opposite side but is less common (fig. 2.1.5. — 60).

Symptoms and Diagnosis. The clinical picture is like that of a mild case of colonic torsion or left dorsal displacement of the large colon over the nephrosplenic ligament. There may be considerable extravasation of blood if venous stasis develops and gas formation is rapid. This leads to severe systemic signs due to the large segment of colon that is affected.

On rectal examination the distended colon is palpated in place of the cecum, which is located farther cranially. If the colon is additionally twisted 180° at the strangulation site, the edematous mesocolon can be felt.

Treatment. Surgical correction offers the only prospect for recovery. After performing a midline laparotomy, the surgeon first attempts to exteriorize the pelvic flexure in order to empty the colon of gas and ingesta. Only then is the reduction carried out. This can be facilitated by evacuating the cecum so that it can be displaced as needed. The reduction is difficult in any case.

Intussusception

Definition and Occurrence. Intussusception refers to a longitudinal displacement of an intestinal loop in which one segment of intestine invaginates into the lumen of an adjacent segment and continues to move caudad in the direction of peristalsis. This causes three tubes of intestine to become telescoped together: An outer tube, called the intussuscipiens, and an inner and middle tube, called the intussusceptum. There is contact between the mucosal surfaces of the outer and middle tubes, and between the serosal surfaces of the middle and inner tubes. A portion of the mesentery also becomes indrawn between the middle and inner tubes. The length of the in-

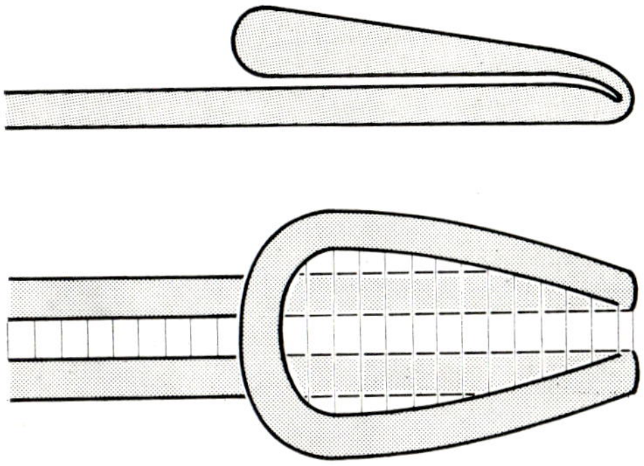

59

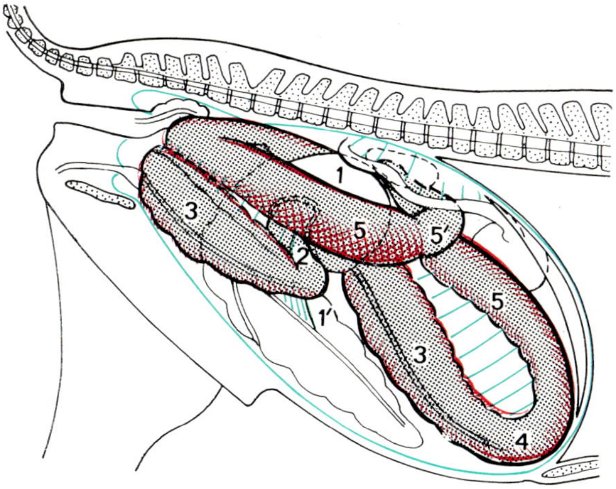

60

Fig. 2.1.5. — 59. Retroflexion of the large colon (modified from Wall). Top: lateral view; bottom: top view.

Fig. 2.1.5. — 60. Right dorsal displacement of the large colon as viewed from the right side:
1 base of cecum; *1′* cecocolic fold; *2* neck of colon; *3* ventral colon; *4* pelvic flexure; *5* dorsal colon; *5′* junction of colic ampulla with transverse colon.

tussusception depends on the length of the involved segment of mesentery: The average length in the horse is between 50 and 70 cm. Considerably longer intussusceptions can occur if the mesentery becomes torn, thus allowing larger excursions of the bowel.

The disorder is relatively uncommon. It usually affects foals or small horses and very rarely affects larger or older horses. Intussusceptions may involve the large or small intestine and are designated as follows according to the area of the bowel affected:
— jejunal intussusception (jejunum into jejunum)
— jejunoileal intussusception (jejunum into ileum)
— ileocecal intussusception (ileum into cecum, fig. 2.1.5. — 61)
— cecal intussusception (cecum into cecum, fig. 2.1.5. — 62, left)
— cecocolic intussusception (cecum into large colon, fig. 2.1.5. — 62, right)
— colonic intussusception (small colon into small colon)
— colorectal intussusception (small colon into rectum).

Intussusceptions are thought to be precipitated by excessive peristalsis like that caused by physical and toxic stimuli (enteritis). Because intussusceptions of the small intestine also occur during physiologic digestion, it is assumed that they are the result of hyperperistalsis.

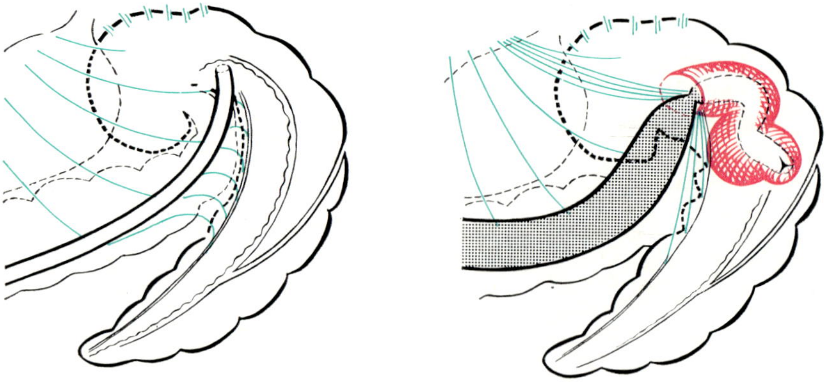

61

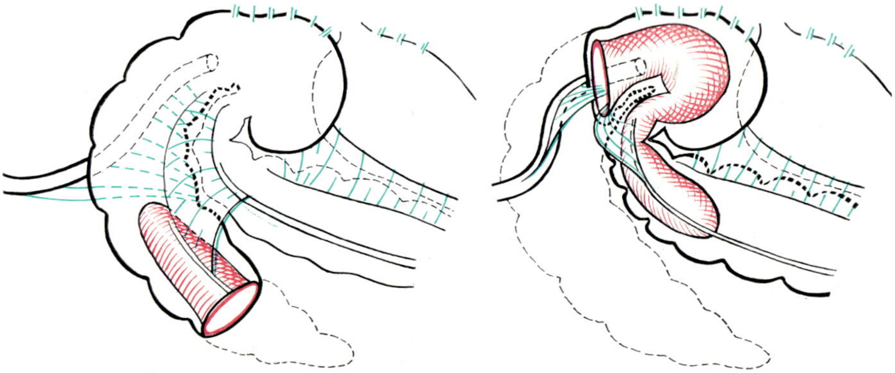

62

Fig. 2.1.5. — 61. Ileocecal intussusception.
Left: normal situation; right: intussusception (medial view).
Fig. 2.1.5. — 62. Left: cecal intussusception; right: cecocolic intussusception (lateral view).

In one laparotomized foal we observed an intussusception about 40 cm long in the exteriorized small intestine in which the intussusceptum repeatedly slid in and out of the intussuscipiens! The cycle lasted about one minute. It appeared as if the intussuscipiens and intussesceptum were actively moving in opposite directions. It may be that local spasms of the circular muscles, small neoplasms, ring-shaped stenoses (like those following end-to-end anastomoses), parasites, etc. lead to a transient incarceration of the invaginated bowel, which is then fixed by a local spasm. The antimesenteric border of the intussusceptum is convexly curved by the pull of the mesentery. At first it is not entirely obstructed. The compression of the mesentery at the neck of the intussusception interferes with venous drainage, leading to congestive hyperemia and stasis edema of the intussusceptum. The submucosa becomes edematous and shows a dark-red to reddish-black discoloration. A vicious cycle is established in which the swellings exacerbate the occlusion of the blood vessels, leading to complete obstruction of the intestinal lumen and finally of the arteries. This is accompanied by a prestenotic stagnation of ingesta with its familiar consequences (e.g., secondary gastric dilation).

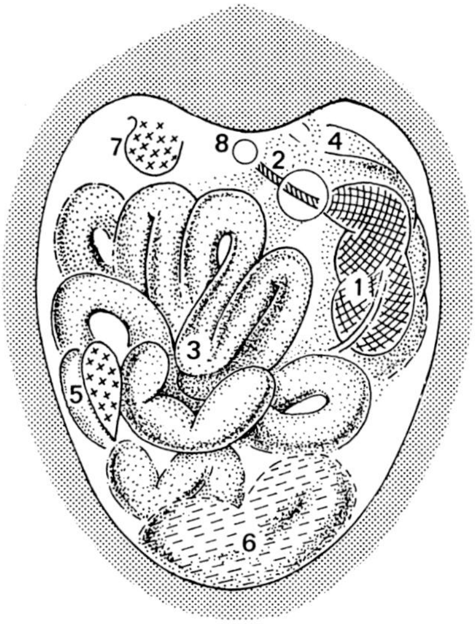

Fig. 2.1.5. — 63. Ileocecal intussusception. *1* pendulous mass of fleshy consistency (intussusceptum); *2* tense, painful mesoileum: *3* tympanitic loops of small intestine; *4* distended duodenum; *5* displaced spleen (sign of secondary gastric dilation); *6* inspissated feces in large colon; *7* left kidney; *8* abdominal aorta. Findings on arm-deep rectal exploration.

While the intussusceptum is dying from necrosis, fibrinous adhesions develop at the site of the invagination. Spontaneous remission may occur if the necrotic intussusceptum is sloughed and the fibrinous adhesions are sufficiently impermeable to bacteria to prevent peritonitis. Otherwise a general, fatal peritonitis will develop, assuming that gastric rupture or a lethal endotoxemia (gangrenous intussusceptum) has not supervened.

Intussusceptions of the large intestine are not accompanied by reflux into the stomach. They cause little interference with water absorption in the large colon. Accordingly, systemic signs are slow to appear. As in the small intestine, spontaneous healing is possible.

Symptoms and Diagnosis. In intussusceptions of the small intestine, the clinical picture is that of a small intestinal ileus. Often the entire intussusception is felt rectally as a painful, freely-movable, coiled bowel segment that has a fleshy consistency.

In ileocecal intussusception a concave, fleshy, sausage-shaped segment is felt in the area of the cecal base (fig. 2.1.5. — 63).

In cecal and cecocolic intussusceptions, a fleshy, knobby, tumor-like mass is palpated in the area of the junction between the body and base of the cecum.

In these diseases systemic signs remain mild for some days, and the colicky pains may subside, mimicking a spontaneous recovery. Blood will be present in the stool if the large intestine is involved.

Intussusceptions of the small colon are easily detected on rectal examination, the involved segment being marked by its fleshy consistency and relative mobility anterior to the pelvis, as well as by its prominent longitudinal band.

The colorectal intussusception is marked externally by a prolapsed rectum. If the rectal prolapse is more than 30 cm long, it may be assumed that the descending mesocolon is torn, with associated blood flow disturbances and consequent intestinal necrosis.

Treatment. Small intestine: The intussusception is surgically exposed. It is seldom possible to manually reduce the intussusception by pulling the involved segments apart.

In most cases surgical resection is necessary, followed by a side-to-side juno-jejunostomy or jejunoileostomy. In ileocecal intussusceptions a jejunocecostomy should follow the resection.

Large intestine: In advanced cases of cecal or cecocolic intussusception, the intussusceptum is left alone, and the site of the invagination is simply oversewn with a continuous suture.

If the ileum is involved, a typhlectomy should be considered following a right lateral flank laparotomy and rib resection. The ileum is then anastomosed to the colon.

In necrosis of the small colon following the reduction of a colorectal intussusception, resection of the necrotic bowel segment is followed by a colorectostomy. This end-to-end anastomosis is done either through a midline approach or transrectally.

Prognosis. Recovery is possible with good surgical technique, provided shock and paralytic ileus can be controlled and diffuse peritonitis can be prevented.

Intestinal Blood Flow Disturbances, Thromboembolic Colic

Definition and Occurrence. Thromboembolic colic generally involves the occlusion of one or more intestinal arteries; the veins are rarely affected. Despite the prevalence of parasitic disease in the horse population, the disease is rare. It mainly affects older foals.

Etiology and Pathogenesis. The lesions of the mesenteric artery are caused by 4th-stage larvae of *Strongylus vulgaris*. According to Enigk [1951], they penetrate the mucosa of the large intestine and enter the arterioles of the bowel wall, where they cause thrombus formation. Endarteritis accompanied by aneurysm and thrombus formation takes place in the cranial mesenteric artery and its branches, and thrombi originating from this site can obstruct larger mesenteric arteries [Marek].

Our own surgical experience has confirmed the occurrence of arteriolar obstruction in the small and large intestine as described by Enigk, but in most cases these findings were secondary or incidental. Therefore, we agree with Marek's assertion that thromboembolic colic in the horse is caused essentially by the thrombosis of larger intestinal arteries. The occlusion of arterioles produces no symptoms in most cases.

The effects of emboli on the microcirculation of the bowel wall depend on the location and extent of the vascular occlusion and on the number, size and anastomoses of the occluded vessels. A slowly developing stenosis may allow time for the development of adequate collaterals, especially in the arteries of the large intestine.

If an intestinal embolism develops suddenly, the progress of the disease depends upon whether

— the microcirculation can be maintained by a well-developed collateral circulation,
— the oxygen supply will diminish to critical levels due to a deficiency of collaterals, or
— the microcirculation and thus the oxygen supply will be lost entirely due to an absence of collateral circulation.

If the deprived region is small, the anastomotic capillaries will assume the blood-supply function following initial ischemia. In this process the capillaries become widely dilatated, and their wall becomes permeable to blood constituents, including the red blood cells. The surrounding tissue becomes infarcted. The submucous layer becomes edematous, and the intestinal wall swells, further compromising the microcirculation. The hemorrhagic infarction, together with intestinal bacteria and toxins, causes necrosis to develop. The damaged tissue can still regenerate at this point if circulatory conditions improve. Because the mucosa is the first layer to become necrotic, intestinal ulcers may form that later cicatrize during healing. Scars of this type in the small intestine can contract and cause stenosis. If the location or size of an embolus are such that a collateral circulation cannot develop, ischemic necrosis of the intestinal wall is inevitable, characterized by a grayish-white and later greenish discoloration of the bowel wall surrounded by a well-defined border of hemorrhagic infarction. This gives rise to a peritonitis which, together with intestinal rupture, leads rapidly to death from endotoxic shock. If the necrosis is extensive, peritonitis and endotoxemia can cause death even in the absence of intestinal rupture.

Symptoms and Diagnosis. In early cases of thromboembolic colic the clinical picture is similar to that of spasmodic colic. Intestinal sounds are increased, and a loose stool is passed at frequent intervals. Systemic signs initially are absent or mild. Rectal examination is negative in many cases.

Thrombosis of the large intestine leads to profuse diarrhea as a result of impaired absorption. If the thromboembolic lesion is localized in the small intestine, the loss of motility leads to signs of ileus with prestenotic impaction and secondary gastric dilation. Sometimes local tympany is also detected in the large intestine. If spontaneous resolution occurs as a result of circulatory anastomosis, colicky signs will improve. If necrosis develops, the disease worsens, and the clinical picture is dominated by peritonitis. Peristalsis decreases progressively and is finally abolished. Fever is present. Marked abdominal distension will be noted in cases of general tympany. Feces are evil-smelling and are passed infrequently and in small amounts. As the peritonitis becomes more severe, there is a marked increase in the pulse rate and respiration. Abdominal paracentesis yields a creamy fluid that is rich in leukocytes and low in erythrocytes. The animal dies from the effects of the peritonitis or rupture of the necrotic bowel wall.

Antibiotics can mask the symptoms for several days. In thromboembolic necrosis of the small intestine, the diagnosis is based upon the characteristic symptoms of small intestinal ileus; in thromboembolic necrosis of the large intestine, it is based on the development of a severe peritonitis. Mild cases that regress spontaneously present a clinical picture of spasmodic colic that is either recurrent or unremitting. The main diagnostic criterion is the peritoneal fluid which, when collected at intervals of a few hours, provides a clear indication of the stage and degree of intestinal damage and peritonitis. The demonstration of a verminous aneurysm or mesenteric abscess on rectal examination has no bearing on the actual diagnosis.

Differential Diagnosis. All other forms of small bowel ileus must be differentiated. In necroses of the large bowel due to strangulation or incarceration, the course is usually peracute, and coprostatis is complete.

Treatment. Treatment with spasmoanalgesics is sufficient in mild cases. If it is suspected that a recurrent colic has a thromboembolic cause, repeated antiparasitic treatments combined with anticoagulant therapy are recommended. The latter should be continued over a period of several months. Depending on body weight, 5—20 mg warfarin (e.g., Coumadin, Falithrom) per day is administered while monitoring coagulation times. The prothrombin time should increase from 12—13 to 15—18 s. In severe cases surgical correction often is successful. Surgical measures are aimed at resecting the necrotic bowel segment far into healthy tissue while restoring the intestinal lumen (see Operative Technique for details).

Internal Injuries

Definition and Occurrence. Crushing injuries of the intestinal tract can not only damage the bowel wall as a result of compression, but can also exert traction on its mesentery sufficient to produce a mesenteric tear. If the intestinal blood supply is preserved, the contusion and tear will heal, leaving behind a defect that predisposes to intestinal incarceration. If the blood supply is disrupted, the affected bowel segment will become necrotic, leading to obstruction and peritonitis.

Perforations are forceful penetrations of the intestinal wall caused by gunshot wounds, impalements, or endogenous causes such as parasites, foreign bodies, ulceration or necrosis. Internal perforations may occur from within the intestinal lumen or from the area immediately surrounding the intestine.

Ruptures of the intestine may result from trauma (hoof strike, parturition, fall, traffic injury) or from an internal mechanism that causes *overstretching* of the bowel (acute and chronic intestinal dilation, acute gastric dilation, rectal examination). All parts of the intestine are susceptible to ruptures of this type.

Sites of predilection are: Cecum: border of cecocolic fold, area of attachment of cecal base. Large colon: area of attachment of colic ampulla. Small colon: antimesenteric border at junction of small colon and rectum.

The 'stretch' rupture starts in the muscular and serous layers, followed by prolapse and rupture of the mucosa. Hence, the mucosal tear is the smallest.

The symptoms vary with the degree and extent of the internal injury. Thus, simple contusions of the bowel may cause no symptoms or produce transitory, mild colicky signs; they usually go unrecognized, therefore. Smaller perforations or ruptures with minimal leakage of intestinal contents into the peritoneal cavity cause a local peritonitis and in exceptional cases may resolve through adhesion formation with neighboring tissues (see section on Peritonitis). With more extensive injuries, large amounts of intestinal contents are spilled into the peritoneal cavity, causing a diffuse peritonitis (fecal peritonitis) that leads rapidly to death from endotoxic shock. If the spilled ingesta become walled off by loops of omentum and bowel, an intra-abdominal abscess will form, leading to multiple adhesions. The majority of perforations and ruptures occur as complications of other intestinal diseases (chronic impactions, obturations, foreign bodies, gastric overload, etc.). Of particular importance are internal injuries associated with parturition and rectal injuries caused by rectal examination.

Internal Intestinal Injuries Associated with Parturition

Intestinal injuries caused by parturition are relatively common in the mare. The following lesions are typical:

— intestinal and mesenteric contusions in the area of the small intestine or small colon without disruption of continuity, in which an adequate blood supply is preserved.
— lesions of these areas in which part of the mesentery is separated from the intestine leading to (a) ischemic necrosis of the bowel or (b) healing with the formation of a defect.
— intestinal and mesenteric contusions in which there is a breach of the intestinal lumen.

Symptoms and Diagnosis. Soon after parturition the mare becomes restless, paws the ground, and lies down and gets up repeatedly. The appetite is reduced or absent. The clinical picture varies with the extent and severity of the intestinal lesions. In the absence of necrosis, the mild colic will usually pass in a few hours without treatment.

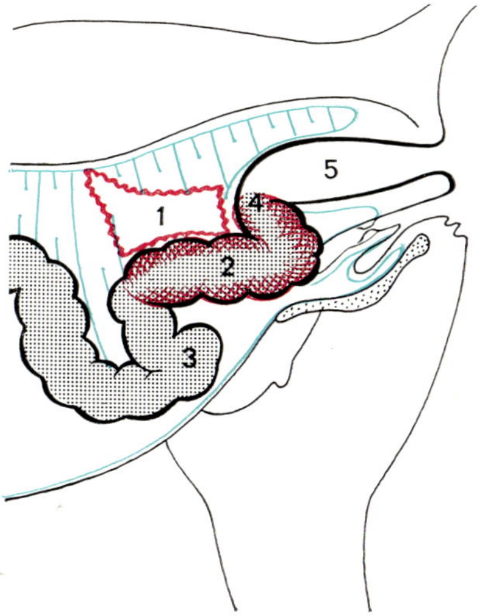

Fig. 2.1.5. — 64. Necrosis of the small colon following a mesenteric tear.
1 mesenteric tear; *2* necrotic zone with impaction; *3* prestenotic coprostasis: *4* kink; *5* rectal ampulla.

Intestinal necrosis is accompanied by extreme colicky signs during the first few hours. The acute colicky stage is sometimes followed by a calm period with continued anorexia and a marked elevation of body temperature. Bacteria migrate from the necrotic bowel segment into the abdominal cavity, causing peritonitis. At this point (24—48 h postpartum) there is a rapid exacerbation of systemic signs. The loss of peristalsis in the necrotic bowel leads to an acute obstruction, causing renewed colic. Two to four days may pass before a perforation develops in the necrotic area. The intestinal contusion can be detected rectally only if it is located in the terminal small colon. Otherwise positive findings are obtained only when the ileus produces characteristic secondary signs (distended or impacted prestenotic bowel segment, pain on palpation of affected bowel segments, fibrinous exudation). In a few cases the traumatized loop of bowel can be felt in the pelvic cavity, where it is bound up in fibrinous adhesions.

Abdominal paracentesis is the most important diagnostic aid if an intestinal contusion is suspected and should be repeated every 6—8 h. Initially the fluid is slightly turbid and contains only erythrocytes, but if the bowel becomes necrotic the fluid takes on a viscous, creamy consistency due to the presence of leukocytes. Samples collected at different times are stored in upright tubes to provide a visible (and often dramatic) record of the rising leukocyte content in early peritonitis. Fluid that is only slightly reddened initially, and later normalizes, indicates regeneration of the contused intestine. Because this disease always occurs in connection with foaling, a prompt diagnosis is not difficult.

A special case is the mesenteric tear at the junction of the descending mesocolon and mesorectum. This lesion is a result of rectal prolapse and, as such, occurs frequently during parturition when there is a prolapse of more than about 30 cm of rectum. This is accompanied by an intussusception of the small colon, and a mesenteric tear issues from the extremely short mesorectum (fig. 2.1.5. — 64).

Only 2—3 h after a successful 'reduction' of the prolapse, an initially mild colic appears, caused by the accumulation of digesta proximal to the necrotic bowel. The necrotic segment is usually from 50 to 80 cm long. On rectal examination the sausage-shaped impaction can be palpated in the small colon. Often the necrotic tissue can also be felt, marked by its dry, velvety surface texture. The impacted feces are strongly adherent to the dry mucosa and are difficult or impossible to dislodge. In doubtful cases the impacted, prestenotic, loops of small colon can be discerned anterior to the pelvis by palpation from within the uterus.

Occasional anal tenesmus is observed initially. Small amounts of feces may be passed. As the disease progresses, the signs of small colonic impaction become predominent. Unremitting mild colicky episodes, gradual onset of tympany, elevations of the pulse rate, respiratory rate and body temperature are characteristic. These symptoms should be looked for if there is an immediate history of rectal prolapse.

Treatment. Conservative treatment is of no value. Operative treatment is difficult and ordinarily requires at least two and preferably three experienced surgeons. Following a postumbilical midline laparotomy, the necrotic bowel segment is resected and a colorectostomy (q.v.) is performed. If a small portion of the rectum is involved, the colorectostomy must be done transanally.

Prognosis. The prognosis is favorable if the operation is performed within the first 24—48 h by capable, experienced surgeons. Peritonitis usually responds well to antibiotic therapy.

Rectal Injuries

Definition and Occurrence. Occasionally the rectum will become perforated during a rectal examination despite precautions. MERKT estimates that the risk is less than 1 : 10,000. This may be correct in gynecological examination. But our experience suggests that this risk is several times greater in cases where there has been deep rectal exploration in the colicky horse. Similar injuries can result from breeding errors in which the stallion's penis enters the rectum of the mare. These injuries typically occur on the dorsal, mesenteric border of the rectum at its junction with the small colon. The perforation may extend to the abdominal cavity in extreme cases, but ordinarily the injury is confined to the mucosa and the muscularis while sparing the serosa.

Symptoms and Diagnosis. Blood on the rectal sleeve first alerts the examiner to the injury in most cases. The ungloved hand is then carefully reinserted, and the size and depth of the injury are ascertained. The next step is to advise the owner or attendant of the situation and jointly decide upon the best course of action: slaughter, immediate surgery or, if facilities or expertise are inadequate, referral to a hospital close by.

Treatment. The rectal ampulla is emptied (assuming this was not done before the injury), and epidural anesthesia is administered. While the anesthetic is taking effect, the necessary instruments are laid out. A small needle holder, a medium-size, curved, sharp needle and several long No. 5 Dexon sutures should suffice for the repair. In most horses both arms can be introduced simultaneously through the anus, one hand approximating the wound edges to form a ridge, and the other guiding the needle. If the anus is narrow, the sharp needle must be passed through the wound edges with one hand, without using a needle holder. Repair starts by placing a simple interrupted suture at the anterior end of the wound. The knots are preplaced outside the anus and advanced to the wound line. An assistant shifts the rupture farther caudad by exerting gentle traction on the threads in order to improve access. Repair is effected most simply with several interrupted horizontal mattress sutures. If the veterinarian feels that his technical proficiency is inadequate for the job, he should prepare the animal for transportation to a hospital. A single dose of 30 mg atropine sulfate is sufficient to abolish bowel motility and thus halt the progression of feces from the small colon to the rectum for several hours. However, the drug does not take effect for about 50 min, and until then fecal balls should be manually removed through the rectum to prevent contamination of the wound and abdominal cavity. MERKT recommends 30 mg of propantheline bromide (e.g., Pro-Banthine), whose onset of action is immediate on intravenous application. Its duration of action is only 2 h, however. 'Cleansing enemas' (with ethacridine lactate, alum, etc.) should be strictly avoided, as they promote the spread of fecal particles to the peritoneal cavity.

Before the intestinal wound is closed, penicillin-streptomycin or terramycin emulsion (50—100 ml) should be deposited in the abdominal cavity through the wound. Large antibiotic doses should also be administered for several days postoperatively. In the case of large tears, fecal balls lodged anterior to the wound ridge must be carefully removed manually at frequent intervals. Food deprivation and the daily administration of 2 l mineral oil by nasogastric tube are important adjunctive measures. Spontaneous defecation may occur surprisingly soon, after only 2 to 3 days, or may be deferred for some time as a result of local inflammation.

Prognosis. The prognosis is poor. The chance of recovery depends on the degree of contamination of the abdominal cavity, the timing of the operation, and the surgical repair. Uneventful healing is always possible, however. Incomplete tears in which the serosa is intact should also be repaired due to the risk of subsequent perforation by impacted feces in the pseudodiverticulum and by gangrene.

Grass Sickness

Definition and Occurrence. Grass sickness is a neurogenic intestinal disease of horses whose cause is unknown. It has been reported mainly in Great Britain, though cases have also occurred in West Germany. It is unknown in North America. Horses of any breed, age and sex, including ponies, are susceptible, but the incidence is highest in the 4- to 7-year age group.

Symptoms and Diagnosis. Affected horses show signs of unremitting colic that is especially severe in peracute cases. In subacute cases the animal's behavior alternates between depression and excitement. There is difficulty in swallowing, and saliva is drooled. If the appetite remains the horse may attept to eat but will be unable to do so. The passage of a nasogastric tube will meet with resistance over the entire length of the esophagus. Affected horses curl and purse the lips a great deal, and their nostrils are usually caked with a greenish vomitus. The visible mucosae are dark red, breathing is rapid, and the pulse rate is usually above 100. Elevated hematocrit values of 60—70 or higher are the rule. The internal body temperature is normal or slightly elevated. Peristalsis is markedly reduced and later is entirely absent. There is patchy sweating, and trembling of the shoulder muscles is sometimes observed. Within a short time secondary gastric dilation appears, and colicky symptoms subside temporarily when this is relieved.

During rectal examination the horse strains vigorously, the small colon is empty, and the rectum is coated with sticky mucus.

The ingesta in the large colon are inspissated, but tympanitic loops of small intestine are never found (this differentiates grass sickness from small intestinal ileus). As the disease progresses, the horse makes repeated attempts to vomit. These are only partially successful but sometimes are sufficient to forestall gastric rupture.

Acute cases die in 1—3 days. If the disease reaches the chronic stage, all the clinical signs are present but are not so pronounced. Secondary gastric dilation is absent in chronic cases. The horse is able to ingest soft feeds but regurgitates frequently. Emaciation is rapid, and death follows in a few weeks.

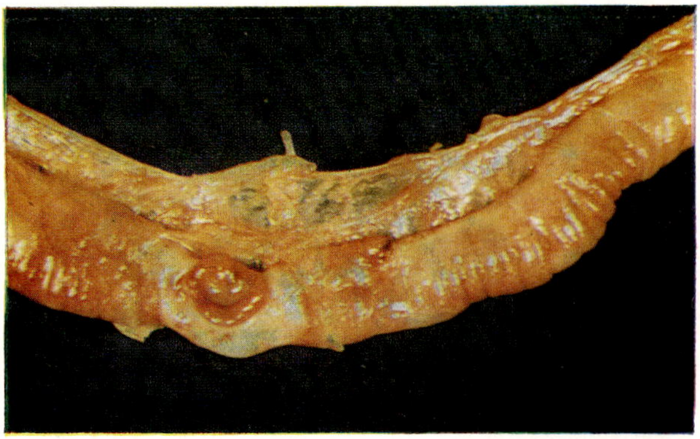

Fig. 2.1.5. — 65. Perforation at the junction of the rectum and small colon caused by irrigation therapy with a rubber tube in meconium retention.

Etiology and Pathogenesis. The disease is geographically limited and occurs in horses that are at pasture. Although no etiologic agent has yet been identified, it is suspected that a neurotropic virus or neurotoxin is responsible. Histologic studies have shown degenerative changes in the sympathetic ganglia with necrosis of neurons, especially in the celiac ganglia. A sustained spasm of the pylorus is also typical, which impedes gastric emptying and leads to secondary gastric dilation and severe disturbances of fluid balance.

Course. Untreated cases usually die within a short time from gastric rupture. A few cases have recovered with intensive care, but this is exceptional.

Treatment. Stomach fluid is siphoned at least every 3 h with an indwelling tube. This is accompanied by continuous intravenous fluid replacement (3—4 l Ringer's solution per hour). The repeated use of spasmoanalgesics and atropine is indicated. Affected horses may survive for days under this intensive regimen. If no marked improvement is noted after 3 days, euthanasia should be considered.

Differential Diagnosis. Other inflammatory conditions of the small intestine must be differentiated. These are generally accompanied by diarrhea. The characteristic symptoms of grass sickness — gastric dilation, empty small bowel, inspissated ingesta in the large bowel — generally enable a diagnosis to be rendered with reasonable certainty.

Prognosis. The prognosis is highly unfavorable, and recovery is rare even with intensive therapy.

2.1.5.10.7. Colic in Foals

Meconium Retention (cf. Sec. 2.7.5.)

Meconium, which is composed of inspissated amniotic fluid, intestinal epithelial cells, intestinal mucus and bile, frequently becomes impacted in the foal and cannot be expelled.

Affected newborn foals are unable to defecate and manifest this by straining, becoming restless and exhibiting mild colicky signs. Later they stop nursing, and a mild to moderate tympany develops.

Rectal examination with the index finger reveals a hard meconium plug just anterior to the cranial pelvic brim that is unable to enter the narrow pelvis. The condition may persist for several days and increasing tympany may occur.

Treatment consists in giving enemas with warm water, soapy solutions or, preferably, with commercially available ready-to-use enemas whose active components are sodium dihydrogen phosphate (16.0 g) and sodium monohydrogen phosphate (6.0 g) (fig. 2.1.5. — 65). The object of this treatment is to soften the meconium plug. It may be supplemented by giving 50 ml castor oil or 50 g sodium sulfate in 1,000 ml water by mouth. The foal's milk consumption should be closely watched. If it is not nursing enough, the dam should be milked and the milk administered by nasogastric tube. The enemas may be repeated after several hours. If this treatment fails to stimulate defecation, a long rectal spoon can be used to free the plug lodged anterior to the pelvis. Alternately, a strong, smooth wire loop can be bent to the necessary shape and inserted to free the obstructing plug.

Operative treatment, though seldom necessary, consists of a laparotomy followed by massage and simultaneous irrigation per rectum to eliminate the impaction. A colotomy is rarely done.

Atresia of the Anus (cf. Sec. 2.8.4.3.)

In this congenital malformation the rectum, anal groove and anal sphincter are present and well developed. The rectum ends blindly a short distance below the outer skin, and all that is lacking is an anal opening. This opening can easily be created by means of a crucitate incision under local anesthesia. Suturing is unnecessary.

Atresia of the Rectum (cf. Sec. 2.8.4.3.)

In this malformation the anal groove and opening are normally developed, but they end blindly. The rectum also ends in a blind pouch. Treatment consists of surgically implanting the rectum in the anal opening peranally under general anesthesia.

Atresia of the Anus and Rectum (cf. Sec. 2.8.4.3.)

The anal groove and anal opening are absent. The rectum terminates farther anteriorally in a blind pouch. Between the absent anal groove and blind rectum is a bridge of connective tissue. Again, a peranal rectopexy may be attempted if treatment is desired.

Partial Agenesis

A blind-pouch atresia of the colon is also encountered in foals, being inherited as a recessive trait. The pelvic flexure is usually absent in this malformation. Clinically the foals exhibit colicky signs shortly after birth, and the rectum is empty or contains a small amount of grayish-white mucus. No meconium can be felt. Because the large colon ends in a blind pouch, affected foals usually succumb to peritonitis 1 to 2 days after birth (figs. 2.1.5. — 66 and — 67). A similar disease of the small colon was described by CROWHURST, who also saw isolated cases of *pyloric and duodenal stenoses*. Affected foals show a reluctance to nurse, malaise and signs of secondary gastric dilation a few hours post partum. The diagnosis is presumptive but can be confirmed by contrast radiographs. CROWHURST recommends Ramstedt's operation for correcting the defect.

Basically all forms of intestinal obstruction that affect the mature horse can occur in the foal. The most frequent are:

— volvulus of the ileum and jejunum,
— impaction by ascarid worms,
— necroses of the cecum and large colon from thromboembolic causes.

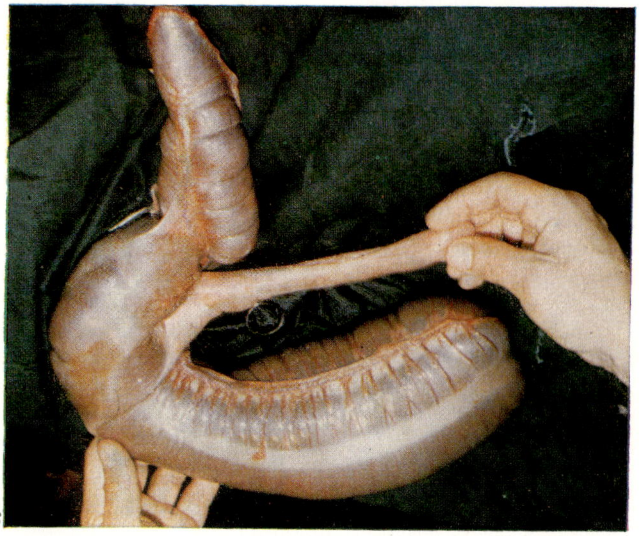

66

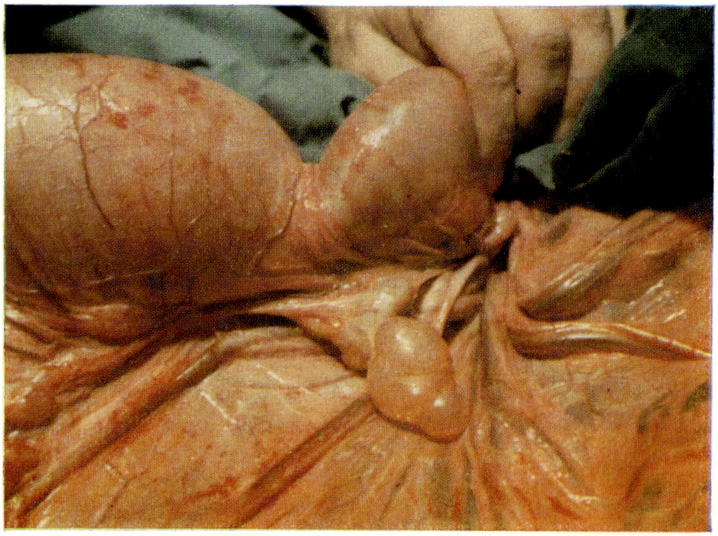

67

Fig. 2.1.5. — 66. Agenesis, atresia of the large colon. The ventral colon ends in a blind pouch, the right dorsal colon is underdeveloped, and the pelvic flexure is absent.

Fig. 2.1.5. — 67. Congenital descending megacolon due to stenosis at the junction of the small colon and rectum caused by fusion with the uterine ligament. The surgeon is holding the poststenotic bowel segment. Below the stenosis is the ovary, and at left is the terminal segment of the hypertrophied small colon (megacolon).

2.1.5.10.8. Diseases of the Abdominal Cavity

Peritonitis

Definition and Pathogenesis. Peritonitis refers to inflammatory changes of the peritoneal lining of the abdominal wall and abdominal organs. The cause is usually bacterial contamination. The peritonitis may be *local* or *diffuse* in its extent. The peritoneum possesses extraordinary defense mechanisms against infection, and smaller infectious foci are rapidly encapsulated by granulocytes, macrophages and fibrin. The greater omentum, which reputedly has the properties of a lymphoid organ, is instrumental in this 'walling-off' process. Thus, for example, smaller defects of the intestine and abdominal wall are effectively sealed off by parts of the omentum. A *local peritonitis* that resolves in this manner generally leads to adhesion formation in the area of the lesion.

In *diffuse peritonitis* the causal organisms have spread throughout the entire abdominal cavity, causing a corresponding spread of the inflammatory process. Following an intestinal rupture, for example, there is an intensive exudation of bloody fluid with fibrin release. The peritoneum becomes coated with blood. The serous coat acquires a dull appearance, and fibrinous adhesions develop between the intestinal loops within 4—6 hours.

Symptoms and Diagnosis. Horses with *local peritonitis* show signs of mild pain with slight abdominal wall tension and have little or no appetite for food. An elevated temperature is the rule. The leukocyte count is mildly to severely increased.

The rectal examination is negative in cases involving the anterior region of the abdominal cavity. In some cases an attachment of intestine to the omentum or abdominal wall can be palpated.

Diffuse peritonitis takes a peracute to acute course and its symptoms are much more severe. Affected horses show signs of extreme pain, accompanied by colic in some cases with abdominal wall rigidity and high fever. Exudation, if severe, can lead to ascites, in which case the peritoneal fluid is turbid, contains erythrocytes and leukocytes, and clots rapidly owing to the presence of fibrin. It will also contain food particles if the gastrointestinal tract has been ruptured. In peracute, diffuse peritonitis, leukopenia develops due to the marked migration of leukocytes into the abdominal cavity (less than $4 \times 10^9/l$). A leukocytosis develops in acute cases that survive 12 h or longer. Signs of severe shock may be evident.

On rectal examination, the accessible peritoneum has a dull, 'dry' texture, the intestinal loops feel immobilized. Palpation causes the animal obvious pain. Respiration is purely costal, rapid and shallow. Groans are often heard during expiration.

Etiology. Peritonitis may result from perforating lesions of the abdominal wall (stab wounds, impalements). Blunt abdominal trauma can lead to peritonitis via an intestinal rupture. One traumatic cause is rectal perforation during a rectal examination or during breeding. Another is vaginal perforation that occurs as a result of breeding or sadism.

Enterocentesis for the purpose of gas release in colic cases or the accidental punture of a loop of bowel during paracentesis can cause intestinal contents to spill into the abdominal cavity especially if tense or paralytic bowel segments are pierced. A local or diffuse peritonitis can result depending on the amount of material spilled. The most frequent cause is rupture of the stomach or intestine as a result of gastric dilation or paralytic ileus. With the exception of small gastric tears, which leak only into the omental bursa, or intestinal tears that open between the mesenteric layers, the resultant peritonitis is always diffuse and takes a peracute, fatal course of several hours' duration. It is accompanied by signs of endotoxic shock.

Foreign body peritonitis is rarely observed in horses, for these animals seldom ingest materials that could have such an effect. However, we have observed several cases in which pieces of wire or wood had perforated the small intestine, leading to a more or less severe local peritonitis. A more frequent cause of peritonitis is extensive intestinal necrosis, especially of the large intestine, secondary to vascular thrombosis. Occasionally peritonitis is seen after castration.

Peritonitis occurs as a metastatic disease during the course of actinobacillus infection in foals ('sleepy foal' syndrome) as well as in abdominal strangles and following navel infections.

The once-dreaded diffuse postoperative peritonitis is rare today due to the proper use of modern surgical technique and antibiotics. Adhesions resulting from local peritonitis still constitute a risk if an extensive intestinal resection is performed (late complications).

Differential Diagnosis. The diarrhea that is occasionally present requires that peritonitis be differentiated from salmonellosis. Salmonellosis is also accompanied initially by leukopenia and signs of shock. Foals with Actinobacillus infection develop renal disorders that are associated with similar clinical pictures.

Course and Prognosis. Peracute or acute cases of diffuse peritonitis rarely survive. Actinobacillus infection in foals also carries a very high mortality. A small-sized local inflammation usually resolves with appropriate therapy, although adhesions always remain and may lead to obstruction later on due to strangulation by fibrous bands, adhesion formation on intestinal loops, etc., q.v.

In advanced cases of intestinal necrosis, peritonitis is often found at surgery (hyperemia, fecal odor). This can be controlled with parenteral and intra-abdominal antibiotics, though a high risk of adhesion formation remains.

Treatment. Treatment is useless following a rupture of the gastrointestinal tract, and the horse should be killed at once. Rectal perforation may heal well if peristalsis is inhibited and the rectum is promptly emptied (q.v.). In vaginal perforation with an associated breach of the abdominal cavity, the chance of recovery is good. Peritonitis following abdominal wall perforations can be contained or prevented by appropriate surgical treatment and antibiotic therapy.

The treatment of peritonitis in the 'sleepy foal' syndrome is rarely successful despite intensive antibiotic therapy.

Intra-Abdominal Hemorrhage

Definition and Etiology. Bleeding into the abdominal cavity with no visible blood loss is rare in the horse and may have various causes.

Blunt abdominal trauma can cause ruptures of the spleen, liver or blood vessels with death from blood loss ensuing rapidly.

Minor hemorrhage may be expected from tears of the mesentery or injuries of the broad ligament of the uterus, especially if there is bleeding *between* the two layers of the visceral peritoneum. Hematomas in the broad uterine ligament are not uncommon in mares near foaling time. In a few cases of long-standing incarcerations in the epiploic foramen, a pressure necrosis of the portal vein has been seen that led to vascular rupture and a rapidly fatal hemorrhage. Castrations, especially when done in the standing horse, may be accompanied by bleeding into the abdominal cavity. In one such case the hemorrhage occurred 10 days after castration. Intramural hematomas of the intestine can also be a source of considerable intra-abdominal bleeding.

Symptoms and Diagnosis. The severity of colicky signs varies according to the nature of the primary disease. When hemorrhage occurs from larger vessels or parenchyma, there is a rapidly progressive weakness with rapid pulse, marked dyspnea, and pallor (sometimes extreme) of the mucosae. Death is caused by hemorrhagic shock. Abdominal paracentesis (q.v.) is the chief diagnostic aid.

Hematocrit, hemoglobin and erythrocyte determination are of little value in cases of fresh, occult blood loss, for these values do not fall until about 8—10 h. Nevertheless, the hematocrit should be determined to provide a basis for a later estimation of lost blood volume. In prolonged hemorrhage the hematocrit may fall below 15. Hemorrhage into the abdominal cavity produces no significant rectal findings, but in cases of hemorrhage into the broad uterine ligament or parts of the mesentery, the hematoma can be palpated rectally as a fluctuant mass.

Prognosis. The prognosis is grave in ruptures of the spleen, liver or blood vessels, for treatment is usually too late. Hemorrhages into the broad uterine ligaments often stop spontaneously if the peritoneum is intact and the bleeding is not too severe. With tears of the mesentery, the prognosis of the primary disorder is the deciding factor, but surgical intervention must be undertaken without delay.

Treatment. Commercially available hemostatic agents are of dubious value. The best treatment and safest is a blood transfusion. If intra-abdominal bleeding has not been arrested within the first 12 h (hematocrit check, pulse rate), a laparotomy should be performed and an attempt made to control the bleeding surgically. Hemorrhage into the broad ligaments during late pregnancy are first treated conservatively. The surgical management of such hemorrhages is difficult and is indicated only in emergencies. In intra-abdominal hemorrhage associated with castration, a prompt laparotomy followed by a search for and ligation of the spermatic cord stump is indicated.

Intra-Abdominal Tumors and Abscesses

Etiology and Pathogenesis. Neoplastic diseases of the abdominal cavity are rare in horses. DOBBERSTEIN found malignant tumors in 0.5—0.8 % of all necropsies. In the abdominal cavity as elsewhere, a distinction is made between primary tumors and metastases. We place mesenteric lymph node abscesses in the same general category on clinical grounds. The principal neoplastic lesion is lymphosarcoma with invasion into some or all lymphatic organs of the abdominal cavity (lymph nodes, bowel wall, omentum, spleen, etc.). The disease takes a leukemic or aleukemic course, usually accompanied by anemia and emaciation. Other types of neoplasm are less common. Adenocarcinomas and reticulosarcomas in the abdominal cavity usually represent metastases of a primary tumor (e.g., of the adrenal gland). Squamous cell carcinomas have been observed on the parietal and visceral peritoneum. Ovarian tumors can reach an extraordinary size, and most are granulosa cell tumors or teratomas. Benign lipomas of the type that cause intestinal strangulations are rare.

Symptoms and Diagnosis. Every neoplastic disease initially takes an insidious course that produces no specific symptoms. The first signs to be noted are emaciation and reduced appetite, depression and a reduction of stamina. Other common external signs are edema of the limbs and prepuce. As well, there may be edema of the lower chest with space-occupying lesions of the precardial mediastinum (primary or metastatic growth). These are usually accompanied by a pronounced ascites. There is a progressive anemia, and the leukemic form of lymphosarcoma leads to a leukocytosis. This leukocytosis is less marked than that in bovine leukosis. Both forms are characterized by a considerable increase of lymphocytes in the differential blood count. Obstruction of the intestinal lumen or adhesions (e.g., from abscesses in strangles) are evidenced by recurring attacks of colic. Larger tumors in the intestinal or mesenteric region, as well as ovarian tumors can be detected on rectal examination.

Abdominal paracentesis is usually rewarding in doubtful cases; the fluid is always increased in volume, is yellow or red-tinged. It may contain lymphocytes, granulocytes and erythrocytes in late stages and in the presence of abscesses.

The diagnosis of squamous cell carcinoma of the stomach is especially difficult. Characteristic symptoms are absent in the early stage of the disease. Older horses are most commonly affected and show swallowing difficulties, signs of esophageal obstruction such as choking and regurgitation and are preceded by weeks of emaciation. When a stomach tube is passed, resistance is met cranial to the cardia.

Differential Diagnosis. Diseases of other organ systems must be excluded as the cause of the edema and ascites. In peritonitis and intestinal necrosis, the changes in the peritoneal fluid are more prominent, and the course is considerably more acute.

Course and Prognosis. Initially, all neoplastic diseases take a protracted course until, usually in the terminal stage, severe changes in metabolism, intestinal function or the other affected organ systems appear.

The prognosis is grave, if a malignant neoplasm is present. Often intra-abdominal abscesses also go undiagnosed until they have reached inoperable proportions. The prognosis is favorable for lipomas and ovarian tumors, for the tumor or affected organ can usually be removed without complications. In addition, metastases in such cases are rare. If a neoplasm of the abdominal cavity is suspected, we recommend an exploratory laparotomy. This will confirm the diagnosis and avoid further unnecessary diagnostic and therapeutic measures. In favorable cases the laparotomy is combined with surgical treatment, e.g., removal of the ovary or an isolated lipoma. Tumor growth at many sites is a sign of metastases. Treatment is useless, and the operation should be terminated.

Ascites

Definition, Etiology and Pathogenesis. Ascites refers to an abnormal accumulation of fluid in the abdominal cavity. The accumulated fluid may be transudate (density < 1.015, protein content < 10 g/l) or exudate (density > 1.015, protein content up to 60 g/l), depending on the cause of the ascites. Mixed and transitional forms are also known.

Transudation due to congestion in the area of the portal vein or vena cava may occur in liver disease, kidney disease, congestive heart failure and tumors of the anterior mediastinum. Exudation is observed in neoplastic and inflammatory lesions of the abdominal cavity and gastrointestinal tract. The most common cause is peritonitis (q.v.).

Intestinal necroses due to mesenteric tears and thrombosis produce a bloody exudate that is high in erythrocytes and leukocytes and is usually low in volume. Larger fluid volumes are associated with neoplasms of the abdominal organs, intestine and peritoneum. A special form of ascites is uroperitoneum following bladder rupture in newborn foals (q.v.). Long-standing mechanical ascites is invariably associated with inflammatory changes of the peritoneum. The initially pure transudate contains increasing amounts of protein and cellular constituents as the disease progresses.

Symptoms and Diagnosis. The most striking symptom is the increasing abdominal circumference. In horses with a very large abdomen (e.g., broodmares) this symptom is often overlooked until late in the disease. Because ascites usually occurs as a complication of a serious illness, it is almost always accompanied by emaciation and anorexia. The abdomen acquires a pear-shaped appearance, and edema of the limbs, prepuce and ventral abdomen is frequently present. The main diagnostic aid is paracentesis. Differential diagnosis is facilitated if this is done after the rectal examination. With a large-volume fluid accumulation, the loops of intestine will seem to float on rectal examination, and fibrin deposits and adhesions will be felt if inflammatory exudate is present. Neoplasms are palpable if located within the area of examination. The fluid collected by paracentesis is tested for density and protein content, and its cellular content is differentiated by examining a stained sediment smear.

Differential Diagnosis. Whenever acute abdominal distension appears, affections of the bowel should always be considered (e.g., tympany, dilation or torsion of the large colon). In pregnant mares hydramnion must be excluded by rectal examination. The fluid-filled uterus will then be felt rising dorsad; often the fetus cannot be discerned.

Course, Prognosis and Treatment. These depend on the primary disorder. In most cases treatment is useless due to the severity of the underlying disease. A ruptured bladder in the newborn foal can be successfully treated surgically if the anuria is noticed in time.

2.1.5.10.9. Ileus

Definition. Ileus is the term applied to an intestinal obstruction and its local and general consequences. The obstruction may be *partial*, in which case the term subileus or preileus is used (e.g., impaction, tonic bowel spasm, intestinal stenosis), implying that some gas and fluid can still traverse the obstruction, while solid ingesta become lodged. The term ileus is reserved for *complete obstruction* in which the symptoms and course are more severe.

The following types of ileus are distinguished:
— mechanical ileus
— dynamic ileus
— mixed ileus.

Mechanical ileus may be caused by an occlusion of the intestinal lumen or by extrinsic lesions that constrict the bowel and its blood vessels (strangulation ileus).

Dynamic ileus may be paralytic or spastic in nature. One form of ileus may be superseded by another, as for example when a *spastic ileus* progresses to paralysis or to an intestinal obstruction or displacement. Similarly, a *paralytic ileus* in the horse may become a *mixed ileus* if the fluid-filled, inactive small bowel undergoes secondary twisting or torsion that creates additional mechanical obstruction. This occurs most frequently in the terminal third of the small intestine, which has an especially long mesentery.

Paralytic ileus, called also *atonic ileus*, occurs as a primary disorder of bowel motility and may have reflex (e.g., postoperative ileus), toxic (peritonitis), metabolic (acidosis, hypokalemia) or ischemic causes (embolism, mesenteric tear).

Paralytic ileus can also arise secondarily during the terminal stage of a mechanical ileus, when atony develops due to an overstretching of the bowel wall by accumulated ingesta.

Pathophysiology of Ileus. Ileus can occur in both the small intestine and colon. The strangulation of an incarcerated loop of intestine initiates a local reaction that first produces a reflex inhibition of bowel motility due to sympathetic tone, accompanied by a dilatation of the intestinal lumen. This is followed by a vagal response that produces a hyperperistalsis, or 'resistance peristalsis', in an attempt to overcome the obstruction. In *small intestinal ileus* the fluid that enters the small intestine as a result of secretion and extravasation cannot drain into the large intestine, where it would be absorbed, and so it accumulates. In ileus of the colon large amounts of gas become sequestered in the larger areas of the colon. *Obturative ileus* generally involves a simple blockage of the intestinal lumen, the dilated section of bowel proximal to the obstruction being called the *prestenotic segment* and distal the empty *poststenotic segment*. Most forms of *strangulation ileus* involve the *incarceration* of a loop of bowel, so that a double stenosis is created. Thus, in addition to a pre- and poststenotic segment there is a *stenostenotic segment* located between the two constrictions.

In each case there is an interruption of the aboral progression of ingesta that leads to an overstretching of the prestenotic and in some cases the stenostenotic bowel segment. This leads to a progressive circulatory impairment that is especially marked in the stenostenotic segment due to the strangulation of mesenteric vessels. Initially there is an interference with venous outflow that may progress to a complete interruption of the venous return (venous stasis). The arterial supply remains at normal levels for some time. A stasis edema develops in the submucous layer, causing the mucosa to become raised from the underlying tissues. Venous stasis edema develops within a few hours and causes local hypoxia or anoxia of the bowel wall, accompanied by a leakage of electrolyte- and protein-rich transudate into the intestinal lumen and abdominal cavity. The vascular walls are initially permeable only to the fluid component of blood but later become permeable to cellular elements as well. At this point hemorrhagic infarction of the affected bowel segment begins (diapedetic hemorrhage).

Up to this time the gross appearance of the incarcerated loop of intestine is as follows: bluish-red discoloration of the outer wall, marked edema of the intestinal wall, gross dilatation and engorgement of the blood vessels, and medium- to dark-red discoloration of the mucosa; arterial pulsation is still present. With the passage of time there is an increasing hemorrhagic infarction of the affected segment and a continuing sequestration of fluid in the intestinal lumen and abdominal cavity (the 'third space'); the increasing swelling of the intestine causes interference with the arterial supply. Further damage to the intestinal wall makes it permeable to toxins and bacteria, which seep into the peritoneal cavity. Gas and toxin formation by bacteria in the stenostenotic loop exacerbate the situation. The result is an intestinal necrosis that starts in the mucosa on the antimesenteric side.

An increased lactic acid formation and catecholamine release takes place in the hypoxic intestinal wall. The decrease in the ratio of intra- to extracellular potassium depresses the excitability of the intestinal musculature, leading to atony of the bowel. Finally the arteries become thrombosed, and intestinal necrosis progresses. Grossly there is a reddish-black discoloration of the mucosa, which acquires a gray, friable coat (villous denudation). Fibrinous exudate appears on the serosa. A hemorrhagic gangrene is produced by bacteria that have invaded the intestinal wall.

In the rare cases where the strangulation or thrombosis blocks the arterial supply immediately and completely, ischemic necrosis is swift to develop. Grossly the intestinal wall appears somewhat thinner than normal, has a parchment-like surface and is pale gray in color, later becoming a green (dry gangrene). Usually a zone of hemorrhagic infarction occurs at the junction between healthy and diseased tissue.

In addition to its immediate local effects on the intestine, ileus also has profound systemic effects. The first is a peripheral circulatory insufficiency. The fluid losses give rise to a *dehydration shock*, which may be combined with *hemorrhagic shock* if blood loss into the intestinal lumen is severe. The body responds to the hypovolemia with an elevation of the *pulse rate*. In addition, the breakdown products of the stagnated ingesta and damaged tissue and the bacterial toxins produce endotoxemia.

This increases the rate at which the vessel walls become permeable to blood constituents (endotoxic shock). The blood flow deficit (hypoxia) and metabolic derangements lead to an *acidosis* which acts with the endotoxin to accelerate damage to the parenchymal organs. With severe tympany, there will also be an *embarrassment of respiration* (elevated diaphragm) and of the venous return to the heart (compression of caudal vena cava). (See Sec. 1.6.2. for details.)

Diagnosis of Ileus

Early Diagnosis. Honoring the age-old rule that the sun should not rise or set on an intestinal obstruction, it is best to perform the operation within 8 to 10 hours after the onset of the obstruction. This means that the equine practitioner must be content with a presumptive diagnosis of some sort of obstruction and defer a final diagnosis until the animal has been hospitalized.

Early referral for hospitalization is the practitioner's most important contribution to a successful surgical outcome. A presumptive diagnosis of obstruction may be made if:

in the early stage

— colicky signs are severe and unremitting, and response to spasmoanalgesics is poor, transitory or absent;

— rectal findings are definite (bowel incarcerated in inguinal ring or incarcerated over the nephrosplenic ligament, small bowel impaction);

in later stages

— colicky signs persist, or cease while systemic signs deteriorate (indolence);

— rectal findings are *characteristic* (constant, topographically fixed pain spots, demonstrable obstruction); or

— rectal findings are *ambiguous* (bowel loops tense and painful, edematous, gas- and fluid-filled);

— peritoneal fluid is increased in volume and/or discolored;

— respiratory and pulse rates and hemoconcentration are significantly increased.

Rectal examination, nasogastric intubation and abdominal paracentesis should be carried out repeatedly, for sequential changes over time provide the best evidence for or against an intestinal obstruction.

Additional signs of ileus are:

— discoloration of the conjunctivae (red, muddy red, dark red, anemic icterus),

— delayed venous return,

— prolonged capillary refill time,

— secondary gastric dilation.

Because the chances for the successful surgical treatment of obstruction are very good during the first hours of the disease but decline later in direct proportion to the duration of the illness, the decision for or against referral and hospitalization should be made within 5 h after the onset of the disease if possible.

Preparation for Transportation to a Hospital. Prior to transportation the stomach contents are siphoned off with a nasogastric tube. *The tube is left in place during transportation,* being fixed to the halter with adhesive tape. Very fractious horses should be premedicated with analgesics and sedatives. Antihypertensive drugs are contraindicated, and drugs or fluids should not be given by mouth.

Parenteral fluids should be administered if early signs of hemoconcentration are noted, bearing in mind that the positive effect of fluid therapy on the circulatory status may temporarily mask the disease process. In horses with a very poor circulatory status that must be transported long distances, the veterinarian should see to it that the fluid therapy is maintained in transit by accompanying personnel.

In emergencies this may even be done by laymen if a catheter has previously been sutured in place. For the practitioner who lacks the means for a qualitative or quantitative assessment of fluid and electrolyte losses, we recommend the administration of high-molecular weight dextran solution (rel. mol. wt. 60,000 to 70,000) and Ringer's solution in a ratio of 1 : 3. In addition, a single administration of 1,000 ml of a 5% sodium bicarbonate solution immediately before transportation may be beneficial.

Severe gaseous distension of the large intestine should be relieved by cecal trocarization before the animal is transported.

A large dose of antibiotics is also recommended for the prophylaxis of bacteremia and peritonitis.

A written record accompanies the animal to the hospital. It should include:

— history (e.g., dietary changes)
— previous episodes of colic
— time of onset of colic
— course of colic
— all administered drugs and dosages
— rectal findings
— results of abdominal paracentesis (specimen may accompany patient if desired).

Following the animal's departure, the hospital should be notified by telephone of the prospective arrival time so that all necessary preparations can be made.

The Fundamentals of Ileus Surgery

Midline Laparotomy

The midline or median laparotomy affords good access to the small intestine (except for the duodenum) as well as to the cecum, large colon and small colon. It has become the standard surgical approach to the abdominal cavity. It is usually done in the umbilical area, although division of the linea alba may be carried to the xiphoid or to the pelvis as needed. From the ventral surface the abdominal cavity is opened quickly and easily with minimal bleeding, and an extensive exploration can be achieved. For this reason the midline laparotomy has become the procedure of choice for exploratory and therapeutic operations.

Anesthesia and Positioning. The patient is placed in dorsal recumbency on the operating table with the hindlegs loosely flexed and tied to the sides of the table and the forelegs suspended on ropes tied overhead. Anesthesia is induced and maintained with halothane and nitrous oxid-oxygen mixture administered by endotracheal tube. Respiratory acidosis always develops after prolonged dorsal recumbency and may reach hazardous levels if the operating time exceeds 1 to $1^1/_2$ h. The technique of assisted ventilation is desirable but has not solved the problem of respiratory acidosis because of its inability to improve the poor perfusion of the ventilated lung regions. Therefore, the best solution is to adopt various measures that will help to shorten the operating time (fig. 2.1.5. — 68).

Operating Technique. The more cranially the incision is placed, the greater the risk of herniation. Therefore the incision is placed as far caudally as possible, making it necessary to divide the umbilicus (umbilical midline laparotomy).

For resections of the caudal portion of the small colon and for a colorectostomy, a postumbilical laparotomy is performed.

In all other intestinal operations the longitudinal incision is started several centimeters caudal to the umbilicus and is extended just far enough to enable the surgeon to insert one arm for exploring the intra-abdominal organs. Afterwards the incision may be extended as far cranially or caudally as necessary.

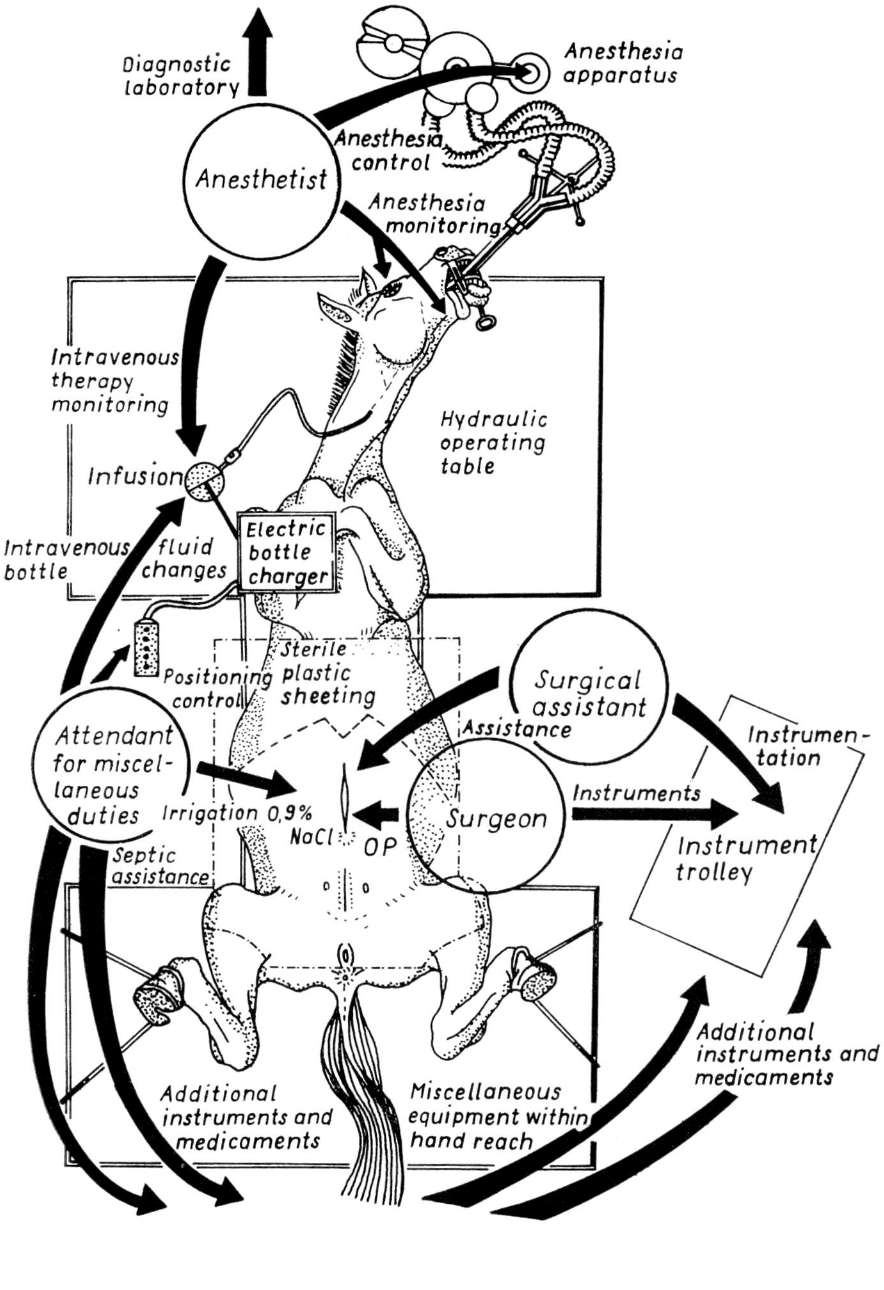

Fig. 2.1.5. — 68. Positioning of the horse and stationing of the surgical team for a midline laparotomy.

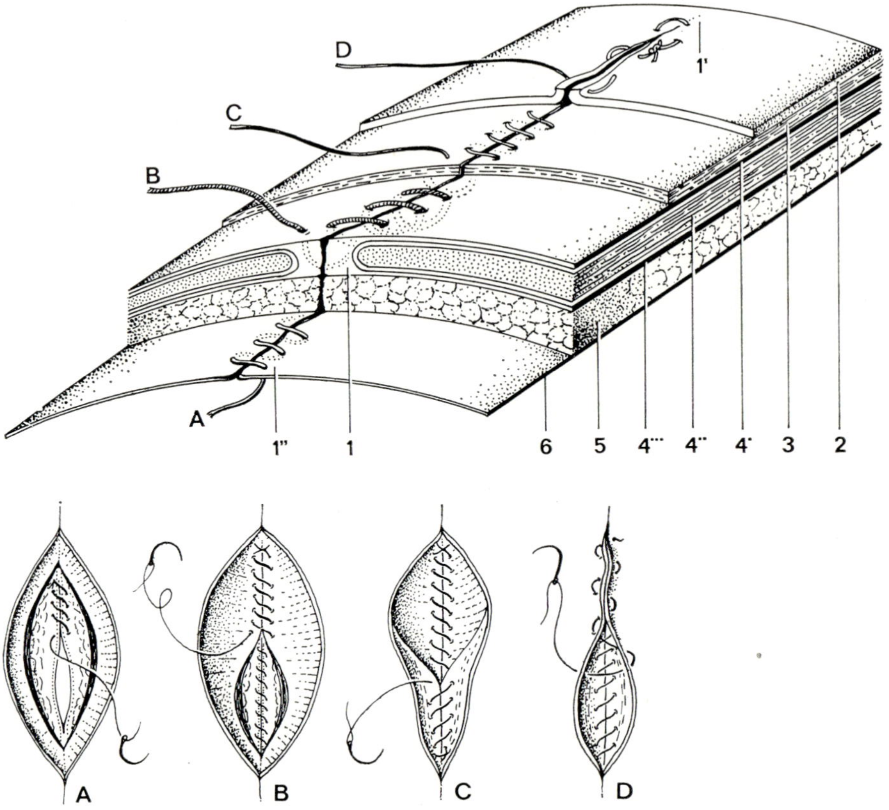

Fig. 2.1.5. — 69. Suturing the abdominal wound in the linea alba.
A suture of the peritoneum; *B* suture of the linea alba; *C* subcutaneous suture; *D* skin suture; *1* linea alba; *1'* midline; *1''* round ligament of the liver; *2* skin; *3* subcutaneous connective tissue; *4'* outer layer of rectus sheath; *4''* rectus abdominis muscle; *4'''* inner layer of rectus sheath; *5* subperitoneal fatty tissue; *6* peritoneum.

The abdominal incision is made precisely through the linea alba. The subperitoneal fatty tissue is divided to expose the round ligament of the liver (lig. teres hepatis), which, after piercing with a stab incision, is divided with a quick craniad and caudad movement of the finger inserted into the peritoneal cavity. Closure of the wound is carried out in layers. No. 3 chromic catgut is used for the continuous peritoneal and subcutaneous sutures, and a No. 5 Dexon suture (doubled) for the suturing of the linea alba. The double Dexon suture is now preferred by us over the No. 6 multifilament steel wire formerly used. Dexon is strong yet absorbable and so greatly reduces the chance of fistula formation. The skin is sutured with No. 5 Supramid Vetafil. The three deepest layers are approximated with simple continuous suture (fig. 2.1.5. — 69).

Lateral (Flank) Laparotomy

The lateral right-flank laparotomy affords good access to the duodenum, jejunum, ileum and cecum.

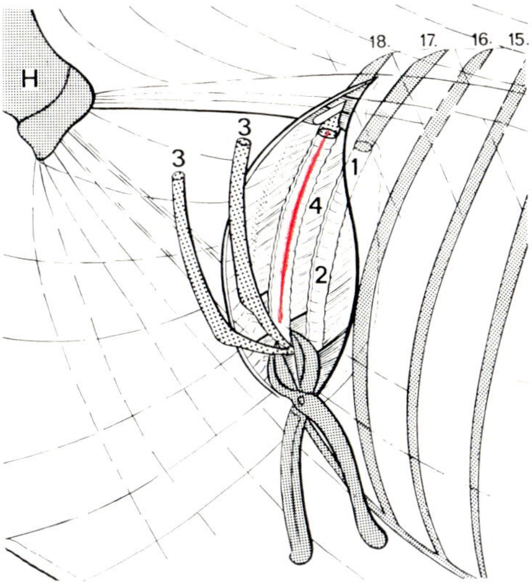

Fig. 2.1.5. — 70. Lateral laparotomy with rib resection. Horse positioned in lateral recumbency. *1* curved skin incision; *2* periosteum; *3,3* 17th and 18th ribs with costal cartilage; *4* intercostal musculature.

A left-flank laparotomy is recommended for manipulation of the large and small colon and for surgical closure of the nephrosplenic space.

Surgical Technique. The horse is positioned in lateral recumbency. The skin incision is made between the 17th and 18th ribs, follows the course of these ribs and extends distally from the lateral border of the ileocostal muscle 25—30 cm ventrally and cranially to the costal cartilage. The muscles overlying the ribs and the periosteum are divided in the direction of the incision. After the 18th and if necessary the 17th rib have been freed from their periosteum with a periosteal elevator, they are resected with a Gigli wire saw or rib shears in the dorsal and ventral wound angles. The base of the costal bed is formed by the inner abdominal fascia and the peritoneum adherent to it. The abdominal cavity is opened with stab incisions, the wound is extended with the scissors along the course of the costal bed. The dorsal and ventral wound angles are developed in step-shaped fashion (fig. 2.1.5. — 70).

When the operation is completed, the peritoneum and transverse fascia are closed with simple continuous sutures of No. 3 chromic catgut. The abdominal wall is closed with interrupted sutures of No. 5 Dexon. The periosteum of the costal bed will afford a good hold for the sutures, and so special care should be taken to preserve it during the rib resection. The subcutis is closed with a continuous suture of No. 3 chromic catgut, and the skin with interrupted Donati-type vertical mattress sutures. A suction drain placed for the first 3 postoperative days will considerably improve healing and, in contrast to the classic flank incision, will minimize fluid accumulation.

Intraoperative Exploration. Operations on the small and large intestine are conducted according to the following scheme: (1) The stenosis or obstruction is located; (2) The prestenotic and stenostenotic bowel segments are evacuated; (3) The stenosis is corrected by a) reposition and/or b) resection.

We recommend using the cecum as a landmark, for it can be easily located and exteriorized and provides a good starting point for locating both the large and small intestine.

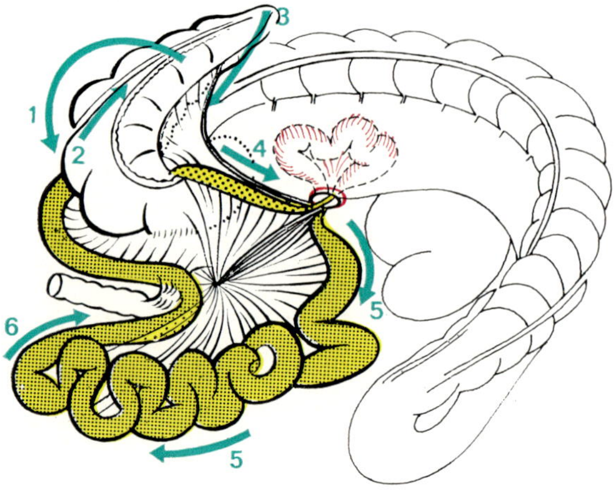

Fig. 2.1.5. — 71. Intraoperative exploration of the small intestine. *1* locating the caudal duodenal flexure (base of cecum); *2* ventral band of cecum; *3* apex of cecum and ileocecal ligament; *4* ileocecal ligament, ileum, incarceration; *5* prestenotic loop of intestine.

Small Intestinal Ileus

In small intestinal ileus the cecum generally is empty or only moderately filled. The base of the cecum is located by standing on the left side of the horse and inserting the left hand into the abdominal cavity in a lateral and dorsal direction. The cecal base is bounded caudally by the caudal flexure of the duodenum, which is identified by its extremely short mesentery. The ventral band of the cecum, which is devoid of ligaments, fat and blood vessels, is reached by passing the hand craniad from the most caudal point of the duodenum. This band is palpated in a ventral direction along the body of the cecum until the apex is reached, which is then exteriorized. The cecum is laid against the right side of the horse, away from the surgeon. The only free longitudinal band of the apex (the dorsal band) is traced to the thin ileocecal fold, which is grasped and held under tension with the left hand. The right hand utilizes the tense ileocecal fold as a guide to reach the ileum. Sometimes this is difficult, because the tense fold is so scanty that it is easily lost unless one is practiced in exploration. If the ileum is freely movable, it is exteriorized. If it cannot be exteriorized, it must be involved in an incarceration and can be traced to the site oj the strangulation (abnormal fixation; fig. 2.1.5. — 71).

It is useful to note that the poststenotic segment of bowel can always be traced back to the strangulation site!

If the poststenotic loop of ileum or jejunum leads to the epiploic foramen, the direction of the incarceration will determine the further course of the operation. In a *lateral incarceration* it is necessary first to locate the stenostenotic loop in the middle of the abdominal cavity. Only after it has been emptied may the incarceration be reduced by traction on the pre- and poststenotic segments.

In a *medial incarceration* through the torn omental bursa, the procedure is reversed. The incarcerated loop is located lateral to the cecum below the right abdominal wall. Traction on the wrong loop of bowel in such circumstances causes even greater incarceration, while traction on the correct loop, without evacuation, may result in profuse, uncontrollable bleeding in the area of the epiploic foramen (portal vein, caudal vena cava rupture!).

Digital enlargement of the epiploic foramen is dangerous and should not be performed. The entire prestenotic small bowel may be dilated with gas and fluid, in which case the intestinal loops will protrude from the peritoneal cavity as soon as

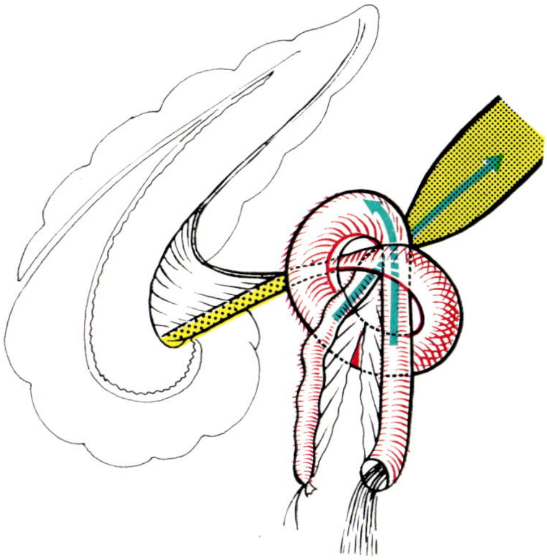

Fig. 2.1.5. — 72. Volvolus of the small intestine. Reduction of the twist after division and evacuation of the stenostenotic loop.

the abdomen is opened. The intestine must then be opened on the antimesenteric border at about the midpoint of the prestenotic segment. A 2-cm incision is made at that point, through which the intestine is drained with the aid of the surgical assistant. The bowel is emptied from the stomach to the stenosis by sequentially raising the loops of bowel so that the fluid is propelled by gravity toward the enterotomy wound. The small intestine is opened with a longitudinal incision and closed by a transverse repair. Evacuation through a catheter is too unproductive and time-consuming. Decompression not only facilitates exploration of the peritoneal cavity but also is an effective measure for the prevention of postoperative paralytic ileus.

The degree of gastric filling is ascertained from the right side of the abdominal cavity rather than from the left, due to interference from the omentum in the latter approach. If the stomach is impacted with dry ingesta, an attempt should be made to remove the material by gastric lavage through a stomach tube. If the duration of the operation or personnel limitations make it impossible to do this right away, the lavage may be deferred.

After an ileal impaction has been freed by massage and irrigation, the entire contents of the small bowel are emptied into the cecum in the manner described. This will enable the sequestered fluid volumes to be reabsorbed in the large intestine.

An ileal impaction cannot always be readily massaged into the cecum. The fecal plug can be softened if necessary by massaging in a cranial direction, thus causing the ingesta to become mixed with the accumulated fluid. In paralytic ileus the sequestered bowel contents also should be emptied into the cecum.

In cases of extensive volvulus of the jejunum or mesenteric herniation, it may be impossible in large horses to exteriorize the twisted bowel. To reduce the twist rapidly without loss of time, a stenostenotic loop of bowel is exteriorized. If it is necrotic, it is transected, drained and the stumps doubly ligated; if it is viable, it is opened with a stab incision and drained. After thorough cleansing with sponges and irrigating fluid, the stumps are returned to the abdominal cavity. This relieves tension on the volvulus while facilitating reduction of the lesion. This technique obviates the risk of intestinal or mesenteric rupture that might result from traction on the wrong loop. If the intestine is necrotic, the mesenteric defect may be left alone initially during the reduction, for its vessels are thrombosed (fig. 2.1.5. — 72).

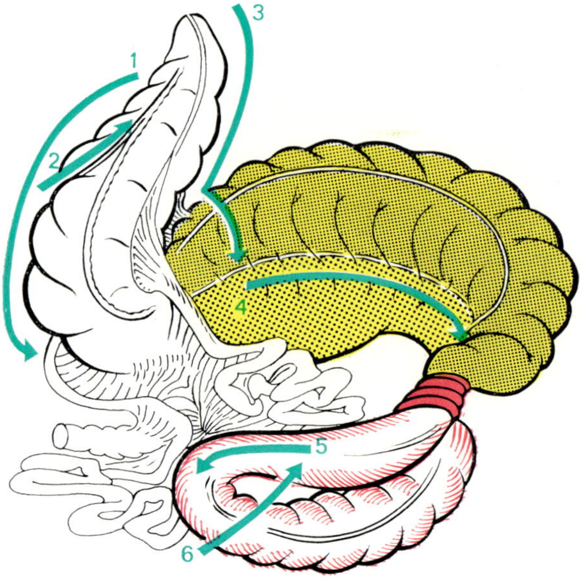

Fig. 2.1.5. — 73. Intraoperative exploration of the large intestine.
1 and *2* same as in figure 2.1.5. — 71; *3* apex of cecum followed to cecocolic ligament; *4* mesocolon of large colon and seat of torsion; *5* and *6* pelvic flexure.

Colonic Ileus

The cecum again serves as a landmark for orientation. If it cannot be located by the method described, a cecal or cecolic intussusception must be present, or else the cecum is grossly displaced (complete colonic torsion).

The cecum is exteriorized, and the cecocolic fold is located and followed to the right ventral colon. The surgeon then passes his right hand along the medial side of the loops of right colon to reach the mesocolon, which is located between the ventral and dorsal colon and contains fat and blood vessels. He follows this to reach the loops of left colon. In this way any torsions or constrictions can be located and identified (fig. 2.1.5. — 73).

The small colon, including the transverse colon, are explored starting from the rectum.

In torsions of the large colon, the procedure may be reversed and the site of the torsion located by starting the exploration from the pelvic flexure.

In displacements or torsion of the large intestine, the first step is to ascertain the extent and location of accumulated gas and impacted ingesta in the stenostenotic and prestenotic segments. The distended bowel is carefully brought up to the laparotomy wound, exteriorized as far as possible, fixed and then punctured with the tip of a scissor to enable the gas to escape.

The small incision is closed immediately by means of a double stitch in a Z or cruciate pattern. Next an attempt is made to exteriorize the pelvic flexure. This must be done with great care and patience and should not be forced, as the intestine is friable and usually edematous and therefore highly prone to rupture. The exteriorized colon is laid between the patient's hind legs. Assistants should be available in the septic area. The colon is then opened near the pelvic flexure and evacuated by irrigation through two tubes (fig. 2.1.5. — 54).

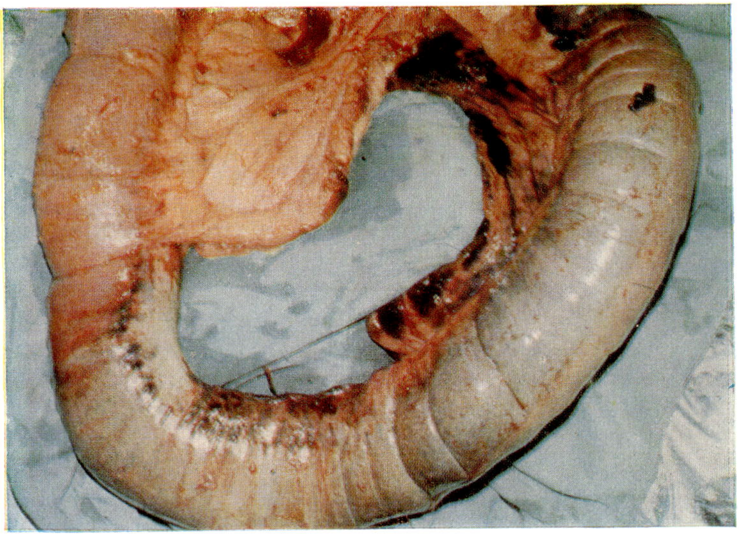

Fig. 2.1.5. — 74. Tear of the mesocolon in a mare. The involved segment of small colon shows a pale olive-green discoloration as a result of ischemic necrosis.

Counter-rotation should never be attempted if the large colon is filled, and the accumulated ingesta proximal to the stenosis must always be removed before such a manipulation is undertaken.

The colonic incision is closed with two layers of continuous inverting sutures. The surface of the colon is then flushed with physiologic saline and returned to the peritoneal cavity, at which time the reduction of the torsion may be performed.

Intestinal Resections and Anastomoses

Jejunojejunostomy

A resection of the jejunum is usually followed by a side-to-side jejunojejunostomy, and in rare cases by a jejunoileostomy. End-to-end and end-to-side anastomoses have proved unsatisfactory in the horse in our experience because they predispose to postoperative impaction and intussusception in the area of the anastomosis. The side-to-side anastomosis may be done using any technique desired. It is important to avoid creating a blind pouch, especially in the afferent bowel segment, for even a very small blind sac can lead to an impaction. Because it is often necessary to resect long lengths of small intestine (up to 10 m) in the horse, an extensive stump of mesentery is left in which some necrotic tissue remains ventral to the ligatures. To avoid adhesion formation in this region, the stump is covered by oversewing an adjacent fold of mesentery on each side (fig. 2.1.5. — 75). For all ligatures and sutures, Dexon is the material of choice.

Ileal Resection and Jejunocecostomy

After the strangulated bowel has been freed, the body of the cecum, the necrotic ileum and the necrotic portion of the jejunum are exteriorized to ascertain the necessary extent of the resection. A right-angle clamp is placed across the terminal ileum

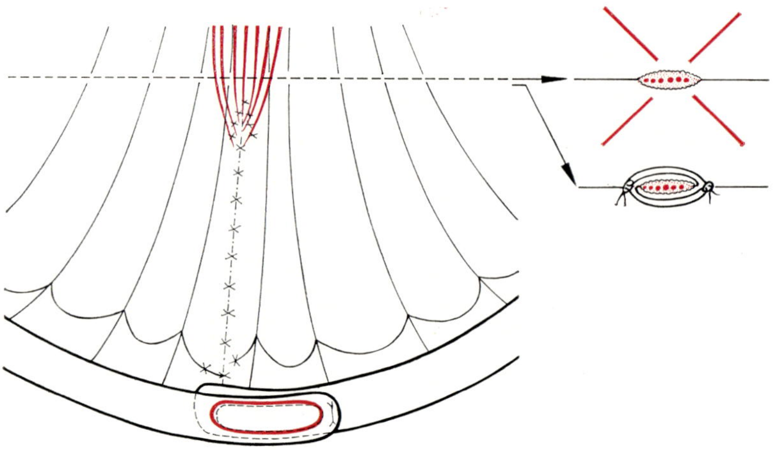

75

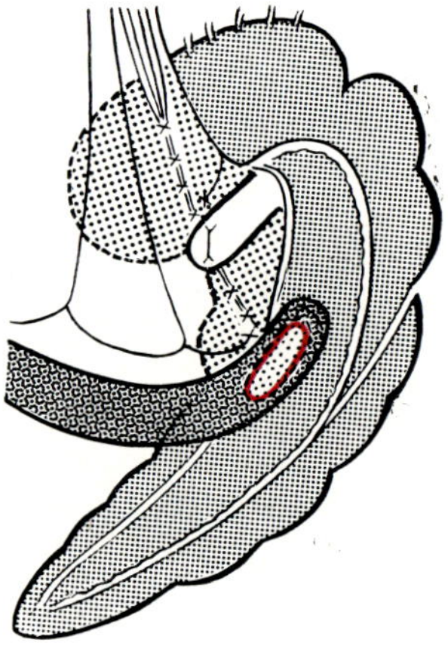

76

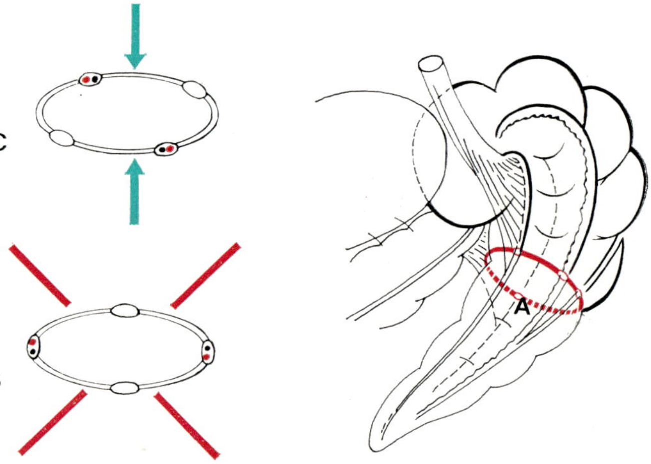

77

Fig. 2.1.5. — 75. Side-to-side jejunojejunostomy. Closure of mesenteric tear and stump by oversewing with adjacent mesentery.

Fig. 2.1.5. — 76. Jejunocecostomy (medial view). The ileal stump (unshaded) is not included in the suture used to repair the mesenteric defect. The jejunum and cecum are joined by a side-to-side anastomosis.

Fig. 2.1.5. — 77. Partial typhlectomy. Medial view of body of cecum. *A* line of resection; *B* incorrect positioning; *C* correct positioning of stump for closure by suture.

at its junction with the diseased segment. Then the ileal artery is doubly ligated using a ligature needle, and the jejunal arteries are occluded dorsal to the proposed line of resection. After completely freeing the proximal loop of bowel of its mesentery, it is tied off tightly with a Nylon thread. Crushing clamps are applied at each end of the necrotic segment, and the resection is carried out. A two-layer closure is used for the ileal stump. The closure should be performed with extreme care in order to prevent later wound dehiscence when ileal motility is restored. Four to five interrupted sutures (Nylon No. 4) are placed in vertical mattress fashion through the serosa, muscularis and mucosa aboral to the right-angled clamp. After the preplaced sutures are drawn tight, the clamp is removed, accurate inversion is secured with a dissecting forceps, and the sutures are tied. A continuous mattress suture is placed through the serosa and muscularis to form a second row. The suture that joins them begins in the dorsal angle of the mesenteric defect. Beyond the ileal stump the mesenteric segment of the afferent loop of jejunum is joined to the ileocecal ligament and to the cecum. The jejunal stump is closed, and the terminal jejunum is carried to its site of anastomosis with the cecum medial to the dorsal band. Anatomic circumstances require that the jejunum be implanted at the junction of the dorsal and middle thirds of the cecum.

The side-to-side anastomosis is carried out in such a way that the jejunum points toward the base of the cecum, thereby mimicking normal anatomic relations (fig. 2.1.5. — 76).

Partial Typhlectomy

Following a midline laparotomy, the cecum is first emptied of gas and ingesta. At the junction between the necrotic part of the cecum, which usually is discolored, and the healthy part is a zone of hemorrhagic infarction that is included in the resection.

The medial and lateral cecal arteries and veins are ligated in their course along the lateral and medial bands. The diseased part of the cecum is excised, and closure is carried out in two layers (e.g. Connell, Cushing), taking care to start the suture such that the individual longitudinal bands are arranged in proper succession and do not come in contact with the start or end of the suture. Only in this way can a good inversion of the bands be achieved at the end of the stump (figs. 2.1.5. — 77 through — 80).

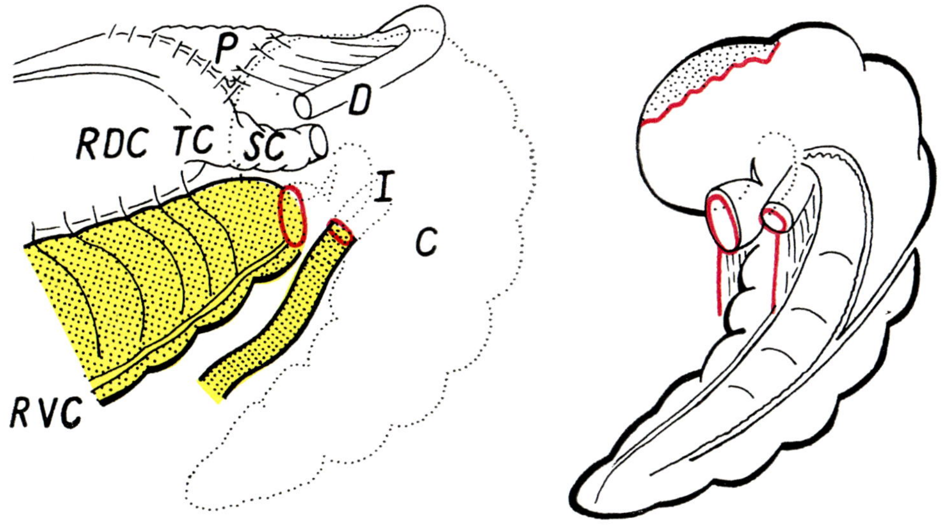

Fig. 2.1.5. — 78. Typhlectomy. RVC = right ventral colon; RDC = right dorsal colon; TC = transverse colon; SC = small colon; P = pancreas; D = duodenum; I = ileum, C = cecum.

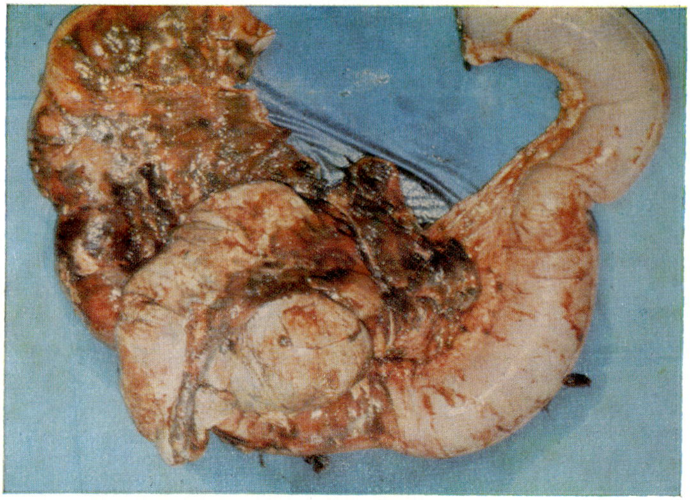

79

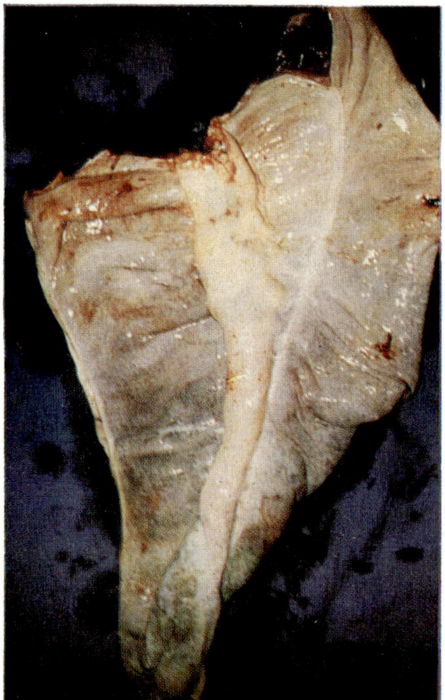

80

Fig. 2.1.5. — 79. Resected portion of mesenteric hernia of the small colon with incarcerated cecum. The involved bowel exhibits signs of ischemic necrosis.

Fig. 2.1.5. — 80. Resected portion from a partial typhlectomy. Ischemic necrosis of the cecal apex (olive-green discoloration), hemorrhagic infarction of the body (blackened mucosa).

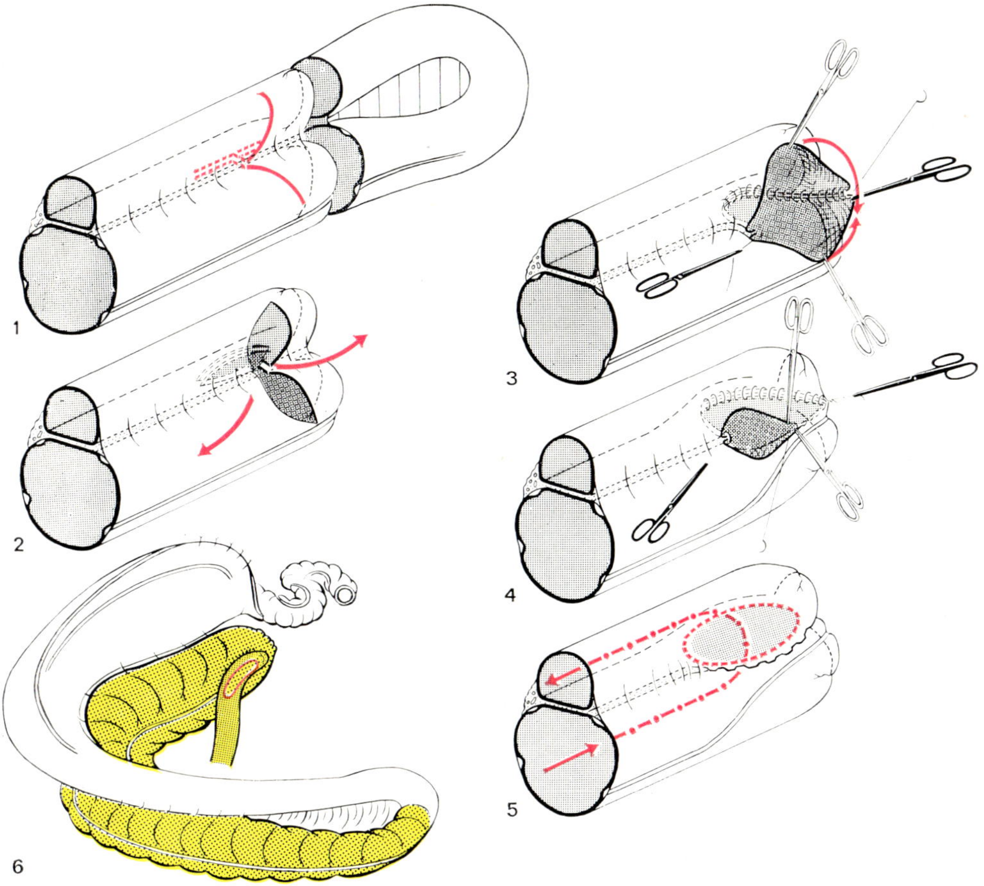

Fig. 2.1.5. — 81. Colocolostomy. Technique of anastomosis after HUSKAMP (1971). Craniolateral view from the left side.

1 After the necrotic loops of left colon have been resected along with the pelvic flexure, and the stumps have been closed with a two-layer continuous inverting suture, each segment is opened from the lateral side with an incision made at a 60° angle to its long axis (red lines). Each incision is extended a short distance transversely through the bowel wall in the mesocolic area, and then a longer distance longitudinally. The connective tissue between the dorsal and ventral segments will maintain their anatomic relation.

2 The resulting enterotomy wound can be widely opened by pulling apart the sides of the primary incision in a longitudinal direction (red arrows).

3 The contiguous bowel walls are united by continuous over-and-over suture in the area of the mesocolon, while the primary incision is held open in both a longitudinal (black clamps) and transverse direction (white clamps). Then the antimesenteric wound edges of both segments are apposed (red arrows).

4 The outer wound edges are held together (white clamps) and united with two layers of continuous sutures.

5 The resulting stoma is widely distensible in all directions and creates a free communication between the ventral and dorsal colon (red arrow).

6 Situation after colocolostomy.

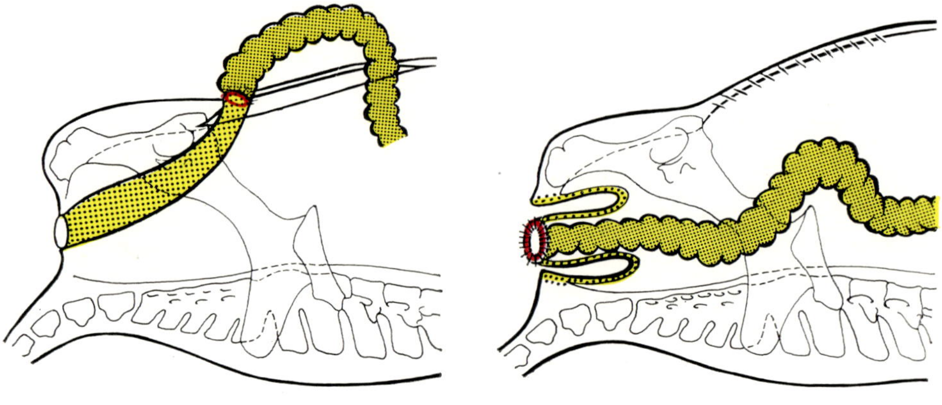

A B

Fig. 2.1.5. — 82. Colorectostomy. *A* end-to-end anastomosis in the area of the laparotomy wound; *B* end-to-end anastomosis following transanal exteriorization.

Typhlectomy and Ileocolostomy

Operation: The cecum is approached through a lateral right-flank laparotomy in which the 17th and 18th ribs are resected. This gives good exposure of the base of the cecum, caudal duodenal flexure, initial part of the right ventral colon, and the ileum.

It may be sufficient to perform an ileocolostomy bypass with exclusion of the cecum, but in cases of chronic cecal dilation with a danger of cecal rupture, a typhlectomy and primary anastomosis are preferred. The reader is referred to the specialized literature for details (fig. 2.1.5. — 78).

Partial Colectomy and Colocolostomy of the Large Colon

The diseased colon is exteriorized, and the dorsal and ventral colonic arteries and veins are doubly ligated on the medial side. The colon is divided along the proposed line of resection, and the resected segment is discarded. Then the stump of the ventral colonic segment is closed in two inverting layers, followed by a similar closure of the dorsal segment.

The closed stumps are positioned such that their lateral side is toward the surgeon. Starting at the line connecting the dorsal and ventral colonic segments, at a distance of 3—5 cm from the closed stumps, each segment is opened with sharp-pointed scissors at an angle of about 60° to its long axis, taking care to spare the larger vessels. The incision extends to the periphery of the dorsal colon and to the lateral band of the ventral colon. The wound edges are fixed with hemostatic clamps. A third incision of equal length is made along the line of attachment of the colonic segments. A continuous suture is started at the end of this incision, using a simple continuous pattern. This suture will secure and define the posterior wall of the stoma in the area of attachment of the colonic segments. For the anterior suture, an inverting suture is started at the oral part of the simple continuous suture and continued to the aboral part. This suture is buried with a Cushing suture placed in the opposite direction. The result is a large, oval stoma that is distensible in all directions and presents no postoperative risks (fig. 2.1.5. — 81).

Colectomy and Colorectostomy of the Small Colon

The approach through the linea alba has proved useful for this operation. In the mare the abdomen is opened with a postumbilical incision placed between the umbilicus and cranial border of the pelvis, followed by a broad dissection into the intermammary sulcus.

In male horses it is necessary first to dissect free the prepuce and retract it laterally so that a midline approach can be carried out. The diseased segment of colon is resected, and an isoperistaltic end-to-end or side-to-side anastomosis is performed.

The colorectostomy must always be done in end-to-end fashion, because the rectal stump cannot be exteriorized far enough for a side-to-side anastomosis (fig. 2.1.5. — 82 A).

If part of the rectum also has to be resected, the anastomosis must be done in two stages following stump closure, abdominal closure and transanal exteriorization (fig. 2.1.5. — 82 B).

In mares the anastomosis can be facilitated by transecting the perineum from the vestibule of the vagina to the rectum if evagination proves difficult.

With all anastomoses in this region of the bowel, fecal inspissation and impactions may be expected to develop anterior to the anastomosis. Careful postoperative treatment with sodium sulfate solutions and mineral oil over a 6-day period is therefore essential.

References

Bolz, W.; Dietz, O.; Schleiter, H.; Teuscher, R.: Lehrbuch der Speziellen Veterinärchirurgie, 2. Aufl. (VEB Gustav Fischer Verlag, Jena 1975).

Bone, J. F.; Catcott, E. J.: Equine medicine and surgery, 1st ed. (Amer. Vet. Publications Inc. 1963).

Carlström, B.: Experimentelle Untersuchungen und klinische Beobachtungen über Veränderungen der Lage der Bauchorgane im Zusammenhang mit Magenüberladung beim Pferd. Arch. wiss. prakt. Tierheilk. *55:* 361, 381, 386 (1927).

Coffman, J. R.; Garner, H. E.; Nelson, S. L.: Lymphoma in the horse: a diagnostic perspective. Vet. Med. and Small Animal Clinician *68:* 401 (1973).

Cotchin, E.: A general survey of tumors in the horse. Equine Vet. J. *9:* 16 (1977).

Crowhurst, R. C.: Abdominal surgery in the foal. Equine Vet. J. *2:* 22 (1970).

Crowhurst, R. C.; Simpson, D. J.; McEnery, A.; Greenwood, R. Es.: Intestinal surgery in the foal. J. South African Vet. Med. Assoc. *46:* 59 (1975).

Dahme, E.; Weiss, E.: Grundriß der speziellen pathologischen Anatomie der Haustiere (Enke, Stuttgart 1968).

Daniels, H.: Die Bauchhöhlenpunktion beim Pferd — Technik und Interpretation. Prakt. Tierarzt *59:* 268 (1978).

Deegen, E.: Kreislaufbehandlung bei Kolik. Collegium Veterinarium, p. 68 (1975).

De Moor, A.; Hende, C. van der: Inspiratory concentrations of O_2, N_2 and N_2O, arterial oxygenation and acid-base status during closed Halothane anaesthesia in the horse. Zbl. Vet.-Med., R. A *19:* 1 (1972).

Doenecke, H.: Beiträge zur Ätiologie, Diagnose und Therapie der Kolik des Pferdes. Tierärztl. Rdsch. *38:* 543, 564, 579, 719, 749, 765 (1932).

Donawick, W. J.; Christie, B. A.; Stewart, J. V.: Resection of diseased ileum in the horse. J. Amer. Vet. Med. Assoc. *159:* 1146 (1971).

Donawick, W. J.; Hiza, M. A.: Metabolic care of the horse with acute intestinal obstruction. Tijdschr. Diergeneesk. *98:* 980 (1973).

Eikmeier, H.: Therapie innerer Krankheiten der Haustiere (Enke, Stuttgart 1970).

Eikmeier, H.: Diagnostik und Therapie der Koliken beim Pferd. tierärztl. praxis *1:* 61 (1973).

Enigk, K.: Die Pathogenese der thrombotisch-embolischen Kolik des Pferdes. Mh. prakt. Tierheilkunde *3:* 65 (1951).

Ferraro, G. L.; Evans, R. R.; Trunk, D. A.; Roberts, T. T.: Medical and surgical management of enteroliths in equidae. J. Amer. Vet. Med. Assoc. *162:* 208 (1973).

Freytag, K.: Prognose und Behandlung bei Obstipationen des Pferdes. Collegium veterinarium, p. 84 (1975).

Feyc, J.: Manche Fragen aus dem Gebiet der Laparotomie und der Behandlung der Darmverstopfungen bei Pferden. Med. vet. *21:* 736 (1965).

Gratzl, E.: Die Punktion der Bauchhöhle des Pferdes von der Linea alba aus mit einem neuen Instrument. Wien. tierärztl. Mschr. *17:* 634 (1930).

Gratzl, E.: Die Behandlung der Blinddarmverstopfung des Pferdes. Wien. tierärztl. Mschr. *21:* 721 (1934).

Gratzl, E.: Beiträge zum Kolikproblem. I. bis IV. Mitt. Wien. tierärztl. Mschr. *23:* 129, 257, 417, 619 (1936); V. u. VI. Mitt. Wien tierärztl. Mschr. *24:* 33, 131 (1937).

Gratzl, E.: Novalgin — ein Kolikmittel. Wien. tierärztl. Mschr. *25:* 402 (1938).

Gratzl, E.: Entstehung und Behandlung der Koliken des Pferdes. Dtsch. tierärztl. Wschr. *50:* 141 (1942).

Gross, R.; Jahn, D.: Lehrbuch der Inneren Medizin (Schattauer, Stuttgart 1966).

Hapke, H.-J.: Pharmakologische Grundlagen der Koliktherapie. tierärztl. prax. *6:* 777 (1978).

Hertsch, B.; Eidt, E.: Zur klinischen Diagnose des Magenkarzinoms beim Pferd. Dtsch. tierärztl. Wschr. *83:* 92 (1976).

Huskamp, B.: Beitrag zur Diagnose und Therapie der beim Rind durch die Geburt entstandenen Darmverletzungen. Vet.-med. Diss., München (1960).

Huskamp, B.: Zur Kolik des Pferdes. Opuscula veterinaria, Hochmoor-Nachr. *4:* 2—7 (1970).

Huskamp, B.: Zur Chirurgie der Torsio coli des Pferdes. Dtsch. tierärztl. Wschr. *78:* 533 (1971).

Huskamp, B.: Zur operativen Koliktherapie beim Pferd. Vortrag vor der Österr. Gesellschaft der Tierärzte in Wien am 25. 10. 1973, auszugsw. in: Opuscula veterinaria, Hochmoor-Nachr. *8:* 7 (1973).

Huskamp, B.: Ileum-Resektion und Jejunocaecostomie beim Pferd. Berliner Münchener tierärztl. Wschr. *86:* 161 (1973).

Huskamp, B.: Ileusdiagnose beim Pferd. Tierärztl. Prax. *1:* 67 (1973).

Huskamp, B.: Die mediane Laparotomie beim Pferd — Technik und Ergebnisse. Dtsch. tierärztl. Wschr. *83:* 276 (1976).

Huskamp, B.: Die Kolik der Stute im Zusammenhang mit der Geburt. Prakt. Tierarzt *3:* 152 (1976).

Huskamp, B.: Some problems associated with intestinal surgery in the horse. Equine vet. J. *9:* 111 (1977).

Huskamp, B.: Kolik beim Pferd. II. Die operativ zu behandelnden Erkrankungen. In: Handlexikon der tierärztlichen Praxis. Med. Book Comp., Kopenhagen 1978, p. 4711.

Huskamp, B.; Kopf, N.: Typhlektomie beim Pferd — Experimentelle und klinische Erfahrungen. Dtsch. tierärztl. Wschr. *85:* 1 (1978).

Huskamp, B.; Kopf, N.: Die Verlagerung des Colon ascendens in den Milznierenraum beim Pferd. tierärztl. praxis *8:* 327, 495 (1980).

Hutyra, F. v.; Marek, J.: Spezielle Pathologie und Therapie der Haustiere (VEB Gustav Fischer Verlag, Jena 1954).

Jaksch, W.: in: Glawischnig/Jaksch: Klinische Propädeutik der Inneren Krankheiten und Hautkrankheiten der Haustiere (Parey, Berlin [West] und Hamburg 1976).

Kalsbeek, H. C.: Colic in the horse. Indications for laparotomie in horses with colic. Tijdschr. Diergeneesk. *98:* 963 (1973).

Kelly, W. R.: Tierärztliche klinische Diagnostik (VEB Gustav Fischer Verlag, Jena 1971).

Kersjes, A. W.; Bras, G. E.: The surgical treatment of ileus in the horse. Tijdschr. Diergeneesk. *98:* 968 (1973).

Kopf, N.: Beitrag zur rektalen und intraperitonealen Diagnostik des chirurgisch behandelten Kolikpferdes. Vet.-med. Diss., Wien (1976).

KOPF, N.: Intraoperative Diagnostik beim chirurgisch behandelten Kolikpferd. Proc. XIIth Congress of the European Society of Veterinary Surgery, Košice, *1:* 30 (1977).

KOPF, N.; HUSKAMP, B.: Die rektale Untersuchung beim Kolikpferd. Prakt. Tierarzt *59:* 259 (1978).

KOPF, N.; NIEBAUER, G. W.; RETTENBACHER, G.: Innere Verletzungen als Ursache oder Folge von Ileus beim Pferd. Wien. tierärztl. Mschr. *66:* 233 (1979).

LAGERWEIJ, E.; VAN DIETEN, J. S. M. M.: Anaesthesia and care during operation. Tijdschr. Diergeneesk. *98:* 975 (1973).

LITTLEJOHN, A.; RITCHE, J. D. S.: Rupture of the caecum at parturition. J. South African vet. Med. Assoc. *46:* 87 (1975).

LOWE, J. E.: Intussusception of the ileum in a horse. A case report. Cornell Vet. *56:* 51 (1966).

LOWE, J. E.: Intussusception in three ponies following experimental enterotomy. Cornell Vet. *58:* 288 (1968).

MAREK, J.; MÓCSY, J.: Lehrbuch der klinischen Diagnostik der Inneren Krankheiten der Haustiere (VEB Gustav Fischer Verlag, Jena 1956).

MAYER, H.; VALDER, W. A.: Graskrankheit in Deutschland. Berliner Münchener tierärztl. Wschr. *91:* 147 (1978).

MERKT, H.; GRASER, A.; SACKMANN, H.; GÜNZEL, A.-R.: Mastdarmperforation beim Pferd — Versuche zur temporären, medikamentösen Peristaltikhemmung. Prakt. Tierarzt *60:* 189 (1979).

MERRITT, A. M.: Treatment of diarrhoea in the horse. J. South African Vet. Med. Assoc. *46:* 89 (1975).

MERRITT, A. M.; BOLTON, J. R.; CIMPRICH, R.: Differential diagnosis of diarrhoea in horses over six months of age. J. South African Vet. Med. Assoc. *46:* 73 (1975).

MEYER, H.: Bedeutung von Futter und Fütterungstechnik bei Koliken des Pferdes. tierärztl. prax. *7:* 221 (1979).

NEUFELD, J. L.: Lymphosarcoma in the horse — a review. Canad. Vet. J. *14:* 129 (1973).

NEUFELD, J. L.: Lymphosarcoma in a mare and review of cases at the Ontario Veterinary College. Canad. Vet. J. *14:* 149 (1973).

PALFNER, D.: Die Kolik des Pferdes, dargestellt unter Berücksichtigung der Fachliteratur aus den Jahren 1920—1970. Vet.-med. Diss., Berlin-Dahlem (1972).

PETERSON, F. B.; DONAWICK, W. J.: Gastric stenosis in a horse. J. Amer. vet. med. Assoc. *160:* 328 (1972).

PUNZET, G.: Grundlagen und Praxis der Infusionstherapie. Wien. tierärztl. Mschr. *63:* 82 (1976).

RICKETTS, S. W.; PEACE, C. K.: A case of peritoneal mesothelioma in a thoroughbred mare. Equine Vet J. *8:* 78 (1976).

ROUS, R. C.: Mesenteric thrombosis. J. South African Vet. Med. Assoc. *46:* 79 (1975).

SCHEBITZ, H.: Zur Ileus-Chirurgie beim Pferd. Berliner Münchener tierärztl. Wschr. *74:* 165 (1961).

SCHLEITER, H.: Beitrag zur operativen Kolikbehandlung der Pferde. Berliner Münchener tierärztl. Wschr. *62:* 157 (1949).

SPÖRRI, H.; STÜNZI, H.: Pathophysiologie der Haustiere (Parey, Berlin [West] und Hamburg 1969).

ÜBERREITER, O.: Innere Einklemmung des Dünndarms durch den Ductus deferens beim Pferd. Wien. tierärztl. Mschr. *26:* 321 (1939).

ULLRICH, K.: Grundriss der speziellen Pathologie und Therapie der Haustiere (Enke, Stuttgart 1966).

WALL, S.: Die Kolik des Pferdes (Ivar Haegströms Boktryckeri, Stockholm 1908).

WESTHUES, H.: Über die Laparotomie bei grossen Haustieren. Berliner Münchener tierärztl. Wschr. *63:* 202 (1950).

WIERUP: Equine intestinal clostridiosis. Acta vet. scand. *18* (1977).

WISEMAN, A.; PETRIE, L.; MURRAY, M.: Diarrhoea in the horse as a result of alimentary lymphosarcoma. Vet. Rec. *95:* 454 (1974).

ZELLER, R.: Die Untersuchung bei Kolik des Pferdes. Collegium veterinarium, p. 81 (1975).

ZELLER, R.: Prognose und Therapie bei sekundärer Magenüberladung und Tympanie. Collegium veterinarium, p. 86 (1975).

2.1.5.11. Diseases of the Liver

2.1.5.11.1. Metabolic Disorders

Degeneration of the Liver (Hepatodystrophy)

Definition. This disease encompasses a range of etiologically diverse degenerations that are associated with varying degrees of hepatic necrosis.

The destruction of liver parenchyma leads to autolysis and resorption, which in severe cases causes a marked reduction of liver size (acute yellow atrophy). A loss or impairment of the detoxifying function of the liver and the associated metabolic derangements can lead to diseases of other organs as well as to signs of central nervous dysfunction (hepatoencephalopathy syndrome)! Terms such as hepatodystrophy, liver degeneration, hepatic necrosis and hepatosis are pathoanatomic concepts. Regardless of the inciting cause there is always some degree of damage to the liver cells. For this reason these terms should be gradually dropped from clinical usage and replaced with the term *hepatic insufficiency syndrome*.

Symptoms. In the milder forms of liver damage, such as those of dietary origin, the manifestations are nonspecific. This is especially true if jaundice is absent. But even if jaundice is present it does not reflect the severity of the disease unless accompanied by a high serum level of bilirubin, indicating hepatic cell damage of significant degree. Painful defecation is often observed in such cases [Mócsy, 1971].

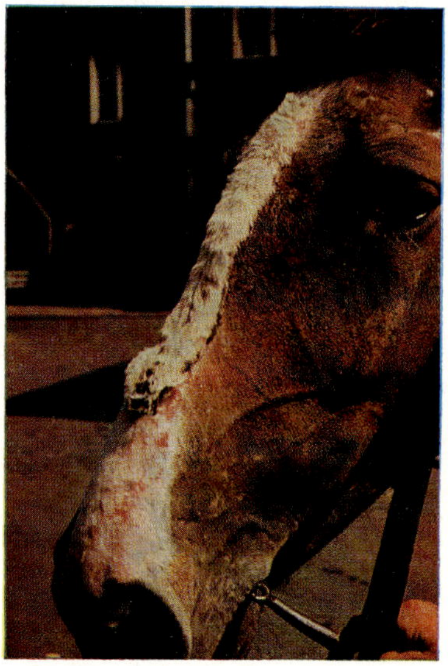

83

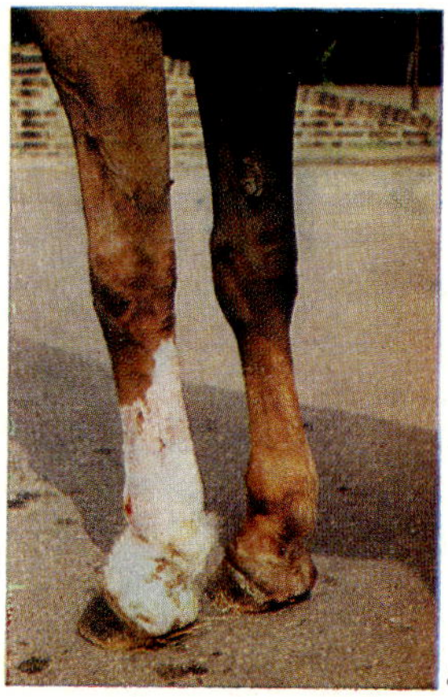

84

Fig. 2.1.5. — 83. Photosensitization in hepatic insufficiency syndrome. Mummification of unpigmented facial skin.

Fig. 2.1.5. — 84. Photosensitization in hepatic insufficiency syndrome. Mummification of unpigmented extremital skin.

In severe cases there are marked signs of intoxication manifested by depression, muscular weakness, an unsteady gait and in some cases excitement (hepatoencephalopathy). In intoxication by poisonous plants, such as *Senecio* species, there is persistent diarrhea with severe straining (even to the point of anal prolapse) and colicky signs. This is accompanied by petechiation of the nictating membrane, a rise in the pulse rate to 100—120, dark discoloration of the urine, proteinuria, and in some cases hemoglobinuria. Fowler [1965] describes the following manifestations of a primary hepatic insufficiency and hepatoencephalopathy based on his observations in 16 horses: depression, aimless walking, head pressing, ataxia, leaning, drooping of the head, quivering of the facial and lip muscles, and a disinterest in eating and drinking. Further manifestations are: icterus, weight loss, colicky signs, photosensitization, reddish-brown discoloration of the urine, heavy sweating, and temperature elevation in the early stages (figs. 2.1.5. — 83 to — 86).

Etiology. Injurious agents can gain access to the liver via the intestinal tract, circulatory system or lymphatic vessels. Damage may be caused by alimentary toxins, bacterial toxins, chemical toxins, or by a protein, vitamin or trace-element deficiency. In each case the severity of the hepatic lesions depends upon the severity of the causal agent or the degree of the deficiency. The major causes of liver degeneration can be classified into three groups: alimentary, toxic and infectious.

Degeneration due to Alimentary Causes. This form of liver damage occurs during the course of nutritional myopathy (White Muscle disease) in foals caused by a selenium deficiency [Pinkiewicz et al., 1974]: dietary hepatosis (cf. Sec. 2.4.1.2.6.).

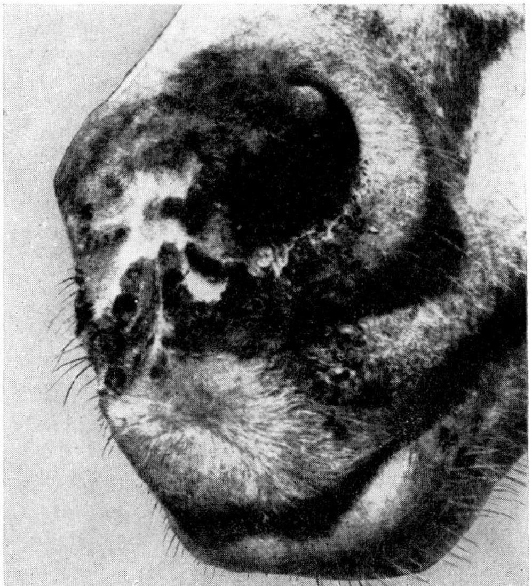

85

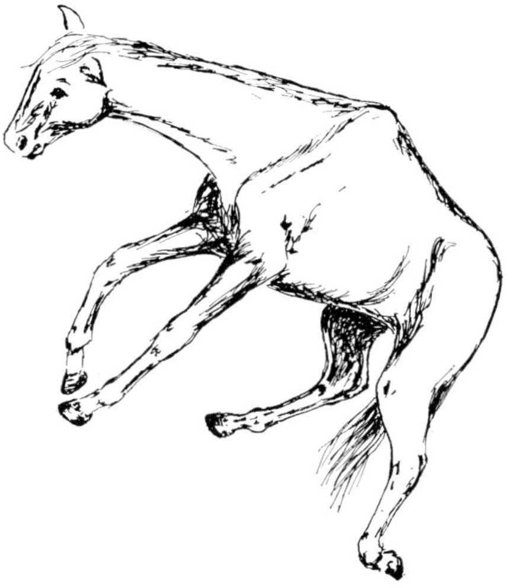

86

Fig. 2.1.5. — 85. Photosensitization lesions on the muzzle in hepatic insufficiency syndrome [after Fowler].

Fig. 2.1.5. — 86. Ataxia resulting from hepatic insufficiency syndrome [after Fowler].

Although the changes in the liver of the foal are minimal (Wolf [1963] states that no changes occur in the foal liver), they should nevertheless be mentioned in view of the pronounced changes in other species, especially swine.

The changes described in foals must be ascribed mainly to circulatory insufficiency (hypoxia of the liver). Vitamin E deficiency, excessive sulfur in the feed, and succinoxidase inhibitors (clover) must be considered in the differential diagnosis of nutritional myopathy, for all these factors can interfere with the utilization of selenium by the body.

Other possible causes are anemia, hemolysis, and a lack of certain sulfur-containing amino acids in the diet (methionine, cystine). It appears that these factors do not play a major etiologic role in this form of liver degeneration in foals. Alimentary endotoxemia as a result of intestinal obstruction also has been incriminated in hepatic degeneration [Hejlasz and Janiak, 1963].

Degeneration due to Toxic Causes. The main cause is the ingestion of spoiled feeds (hay that is dirty or contaminated with fungi). Another frequent cause is the ingestion of poisonous plants, such as *Senecio vernalis*, *Senecio jacobaea* and other *Senecio* species, *Crotalaria* species (legumes), and seeds of *Amsinckia intermedia*. The toxic substances in the *Senecio* species are pyrrolizidine alkaloids. These poisonings have become known under a variety of names in many parts of the world: walking disease, bottom disease (U.S.), pictou cattle disease (Canada), dunziekte (South Africa), sirasyke (Norway), Zdar disease (Czechoslovakia), Molteno disease, straining disease (Australia) and Schweinsberg disease (Germany). All these names refer to diseases that are similar or identical. Cirrhosis of the liver invariably develops in chronic cases.

Poisonings can also result from the ingestion of straw, peas, vetch, alfalfa and hay mixed with large amounts of weeds. Matthiakis attributes the effect of alfalfa to the fact that proteins contained in the plant undergo putrefaction in the large bowel, leading to the liberation of toxic compounds (toxic amines produced by the decarboxylation of amino acids). In Australia, 'Kimberley horse disease' has been described in horses fed plants of the genus *Crotolaria.*

Yet another cause of liver degeneration in the horse is stachybothryotoxicosis caused by the ingestion of *Stachybotrys atra* and *Stachybotrys alternans* (cf. Sec. 2.5.1.3.).

The injurious effect of feedstuffs cannot derive entirely from toxic substances that may be contained in them or from the toxins produced by fungi. The effect must depend in part on abnormal metabolic products that are formed from them as a result of digestive disorders — most notably foreign proteins and their high-molecular breakdown products. If the intestinal epithelium is damaged, these products can be absorbed and cause liver damage through allergic mechanisms. Derangements of the acid-base balance are conducive to liver damage of this type.

Liver degeneration can also be caused by chemical poisons, most notably phosphorus, arsenic, antimony and carbon tetrachloride. Carbon tetrachloride is especially toxic to horses, particularly when administered as an antihelmenthic without mineral oil. Poisonings can also result from the accidental ingestion of chlorine derivatives of the aromatic hydrocarbons (e.g., 6-chloroethane). The cresols and their derivatives contribute significantly to the occurrence of liver degeneration in horses. Finally, the toxic action of intestinal parasites must not be overlooked in the etiology of such liver pathology.

Degeneration due to Infectious Causes. This form is caused by various agents that produce a clinical picture of inflammation. However, the disease has a tendency to take a rapid systemic course in which the development of inflammatory changes is suspended in favor of degenerative, necrotic hepatic lesions. Most important in the horse is viral hepatitis, which is described in the section on Hepatitis. The present section also deals with focal hepatic necrosis as a result of infectious abortion in mares, necrobacillosis, and specific necroses associated with various infectious processes.

Pathogenesis. The liver performs a vital function as an organ of detoxification. This function is based upon conjugation, oxidation, acetylation, methylation and other processes that inactivate toxic decomposition products, infectious agents and indirect metabolic products that are absorbed from the digestive tract. The products of this detoxification are nontoxic.

If the hepatic cells are significantly damaged by toxic substances, degenerative processes are initiated which are perpetuated and potentiated by the injurious effect of endogenous (mainly proteolytic) enzymes. The central or peripheral portions of the hepatic lobules or the reticular fibers may be affected, depending on the mode of invasion of the injurious substances. Poisons such as carbon tetrachloride, phosphorus, arsenic, antimony and bacterial toxins cause direct damage to the hepatic parenchyma and lay the groundwork for proteolytic autolysis. If the hepatic cells have become hypersensitized as a result of emaciation, fatty degeneration, pregnancy or a heavy milk output, poisons of even moderate toxicity can produce the same effect. The damage to the liver cells may be degenerative or necrotic, depending on the quantity and nature of the toxins.

If the glycogenolytic function of the liver has been damaged by toxins such as carbon tetrachloride, a clinically manifest jaundice will develop [BAUMGÄRTEL]. In other cases, icterus may be absent despite severe hepatic damage.

When the detoxifying function of the liver becomes compromised, a hepatogenous autointoxication develops that usually is accompanied by neurologic signs (hepatoencephalopathy).

Metabolic derangements are associated with hypoglycemia and aminoacidemia. This state leads to acidosis and ketosis, as does an increased lipolysis in the presence of hypoglycemia.

Evidence from recent investigations indicates that disturbances in the enzymatic cell system play a significant role in hampering the detoxifying function of the liver. CHERNICK et al. [1955] claim that the primary disorder in cases of liver damage is one of cellular respiration, more specifically the formation of nicotinamide adenine dinucleotide (NAD).

Hepatic coma represents the extreme form of hepatic necrosis from a clinical standpoint. Until fairly recently it was thought that extreme forms of liver disease were accompanied by a triad of deficiency symptoms involving a fall in the blood levels of glucose, urea and cholesterol. These views have not been confirmed, however.

Today it is generally believed that the prime factor in the pathogenesis of hepatic coma is *ammonia* intoxication. The ammonia may originate from three sources: from the deamination of amino acids in the bowel, from the breakdown of amino acids in the various organs, and from the deamination of free and conjugated (direct) purine bases. Under normal circumstances ammonia is converted in the liver to nontoxic urea, which is excreted in the urine in monogastric animals. Optimum oxidation is necessary for the synthesis of urea. Any factor that contributes to hepatic anoxia simultaneously raises the concentration of ammonia in the blood. According to RIDDEL and McDERMOTT the toxic effect of ammonia is based on its binding with α-ketoglutaric acid. Ammonia binds a large amount of this acid and excludes it from the Krebs cycle, thereby interfering with the renewal of oxaloacetic acid and with further reactions in the citric acid cycle. These reactions can take place only in the presence of ATP and lead to a reduction in the oxygen content of the tissues, especially in the brain. This 'intoxication' is manifested by muscular tremor and in some cases by muscular rigidity [HOOPER, 1972]. It has been shown in experiments with sheep [HOOPER, 1972] that the i.v. administration of 2 ml of ammonia per kg BW produces the same clinical picture and pathohistologic changes in the optic thalamus as those produced by the experimental poisoning of sheep with *Senecio* alkaloids. Clinical signs included severe depression, muscular fibrillations, hepatic necrosis and vacuolization of the nerve cells. The research demonstrates that *ammonia poisoning* provides a satisfactory model for hepatic encephalopathy. The facts that prove that hepatic coma is due to hyperammonemia are very closely related to the metabolism of glutaminic acid and its amide, glutamine, in the body. On the one hand these compounds form the basis for metabolism in the brain, and on the other they play a role in the direct transfer and detoxification of ammonia. Besides hyperammonemia, hepatic coma is accompanied by respiratory difficulty leading to metabolic alkalosis, a disturbance of the carbohydrate, protein and fat metabolism (α-ketoglutaric acid deficit, pyruvic acid excess), and to potassium, phosphorus, calcium, magnesium and arginine deficiencies. All these disturbancess seriously disrupt the Krebs cycle [KUBICKI, 1966; ROSSOW and URBANECK, 1962; TENNANT et al., 1972, 1973; THOMSETT, 1971].

Lesions [DAHME and WEISS, 1973; NIEBERLE and COHRS, 1975]. In milder cases involving degenerative lesions of the parenchyma, the liver is slightly enlarged, its borders are rounded, and the changes are evenly distributed over the organ. The liver is soft and friable. The changes usually involve the central portions of the lobules, which show a dark, gray-white, yellow-white, gray-blue or gray discoloration. A bluish-red discoloration signifies that the capillaries are dilated and engorged with blood. The presence of tiny necrotic foci is characteristic of various infectious diseases.

In cases of moderate intensity, especially following the ingestion of plant toxins *(Senecio, Lupinus)* or chemical poisons (e.g., carbon tetrachloride), the liver shows a greater degree of enlargement and is very hard. The lobulation is more pronounced, the central veins are dilated, and the peripheral or central portions show a yellow discoloration.

Microscopic examination reveals dilatation of the central veins and nearby capillary vessels, as well as parenchymal degeneration; a necrobiotic fatty infiltration, vacuolization and atrophy of the hepatocyte trabeculae surrounding the capillary vessels; infiltrations of round cells; and new bile-duct formation. In acute liver atrophy, the liver is reduced in size by the autolysis of hepatic cells and the absorption of decomposition products. It is soft, pale-yellow and covered with petechiae that give it a mosaic-like appearance.

Laboratory Diagnosis. All authors, including ALLEN and ARCHER [1972], CARGILL and SHIELDS [1971], CARPER [1967], FREEDLAND et al. [1965], MCGUIRE et al. [1974], GERBER [1963—1966], HOMOLKA [1961], MARKIEWICZ [1967], STANKIEWICZ [1973], THOMA [1973], WEBER [1969], ZAPRZAL [1969], ZELLER and KELLER [1964], agree that it is impossible to differentiate degenerative liver disease from hepatitis on the basis of laboratory tests alone. A needle biopsy is best suited for this purpose.

As a rule, the laboratory evaluation includes the following battery of tests (exact techniques will vary from one laboratory to the next):

1. Urinalysis
2. Serum bilirubin determination
3. Serum colloidal reactions ('liver tests')
4. Serum protein electrophoresis
5. Serum enzymes

a) Secretory enzymes
b) Indicator enzymes ('necrotic' enzymes)
c) Excretory enzymes
6. Bromsulphalein test
7. Glucose tolerance test
8. Blood cholesterol and lipids
9. Erythrocyte sedimentation rate.

Urinalysis: Specific gravity: 1,015—1,045; color: yellow to amber, dark-brown to reddish-brown; pH: 5.0—8.5; protein: trace to 4 +; bilirubin: 0 to 4 +; urobilinogen: trace to 3 +; blood: 0 to 4 + [Fowler, 1965]. It must be emphasized that the correlation between the individual parameters is relatively poor in any given case. In cases with a severe course and unfavorable outcome, all values are elevated.

Bilirubin [Cornelius et al., 1965; Eikmeier, 1959; Ford and Gopinath, 1974; Grassnickel, 1959; Konrad, 1968; Pribyl, 1967; Sova, 1964, 1968, 1969; Sova et al., 1965; Wunderlich and Prösch, 1963; Zeller and Keller, 1964]: In mild cases (diatetic hepatitis) the total bilirubin is between 25.6 and 51 μmol/l. Thus, Konrad [1968] reports the following values for equine colics: mean total bilirubin 41.2 μmol/l, direct bilirubin 13.8 μmol/l, indirect bilirubin 22.9 μmol/l. For alimentary intoxication he reports a total bilirubin of 41.7 μmol/l, a direct bilirubin of 12.3 μmol/l and an indirect bilirubin of 4.4 μmol/l.

Reksa [1968] made interesting observations in his analysis of bilirubin levels in horses with alimentary autointoxication secondary to intestinal obstruction. Determining the bilirubin levels for successive disease stages, he found that while the total bilirubin continued to rise, the level of direct (bound) bilirubin decreased with time (regression of the obstruction). This was accompanied, however, by a rise in the indirect bilirubin. In his investigations, the total bilirubin on day 2 of the intestinal obstruction (mean value for 21 cases) was 34.2 ± 6.7 μmol/l (25.6—47.9), the direct bilirubin was 10.3 μmol/l, and the indirect bilirubin 24.0 μmol/l. On day 5 the total bilirubin was 39.3 ± 10.3 μmol/l (30.8—54.7), the direct bilirubin 3.4 μmol/l, and the indirect bilirubin 35.9 μmol/l.

Reksa [1968] reports the following normal values for the horse: total bilirubin 20.2 ± 1.2 μmol/l (4.4—35.9), direct bilirubin 5.1 μmol/l (3.4—10.3), and indirect bilirubin 15.0 μmol/l (6.8—19.8).

Acute hepatosis [after Sova, 1968]: In this disease the arithmetic mean for the total bilirubin (for 97 cases) is, according to Jirgl, 58.8 ± 24.3 μmol/l. A rise above 34.2 μmol/l was recorded in 52.9 % of cases, and a rise above 155.6 μmol/l in 8 % of cases.

Kuchar found in his study of 32 horses a moderate elevation of the direct bilirubin in 53.1 % of cases and a significant elevation in 6.3 %. For the indirect bilirubin he found a moderate rise in 72 % and a significant rise in 21.7 %.

Diffuse hepatic necrosis: Jirgl reports a total bilirubin (mean value for 37 cases) of 244.5 ± 82.1 μmol/l (87.2—547.2). Kuchar found a significant elevation of direct bilirubin in 40 % of cases and an extremely high increase in 60 % of cases. The indirect bilirubin showed a moderate rise in 20 %, a significant rise in 20 % and an extreme rise in 30 %.

The results presented above are consistent with the findings of other authors [Blazek, 1966; Forenbacher, Grassnickel, 1959; Konrad, 1968; Neumann].

In interpreting the results, it must be borne in mind that the total bilirubin may reach a value of 119.7 μmol/l in anorexic animals. Values up to 34.2 μmol/l are characteristic of subicteric states.

Serum colloidal reactions [Sova, 1963, 1968, 1969]:

Diffuse hepatosis: Weltmann reaction (166 cases). Complete flocculation
in test tube 4 in 0.6 % of cases,
in test tube 5 in 5.2 % of cases,
in test tube 6 in 8.0 % of cases,
in test tube 7 in 8.7 % of cases,
in test tube 8 in 30.4 % of cases,
in test tube 9 in 37.8 % of cases,
in test tube 10 in 8.7 % of cases,
in test tube 11 in 0.6 % of cases.

Diffuse hepatic necrosis: Weltmann reaction: Of 27 cases, a left shift was found in 7 % and a right shift in 17 %. This reaction accurately reflects the status of the globulin fractions of the serum proteins.

The Takata reaction, Hejda reaction, Gross reaction, copper acetate test and cadmium sulfate turbidity test are entirely unsuitable for the diagnosis of hepatic necrosis. In addition, electrophoresis and total protein assays do not yield characteristic values for acute hepatosis or hepatic necrosis.

Serum enzymes:

	Number of cases	Results
Acute hepatosis		
Serum glutamic oxylactic transaminase (SGOT) (μkat/l)[1]	84	3.76 ± 2.08
Serum glutamic pyruvic transaminase (SGPT) (μkat/l)	64	0.32 ± 0.28
Lactic acid dehydrogenase (LDH) (mM)	32	15 ± 6.7
Malic acid dehydrogenase (MDH) (mM)	31	5.1 ± 4.2
Sorbitol dehydrogenase (SDH) (mM)	22	0.046 ± 0.123
Acid phosphatase (μkat/l)[2]	34	0.02 ± 0.018
Alkaline phosphatase (μkat/l)[2]	34	0.20 ± 0.11
Diffuse hepatic necrosis		
Serum glutamic oxylactic transaminase (SGOT) (μkat/l)	14	9.92 ± 1.95
Serum glutamic pyruvic transaminase (SGPT) (μkat/l)	14	0.35 ± 0.17
Lactic acid dehydrogenase (LDH) (mM)	1	33.2
Malic acid dehydrogenase (MDH) (mM)	1	2.0

As the above values indicate, SGOT (aspartate amino transferase, ASAT) is the most important of the enzymes investigated, especially in the diagnosis of diffuse hepatic necrosis.

The determination of SGPT is of less importance in view of the sizable scatter of values (acute hepatosis).

The assays of LDH, MDH and SDH are of practically no importance, for all values are within normal limits. Sova states that the activities of these enzymes are elevated only in the early stage of the disease.

The value of acid and alkaline phosphatase assays is limited by the fact that elevations are also present in a number of other internal diseases.

[1] Conversion: 1 U/l × 0.01667 = μkat/l; 1 μkat/l × 60.0 = 1 U/l.

[2] Horses > 5 years.

Bromsulphalein test [Sova, 1964, 1968, 1969]:

	Acute hepatosis	Diffuse hepatic necrosis
5 mg/kg BW 5%		
3 min	54.1% ± 11.6%	82.8% ± 12.4%
5 min	44.8% ± 9.1%	71.6% ± 11.3%
7 min	30.9% ± 5.2%	61.9% ± 10.3%
10 min	21.0% ± 5.2%	47.9% ± 9.4%
12 min	16.4% ± 13.7%	44.5% ± 6.5%
15 min	11.9% ± 3.6%	41.1% ± 8.3%
Retention index (3—15 min) (in %)	22.5% ± 6.4%	49.4% ± 4.9%
Elimination constant k (3—15 min)	0.057	0.029
Fractionated elimination K	0.121	0.067
BSP clearance tot/min/ml	3,161 ml	2,325 ml
BSP clearance tot/min/ml/kg	6.3 ml	4.7 ml
Biologic elimination half-life (t 1/2 in min)	5.7 min	10.3 min
Percentage elimination rate in %/min	12.1%	5.7%

A comparison of the values for both degrees of liver damage demonstrates the great value of the BSP test. In both groups the retention values are significantly higher than in normal animals. In acute hepatosis the retention index is twice the normal value, and in hepatic necrosis four times as high. The rest of the values also attest to the usefulness of this test in the diagnosis of hepatic disease.

Sova considers retention values above 15% to be positive and values of 12—15% to be borderline.

Blood lipids and sterols:

	Acute hepatosis	Diffuse hepatic necrosis
Total cholesterol (mmol/l)	3.11 ± 0.90	3.37 ± 1.03
Free cholesterol (mmol/l)	1.35 ± 0.30	1.71 ± 0.30
Esterified cholesterol (mmol/l)	1.80 ± 0.53	1.86 ± 0.60
Phospholipids (mmol/l)	2.64 ± 1.96	2.14 ± 1.32
Total esterified fatty acids (mmol/l)	138 ± 67	235 ± 245.5

Most significant is the elevation of free and total cholesterol. It must be considered, however, that the rise of total cholesterol occurs at the expense of free cholesterol. While the increase in phospholipids and esterified fatty acids is noteworthy, the diagnostic importance of these parameters is limited by the large scatter of values. The fall of esterified cholesterol that is characteristic of hepatic coma in human medicine is not especially marked in the horse.

Erythrocyte sedimentation rate [Westergren; Sova, 1963, 1968, 1969]:

	Acute hepatosis	Diffuse hepatic necrosis
Sedimentation rate 15 min		
< 5 mm	5.8%	80%
5—19 mm	20.7%	15%
20—60 mm	46.6%	0%
61—100 mm	26.1%	5%
> 100 mm	0.8%	0%

The sedimentation rates behave differently in the two disease groups. The ESR is increased in hepatosis, while it is decreased in diffuse hepatic necrosis; this decrease is particularly evident in the figures presented above.

In summary, it must be concluded that only a *liver biopsy* yields reliable results in diffuse hepatic diseases. However, it too may fail if the changes are *focal* in nature. The most useful laboratory studies are the following: serum SGOT (ASAT), serum bilirubin, BSP test, blood glucose curve and ESR.

Hematologic values in primary hepatic insufficiency and in 'hepatoencephalopathy syndrome' based on the material of FOWLER [1965] (mean values for 16 horses).

RBC (10^{12}/l)	Hematocrit (%)	Hemo globin (g/dl)	Leuko-cytes (10^9/l)	Lympho-cytes (%)	Neutrophils (%)	Segmented nuclei (%)
9.59	4.8	17.8	18.3	15.6	66.6	
(4.95···13.1)	(3.2—6.1)	(15.7···22.0)	(11.3···25.6)	(5.0···33.5)	(58.0···95.5)	(0.3···13.0)
vs. normal values of						
7.0···13.0	3.2···55	10.0···18.0	7.0···14.0	25···70	30···65	0···2.0

As the above data indicate, the hematocrit, leucocyte and neutrophil counts are increased in hepatic insufficiency. The high hematocrit and hemoglobin values are obviously a consequence of dehydration. FOWLER's icteric index exceeded 100 units in all cases reviewed (normal = 1—25 units). If the icteric index is known, the bilirubin value can be calculated in μmol/l by dividing the index by 5. The determination of ammonia and α-amino acid nitrogen in the blood and the chromatographic assay of amino acids in the serum and urine are also important in the diagnosis of degenerative liver disease.

Clinical differential diagnosis of primary hepatic insufficiency [after FOWLER, 1965]:

	Hepatic insuffi-ciency	Encephalo-myelitis	Rabies	Intestinal obstruction	Infec. anem.	Pheno-thiazine poisoning	Lepto-spirosis
Ataxia	+	+	+	±	±	—	—
Aimless walking	±	±	±	—	—	—	—
Depression	+	+	slight	slight	—	—	slight
Hypertonic face and lip muscles	±	±	±	±	—	—	—
Yawning	±	—	—	±	—	—	—
Colicky signs	±	—	—	+	—	—	—

Fever	rarely	in early stage	—	only terminally or after colic	±	—	+
Icterus	usually	—	—	+	+	+	+
Discolored urine	±	—	—	±	±	+	+
Head pressing	±	±	±	—	—	—	—

Treatment. Treatment is the same for acute hepatosis and diffuse hepatic necrosis. The goal is the preservation of viable hepatic tissue. Success depends on the cause of the disease and the intensity of the therapy. In each case treatment starts by giving a laxative, preferably sodium sulfate in a dose of 500.0 g in 5% aqueous solution. This should be followed by several doses of charcoal in doses of 100—200 g by nasogastric tube. Antibiotics should also be administered via the tube. In cases of alimentary autointoxication secondary to colicky diseases [Hejlasz and Janiak, 1963], good results are obtained with 10.0 g chloramphenicol. Fowler [1964] administers broad-spectrum antibiotics i.v., for the damaged liver is prone to secondary infection. Götze [1953] injects sodium acetyl methionine in a dose of 3.5 to 4.0 g/100 kg BW i.v. for the purpose of protecting the liver parenchyma. Recently, intravenous administration of amino acids has also been recommended. The Polish product 'Amino Acids for Infusions Polfa' is a hydrolysate of animal protein that contains a complete range of free amino acids and approximately 7% peptides. The infusion of one liter provides all amino acids essential for urea synthesis (arginine, citrulline, ornithine). If methionine or other amino acids are unavailable, an alternative is to administer milk by stomach tube in a dose of 1—2 liters, for methionine is a constituent of casein. Choline is also beneficial owing to its lipotropic action and its ability to act as a methyl group donor, thereby promoting methionine synthesis. Vitamins are also used therapeutically, especially B-complex, A, K, E and C. Vitamins E, C and selenium are useful in the prophylaxis of hepatic necrosis. The i.v. infusion of glucose with vitamin C and the use of cholinergic drugs are helphul in the treatment of degenerative liver disease. Sugar may also be given via the stomach tube.

If significant dehydration has developed as a result of sweating (hypertonic water depletion), it is essential that hypo- or isotonic polyelectrolyte solutions be administered.

In states of psychomotor excitement and especially during manic episodes, treatment with sedatives is indicated, chloral hydrate being the agent of choice. Barbiturates, phenothiazine derivatives and morphine preparations are contraindicated.

Cases which take a very severe course (e.g., hepatic necrosis or hepatic coma) may respond to the i.v. administration of hydrocortisone in a dose of 1.0—1.5 g (given daily until improvement is noticed), as well as to i.v. doses of sodium glutamate.

Fowler [1964] reported no particular benefit from 26.0 g sodium glutamate administered in a 10% glucose solution 3 times daily. Hepatic coma is a very severe and dramatic clinical syndrome. A multidirectional therapeutic approach is justified in such cases, and the treatment of hepatic coma must take into account all demonstrable or presumed metabolic derangements.

Amyloidosis of the Liver

Definition. Amyloidosis is a degenerative disease based upon an abnormal deposition of amyloid in the tissues. It is the result of a defect in the protein metabolism.

Symptoms. In mild cases of hepatic amyloidosis, which can be diagnosed on the basis of liver function tests, clinical manifestations are seldom present. Enteritis may be observed. In severe cases, the liver is enlarged two to four times its normal size and is palpable. Additional symptoms are mainly referable to the underlying disease and include digestive disturbances, emaciation and splenomegaly. In other cases, ascites may be present due to the obstruction of blood flow in the portal circulation. More frequent is a rupture of the liver due to external trauma, leading to a potentially fatal internal hemorrhage.

Other reported symptoms include dyspnea due to enlargment of the regional lymph nodes. In horses used for commercial serum production, MARKIEWICZ [1965] observed edema, pallor of the mucosae, circulatory insufficiency and superficial suppurative foci. He attributed the presence of anemia to the periodic drawing of blood, to hepatic insufficiency, and to a reduction in the liver's ability to store copper and iron.

Etiology. Amyloidosis is a secondary disease. It is most commonly associated with chronic wasting diseases, suppurative processes, and recurrent or long-term insult by bacterial toxins. It also arises during the course of specific inflammatory diseases such as tuberculosis, as well as in neoplastic diseases. Of all animal species, amyloidosis is most frequently observed in horses used for serum production. ARNDT and DIRKEN found a 56.7 % prevalence of amyloidosis in that population. The spleen was involved in every case, the liver in half the cases, the adrenal glands in 25 %, and the kidneys in about 15 %. Amyloid changes rarely occur in the intestinal tract. In horses that are used continuously for serum production, amyloid degeneration of the liver takes about 6—8 months to appear. In horses used for the production of tetanus antitoxin, the titer is 1 : 350 [SZPAIER, 1957; MARKIEWICZ, 1965], and 1 : 600 in the third year of immunization. The prevalence of the disease depends on the nature of the antigen. The principal antigenic factors are, in descending order: diphtheria, scarlet fever, chicken pasteurellosis, and inoculations with toxins [SIPOS].

Pathogenesis. Amyloid is a compound made up of protein substances (globulins, tryptophan and other amino acids) and glycoproteins that are combined with acid mucopolysaccharides. The carbohydrate component determines the staining reactions of the amyloid in histologic specimens. Moreover, different varieties of amyloid have different staining properties owing to their diverse chemical structures. At present it is believed that amyloid is elaborated by the cells of the reticuloendothelial system (RES).

The prevalence of amyloidosis among horses used for immune serum production supports the view that amyloid represents an aberration of protein formation. This results in an allergic-hyperergic cell reaction with associated cellular damage. Inflammatory diseases of the bowel may also cause amyloidosis in horses.

Amyloid shows a double refraction when illuminated with polarized light. It typically appears in the form of homogenous flake- or trabecula-like masses. On electron microscopic examination, amyloid is found to be a conglomerate of fine filaments that are arranged in bundles or form an irregular meshwork.

Lesions. In mild cases the liver is mildly enlarged and slightly pale. In advanced cases the liver may be enlarged 2 to 4 times its normal size, is light brown, yellowish, gray or claylike in color, and its normal weight of 5 kg may be increased to 10—25 kg. In the horse it is often soft and friable, but it may also be hard and firm. Initially the lobular pattern is often distinct as in peripheral fatty infiltration, but the light peripheral zone is glassy with a dull luster. The cut surface presents a dull, waxy appearance throughout. Hjärre and Nordlund [quoted in Hutyra et al., 1962] recognize three forms of amyloidosis:

1. Typical form: The amyloid shows a metachromatic staining reaction, and all the organs typical of the affected species are equally involved; in the horse the liver and spleen are mainly affected.

2. Atypical form: The typical organs and tissues are not equally involved, and lesions are seldom confined to those tissues. The staining reaction is hypo- or achromatic.

3. Transitional form: The picture of 'typical' amyloidosis is combined with numerous deposits of amyloid showing little or no staining reaction. One or more organs may be involved.

Microscopically, amyloid deposits are observed between the capillary vessels of the portal vein and between the hepatocellular trabeculae at the periphery of the lobules. From there they spread in stages toward the center of the lobules. Thus, connections are established early between the individual lobules, and this accounts for the friable consistency of the diseased organ. Johne also observed amyloid deposits within the liver cells of horses.

Diagnosis. The Congo red test of Bennhold is of most value. A measured amount (80—100 ml) of a 1% solution of Congo red is injected intravenously. In advanced cases the dye binds so rapidly to the amyloid that one hour later it can no longer be detected in the bloodstream. In doubtful cases a needle biopsy may be performed. If albuminuria is demonstrated, it must be assumed that the kidney is also involved in amyloidosis.

Markiewicz [1965] investigated the liver function of horses used for serum production and in each case observed the following syndrome: hypochromic anemia, leukocytosis, increased ESR, a decrease in albumin, an increase in β- and γ-globulins, a positive cadmium test, a broadened coagulation band in the Weltmann reaction, a positive galactose test and a fall of urea levels.

Determination of the serum bilirubin is of only relative value.

It is significant that these blood changes appear during the first months of immunization, at a time when no clinical abnormalities are apparent. The changes become more intense during the first year and maintain a constant level thereafter [Preger and Albickaja, 1971].

Prognosis. Remission can occur in the early stage of hepatic amyloidosis, but in late stages the prognosis is poor. Affected animals die from the primary disease, a supervening disease, cachexia or hepatic rupture.

Treatment. The treatment of hepatic amyloidosis is mainly directed toward the underlying disease. Affected horses must be fed intensively, taking care to limit their intake of protein-rich feeds, because amyloid is the product of an aberrant protein metabolism. If the amyloidosis is very extensive, treatment is of no value. Mild cases should receive the standard supportive therapy for degenerative liver disease.

Fatty Liver (Fatty Degeneration of the Liver, Hepatic Lipoidosis)

Definition. The liver plays a central role in fat metabolism, the periphery of the lobules representing the most active zone. It is normal for the liver cells to contain droplets of fat (physiologic fatty infiltration). Rievel [1906] reported an incidence of 2—2.5% in the horse. 'Fatty liver' develops when fat accumulates in the liver to an abnormal degree. Two types of changes can occur: (1) a simple, pathologic fatty infiltration, generally called simply 'fatty infiltration', and (2) a degenerative (necrosing) fatty infiltration, known as 'fatty degeneration'. Only the latter condition is of clinical importance. Its principal causes are toxins and anoxia.

Symptoms. The clinical picture of fatty liver is nonspecific, and so the disease is frequently overlooked. In simple pathologic fatty infiltration and general obesity, no signs of hepatic insufficiency are present apart from a low exercise tolerance. In fatty degeneration secondary to an infectious disease, the syndrome is reasonably specific for this disease. In the case of toxic degeneration, the detoxifying function of the liver is lost as a result of damage to the liver cells. Large amounts of toxins, including those originating from the destruction of liver cells, produce a picture of general intoxication. The decrease in hepatic glycogen results in ketosis. This syndrome may be accompanied by signs of heart and renal disease which exacerbate the state of general intoxication. Petechiae are commonly present. In cases that take a rapid course, neurologic signs may also be observed (hepatic encephalopathy). Jaundice is common. In both the simple and degenerative forms of fatty infiltration, sudden death can result from internal bleeding due to rupture of the liver.

Etiology. Fatty liver can result from a number of causes. The most important are malnutrition, protein deficiency, oxygen 'deficiency' (hypoxemic fatty degeneration), hepatotoxic substances, and the loss of the lipolytic functions of the liver cells (toxic fatty degeneration). Fatty degeneration due to malnutrition generally develops as a result of chronic enteritis or other systemic diseases. Liver damage in such cases is due mainly to protein deficiency. An adequate supply of dietary protein is crucial to the maintenance of normal hepatocellular function. A protein deficit like that associated with starvation damages the active cytoplasm of the hepatic cells. This in turn leads to disturbances in the synthesis of basic protein enzymes that are instrumental in fat digestion.

Hypoxemic fatty degeneration of the liver can result from circulatory insufficiency with consequent vascular congestion or may develop as a result of anemia.

The toxic form of fatty degeneration is the most frequent, however. Of greatest etiologic importance are such toxins as phosphorus, antimony and arsenic compounds, chloroform, iodoform, carbon tetrachloride, certain plant toxins (from lupines, vetches, etc.), pathogenic fungi, and toxic or infectious products.

Overfeeding, i.e., a higher-than-normal fat assimilation, also has causal significance. When an animal is overfed or overfattened, the fat load presented to the liver exceeds the organ's capacity to metabolize it. Diabetes mellitus is a very rare cause of fatty liver in horses.

Pathogenesis. The pathogenesis of fatty liver is greatly complicated by the fact that multiple factors are involved. As a general rule, it may be said that fatty liver is the result of an excessive fat load presented to the liver, combined with the inability of the liver to metabolize it further. In the hypoxemic as well as toxic forms, the main cause of the fatty infiltration presumably lies in a failure of enzyme function (EGER: 'dysenzymemia'). For example, experiments with induced toxic liver damage have demonstrated a reduction in the activity of succinic dehydrogenase.

Attention has also been focused on the toxic effect of certain antibiotics (except penicillin) as a cause of fatty liver. It has been shown in experiments on animals and bacteria that antibiotics inhibit the incorporation of amino acids into proteins, thereby interfering with protein synthesis in the liver. Closely related to these problems and to a general protein deficit (which also occurs in wasting diseases) is a deficiency of the lipotropic factors that are necessary for the transport of fats.

It is known that the functional capacity of the liver with regard to the excretion and utilization of fats is closely linked to the quantity of glycogen present in the organ. When the glycogen is consumed as a result of malnutrition or wasting disease, the liver takes the fat it needs from storage sites in the body, especially from the adipose tissue (depot fat), and accumulates it in increasing quantities. In such cases, the reduced carbohydrate metabolism and the associated absence of pyruvic acid, which is transformed by carboxylase into the oxaloacetic acid necessary for normal Krebs cycle function, lead to an accumulation of ketone bodies in the body, or ketosis.

Diabetes offers a model for clarifying the pathogenesis of fatty liver. The energy deficit that results from reduced glucose utilization interferes with the synthesis of ATP, which in turn inhibits the synthesis of phosphocholine and consequently of the phospholipids. The result is a reduction in the transfer of fats from the liver. A decrease in cholesterol synthesis is a further cause of reduced phospholipid synthesis.

Lesions. In diffuse fatty infiltration the liver generally is increased in size and weight. In severe cases the liver weight may increase to 14 kg (normal $\sim$ 5 kg). The anemia caused by pressure from the enlarged liver cells on the capillary system of the portal vein causes the liver to acquire a pale-yellow color, or a reddish-yellow color if the vessels are congested. Its edges are rounded, its surface smooth, and the lobular pattern is indistinct in cross-section. In toxic fatty degeneration the liver may be shrunken as a result of cell destruction. When jaundice is present the organ acquires a saffron-yellow color ('hepar crocatum'). A fatty infiltration that is grossly visible in the liver of an herbivorous animal is always pathological.

Histologic Changes. The deposition of fat in the liver cell may be central, intermediate, peripheral or diffuse. Fatty degeneration of the centrilobular regions is characteristic of hypoxia and anemia, chronic nutritional deficiencies, and certain intoxications in which the oxygen demand at the periphery of the lobule is so high that central regions are deprived. A centrilobular hypoxemic fatty infiltration is also observed in stasis liver in which there is atrophy of the centrilobular cells. Peripheral fatty degeneration is usually the result of blood-borne toxins. The degeneration is most rapid and severe in the cells at the periphery of the lobule, which are the first to come in contact with the arterial and venous blood of the portal circulation.

In milder cases where no microscopic structural changes are visible in the cell body or its nucleus, the cell can regain its normal function once the cause has been corrected. In severe cases with visible changes such as pyknosis, karyorrhexis and karyolisis, cell death is inevitable. If the action of the causal agent is rapid and severe, small fat droplets will completely fill the cell.

Diagnosis (Laboratory Diagnosis). In uncomplicated cases of fatty liver, the majority of function tests are negative. Positive results are more characteristic of later stages in which elements of the RES become more active. Protein disturbances may arise with hypalbuminemia and an increase of α- and β-globulins. The Bromsulphalein test and glucose tolerance test are considered to be the most sensitive.

Treatment. Dietary fats and carbohydrates should be restricted in favor of high-protein feeds. Medical treatment is the same as for hepatic dystrophy and degeneration. Lipotropic factors such as methionine, casein, vitamin B_{12}, etc., liver extracts, glucose, vitamin C, vitamin K, vitamin E and amino acids should be administered. If the etiology is known, treatment of the cause is indicated.

2.1.5.11.2. Hepatitis

Definition. A strict differentiation between inflammatory liver disease, or hepatitis, and degenerative liver disease, or hepatosis, is clinically difficult or even impossible. This is particularly true in the case of 'abortive forms' of liver disease in which the signs of a full-blown inflammation are unable to develop. Inflammation of the liver may be caused by toxic, infectious or parasitic agents that gain access to hepatic tissue by way of the blood stream or biliary tree. Clinical experience and experimental results confirm that the various changes in the liver cannot be the result of any one of these factors alone. The severity of the lesions is influenced by numerous factors such as circulation, nutritional status and coexisting disease.

The term hepatitis used here refers to diffuse hepatic diseases in which regressive or catabolic changes in the liver cells are of greater significance than the concurrent vascular and mesenchymal changes.

Hepatitis may be acute or chronic, local or diffuse, purulent or nonpurulent, and classified into specific etiologic forms.

Acute Nonpurulent Hepatitis

Etiology. This disease may occur as a clinical manifestation of many infectious diseases and toxicoses. This class of diseases includes all cases that directly involve the liver, such as enzootic hepatitis of horses, serum hepatitis and septic diseases with secondary liver inflammation such as equine infectious anemia, leptospirosis, infectious bronchopneumonia, Wesselbron disease and viral abortion in mares.

THEILER in 1918 described a hepatitis in horses that had been passively immunized against African horsesickness. In Finland 1,600 cases of hepatoencephalopathy were reported in horses during the period from 1866 to 1940. Attempts to transmit the disease experimentally to healthy horses have been unsuccessful. Neither has it been possible to identify the etiologic agent. Information is also lacking on the inoculation of horses with biologic material. Nevertheless, it may be assumed that both diseases have the same etiology as experimentally induced serum hepatitis. This is observed following the administration of anti-anthrax serum, pregnant mare serum, tetanus antitoxin and after immunization against tetanus, equine encephalomyelitis and viral rhinopneumonitis. Today it is generally believed that the primary cause of this disease is *biologic material of equine origin* [PANCIERA, 1969]. REISINGER [1969], on the other hand, argues that this disease is more *toxic* than serologic in nature. When the liver is damaged, a type of endotoxic shock develops following the administration of an equine-origin biologic. If hepatic damage is negligible, the course of the disease is mild.

HELBROOK believes that serum hepatitis is a result of multiple parenteral injections.

Pathogenesis. According to EPPINGER, the infectious agent in nonpurulent hepatitis damages the capillary vessels in the centrilobular zone, giving rise to a serous inflammation ('serous hepatitis'). The damaged capillary vessels become dilated and more permeable to the protein-rich blood plasma. Large amounts of plasma enter the spaces of Disse and expand them. The liver cells become depleted of oxygen and degenerate. This degeneration may be partly due to the direct action of toxins on the liver cells. As a result of these changes, there is a disintegration of the architecture of the lobules, and the channels that communicate directly with the spaces of Disse. This allows bile to mix with the blood, and icteric signs appear. Besides degeneration, a cellular proliferation is also observed. This includes the cells of the RES. Degenerative processes are especially marked in a 'parenchymal' inflammation. The outcome of the disease is variable, depending on the quantity of the serous exudate and the amount of protein it contains. If the exudate is minimal in quantity and contains little protein, then resolution is possible through absorption of the exudate via the lymph. However, if exudation is extensive and takes a fulminant course, the liver parenchyma may be severely damaged. The exudate can cicatrize, leading to cirrhosis of the liver or acute yellow atrophy.

Lesions. In nonpurulent inflammation, small foci of cellular infiltration are present that ordinarily are visible only under the microscope. The infiltrate consists of varying proportions of lymphocytes, leukocytes, plasma cells and eosinophils, which are located between the lobules. Accompanying these changes is an unrelated diffuse, serous hepatitis that is characterized by an inflammatory edema. This includes a filling of the pericapillary spaces of Disse with serous fluid and neutrophils and a mobilization of the Kupffer cells. A parenchymal degeneration of the hepatocytes is also observed.

In serum hepatitis, the liver may be of normal size, enlarged or shrunken. It is friable, and yellow or greenish in a lobular pattern. Fibrin strands may be adherent to the hepatic capsule. The serosa may show numerous petechiae. Icterus is always present. There may be congestion and hemorrhage in the renal and adrenal cortices and the gastrointestinal mucosa. The spleen is occasionally congested.

The histologic changes are similar to those described previously. In equine infectious anemia, significant swelling of the spleen and lymph nodes is accompanied by a marked enlargement of the liver. In longstanding cases the liver acquires a striking nutmeg-like appearance with a brownish discoloration of the parenchyma. Histologically there is an accumulation of hemosiderin in the Kupffer cells, and lymphohistiocytic reactions occur in the interstitial tissue. There is frequently a marked swelling of the medullary substance of the hepatic lymph nodes. Intranuclear inclusion bodies are typical of viral abortion of mares (rhinopneumonitis). They are located at the margins of the necrotic foci, in the epithelium of the bile ducts, the endothelial cells of the blood vessels, the smooth muscle cells and fibroblasts of the vascular walls and hepatic capsule. They are also located in the epithelium of the bronchi, bronchioles and pulmonary alveoli, but rarely in the thymus, spleen, lymph nodes and Peyer's patches.

Multiple hepatic necrosis is observed in aborted foals.

Purulent Hepatitis

Etiology. Purulent hepatitis may take an acute or chronic course and usually occurs in the form of abscesses caused by any of a number of pyogenic bacteria. The main causative organisms in the horse are *Streptococcus equi* and *Str. zooepidemicus*, and actinobacillosis in the foal.

Symptoms. Small abscesses that form slowly and often in large numbers produce minimal disease symptoms and may cause only a moderate degree of emaciation. In cases of pyemia, the clinical picture may be altered by the primary disease. In other cases there is significant fever that may be intermittant or sustained. Emaciation, icterus and bilirubinemia, combined in some cases with leukocytosis, may also be present.

The presence of a large number of abscesses may lead to death as a result of toxin absorption. Serum hepatitis occurs within 27 to 165 (usually 40 to 70) days following the administration of affected serum. Acute cases are characterized by a sudden onset and rapid course. Fever is usually absent, the pulse is rapid, and icterus is usually present. Additional signs are profuse sweating, unsteady gait, staggering, muscular tremors, head pressing, and excitement alternating with depression. Anorexia, yawning and constipation complete the clinical picture. Hematologically there is leukocytosis, bilirubinemia and hypoglycemia. Blood, protein and bilirubin are detected in the urine. Fatal cases usually die within 12 to 48 hours. The mortality rate is as high as 90 %.

Blazek [1956] described an enzootic hepatitis of horses that was very similar to viral hepatitis in man. The course is marked by icterus, hemoglobinuria and neurologic signs. Wesselbron disease, which affects mainly sheep, has also been observed in horses. It is characterized by icterus, anemia and hemorrhagic enteritis.

Pathogenesis. Primary hepatic abscesses can result from the direct seeding of infectious organisms in the liver by a perforating foreign body. Secondary abscesses can develop from an infection carried by the blood, bile or lymph. They may also spread from neighboring tissues. Blood-borne infections usually arrive via the portal vein or umbilical vein (in neonates) and less frequently via the hepatic artery and hepatic vein. The portal vein also provides a pathway by which abscesses can metastasize to the liver from the mesentery, intestine or spleen. Pyogenic bacteria can also be introduced into the liver by the larvae of certain parasites. In some cases a purulent infection can arise in connection with bilestones, parasites or foreign bodies such as sand or vegetable spicules, that have become lodged in the bile ducts. This can in turn cause a purulent inflammation. Suppurative processes can also develop around hydatid cysts, tuberculous and botryomycotic foci, and in rare cases around necrotic mycotic foci. Numerous abscesses can cause death from toxin absorption, although some form of recovery is more frequently observed. Smaller abscesses may cicatrize following the absorption of their contents. Large abscesses can become encapsulated and may be harmless.

Lesions. Recently formed abscesses appear as sharply-circumscribed foci that are pale green, grayish green or dark gray in color and contain a soft, odorless, creamy pus. In some abscesses the pus is foul-smelling.

Older abscesses usually range in size from a pea to a hazelnut but may grow considerably larger. The capsule is of variable thickness depending on the size of the abscess. In old abscesses the pus has acquired a thick, heavy consistency as a result of calcium salt deposition. Hematogenous abscesses are generally multiple and may produce slight hepatic enlargement with associated fatty or parenchymal degeneration. Abscesses may resemble soft necrotic, tuberculous and botryomycotic foci. The latter are very often accompanied by infection with pyogenic bacteria.

Hepatic tuberculosis in horses is marked by the presence of lesions that may reach the size of a fist. They are grayish-white in color and are usually similar in appearance to certain tumors. Often they have acquired a hard consistency as a result of fibrous tissue proliferation.

Botryomycosis occurs as a metastatic condition in horses. In these cases a number of fibrous, cicatrized nodes ranging in size from a pea to a fist or larger are observed. The lesions are grayish-white in color and contain yellow-orange to yellow-brown purulent foci. Necropsy findings depend on the underlying disease and are described in other sections of this book.

Diagnosis of Hepatitis:

Liver Biopsy [Sova, 1965]. According to Griffault, a liver biopsy provides the best means of localizing the abscess in purulent hepatitis. It should be done in the 16th intercostal space on the first percussion line of the lung. An alternate site is the 13th, 14th or 15th intercostal space, 2 to 3 fingerbreadths anterior to the caudal lung border. The biopsy is done with an appropriate trocar/stylet instrument. When the organ is reached, the stylet is withdrawn, and the cutting sheath is passed into the liver to a depth of 4—5 cm and rotated to the right or left to excise a core of tissue. The biopsy can also be done with the Vim-Silverman needle, which consists of an outer cannula with a beveled tip and an inner split needle. After the liver is reached, the inner needle is advanced to the desired depth, and then the outer needle is inserted to the same depth. The entire arrangement is then rotated 180° to excise a core of tissue, and both needles are withdrawn simultaneously.

Laboratory Diagnosis [after SOVA, 1968]. The following forms of acute hepatitis can be diagnosed on the basis of laboratory findings:

1. Hepatitis secondary to septic diseases.
2. Enzootic hepatitis, unless hepatic necrosis has developed.
3. Cases where hepatitis has been demonstrated histologically.
4. Cases of cholangitis that have also been diagnosed by liver biopsy, with associated bile duct lesions and acute hepatitis.

Serum bilirubin (method of JENDRASSIK and CLEGHORN; values in mol/l):

	Acute hepatitis			Normal values		
	n	x̄	s	n	x̄	s
Bilirubin (after JIRGL)	125	95.2	30.4	33	22.7	0.85
	Results:					
		0— 34.2	13.3 %			
		35.9— 85.5	42.4 %			
		87.2—153.9	24.8 %			
		155.6—256.5	16.0 %			
		258.2—376.2	1.6 %			
Bilirubin (after FOUCHET)	137	negative	14.9	110	negative	100 %
		1 +	49.2			
		2 +	23.8			
		3 +	21.1			
Bilirubin (after FOUCHET) (direct)	21	negative	14.3 %	20	negative	95 %
		1 +	61.9 %		+	5 %
		2 +	23.8 %			
(indirect)	21	negative	4.9 %	20	negative	46 %
		1 +	61.9 %		positive	55 %
		2 +	32.2 %			

As the data above indicate, total bilirubin values (after JIRGL) in excess of 154 μmol/l were found in 17.6 % of cases, as compared to only 8 % in acute hepatosis, values never exceeding 155.6 μmol/l. An elevated direct bilirubin was found in 85.7 % of horses with acute hepatitis and in only 59.4 % with acute hepatosis. It should also be noted that total bilirubin values below 34.2 μmol/l were found in only 13.3 % of cases, versus 47.1 % in acute hepatosis.

Serum colloidal reactions:

	Hepatitis			Normal values		
	n	Result		n	Result	
WELTMANN reaction	166	tube 4	3.1 %	130	tube 7	4.7 %
		5	5.7 %		8	43.0 %
		6	5.7 %		9	51.0 %
		7	15.6 %		10	0.8 %
		8	45.2 %			

The WELTMANN reaction showed a left shift in 14.5 % of cases (vs. 13.8 % in acute hepatoses). A right shift was observed only in acute hepatosis, and no such shift occurred in acute hepatitis. In the electrophoretic separation of serum proteins a left shift corresponds to higher values of α-globulins, while a right shift reflects higher values of γ-globulins.

Because a relatively high percentage of the electrophoresis migration patterns showed a normal breakdown of serum proteins (11.5 %) and a slight elevation of α-globulins with a simultaneous increase in α- and γ-globulins (15.2 %), this test appears to be of limited value in the diagnosis of acute hepatitis. The same applies to acute hepatoses.

Serum enzymes:

	Acute hepatitis			Normal values		
	n	x̄	s	n	x̄	s
Serum glutamic oxaloacetic transaminase (SGOT) (μkat/l) (ASAT)	12	6.13	2.03	22	3.50	0.67
Serum glutamic pyruvic transaminase (SGPT) (μkat/l)	11	0.22	0.22	22	0.10	0.07

Of all the enzyme tests that demonstrate damage to the liver parenchyma, the determination of SGOT (ASAT) activity is the most important, especially in view of the fact that the rise in its activity is proportional to the degree of ischemic necrosis. The SGPT determination, on the other hand, is of less value owing to the large scatter of the results.

Determinations of other enzyme activities, such as LDH and MDH, are of limited value, because the differences relative to healthy horses are not statistically significant. A rise in SDH activity is observed only during the first three days of the disease.

Bromsulphalein test (Bromsulphalein liver function test):

	Acute hepatitis			Normal values		
	n	x̄	s	n	x̄	s
BSP test 5 mg/kg in 5 % Concentration						
3 min	2	51.1 %	2.1 %	14	37.3 %	10.8 %
5 min	2	43.9 %	2.1 %	14	26.6 %	11.1 %
7 min	2	37.2 %	3.95 %	14	15.2 %	9.8 %
10 min	2	29.1 %	1.7 %	14	9.8 %	4.1 %
12 min	2	25.8 %	1.3 %	14	5.6 %	2.9 %
15 min	2	22.9 %	1.7 %	14	3.4 %	2.0 %
Retention index (3—15 min) in %	2	45.1 %	6.4 %	14	11.1 %	4.9 %
Elimination constant (k) (3—12 min)	2	0.033		14	0.138	0.017
Fractionated elimination (K)	2	0.076		14	0.317	0.04

	Acute hepatitis			Normal values		
	n	$\bar{x}$	s	n	$\bar{x}$	s
BSP clearance tot/min/ml	2	2,804 ml		14	7,925 ml	2,118 ml
BSP clearance tot/min/ml/kg	2	5.6 ml		14	15.9 ml	4.1 ml
BSP/biologic elimination half-life ($t_{1/2}$)	2	9.1 min		14	2.2 min	0.5 min
Percentage elimination rate (in %/min)	2	7.6 %		14	31 %	9 %

The Bromsulphalein test is the most valuable for the assessment of liver function. The retention index in acute hepatitis is 3 to 4 times higher than in healthy horses. Determination of the other parameters of indirect Bromsulphalein clearance is also very useful. For example, the elimination constant in healthy horses is 0.138, compared to only 0.033 in diseased horses. Similar marked differences are found in the BSP clearance (tot/min/ml and tot/min/ml/kg) and the BSP/biologic elimination half-life ($t_{1/2}$).

Blood lipids and sterols (lipoids):

	Acute hepatitis			Normal values		
	n	$\bar{x}$	s	n	$\bar{x}$	s
Total cholesterol (mmol/l)	21	2.97	0.83	16	2.82	0.37
Free cholesterol (mmol/l)	2	1.81	0.74	16	0.92	0.33
Esterified cholesterol (mmol/l)	2	1.93	0.60	16	1.92	0.43
Phospholipids (mmol/l)	7	2.83	1.55	16	1.90	0.40
Total esterified fatty acids (mmol/l)	7	228.0	133.0	22	174.0	51.7

Of all the specific lipoids, the rise of free cholesterol is the most pronounced. It results from the reduced binding ability of the esterified cholesterol that is a consequence of hepatic disease. The remaining compounds, while displaying significant differences relative to normal animals, are limited in their diagnostic value due to wide ranges of values.

Glucose tolerance test:

	Acute hepatitis			Normal values		
	n	$\bar{x}$	s	n	$\bar{x}$	s
Glycemia (mmol/l)[1]	5	5.48	0.92	50	5.48	0.78
Glycemic curve	Glycemia (mmol/l)			Glycemia (mmol/l)		
0.25 g in 40 % glucose solution per kg BW fasting	1	5.99		5	4.72	
30 min		8.82			6.66	
90 min		7.71			5.11	
120 min		6.45			4.77	
270 min		4.50			5.11	

[1] Glucose conversion: mg/100 ml × 0.0555 = mmol/l; mmol/l × 18.02 = mg/100 ml.

The glucose determination is virtually useless due to the variability of normal values. By contrast, the 'glycemic' curve exhibits a distinct peak after 30 min, indicating a decline in the glucogenogenesis process. This curve is therefore of potential diagnostic importance.

Erythrocyte sedimentation rate [WESTERGREN]:

	Acute hepatitis		Normal values	
	n	Result	n	Result
ESR	216		293	
15 min				
< 5 mm		27.1 %		4.2 %
5—19 mm		16.4 %		22.4 %
20—60 mm		37.8 %		66.2 %
61—100 mm		16.4 %		6.5 %
> 100 mm		2.3 %		0.7 %

Although the ESR is normally decreased in cases of acute hepatitis, a marked increase was also found after 15 min in 16.4 % (range of 61—100 mm) of affected horses and 6.5 % of normal horses. It will be recalled that in acute hepatosis, an increased ESR was demonstrated in 26.1 % of cases. A decrease of the ESR was found in 27.1 % of acute hepatitis cases. In interpreting these results, it must be remembered that the ESR is decreased by strong bilirubinemia and increased by high gammaglobulinemia.

In summary, the following tests are of diagnostic importance in acute hepatitis: ESR, total and direct bilirubin, SGOT (ASAT) activity, free cholesterol, and the BSP test. It should be emphasized, however, that these reactions are also suitable for the diagnosis of acute hepatosis. The liver biopsy is of decisive importance, although the demonstration of liver damage by laboratory studies always provides a useful guideline for therapy.

Treatment. If the cause of the hepatitis is known, initial effort must be directed toward correction of the underlying disease. If the cause is unknown, treatment is symptomatic. This also applies to cases having a viral etiology. For this reason the prophylaxis against secondary bacterial infections is an essential part of the treatment of so-called enzootic hepatitis in horses.

Another essential aspect of treatment is supportive therapy. The goal is preservation of hepatic tissue. This has already been mentioned in the treatment of hepatic dystrophy and degeneration. The object is to correct any icterus resulting from the hepatitis while preventing an acute inflammation from progressing to a chronic one or to hepatic cirrhosis. The key to this treatment are the cortisone compounds. These significantly shorten the duration of icterus, especially when administered early. Presumably the anti-inflammatory effect of the cortisone derivatives is complemented by their ability at reducing the permeability of the cell membranes.

Treatment with steroids has both positive and negative aspects. Negative aspects include activation of chronic inflammatory processes and the inhibition of immune mechanisms. This results in signs of icterus recurring after discontinuance of the steroid therapy. When glucocorticosteroids are given, a course of broad-spectrum antibiotics is indicated.

The antibiotics of choice for the prevention of secondary infections as well as for protection during glucocorticosteroid therapy are penicillin (shown to be non-hepatotoxic) and possibly streptomycin. Unlike other broad-spectrum antibiotics, streptomycin exhibits a certain lipotropic property. It acts as a precursor of inositol owing to its content of streptidine. Other aspects of treatment are similar to that for liver degeneration.

Cirrhosis of the Liver

Definition. Cirrhosis of the liver is a nonspecific syndrome that represents only one reaction of this organ to chronic insult by various agents. Hepatic cirrhosis has the character of a systemic disease producing complete disruption of lobular architecture as a result of the focal loss of parenchyma, fibrosis, nodular regeneration and compensatory hyperplasia. If just one of these changes is lacking, the disease process cannot be assigned to the group of true cirrhoses. Variations may occur only in the histologic changes, and the development of these changes is similar regardless of the precipitating factors. The minor variations that exist in the nature of the changes enable us to classify the disease into three forms:

1. Portal cirrhosis (venous, diffuse, finely-nodular, deficiency cirrhosis).
2. Postnecrotic cirrhosis (toxic, infectious, coarsely-nodular cirrhosis). Forms 1 and 2 represent the main forms of atrophic cirrhosis, also called Laennec's cirrhosis.
3. Biliary cirrhosis (hypertrophic cirrhosis).

This classification is not always applicable, however, because the liver frequently exhibits multiple forms at one time.

Symptoms. Konrad [1968d] presented a complete review of diffuse hepatic cirrhosis. Drawing on the histopathologic results of liver studies in horses obtained from regions in Czechoslovakia affected with a disease called Zdar disease, or hepatic cirrhosis of horses, he identified three stages in the natural history of the disease:

1. Initial stage (stage of hepatic irritation)
2. Preclinical stage of hepatic cirrhosis
3. Stage of clinical manifestation of so-called Zdar disease.

Konrad states that the onset of the disease is unaccompanied by any clinical symptoms and can be diagnosed only by the histologic examination of biopsy material. The various signs of disease that sometimes appear during this stage are incidental in nature.

In Konrad's classification, the interval between stage 1 and stage 3 of the cirrhosis may be as much as several years. Konrad observed horses in which stage-1 changes persisted over a period of 3 years without remission or exacerbation. The 'latent' period before the appearance of a diffuse cirrhosis is 2 to 2½ years on the average.

The appearance of cirrhosis symptoms and neurologic signs characteristic of the 'hepatoencephalopathy syndrome' is ordinarily preceded by nonspecific digestive disorders (in the absence of feeding errors). These include changing appetite; chronic inflammation of the gastric mucosa; frequent yawning; occasional diarrhea alternating with constipation; and attacks of colic. Other signs are rapid fatigability, weight loss and dullness of the haircoat. In later stages there are ulceration of the buccal and labial mucosa, aimless walking, staggering, profound apathy, pushing against obstacles, etc. The appearance of these signs heralds the terminal stage of hepatic cirrhosis, and treatment at this point is of no value.

If the liver is greatly enlarged, an area of dullness will be noted on the right side immediately posterior to the caudal lung border in the region of the 10th to 17th intercostal space. Occasionally the enlargement is so great that a bilateral swelling will be visible in the subcostal region.

The results of the histologic studies of KONRAD in Zdar disease, KÖHLER [1950] in Schweinsberg disease (which is identical), HUPKA [1955], and VANEK [1956] confirm that plants of the genus *Senecio* are instrumental in equine hepatic cirrhosis.

Etiology. Hepatic cirrhosis is rarely caused by an isolated etiologic agent. It is caused by irritants that produce degenerative changes in the parenchyma and proliferative changes in the mesenchyma. In the majority of cases it is the result of multiple influences or represents the end stages of some other disease. Very often the causes of a cirrhosis are so closely interrelated that it is difficult to assign a primary causal role to any particular factor. In other cases one may fail to disclose any of the causes. The most frequent causes in animals are toxic, infectious and parasitic agents. The main precipitating factors are chronic intoxication caused by the ingestion of spoiled feeds or poisonous plants, as well as all other factors that lead to liver degeneration (secondary cirrhoses). Endemic hepatic cirrhosis of horses is known by various names in many countries: Schweinsberg disease (which occurs in the Ohm River Valley in Hessen), Zdar disease (southern Czechoslovakia), Winton disease (New Zealand), Walking disease (West Coast of North America), danziekte (South Africa), and bottom disease (South Dakota). Despite much research, the etiology of this disease is still not fully understood (cf. Sec. 2.1.5.11.1.). KRAL [1922] and HERAN [1926] reported strongylosis as a cause of the cirrhosis; LUKES and CECG [1948, 1950] attributed it to the late stage of leptospirosis and to the effect of plant feeds or soil composition; HJÄRRE and CALSTRÖM to the heavy feeding of clover *(Trifolium hybridum);* STROH and ZIEGLER to autointoxication or the terminal stage of infectious anemia; and many authors such as REYNOLDS [1936], VANEK [1956] and BULL [1961] to chronic intoxication by various *Senecio* species. The disease is enzootic in character and occurs mostly in marshy or swampy regions. Here indiginous poisonous plants play the main causative role.

Pathogenesis. The development of anatomic changes depends upon the *route* by which the pathogenic agent has gained access to the liver. If the toxins are carried to the liver by the arterial blood, the lesions are confined mainly to the periphery of the lobules and the interstitial tissue, similar to a cirrhosis following inflammation of the bile ducts. If the toxins reach the liver with the venous blood by way of the intestinal tract, the lesions are mainly centrilobular. Parasites that have invaded the liver through the capsule cause an irregular destruction of hepatic tissue at various sites in the organ. In turn, toxic products released as a result of the parasitic invasion, gain access to other parts of the liver by way of the lymphatic vessels. Depending on the nature of the damage and the affinity of the individual hepatic tissue elements for the toxic products, either a primary atrophy of liver cells with compensatory hyperplasia of the connective tissue of the remaining, undamaged liver cells and bile ducts occurs, or a primary growth of mesenchymal tissue with a secondary, pressure-dependent degeneration or atrophy of hepatocytes occurs. In some cases both processes occur simultaneously from the outset of the disease. Occlusion of the many branches of the portal vein as a result of the advancing cirrhosis leads to congestion in the areas supplied by that vessel and an accumulation of exudate in the abdominal cavity. With simultaneous blockage of the bile ducts, cholestasis and icterus will develop. The consequences of a significant atrophy of hepatic cells are disturbances in the detoxifying function of the liver and metabolic derangements. The disturbances of digestion and absorption that appear at this time are attributable to venous congestion in the intestinal tract, liver and pancreas (decreased pancreatic secretion).

The breakdown of the hepatic barrier to toxins from the intestinal tract and the consequent metabolic disturbances enable toxic substances to gain access to the

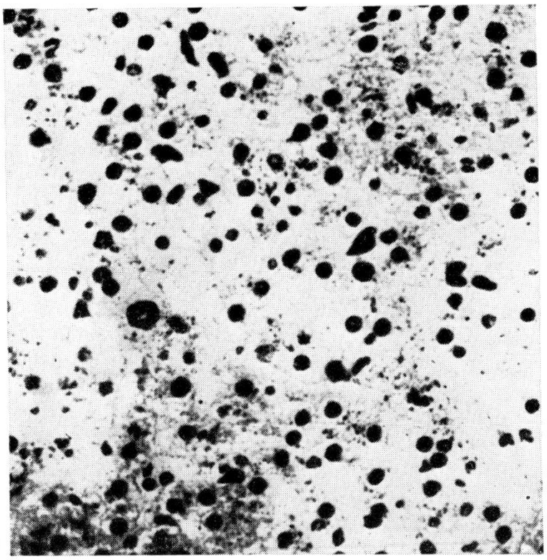
87

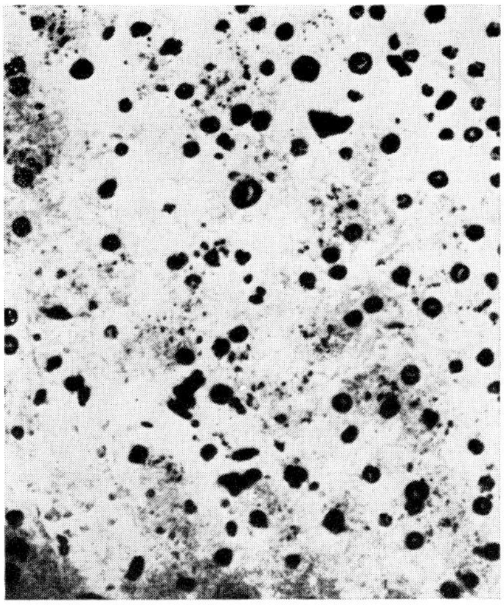
88

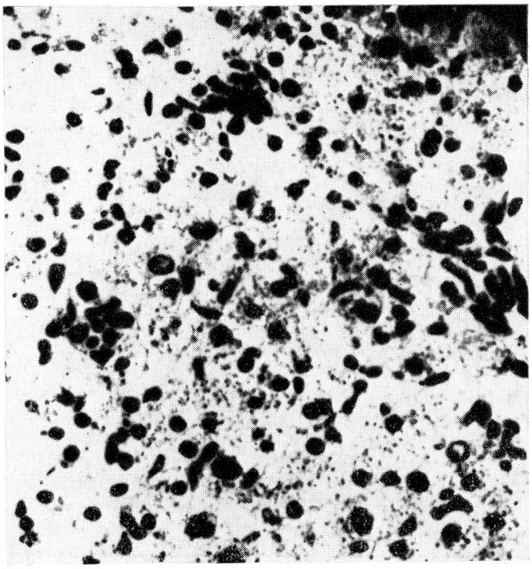
89

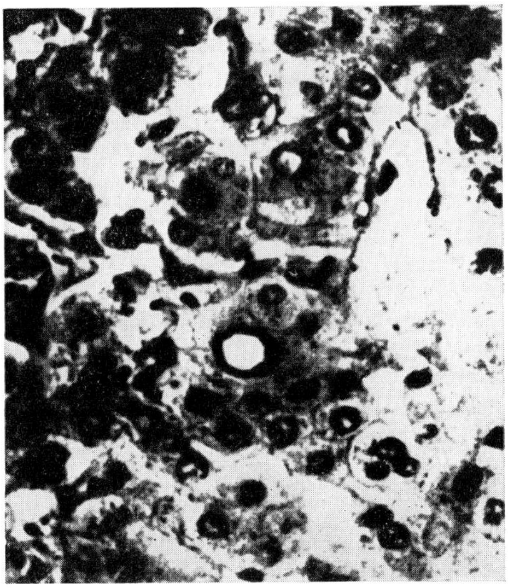
90

Fig. 2.1.5. — 87. Early stage of hepatic cirrhosis (biopsy specimen): karyomegaly and marked activation of reticuloendothelial cells [after KONRAD, 1968].

Fig. 2.1.5. — 88. Early stage of hepatic cirrhosis (biopsy specimen): bizarre nuclear forms in swollen endothelial cells of the sinusoid. Sporadic liver cells with large nuclei are seen [after KONRAD, 1968].

Fig. 2.1.5. — 89. Early stage of hepatic cirrhosis (biopsy specimen): The nuclei of some liver cells are slightly enlarged and vacuolated. Marked reticuloendothelial cell hyperplasia, small cellular aggregations. A meshwork of newly-formed reticular fibers tends to occur at these sites [after KONRAD, 1968].

Fig. 2.1.5. — 90. Terminal stage of hepatic cirrhosis: Detail of a highly magnified nucleus of a liver cell with a large vacuole. The activity of the endothelium of the hepatic sinusoid is clearly visible [after KONRAD, 1968].

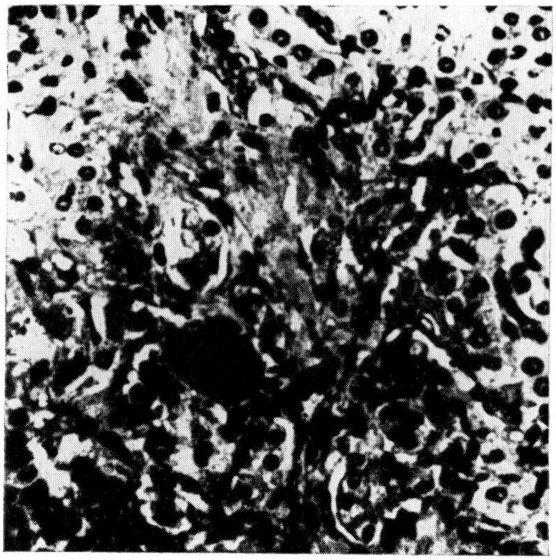

Fig. 2.1.5. — 91. Terminal stage of hepatic cirrhosis: The lobules are irregularly subdivided by fibrous tissue strands. The lobular architecture is completely disrupted [after KONRAD, 1968].

central nervous system. This leads to the degeneration of ganglion cells, changes in the Nissl bodies, degeneration of the myelin sheaths, and later to phagocytosis and proliferation of finely-granular glial cells, in which scar tissue is later observed [DOBBERSTEIN; HEIDEGGER].

Lesions. The following forms of hepatic cirrhosis may be distinguished from a morphologic standpoint: atrophic, hypertrophic, and an intermediate or atrophic-hypertrophic form (fatty cirrhosis).

Atrophic Cirrhosis (Laennec's Cirrhosis)

Atrophic cirrhosis is rarer in the horse than in the dog and pig. The liver is decreased in size and presents a finely or coarsely granular surface. The consistency is very firm, and the hepatic tissue is usually difficult to cut and crunches under the knife. It may also be covered with nodules that may be the size of a hen's egg. On the cut surface the lobules appear as small granules embedded in a pale-pink to gray connective tissue matrix. Atrophic cirrhosis is usually accompanied by ascites and by congestion of the portal circulation. There is little or no splenic enlargement, and icterus is usually mild or absent.

Hypertrophic Cirrhosis (Hanot's Hypertrophic Cirrhosis)

This form is characterized by a marked proliferation of interlobular and pericellular connective tissue. The liver is greatly enlarged and may reach a weight of 20 kg in large horses. The consistency is flabby to hard, the color yellow to yellow-green, and the surface smooth or finely granular. In the so-called regenerative form of Joest, the liver is very often coarsely granular or knobby. Hypertrophic cirrhosis is typical of Schweinberg disease and related or identical enzootic equine hepatic diseases. In these diseases DOBBERSTEIN distinguishes two types of cirrhosis according to the nature of the hepatic lesions: (1) a pericellular cirrhosis in which connective tissue proliferation and bile duct hypertrophy are predominant. Here the hepatocellular changes are confined at most to those of pressure atrophy, and inflammatory infiltration is minor; and (2) a cirrhosis with little or no connective tissue proliferation, the most salient features being regenerative changes or hypertrophy and regeneration of the liver cells and inflammatory cellular infiltration.

In some of the aforementioned diseases that are of the pericellular cirrhosis type, there is splenomegaly in addition to the hepatic enlargement. Icterus is frequently present. In other diseases of this type the spleen is unaffected, and jaundice is an inconsistent feature.

The second type of cirrhosis according to DOBBERSTEIN's classification displays an obvious relation to the reticuloendothelial system (RES). The spleen is unchanged. STROH and ZIEGLER consider this form to be typical of chronic, static anemia in horses.

Histologic Changes [after KONRAD]. The early stage of the disease is characterized by frequent appearance of large liver cells with large, sometimes vacuolated nuclei, and by a proliferation of the RES (megalocytosis, karyomegaly). Simultaneously the fibrous tissue thickens and spreads amongst the individual liver cells. At this point the integrity of liver function depends on the degree and extent of changes in the hepatic architecture. Later scarring develops, the disease process increases in severity, and in the terminal stage there is degeneration of the intercellular spaces (fig. 2.1.5. — 87 to — 91).

According to DOBBERSTEIN, the changes in the brain consist of a reduction in the ganglion cells, a degeneration of the myelin sheaths, a mobilization of the glial cells and a transformation of glia into granular and pale multinucleate cells.

Laboratory Diagnosis [after SOVA].
Hematologic Studies:

	Diffuse hepatic cirrhosis			Normal values		
	n	$\bar{x}$	s	n	$\bar{x}$	s
Erythrocyte sedimentation [WESTERGREN]						
5 min	28	12	11	200	3.7	3.6
10 min	28	38	26	200	14.7	8.3
15 min	28	68	27	200	33.5	24.0
30 min	28	107	19	200	69.3	36.9
24 h	28	133	8	200	126.0	33.5
Erythrocytes (10^{12}/l)	29	7.71	0.926	200	8.537	1.553
Leukocytes (10^9/l)	29	9.06	2.98	200	8.36	1.55
Hemoglobin (g/dl)	29	9.6	1.1	200	10.2	1.7
Hematocrit	21	3.7	0.4	200	4.1	0.7
Differential blood count						
Monocytes %	29	1.7	1.5	200	1.5	0.2
Lymphocytes %	29	14.7	7.0	200	37.0	10.6
Eosinophils %	29	2.2	2.8	200	4.6	2.9
Basophils %	29	0.5	0.8	200	0.26	0.15
Segmented neutrophils %	29	78.5	9.4	200	54.6	10.3
Nonsegmented neutrophils %	29	1.6	1.5	200	1.3	1.1

The results show that the ESR is increased and is correlated with the increase in the γ-globulin fraction. The red blood count, hemoglobin level and hematocrit are in the normal range or slightly subnormal. The leukocyte count is in the high-normal range. The relative neutrophilia, lymphopenia and eosinopenia are marked, however.

Serum Proteins (See Hepatitis for normal values):

	Diffuse hepatic cirrhosis		
	n	x̄	s
Total protein (g %)	21	8.1	0.6
Paper electrophoresis			
Albumins %	20	34.2	5.1
Globulins %			
α	20	20.6	3.8
β	20	15.5	2.9
γ	20	30.5	6.5
Mucoproteins (mg % tyrosine)	6	1.6	0.4
Mucoproteins (normal)	16	1.4	0.2

The total protein values are somewhat higher than in normal horses. They agree with the values reported by Konrad [1959] and Hudacek [1960]. Forenbacher [1957] indicates subnormal values for horses.

Electrophoresis reveals a marked gammaglobulinemia.

Turbidity and flocculation tests: Turbidity and flocculation tests are of little or no value in the diagnosis of hepatic cirrhosis. The only significant abnormality is a right shift in the Weltmann coagulation band.

	n	Result	
Weltmann reaction	28	tube 7	1 (4 %)
		8	5 (18 %)
		9	16 (57 %)
		10	6 (21 %)

The results of the *bilirubin* determination are also ambiguous.

Glucose Tolerance Test:

	Diffuse hepatic cirrhosis	
	n	Glycemia in mmol/l
0.25 g glucose in 40 % solution per kg BW	11	
fasting		4.83
30 min		7.44
90 min		5.83
120 min		4.55
270 min		5.44

Characteristic in this test are the appearance of hyperglycemia after 30 minutes and a gradual return to the fasting level after 90 minutes.

Enzymes:

	Diffuse hepatic cirrhosis		
	n	x̄	s
Serum glutamic oxaloacetic transaminase SGOT (ASAT) (μkat/l[1])	14	4.82	0.88
Serum glutamic pyruvic transaminase SGPT (μkat/l)	19	0.24	0.16
Alkaline phosphatase (μkat/l)	14	0.38	0.14
Acid phosphatase (μkat/l)	14	0.025	0.018

[1] Conversion: E/l × 0.01667 = μkat/l; μkat/l × 60.0 = E/l.

Of the enzymes presented, SGOT (ASAT) and alkaline phosphatase show especially high activities, and SGPT shows a low activity.

Lipoids[1]:

	Diffuse hepatic cirrhosis		
	n	x̄	s
Total cholesterol (mmol/l)	21	3.28	1.04
Free cholesterol (mmol/l)	15	1.39	0.30
Esterified cholesterol (mmol/l)	15	1.99	0.83
Total esterified fatty acids (mmol/l)	14	137.5	78.5
Phospholipids (mmol/l)	15	2.05	0.94

In the determination of serum lipids, special attention should be given to the rise of free cholesterol and the fall of the total esterified fatty acids. Some elevation of the total cholesterol and phospholipids is also present.

The results of the various laboratory investigations indicate that the following findings are of significance in the diagnosis of hepatic cirrhosis: elevation of the ESR, relative neutrophilia, lymphopenia and eosinopenia, gammaglobulinemia and a negligible elevation of total and direct bilirubin. In addition there is hyperglycemia and delayed return to normal in glucose tolerance test, significant SGOT (ASAT) and alkaline phosphatase activity, rise of total cholesterol, free cholesterol and phospholipids, and fall of total esterified fatty acids.

Treatment. The disease process is irreversible once clinical signs of the cirrhosis have appeared, and so treatment is useless in the vast majority of cases. If it is nevertheless decided to treat the condition, the most that can be hoped for is an arrest of further deterioration.

Diet is of particular importance. Icterus is treated by administering choleretics, such as Carlsbad salt in a dose of 25—100 [sic], and glucocorticoid preparations as described under the treatment of hepatitis. An advantage of glucocorticoids is that they may retard the process of connective tissue formation. Recently testosterone has found use in human medicine by virtue of its positive influence on hepatocellular function and its diuretic action. Lipotropic substances and preparations mentioned in the context of hepatitis therapy are always useful.

In endemic areas, periodic needle biopsies of the liver provide the best means of early diagnosis.

[1] Conversion for cholesterol: mg% × 0.0259 = mmol/l; mmol/l × 38.66 = mg%;
for phospholipids: mg/100 ml × 0.01292 = mmol/l; mmol/l × 77.4 = mg%.

2.1.5.11.3. Parasitic Liver Diseases

A number of parasites whose epizootiology, symptoms, diagnosis, treatment and prophylaxis are reviewed in Sec. 2.3. can invade the liver and produce lesions.

Fascioliasis (cf. Sec. 2.3.2.1.)
Fascioliasis, or liver fluke disease, is an acute, necrotizing disease of the hepatic parenchyma resulting from the migration of young liver flukes and from chronic inflammation caused by the residence of mature flukes in the bile ducts. Young flukes can gain access to the liver by way of the portal vein or through the peritoneal cavity. They initially migrate through the intestinal wall.

Dicroceliasis (cf. Sec. 2.3.2.2.)
Unlike the liver fluke, the 'lancet' fluke exists almost exclusively on warm, dry meadows and pastures that are rich in calcium. Their eggs tolerate feces, dung and liquid manure as well as the effects of frost and dryness for a year or more. In fresh water they remain infective for up to 80 days. *Dicrocoelium* flukes are an incidental finding in the horse.

Hydatidosis (cf. Sec. 2.3.2.4.)
Hydatidosis, or infection with tapeworms of the genus *Echinococcus*, is much less common in horses than in ruminants and swine. According to LICHTENBERG, 95.5 % of cases affect the liver and 5.5 % the lungs. Infestation with the parasites initiates a well demarcated inflammatory reaction that forms a host capsule (adventitious membrane) about the parasite. This is treated as a foreign body by the host. If these primary foci gain entry to the blood vessels, they can lead to a secondary hydatidosis of the liver or other organs. In these cases, pieces of the capsule, tapeworm heads or daughter cysts can act as emboli. Dislodged cystic material may seed the hydatidosis to the peritoneum. The cysts produce clinical symptoms only if the infestation is very heavy.

Strongylosis (cf. Sec. 2.3.2.10.)
All strongyle species pass through several larval stages during their life cycle. The horse is infected by the 3rd-stage larvae, known also as 'infective larvae'. In the digestive tract they form submucosal or subserosal nodules in the wall of the cecum and molt after 11 days to become 4th-stage larvae. Some of these larvae enter the peritoneal cavity, through which migration to the liver is possible (cf. Sec. 2.3.).

Ascariasis (see Sec. 2.3.2.8.)

Leishmaniasis
Horses become infected with the protozoan *Leishmania donovani* when they are bitten by the fly *Phlebotomus papapatasi*, the intermediate host of this organism. The parasites live in the endothelium of the blood and lymph vessels and various parenchymal organs. They are round or oval and measure 2—4.5 μm in size. Gross changes in infected horses include enlargements of the liver, spleen and lymph nodes. The disease known as 'kala-azar' occurs mainly in large parts of Asia, the Mediterranian, in Africa and in South America. Heavy infestations lead to emaciation with atrophy of the bone marrow, conjunctivitis and keratitis. Ascites and hindquarter paralysis may also appear.

Linguatuliasis

Infection results from ingesting the eggs of the tongueworm, *Linguatula serrata*. The horse serves as an intermediate host. The 1st-stage larvae develop in the equine intestinal tract. They are equipped with two pairs of hook-like limbs and a boring apparatus which they use to penetrate the intestinal wall and travel with the blood and lymph to the lymph nodes, lungs, kidneys and other organs. They travel particularly to the liver, where they become encapsulated in the capillary system. The larvae form small, nodular, glassy, grayish-white foci that are most frequently found beneath the hepatic capsule and serous surfaces. They cause subcapsular hematomata and local fibrinous inflammation of the serous capsule (perihepatitis).

Other intermediate hosts for this parasite are the sheep, goat, and in rare cases man. The final host is the dog.

References

ALLEN, B. V.; ARCHER, R. K.: A blood coagulation test (Normotest) as another measure of liver function in the horse. Equine vet. J. *4:* 217 (1972).

BLAKELY, J. A.: An unusual case of neonatal-jaundice in a thoroughbred foal. New Zealand vet. J. *21:* 6, 123 (1973).

BLAZEK, K.; KONRAD, J.: Beitrag zur Ermittlung von Frühstadien der Zdárer Pferdekrankheit. Arch. exp. Vet.-Med. *20:* 865 (1966).

BULL, L. B.: Liver disease in livestock from intake of hepatotoxic substances. Austral. vet. J. *37:* 126 (1961).

CAMERON, TH. W. M.: The parasites of domestic animals (Adam & Charles Black, London 1951).

CARGILL, C. F.; SHIELDS, R. P.: Plasma arginase as a liver function test. J. comparat. Pathology *81:* 447 (1971).

CARPER, H. A.: The laboratory diagnosis of liver disease in the horse and cow. Amer. J. vet. clin. Path. *1:* 77 (1967).

CORNELIUS, C. E.; GARMURI, G.; GRONWELL, R.; RHODE, E. A.: Preliminary studies on experimental hyperbilirubinemia and hepatic coma in the horse. Cornell Vet. *55:* 110 (1965).

DAHME, E.; WEISS, E.: Podstawy szczegołowej anatomii patologicznej zwierzat domowych. P.W.R.iL., Warszawa 1973.

DZIAŁOSZYNSKI, L.; MACIEJEWSKA, M.: Frakcje białkowe surowicy krwi konskiej. Med. Weteryn. *13:* 173 (1957).

EIKMEIER, H.: Untersuchungen über den Serumbilirubinspiegel des Pferdes. Berliner Münchener tierärztl. Wschr. *72:* 48 (1959a).

EIKMEIER, H.: Untersuchungen über den Serumbilirubinspiegel des Pferdes. Berliner Münchener tierärztl. Wschr. *72:* 446 (1959b).

FORD, E. J. H.: Clinical aspects of ragwort poisoning in horses. Vet. Annual *14:* 86 (1973).

FORD, E. J. H.; GOPINATH, C.: The excretion of phylloerythrin and bilirubin by the horse. Res. Vet. Sci. *16:* 168 (1974).

FOWLER, M. E.: The clinical syndrome of liver disease in the horse. Proc. 10th Amer. Assoc. Equine Pract. Conv., Denver (1964), p. 113.

FOWLER, M. E.: Clinical manifestations of primary hepatic insufficiency in the horses. J. Amer. vet. med. Assoc. *147:* 55 (1965).

FREEDLAND, R. A.; HJERPE, C. A.; CORNELIUS, C. E.: Comparative studies on plasma enzyme activities in experimental hepatic necrosis in the horse. Res. vet. Sci. *6:* 18 (1965).

GERBER, H.: Aktivitätsbestimmungen von Serumenzymen in der Veterinärmedizin. Schweiz. Archiv Tierheilk. I. Inhaltsbericht. *105:* 529 (1963); II. Klinische Anwendung. *106:* 85 (1964); III. Eigene Untersuchungen bei Pferden

a) Alkalische Serumphosphatase (SAP). *106:* 354 (1964).
b) Bestimmungen der GOT-, GPT- und GPK-Aktivitäten in einigen Organen des Pferdes als Grundlage für die klinische Verwendung von Serumenzym-Aktivitätsbestimmungen. *106:* 410 (1964).
c) Bestimmung der SGOT-, SGPT- und SCPK-Aktivität bei Myopathien und Cardiopathien des Pferdes. *106:* 478 (1964).
d) Bestimmung der LDH-, MDH-, GLDH-, ALD- und der α-Amylase-Aktivität in einigen Organen des Pferdes als Grundlage für klinische Interpretation von Serumenzym-Aktivitätsbestimmungen. *107:* 626 (1965).
e) Serum-Enzymmuster bei paralytischer Myoglobinämie des Pferdes. *107:* 685 (1965).
f) LDH-Isoenzyme in einigen Organen und im Serum kranker und gesunder Pferde. *108:* 33 (1966).

Grassnickel, W.: Zur Bilirubinspiegelbestimmung und seiner Auswertung beim Pferde. Berliner Münchener tierärztl. Wschr. *72:* 443 (1959).

Hejłasz, Z.; Janiak, T.: Skutecznośc chloromycetyny w leczeniu autointoksykacji pokarmowych u koni. Med. Weteryn. *19:* 92 (1963).

Homolka, J.: Diagnostyka biochemiczna. P.Z.W.iL., Warszawa 1961.

Hooper, P. T.: Spongy degeneration in the brain in reaction to hepatic disease and ammonia toxicity in domestic animals. Vet. Res. *90:* 37 (1972).

Hutyra, F.; Marek, J.; Manninger, R.; Mócsy, J.: Szczegołowa patologia i terapia chorob zwierzat. II. tom. P.W.R.iL., Warszawa 1962.

Konrad, J.: Hämatologische Studien bei der Cirrhosis hepatis fasciolosa bovum im Vergleich zur Zdárer Leberzirrhose der Pferde. Tierärztl. Umschau *23:* 108 (1968a).

Konrad, J.: Dynamik der Eiweissfraktionen des Blutserums bei akuten Leberkrankheiten des Pferdes. Zbl. Vet.-Med. R. A. *15:* 123, 134 (1968b).

Konrad, J.: Die Bilirubinämie im Verlaufe der Leberzirrhose der Pferde. Wien. Tierärztl. Mschr. *55:* 84 (1968c).

Konrad, J.: Ergebnisse der Studien über das sogenannte Anfangsstadium und die Pathogenese der Zdárer Krankheit (Cirrhosis hepatis diffusa). Dtsch. Tierärztl. Wschr. *75:* 40 (1968d).

Kubicki, St.: Choroby watroby i dróg zółciowych. P.Z.W.iL., Warszawa 1966.

Markiewicz, K.: Badania czynności watroby u koni uzywanych do produkcji surowic odpornościowych. Polskie Archiv Weteryn. *8:* 651 (1965).

Markiewicz, K.: Aktywnośé aminotransferazy asparaginowej i alaninowej oraz esterazy cholinowej nieswoistej w ocenie stanu czynnościowego watroby u koni. Med. Weteryn. *23:* 343 (1967).

McCollum, W. H.: Comments on serum hepatitis in the horse. J. Amer. vet. med. Assoc. *155:* 410 (1969).

McGuire, T. C.; Poppie, M. J.; Banks, K. L.: Combined (B- and T-lymphocyte immunodeficiency: a fatal genetic disease in Arabian foals. J. Amer. vet. med. Assoc. *164:* 70 (1974).

Mócsy, J.: Weterynaryjna diagnostyka kliniczna. Wyd. II. P.W.R.iL., Warszawa 1971.

Nieberle, K.; Cohrs, P.: Lehrbuch der speziellen pathologischen Anatomie der Haustiere, 5. Aufl. (VEB Gustav Fischer Verlag, Jena 1975).

Panciera, R. J.: Serum hepatitis in the horse. J. Amer. vet. med. Assoc. *155:* 408 (1969).

Pinkiewicz, E.; Grzebuła, S.; Rubaj, B.: Badania nad pokarmowa dystrofia mieśni u zrebiat. I. Kliniczny oraz anatomo-histologiczny obraz choroby. Biuletyn V Zjazdu P.T.N.W., Olsztyn, 12—14. IX. 1974, str. 114—115.

Preger, S. N.; Albickaja, N. D.: Diagnostika i leczenje gepatita u łoszadiej-producentow. Weterinarija (Moskva) *12:* 74 (1971).

Pribyl, S.: Choroby młodych zwierzat gospodarskich. P.W.R.iL., Warszawa 1967.

Reksa, M.: Sprzezone badania czynności watroby w autointoksykacjach pokarmowych u koni. Dyssertacja doktorska, Wrocław (1968).

Reynolds, A. J. S.: Ragwort poisoning in Pembrokeshire. Vet. Rec. *48:* 1407 (1936).

Rossow, N.; Urbaneck, D.: Untersuchungen zur Beurteilung des Verlaufes von Leberparenchymschäden. Mh. Vet.-Med. *13:* 175 (1962).

Sova, Z.: Die von Domynsky modifizierte Probe nach Gros und ihre Verwendbarkeit in der Diagnostik der Hepatopathien bei Pferden. Arch. exp. Vet.-Med. *17:* 703 (1963a).

Sova, Z.: Über die Eignung der Reaktion nach Takata zur Diagnostik der Hepatopathien bei Pferden. Arch. exp. Vet.-Med. *17:* 709 (1963b).

Sova, Z.: Die Verwendbarkeit des Kupferazetattests in der Veterinärmedizin bei Pferden mit besonderer Berücksichtigung der Diagnostik der Hepatopathien. Dtsch. Tierärztl. Wschr. *70:* 357 (1963c).

Sova, Z.: Die Trübungsreaktion nach Hejda bei gesunden, leberkranken und an anderen Krankheiten leidenden Pferden. Mh. Vet.-Med. *18:* 416 (1963d).

Sova, Z.: Die Blutkörpersenkungsreaktion in der Diagnostik der Leberkrankheiten des Pferdes. Zbl. Vet.-Med. R. A. *10:* 584 (1963e).

Sova, Z.: Die Verwendung der Trübungsreaktion mit Kadmiumsulfat in der internen Veterinärmedizin mit besonderer Berücksichtigung der Diagnostik der Hepatopathien bei Pferden. Schweiz. Archiv Tierheilk. *105:* 165 (1963f).

Sova, Z.: Die Reaktion nach Weltmann bei inneren Krankheiten der Pferde mit besonderer Berücksichtigung der Diagnostik der Hepatopathien. Wiener Tierärztl. Mschr. *50:* 761 (1963g).

Sova, Z.: Die Ermittlung des Gesamtproteins im Pferdeserum bei der Diagnostik der Leberkrankheiten. Arch. exp. Vet.-Med. *18:* 861 (1964a).

Sova, Z.: Die Bedeutung der Ermittlung der Bilirubinämie für die Diagnostik der Hepatopathien bei Pferden. Zbl. Vet.-Med. R. A. *11:* 760 (1964b).

Sova, Z.: Das hämatologische und biochemische Bild des Versagens der Leber bei Pferden im Endstadium der Zdárer Krankheit (Fibrosis hepatis diffusa). Zbl. Vet.-Med. R. A. *12:* 653 (1965a).

Sova, Z.: Die Leberbiopsie beim Pferd, ihre Technik, Ergebnisse und Bedeutung in der Labordiagnostik der Hepatopathien. Prakt. Tierarzt *46:* 447 (1965b).

Sova, Z.: Die Leberbiopsie beim Pferd, ihre Technik, Ergebnisse und Bedeutung in der Labordiagnostik der Hepatopathien. Prakt. Tierarzt *46:* 498 (1965c).

Sova, Z.: Zehnjährige Erfahrungen in der Diagnostik akuter Hepatitiden und akuter Hepatose bei Pferden. Prakt. Tierarzt *48:* 351, 452 (1968).

Sova, Z.: Laborbefunde bei Pferden mit diffuser Lebernekrose und Leberkoma. Prakt. Tierarzt *50:* 311 (1969).

Sova, Z.; Jicha, J.: Die Aktivität der Serumglutaminoxalessigsäure- und Serumglutamin-Brenztraubensäure-Transaminase in der Diagnostik der Leberkrankheiten des Pferdes. Zbl. Vet.-Med. R. A. *10:* 295 (1963a).

Sova, Z.; Jicha, J.: Die Aktivität der Apfelsäure- (MDH-), Milchsäure- (LDH-) und Sorbitdehydrogenase (SDH) im Serum gesunder und leberkranker Pferde. Zbl. Vet.-Med. R. A. *10:* 305 (1963b).

Sova, Z.; Jicha, J.: Die Ermittlung der Aktivität der alkalischen und sauren Phosphatase in der Diagnostik der Hepatopathien bei Pferden. Zbl. Vet.-Med. R. A. *10:* 314 (1963c).

Sova, Z.; Jicha, J.: Die Ermittlung des Gesamtcholesterols (TCH), des veresterten Cholesterols (FCH), der Phospholipide (PL) und der gesamten veresterten Fettsäuren in der Diagnostik der Hepatopathien bei Pferden. Zbl. Vet.-Med. R. A. *11:* 461 (1964).

Sova, Z.; Jicha, J.; Komarek, J.: Die hämatologischen und biochemischen Normalwerte beim Pferd. Berliner Münchener tierärztl. Wschr. *78:* 144 (1965).

Sova, Z.; Komarek, J.: Die Bromsulphalein-Leberfunktionstests beim Pferd. I. Mitt. Die direkte Bestimmung der Farbstoffretention. Zbl. Vet.-Med. R. A. *11:* 448 (1964a).

Sova, Z.; Komarek, J.: Der Bromsulphalein-Leberfunktionstest beim Pferd. II. Mitt. Indirekte Bestimmung der Eliminationswerte bei gesunden und kranken Pferden. Zbl. Vet.-Med. R. A. *11:* 502 (1964b).

Sova, Z.; Komarek, J.: Die Papierelektrophorese in der Diagnostik inneren Krankheiten bei Pferden mit besonderer Berücksichtigung der Hepatopathien. Arch. exp. Vet.-Med. *18:* 869 (1964c).

Stankiewicz, W.: Hematologia Weterynaryjna. P.W.R.iL., Warszawa 1973.

Stöckl, W.: Elektrophoretische Serumuntersuchungen bei Haustieren unter normalen Bedingungen und nach Antigenzufuhr. (Mit einem Beitrag über die Wirkungsweise von Adsorbatvaccinen.) Wiener Tierärztl. Msch. *43:* 150 (1956a).

IV. Untersuchungen über das normale Verhalten der Serumproteine bei Pferd, Rind, Schwein, Schaf und Huhn. *43:* 226 (1956b).

VI. Eiweißchemische Serumuntersuchungen nach Antigenzufuhr bei Haustieren. *43:* 402 (1956c).

TENNANT, B. U.; EVANS, C. D.; KANEKO, J.; SCHALM, I. W.: Intravascular hemolysis associated with hepatic failure in the horse. California Vet. *27:* 15 (1972).
TENNANT, B. U.; EVANS, C. D.; SCHWARTZ, L. W.; GRIBBLE, D. H.; KANEKO, J. J.: Equine hepatic insufficiency. Veterinary Clinics of North America *3:* 279 (1973).
THOMA, H.: Blutgerinnungsstörungen bei Pferd und Hund und deren Beeinflussung durch unspezifische Therapie. Vet.-med. Diss., München (1973).
THOMSETT, L. R.: Acute hepatic failure in the horse. Equine Vet. J. *3:* 15 (1971).
VESSELINOVITCH, S. D.: The analysis of serum proteins of domestic animals by filterpaper electrophoreses. Cornell Vet. *49:* 82 (1959).
WEBER, M.: Untersuchungen über die Blutgerinnung bei Pferd und Hund. Retraktion, Faktor II, V, VII, Hitzefibrin, Trombocytenzahl. Vet.-med. Diss., München (1969).
WÜRZNER, P.; LEEMANN, W.; WEBER, H.: Die l-Phosphofructaldolaseaktivität beim akuten Leberschaden des Pferdes. Zbl. Vet.-Med. R. A. *14:* 208 (1967).
WUNDERLICH, H.; PRÖSCH, CH.: Ikterus, Hyperbilirubinämie und Leberfunktion bei Darmerkrankungen der Pferde. Mh. Vet.-Med. *18:* 527 (1963).
ZAPRZAŁ, K.: Kaminie zółciowe u konia. Med. Weteryn. *25:* 743 (1969).
ZELLER, R.; KELLER, H.: Icterus, Bilirubinämie und über Leberfunktion bei Darmerkrankungen der Pferde. Mh. Vet.-Med. *19:* 465 (1964).

2.1.6. Diseases of the Urinary System

Diseases of the kidneys and urinary tract are infrequently diagnosed in the horse. They hardly ever occur as separate entities. Involvement of the kidneys is a feature of many infectious diseases, intoxications, etc. Unfortunately, secondary renal disease produces few specific symptoms, and so it usually goes unrecognized or is masked by the symptoms of the underlying disease. Such significant extrarenal signs as edema formation, renovascular hypertension and left ventricular hypertrophy are seldom observed in horses, or their relation to possible renal disease is not appreciated. The main diagnostic tool is urinalysis, which must take into account the peculiarities of the equine urine (turbidity and high viscosity).

2.1.6.1. Diseases of the Kidney

2.1.6.1.1. Nephritis

Inflammations of the kidneys encompass a group of purulent and nonpurulent renal diseases that may be diffuse or focal in extent and may take an acute or chronic course. Nephritis is of minor importance in the horse as compared to other species. It occurs almost exclusively as a result of infectious or other systemic diseases.

Symptoms. In *acute diffuse nephritis* there are marked systemic signs with fever, depression and anorexia. Affected horses frequently exhibit mild signs of unrest that are reminiscent of colic, and they are reluctant to move (stiff gait). Tenderness and enlargement of the kidney are frequently noted on rectal examination.

The pulse rate is often elevated. The 2nd heart sound may be accentuated or split. Edema of the ventral abdomen is occasionally present. Less urine is voided than normal, even though the animal may have an increased desire to urinate.

The urine itself has a high density and contains varying amounts of protein and cellular constituents — red cells, renal epithelial cells and casts. The urea content of the blood (BUN) is significantly increased only in severe cases. Aside from the urinary findings, the clinical manifestations of the disease are often vague and nonspecific. This applies in particular to *acute focal nephritis*, which is also characterized by a less remarkable urinary sediment and a very mild proteinuria.

The course of *chronic nephritis* is subtle. The most salient features are emaciation over a period of weeks or months and constant proteinuria in the absence of significant cellular constituents. The clinical picture of chronic cardiac failure may emerge as the disease progresses.

Purulent nephritis or *renal abscesses* occur mainly in younger horses and foals. The symptoms may be those of an acute nephritis but tend to go unnoticed in the development of the primary infectious disease. The urine may contain large concentrations of leukocytes, epithelial cells and casts as well as bacteria. In the presence of a renal abscess, the urine is changed only if the process has invaded the urinary tract. In most cases renal abscesses are not detected until necropsy.

Pyelonephritis is of no practical importance in horses.

Etiology and Pathogenesis. The kidneys, being the most important excretory organs, are susceptible to damage by various microorganisms and their products during the course of infectious diseases. Toxic substances and metabolic products can also evoke an inflammatory reaction, which in many cases cannot be strictly differentiated from degenerative change.

Sensitization with *Streptococci spp.* and allergens is of special importance in the pathogenesis of glomerulonephritis. Antigen-antibody reactions can produce lesions of the renal parenchyma that give rise to a chronic inflammation.

Not infrequently, renal abscesses arise from a metastasis in strangles. The purulent nephritis that occurs in foal septicemia is caused by *Actinobacillus equuli*. By contrast, ascending renal inflammations with *Corynebacterium renale* and other organisms are rare in horses.

The *differentiation* of acute and chronic, purulent and nonpurulent nephritides from one another and from nephrosis often proves difficult. Diseases of the urinary tract and genital system can be excluded with certainty on the basis of the history, clinical manifestations and especially the urinary findings.

Diagnosis. Because the clinical manifestations are often subtle and nonspecific or are masked by the primary disease, a urinanalysis should be performed whenever nephritis is suspected, especially if the rectal examination demonstrates renal tenderness or enlargement. Proteinuria, cylindruria, and the presence of varying amounts of red cells, white cells and renal epithelial cells are the principal changes. Determination of the BUN gives information on the functional state of the kidneys and the degree of any renal failure that has developed.

Prognosis. Acute diffuse inflammation with evidence of anuria usually progresses to death in 1—2 weeks. The other forms of nephritis also carry an unfavorable prognosis as far as a complete recovery is concerned. Chronic as well as purulent nephritides may persist for months, during which time the animal's exercise ability is impaired, and its condition will deteriorate if it is forced to do work.

Treatment. Treatment centers on the primary illness. If the disease has a bacterial etiology, it is controlled with large doses of a suitable antibiotic. This is combined with rest and diet change. In acute cases water intake should be restricted, and vitamin- and carbohydrate-rich feeds should be offered. Intravenous infusion of glucose solutions with ascorbic acid as well as calcium chloride solutions may be beneficial.

Hydrochlorothiazide may be administered to promote diuresis, but because renal edema is rarely observed, it is often more important to administer a cardiac stimulant such as strophanthin at the first sign of cardiopathy.

Glucocorticoids are also used in combination with antibiotics.

2.1.6.1.2. Nephrosis

Definition. Nephrosis is a degeneration of the kidney involving metabolic disturbances of the renal parenchyma that mainly affect the tubule cells, leading to their degeneration and necrosis. Nephrosis generally occurs secondarily to other diseases that lead to renal damage from endogenous or exogenous toxic substances. The degeneration may be acute or chronic.

Symptoms. The signs of nephrosis usually are obscured by those of the primary disease.

The major changes are demonstrable by urinalysis. Marked proteinuria is present, especially in acute cases. The urinary sediment contains degenerated epithelial cells as well as hyaline and epithelial casts.

If renal damage is severe and long-standing, signs appear that are similar to the nephrotic syndrome in man: a fall of the serum proteins to 4 or even 3 g/100 ml, and extensive edema formation. Our own observations confirm that hypochromic anemia is consistently present. On the other hand, pronounced uremia is rarely seen. Elevated BUN levels are most frequently observed in cases of paralytic myoglobinuria (tying-up syndrome). The blood lipid content and chloride concentration are markedly elevated in nephrosis [Chrustalev, 1976].

Etiology and Pathogenesis. Degeneration of the kidney is usually the result of toxic damage to the renal parenchyma. The causes include poisonings with heavy metals (mercury, bismuth, copper), arsenic, phosphorus, chlorinated hydrocarbons and phenothiazine, as well as the ingestion of plants that contain toxic compounds, such as oak leaves (our observations). Similar damage can be caused by bacterial toxins and by autointoxication associated with gastrointestinal disease. Severe degenerative changes of the kidney are commonly associated with paralytic myoglobinuria and hemolytic anemias.

A special form is amyloid nephrosis, in which amyloid, an endogenous antibody globulin, is deposited in the renal tissue. Amyloidosis of this type, combined with involvement of other organs (liver, spleen), is encountered in horses used for commercial serum production as well as in chronic infectious diseases.

Diagnosis can be a difficult matter, owing to the secondary nature of the disease. Often nephrosis is detected only through a routine urinanalysis.

The *differential diagnosis* of renal inflammation is seldom possible, because degenerative damage frequently initiates inflammatory change.

The *prognosis* depends on the character of the primary disease and the degree of renal damage. Mild cases recover without special treatment when the primary condition is resolved. If extensive necrotic damage has occurred, the prognosis is unfavorable to poor.

Treatment. Main emphasis is on identifying the causal toxin and administering the appropriate treatment. It is vital that the functional state of the kidneys be closely watched. With large protein losses a high-protein feed should be provided, and water intake should not be restricted. The water, electrolyte and acid-base balance should be regularly checked and corrected as needed by infusions or by administering diuretics or hormone preparations (see Nephritis).

2.1.6.2. Diseases of the Bladder

2.1.6.2.1. Cystitis

Cystitis is an acute or chronic, superficial or deep inflammation of the mucosa of the urinary bladder. It occurs only sporadically in the horse, usually as a sequel to other pathologic conditions of the urinary system. However, NATSCHEFF [1957] mentions an asymptomatic, catarrhal cystitis that occurs with some frequency in the horse. There are also reports from Australia on a usually fatal bladder inflammation in horses that has assumed epizootic-like proportions [HOOPER, 1968].

Symptoms. The disease is observed more frequently in mares than in stallions or geldings. Acute cases are characterized by frequent, painful urination (pollakiuria, stranguria). Although the flow of urine is greatly restricted, and usually only drops are voided, the horse may continue to stand in a urinating posture for some time after the flow has ceased. Mild or even severe colicky signs may be exhibited during this time.

The bladder is usually found to be empty and tender on rectal examination.

Blood, mucus or shreds of pus often will be evident on gross examination of the urine. The sediment is large in volume and consists of leukocytes, squamous cells from the various layers of the bladder wall, as well as triple phosphate crystals and bacteria.

In chronic cases the abnormalities tend to be less marked than in acute cystitis. The frequent dribbling of urine leads to discoloration of the hair, hair loss, and inflammation of skin areas that come in contact with the urine. But most chronic cases show no obvious clinical signs and can be recognized only by an increase in urinary sediment, which consists mainly of squamous epithelial cells.

Etiology and Pathogenesis. Primary cystitis is reported only in horses that graze on Sudan grass. Mechanical irritation associated with urolithiasis or catheterization of the bladder is the principal cause of cystitis. Moreover, inflammations of the vagina or uterus can sometimes spread to involve the bladder.

The inflammation is perpetuated by *Escherichia coli*, *Pseudomonas aeruginosa*, streptococci, staphylococci and other organisms that reach the bladder from various sources (introduced from the outside, hematogenous, lymphogenous, descending). *E. coli* in particular is responsible for breaking down the urea contained in the bladder urine into ammonia. This ammonia exacerbates the inflammation and promotes further bacterial invasion; also, this highly toxic product is absorbed to some degree by the bladder wall, which ordinarily is impermeable to urinary constituents.

Differential Diagnosis. Cystitis must be differentiated from urolithiasis and paralysis of the bladder, which are coexisting conditions and predispose to cystitis.

Diagnosis. The animal's behavior during urination, the palpatory findings and the results of the urinalysis form the basis for diagnosis. In acute cystitis the urine is nearly always alkaline, very turbid, and has an ammonia smell. The sediment is increased in volume and contains squamous cells, erythrocytes and leukocytes. Proteinuria is also present. In chronic cases the urine changes usually are limited to an increased cellular content.

Prognosis. If the predisposing cause can be removed and the infection controlled, acute cases can recover in 1 to 2 weeks, and marked improvement usually is noted within a few days. Chronic cases and deep inflammation, on the other hand, can be highly refractory to treatment.

Treatment. Besides treating the primary condition, it is necessary to administer a prolonged course of systemic antibiotics, having first cultured the midstream urine to identify the pathogen and determine its drug sensitivity. Treatment is supported by increasing the fluid intake and giving warm enemas or vaginal irrigation as needed.

Though popular, the urinary antiseptic hexamethylenetetramine (10.0—15.0 g) should not be overrated in its effect, for an acidic milieu must be present before it can liberate formaldehyde and become effective. Irrigation of the bladder with antiseptic solutions is of little value!

2.1.6.2.2. Paralysis of the Bladder

Paralysis of the bladder is marked by an inability to hold the urine or empty the bladder voluntarily.

Symptoms. With overstretching of the detrusor muscle of the bladder, the fibers lose some or all of their contractile ability. The result is retention of urine with increasing fullness of the bladder, leading to unrest and unsuccessful attempts at urination. On rectal examination the bladder is palpably distended. If incontinence is present, on the other hand, no urgency is apparent, and an involuntary dribbling of urine occurs. The skin over which the urine is dribbled soon becomes inflamed. The flaccid bladder is palpable on rectal examination and can be evacuated by manual compression.

Etiology. The disturbances of micturition may have a myogenic or neurogenic origin. If the horse cannot void urine properly because of long-sustained exertion or obstruction of the urethra, damage to the detrusor muscle may result (overstretching, paresis, or even paralysis). This is frequently accompanied by a spasm of the sphincter muscle. Inflammation of the vesical mucosa or peritoneum can also be a precipitating cause.

Bladder paralysis is most commonly the result of spinal cord lesions. Malformations are an infrequent cause (e.g., a ureter that bypasses the bladder and empties directly into the urethra).

The *diagnosis* is readily made on the basis of the history and clinical examination (coexisting rectal paralysis is usually present in neurogenic cases). If urinary retention is present, spasm of the bladder sphincter and especially mechanical obstruction of the urinary tract must be ruled out.

The *prognosis* depends on the primary disorder and is less favorable in neurogenic bladder dysfunction. Myogenic disturbances usually pass quickly following evacuation of the bladder. Cystitis is always a potential complication.

Treatment. Main emphasis is placed on regular evacuation of the bladder by massage, which may be combined with catheterization. Paralysis is treated with vitamin B preparations, strychnine injections and physiotherapeutic measures. Due to the risk of cystitis, particularly when frequent catheterization is performed, the retrograde administration of prophylactic antibiotic- or sulfonamide-containing preparations is also recommended.

2.1.6.2.3. Eversion and Prolapse of the Bladder

This condition occurs only in mares and generally as a consequence of dystocia. Through heavy straining, the bladder is everted and forced through the urethra into the vagina. It may even protrude from the pudendal fissure, presenting its mucosal lining as an outer surface.

A prolapse in the true sense can result from injuries of the abdominal wall or vagina (bladder prolapse without eversion), but this is uncommon.

Treatment for both lesions consists in careful replacement of the bladder, which is first thoroughly cleansed with a mild antiseptic. It may be necessary to irrigate the bladder with cold physiologic saline to reduce swelling. In a simple prolapse, closure of the wound is sufficient to prevent recurrence. In eversion, it is advisable to place a pursestring suture about the opening of the urethra.

2.1.6.3. Diseases of the Urethra

Diseases of the urethra are rare in horses, and only urethritis is of importance. It usually occurs in conjunction with cystitis. Mechanical irritation associated with catheterization or urethral calculi can also cause inflammation. Rough manipulation can cause even more severe injuries of the urethra. The bend of the urethra at the ischial arch of the stallion or gelding is particularly prone to such injuries.

The main clinical sign of urethritis is painful urination. Treatment is like that for cystitis, except that irrigation with warm antiseptic solutions as well as oil-based antibiotics or sulfonamides is indicated. With more severe damage, residual stricture of the urethra may result.

2.1.6.4. Urolithiasis

Urolithiasis refers to the formation of calculi of varying composition (uroliths) in the urinary tract and the consequent mucosal damage or loss of patency. The calculi may be described as renal, ureteral, vesical or urethral depending on their localization in the urinary system.

The bladder is the most common site for urinary calculi in the horse, which range from the size of sand grains to 'macroliths' weighing up to 16 kg [Chrustalev, 1976].

Symptoms. The disease is usually chronic in nature and can exist for some time without causing symptoms. It may be brought on suddenly by a mechanical irritation of the mucosa or a urinary tract obstruction. At this point colicky episodes constitute the main symptoms of urolithiasis. These may consist of severe attacks lasting several hours, or evidence of pain manifested by stiffness of gait and refusal to move at fast gaits.

Stranguria is frequently observed during rest, and straining is either ineffectual or expels a urine that contains clotted blood. The urine also has a high content of erythrocytes or, if secondary inflammation has developed, leukocytes and protein.

The clinical picture depends on the location of the calculi. Stones in the renal pelvis seldom cause problems. Even if the calculus enters the ureter and obstructs it, the symptoms remain nonspecific. Hydronephrosis can result from the damming back of urine, in which case normal renal function is maintained by the healthy kidney. Tenderness and enlargement of the kidneys is sometimes noted on rectal examination.

Rectal palpation is mainly of value in the diagnosis of vesical calculi, which are detected most easily when the bladder is empty. Hematuria and cystitis dictate the rest of the picture of vesical calculi, though symptoms may be entirely absent. The entry of a calculus into the urethra leads to marked clinical signs associated with disturbed micturition. Besides evidence of pain and frequent, unsuccessful attempts to urinate, distension of the bladder is palpable per rectum. The location of the calculus can be ascertained by passing a catheter.

Etiology and Pathogenesis. The influence of alimentary factors is evidenced by the fact that the calculi are composed mostly of calcium carbonate when the diet consists largely of green feeds and roughages, and of phosphate when concentrates and bran are fed. The ingestion of large amounts of the mineral in question is only one prerequisite for the formation of uroliths. The salts must be deposited about an *organic matrix* or nucleus whose origin and development is not fully understood. Presumably they are comprised of polysaccharide-protein complexes that originate from the renal tubule cells. The concentric deposition of inorganic materials about these crystallization nuclei usually begins in the calyces or pelvis of the kidney and is continued there or in the bladder.

Factors include: dehydration with the formation of a highly concentrated urine, stagnation or decomposition of the urine, and vitamin A deficiency and consequent sloughing of epithelium. Also included are inflammatory or degenerative changes of the glomerula and tubules that can reduce the efficiency of the protective colloids in the urine or alter their quantitative ratio to the crystalloids, leading in turn to precipitation and urolith formation.

Urolithiasis must be *differentiated* from inflammatory renal and urinary tract diseases (nephritis, pyelitis, cystitis, urethritis). This differentiation is based chiefly upon the clinical evaluation. Urine changes provide an uncertain basis for determining whether the inflammatory reaction represents a complication of the urolithiasis or is an expression of a separate disease process.

Diagnosis. Vesical calculi, the most common urolith in the horse, can often be palpated on rectal exploration. This is most easily done when the bladder is empty and the horse has been premedicated with a tranquilizer.

Urethral calculi lead to the most pronounced clinical signs. Often they can be palpated directly or indirectly (by tenderness) in the perineal part of the urethra. Passage of a catheter enables a precise localization to be made.

Renal calculi, on the other hand, are rare in horses. They often go unrecognized because the attendant colicky signs and urine changes are difficult to interpret, while special diagnostic studies such as excretory urography are impractical.

The *prognosis* is doubtful to unfavorable. Even if a vesical calculus is spontaneously expelled with the urine, a recurrence is probable. Sudden obstruction of the urinary tract, possibly resulting in complete renal failure (uremia) or bladder rupture, is always possible.

Treatment. Urinary calculi are removed surgically. Vesical calculi in mares can be extracted directly through the urethra. The urethra is carefully dilated after the stone has first been fragmented with a lithotome. In male horses the calculus must be removed through a urethrotomy at the ischial arch under epidural anesthesia. If a calculus has entered the urethra, expulsion can sometimes be achieved by administering a central-acting muscle relaxant, otherwise a urethrotomy is indicated. This is done in the area of the ischial arch. It is important to note that the removal of a urinary calculus does not necessarily cure urolithiasis. Surgery should be followed by the administration of hyaluronidase, ample water should be provided with allowance for fluid losses from sweating, and the ration should be modified in accordance with the results of the chemical analysis.

References

Carthe, D.; Ansay, M.; Lomba, F.; Bienfet, V.; Chauvaux, G.: Myoglobinurie chez les poulains demi-song de selt mois. Ann. Méd. Vét. *120:* 325 (1976).

Chrustalev, A. S.: Bolezni močevoj sistemy. In: Scharabrin, I. G.: Vnutrennie nezaraznye bolezni sel'skozjajstvemnych zivitnych, 5. Aufl. (Kolos, Moskva 1976).

GIBBONS, W. J.: The urinary system. In: CATCOTT, E. J.; SMITHCORS, J. F.: Equine medicine and surgery, 2nd ed. (Amer. Vet. Publ. Inc., Wheaton, Ill. 1973).
HOOPER, P. T.: Epizootic cystitis in horses. Austral. vet. J. *44:* 11 (1968).
JACKSON, L. L.: Equine azoturia, a clinical review. Iowa State Univ. Vet. *32:* 16 (1970).
KAMPEN, K. R. VAN: Sudan grass and sorghum poisoning of horses — A possible lathyrogenic disease. J. Amer. Vet. med. Assoc. *156:* 629 (1970).
LOMBA, F.: La glomérulo-néphrite chez l'animal. Ann. Méd. vétérin., Bruxelles *113:* 232 (1969).
MARTIN, J.; KETZ, H.-A.: Pathophysiologie der Harnorgane. In: POTEL, K.: Lehrbuch der Pathologischen Physiologie der Haustiere (VEB Gustav Fischer Verlag, Jena 1969).
NATSCHEFF, B.: Vătrešni nezarazni bolesti na domašnite životni. Bd. 2, Zemizdat, Sofia 1957.
ORDIDGE, R. M.: Urinary incontinence due to unilateral ureteral ectopia in a foal. Vet. Rec. *89:* 384 (1976).
RAJASEKHAR, M.; KESHAVAMURTHY, B. S.: Acute cystitis due to Pseudomonas aeruginosa in a race-horse. Vet. Rec. *89:* 214 (1976).
TOMOV, A.; NIKOV, S.; PRODANOV, P.; NAJDENOV, N.; SCHOSCHKOV, D.; KAMBUROV, G.: Otravjanija pri domašnite životni, ribiti i pčelite. Zemizdat, Sofia 1970.
UDALL, R. H.; CHOW, FU HO CHEN: The etiology and control of urolithiasis. Advances vet. Sci. *13:* 29 (1969).
ZELEV, V.: Slučaj na ogništen glomerulonefrit pro konski fetusi. Izvest. Inst. svavnit. patol. životni Sofia *15:* 199 (1973).

2.1.7. Hernias

2.1.7.1. Diaphragmatic Hernia

Occurrence. Diaphragmatic hernia is rarely diagnosed in the horse. The sporadic cases reported in the literature were mainly discovered at necropsy or during a laparotomy [BUYUKMIHCH, 1973; FIRTH, 1976; PEARSON et al., 1977; POTTER, 1964; SCOTT and FISHBACK, 1976; WILLIAMS, 1963]. The condition was diagnosed ante mortem by clinical and radiographic studies in one case [SASSE and KALSBEEK, 1965; SPEIRS and REYNOLDS, 1976], and there are reports of similar diagnoses in four other horses. The prevalence of the condition is probably greater than has been previously assumed.

Symptoms. The cardinal symptom is colic, which sometimes is recurrent over a prolonged period. The incarceration and torsion of intestinal loops cause very severe colic, and shock develops rapidly. Respiratory symptoms are usually less dramatic. With careful examination, however, indications for thoracic radiography may be present. The respiratory rate is usually elevated. If a very large rupture is present, large portions of the viscera will herniate into the thorax, and there will be a dorsad compression of the lungs. Marked polypnea and dyspnea on exertion may then be noted [SPEIRS and REYNOLDS, 1976]. Respiratory sounds over the thorax may be much attenuated or even absent, and intestinal sounds or crepitant noises may be heard, depending on the localization of the lesion. If intestine has herniated into only half of the thorax, increased respiratory sounds may be auscultated over the contralateral side. A horizontal line of dullness is sometimes demonstrated by percussion. If the rupture is associated with fluid accumulation in the thorax, then fluid will be obtained on thoracocentesis [VERSCHOOTEN et al., 1977]. This fluid may consist of intestinal contents. Distended loops of intestine will be found on rectal exploration.

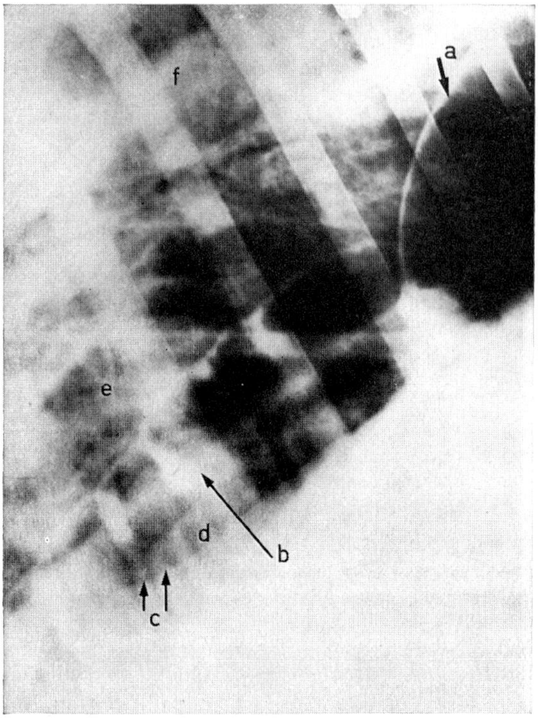

1

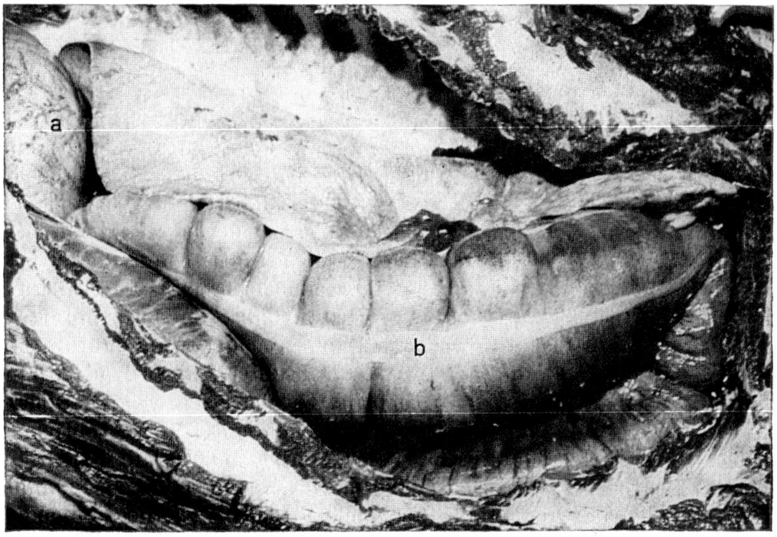

2

Fig. 2.1.7. — 1. Diaphragmatic hernia. Lateral chest film. Stomach (a), colon (b), vena cava (c) and loops of intestine (d), which show an alternating, striate pattern of light and shadowy areas. Partial septae formed by walls of small intestine (e) are seen dorsal to the colon. The pulmonary arteries (f) are displaced far dorsad.

Fig. 2.1.7. — 2. Diaphragmatic hernia. Same case as in Fig. 2.1.7. — 1. A portion of the stomach (a) and the pelvic flexure of the large colon (b) have herniated into the thoracic cavity; the small intestine has already been removed.

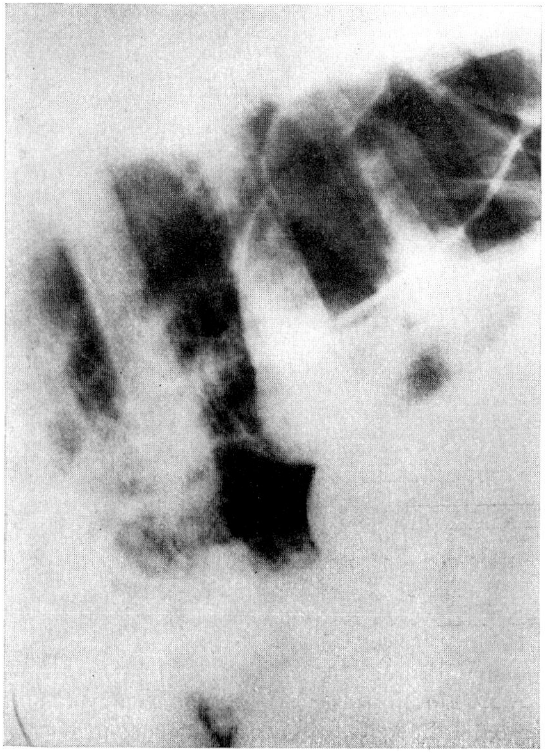

3

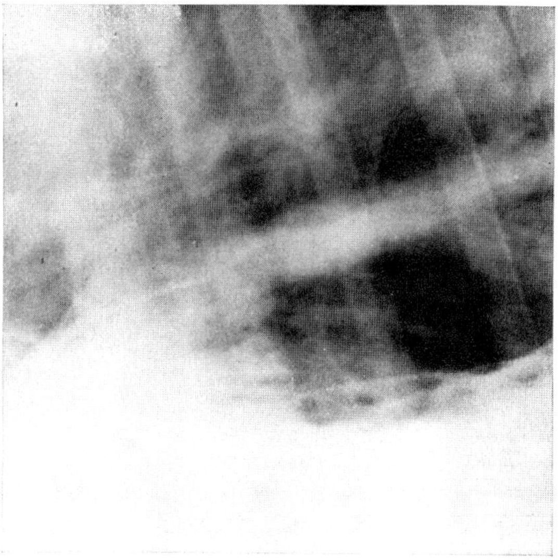

4

Fig. 2.1.7. — 3. Diaphragmatic hernia. Right laterolateral chest film: The thorax is largely filled with loops of small intestine.

Fig. 2.1.7. — 4. Diaphragmatic hernia. Right laterolateral chest film. The caudal vena cava is thickened by a density occupying the ventral lung field cranial to the diaphragm. The contour of the diaphragm is not visible.

Etiology. It is not always possible to identify the exact cause. Sometimes, the hernia will be preceded by severe trauma or by parturition [Verschooten et al., 1977]. The hernia may also develop concurrently with a rib fracture, in which case the omentum may be fused with the fracture callus [Sasse and Kalsbeek, 1965]. The traumatic etiology in such cases is obvious. Congenital cases involving a diaphragmatic defect are rare.

Pathology. The location and extent of the rupture are highly variable. Its length may range from 3 to 40 cm. The nature and mass of abdominal viscera that herniate into the thorax are largely dependent on the length of the tear. Small tears, which occur mostly in the dorsal part of the diaphragm, can only admit portions of the small intestine, especially loops of jejunum, into the thorax. The danger of incarceration in such cases is great. Large ruptures can allow large portions of the stomach, small intestine, colon and even the liver and spleen to enter the thoracic cavity. Ruptures of this size usually occur in the ventral and midportion of the diaphragm and are often shifted somewhat toward one side. Large tears do not usually lead to intestinal incarceration, although torsion or volvulus may develop.

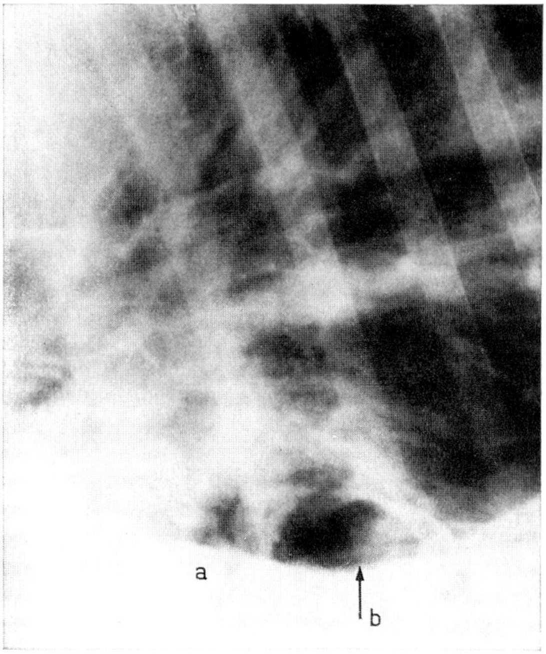

5

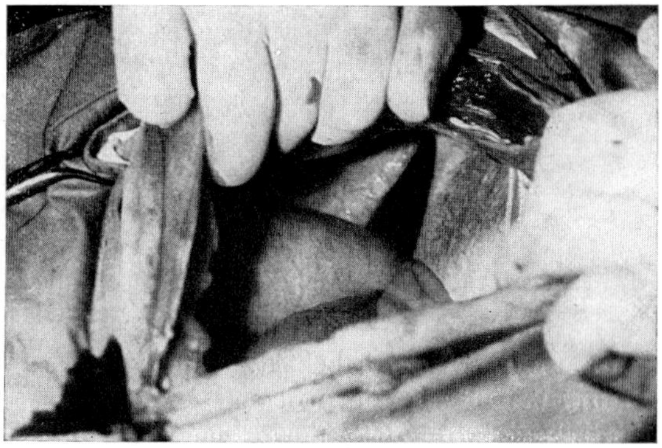

6

Fig. 2.1.7. — 5. Diaphragmatic hernia. Same case as in fig. 2.1.7. — 4 following the removal of one liter of serous fluid from the thorax. A curved segment of colon (a) and gas-filled loops of intestine (b) are visible.

Fig. 2.1.7. — 6. Diaphragmatic hernia. 25-cm-long rupture in the ventral midportion of the diaphragm.

Diagnosis. The clinical examination often provides sufficient grounds for making a presumptive diagnosis of diaphragmatic hernia. A ruptured diaphragm should always be suspected in animals that show colicky signs after a trauma and in which percussion and auscultatory findings are abnormal. Radiographic examination often confirms the diagnosis (fig. 2.1.7. — 1, 3, 4, 5). An image intensifier is excellent for this purpose, for it provides very clear visualization of intestines that have entered the thorax. Although these structures are often more difficult to discern on individual radiographs, an accurate diagnosis can usually be made on the basis of several films.

Bilateral films are essential, for they can show which half of the thorax the intestines occupy in cases of unilateral herniation. If findings are equivalent in both projections, it is likely that the rupture is located on or near the midline. Accurate localization is essential if surgical repair is contemplated. If the tear is ventral in location and a loop of colon has herniated more or less horizontally into the thorax, and fluid is simultaneously present in the thoracic cavity, the fluid must be aspirated before good radiographs can be obtained.

Prognosis. The prognosis depends largely on the size and location of the rupture, on the nature and mass of herniated intestine, which may be strangulated or incarcerated, on the possible development of shock, and on traumatic injuries. Respiratory problems are less critical.

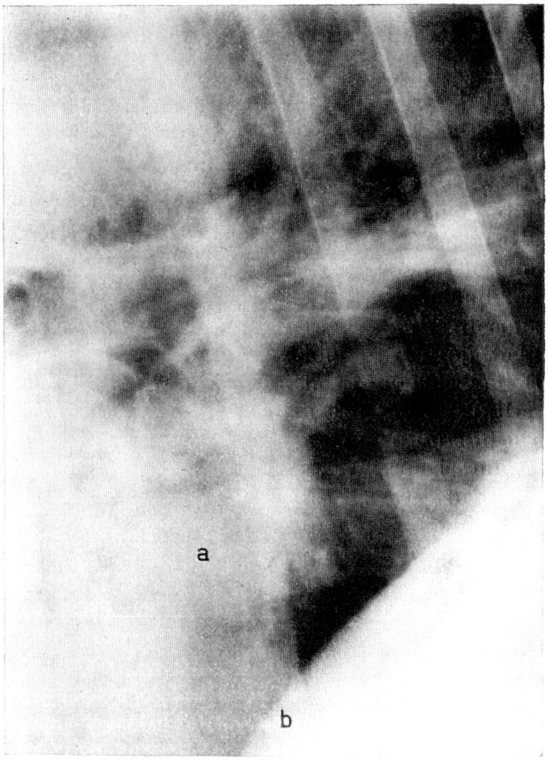

Fig. 2.1.7. — 7. Diaphragmatic hernia. Same case as in fig. 2.1.7. — 6, 21 days after surgical correction. The caudal vena cava (a) and diaphragm (b) are clearly demonstrated in the distal part of the diaphragm.

Treatment. Surgical correction of the hernia is possible in certain cases [Scott and Fishback, 1976; Verschooten et al., 1977; Williams, 1963]. Operability is determined essentially by the general condition of the animal at the time the diagnosis is made. Immediately after the induction of anesthesia, artificial ventilation must be started with a bellows or automatic respirator. Ventromedial ruptures are the easiest to treat from the standpoint of reduction and repair.

The incision is usually made on the linea alba and is extended up to 30 cm caudad from the xyphoid. A paracostal incision may be more favorable for certain localizations. In the case of a ventral rupture, replacement of the colon may prove extremely difficult with the animal in dorsal recumbency, because the heavy parts of the bowel lie deep to the rupture site. Reduction is greatly facilitated by placing the animal in an oblique position intermediate between dorsal and lateral recumbency. The rupture is repaired with interrupted sutures. Before the last stitch is placed, the lungs are fully inflated with the respirator to expel all air from the thorax. If the diaphragmatic wound is unusually large, additional strength can be obtained by suturing a piece of mesh over the defect [Scott and Fishback, 1976].

References

BUYUKMIHCI, N.: Diaphragmatic hernia in a horse. (Clinical Item.) J. Amer. vet. med. Assoc. *162:* 898 (1973).

COFFMAN, J. R.; KINTNER, L. D.: Strangulated diaphragmatic hernia in a horse. Vet. Med. *13:* 423 (1972).

FIRTH, E. C.: Diaphragmatic hernia in horses. Cornell. vet. *66:* 353 (1976).

PEARSON, H.; PINSENT, P. J. N.; DENNY, H. R.; WATERMAN, A.: The indications for equine laparatomy. An analysis of 140 cases. Equine Vet. J. *7:* 131 (1975).

PEARSON, H.; PINSENT, P. J. N.; POLLEY, L. R.; WATERMAN, A.: Rupture of the diaphragm in the horse. Equine Vet. J. *9:* 32 (1977).

POTTER, R. H.: Colic caused from diaphragmatic hernia. Southwestern Vet. *17:* 235 (1964).

SASSE, H. H. L.; KALSBEEK, H. C.: Enkele gevallen van hernia diaphragmatica traumatica bij het paard. Tijdschr. Diergeneesk. *90:* 1327 (1965).

SCOTT, E. A.; FISHBACK, W. A.: Surgical repair of diaphragmatic hernia in a horse. J. Amer. vet. med. Assoc. *168:* 45 (1976).

SPEIRS, V. C.; REYNOLDS, W. T.: Successful repair of a diaphragmatic hernia in a foal. Equine Vet. J. *8:* 170 (1976).

VERSCHOOTEN, F.; OYAERT, W.; MUYLLE, E.; MOOR, A. DE; STEENHAUT, M.; MOENS, Y.: Diaphragmatic hernia in the horse. 4 case reports. J. Amer. Vet. Rad. Soc. *45:* 18 (1977).

WILLIAMS, D. J.: Diaphragmatic hernia in a pony. Mod. Vet. Pract. *44:* 54 (1963).

WIMBERLEY, H. C.; ANDREWS, E. J.; HASCHEK, W. M.: Diaphragmatic hernias in the horse: A review of the literature and analysis of six additional cases. J. Amer. vet. med. Assoc. *170:* 1404 (1977).

WYN-JONES, G.; BAKER, J. R.: A probable congenital diaphragmatic defect in an adult pony. Vet. Rec. *105:* 251 (1979).

2.1.7.2. Umbilical Hernia

Definition. In umbilical hernia there is a median ring or defect in the abdominal wall at the umbilicus which allows the viscera to pass through the umbilical opening into an inner hernial sac without injuring the skin or peritoneum.

Symptoms. A fully developed umbilical hernia is seldom seen in newborn foals. From 10 to 14 days after birth a palpable defect appears on the midline cranial and caudal to the umbilical scar, from which protrudes a flattened oval of skin, fascia and peritoneum. In the 3rd to 4th postnatal week the hernia increases in size as a result of rising intra-abdominal pressure, producing a conspicuous, dependent hernial sac. It may be hemispherical, oval or egg-shaped (fig. 2.1.7. — 8). This enlargement at the umbilicus is cool and nontender and initially is associated with no systemic signs. The hernial contents are soft and are manually reducible. Passing the hernial sac between the fingertips, two layers can be discerned: the skin, forming the outer hernial sac, and the everted peritoneum with a subcutaneous layer of connective tissue, forming the inner sac. The layers are firmly adherent to each other in the area of the umbilical scar. In some cases the hernial contents cannot be completely returned to the abdominal cavity, even in the absence of systemic signs. This indicates the presence of adhesions in the inner sac. The adhesion may be formed by a strand of omentum, or the bowel may be adherent to the parietal peritoneum. If little or no displaceable contents are found between the inner and outer sac on one side by digital palpation, an *interstitial hernia* is present. This is a very rare condition in foals. The hernial ring is palpable in the abdominal wall, is circular or slitlike, and

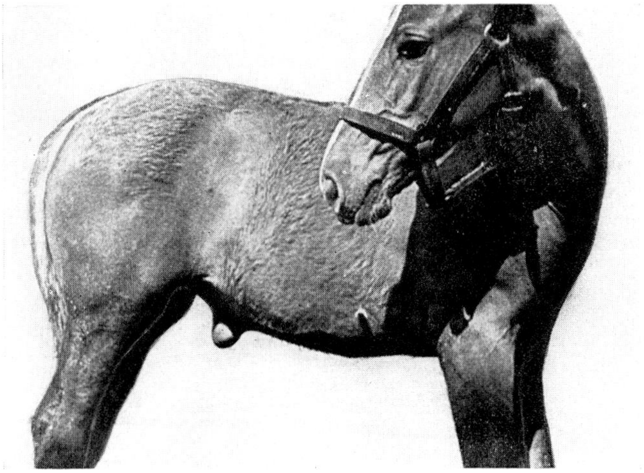

Fig. 2.1.7. — 8. Umbilical hernia.

its edge may be sharp or rounded. It may be possible to insert a fingertip or one or more fingers into the ring. If the hernial contents are hard and tender, the wall of the hernial sac is edematous, and the hernia is irreducible, an incarceration is indicated. This is accompanied by colicky signs, sweating, trembling, fever and depression. Affected animals often roll and may remain in dorsal recumbency for some time. Sometimes it is possible to return the hernial contents to the abdominal cavity by careful massage. If not, intestinal necrosis will develop. Death from peritonitis, systemic infection or endotoxemia follows within 24 hours after the onset of the incarceration.

Etiology. The predisposition to umbilical hernia is probably inherited. The actual hernia does not usually appear until several days or even weeks after birth, however. The presence of a defect at birth is a condition known as *hernia umbilicalis preformata.* Acquired umbilical hernias are rare but may occur at any age as a result of trauma.

Differential Diagnosis. Umbilical abscesses show increased warmth, are tender, and are irreducible yet fluctuant. A tumor in the umbilical region may resemble an umbilical hernia but is irreducible. A hematoma in this region appears suddenly, is fluctuant and irreducible. Umbilical cysts are rare in foals and can be shifted about within the abdominal wall. Ventral hernias near the umbilicus can occur in horses as a result of trauma and may be mistaken for an umbilical hernia by virtue of their location.

Prognosis. The smaller the hernial ring, the more favorable the prognosis, provided the hernial contents can be reduced. In foals that exhibit no colicky signs that might suggest an incarceration, it is best to wait until the animal is 8 to 9 months old before doing surgery, as this is the most favorable time for operative intervention. Incarcerated hernias should be operated on immediately, preferably within the first 6 hours. Intestinal necrosis will progress requiring that a bowel resection be carried out in addition to the hernial repair.

Treatment. Horse owners are fond of using trusses or corsets. These are indicated only if the hernial ring is no larger than finger-size. Treatment with a truss can reduce the size of the hernial ring and even bring about a definitive closure, although this is not the rule. There is always a danger that the band will slip and compound the problem by causing inflammatory changes in the area of the hernia.

The practice of applying irritants to the outer hernial sac or brushing the sac with acids or other caustic chemicals is not without risk. It can result in necrosis of the outer sac or the development of adhesions between the inner hernial sac and intestines, without effecting closure of the hernial ring. Another method is to inject sterile hypertonic saline solution or 75—90 % alcohol around the ring between the inner and outer sac. Instead of hypertonic saline or alcohol, agents that stimulate fibrous tissue growth have also been employed. The object in each case is to reduce the size of the hernial ring or effect a definitive closure. These methods, too, are not without risks due to uncertainties with respect to dosage.

Surgical treatment is deferred until the animal is 6—12 month old. Bloodless methods include clamping off the hernial sac or isolating it by sutures or ligatures in the dorsally recumbent foal, with the object of stimulating scar tissue formation in the ring. Aside from the fact that these methods are not entirely safe, they carry a risk of peritonitis or sloughing of the hernial sac and consequent intestinal prolapse. Open reduction is preferred for hernial rings that are more than 2—3 fingerbreadths in diameter. In all surgical techniques the foal is cast in dorsal recumbency, placed under general anesthesia, and the inner hernial sac is dissected free of the outer sac. At this point various techniques may be used: The inner sac may be returned to the abdominal cavity and the hernial ring closed with interrupted horizontal mattress sutures of a material that is slow to absorb. Another method is to resect the inner sac at the ring, which is then closed by suturing peritoneum to peritoneum. In another technique the inner sac is dissected free, twisted, ligated near the ring and resected peripheral to the ligature. The stump is oversewn, and then the skin is closed in the usual fashion. The stump of the inner hernial sac will slough in 10 to 14 days. With an unusually large hernial ring that can accommodate 4, 5 or more fingers, the best repair method is to suture a mesh made of synthetic suture material over the exposed inner sac. The mesh will stimulate granulation tissue formation during healing, and this tissue will completely invade the mesh to form a fibrous tissue plaque. This will permanently seal the defect.

Occasionally when the inner sac of a reducible umbilical hernia is dissected free, it is found to be adherent to parts of the gut or omentum. It is necessary in such cases, regardless of the surgical technique being used, to open the inner sac and separate the adhesions between the parietal peritoneum and the omentum or intestine. Then the opening in the sac is closed, and the operation is continued in accordance with the method chosen.

Treatment When an Incarceration is Present. Surgery should be performed without delay. General anesthesia is induced, and a continuous intravenous drip is started with a weak glucose solution and sodium bicarbonate solution. Again, the inner hernial sac is dissected free, and an attempt is made to reduce the hernial contents by massage. If this is successful in the anesthetized foal, it may be assumed that the previously incarcerated bowel will recover. If this attempt fails, it is necessary to open the inner sac. This must be done with great care to avoid injury to the incarcerated bowel. The afferent loop of intestine will be distended with gas. First an attempt is made to reduce this loop, and if this succeeds the entire reduction may be done without a herniotomy. Otherwise the hernial ring must be enlarged from the inside outward in the area of the linea alba. The resection of a necrotic bowel segment is necessary only in extreme cases and should be followed by an end-to-end anastomosis. The operation is concluded in the usual fashion. Prophylactic antibiotics are administered for 5—6 days postoperatively.

Postoperative Care. The animal is confined to a small space during the first postoperative weeks to prevent excessive movement. Only moderate amounts of food should be offered during this time.

2.1.7.3. Funicular Umbilical Hernia

Definition. In this condition a loop of intestine is present in the umbilical cord at birth or enters the cord during the first weeks of life.

Symptoms. The umbilical cord is thickened and tapers to a conical point at its lower end. The contents are reducible. If the umbilicus has sloughed, sometimes a granulating surface is left which later forms a fibrous-tissue hernial sac.

Differential Diagnosis. The possibility of a urachal fistula must be considered. In this condition, however, urine is observed dribbling from the thickened, inflamed umbilical cord. The cord itself takes on a slimy consistency. Umbilical abscess, omphalophebitis and omphaloarteritis are distinguished by painful inflammatory swellings that are sometimes fluctuant. Omphalitis, moreover, is usually associated with systemic signs or even polyarthritis.

Treatment. Funicular umbilical hernia in the newborn foal should be treated without delay. The foal is cast in dorsal recumbency, the hernial contents are returned to the abdominal cavity by careful massage, and a wide bandage is wrapped about the thickened umbilical cord. This bandage is left in place until the umbilical stump sloughs.

2.1.7.4. Inguinal Hernia, Scrotal Hernia

Definition. In an inguinal hernia, loops of omentum, intestine or both protrude through the vaginal ring into the processes vaginalis and come to lie in the inguinal area. In scrotal hernia loops of intestine occupy the cavity of the tunica vaginalis along with the testis. Accordingly, the hernial opening in both inguinal and scrotal hernia is always formed by the vaginal ring. At this site the processes vaginalis passes obliquely downward into the inguinal canal, where it forms an hourglass-like constriction. The more frequent form in the horse is the congenital scrotal hernia, which usually appears in male foals that are a few days old. Its occurrence may be uni- or bilateral. Acquired scrotal hernia, usually with incarceration, is most common in the breeding stallion but is being seen with increasing frequency in Standardbreds in training. The hernias occasionally occur in mares, where they may be mistaken for ventral hernias.

Symptoms. Descent of the testis is sometimes not complete until 8 to 14 days after birth. A fullness of one or both halves of the scrotum may be evident at this time or earlier in rare cases. This is most obvious when the foal is viewed from behind. Cases are known in which the enlarged scrotal halves hung to the level of the hock in suckling foals. On palpation the contents of the scrotum can easily be pushed back into the abdominal cavity. Intestinal sounds are usually audible due to the presence of fluid in the gut. The inguinal ring in such foals is usually large enough to accommodate 3 or 4 fingers. Manual reduction of the hernia is of only temporary benefit in the standing animal, for the loops of bowel quickly slip back into the scrotum. In rare cases scrotal hernia in the suckling foal will lead to an incarceration, at which point colicky signs become evident. The affected foal begins to roll and quickly becomes depressed.

Suckling foals that present with uni- or bilateral scrotal hernia should not be operated on immediately. Small scrotal and inguinal hernias frequently reduce spontaneously during growth in the first year of life. The formation of adhesions between the tunica vaginalis and the herniated gut or omentum is very rare during the first year of life. This is apt to occur only if the enlarged scrotum has been unwisely treated with irritant solutions.

Mature stallions, breeding stallions as well as racing horses (especially Standardbreds) usually present with severe colicky signs that appeared a short time after breeding, training or racing. The cause is an incarceration, i.e., a loop of bowel has entered the hernial sac and become strangulated. Occasionally such signs are associated with congenital scrotal hernia in the male foal. The colicky signs are very severe, and affected animals will roll and stand up again, stamping with the feet. Whenever colicky signs are exhibited by male horses of any age, the inguinal and scrotal area should be carefully examined. In the presence of an incarcerated inguinal or scrotal hernia the scrotal area usually will feel hard, firm and tender on palpation. The scrotum itself is enlarged for some time after the onset of the incarceration, and the scrotal skin shows edematous swelling. The contents, which are tender to pressure, are irreducible during palpation. On rectal examination, two segments of intestine are felt entering the inguinal canal. The afferent segment is filled with gas, while the segment exiting the vaginal ring is empty. Palpation of these loops at the internal inguinal ring is noticeably painful. On external palpation the hernial contents cannot always be distinguished from the testis. Two to three hours after the onset of colicky symptoms, marked systemic signs appear in the foal or mature stallion with an incarcerated scrotal hernia. Necrosis of the strangulated loop of bowel will develop within 6—10 hours, at which time colicky signs and sweating subside. The pulse becomes weak and rapid, rising to as much as 120 beats/min. Twelve to 14 hours after the onset of colicky signs, cold sweating occurs and the conjunctivae become pale. Food and water are refused. Death usually occurs 20—24 hours after the first symptoms appear.

In mares with inguinal hernia, a hemispheric swelling is noted in one half of the udder, which sometimes extends around to the fold of the stifle. The swelling is about twice the size of a fist, soft and partially reducible. Incarcerations are practically unknown.

Differential Diagnosis. Traumatic ventral hernias located in the region of the stifle fold can be excluded by their localization. Traumatic orchitis or testicular torsion should be considered in mature stallions. Inguinal hernia in mares must also be differentiated from abdominal hernias and uni- or bilateral mastitis.

Treatment. In congenital scrotal hernia of the male foal, a wait-and-see approach is taken. If within a year the inguinal ring has not narrowed and the hernial contents have not reduced spontaneously, then closed castration is performed on the affected side. The healthy side is not castrated right away. If an incarceration is diagnosed in the male foal, immediate surgery is indicated. The outer hernial sac is dissected free, and the inner sac is widely opened. An attempt is then made to return the hernial contents to the abdominal cavity by careful massage. This is nearly always possible in male foals without a herniotomy. The next step is a closed castration on the affected side.

For incarcerated scrotal hernia in breeding stallions or racing animals, it is desirable to operate within 6—10 hours after the onset of the disease; otherwise intestinal necrosis will necessitate a bowel resection. The operation is best performed under halothane anesthesia. Intravenous therapy is also started with 2 to 3 liters of a 5% glucose solution and 5% sodium bicarbonate solution. With the animal in dorsal recumbency, the outer hernial sac is opened with a long incision. The inner sac is bluntly dissected free down to the external inguinal ring. This sac is then opened while the testis is fixed with a forceps. An attempt is now made to massage the hernial contents back into the peritoneal cavity while the inner hernial sac is fixed with the aid of peritoneal clamps. An hourglass-like constriction will always be present at the inguinal ring. If the first attempt at reduction is unsuccessful, the next step is to carry out a unilateral castration on the affected side. After this, the surgeon attempts to return the stump of the spermatic cord to the abdominal cavity. If reduction is still not possible at this time, a herniotomy should be done under digital control, a 1- to 1½-cm incision being made in the inguinal ring from its lumen outward. This is usually sufficient to enable a reduction, after which the incision is closed with simple interrupted preplaced sutures. Finally the entire inner hernial sac is ligated directly at the external inguinal ring using heavy surgical gut. If a dark red discoloration of the bowel is noted, a thrombosis has occurred within the mesentery or the mesenteric vessels, and resection should be performed. For this the small intestine is brought out of the abdominal cavity bilaterally until the resection can be carried out in healthy tissue. This is followed by an end-to-end anastomosis. Then the exteriorized bowel is returned to the abdominal cavity, employing a herniotomy if necessary. Intravenous therapy is helpful in preventing intra- and postoperative shock. If a 5—10 % glucose solution and sodium bicarbonate solution are not available, dextran preparations are a suitable alternative for slow drip infusion. Large doses of antibiotics should be administered for 6—7 days postoperatively. In Standardbreds and breeding stallions, the testis on the unaffected side should not be removed. A stallion with one testicle can still breed. The unilaterally castrated Standardbred stallion can continue to compete in races for stallions.

2.1.7.5. Femoral Hernia

Definition. Femoral hernia involves the herniation of a loop of small intestine into the femoral canal, the hernial sac being formed by the medial femoral fascia. A partial rupture of the femoral fascia may be present.

Symptoms. Femoral hernia is marked by constant unrest or colicky signs of sudden onset. The animal adopts a straddling position with the hind legs and will move forward only if forced to do so. External inspection and palpation will reveal a somewhat flattened, apple- to fist-size swelling on the inside of the thigh, specifically at the site where the great saphenous vein disappears in the femoral canal as it courses toward the pelvis. On rectal exploration a cord-like loop of intestine will be felt entering the femoral canal.

Etiology. Femoral hernia can occur in draft horses that attempt to move a heavy load by planting the hind legs in the ground with the legs spread apart. It is especially likely to occur if the load is very heavy and the ground is soft.

Treatment. Reduction is attempted per rectum by exerting constant, gentle traction on the palpable cord. The horse should be in dorsal recumbency and deep general anesthesia for this procedure. Good relaxation with the aid of halothane anesthesia or the additional use of muscle relaxants is necessary during the reduction attempt, with both hind legs secured in wide abduction. If the reduction is successful, an interrupted suture is placed between the inguinal ligament and the sartorius muscle. This suture must be placed very carefully to avoid injury to the femoral arteries and veins.

2.1.7.6. Ventral Hernia (Abdominal Hernia)

Definition. Ventral hernia is the term applied to hernias of the abdominal wall that occur as a result of blunt trauma. The skin and peritoneum may remain intact, creating both an inner and outer hernial sac. In this case a 'true' hernia is present, as opposed to the subcutaneous or 'false' hernia that occurs when the skin is intact but the musculature and peritoneum are torn. Common to all abdominal hernias is the absence of a preformed hernial opening.

Ventral hernias in the horse may be classified according to etiology as traumatic abdominal wall ruptures, postoperative hernias and incisional hernias. They may be classified according to location as follows:

1. *Iliac hernias* occur above the stifle fold in the horse and are usually caused by a kick from another animal (fig. 2.1.7. — 9).
2. *Hypogastric hernias* occur below the stifle fold and are generally caused by trauma from the shaft of a cart or the dividing bar between two stalls.
3. *Interstitial inguinal hernias* follow a perforation of the internal obliquus abdominis muscle during surgery for abdominal cryptorchism.
4. *Paraumbilical hernias* are located at the periphery of the umbilicus and are the result of blunt trauma.
5. *Rupture of the prepubic tendon* of the rectus abdominis muscle occur during late gestation in mares (fig. 2.1.7. — 10).
6. *Hernias of the linea alba* occur as a malformation between the umbilicus and sternal manubrium.
7. *Epigastric hernias* usually develop from kicks and are located near the midline.
8. *Hypochondriac hernias* present as a bulge in a slit between the two obliquus muscles and the transversus abdominis muscles at about the level of the 13th to 14th ribs in the 'interval of Schmaltz'. They are attributed to a congenital defect that becomes a hernia only in older horses that are overexerted.

Symptoms. When the abdomen is subjected to a trauma, the area surrounding the hernia swells quickly, and dependent edema may appear on the ventral abdomen. If the peritoneum is torn and the hernial sac consists of skin only, the peristalsis of the prolapsed bowel can often be detected through the skin. In the presence of acute inflammatory swelling, it may be difficult to palpate the hernial ring initially. The examination will be easier after a few days have passed. The typical hernial ring is circular and has rounded edges. It is not unusual for prolapsed loops of intestine to become fused to the subcutaneous tissue or outer hernial sac.

Postoperative incisional hernias are encountered after laparotomies in cases where an increased intra-abdominal pressure combined with undue stress on the abdominal wall has led to partial suture dehiscence. Hernias of this type generally appear between 6 and 10 days postoperatively. Incisional hernias usually occur several weeks postoperatively and are due to overstretching of the scar tissue, producing a slitlike hernial ring.

Iliac and other ventral hernias that occur on the sides of the abdominal wall and ventral abdomen are usually quite large. They are reducible immediately after their occurrence and particularly for the first few days thereafter. If such hernias remain unreduced for several weeks after the trauma, the hernial ring becomes oval or slitlike. Sometimes even three elliptical rings can be palpated in the abdominal wall, one atop the other. A layered ring configuration of this type indicates that the abdominal muscles have become divided in the direction of their fibers. On rectal examination not all the rings can be palpated, especially those located far anteriorally. Incar-

9
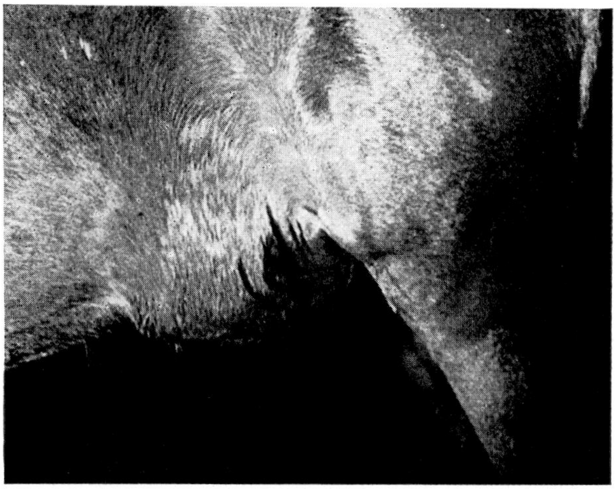

10
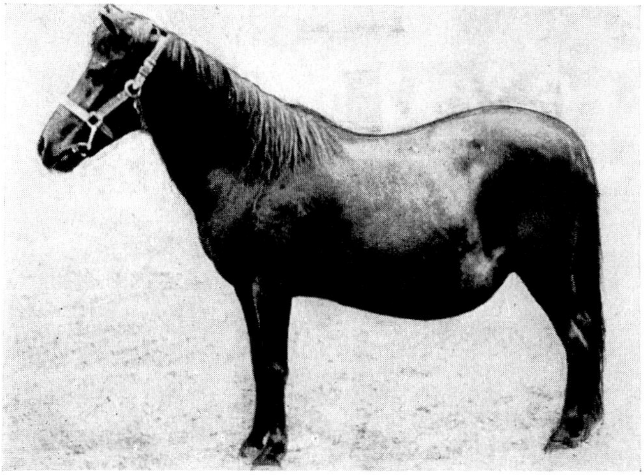

Fig. 2.1.7. — 9. Iliac hernia ('flank rupture').
Fig. 2.1.7. — 10. Ventral hernia; rupture of the prepubic tendon.

ceration is uncommon and is associated only with iliac hernias and other abdominal hernias that involve the flank.

A tendinous rupture of the rectus abdominis muscles can occur in mares during late gestation. An external trauma may be the precipitating cause. The contour of the ventral abdomen drops to the level of the hock, accompanied by edematous swelling of the subcutaneous connective tissue (fig. 2.1.7. — 10). The large hernial ring runs transversely just anterior to the pelvis. All of the ring cannot be palpated per rectum. The ring is palpable externally only in the dorsally recumbent animal.

Interstitial inguinal hernia occurs as a complication of abdominal cryptorchism surgery. A common history was that the operative wound was extended so that the entire hand or forearm could be inserted into the abdominal cavity to locate the undescended testis. Between 2 and 3 weeks postoperatively a hernial sac about twice the size of a fist is noticed in the inguinal region. The hernial ring is palpable rectally. The hernial sac usually contains omentum but may contain intestine in rare cases. The localization of the hypochondriac hernia is quite typical. The hernia is a true one, possessing an internal sac. Hernias of this type are about the size of a handball, with a small, slitlike ring that usually can accomodate 3 or 4 fingertips.

Treatment. Small, slitlike abdominal hernias secondary to injuries sometimes will reduce spontaneously. In the surgical treatment of ventral hernias in the horse, the following guidelines are followed:

— First the outer hernial sac is opened just far enough that the hand or fingers can be inserted to determine whether an inner sac is present. If so, the inner sac should not be opened right away.

— If there is no inner hernial sac, as is generally the case in traumatic iliac hernias, the surgeon looks through the opening in the outer sac to ascertain the nature and condition of the prolapsed viscera. If the gut is badly contused, shows signs of incipient necrosis or presents a visible wound, it must be decided whether an intestinal resection, intestinal suture or partial amputation of the omentum is indicated. Any adhesions that have formed between loops of intestine must be carefully separated. The chronically inflamed serosa may be treated topically with prednisolone emulsion.

— If an inner hernial sac is present and loops of intestine or omental tissue are adherent to it, they, too, must be carefully freed and returned to their normal position. In doing this, it may prove necessary to tie off and resect portions of the omentum.

— A close scrutiny is made of the hernial ring and its edges. If the hernia is already several weeks old, the edges of the hernial ring will be thick and rounded — a situation ideal for closure by suture. The surgeon checks again to see whether several overlying hernial rings are present in the form of muscular tears in the direction of their fibers. In such cases, preparation is made for a layered closure of the hernial opening, which sometimes can be done without tension.

— If an inner sac is present, it is opened and fixed at its edges with grasping forceps. The parts that were the last to herniate are always the first to be reduced. If it is not possible to separate adhesions between the hernial contents and the inner lining of the internal sac, portions of this sac may be left adherent to the intestinal wall.

— Closure of the hernial ring is done with simple interrupted sutures. Heavy chromic catgut or slow-absorbing synthetic absorbable suture materials should be used in the horse. If complete closure cannot be effected, a mesh made of Perlon or some other synthetic, nonabsorbable suture material can be sewn over the defect to create an effective seal. First, the peritoneal sac must be inverted into the peritoneal cavity and secured there with sutures. Multiple-layer hernial rings are closed in appropriate fashion. It is seldom necessary to resect skin from a large outer hernial sac. Drainage through a separate incision is recommended.

— The placement of tension-relieving sutures has proved beneficial in the horse.

— Following operations for hernias in the posterior portion of the abdominal wall, it may be necessary to keep the horse standing with cross-ties for several days or place the hindquarters on an inclined plane to reduce stress on the operated area. Antibiotics are administered for 6—7 days postoperatively. The outer hernial sac should be watched for drainage.

Prognosis. The prognosis is good for all types of abdominal hernia, provided the hernial ring is not so large that closure is made under tension. Ventral hernias resulting from a rupture of the rectus abdominis muscles carry an unfavorable prognosis or are inoperable. Even after foaling or a cesarean section, repair of the torn rectus muscle is generally impossible.

Comments. Equine abdominal hernias should be operated within the first 24 hours if possible, and thus before strong muscular retraction has occurred. Closure of the ring usually presents no difficulties in such cases. If the ventral hernia is already several days old when the animal is seen, and the patient exhibits no colicky signs that might signify an incarceration, surgery should be postponed for 3 to 4 weeks. By that time the edges of the hernial ring will be thick and rounded and better able to hold sutures. Racing animals may be returned to work only if the hernial ring was a small one. Horses with very large hernias may be suitable only for breeding purposes.

2.1.7.7. Perineal Hernia

Definition. Perineal hernia in the horse is generally subcutaneous. It results from a tear of the peritoneum in the rectogenital, vesicogenital or pubovesical excavation. The contents of the hernia lie in the retroperitoneal pelvic cavity. The skin of the inguinal region is outpouched next to or below the anus, forming the outer hernial sac. Isolated cases of perineal hernia have been observed in the mare.

Symptoms. The hernia usually occurs as a complication of dytocia and presents as a sac about the size of a soccer ball located lateral to and somewhat below the anus and extending to the lateral vaginal region. Hernial contents may be palpable on rectal or vaginal examination and consist of small intestine, omentum, and sometimes portions of the bladder.

Differential Diagnosis. Perianal cellulitis (phlegmons) or abscesses should be considered. External palpation and rectal examination in such cases reveals severe tenderness and systemic signs. In extreme cases malignant melanoma should be considered, especially in gray horses.

Treatment. The mare is positioned in lateral recumbency under halothane anesthesia with the affected side uppermost. The head is positioned lower than the pelvis so that the hernial contents will slip back into the abdominal cavity. An incision is made next to the anus and parallel to the vagina, extending past the outer hernial sac. Omentum and bowel are returned to the abdominal cavity, with care taken to free all adhesions in the retroperitoneal pelvic space. The hernial ring (peritoneal rupture) must be sutured as far anteriorally as possible in the pelvic cavity. Natural silk has been used by the author. The inferior and lateral tail muscles are joined to the internal pelvic muscles with simple interrupted sutures. These sutures, which are placed in layers from within outward, include the sacrotuberal ligament. The arteries and nerves coursing through the pelvis should be carefully spared. The operation is concluded by packing the wound and closing the skin. The patient should be kept standing with cross-ties and with the hindquarters elevated for several days, as after spaying. Antibiotics are given for 5—6 days postoperatively.

Comment. If the perineal hernia has been successfully repaired, the mare should no longer be used for breeding if at all possible, for the hernia is likely to recur during the next parturition.

References

Hamilton, D. P.; Nelson, D. R.; Hardenbrook, H. J.: Repair of ventral abdominal hernia in a horse, using tantalum mesh. J. Amer. vet. med. Assoc. *164:* 1204 (1974).

Johnson, J. H.: Use of polypropylene mesh as a prosthetic material for abdominal hernias in horses. J. Amer. vet. med. Assoc. *155:* 1589 (1969).

JOHNSON, J. H.: A surgical technic for umbilical herniorrhaphy. Vet. Med. Small and Animal Clinician *65:* 967 (1970).
LOOMIS, W. K.: A ventral hernia with incarceration in the horse. A case report. Cornell Vet. *57:* 119 (1967).
MEIER, P.: Zur Sklerotherapie von Hernien bei Haustieren. Schweiz. Arch. Tierheilk. *105:* 429 (1963).
NOONE, J. P.: Scrotal herniation of the urinary bladder in the horse. Irish vet. J. *2:* 11 (1966).
NUMANS, S. R.; WINTZER, H. J.: Zur Alloplastik in der Hernienbehandlung bei grossen Haustieren. Wien. tierärztl. Mschr. *51:* 433 (1964).
WOLTER, J.: Die operative Nabelbruchversorgung mit Hilfe eines flexiblen Pilzes und Technovit. Tierärztl. Umschau *22:* 243 (1967).

2.1.8. Diseases of the Male Genital Organs and Hermaphroditism

2.1.8.1. Cryptorchidism

(cf. Sec. 2.8.11.1.)

Definition. Cryptorchidism refers to the failure of one or both testicles to descend normally.

Forms. A distinction is made between inguinal, abdominal and partial abdominal cryptorchidism in the horse. In the inguinal form the testicle and epididymis lie inside the inguinal canal, contained within a rudimentary sac of tunica vaginalis (vaginal process). In abdominal cryptorchidism the testicle and its adnexa are located *within* the abdominal cavity, in which case the retained testicle will be located either caudal to the kidneys or directly at the vaginal ring. Partial abdominal cryptorchidism is present when the tail of the epididymis and the vas deferens are contained within the vaginal process, while the testicle itself lies within the abdomen at the vaginal ring.

All breeds of horse are susceptible to cryptorchisdim. One or both testicles may be involved. According to BRANDSCH [1964], abdominal or inguinal cryptorchidism occurs on the left side in 47.7 % of cases, on the right side in 36.3 %, and is bilateral in 16 %. A similar ratio occurs in ponies.

SILBERSIEPE, BERGE and MÜLLER [1976] state that abdominal and partial abdominal cryptorchidism are considerably more frequent than the inguinal form, citing a ratio of 152 : 77. Mono- and polyorchidism have not yet been described in the horse.

Symptoms. Cryptorchidism is recognized by the absence of one or both testicles in the scrotum. The undescended testicles continue to secrete male hormones, and so even bilateral cryptorchid stallions exhibit libido and are able to copulate. However, spermatogenesis never develops in these testicles, and the animal is infertile. Cryptorchid testicles are usually small and have a flabby consistency. The testicular mesentery is often long and broad. The testicle and epididymis may be firmly adherent. The weight of the cryptorchid testicle is considerably less than that of the normal testicle. MÜLLER [1976] reports that the cryptorchid testicle has a weight of only 15—50 g, as compared to the 100—150 g weight of the normal juvenile testis. Abdominal testicles may undergo cystic or neoplastic change. Besides dermoid and follicular cysts, teratomas may develop and reach a weight of up to 3 kg [MÜLLER, 1976].

Etiology. Normally, testicular descent takes place at birth and is complete shortly thereafter. In the cryptorchid individual, testicular descent is hampered due to a shortening of the gubernaculum testis. Cryptorchidism, be it of the abdominal, partial abdominal or inguinal variety, is the result of genetic and hormonal factors as well as mechanical factors that arise during the descent of one or both testicles (e.g., a too narrow vaginal ring). Arthur [1961] found that testicular descent in the stallion occurs some time later than in ruminants. He attributes this to a high level of circulating estrogen in the pregnant mare, which causes a retardation of testicular growth in the male fetus.

Differential Diagnosis. Special attention should be given to horses that display primary and secondary sex characters despite demonstrable castration. The differential diagnosis is based upon the history and clinical examination; a rectal examination and special tests may be indicated in some cases. Hermaphroditism (presence of external male and female genital organs) and hypospadias must be excluded.

Diagnosis. Diagnosis is not always easy, and close attention should be given to the history and special signs. Often the presence of 'studdish' behavior combined with information furnished by the owner or attendant and an external examination by the veterinarian are sufficient to suggest a diagnosis. When it is known that previous attempts to castrate the animal have failed, diagnosis is a relatively simple matter and an examination of the inguinal region will usually suffice. The scrotal area is inspected on both the left and right sides. If a normal testicle has been removed on one side, a loosely-hanging double fold of skin will be present, representing the scrotal remnant. The scrotum must be checked for the presence of scars. The skin fold is grasped and pulled taut with the thumb and index finger of one hand. In bilaterally castrated horses a cutaneous scar can usually be found on each side of the scrotum, sometimes running obliquely across the median raphe; often there is a funnel-like indrawing of the skin at the scar. The demonstration of scars is never sufficient in itself, however. The cutaneous scars in castrated horses may be attached to a cord of fibrous scar tissue that widens to several centimeters in a dorsal direction and enters the inguinal canal as a spermatic cord stump. The cord stump, if present, can be felt between the fingers when the scrotal skin is grasped and can be followed into the inguinal ring. If a gelding with abdominal cryptorchidism has already been castrated on the affected side, a large, bulging cutaneous scar can usually be found. If a skin incision was placed on one side with the object of performing a castration, but the testis was not actually removed, no spermatic cord stump will be felt entering the inguinal ring when traction is exerted on the cutaneous scar. It should be remembered, however, that a thorough, bilateral external palpation of the inguinal region is essential, and one should never rely solely on the demonstration of a spermatic cord stump. A tangled mass of veins can sometimes be mistaken for a testicle retained in the inguinal canal.

An abdominal testicle is palpable on rectal examination as a smooth, flaccid but well-defined structure about the size of a small hen's egg lying to the right or left of the midline, generally anterior to the pelvic brim [Müller, 1976]. The animal may object somewhat when the retained testicle is touched. Small testicles cannot always be located during rectal exploration. A period of at least 36 hours should elapse between the rectal examination and the operation.

The vasa deferentia provide additional important diagnostic clues during rectal exploration. A vas deferens entering the inguinal canal is a sign that the horse has been castrated on that side or is an inguinal cryptorchid. If there is no vas deferens in the canal, it may be inferred that a condition of abdominal cryptorchidism exists on the side in question, provided the retained testicle has not previously been removed. One additional point should be noted in the diagnosis of equine cryptorchidism: A horse may be classed as a gelding only if a spermatic cord stump can be found in the inguinal region on each side, and the scrotum presents a corresponding cutaneous scar. Occasionally a cord may be found that is similar to, but considerably larger than, the stump of the spermatic cord, in a horse that continues to display studdish behavior. The explanation is that the animal was a partial abdominal cryptorchid at the first castration attempt, and only the tail of the epididymis and a portion of the vas deferens were excised, leaving behind the undescended testicle at the vaginal ring.

According to WOLLRAB [1971], the estrogen content of the urine is useful in the diagnosis or differential diagnosis of cryptorchidism, for estrogens are formed only if the internal secretory function of the testicle is intact.

Most cryptorchids are presented for operation when 2 to 3 years of age. In most cases the owner still believes that the retained testicle will eventually descend as the animal grows, but this is possible only in yearling stallions with an inguinal retention.

Prognosis. The prognosis is good with removal of the undescended testis.

Treatment. Inguinal, abdominal and partial abdominal cryptorchidism are treated by surgical removal of the retained testicle. Various methods may be used:

— inguinal or Belgian method after MERRIAM [1972], VALDEZ et al. [1979], etc.;

— left flank approach in the standing position after BURGER [1959] or SWIFT [1972] (pony);

— para-anal approach in the standing position after DIETZMANN and MÖLLER [1959];

— paramedian approach after WRIGHT [1960], DEMOOR and VERSCHOOTEN [1967], LOWE and HIGGINBOTHAM [1969], COX [1979], ARCULARIUS [1974];

— median approach, best suited for bilateral abdominal cryptorchidism, after BLENDINGER [1958] and HUSKAMP [1976].

The reader should consult the various surgery textbooks for further details on the different operative techniques.

Comments. An inherited predisposition to cryptorchidism cannot be ruled out. Correction of the condition in horses is a matter of economic necessity, and successfully operated horses are suitable for work or riding.

2.1.8.2. Diseases of the Testicle

2.1.8.2.1. Aseptic and Purulent Orchitis and Epididymitis

Definition. These are inflammatory conditions of the testicle and epididymis that result in a loss or reduction of fertility. Acute aseptic and pyogenic forms exist.

Symptoms. Acute aseptic orchitis and epididymitis are characterized by a cautious gait, unilateral lameness and sometimes fever. The libido is depressed. The scrotal skin is tense. The testicle and epididymis are tender, swollen, have a firm consistency and are warm to the touch. The mobility of the testicle and epididymis within the tunica vaginalis is reduced.

Acute pyogenic orchitis and epididymitis have essentially the same clinical features as the aseptic forms. There is considerable swelling and edema of the testicular interstitial tissue and vaginal tunics with tenderness of the testicle, epididymis and spermatic cord. A perforating wound of the scrotum may be demonstrable in some cases (riding accident, fall on sharp object), resulting in testicular cellulitis and abscessation. Fever, depression and anorexia are accompanying signs. Testicular fibrosis and adhesive periorchitis may later develop.

Etiology. Acute aseptic and pyogenic orchitis and epididymitis result from contusions, perforating wounds and consequent pyogenic infection.

Differential Diagnosis. The reduced testicular size and enlarged, fluctuant and painless scrotum seen in hydrocele serve to differentiate this condition from orchitis and epididymitis. In hematocele there is generally a balloon-like swelling of the tunica vaginalis, and the scrotal skin is tense. In unincarcerated scrotal hernia there is a considerable enlargement of one scrotal half, and the testicle feels smaller than normal, especially in foals. The contents (intestine or omentum) are reducible.

Diagnosis. It is important to draw a distinction between acute aseptic, pyogenic and specific orchitis and epididymitis. The diagnosis is made by exclusion and is based on the history, clinical findings, and allergic and serologic examinations. Sometimes an organism can be demonstrated or the cause ascertained by means of bacteriologic and serologic examinations of the ejaculate.

Prognosis. A complete recovery is unlikely, for spermatogenesis is nearly always impaired.

Treatment. Heat and deep-acting medicaments should be avoided in the local treatment of testicular diseases, owing to the extreme delicacy of the testicle and epididymis and the susceptibility of the testicular parenchyma to degenerative change.

In acute testicular inflammation, systemic signs can be controlled with parenteral doses of sulfonamides, antibiotics and glucocorticoids.

Acute aseptic orchitis and epididymitis resulting from closed injuries respond favorably to rest and cold compresses (acetate mixtures) as well as to weakly-penetrating ointments that do not irritate the scrotal skin; 1—1.5 % prednisolone ointment is good for this purpose. Acute, perforating scrotal wounds that involve the testicle are treated by suturing the tunica albuginea and scrotum in layers, while ensuring adequate antibiotic protection for the cavity of the tunica vaginalis (the vaginal cavity). If testicular cellulitis and abscesses are present, unilateral castration is indicated.

Comments. In view of the associated disturbance of spermatogenesis, unilateral aseptic or pyogenic orchitis and epididymitis reduce the breeding value of the affected stallion, while bilateral orchitis and epididymitis make the animal completely unsuited for stud use.

2.1.8.2.2. Testicular Tumors

Definition. Tumors of the testicle may be benign or malignant. Benign tumors include fibromas, adenomas and chondromas. The principal malignant neoplasms are carcinomas and sarcomas. Dermoid cysts and teratomas occur sporadically.

Symptoms. The testicle is enlarged, and the weight of the mass causes the scrotum to hang unusually low. A *fibroma* arising from the tunica albuginea or testicular connective tissue develops slowly and varies in size from a chestnut to an apple. It is round, hard (fibroma durum), nontender, and has a knobby surface texture. The scrotal skin and tunica vaginalis overlying the diseased testicle are tense. Generally the testicle cannot be moved about within the tunica.

Testicular *adenomas* usually present as circumscribed, nodular masses that may contain cysts. The scrotal skin is normal in appearance and can be readily moved about over the affected testis.

Chondromas are found incidentally during castrations, especially of abdominal testicles. The involved testicle is hard and nontender. Slow-growing tumors can form lobulated masses within the testicular connective tissue.

Testicular sarcoma is characterized by a gradually progressive enlargement of the testicle and epididymis. This tumor arises from the connective tissue of the testicle (fibrosarcoma). It permeates the entire organ, causing a tissue destruction that obliterates normal testicular contours. The scrotal skin is fixed over the testicular neoplasm. Little or no tenderness is associated with the lesion, which initially feels soft and later hard. Sarcomatous change is occasionally observed in abdominal testicles, in which case the spermatic cord shows a dark bluish-red discoloration and considerable swelling [Silbersiepe and Meyer, 1936].

Testicular carcinoma is most common in older horses and usually occurs as an adenocarcinoma. It develops as a solitary lesion and has a tendency to metastasize. Testicular enlargement is rapid, and a hard mass is felt through the tense scrotal skin. Infiltrative growth soon leads to vegetations, ulcerous degeneration or fistulization of the scrotal skin. The tumorous tissue has a tendency to spread by way of the spermatic cord to the deep inguinal ring. The associated regional lymph nodes may also be involved. A swinging-leg lameness often results.

Teratomas, or tumors comprised of cells derived from all three germ layers ('mixed tumors'), are characterized by testicular enlargement. They have been known to reach the size of a soccer ball in cryptorchid testicles. They are hard, have a knobby surface, and sometimes are permeated with cysts. Horn-like structures, hair or even teeth may be contained in these cysts.

Dermoid cysts are uni- or multilocular retention cysts in degenerated abdominal testicles that may reach the size of a coconut. Their contents usually consist of hair, teeth and bone chips. Generally they are adherent to the abdominal wall or intestine.

Etiology. The origin of benign and malignant tumors is poorly understood. For the clinician, there are several factors that are thought to be instrumental in the causation of tumors. Experiments have shown that benign tumors can be transmitted to other animals through cell-free filtrates. Malignant tumors can be produced by certain chronic irritants. Thus, it is likely that the higher ambient temperature to which inguinal and abdominal testicles are exposed is a factor in the development of tumors (teratomas) in these structures. In the case of spontaneous tumors, a predisposition to neoplastic disease may be inheritable. Congenital predisposition of this type is known for teratomas as well as for dermoid and other cysts. In addition, an age disposition is known to exist in certain animal species (papillomas affecting primarily the young, and carcinomas the old).

Differential Diagnosis. Testicular tumors have to be differentiated from hematomas, hernias, abscesses and orchitis.

Diagnosis. 'Testicular tumor' is often the only diagnosis possible. Rapid, infiltrative growth, recurrence or metastases with progressive emaciation (cachexia) are good signs of a malignancy. The diagnosis is established by histologic examination of the surgically removed testicle.

Prognosis. The prognosis is good for a fibroma or adenoma that is solitary in occurrence and can be removed entirely by unilateral or bilateral castration. The prognosis is guarded in cases of extensive tumor growth and poor if the neoplasm is inoperable. Sarcomas and carcinomas of the testis carry a guarded to poor prognosis, and the outlook is hopeful only if there has been no metastasis, and the excision is carried into healthy tissue to forestall a recurrence [Bolz, 1980].

Teratomas and dermoid cysts of abdominal or inguinal testicles have a favorable prognosis owing to their good operability.

Treatment. Tumors that are confined to the testicle within the scrotum are removed by castration. Tumors with extension to the spermatic cord should be removed as far into the inguinal canal as possible. Tumors situated within the peritoneal cavity are removed by cryptorchidectomy.

2.1.8.3. Hermaphroditism

Definition. Hermaphroditism is a state characterized by the presence of both male and female structures and by a combination of male and female sex characters in the same animal. The gonads and the rest of the genital tract are affected in various ways.

Forms and Symptoms. The hermaphroditism may be of the bilateral glandular form or the testicular form. Affected animals are restless and display abnormalities of sex drive and micturition. While the behavior usually is more or less female, the hermaphrodite exhibits studdish behavior when exposed to mares. However, the morphologic criteria may be characteristic of a female (mammary development) or male (testicle just below the skin, a hand's breadth below the external angle of the ilium). Examination of the external genitalia reveals a vulva-like prepuce below the anus directly anterior to the ischial incisure. Within the prepuce is a penis-like structure with a well developed glans and prominent urethral orifice that can extend posteriorally during erection. Rectal examination is not always diagnostic, and some cases are not amenable to an antemortem diagnosis.

Differential Diagnosis. The presence of normal primary sex characters in cryptorchidism distinguishes this condition from hermaphroditism.

Diagnosis. In most cases a diagnosis can readily be made on the basis of external signs.

Treatment. Cosmetic surgery may be successful in creating a normal female habitus.

Prognosis and Comments. Hermaphroditic horses that have undergone cosmetic surgery are suitable for all types of non-breeding work.

2.1.8.4. Diseases of the Spermatic Cord

Suppurative and Fibroplastic Funiculitis and Vaginitis

Spermatic Cord Fistula

Definition. *Acute funiculitis* is a pyogenic inflammation of the spermatic cord. *Spermatic cord fistula* is a chronic, pyogenic inflammation of the cord stump and tunica vaginalis with a tendency toward abscessation and fistulization.

Symptoms. Acute pyogenic funiculitis develops a few days following castration. The scrotum is tender and warm to the touch. The inflammatory swelling extends upward from the scrotum, producing enlargement of the spermatic cord (fig. 2.1.8. — 1). The cause lies in a rapid, premature adhesion of the castration wound edges, causing an incarceration and congestion of the cord stump and tunica vaginalis. Wound healing is impaired. Exuberant granulation tissue can lead to the formation of rapidly-growing, mushroom-like granulomas on the cord stump.

Spermatic cord fistula develops gradually over a period of 6—8 weeks, or in rare cases even years, after castration and is characterized by a uni- or bilateral, bottle-size thickening of the spermatic cord. The fistulous openings are usually found in the area of the castration scars and represent tubular wound openings about the

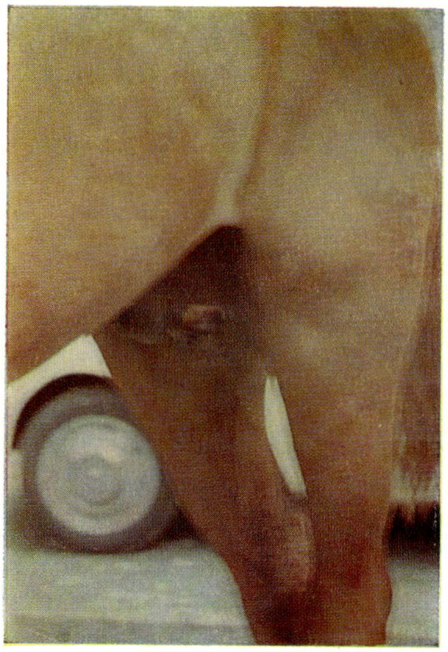

1

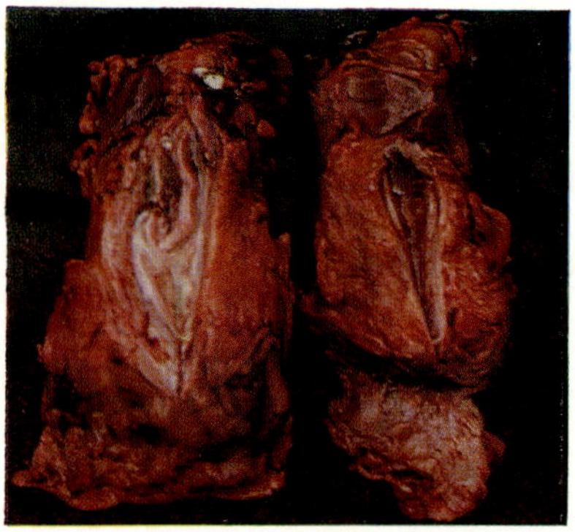

2

Fig. 2.1.8. — 1. Spermatic cord fistula.

Fig. 2.1.8. — 2. Bilateral spermatic cord fistula: resected stumps with necrotic cavities following ligation of the spermatic cords.

diameter of a knitting needle. The fistulous tracts are tortuous, of variable length, and generally are too narrow to permit the insertion of a probe. The fistulous openings exude a creamy, yellowish or greenish, sometimes foul-smelling pus which soils the area surrounding the fistulous opening and the inside of the thigh. The thickened spermatic cord feels hard on palpation and is usually nontender. It initially reaches the size of a pigeon egg or goose egg but may grow very much larger, especially if specific wound infections supervene. The mass tapers in bottle-shaped fashion toward the inguinal region, remnants of the spermatic cord and tunica vaginalis forming the neck of the 'bottle'.

Etiology. Sometimes an excessively long spermatic cord stump or prolapsed portions of the tunica vaginalis can give rise to an *acute pyogenic funiculitis and vaginitis.*

Spermatic cord fistulas result mainly from faulty ligation of the uncovered spermatic cord with silk or nylon threads, as well as from repeated crushing of the spermatic cord during emasculation, opening the way for micrococcal infection. Infection with various organisms can be picked up from straw bedding. In addition, poor sanitation and breaks in aseptic technique during and after the castration are a potential cause of funiculitis and vaginitis.

Differential Diagnosis. Retained wound secretions, scrotal edema and cellulitis during the first days after castration, combined with systemic signs, may be mistaken for pyogenic inflammations or fistulas of the spermatic cord.

Prognosis. The prognosis is good, except in the case of spermatic cord fistulas that extend far up into the inguinal canal. These may have already led to adhesions as a result of scrotal botryomycosis or reach beyond the vaginal ring to the abdominal wall.

Treatment. Funiculitis should be treated conservatively in the early stages. The daily application of penetrating ointments is the therapy of choice. Stall confinement is indicated until signs of inflammation subside. As a rule, even severe spermatic cord inflammation will regress spontaneously under such therapy. Avoid premature operative intervention! If a unilateral or bilateral granuloma has formed as a result of the castration, at least 4 weeks should pass before additional surgery is done.

The treatment for spermatic cord fistulas is surgery. With the animal in dorsal recumbency and under general anesthesia, the surgeon first cuts around the fistulous opening in spindle-shaped fashion, then dissects free the altered cord stump and associated parts of the tunic and resects them, carrying the excision into healthy tissue (fig. 2.1.8. — 2). We follow the rule that it is better to remove too much than too little diseased cord tissue, including the surrounding tunica vaginalis.

Müller [1976] describes a standing procedure, suitable for calm horses, in which spermatic cord fistulas that are only 2—3 months old are split with a probe-ended knife. In several cases a curette was used to remove necrotic tissue at the base of the fistula, a piece of tunica vaginalis, portions of the epididymis or an ingrown ligature. Treatment was followed by uneventful healing.

Comments. The operation for spermatic cord fistula is contraindicated if lesions extend to the vaginal ring and abdominal wall or to the regional lymph nodes.

2.1.8.5. Hydrocele

Definition. A hydrocele is a cyst of the tunica vaginalis that is caused by serous effusion, less frequently by hematomas. They are characterized by watery secretions and testicular atrophy. The condition may be acute or chronic.

Symptoms. Hydrocele presents as a soft, warm scrotal mass that is moderately tender in acute cases. The contents are fluctuant and may completely fill the vaginal cavity or may form cysts confined to the spermatic cord (spermatocele) or testis. Most hydroceles enlarge the scrotal cavity to 3—4 times normal size. The testicle is almost always smaller than normal and may be completely atrophic.

Etiology. Müller [1976] states that hydrocele can be congenital in the horse, for it has been encountered during the castration of stallions. As a rule, however, it is a result of trauma, especially contusions of the testicle or cord. The migration of certain parasites through the vaginal ring (*Setaria equina, Strongylus edentatus, Fasciola hepatica, Parafilaria multipapillosa*, etc.) has also been implicated.

Differential diagnosis must be made from scrotal hernia, in which the scrotum contains portions of the bowel or omentum in addition to varying amounts of accumulated fluid. Inguinal and scrotal hernia can be excluded by rectal exploration (free inguinal ring).

The *diagnosis* is verified by aspiration of the scrotal cavity, which in hydrocele will yield a serous, slightly stringy, amber-colored fluid.

Treatment consists in operative removal of the contents (castration) combined with excision of the tunica vaginalis (scrotal hernia operation).

Comments. A hydrocele rarely is a debilitating problem. Surgery is necessary only if the sac is very large; with unilateral castration, fertility will be preserved.

2.1.8.6. Varicocele

(Dilatation of the Pampiniform Plexus)

Varicocele is based upon a varicose dilatation of the internal spermatic vein in the pampiniform plexus. The plexus becomes greatly distended and feels like a 'bag of worms' on palpation. Varicocele is thought to be a congenital disorder. The definitive treatment is castration, although therapy is unnecessary in the majority of cases.

2.1.8.7. Hematocele

Definition. Hematocele is an accumulation of blood in the tunica vaginalis.

Symptoms. Hematocele develops suddenly and is characterized by a unilateral or bilateral ballooning of the scrotal sac, the scrotal skin becoming tightly stretched. The swelling is fluctuant and generally nontender.

Etiology. The most frequent causes are blunt trauma from kicks, blows or collisions.

Treatment is initially conservative, employing absorption-enhancing ointments, and is later surgical (procedure same as that for spermatic cord fistula).

Comments. Hematocele can impair or destroy the breeding soundness of stallions (testicular atrophy).

2.1.8.8. Postcastration Hydrocele

Definition. This is a special category of hydrocele that is observed only in castrated animals and involves an accumulation of serous exudate in the vaginal cavity (hydrocele or omental hernia of the gelding). A strand of omentum is adherent to the castration scar in the vaginal cavity.

Symptoms. On superficial examination of the gelding several weeks or months after castration, the scrotum appears much as it does in a noncastrated animal. Secondary sex characters are absent. A castration scar is present. The cyst of the tunica vaginalis is conspicuous by its size, especially in the gelding. The mass feels tense, is seldom warm and is sometimes fluctuant. The scrotal contents are irreducible. On rectal examination a strand of omentum can nearly always be felt entering the inguinal ring.

Etiology. The main cause is a rapid sealing of the edges of the surgically opened vaginal cavity following castration. However, an excessively large vaginal ring with prolapse of omental tissue during or after castration may also be responsible. The prolapsed or excised piece of omentum tends to become fused to the castration scar (omental hernia). This prevents the scrotal involution that normally follows castration. The vaginal sac and scrotum undergo an enlargement and contain portions of the omentum. A permanent communication is established with the peritoneal cavity through the vaginal canal.

Differential diagnosis is made from scrotal hernia and testicular hydrocele, which occur only in stallions.

The *prognosis* of postcastration hydrocele is good.

Treatment. Surgery is done in dorsal recumbency. The tunica vaginalis is opened either bluntly or sharply, and the adherent omental tissue is separated and returned to the abdomen. Then the vaginal sac is ligated at the external inguinal ring. Usually a vaginal sac containing only one strand of omentum can be bluntly separated from surrounding tissues up to the external inguinal ring, where it is ligated and excised.

2.1.8.9. Diseases of the Scrotum and Prepuce

2.1.8.9.1. Wounds, Cellulitis and Abscesses of the Scrotum and Prepuce

Definition and Occurrence. These are fresh wounds that may be followed by local pyogenic infection with cellulitis (phlegmon) and abscessation of the scrotum and prepuce.

Symptoms. Usually a slit wound, flap-shaped wound or contusion is evident; pouch-shaped wounds are rare. Perforating wounds present as tubular tracts or cavities. Extensive perforating wounds of the scrotum can cause a breach of the processes vaginalis, with prolapse of the testicle and spermatic cord. Thus, perforating wounds of this type may be accompanied by cellulitis.

Acute subcutaneous cellulitis is easily recognized on inspection and palpation by the marked swelling of the scrotal and preputial skin and the subcutis. The skin feels firm and slightly elastic and initially does not pit on pressure. It is tender and warm to the touch. Inflammatory edema is present, often with prolapse of the inner prepuce that may be mistaken for penile prolapse. Chronic cellulitis of the scrotum and prepuce, termed scleroderma or pachyderma, is not warm to the touch, is nontender and does not pit easily on pressure.

Abscesses in areas of cellulitis present as bulges of the scrotal and preputial skin. They erupt toward the exterior.

Specific infections are uncommon in the scrotum but are relatively frequent in the prepuce. They are characterized by a necrosis of the skin and subcutis, and in some cases by the formation of ulcerous, plaquelike lesions on the prepuce.

Etiology. Most wounds of the scrotum and prepuce occur when horses become entangled in fences, fall onto sharp objects, fail to clear an obstacle when jumping, become hung up on stall partitions, etc.

Cellulitis of the scrotal skin and prepuce results from pyogenic infections of the subcutaneous connective tissue secondary to traumatic or castration wounds or other operative procedures in the inguinal region. According to MÜLLER [1976], spermatic cord fistulas are also a frequent cause. Sclerodermas (pachydermas) develop secondarily to cellulitis and chronic congestive edema.

Differential Diagnosis. Acute cellulitis of the scrotum can occasionally be mistaken for orchitis, epididymitis, cellulitis of the spermatic cord and tunica vaginalis, as well as epitheliomas (spinocellular epithelioma) [TREFOGLI et al., 1974].

Preputial cellulitis with prolapse of the inner fold can mimic penile paralysis.

Prognosis. Superficial wounds of the scrotum and prepuce carry a good prognosis. Deeper wounds and wounds coming in contact with specific infectious organisms have a guarded prognosis.

Perforating wounds of the scrotum often carry a danger of systemic pyogenic infection. Testicular abscesses and peritonitis are possible complications. Cellulitis of the scrotum and prepuce will heal with proper therapy and hence carries a good prognosis, although residual scarring of the prepuce is frequent.

Treatment. Superficial and deeper, non-perforating wounds of the scrotum and prepuce heal well with nonsurgical treatment. This includes the application of antibiotic ointments or sulfonamide-containing powders. Perforating wounds are surgically repaired in layers. When the tunica vaginalis has been breached causing prolapse of the testicle, epididymis and spermatic cord, castration is sometimes necessary in the stallion. The relatively uncommon transverse tear injury of the prepuce immediately behind the preputial orifice may create strictures that hamper penile extension. Treatment in such cases consists in excising a sufficiently large tissue wedge from the inferior (ventral) prepuce.

Cellulitis of the scrotum is treated conservatively with diluted, penetrating ointments (e.g., camphor ointment, ichthammol ointment, carbol mercury ointment). Castration wounds are opened to permit drainage of secretions before ointment is applied. If systemic signs are present, supportive parenteral treatment with sulfonamides or antibiotics is indicated.

Cellulitis of the prepuce is also treated conservatively. After the area is washed with warm, mild disinfectant solutions and dried, ointments are applied for several days. Mild exercise is desirable. Abscesses should be incised after conservative treatment, and drainage is advised in some cases.

Comments. Wounds, inflammations and abscesses of the scrotum and prepuce are of economic importance in that they can compromise the working and breeding ability of the affected horse.

2.1.8.9.2. Tumors of the Scrotum and Prepuce

Occurrence. Benign tumors occur on the scrotum and prepuce in the form of fibromas and papillomas. Malignant tumors of these tissues include sarcomas, sarcoids and carcinomas, which affect mainly the prepuce.

Specific granulomas are rare and appear on the scrotum as botryomycosis.

Symptoms. Papillomas and the less frequent *fibromas* appear on the scrotum and prepuce as firm, solitary or multiple, sometimes pedunculated neoplasms varying in size from a hazelnut to a pigeon egg.

Sarcoids and *sarcomas* occur mainly on the ventral aspect of the prepuce but may develop on the lateral aspects as well. They may be solid or may ulcerate. They are firmly adherent to the cutis but may spread to the subcutaneous connective tissue by infiltration.

Not infrequently, *carcinomas* arise from the wall layer of the prepuce, erupting both toward the exterior and inward toward the penis. They are recognizable by their size, ulceration and their ragged, proliferative margins.

Melanosarcomas are peculiar to gray horses. Extension to the inguinal lymph nodes is known (cf. Sec. 2.1.1.4.3.).

Botryomycomas, observed as primary botryomycosis of the scrotum by Überreiter (quoted in Müller [1976]) and also affecting the prepuce, are distinguished by their irregular, knobby, clefted form. They can reach a substantial size.

Differential Diagnosis. It is not always possible to distinguish clinically between benign and malignant tumors, unless the lesion has reached an advanced stage. In some cases it will be necessary to submit biopsy material for histopathologic evaluation.

Diagnosis and Prognosis. The diagnosis will be limited to 'tumor' in the majority of cases. Papillomas and fibromas carry a good prognosis with operative removal. The prognosis for sarcoids, sarcomas and carcinomas is grave, as metastasis or local invasion is likely.

Treatment. Given a favorable location, size and extent, early-stage benign and malignant tumors as well as botryomycomas of the scrotum and prepuce are treatable by surgical excision. Unilateral castration may occasionally prove necessary in the stallion, although this method has obvious disadvantages from a breeding standpoint. Penile amputation may be considered in the gelding, although nowadays this measure is rarely adopted.

2.1.8.9.3. Posthitis

Definition. Posthitis is a chronic mucosal inflammation of the internal surface of the prepuce. It occurs in both stallions and geldings.

Symptoms. The condition is marked by inflammatory strictures of the prepuce. These strictures contain connective-tissue septa and are often prone to necrosis. The accumulated, decomposing smegma can form dense structures (preputial calculi) that obstruct the urethral process and interfere with urination. Inflammation due to the accumulated smegma can cause thickening of the prepuce with the formation of flap-like, annular fibrous septa. These produce a gradual occlusion of the prepuce with a danger of urine retention, cystitis and nephritis. Some degree of atrophy of the penis may even occur in neglected cases.

Etiology. The cause of posthitis is excessive smegma formation by the sebaceous glands in the area of the fossa glandis within the preputial sac.

The *prognosis* is good to guarded.

Treatment consists in removing the accumulated smegma following repeated lukewarm irrigation of the preputial cavity with a mild soapy solution. Cleansing is followed by irrigation with low-strength antiseptic solution and additional washing with acridine dye solutions. Chronic inflammatory strictures, including abnormal rings and compartments, are surgically corrected by removing a wedge-shaped piece of prepuce and extirpating the septum. Alternatively one may have to perform a total circumcision of the prepuce.

Comment. Posthitis is of economic significance in both stallions and geldings. A stallion with chronic posthitis may be unsound for breeding.

2.1.8.9.4. Phimosis

Definition. Phimosis is a rare, acquired and sometimes congenital constriction of the preputial orifice that hampers or prevents penile extension.

Symptoms. Extensive mucosal swelling is seen in the preputial orifice that may spread to the visceral layer of the prepuce and the glans. Urine is expelled in an intermittent, usually thin stream. This leads to a retention of urine and secretions. The decomposing urine has a foul odor and is mixed with concretions of varying size. In most cases penile extension is prevented. Phimosis may be accompanied by edema that extends to the scrotum.

Etiology. Acquired phimosis is the result of inflammatory and cicatricial lesions of the prepuce. Trauma, preputial calculi and tumors such as an epithelioma [TREFOGLI et al., 1974] may be the primary cause. Post-traumatic scarring leads to adhesions and thus to possible occlusion of the preputial orifice.

Treatment. Conservative methods such as irrigation with mild antiseptic solutions are beneficial only in cases where the preputial orifice retains some patency. The first line of treatment is surgical and includes incision, circumcision or the excision of a wedge of preputial skin based toward the preputial orifice, with exposure of the penis. Then the parietal layer of the prepuce is joined to the outer skin with a row of closely-spaced interrupted sutures.

Comments. Acquired phimosis in the stallion can impair breeding soundness, even with appropriate therapy.

2.1.8.9.5. Paraphimosis

Definition. Paraphimosis is a state in which the affected prepuce has retracted behind the glans, preventing penile retraction due to constriction or swelling of the preputial ring.

Symptoms. The prepuce is swollen. The inflamed and swollen penis feels warm to the touch, although it will feel cold if the strangulation is longstanding. Severe edema formation accompanies the penile swelling.

The 'penile prolapse' that occurs several days after castration should not be confused with paraphimosis. It merely represents a prolapse of the inflamed and swollen internal layer of the prepuce [MÜLLER, 1976].

Etiology. The cause is variable and includes various inflammatory stimuli. Trauma and neoplasms may be responsible.

The *prognosis* is guarded and depends on the stage and severity of the disease. In longstanding paraphimoses with associated diphtheritic membranes and necrosis of the penis, recovery is unlikely.

Treatment. With the animal in dorsal recumbency, an attempt can be made to reduce the penis after lubricating the glans and surrounding tissues. The prolapse that follows penile paralysis can be corrected only by surgery. The application of a well-fitting suspender device to the ventral abdomen is necessary only if initial attempts at reduction are unsuccessful.

Chronic cases with ulceration and necrosis are treated surgically, with careful excision of the diseased tissues. Subsequent irrigation with mild antiseptic solutions and the application of cod-liver-oil ointment are beneficial. Often it will be necessary to temporarily close the preputial orifice for 3—6 days with simple interrupted sutures.

2.1.8.10. Diseases of the Penis

2.1.8.10.1. Wounds, Closed Injuries and Inflammation of the Penis

Occurrence. Wounds, contusions and inflammations of the penis are occasionally seen; penile hematomas are less common.

Symptoms. Affected stallions continue to exhibit libido but rarely engage in copulation because of pain. The nature, appearance and extent of the penile wound (fig. 2.1.8. — 3) vary with the injury. Most common are transverse tears of the mucosa, but jagged tears extending into the submucosal connective tissue are not infrequent. Bleeding from the preputial orifice is the salient feature of superficial and deeper wounds. In the case of perforating wounds, which are less frequent, blood mixed with urine trickles from the preputial orifice or wound opening. The bleeding may be profuse, depending on the extent and depth of the wound. When the injured penis is withdrawn from the prepuce, areas of extravasated blood up to several centimeters across will be seen in the mucosa in the vicinity of the wound. Deeper wounds sometimes give the penis an 'incised' appearance, in which case urethral involvement is possible. PASCOE [1971] found deep, bleeding wounds in the upper fossa glandis of stallions with a direct access through the tunica albuginea to the corpus cavernosum. Improperly cared for, penile wounds commonly result in cellulitis and necrosis. Disturbances of micturation are also frequent [MÜLLER, 1976].

Healed penile wounds are sometimes associated with adhesions of the glans penis and preputial mucosa. These adhesions may be solitary or multiple and sometimes encircle the penis. Fibrous adhesions of this type are of about pencil thickness, are band-like in some cases, and have a pale color.

Closed injuries of the penis can take the form of contusions, ruptures or hematomas. Contusions produce a bluish-red or dark-red discoloration and localized swelling of the penis due to the extravasation of blood. Sometimes more extensive hemorrhages are noted in the mucosa and underlying connective tissue. Ruptures and hematomas are frequently extensive, in which case the penis is partially or completely prolapsed and shows a sickle-shaped, caudad curvature. The tube-shaped hematoma, which often extends to the ischial arch, is dorsal in location.

Inflammation of the penis affects its mucous membrane and is usually associated with inflammation of the preputial mucosa. The picture corresponds essentially to that of a posthitis. The mucosa is reddened, swollen and tender.

Etiology. Wounds of the penis can occur during attempts to cross low stall partitions or fences or as a result of falls on sharp objects. Often injuries are sustained during the act of breeding due to sudden movement by the mare, a too narrow vulvar fissure, or cuts from sharp tail hairs of the mare. Injuries can also result from the use of a poor-quality artificial vagina during semen collection.

Inflammation of the penile mucosa is due mainly to the irritating action of decomposing urine and/or smegma.

Differential Diagnosis. Hematomas must be differentiated from abscesses. Aspiration confirms the diagnosis.

Prognosis. Superficial wounds have a good prognosis, while deep or perforating wounds with associated urethral damage carry a high risk of stricture or urethral fistula. Contusions of the penis have a guarded prognosis.

Treatment. Fresh incised wounds of the penile mucosa that are smooth and superficial and do not require suturing may be treated topically with sulfonamide- or antibiotic-containing ointments, powders, emulsions or suspensions. These are used once hemostasis has been achieved. Older superficial wounds should be managed conservatively after they have been cleansed and irrigated with diluted acridine dye or potassium permanganate solutions. Parenteral antibiotic or sulfonamide therapy should be considered for the prevention of bacterial infection.

Fresh perforating wounds that do not involve the urethra should be repaired with closely-spaced sutures of non-absorbable suture material. Neglected perforating wounds must heal by second intention, all necrotic tissue having first been carefully removed from the wound interior. Suturing can sometimes be attempted after freshening the wound edges; this will be possible in some situations and impossible in others.

Transverse tears of the penis with damage to the urethra usually necessitate amputation of the penis. Le Gall and Durbal [1973] describe an amputation technique that does not destroy the breeding value of the stallion. The simultaneous creation of a urethral fistula, in which the urethral mucosa is sutured to the outer skin, may prove necessary depending on the location of the penile wound.

Contusions of the penis are treated topically with cod-liver-oil ointments. A suspender device is also attached in most cases.

When a penile hematoma is present, the penis must be immobilized with the aid of a suspender. Drainage sometimes proves necessary, but this should not be done before day 7.

In the case of mucosal inflammation, the adhering smegma is first removed by multiple irrigation with warm, low-strength astringent solutions, the area is washed repeatedly with acridine dye solutions, and finally antibiotic or sulfonamide-containing ointments, emulsions or suspensions are applied.

Comments. Deep wounds, perforating wounds, contusions, hematomas and inflammations of the penis, infectious or otherwise, can prove refractory to treatment in some instances and cause damage that lessens the breeding value of the affected stallion.

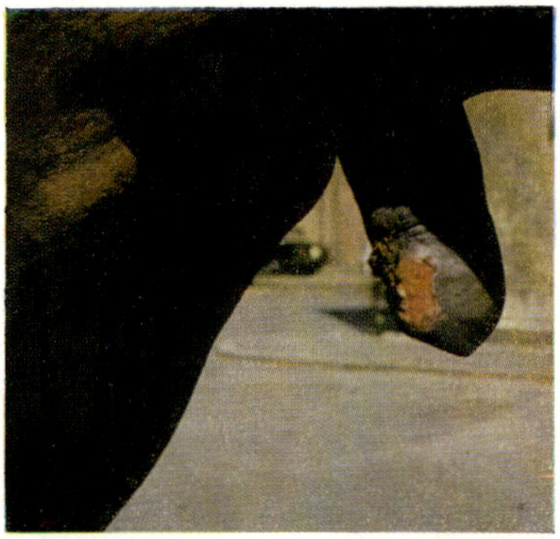
3

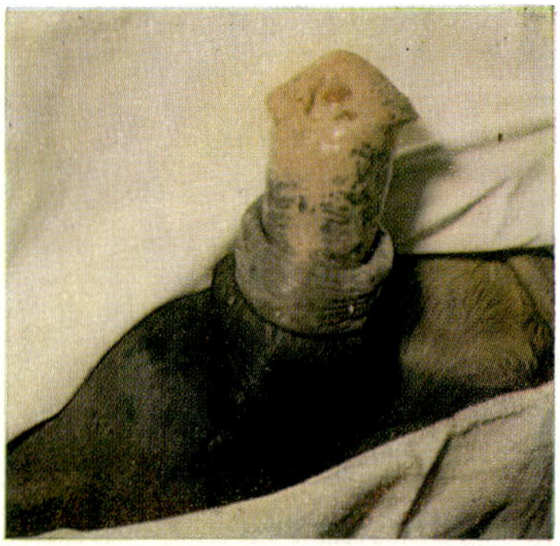
4

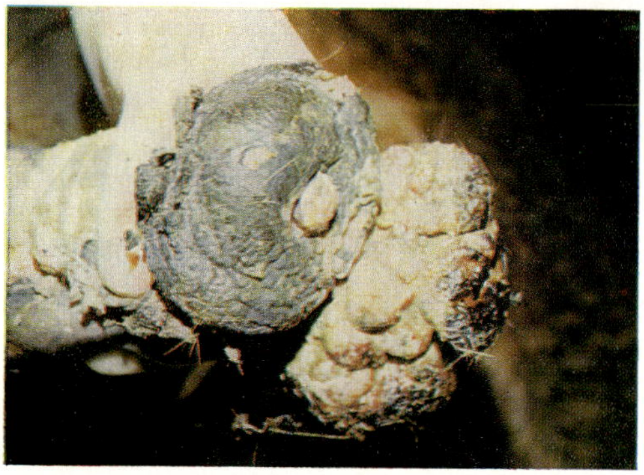
5

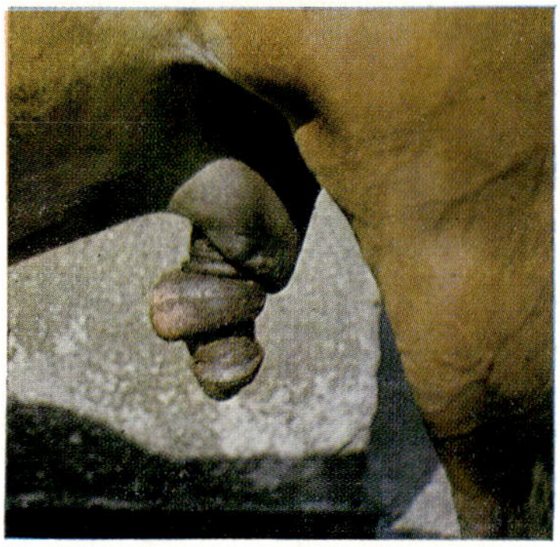
6

Fig. 2.1.8. — 3. Wound of the glans penis.
Fig. 2.1.8. — 4. Tumor of the glans penis.
Fig. 2.1.8. — 5. Degenerating papilloma of the glans penis.
Fig. 2.1.8. — 6. Prolapse of the penis with ring-shaped swelling of the inner prepuce.

2.1.8.10.2. Tumors and Malformations of the Penis

Forms and Occurrence. Tumors are most commonly situated on the glans but may also occur on the body or at other locations (fig. 2.1.8. — 4). Neoplasms of the penis may be benign (papilloma) or malignant (squamous cell carcinoma, epithelioma) [Trefogli et al., 1974].

Symptoms. The tumor may be visible when the penis is extended, or its presence may be signaled by a bloody discharge from the preputial orifice. A swelling of the prepuce that extends deep into the inguinal region may also be indicative of a penile neoplasm.

Papillomas of the penis appear as round or oval masses and may be pedunculated, though most are sessile. The tumor surface is smooth and rarely shows fissuring. Papillomas range in size from minute to large growths that involve the penis and glans. They tend to bleed easily on account of their thin epithelium. Heavy exudation can occur on contact with smegma (fig. 2.1.8. — 5).

Malignant tumors of the penis can occur as *sarcomas*, *squamous cell carcinomas* and *epitheliomas* and are most commonly seen in older horses. They may be pedunculated or sessile and can grow to softball-size or larger, covering the entire glans. The typical mass is cauliflower-like, often ulcerating, is accompanied by a slight caseous exudation, and bleeds easily. Metastasis, especially to the superficial and deep inguinal lymph nodes, is common [MÜLLER, 1976]. 'Contact metastases' can occur as a result of mucosal irritation due to prolonged contact with the visceral and parietal layers of the prepuce, the area of the preputial orifice forming the site of predilection for such lesions. A search should be made for these foci (which often are minute) during examination of the preputial layers.

Etiology. See Sec. 2.1.8.2.2.

Differential Diagnosis. See Sec. 2.1.8.2.2.

Prognosis. The prognosis is guarded to poor for all malignant tumors, although MÜLLER [1976] reported good results with local hyperthermia in the treatment of squamous cell carcinoma. Papillomas carry a guarded prognosis due to their potential transmissibility and liability to recur; the severity of the prognosis depends on the location, extent and number of neoplasms. Extirpation frequently gives rise to increased smegma secretion and to adhesions of the penile mucosa.

Treatment. The treatment of choice depends on the nature, location and extent of the tumor as well as on the desire to maintain the animal's breeding value. Amputation of the penis may be rejected on economic grounds. If this operation is done, however, it is essential that a urethral fistula be created in order to prevent cicatricial strictures of the penile stump and urethral stenosis. According to LE GALL and DURBAL [1973], it is possible to carry out penis amputation and still preserve the breeding soundness of the stallion. MÜLLER [1976] reports a favorable response of squamous cell carcinoma to local hyperthermia (45 °C).

Comments. Neoplasms of the penis are of economic interest owing to their impact on breeding soundness. As a general rule, penile neoplasia effectively destroys breeding soundness due to the probable need for penile amputation, although soundness for other types of work can be preserved.

2.1.8.10.3. Paralysis of the Penis

Definition. Penile paralysis involves a partial or complete prolapse of the penis from the preputial orifice coupled with a failure of penile retraction (fig. 2.1.8. — 6).

Symptoms. The penis hangs from the prepuce at all times. It is not retracted either during standing or exercise, during which time it flails about, striking the inner thighs and ventral abdomen. In this condition the penis is highly susceptible to trauma from contact with the stall floor during recumbency, from chafing against the thighs and abdomen during movement, and from temperature effects (heat and cold). The local bacterial infection that usually accompanies such wounds can give rise to extensive congestive and dependent edema and cellulitis. There are two main parts to the prolapsed penis which usually are well-defined: (1) an inferior part that is soft, rounded, presents a conical swelling, and is partially covered by firm skin; and (2) a superior, well-delineated part that is bisected by a sometimes well-defined, circumferential groove. This part forms a hard, ring-shaped cuff that usually cannot be pitted with the fingers. In the majority of cases the cuff and swollen glans make manual reduction impossible. No systemic signs occur, although nutritional condition may deteriorate. Rare cases may be complicated by paralysis of the tail or hindquarters. Micturition is not impaired. In longstanding cases greasy exudate, crusts and bleeding ulcers may appear on portions of the penile mucosa.

Etiology. The etiology varies and is not always obvious. The major cause is general debility with loss of muscle and fatty tissue, allowing the pudendal nerve to become contused or overstretched at the ischiatic arch. Penile paralysis is a neurogenic disease. It can result from direct trauma to the penis in the form of a contusion or stretch injury. Closed injuries that involve damage to the pudendal nerve or dorsal nerve of the penis can occur during drug-induced penile prolapse if the prolapse lasts longer than about 6 hours [Müller, 1976]. Infectious diseases (pleuritis, upper respiratory tract infections and other diseases) can also be a cause of penile paralysis. Spinal cord pathology and fractures of the 2nd through 5th lumbar vertebrae may have causal significance.

Differential Diagnosis. Differentiation from cellulitis, preputial edema and paraphimosis is necessary.

Prognosis. The prognosis is guarded. Acute cases due to closed injuries (contusion, stretch) as well as cases that follow on pleuritis and other diseases can recover within a few weeks. Cases of longer duration associated with cellulitis and eventual chronic fibrosis have a poor prognosis.

Treatment. Treatments vary with the duration, severity and extent of the disease. In cases of only a few days' duration that are uncomplicated by bacterial infection, reduction can usually be achieved through massage of the penis [Müller, 1976]. Then either a well-padded, loose-fitting suspender apparatus (bandage of Bolz [1970]) or 'bolster suture' of Müller [1976] is used to effect partial closure of the preputial opening. Treatment is continued until the edema accompanying the prolapse has subsided and wound surfaces are well epithelialized.

Some authors scarify the edematous parts of the penis and remove accumulated fluid by compression, the aim being to reduce the size of the penis so that it can be returned to the prepuce.

Recovery may possibly be hastened by giving large doses of vitamin-B complex.

If the aforementioned conservative measures fail to correct the penile paralysis and prolapse within 3 to 4 weeks, surgical retraction of the penis is indicated. This can be done using various techniques. In Bolz's [1970] method, penile retraction is achieved by opening the prepuce anterior to the scrotum and suturing the blind end of the invaginated preputial tube to the cutaneous wound. We can also recommend the method of Ludwig as modified by Schebitz [1950], in which the internal prepuce is resected and the prolapsed penis is embedded or sutured into a corresponding opening in the external prepuce. One may also use the method of Mörkeberg as modified by Westhues. These are superior to the techniques of Vennerholm and Forsell. These have the disadvantage of creating large wound surfaces (see surgical textbooks for further details).

Amputation of the penis is rarely practiced any longer as a remedy for penile paralysis.

In all surgical methods of retraction of the penis as well as penile amputations, concurrent castration is indicated.

Comments. Penile paralysis represents a serious disorder in the stallion and implies breeding unsoundness, although other usage of the affected animal is possible for a certain period of time.

References

Arcularius, K.: Die Kastration des abdominal-kryptorchiden Hengstes. Mh. Vet.-Med. *29:* 188 (1974).

Arthur, G. H.: Die Chirurgie des Kryptorchismus beim Pferd. Vet. Rec. *73:* 385 (1961).

Blendinger, W.: Die Kastration des kryptorchiden Pferdes in der Linea alba. Dtsch. Tierärztl. Wschr. *65:* 527 (1958).

Bolz, W., unter Mitarb. von Dietz, O.: Lehrbuch der Allgemeinen Chirurgie für Tierärzte, 4. Aufl. (Enke, Stuttgart und VEB Gustav Fischer Verlag, Jena 1970).

Bolz, W.; Dietz, O.; Schleiter, H.; Teuscher, R.: Lehrbuch der Speziellen Veterinärchirurgie, 2. Aufl. (VEB Gustav Fischer Verlag, Jena 1975).

Burger, Ch. H.: Operation des Kryptorchismus am stehenden Pferd — linke Flanke. J. Amer. vet. med. Assoc. *135:* 379 (1959).

Cox, J. E. et al.: An analysis of 500 cases of equine cryptorchism. Equine Vet. J. *11:* 119 (1979).

De Moor, A.; Verschooten, F.: Paramedianschnitt zur Entfernung von abdominalen Hoden beim Pferd. Vet. Med. and Small. Animal. Clinician. *62:* 1083 (1967).

Dietzmann, U.; Möller, R.: Stehendkastration des abdominal-kryptorchiden Pferdes. Dtsch. Tierärztl. Wschr. *66:* 641 (1959).

Huskamp, B.: Die mediane Laparotomie beim Pferd — Technik — Ergebnisse. Dtsch. Tierärztl. Wschr. *83:* 263 (1976).

Le Gall, A.; Durbal, F. F.: Technique simplifiée d'amputation du pénis chez le cheval. Rec. Méd. Vét. Ecole Alfort *149:* 239 (1973).

Lowe, J. E.; Higginnbotham, R.: Kastration von abdominalen kryptorchen Pferden durch paramediane Laparotomie. Cornell Vet. *59:* 121 (1969).

Merriam, J. G.: Ein inguinaler Zugang bei der Kryptorchidektomie des Pferdes. Vet. Med. and Small. Animal Clinician *67:* 187 (1972).

Pascoe, R. R.: Ruptur des Penisschwellkörpers bei einem Hengst. Austral. vet. J. *47:* 610 (1971).

Silbersiepe, E.; Berge, E.; Müller, H.: Lehrbuch der speziellen Chirurgie für Tierärzte und Studierende, 15. Aufl. (Enke, Stuttgart 1976).

Sikora, Z.: Beitrag zur Kastration des abdominalen Hengstkryptorchiden durch Flankenschnitt. Med. weteryn. *3:* 182 (1968).

Stickle, R. L.; Fessler, J. F.: Retrospective study of 350 cases of equine cryptorchism. J. Amer. Vet. Med. Assoc. *172:* 343 (1978).

Swift, P. N.: Castration of a stallion with bilateral abdominal cryptorchism by flank laparotomy. Austral. vet. J. *48:* 472 (1972).

Trefogli, C. A.; Lucas, E. C.; Barberis, S. J.; Fridkin, A.; Mussi, A. A.: Epithelioma espinocelular y fimosis. Gac. Vet. (Buenos Aires) *36:* 284 (1974).

Valdez, H. et al.: Abdominal Cryptorchidectomy in the horses, using inguinal extension of the gubernaculum testis. J. Amer. Vet. Med. Assoc. *174:* 1110 (1979).

Wright, J. G.: Die Laparo-Orchidektomie beim Pferd bei abdominalem Kryptorchismus. Vet. Rec. *72:* 57 (1960).

2.1.9. Sterilization and Castration of the Stallion

2.1.9.1. Sterilization of the Stallion

Definition and Application. Sterilization involves the surgical interruption of the sperm-conveying structures. The operated stallion is rendered infertile, but the libido is not affected. In addition, the animal retains its masculine behavior and appearance, which may be desirable in riding and carriage horses.

Operative Technique. The stallion is cast onto its left side under general anesthesia, and the uppermost hind leg is tied back as for castration. The field of operation is scrubbed with surgical soap and sprayed with a suitable antiseptic. With one hand the surgeon grasps the scrotal neck of the lowermost, left testicle and presses deep into the scrotum until the club-shaped contour of the tail of the epididymis is visible at the caudal end of the testis. He then makes an incision through the scrotum and tunica vaginalis directly over the tail of the epididymis, taking care that the incision through the scrotum is larger than that through the tunica vaginalis. The cut through the tunica vaginalis should be just large enough to allow the tail of the epididymis to pass through. For resection of the tail of the epididymis, a medium-size artery forceps is clamped across the terminal part of the body of the epididymis, parallel to the direction of the incision, such that the sectioned tunica vaginalis lies within the jaws of the forceps. Now a double strand of surgical gut is carried between the artery forceps and caudal end of the testicle, passing also between the body of the epididymis and initial portion of the vas deferens. Ligatures are placed and tied. The tail of the epididymis is resected parallel to the artery forceps with a scissors or scalpel. The ligated stumps of the spermatic canal and vas deferens are now outside the tunica vaginalis. The edges of the scrotal wound are joined with a double row of continuous surgical gut. Suture removal is unnecessary.

Aftercare. Postoperative swelling of the wound is rare, and so wound aftercare is seldom required. Exercise is desirable during the first postperative days.

2.1.9.2. Castration of the Stallion[1]

Castration of the Stallion with Incision of the Tunica Vaginalis

Indications. These include economic considerations, orchitis, testicular neoplasms, hydrocele, varicocele, hematocele, dermoid cysts, perforating scrotal wounds and fistulas.

Technique. The stallion is cast onto its left side under general anesthesia with a suitable casting apparatus. The uppermost hind leg is secured in flexion, and the scrotum and scrotal region are scrubbed and sprayed with a suitable antiseptic. For stallions that are shedding their hair coat, the insides of the thighs should be wetted to prevent hair contamination of the operative area. Both testicles are grasped firmly from the front with the left hand, and the scrotal skin is tensed so that the median raphe is visable. At this time two superficial 'guide incisions' are made lateral to the median raphe, diverging slightly in a cranial direction. Each incision is made in an anteroposterior direction, and each extends only to the subcutis (dartos). Next, the lowermost (far) testicle is grasped firmly at the scrotal neck from front to back with the left hand, which will cause the primary incision to gape slightly. An incision about 7—10 cm long is now made boldly through all the coats of the testicle, without cutting into the testis itself. In stallions younger than 2½ years, the testicle and spermatic cord should be given a half-twist following the incision in order to put the vascular portion of the spermatic cord in the inner angle of the emasculator jaws. In stallions older than 2½ years, it is unwise to have this much tissue in the emasculator, as this will hamper the crushing action of the instrument. It is better to incise the scrotal ligament with a scissors at the tail of the epididymis, and then push back the mesorchium with the left hand so that the spermatic cord can be isolated and crushed in the manner described, and the testicle removed. The procedure for the near testicle is the same.

For safety, one may elect to use two castration instruments. One method, for example, is to first place a crushing forceps around the spermatic cord and then apply the emasculator distal to it. The dual crushing action combined with the cutting

[1] Taken largely from Dietz, Schaetz, Schleiter and Teuscher: Anästhesie und Operationen bei Gross- und Kleintieren, 3rd ed., 1980, with permission of S. Hirzel Publishers, Leipzig.

action of the emasculator practically eliminates the danger of postoperative bleeding from the cord. Using 4 Pean or similar artery forceps, the cranial and caudal edges and both sides of the wound are grasped and well retracted so that the surgeon can verify that an adequate incision has been made through the coats of the testis, particularly the tunica vaginalis, and that satisfactory hemostasis has been achieved. The incision through the tunics may be extended in a cranial direction if necessary. If bleeding from the cord vessels occurs despite every precaution, the cavity of the wound is packed, and the cord is carefully exteriorized with a dressing forceps and ligated with a loop of surgical gut ('castration loop'). If the castration is done with good aseptic technic, the introduction of sulfonamides or antibiotics into the wound cavity is unnecessary and is not recommended.

Aftercare. The new gelding is either stabled for 24 hours or, preferably, is turned out on pasture immediately after the operation, which usually is performed in the spring or early fall. The animal should at least be placed in a paddock so that free exercise is possible. Tetanus antitoxin is administered to all horses that have not been actively immunized prior to the castration.

Postoperative Bleeding from the Cord Vessels. Such bleeding can occur hours or even days following an open castration. With the hand in a sterile rubber glove, the wound is carefully checked with the animal standing, any clotted blood is removed, and the source of the bleeding is localized. For the actual hemostasis, the animal is sedated, the wound edges are retracted, and one or two long artery forceps (Pean) are placed around the spermatic cord, including its vascular portion, and left in place for at least 24 hours while the animal is kept standing in cross-ties. This method is not always successful. For the less experienced surgeon, therefore, we recommend casting the animal again, extending the wound craniad and caudad to enlarge the operative cavity, grasping the spermatic cord under vision and ligating it with a castration loop of surgical gut.

Prolapse of Omentum. Prolapse of omentum is a rare complication. If it occurs following a castration, about 20—30 cm of the prolapsed tissue should be withdrawn from the wound and resected well into the inguinal canal with an emasculator. An alternate method is to ligate the omentum with surgical gut and resect the distal portion. If omental tissue prolapses during the castration, the procedure is similar to that for a closed castration: The tunica vaginalis is freed from surrounding tissues well into the inguinal canal, it is pulled upward on the spermatic cord with several artery forceps, emasculators are placed around the tunica vaginalis and cord and closed to crush the contained structures, and a ligature is applied at the crushed site. The omentum must not become incarcerated during this procedure, but must be allowed to slip back into the peritoneal cavity.

Castration of the Stallion without Incising the Tunica Vaginalis

Indications. This method, known as the 'closed' technique, is preferred for older stallions. In animals with a large vaginal orifice, this technique will eliminate the danger of omental or intestinal prolapse. It is also indicated in animals with scrotal hernia.

Technique. The animal is cast under general anesthesia and the skin prepared in the usual fashion. The testicle is grasped at the scrotal neck as for an open castration. A longitudinal incision is made through the skin and dartos, slightly diverging from the median raphe; the tunica vaginalis is not incised. By blunt dissection or with gentle, dissecting strokes of the scalpel, the tunica vaginalis is freed from the surrounding loose connective tissue until the lateral contours of the testicle and part of the spermatic cord are visible. Blunt finger dissection of surrounding tissues is continued chiefly in the lateral, cranial and caudal directions until the external cremaster muscle is visualized. The use of curved scissors for separating the aforementioned connective tissue has the advantage of allowing an unrestricted view of the operative field while enabling torn connective tissue to be removed from the wound. The testicle is excised either with emasculators or with a cutting instrument following ligation.

Technique for the Use of Emasculators (HAUSMANN emasculator, Serra or Sand emasculators): The forceps are applied to the covered spermatic cord about a hand's width proximal to the testicle. Considerable force will have to be applied to close the castration forceps if there is much swelling of the cord and the tunica vaginalis is tough. The forceps are left closed until the testicle and distal part of the vaginal process fall away. It should be noted that this technique does not ensure closure of the vaginal canal and is contraindicated in stallions with scrotal hernia or a predisposition to hernia.

Because the vessels are not always well occluded due to the large cross-section of the crushed tissues, it is best to use two castration forceps for the procedure: one proximally and one emasculator distally. The skin incision will have to be extended 2 or 3 cm in a cranial direction when 2 instruments are used.

Technique for Ligation of the Cord. Ligation with surgical gut offers an alternative to the more or less outdated method of emasculation by the closed technique. An emasculator is placed around the exposed, covered spermatic cord as far up in the inguinal canal as possible. At the same time, a forceps with teeth or a BILLROTH toothed forceps is used to exteriorize the testicle and epididymis contained within the tunica vaginalis. The same site is crushed 2 or 3 times, each time rotating the enclosed testicle by about 180°. Then the crushed site is ligated with a loop of medium-size surgical gut. Finally the spermatic cord is divided with a scissors or emasculator about 2—3 fingers' breadth distal to the ligature. The ends of the thread can be passed through the cord distal to the ligature and tied to keep the ligature from slipping. The ends should hang down several inches from the castration wound.

Aftercare. Exercise is beneficial. The ligature will slough spontaneously about 2—3 weeks postoperatively, or it may be removed by carefully pulling on the ends of the thread.

Technique in Animals with a Scrotal Hernia or Predisposition to Hernia. The surgical technique must be modified somewhat in the presence of a scrotal hernia, which is most common in male foals and is unilateral in most cases. It should be remembered that scrotal hernias may still reduce spontaneously in foals that are less than a year old.

The foal is anesthetized and cast in dorsal recumbency. The scrotum is grasped with a toothed forceps, and an incision is carefully made around the outer hernial sac (scrotal skin) in spindle-shaped fashion, taking great care not to open the inner sac (tunica vaginalis). By slow, blunt dissection with the fingertips in the direction of the enlarged inguinal ring, the inner hernial sac is exposed. Excess connective tissue is removed with a curved scissors, taking care to spare the often greatly enlarged and tortuous veins at the constricted neck of the vaginal sac. The inner hernial sac having been completely freed from surrounding tissues, the testicle is immobilized with the right hand, and the sac is twisted such that the hernial contents (omentum, bowel) are gradually returned to the abdominal cavity. At the external inguinal ring, the spermatic cord is singly ligated (the thread ends being passed through the cord) or doubly ligated with heavy surgical gut. The ends of the thread are left hanging from the scrotal wound.

In this procedure as in others, forceps emasculation has become obsolete.
The ligatures will slough in about 8—10 days or may be removed by careful traction along with the necrotic cord stump.

Castration of the Stallion with Incision and Repair of the Tunica Vaginalis [Müller, 1977]

Indications. The goal is an aseptic castration that avoids complications associated with the presence of a wound cavity (hemorrhage, postoperative bleeding, prolapse of omentum or bowel, infection). The technique described below is a practice-applicable procedure that is suitable for stallions in all age ranges.

Technique. The stallion is cast under general anesthesia and positioned in dorsal recumbency. The operative area is prepared in the usual fashion. The testicle is grasped firmly with the left hand and held in such a way that the skin over the scrotum is tense. With the right hand the skin and dartos are divided parallel to the median raphe for a distance of no more than 4—5 cm, taking care not to incise the tunica vaginalis. Gentle pressure is exerted to exteriorize the testicle and enclosing tunica vaginalis, while the connective tissue surrounding the tunica is separated with a few dissecting cuts of the scalpel or scissors. As before, the left hand immobilizes the spermatic cord and testicle. At this time the extremity of the tunica vaginalis is incised for a length of 1—2 cm over the testicle, and 2 or 3 long Pean or similar forceps are applied to the tunica to keep it from retracting (we place 1 forceps at the cranial end of the incision and another at the caudal end). Next, the incision in the tunica vaginalis is extended in preparation for delivery of the testicle, which is done with the aid of a small Billroth or similar forceps. The immobilizing left hand releases its grasp. Traction is now applied to the Pean and Billroth forceps in preparation for excision of the testicle and epididymis and management of the cord, and the tunica is freed of remaining connective tissue by finger dissection. At this point the testicle and tunica vaginalis should project 5—8 cm from the wound. A suitable emasculator is placed around the tunica vaginalis and enclosed spermatic cord at the level of the scrotal wound edges. In this way compression is applied to the cord and cord vessels, and bleeding from the vessels is prevented.

Management of the cord consists of dividing the scrotal ligament with scissors, applying 1 or 2 Pean forceps across the uncovered cord, and transecting the cord with the scissors, thereby emasculating the testis. It is important that the epididymis also be resected! Before the artery forceps are removed, the cord stump is ligated with a loop of surgical gut to prevent postoperative bleeding from the testicular artery and other vessels. Next the incision in the tunica vaginalis is repaired with a continuous gut suture. The edges of the incision should be *inverted* as much as possible when the suture is placed. The reason for repairing the tunica vaginalis is to guard against omental and intestinal prolapse while preventing effusion into the wound from the serous coat of the tunica vaginalis. This may potentially interfere with wound healing. The artery forceps are removed from the spermatic cord, and the cord stump and tunica vaginalis are allowed to retract into the wound cavity. To reduce dead space, the interior surfaces of the loose connective tissue that fills the inguinal canal are apposed with a few interrupted gut sutures. The operation is concluded by closing the skin wound with a double row of interrupted gut sutures. Suture removal is unnecessary. Primary healing is the goal.

Aftercare. Weather permitting, the new gelding should be pastured immediately after the operation. Otherwise the animal should be exercised twice daily for 30 minutes if possible starting on the 2nd postoperative day. The mild wound swelling that appears on postoperative day 5—7 will eventually disappear without treatment.

Intervention should be considered only if fever and anorexia develop. Immunization against tetanus is required.

Castration of the Stallion through an Incised Opening
(after Dietz and Nagel [1961])

Indications. This technique draws on experience in the surgery of spermatic cord fistulas. The course of healing of the surgical wound depends on a relatively dry subcutaneous cavity.

Technique. The stallion is placed under general anesthesia and cast onto its side or back. The scrotum is grasped firmly with the left hand, and the scrotal skin and dartos are opened with an incision lateral to the median raphe. The left hand must hold the scrotum proximally so that the skin over both testicles is tense. The fascia-covered testicle is grasped with a toothed forceps. By careful scraping with the dull edge of the scalpel, the loose attachment between the superficial scrotal fascia and dartos is freed around to the lateral surfaces of the scrotum. From about the middle of the lateral surfaces, the dissection is continued bluntly in a proximal direction in the same layer; finger dissection is best for this purpose, but a curved scissors is sometimes used. As the dissection nears the abdomen, branches of the external pudendal vein or external pudendal artery, which may be up to several centimeters thick, will be encountered laterocaudally. These vessels must be spared and should be carefully retracted away from the vaginal process. At this point the direction of the finger dissection is changed so as to penetrate the fascia that fuse at various levels with the outer abdominal wall, as well as the interfascial tissue. The fascial remnants still enclosing the processus vaginalis are left in place. In the same way, the attachments between the scrotal septum and fibrous layer of the tunica vaginalis are separated. The exposed vaginal process is crushed 2 or 3 times with forceps close to the external inguinal ring and ligated. The forceps is left closed, while a suitable emasculator is placed around the spermatic cord about 2 cm distal to the initial crush site. The cord is then crushed, divided, and the testicle removed. From the same incision, the vaginal process of the opposite side is exposed. Further development of the second tunica- and fascia-covered testicle is carried out in the manner described. After the second testicle has been emasculated, there will be left a large, almost subcutaneous wound cavity that is partitioned only in its dorsal portion by the remnant of the scrotal septum. The wound cavity is left open, and the two skin flaps of the scrotal wound do not require suturing.

Aftercare. Wound healing is uneventful, and so minimal postoperative care is necessary.

Standing Castration of the Stallion

Indications. This method is suitable for stallions up to about 3 years of age whose testicles can be grasped easily. The advantage of the standing method is that the castration can be done more rapidly and in some cases more easily than in the recumbent position. The disadvantages are the limited potential for restraint (the animal may lie down during the procedure) and the danger of omental or intestinal herniation and postoperative bleeding. The procedure calls for intuition and dexterity on the part of the surgeon. Facilities for inducing general anesthesia and a casting apparatus should be on hand in the event that complications arise.

Basic Considerations. The animal should not be supported on either side during the operation, and unnecessary contact with the flank area intraoperatively should be avoided. An assistant should hold the tail to one side without using it as a 'restraint rope'. The tail should be kept wrapped for 2—4 days after the castration.

Technique. After a twitch is applied by an assistant and anesthesia is induced (sedative or narcotic plus local anesthesia), the operative field is scrubbed and the scrotal area sprayed with tincture of iodine or a similar agent. The surgeon approaches the horse from the left side in a slightly stooped position, grasps the scrotum from the front with the left hand and immobilizes the 2 testicles in the scrotum. With the scalpel held in the right hand, a swift, bold incision is made parallel to the median raphe over the right testis, extending in depth through the skin, dartos and tunica vaginalis. An incision is then made over the left testicle in the same manner and from the same side. If no intratesticular anesthesia was administered, bilateral anesthesia of the spermatic cords can be achieved by 'painting' on anesthetic with a sterile gauze pad and dressing forceps until the internal cremaster muscle relaxes and the testicles, including the epididymis and scrotal ligament, protrude completely from the wound cavities. Now, starting on the left side, the testicle is twisted 180°, and the emasculator is placed around the spermatic cord and closed to effect the emasculation. For safety, a long artery clamp should be applied to the spermatic cord a short distance above the emasculator so that the cord can be more easily withdrawn in the event of postoperative bleeding. The same procedure is followed for emasculating the right testicle.

In young stallions (1—2 years) with well-developed testicles, the scrotal ligament and mesorchium should be incised (following local anesthesia) with a snip of the scissors at the site where the ligament attaches to the tail of the epididymis and carefully stripped upward with the fingers toward the abdominal cavity. This is done because if the spermatic cord and the scrotal ligament plus mesorchium were all to come between the emasculator jaws, the large cross-section of the enclosed tissues would greatly diminish the crushing action of the instrument. Therefore, after the scrotal ligament and mesorchium have been separated from the cord, both are excised with the emasculator before the spermatic cord is crushed and the testicle removed. Care should be taken not to make the incision in the tunica vaginalis too short. If necessary the operative wound can be extended with the scissors. The wounds are left open.

Aftercare. Bleeding from spermatic cord veins or from veins supplying the tunica vaginalis or scrotal skin is frequent when morphine is used for restraint of the standing horse, but this bleeding will stop about 20—30 minutes postoperatively when the effect of the morphine subsides. If arterial bleeding persists for more than 15 minutes postoperatively, the cord remnant should be carefully withdrawn with the aid of the artery forceps applied previously and then ligated with surgical gut. Tetanus prophylaxis should be provided.

References

Ban, N. E.: Kastration von Pferden und Komplikationen, die daraus entstehen. Vet. Rec. *87:* 502 (1970).

Berge, E.; Westhues, M.: Tierärztliche Operationslehre (Parey, Berlin [West] und Hamburg 1969).

Dietz, O.; Gängel, H.; Richter, W.: Die Sterilisation des Ebers und des Hengstes. Mh. Vet.-Med. *29:* 906 (1974).

Dietz, O.; Nagel, E.: Beitrag zur Kastration des Hengstes unter Klinikverhältnissen. Berliner Münchener Tierärztl. Wschr. *74:* 189 (1961).

Dietz, O.; Schaetz, F.; Schleiter, H.; Teuscher, R.: Anästhesie und Operationen bei Gross- und Kleintieren, 3. Aufl. (Hirzel, Leipzig, und Enke, Stuttgart 1980).

Heinze, C. D.: Methoden der Hengstkastration. J. Amer. vet. med. Assoc. *148:* 428 (1966).

Hubelcius, D. R.; Rasolinson, R.: Eventration as a sequel to castration of the horse. Austral. vet. J. *5:* 288 (1972).
Johnson, J. H.: Post castration complications. Mod. vet. Pract. *54:* 49 (1973).
Kiley, M.: A review of the advantages and disadvantages of castrating farm livestock with particular reference to behavioural effects. Brit. vet. J. *132:* 323 (1976).
Kostyra, J.: Eigenes Verfahren zur Behandlung des Darmvorfalles bei Hengsten nach der Kastration. Med. weteryn. *73:* 600 (1967).
Lowe, J. E.; Dougherty, R.: Kastration von Pferden und Ponys durch primäre Wundverschlussmethode. J. Amer. vet. med. Assoc. *160:* 183 (1972).
Lübke, M.-J.: Die Kastration des Hengstes unter Antibiotikaschutz und postoperativer Analyse. Tierärztl. Umschau *12:* 170 (1957).
Mikusz, St.: Bemerkungen zum Darmvorfall nach der Kastration des Hengstes. Med. weteryn. *24:* 180 (1968).
Müller, H.: Über Wirkung und Wert der antibiotischen und chemotherapeutischen Wundprophylaxe bei der Heilung der Kastrationswunde des Hengstes. Dtsch. tierärztl. Wschr. *64:* 503 (1957).
Müller, H.: Die Kastration des Hengstes nach heutigen chirurgischen Grundsätzen. Tierärztl. Umschau *32:* 367 (1977).
Riev, A.: Contribution à l'étude de la castration chez le cheval par le cluppe métallique du docteur Schecker. Vet. med. Diss., Paris-Alfort (1957).
Robertson, J. S.: Castration in farm animals; its advantages and disadvantages. Vet. Rec. *78:* 130 (1966).
Schulte zu Sudern, L.: Eine Literaturstudie über die Kastration bei unseren männlichen Haussäugetieren. Vet.-med. Diss., Hannover (1976).
Tamás, L.; Fellner, F.: Allatorvosi Sebészeti Mütéttan. Mezögazdasági Kiadó, Budapest 1960.
Teuscher, R.: Kastration am stehenden Hengst, ihre Entwicklung und Bedeutung für den prakt. Tierarzt. Mh. Vet.-Med. *7:* 223 (1952).
Wriedt, W. D.; Schebitz, H.; Böhm, D.: Zur Kastration des Hengstes. Berliner Münchener tierärztl. Wschr. *92:* 41 (1979).

2.1.10. Reproductive Disorders in the Stallion

To achieve optimum reproductive efficiency in the breeding of horses, it is essential that regular, systematic evaluations be made of the animals' sexual health. This includes a breeding soundness examination of stallions that are used for service.

Besides the disorders such as lack of libido, impotence and poor semen quality, there are a variety of other disturbances in the breeding health of the stallion, some infectious in nature, that prohibit the use of the affected stallion.

2.1.10.1. Anatomy and Physiology of Sexual Potency in the Stallion

Preliminary Remarks on Anatomy

Our anatomic descriptions are limited to the topographic relations that are important in the breeding soundness examination. These are shown in fig. 2.1.10. — 1. Details on anatomy or histology should be sought in the literature.

Preliminary Remarks on Physiology

Stallions reach sexual maturity at about the age of 15 months. The development of sexual potency is breed-dependent and is closely related to environmental factors. 'Studdish' behavior can already be observed in foals before the start of spermato-

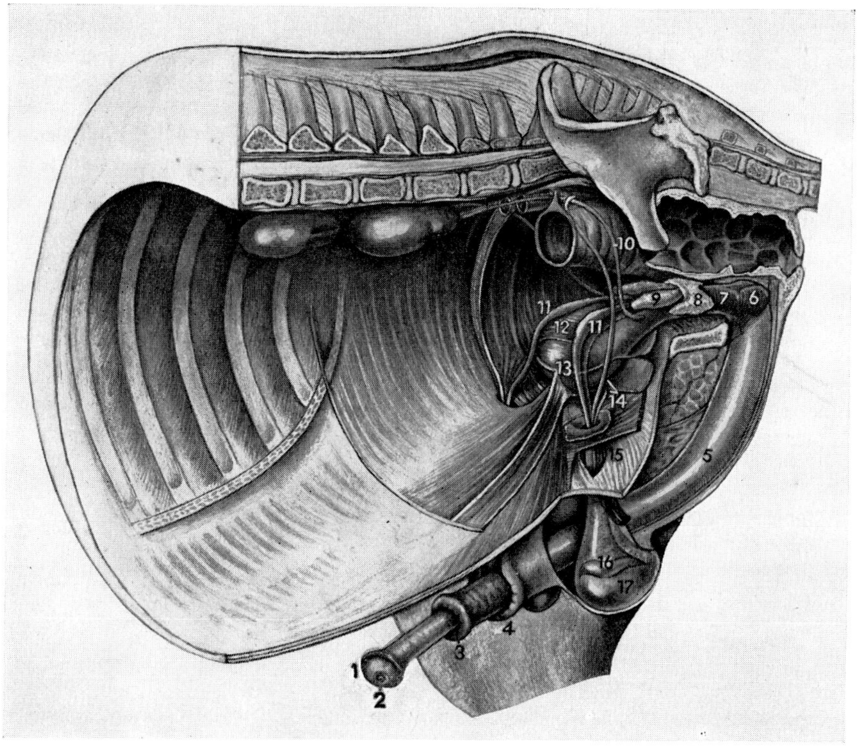

Fig. 2.1.10. — 1. Topography of the male genital tract, craniolateral aspect. 1 = glans penis (extended); 2 = urethral process; 3 = preputial ring (extended); 4 = preputial orifice; 5 = penis; 6 = bulbourethral glands; 7 = pelvic part of urethra surrounded by urethral muscle; 8 = lateral lobes of prostate; 9 = seminal vesicle; 10 = ureters; 11 = vas deferens; 12 = urogenital fold connecting both vasa deferentia; 13 = urinary bladder; 14 = internal spermatic artery and vein; 15 = superficial inguinal ring; 16 = epididymis; 17 = testis [after BIELANSKI].

genesis, and copulation is possible at that time. Warm-blooded stallions reach breeding maturity at 44 months, and cold-blooded stallions at 36 months. 'Old age' occurs at 18—30 years in warm-bloods and at 12—20 years in cold-bloods.

The normal act of breeding is comprised of several reflexly-controlled phases whose intensity is hormone-dependent. These include foreplay, erection of the body of the penis, mounting of the mare by the stallion, searching movements, intromission and pelvic thrusts with accompanying swelling of the glans. This is followed by ejaculation, return of the penis to a flaccid state, dismounting of the stallion, and subsidence of the glans swelling.

Sexual excitement of the stallion occurs chiefly in the presence of an estrous mare, but other circumstances can also bring about sexual arousal and studdish behavior. For example, the majority of stallions will not hesitate to mount a 'phantom' mare (fig. 2.1.10. — 2). Only a small percentage (25 %) require the presence of an estrous mare; very few will reject the phantom altogether. Sexual behavior in the stallion is influenced by temperament as well as experience and ranges from vigorous to subdued, vicious or fearful, and may be marked by peculiarities that are most commonly seen in older horses.

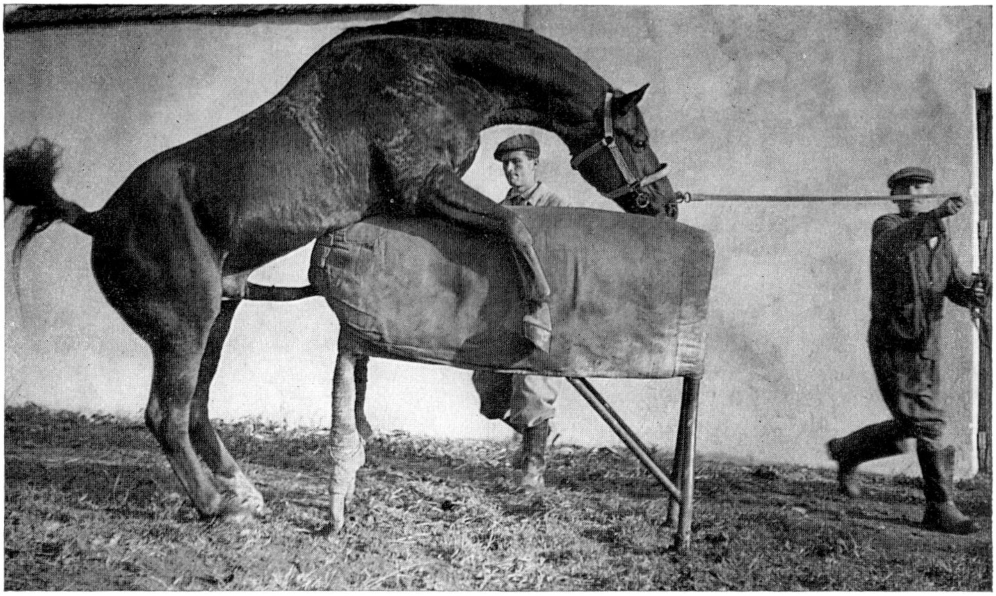

Fig. 2.1.10. — 2. Stallion mounting a 'phantom' [after PLEWINSKI].

Foreplay and sexual drive are very well developed if the stallion has an erection and attempts to mount occur when first exposed to the mare or within about 4 minutes thereafter. If the stallion shows no interest in covering the mare after 15—20 minutes of being presented to her, despite repeated attempts and coaxing, then the libido may be deficient. The stallion with normal sexual behavior will immediately mount and clutch the mare (or phantom) and initiate searching movements with the penis, followed by intromission and multiple strong pelvic thrusts. Intromission is often aided by manually directing the penis into the vagina.

Following intromission and thrusting, the glans penis swells and everts somewhat, tamponading the cranial portion of the vagina and dilating the opening of the cervix. This is highly distensible in the estrous mare. This enables the stallion to ejaculate directly through the cervix and into the uterus.

A period of up to 2 minutes normally elapses between initial insertion of the penis and ejaculation. However, it is not abnormal for the stallion to mount several times before finally ejaculating. An average of 1.4 mounts is necessary per ejaculation. Ejaculation takes place in two phases. A distinction is made between the mucous and the sperm-containing portions of the ejaculate.

The wave-like movements of the urethra that occur during ejaculation are not proof that ejaculation has taken place. Only the demonstration of semen is conclusive. Immediately after ejaculation, which lasts up to 26 seconds, the body of the penis collapses. At this point the stallion dismounts.

Outside the vagina, the swollen glans penis returns to normal size, and the entire penis retracts into the prepuce. Temperamental stallions and those that have not done service for some time can be used again a short time thereafter.

The degree of use of a stallion is dependent on individual circumstances. Young stallions can perform up to 3 covers per week, while older stallions can perform up to 10. The breeding season lasts 4—5 months.

Table 2.1.10. — 1. Seminal Characteristics

	Minimum values	Average values
Color	grayish-white	milky white to milky gray
pH	6.8—7.4	
Percent progressively motile spermatozoa	45 %	
Sperm concentration/mm³	0.1 million	0.08—0.8 million (total = 6 million sperm)
Abnormal spermatozoa	max. 35 %	
Characteristic odor		

The sexual behavior of a stallion can be tested only by exposing the animal to an estrous mare.

Temperamental stallions may become sexually aroused even when exposed to a nonestrous mare or to a gelding.

Masturbation, refusal to breed certain mares, and a predilection for geldings and other animals or objects are examples of abnormal sexual behavior in the stallion. These modes of behavior are considered serious faults and may be hereditary in origin [Götze, 1949]. Peculiar traits such as herd preference or playfulness are often observed in stallions. In the former case the stallion displays a greater interest in mares from other herds than in mares from its own herd.

Some stallions will reject mares that are in foal. Others must be longed or ridden before breeding or may breed only in special surroundings.

Slow breeders will display an interest in the mare for a considerable period of time before finally attempting to mount. Other stallions are easily distracted from the mare by noise or other stimuli. The dividing line between physiologic behavior and pathologic states is difficult to draw.

The average seminal characteristics of the stallion are presented in table 2.1.10. — 1.

The volume in light breeds should be at least 40 ml, and in heavy breeds at least 60 ml.

The semen evaluation is carried out according to the methods and criteria that are customary in artificial insemination. The table of Bretschneider [1963] is used for the assessment of morphologic abnormalities (fig. 2.1.10. — 3).

Reproductive Efficiency

The fertility of a stallion can be measured only by its efficiency in inducing pregnancy. Laboratory methods are capable only of screening out ejaculates or stallions that are unsuitable prior to use.

Reproductive efficiency is influenced by numerous factors, most notably age, breed and intensity of breeding. In a setting of uncontrolled pasture breeding, for example, conception rates of around 50 % are considered acceptable. Expectations are much higher on modern establishments where hygiene and preventive medicine are practiced as a routine part of the breeding program.

In connection with the increasing use of artificial insemination in horse breeding, Nishika and Shinimiya [1972] evaluated the reproductive efficiency of 12 stallions over a 10-year period. The average conception rate with deep-frozen semen was 64.9 %, with a range between 34.3 and 67.2 %. Results were also influenced by preparation of the semen and insemination technique.

Head cap

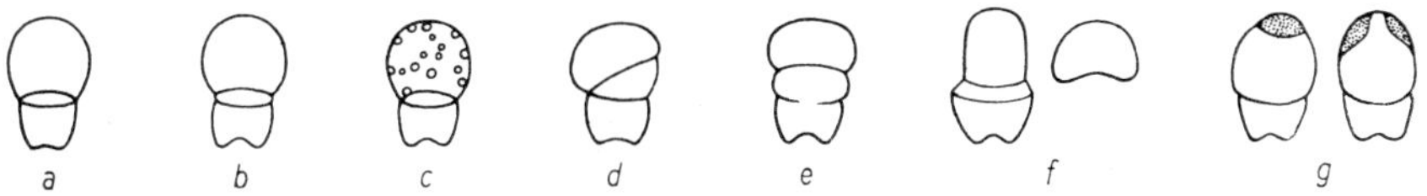

a = normal, b = too wide, c = granular, d = malplaced, e = too small, f = loose, g = malformed

Head shape and size

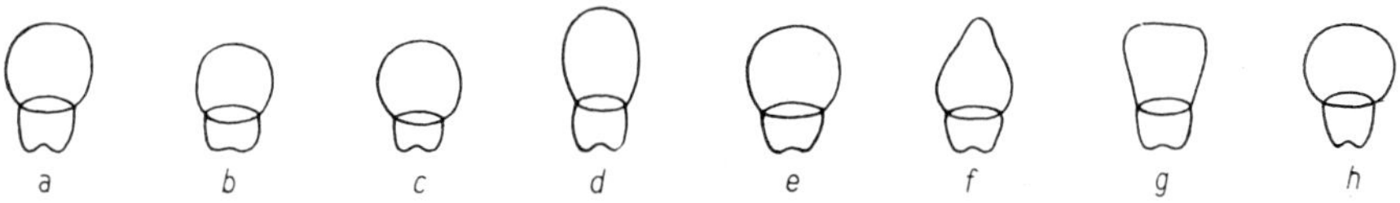

a—c = normal, d = too narrow, e = pear-shaped, f = lance-shaped, g = spade-shaped, h = club-shaped

Head base and neck

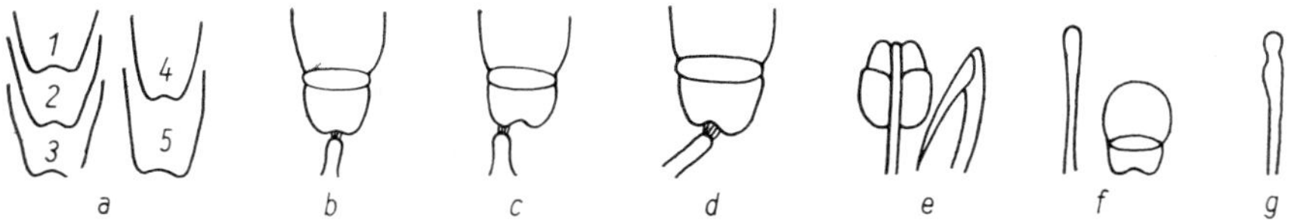

a1 = normal, 2 = too straight, 3 = everted, 4 = too narrow, 5 = too wide; b = symmetrical, c = abaxial, d = paraxial, e = retroaxial, f = broken neck, g = loose tail

Midpiece

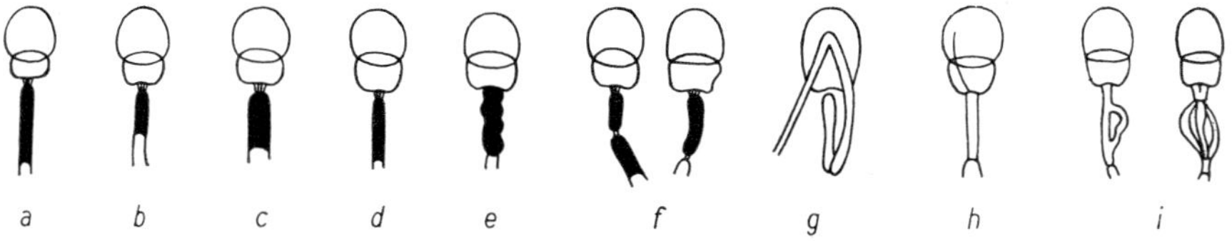

a = normal, b = too short, c = too wide, d = too thin, e = malformed, f = broken, g = plicated, h = axial type, i = fibrillary type

Tail

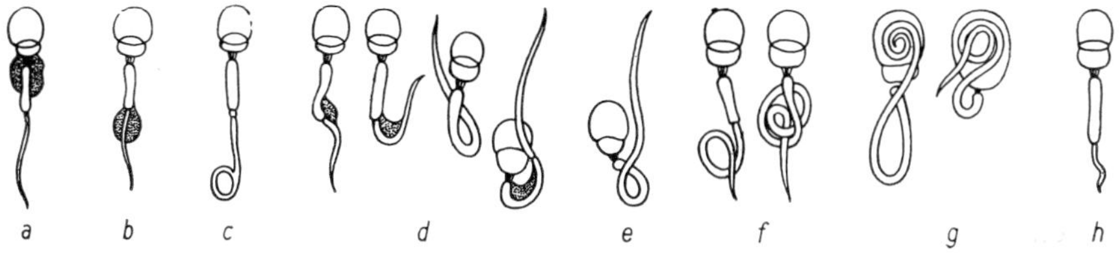

a = persistent plasmic droplets on neck, b = on midpiece, c = on tail, d = plasmic droplets connecting midpiece with tail, e = looped tail, f = convoluted tail, g = tail around head, h = rudimentary tail

Teratoid sperma-tozoa

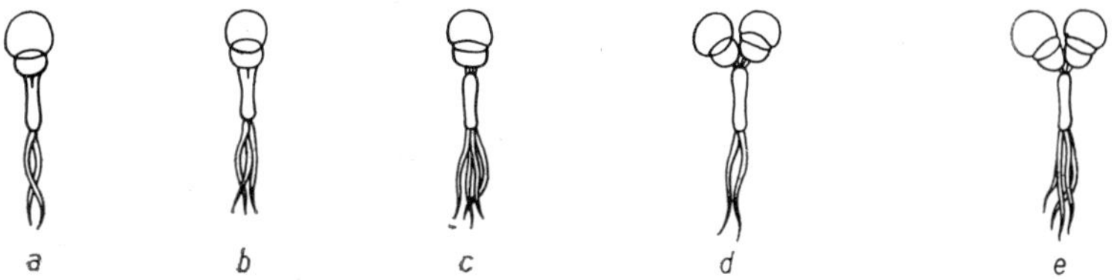

a = 1 head with 2 tails, b = 1 head with 3 tails, c = 1 head with 4 tails, d = 2 heads with 2 tails, e = 2 heads with 4 tails

Fig. 2.1.10. — 3. Normal and abnormal spermatozoan morphology [adapted from BRETSCHNEIDER, 1963].

Soviet researchers PLATOV and FOMINA [1976] reported conception rates in excess of 60 % when specially developed extenders were added to the semen before deep freezing. PICKETT et al. [1976] investigated the effect of the sperm content of the inseminate on conception and concluded that under optimum breeding conditions, 100×10^6 spermatozoa are sufficient to achieve a high conception rate (88.9 %). As breeding conditions become less favorable, a greater percentage of highly motile spermatozoa is required in the inseminate.

When sperm motility is assessed, it is necessary to determine not only the percentage of motile spermatozoa, but also the vigorousness of the motion. HENDRIKS [1972] describes positive correlations between progressive sperm motility and fertility. It is also noteworthy that dilution of the semen restores motility to a great many spermatozoa that appear dead in the untreated sample.

The percentage of abnormal spermatozoa correlates inversely with fertility. In addition, a highly significant connection has been demonstrated between sperm motility and normal sperm morphology.

Semen quality is influenced by many factors [VAN DER HOLST, 1975]. During the off-season, for example, there is a reduction in the percentage of progressively-motile spermatozoa, the volume of ejaculate and the sperm concentration, while the percentage of abnormal spermatozoa is increased. Semen quality also declines in stallions above the age of 15.

Environmental factors can also have an impact on the sexual potency of the stallion. When continuous lighting is maintained in stables during the off-season, an increase is noted in the proportion of progressively-motile spermatozoa. A vitamin- and mineral-rich diet also can enhance sexual potency and seminal characteristics.

HERAK et al. [1976] conducted a series of follow-up examinations over a 10-month period focusing on the biochemical properties of stallion semen. They discovered a seasonal rhythm that is determined by the timing and duration of the breeding season. The activities of β-glucuronidase and LDH in the sperm are highest in the month of May, and the content of β-glucuronidase, LDH and α-HBDH in the total ejaculate increases seasonally.

2.1.10.2. Supervision of Breeding Health in the Stallion

Health supervision of the stallion must be comprehensive enough to detect all conditions that adversely affect fertility, so that prompt corrective measures can be taken. Examinations are usually conducted at regular intervals and in accordance with a specified routine. If a decline in fertility is noted, special examinations should be done to identify the problem, and appropriate corrective measures taken.

For stallions that are used for artificial insemination, preliminary health examinations and regular follow-up examinations are a prerequisite for the unrestricted use of these animals.

The following are essential elements in the breeding soundness examination of the stallion:

1. General physical examination.
2. Special clinical examination of all parts of the genital tract and of breeding behavior.
3. Semen evaluation: sperm motility and morphology, bacteriologic or virologic examination of ejaculate.

The results of the examination are summarized in the form of an assessment of breeding soundness and should be included in the animal's pedigree papers.

In the course of the general examination, the following points should be noted in addition to general condition and nutritional status:

— Dentition: Stallions with parrot or sow mouth are unsuited for breeding.

— Respiration and circulation: Short-windedness, roaring, and similar conditions can constitute breeding unsoundness.

— Limbs, feet, gait: These should be subjected to a critical assessment, for diseases of the limbs can impair breeding ability.

Stallions with serious defects such as canker, grease heal with severe granulation, knuckled fetlocks or interfering are unsound for breeding. Minor defects should be treated.

— Examination for infectious diseases: The blood and semen are examined serologically for brucellosis, and the blood and feces may be tested for the presence of Salmonella.

Unrestricted use of the stallion is possible only if all findings are negative. Suspicious reactions require further clarification.

For the special clinical examination of the genital tract, it is necessary that the stallion be stimulated by an estrous mare or phantom. The following structures are examined:

— Scrotum: Diseases that adversely affect semen quality cause breeding unsoundness. Other lesions should be treated.

— Testicle and epididymis: The testicle should be well developed in relation to body size, symmetry, and have characteristic turgor. Abnormalities such as cryptorchidism, testicular hypoplasia, asymmetry, uni- or bilateral atrophy, orchitis and turgor changes that affect semen quality destroy the breeding value of the stallion.

— Prepuce and penis: Curable lesions mandate temporary sexual rest, while incurable lesions exclude the animal permanently from breeding use.

— Semen: Several ejaculates should be collected for the assessment of semen quality. Abnormalities may warrant a temporary or permanent exclusion of the animal from use.

Bacteriologic Examination

The bacteriologic examination of the preejaculate and semen is an essential part of the breeding soundness examination of the stallion. For collection of the sample the stallion is prepared by sexual stimulation and by washing the penis (1 : 1,000 acridine dye). The collection must be made in an area with solid flooring so that dust will not contaminate the sample. Semen may contain *E. coli*, hemolytic and nonhemolytic streptococci and staphylococci, *Proteus sp.*, *Pseudomonas aeruginosa*, coliform bacteria, and gram-negative and gram-positive diplococci [Aehnelt, 1975; Raynor and Jackson, 1965; Röstel, 1975; Scherbarth et al., 1976].

Raynor and Jackson [1965] found correlation between the presence of *Pseudomonas aeruginosa*, *Proteus sp.* and hemolytic streptococci, a high white cell concentration, and poor semen quality.

The bacterial content is different during the breeding season and off-season. While Röstel [1975] found contamination in 22.1 % of preejaculate samples and 11.2 % of semen samples during the breeding season, the prevalence was only 2 % during the off-season. Scherbart et al. [1976] state that this percentage is considerably higher and corresponds to the prevalence of positive cervical swabs in mares. These authors observed no disease symptoms in the stallion that were referable to the presence of hemolytic bacteria.

Scherbarth et al. [1976] found β-hemolytic streptococci in an average of 53.5 % of contaminated samples. Immediately after the breeding season this value declines due to an increase in β-hemolytic *E. coli* and *Klebsiella sp.* [Merkt et al., 1974; Röstel, 1975; Scherbarth et al., 1976]. A substantial reduction of the bacterial content is observed following 8—12 days' sexual rest. Aehnelt [1950] and Scherbarth et al. [1976] state that the bacterial content of the preejaculate and semen should be evaluated within the context of the clinical picture, semen examination and result of fertilization. In this way any transitory presence of bacteria can be clarified and specific antibiotic therapy facilitated if neccessary.

2.1.10.3. Fertility Disorders in the Stallion

2.1.10.3.1. Lack of Libido

Lack of libido refers to an absence or deficiency of sexual desire in the stallion, characterized by an absence, lack or delay of sexual interest in the mare, as well as deficiencies in all other aspects of sexual behavior.

Young stallions occasionally exhibit disturbances of sexual behavior that are attributable to a lack of experience. Temporary problems can also result from difficulty in adjusting to a new environment, or from simple overuse. In addition, older stallions sometimes require a longer preparation time before they are fully aroused and ready to cover the mare.

Frequently, stallions used for racing are treated with estrogens to inhibit stallion like behavior. The resulting depression of libido often persists for some time after the hormones are discontinued, and one must await the next breeding season before normal sexual behavior is reestablished.

The causes of poor libido include inadequate sexual responsiveness, disturbances of neurohormonal secretion, severe systemic illness, as well as breeding injuries and negative experiences associated with breeding. As a general rule, stallions with poor sexual behavior should be not be used for breeding. Attempts to correct the situation with drug therapy are futile in the great majority of cases.

Only spirited stallions with good libido should be used for breeding. With inexperienced stallions, a wait-and-see approach should be taken. It is helpful if such animals are exposed to spirited stallions in the act of breeding, as this will help them to learn by imitation. The 'acclimatization sterility' that is occasionally seen in stallions following a location change is also best handled with patience and the maintenance of a favorable environment.

Teasers should be used wherever possible as a means of avoiding stallion overuse. Overused stallions should be kept under optimum environmental conditions and placed on a light breeding schedule until normal fertility is restored.

2.1.10.3.2. Impotence

Impotence denotes an inability to engage in copulation, even though the libido may be normal. The following conditions may cause this disorder:

— Surgical diseases of the hind limbs (feet, joints, bones, tendons and tendon sheaths, blood vessels, muscles) which cause pain or prevent the stallion from mounting the mare. Often the stallion will attempt to mount despite the pain but will usually be forced to interrupt breeding. Such situations are potentially hazardous. Even when the disorder has been corrected, the unpleasant experience may have caused irreparable psychologic trauma with a consequent inability to perform.

— Injuries and inflammation of varying etiology affecting the external and internal genital organs can prevent or seriously hamper copulation. Included are lesions of the penis, prepuce, scrotum and testicle. Diseases of the ampulla of the vas deferens and seminal vesicles can also cause interference with copulation.

— Erectile abnormalities of the penis and glans. Sometimes penile erection is absent or incomplete despite a normal libido. In such cases the stallion is unable to insert the penis into the vagina, or can do so only with much assistance.

This condition can also arise if the stallion is permitted to mount the mare immediately after contact is established, before having time to become adequately stimulated.

Failure of penile erection is thought to be based upon an inherited defect. Diseases of the lumbar spine have also been incriminated.

Abnormalities of glans erection are seen in a number of stallions. Either the glans swells fully before intromission, thus hampering entry, or there is a failure of normal glans eversion once intromission is achieved.

— Neoplasms of the glans and prepuce (papilloma, melanoma, hemangioma) are a source of breeding difficulties.

— Impotence is in effect present if the vagina is too narrow, either in maiden mares or as a result of injury during foaling, to permit intromission. This condition may cause the mare to resist violently if breeding is attempted, or may cause misdirected intromission leading to serious injury.

— Central nervous disorders are frequently accompanied by motor disturbances and an unsteady gait and may also cause impotence or penile prolapse.

Paralysis can also develop as a sequel to the disease dourine (see below).

— Disturbances of ejaculation. Ejaculation fails to occur or is achieved only after several covers, with an otherwise normal pattern of sexual behavior. In some cases the stallion may cover the mare but fail to perform pelvic thrusts, while other animals fail to ejaculate despite strong, sustained pelvic thrusts to the point of near-exhaustion. The severity of the disorder ranges from mild to severe.

The condition has been attributed to disturbances of impulse formation and conduction or spasticity of the bulbocavernous muscle. In older stallions, colicky signs with prostration and unrest are sometimes observed after coitus. These are related to temporary pain induced by the sexual act and normally pass without treatment.

2.1.10.3.3. Sterility

The act of copulation is normal and complete, but conception fails to occur. In these cases both the stallion and mare should be given a complete examination. A variety of conditions may be detected in the male. Besides typical changes in the quality of the ejaculate, however, there are also cases where no significant seminal abnormalities can be detected by the usual methods of evaluation. In some instances the ejaculate may have an apparently normal composition, but the survival time of the spermatozoa is extremely short. In other cases a deficient secretion by the accessory glands can be demonstrated. Frequently, however, examination of the semen will yield no demonstrable abnormalities of any kind. Recent biochemical and immunologic tests performed by Balbierz et al. [1976] on the semen and blood of sterile stallions showed no marked differences relative to fertile stallions.

The typical seminal changes that are associated with sterility include:

— An absence of sperm in the ejaculate. The ejaculate consists only of accessory secretions and contains neither spermatozoa nor their precursors (aspermia). This condition, which stems from a developmental defect of the germinal epithelium, is most commonly seen in bilateral cryptorchidism, germinal aplasia and hypoplasia of the testes or as a sequel to atrophic and inflammatory conditions. Occlusion of the sperm-conveying structures can have a similar effect. In azoospermia, only precursors of the spermatozoa (spermatids, spermatocytes and spermatogonia) are present in the semen. The cause of this arrested development lies in profound congenital or acquired defects such as hypoplasia, inflammation and degeneration of the testicular epithelium. When there is a partial dysfunction of the spermatogenic epithelium, spermatozoa are produced in deficient numbers. The sperm concentration of the ejaculate does not reach the level necessary for a satisfactory conception rate (oligospermia). This condition also occurs as a consequence of overuse.

— Disturbances of sperm motility. The number of progressively-motile spermatozoa present in the semen is below the minimum number necessary for reliable fertilization (cf. Sec. 2.1.10.1.). Likewise, the fertility of semem in which a high percentage of the spermatozoa exhibit stationary motion is poor.

The term necrospermia is applied if all the spermatozoa of the semen are dead or motionless.

— Abnormalities of sperm morphology. Experience has shown that the proportion of abnormal spermatozoa in the sample should not exceed 20 %. Beyond this level, even the normal-appearing spermatozoa in the semen will probably have defects of metabolism and structure that will interfere with normal fertilization. In a highly comprehensive study of 539 semen samples from 171 stallions, HENDRIKS et al. [1976] present interesting findings on the question of spermatozoan abnormalities. More than 60 % of the spermatozoa have a normal morphology. The proportion of viable spermatozoa is 75 %. Head changes are found most frequently in dead sperm. Protoplasmic droplets, on the other hand, are most commonly found on live sperm. The percentage of abnormal spermatozoa increases slightly in older stallions due to changes in spermatogenesis (primary) or in the maturation, storage and transport of the spermatozoa (secondary). While changes in the heads of the spermatozoa are characteristic of primary defects, secondary defects tend to be reflected in abnormalities of tail morphology.

— Contamination of the ejaculate with blood (hemospermia) or pus (pyospermia) as well as with numerous types of bacteria (bacteriospermia). Causes include injuries and inflammatory lesions of the testicles or sperm-conveying structures.

Opinions vary as to the impact of hemospermia on semen fertility.

2.1.10.4. Sexually-Transmitted Infections in the Stallion
(cf. Sec. 2.1.11.3.5.)

2.1.10.4.1. Dourine (Paralytic Coital Exanthema)

The causal organism of dourine, *Trypanosoma equiperdum*, is transmitted by copulation. The incubation period varies between 5—6 days and several weeks. The initial sign is a doughy, nontender swelling of the prepuce, glans, penis and urethral orifice. The edema extends to the scrotum and ventral abdomen. Pea-sized nodules appear on the glans, degenerate and coalesce to form ulcers. White scars are left behind when resolution occurs. There is a gray or yellow-red discharge from the urethra. Libido is initially increased in affected stallions. Later in the course of the disease, urticarial plaques appear on the flank, shoulder and neck.

Additional signs are pruritus and vesiculation. Initially the skin is hypersensitive. This stage is followed by hyposensitivity and numbness, which in turn are followed by varying forms of paralysis (facial paralysis, limb paralysis, etc.). A rapid loss of condition is observed. Death usually occurs after several weeks, but chronic cases may survive for 2 years or more.

Once the disease has been detected, strict control measures must be implemented to limit its spread (cf. Sec. 2.1.11.3.5.).

2.1.10.4.2. Coital Exanthema (Herpes Exanthema, EHV-3)

Transmission occurs by coitus. The preputial mucosa is red and swollen. Pain is evidenced if the stallion attempts to breed. Pruritus and frequent urination are present.

Flat, dull, opaque areas appear on the mucosa. The individual vesicles may coalesce, creating a picture of diphtheritic inflammation. It is not long before these areas undergo purulent degeneration and are sloughed, leaving behind crater-like erosions with deeply red, granulating margins. Following resolution, deep red patches that bleed easily are still visible on the preputial mucosa. Later on, white patches can be seen on the glans penis.

The effect of the disease on potency and fertility is both minor and indirect. However, the condition is highly infectious, and affected mares must not be bred until they recover.

It should be added that secondary bacterial infections are a danger in coital exanthema and can lead to persistent mucosal inflammation (cf. Sec. 2.1.11.3.5.).

2.1.10.4.3. Strangles

Strangles can also be potentially transmitted by coitus and causes a sometimes severe inflammation of the external genitalia of the mare.

2.1.10.4.4. Bacterial Infections

The stallion may be clinically normal yet still transmit a bacterial infection to the mare (cf. Sec. 2.1.12.3.).

References

Aehnelt, E.: Das Sperma des Hengstes unter Berücksichtigung von Umwelt und Vererbung. Vet.-med. Habil-Schrift, Hannover (1950).

Balbierz, H.; Nikołajzuk, M.; Kosiniak, K.: Importance of biochemical and immunological tests for estimating semen in stallions with reduced fertility. Proc. 8th Int. Congr. Anim. Reprod. Art. Insemination Kraków *6:* 872 (1976).

Bretschneider, L. H.: Die Morphogenese und Pathogenese der Spermien des Bullen. Cit. in Schaetz, F.: Die künstliche Besamung bei den Haustieren (VEB Gustav Fischer Verlag, Jena 1963).

GÖTZE, R.: Besamung und Unfruchtbarkeit der Haustiere (Schaper-Verlag, Hannover 1949).
HENDRIKS, J.: Einige Bemerkungen zur Fortpflanzung beim Pferd. Proc. 7th Int. Congr. Anim. Reprod. Art. Insemination München *8:* 2186 (1972).
HERAK, M.; SUKALIC, M.; PREMZL, B.; EMANOVIC, D.: Some biochemical characteristics o stallion sperm. Proc. 8th Int. Congr. Anim. Reprod. Art. Insemination Kraków *6:* 904 (1976).
MERKT, H.; KLUG, E.; BADER, H.: Bericht über die Herbstuntersuchung 1973 in der westdeutschen Vollblutzucht. Vollblut, Zucht u. Rennen *57:* 56 (1974).
MERKT, H.; KLUG, E.: Fortpflanzungsprobleme im Rahmen der künstlichen Besamung beim Pferd. Dtsch. tierärztl. Wschr. *83:* 539 (1976).
MERKT, H.; KLUG, E.; KRAUSE, D.; BADER, H.: Results of longterm storage of stallion semen. J. Reproc. Fertility *23:* 105 (1975).
NISHIKAWA, Y.; SHINIMIYA, S.: Gefrierfähigkeit von Hengstsamen ausserhalb der Zuchtsaison. Proc. 7th Int. Congr. Anim. Reprod. Art. Insemination München *8:* 1034 (1972).
PLATOW, E. M.; FOMINA: Freezing stallion semen in the horse breeding of the USSR. 8th Int. Congr. Anim. Reprod. Art. Insemination Kraków *6:* 204 (1976).
RAYNOR, R. E.; JACKSON, R. S.: Bacteriologic examinations of stallions. Mod. Vet. Pract. *46:* 90 (1965).
RÖSTEL, W.: Vorkommen und Antibiotikaresistenz haemolysierender Sterilitätskeime bei Zuchtstuten und Deckhengsten in Schleswig-Holstein. Tierärztl. Umschau *30:* 66 (1975).
SCHAETZ, F.: Die künstliche Besamung bei den Haustieren (VEB Gustav Fischer Verlag, Jena 1963).
SCHERBARTH, R.; KRÜGER, A.; FLÜGE, A.: Zuchthygienische Überwachung der hannoverschen Warmblutzucht. Dtsch. tierärztl. Wschr. *83:* 1 (1976).
VAN DER HOLST, W.: A study of the morphology of stallion semen during the breeding and nonbreeding seasons. J. Reprod. Fertility suppl. 22, p. 87 (1975).
WERHAHN, H.: Andrologische Untersuchungen in einem großen Beschälerbestand — Auswahl von Hengsten als Samenspender für die instrumentelle Samenübertragung mit Tiefgefriersperma. Vet.-med. Diss., Hannover (1978).

2.1.11. Diseases of the Female Genital Organs and Reproductive Disorders

Diseases of the genital organs (fig. 2.1.11. — 1) and reproductive disorders in the mare are the product of much the same influences as in other domestic animals, although there are some more or less species-specific trends in the prevalence of certain forms of sterility. The reproductive potential of the horse is not exploited to the degree that is common in other species, and often, as in the case of the Thoroughbred, it is not exploited at all until other types of service have been rendered. The reproductive cycle of the horse is such that the average broodmare cannot be expected to produce a foal every year. In fact, a barren interval of one or even two years not only does not adversely affect the value of the mare, but is actually calculated into many breeding programs.

Because the care, feeding and use of the mare generally conform to higher standards than in other domestic animals, organic and stress-related sterility is relatively rare. There is a relatively greater incidence of sterility due to poor breeding practices relating to the timing of breeding, compulsory seasonal breeding and other factors. This should be considered apart from individual infertility processes if we are to understand the complete range of interactions between reproductive potential and reproductive efficiency.

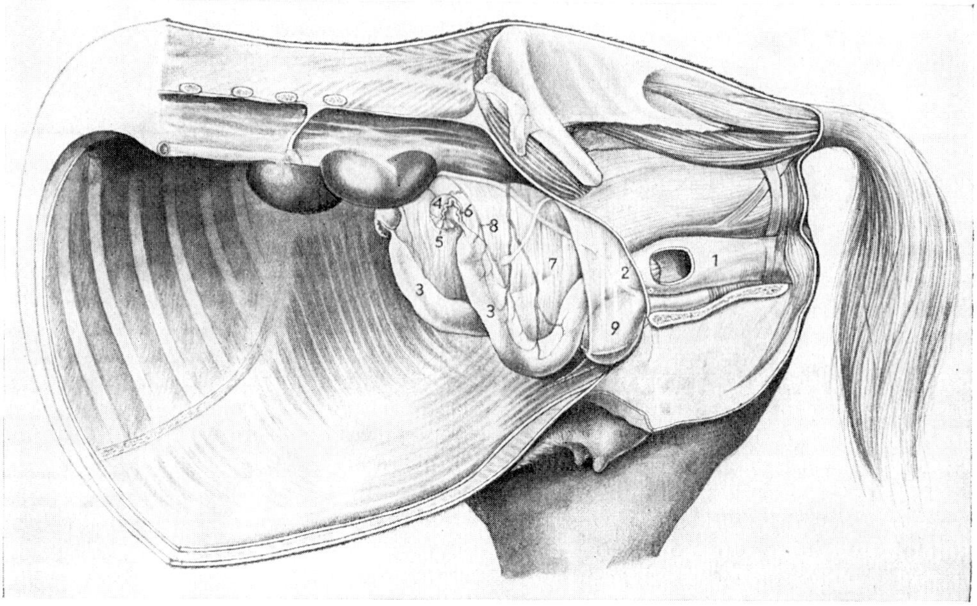

Fig. 2.1.11. — *1.* Topography of the female genital tract. 1 = vagina (fenestrated); 2 = cervix; 3 = corpus uteri; 4 = ovary; 5 = ovulation fossa and infundibulum; 6 = uterine tube; 7 = mesometrium; 8 = mesovarium; 9 = urinary bladder [after BIELANSKI].

2.1.11.1. Reproductive Cycle of the Mare

The first breeding occurs at the age of 2—3 years in cold-blooded mares and at 3—5 years in warm-blooded and Thoroughbred mares. Fertility declines at about the age of 14—16 years in medium and heavy breeds, while Thoroughbred mares generally can conceive until about the age of 18 and may remain fertile for some time thereafter — in some cases up to age 25. Ponies have approximately the same reproductive life as Thoroughbreds.

Some broodmares may not foal each year, but exhibit irregular patterns of conception. Some mares will produce a foal every other year, while others will foal for 2 or 3 consecutive years and then skip a year. These barren intervals may be genetically determined and in part based upon exogenous influences such as environmental conditions, poor breeding practice, or true sterility. It would be wrong to seek a pathogenic cause, and attempt to treat such a cause, whenever a mare fails to conceive. In most cases it is difficult to recognize a barren interval as such. One should resist the temptation to undertake treatment in every case, only to learn from the mare's lack of response that therapy was useless all along.

For mares that are 'pasture-bred' the horse breeder is happy if a given mare produces 2 foals in 3 years, and an 'every other year' pattern of conception is considered to be acceptable. In Thoroughbred breeding, on the other hand, a reproductive efficiency of 80 % per year and herd is strived for. In the final analysis, of course, only the total output that is achieved during the period available for reproduction will establish the true reproductive efficiency of the individual animal.

The estrous cycle of the mare varies between 20 and 23 days in length, with an average length of 21 days. Extreme values of 18 or 30 days are occasionally observed. The estrous period itself lasts an average of 4 to 7 days, so that an average of 16 days pass between the end of one estrus and the start of the next. However, this is subject to much variation, and the boundaries between normal and abnormal estrous cycles are sometimes indistinct, as in early nymphomania. Often the estrous periods are considerably longer at the start of the breeding season and become a great deal shorter during the warm months. In June and July in the Northern hemisphere, ambient conditions relating to temperature and the length of daylight are such that the phases of the cycle are the most precise during this period. In many countries, however, the breeding season is officially concluded by this time due to organizational reasons.

The 21-day cycle is not sustained throughout the year, but is a seasonal phenomenon. Mares of the light breeds have several succesive cycles in the spring and usually several in the fall, while the heavier breeds normally come into heat only a few times in the spring and rarely come into estrus in the fall. The signs of estrus are quite marked in Thoroughbred and warm-blooded mares, while in cold-blooded breeds the evidence of estrus tends to be more subtle.

Detailed studies have shown that cyclic processes need not be absent in the mare during the off-season, but may simply be at a subclinical level. For example, 4 to 6 anovulatory estrous periods lasting only 1 to 2 days and having few or no outward manifestations are often demonstrable during the 'anestrous' period, these short periods of heat occurring at different times within a given band of mares. It is also noteworthy that besides light and temperature, the occurrence of the first estrus depends on nutritional status; other stimulants such as the presence of stallions, the administration of hormones, etc. are of only minor importance.

The signs of estrus are, with some reservations, the criterion for determining breeding times in breeding operations. These signs are detailed below:

— External signs of estrus. The vulva is swollen and congested, and a mucous discharge is present. When exposed to a stallion, the mare will display receptive behavior; she will stand straddle-legged, squirt urine, raise the tail and spread the labia so that the clitoris is exposed ('winking'). Many mares will strike out when touched or nipped by the stallion; this constitutes normal sexual behavior and should not be interpreted as a refusal to breed. Often breeders can recognize estrus simply by the mare's general behavior, and especially by frequent kicking, nickering and urination when the flank and ventral abdomen are touched.

— Internal signs of estrus. The vaginal mucosa has a reddened appearance, and there is a heavy secretion of mucus from the vagina and cervical canal. Rectal palpation is useful for ascertaining the degree of edema of the genital organs, and it is especially useful for assessing the ripeness of the follicle or confirming the occurrence of ovulation, which ideally corresponds to the peak of estrus.

Most breeders still prefer to use a 'teaser' to test the mare's readiness to breed. This is done to protect the stallion from injury by a resisting mare as well as to prevent unnecessary excitement of the stud at a teasing rail or wall.

The mare should be bred as close as possible to ovulation time, which occurs about 24 hours before the end of estrus.

External signs of estrus, especially in the early stage, cannot always be equated with ovulation, and, conversely, ovulation does not always coincide with maximum receptiveness in the mare. Nevertheless, the strongest external signs of estrus coincide with ovulation in more than 80 % of mares. Inasmuch as ovulation occurs 4/5 of the way through the estrous period, the most favorable breeding time for the normally estrous mare is between the 4th and 6th day. Adjustments must be made, of course, depending on the exact length of estrous. For this reason it is unwise to breed the mare on the 1st or 2nd day of estrus, unless the estrus period is quite short, as in the case of certain Thoroughbreds. It is good practice to maintain surveillance at least of problem mares, performing regular rectal examinations until the animal is bred or ovulation occurs.

Results in the breeding of Thoroughbred and warm-blooded mares are approximately as follows:

First fertilization rate	approx. 50 to 55 %
Conception rate, total	80 %
Breeding index (no. of estruses before conception)	1.5 to 2.5
Abortion rate including twins	3 to 10 %
Foal mortality up to 4 weeks	up to 5 %

About 8—12 days after parturition, the mare again comes into heat ('foal heat'). Following a normal delivery and uncomplicated puerperium, the mare should have no difficulty conceiving during this estrus. However, it is argued by some (though contested by others) that the prospect of conception is not favorable during foal heat, for the mare is not in an optimum condition to conceive. The rate of embryonic mortality is higher than in mares bred during the next estrus. The general recommendation, therefore, is to breed a mare in foal heat only if she has had a normal parturition, delivered a healthy foal, expelled the fetal membranes within 2—3 hours, had no discharge during the puerperium, and the birth canal is undamaged and free of inflammation.

2.1.11.2. Congenital and Inherited Infertility Factors

Anatomic or functional-anatomic defects of the sex organs that are either inherited or arise incidentally during intrauterine development are relatively uncommon. They may be recognized when the animal is still a foal or may go undetected until later when breeding is attempted.

A sizable proportion of breeding animals affected with genital abnormalities have an infertility that renders them unable to reproduce and thus unable to transmit their defect. Nevertheless, the delayed recognition of such abnormalities is a source of significant economic and breeding losses. Moreover, factors that are inherited as recessive traits often remain unexpressed for years and so are inadvertantly transmitted to new generations. Hence, when deficiencies of the reproductive organs are encountered, a careful search should be made for the origin and significance of the defects so that the carriers of the traits can be excluded from breeding. Many abnormalities occurring outside the genital tract also justify such an exclusion.

Hermaphroditism (see Sec. 2.1.8.3.) and infantilism are occasionally observed. Their recognition in colts and fillies is not difficult. On the other hand, assessment often proves difficult in conditions such as virilization or problems that are prevalent in certain blood lines, such as nymphomania, pneumovagina and weak estrus with difficult conception. Special attention should also be given to events such as hydramnion, fetal malformations, and unexplained abortions and premature births. Many times these occur at the same point in the pregnancy and under the same circumstances, in an individual animal or in a particular line. The same applies to twin pregnancies and the 'weak foal' syndrome, for which a genetic determination may be made that warrants corrective breeding measures.

2.1.11.3. Diseases of the Vulva and Vagina

2.1.11.3.1. Narrowness of the Vaginal Orifice

In maiden mares the vaginal orifice is often so narrow that, when combined with a tough imperforate hymen, it makes the first breeding very difficult. By being attentive and helpful during the breeding and having the mare serviced by an even-tempered, experienced stallion that is not too strong physically, the breeder should be able to resolve this temporary defect without incident. In older mares, too, scarring and strictures of the vagina secondary to dystocia or inflammatory conditions can cause complications during breeding and so require prompt correction. When these lesions are present, forceful intromission of the penis or 'crooked mounting' by the stallion can occasionally result in perforation of the vaginal wall. In severe cases intestine may eviscerate through the vagina. The prognosis is grave.

In animals with infantile genitalia and in hermaphrodites, poor development of the caudal segment of the genital tract is a common finding. Sometimes examinations for infertility or for unspecified complaints in the abdominal and pelvic region (e.g., mild but persistent colic) will disclose congenital or acquired transverse obstructions of the cranial vaginal segment or cervix. These are often accompanied by a sizable mass of accumulated secretions. In favorable cases the obstruction consists only of a membrane-like septum that can be surgically removed. The accumulated matter is removed and the inflammatory or secretory processes, especially those affecting the uterus, are rectified. Included in this category is closed pyometra, which arises from a complicated puerperium with vaginal lesions.

2.1.11.3.2. Perineal Lacerations

Dystocia or incompetent obstetrical care frequently result in lacerations of the perineum or perforations of the vaginal roof or rectal floor (rectovaginal fistula). If the lacerations do not involve the cervix, then Götze's operation offers a good prospect for recovery and the possibility of continued breeding use.

2.1.11.3.3. Pneumovagina

Definition. Pneumovagina is a condition in which air is aspirated into the vagina due to deficient closure of the vulvar lips. It results from tissue defects associated with foaling injuries and is especially common in cases of perineal laceration. It is also seen in emaciated states and in old age. Pneumovagina is a frequent cause of sterility in mares.

Symptoms. The anus is sunken, causing the vulva to assume a sloped or even horizontal position. The labia often are atrophied and are inverted, allowing air, feces and bacteria to enter the vagina. Pneumovagina is further characterized by the presence of gurgling, sucking sounds when the mare walks, lies down or gets up, as well as during defecation and urination. These more or less marked disturbances lead to chronic irritation of the vaginal mucosa with ascending infections of the cervix and uterus and endometritis.

Treatment. In cases of transitory emaciation, improvement of the nutritional status will probably enable a full recovery. In most cases, however, reconstructive surgery by the method of Götze, Benesch or Caslick is indicated. The chance of recovery is 70—75 % if surgery is done early.

2.1.11.3.4. Neoplasms

Neoplasms are relatively uncommon. Neoplasms of the vagina include benign connective-tissue tumors (fibroma, myoma), as well as infiltrative, metastasizing tumors (carconima, sarcoma, melanoma). In advanced cases these cause a bloody, greasy, malodorous discharge and are inoperable. Intermittent or continuous bleeding from the vagina, usually in small amounts, almost always originates from hemangiectases (varicosities) located cranial to the hymenal ring and is increased during pregnancy. These dilatations of the blood vessels, which are usually superficial and ventral in location, are amenable to surgical removal.

2.1.11.3.5. Infectious Vaginal Diseases

Local infections of the vagina have become relatively rare. The clinical picture is often subtle, yet vaginal infections of this type are highly contagious on sexual contact, often assuming epizootic proportions, and predispose to sterility-causing inflammation of the uterus.

Dourine (cf. Sec. 2.1.10.4.1.)
Following an incubation period of 5 days to several weeks or months, painless, doughy, irregular thickenings appear on the labia, and soft yellow swellings appear on the mucous membranes of the vulva and vagina, which sometimes protrude from the vulvar fissure. Pea-size nodules form on the mucosa of the external genitalia, the labia and the surrounding skin and sometimes extend to the mammary gland. These nodules become ulcers, which resolve leaving behind white patches. There is also a gray, mucoid discharge from the vulva. Affected mares urinate frequently and have a high incidence of abortion.

Coital Exanthema (Infectious Pustular Vaginitis, Herpes Exanthema, EHV-3) (cf. Sec. 2.1.10.4.2.)
Coital exanthema is a sexually-transmitted infection that can reach epizootic proportions. From 3 to 6 days after coitus, tender, deeply-red inflamed areas appear on the mucous surfaces of the vulva and vagina. These lesions soon coalesce and produce a copious discharge. The infection is highly refractory to treatment, but the topical application of a soothing antibacterial medicament is indicated. Resolution occurs in 2—3 weeks, leaving behind characteristic small, unpigmented areas on the vulva and anus. It is unclear whether coital exanthema contributes to early embryonic mortality, but outbreaks in horse populations have been correlated with a definite decline in conception rates among broodmares. Endometritis due to secondary bacterial infection can occur as a sequel to coital exanthema.

Bacterial Vaginal Catarrh (cf. Sec. 2.1.10.4.4.)
Localized bacterial infections of the vagina are seldom observed clinically. However, they are of significance in that bacteria introduced during coitus can lead to sterility-causing endometritis while producing no apparent lesions of the vaginal mucosa. For this reason, it is vital that a clinical and bacteriologic examination be carried out if suspicious signs are noted (e.g., discharge from the vulva) so that sexually-transmitted diseases can be detected, and prompt treatment can be administered for all forms of local disease.

Strangles (cf. Sec. 2.1.10.4.3.)

During breeding, strangles can be transmitted to the mare through the respiratory discharges of the affected stallion (sniffing, snorting, nipping). The initial sign, appearing some time after the act of breeding, is the development of severe inflammation of the mucosa, connective tissue and perivaginal area with abscessation. As the disease progresses, a sequestered, subfascial cellulitis often develops on the insides of the thighs and may extend to the mammary glands, causing liquefaction. *Str. equi* are demonstrated by bacterial culture. Treatment involves the incision and drainage of abscesses and the canalization of cellulitic areas. The progress of vaginal healing should be checked at frequent intervals. Primary involvement of the endometrium is extremely rare.

2.1.11.4. Diseases of the Cervix

The cervix of the mare, unlike that of other animals, is not tightly closed and is easily distended manually from the outside, or when the internal pressure is raised. The cervical os is open during estrus or coitus, and the stallion usually ejaculates directly through the cervix into the uterus. This relative incompetency of cervical closure has disadvantages, however. On the one hand, it means an increased risk of abortion during pregnancy associated with pressure from abdominal musculature, colic, overexertion, etc. On the other hand, in nonpregnant mares it allows pathogenic organisms and air ready access to the uterus, especially in wind-sucking mares; the resulting pneumometra can be a cause of persistent infertility. Thus, even in health, the extreme receptiveness of the cervix, while important to the mare's reproductive system, predisposes to various pathologic states that must not be neglected in fertility management and infertility control.

Diseases of the cervical mucosa rarely occur in isolation and generally are associated with an ascending endometritis. Cysts of the cervical mucosa are also infrequent.

2.1.11.5. Diseases of the Uterus

Definition. At one time, chronic endometritis due to bacterial infection was the 'catch-all' explanation for infertility in the mare. Today this disease is still considered a significant cause of infertility, but a prime role is no longer ascribed to the absolute pathogenic effect of bacterial invaders. It is generally agreed that before resident bacteria can become pathogenic, certain circumstances must be present which alter the local resistance to infection. Foremost among these are systemic stresses, dystocia, mucosal stress in pneumometra, predisposing primary inflammatory conditions, as well as hormone-related mucosal irritations that are conducive to bacterial invasion (e.g., nymphomania). It is also true, however, that certain organisms, such as hemolytic cocci, can exert a direct pathogenic effect without any assistance from other factors. These bacteria can be transmitted back and forth between the broodmare and stallion and can acquire an epizootic character.

Symptoms, Diagnosis and Treatment. Endometritis usually leads directly to infertility, but in some cases it may cause early embryonic death, creating a split estrus that warrants further investigation. The clinical forms are variable, and the boundaries between them are often indistinct. It should be noted that many of the clinically simple uterine diseases do not involve marked inflammatory processes, but rather a functional incompetence with atypical endometrial behavior that can no longer guarantee normal development of the fertilized ovum.

Mares with endometritis will often have a discharge from the genital tract, even during anestrous periods, that forms crusts on and around the margins of the vulvar lips, extending in some cases to the tuber ischii and undersurface of the tail. The color and consistency of the exudate are variable. Other signs of endometritis are an increase in the size and consistency of the uterus and the presence of abnormal uterine contents. Washings and swabs from the vagina and uterus as well as biopsy samples from the uterine mucosa should be obtained for bacteriologic, cytologic and histologic study. Transcervical palpation of the endometrium with the finger is of diagnostic value in some cases.

The various forms of endometritis can be divided into several broadly-defined categories:

Endometritis Sicca

Endometritis sicca (dry e.) is a mucosal inflammation with minimal clinical signs and no secretory activity. It mainly affects older mares that have previously had a catarrhal endometritis or have been barren for several years. The endometrium is firm and flattened; the characteristic soft, velvety surface and physiologic secretion are absent. Returned irrigating fluid shows no evidence of abnormality. The prognosis of endometritis, which usually is diagnosed only after several unsuccessful attempts to conceive, is dependent on the age of the mare and the duration of the disease. It is guarded at best. Irrigation with rubefacient irritants such as iodine preparations or other medicaments that have proved useful in treating affections of the uterine mucosa is occasionally successful.

First-Degree Chronic Catarrhal Endometritis (E_1)

A split estrus is characteristic. Few clinical signs are apparent on examination of the genital tract. Returned irrigating fluid may have a cloudy or dusty turbidity but contains no large flakes. The prognosis is favorable. One or two simple irrigations followed by the infusion of dilute solutions with mild rubefacient properties are usually sufficient. Antiseptic or bactericidal components should also be present in the solution.

Second-Degree Chronic Catarrhal Endometritis (E_2)

This form is characterized by an increased discharge from the vulva and cloudy mucus in the vagina, even outside of estrus. The endometrium is slightly swollen, and numerous flakes are seen swirling in the cloudy irrigating fluid. The uterus feels hard on rectal palpation. Repeated treatment (irrigation with physiologic saline, acridine dye solutions, iodine preparations, etc.) can lead to a recovery and subsequent pregnancy, though this cannot be predicted with any certainty.

Mucopurulent Endometritis (E_3)

There is an intermittent or continuous mucopurulent discharge of variable quantity that soils the area surrounding the vulva, the tuber ischii and the underside of the tail. Streaks of mucus ooze into the vagina from the os uteri. The uterine mucosa is thickened and sometimes exhibits cystic-glandular changes. On rectal examination, the uterine wall is found to be thickened and abnormally firm; occasionally small amounts of purulent exudate fluctuate in its lumen. Returned irrigating fluid is milky and turbid and contains many flakes. If the fluid is allowed to stand, the purulent components will form a thick sediment at the bottom of the glass. Reversal of the suppurative processes is not possible in every case, and conception is rarely achieved. Treatment consists of irrigations and infusions performed every week or so; local treatment with sulfonamides and antibiotics (after sensitivity has been determined) can be beneficial.

Pyometra

Pyometra is an accumulation of purulent exudate within the uterus, often in large amounts, that occurs during the course of suppurative processes. Open pyometra results from atonic conditions of the uterine musculature, while closed pyometra results from intrauterine pus accumulation with a closed cervix and vagina. Often there is a continuous purulent discharge from the vulva, especially during recumbency, that soils the insides of the thighs and even the hind legs and also produces an irritation leading to alopecia and dermatitis. Closed pyometra is in most cases detected incidentally during routine examination of the genital tract or when signs of systemic illness appear such as emaciation, arching of the back, straining and colic.

Infertility is practically an inevitable consequence of pyometra due to the irreparable changes that occur in the uterine mucosa. The goal of treatment is simply to halt the unpleasant and unhygienic discharge. Treatment includes cleansing irrigations, the use of hypertonic infusions, and possibly the local application of specific antibacterial preparations. The discharge cannot be stopped in every case, however.

Other Chronic, Sterility-Causing Conditions of the Uterus

Pneumometra is a complication of dystocia or general emaciation. Attempts at treatment center on the correction or elimination of the pneumovagina that is also present in most cases. The condition of the mucosa is often identical to that seen in endometritis sicca. The prognosis is guarded.

In *urometra* (urine pooling), a sunken vaginal floor allows urine to trickle into the uterus. Often the condition is associated with pneumometra. The prognosis is unfavorable, unless corrective surgery is performed.

Myxometra and *hydrometra* represent hypersecretory states that presumably are based on errors of hormonal regulation. Secondary bacterial invasion is a frequent complication.

The rare *hematometra*, or accumulation of blood in the uterus, is chiefly the result of vascular trauma.

Postpartum Complications as a Cause of Endometrial Disease

Retention of the fetal membranes, injury to the uterine mucosa during parturition, twin pregnancies, abortion, etc. can cause acute metritis and laminitis as well as chronic endometritis with intractable sterility. Simple retention of the membranes and retention at the microscopic level, in which chorionic villi retained in the crypts delay and complicate involution, are marked by the development of a severe leukocytosis and the accumulation of large amounts of liquid detritus. The result is chronic endometritis. This is an important cause of infertility and calls for careful management during the postpartum period. If uterine activity is sluggish after foaling, measures should be taken to stimulate expulsion of the fetal membranes within 4—6 hours. The intravenous or intramuscular injection of oxytocin is not always sufficient to achieve placental separation, even with manual assistance. The veterinary school of Ghent in Belgium reports a 90 % success rate with the i.v. drip infusion of a total of 50 I.U. oxytocin in 1—2 l physiologic saline over about a 2-hour period. The placenta separates completely and can be easily removed from the uterus. Generally the mare can then be bred during the 1st foal heat.

Severe, acute metritis requires vigorous, systematic treatment consisting of irrigation and local application of bactericidal agents. Often this must be continued for some time until a satisfactory response is obtained. The chances for immediate restoration of fertility are guarded, however, and the mare probably cannot be bred again until the following season.

Prognosis. There is no valid scheme for the prognostic evaluation of mares with endometritis based on clinical, bacteriologic, cytologic and other findings. Patience and experience are the best guides in selecting treatment and making a prognosis. A prime concern is restoration of the functional capacity of the endometrium. This is contingent upon several factors. A favorable prognosis can be offered if the mucosa is still unchanged, retains its velvety texture, is smooth and not too dense. A favorable prognosis can also be given if the mare is not too old (especially in heavier breeds), and minimal time has elapsed since the last foaling. The chance of conception decreases by about 25 % every year the mare remains barren.

On the other hand, maiden mares often exhibit a refractory infertility of unknown etiology. Their evaluation and prognosis are more difficult than in the case of multiparous mares, whose functional integrity has been demonstrated by a prior pregnancy.

All *Streptococcus* species and various other pyogenic organisms respond well to treatment if the endometrial lesions are not too deep or the mucosa has not yet undergone significant fibrosis. By contrast, hemolytic staphylococci are often therapy-resistant. The prognosis depends not so much on the degree of the infection as on the difficulty in restoring the functional integrity of the endometrium.

In some cases treatment with specific antibacterial agents will be indicated. When agents are applied directly to the endometrium, the stimulative effect on the mucosa is generally more important than the antiseptic action. The number of irrigations, local mechanical stimulation (mucosal massage), treatment with local and systemic drugs, and adjunctive treatments with hormones will depend upon the individual case. Turning the mare out to pasture along with a high-quality, natural diet are important aids in the restoration of fertility. Sexual rest is indicated for at least 1—2 estrous periods after the final examination.

Remarks on the Problem of Sexually-Transmitted Epizootic Infections

Certain highly-contagious diseases are transmitted chiefly by sexual contact, affect mainly the genital tract, and have a high morbidity. Diseases of this type have various etiologies, but all bear some relation to the reproductive organs, and all cause significant reproductive losses. Many organisms, such as streptococci, can invade various segments of the female genital tract as well as other organs in the mare, can cause abortion, or can produce infection in the newborn foal. A massive outbreak need not be present for a disease to be characterized as epizootic. It is sufficient for the threat of such an outbreak to be present in order to so characterize the disease and institute special measures for prevention and control. Besides the classic equine venereal diseases such as coital exanthema and dourine, infections with bacteria can cause considerable damage in the horse population either on a periodic or relatively permanent basis. A good example of a venereal infection that appears suddenly and spreads rapidly is contagious equine metritis, a disease that is currently found in many countries.

Contagious Equine Metritis (CEM 1977, métrite contagieuse équine 1977)

Definition. CEM is a mutually transmissible infection of the equine genitalia caused by the immobile gram-negative coccus *Hemophilus equigenitalis.* Observed since 1975 and spread by the exchange of Thoroughbreds (France, Ireland, England, U.S., Australia, etc.), this disease has been officially recognized since 1977 as a venereal disease of horses and other equidae. Transmission is mainly by copulation, although the bacteria can also be transmitted through other forms of close contact between animals (e.g., during teasing), through manipulations by attendants during breeding, as well as by the use of contaminated grooming tools, sponges, etc.

Symptoms. An incubation period of 24—48 hours is followed by the appearance of a gray, turbid, mucopurulent discharge from the ventral commissure of the vulva as a sign of bacterial invasion of the mucosae of the vagina, cervix and uterus. This discharge persists for about 11—18 days, although the bacteria sometimes remain in the urethral orifice and area of the clitoris (clitoral fossa) for as long as 100—200 days. The clinical signs may regress spontaneously within 14—42 days. Because these signs are nonspecific, a bacteriologic examination is essential for confirming the diagnosis. In the stallion, no clinical changes are apparent, although the organism can frequently be cultured from the prepuce, urethra, urethral orifice and preejaculate and may reside there for up to 200 days or more. It is possible for the organism to be transmitted from the area of the urethral orifice to the foal during parturition in infected mares.

Diagnosis. The bacteriologic diagnosis is based on an examination of material swabbed from the aformentioned mucosal areas. Due to the great sensitivity of the organisms, the sample should be collected in a vacuum and transferred quickly to the laboratory in a suitable transport medium. Serologic and cytologic tests may also be carried out.

Treatment. In affected mares the uterus is treated several times daily with chlorhexidine 1 : 5,000 for a period of several days, or 3—5 intrauterine applications of nitrofurazone, ampicillin or penicillin. Local treatment may be supplemented by concomitant injections of ampicillin or tetracyclines at 12-hour intervals for 5 days. Disturbances of the intestinal flora may occur in some instances during this therapy. In stallions, the erect penis should be thoroughly washed with chlorhexidine 3 to 5 times at intervals of 1—2 days; 2 % nitrofuran ointment is massaged into the penis after each washing. As in the mare, antibiotics are administered parenterally for about 5 days.

Mares may be bred again only after 2 or 3 negative swabs have been obtained. Stallions should do service only after they have covered a test mare, and a subsequent examination shows that no transmission has occurred.

Prophylaxis. If CEM is suspected or demonstrated, immediate, strict hygienic measures must be instituted with regard to pregnant and nonpregnant mares, stallions, teasers, foals born to suspected mares, as well as stalls, grooming tools, etc. The importation and exportation of horses also must be subject to strict controls. Local laws and regulations will dictate the specific nature of control measures.

2.1.11.6. Disturbances of Ovarian Function

Deficiencies or abnormalities of ovarian function account for the majority of reproductive disorders in the mare. Rarely are these conditions primary in nature. They are controlled mainly by higher neurohormonal centers and are largely the result of stress factors, i.e., the body lacks the ability to withstand imposed stresses and responds by reducing or 'shutting down' the reproductive system. The principal stress factors are overexertion; changes of climate and location; dietary deficiencies of minerals, trace elements and vitamins; chronic diseases, etc. These stress-induced inhibitors of ovarian function vary in their duration and clinical manifestations, and they can cause irreversible morphologic changes. Often, as in nymphomania and masculinity of adrenal origin, it is difficult to idenfity a specific etiologic factor.

In mares that have reproductive disorders due essentially to ovarian dysfunction, it is necessary to determine the cause, eliminate the stress factors, and institute medical care that will help to reestablish a regular cycle. An empirical approach without a detailed diagnosis may well prove successful in some instances, but it will obscure the cause of the stress and thus prevent the prompt correction of the factors.

The ovary of the mare at rest is about the size of a chestnut, is covered with peritoneum up to the ovulation fossa and is highly sensitive to pressure. The ovary is readily palpable, as are the changes that occur in it with the estrous cycle. The ovary rapidly changes its size, shape and surface contours and may reach a diameter of 5—8 cm in the normal state. In old mares the ovary frequently undergoes a progressive atresia, and occasionally it enlarges to the size of a fist or softball, becoming hard, knobby and fibrous. Microcystic degeneration with the appearance of numerous small vesicles is also a consequence of aging and is refractory to treatment.

Breeding should be preceded by a rectal examination (follicle check) and behavioral assessment with a teaser in order to ensure that the mare is in estrus and that a mature follicle is present. This is essential if irretrievable time losses and other costs are to be avoided.

Anestrus

Here the mare fails to come into estrus at the expected time. Rectal examination reveals little or no cyclic activity. Sometimes anestrus occurs in certain years because of a harsh climate or poor feeding conditions, newly-introduced animals being the most affected. Pasturing and sunlight generally will lead to the establishment of estrous cycles.

Anestrus may result from exposure to severe or sustained stress factors, as after strenuous exercise on a race track, or, as mentioned earlier, it may simply arise ideopathically as a feature of the mare's own foaling pattern, in the absence of a demonstrable stress factor.

If a thorough examination indicates that the mare is capable of having estrous cycles but is not, it may be possible to induce estrus through any of a variety of means.

One such means is follicular stimulation with PMSG (FSH), ovulation induction with HCG, or both concurrently at calculated intervals and dosages. The prostaglandins and their synthetic analogs are widely used. An effective method that is especially well suited for use on a herd scale is to increase the exposure to light to about 16—20 hours per day. Experiments have shown that under an increased-light regimen of this type, which may be started as early as December, estrus appears 2—4 weeks earlier than usual, and its onset is more reliable. Such methods are replacing older, outmoded practices such as infusing the uterus with saline solution or iodine preparations, multiple abrupt dietary changes at 4- to 8-day intervals, massage of the ovaries, feeding germinated wheat, etc.

Silent Heat

A mare in silent heat fails to show overt signs of estrus and will initially reject a stallion that is presented to her, even though rectal examination reveals that follicular maturation and ovulation are proceeding normally. Often the mare will accept the stallion after repeated teasing. Sexual excitement, or receptivity, can be promoted by administering small amounts of estrogen. The mare should have no difficulty conceiving if follicular maturation has progressed normally, and the usual estrous changes are present in the uterus and vagina.

Weak signs of estrus are occasionally found in entire herds early in the breeding season as a result of adverse climatic and nutritional factors.

Weak Estrus in Maiden Mares

Weak estrus in young mares is a special problem that can affect large numbers of animals. It is considered to be a result of circumstances rather than a disease entity. It may be ascribed to the still untrained and highly sensitive reproductive system of the maiden mare, but, as in silent heat, it appears that specific exogenous stress factors associated with care, feeding and season play a dominant role. Experience has shown that the following practical guidelines are useful in dealing with weak estrus in the maiden mare:

a) One should not hesitate to skip the very first estrus if need be, for it is usually anovulatory and of short duration, and its signs tend to be weak.

b) Breeding is best done in the late spring when the weather is warm, the animals are on pasture and are exposed to sunlight for much of the day.

c) Breeding during estrus itself (e.g., on the 1st or 2nd day) is useless, inasmuch as ovulation does not occur until several days later. Breeding and rebreeding should not be done before the 3rd or 4th day, although individual as well as breed-dependent factors must be taken into account.

The careful supervision and management of young mares will save superfluous or unnecessary breedings, and will enhance the efficiency of the breeding operation. Palpation of the ovaries is essential for determining the stage of follicle maturation.

Apparently Normal Estrus

Some problem mares show more or less definite signs of estrus, yet ovulation is delayed, i.e., the follicle persists after the regression of clinical estrous signs or after the mare is obviously ready to breed.

Even more often, the mare shows vaginal and other signs of estrus but does not ovulate. The follicles become atretic, while the estrous period is of irregular length.

These phase shifts in the estrous cycle can be detected only through systematic ovarian palpation or ovulatory monitoring. Both abnormalities — delayed ovulation and failure to ovulate — pose a significant threat to the orderly running of a breeding operation. Seasonal conditions have been found to be of significance, and studies have shown that such disturbances are most likely to arise at the *start* of the breeding season and tend to decrease as the weather becomes warmer. It is clear that the disorder is based upon a time-related derangement of the complex, neurohormonally-controlled cycle mechanism. The relative importance of individual susceptibility to stress factors or exposure to an undue complex of stresses can be ascertained through analysis of the individual situation. Corrective measures are similar to those for anestrus and should be preceded by a detailed evaluation. This is much more superior to an empirical approach.

The *treatment* of deficient estrus or anestrus is based upon the same guidelines and measures that were outlined in previous sections. Identifying the cause is of major importance in the selection of corrective measures. As mentioned earlier, prostaglandin $F_{2\alpha}$ and its analogs are widely used owing to their luteolytic, estrus-inducing action. The analogs are preferred, because they do not produce the severe side-effects associated with the natural prostaglandin. The dosage for the correction of silent heat, weak estrous processes or for the purpose of synchronization is a single dose of 5 mg injected intramuscularly. Mares that have just foaled are skipped during the first estrus (foal heat) due to the uncertainty of conception at that time. Prostaglandins are administered 5 or 6 days later. The mares will come into estrus in 2—4 days and will ovulate 2 days thereafter. Thus, about 8—10 days are gained in the reproductive cycle, while the chance of conception is materially enhanced. In mares that are not cycling and have had no previous estrous periods or have no demonstrable ovarian activity, the prognosis is not so favorable (70 % or less). Response to therapy is poor owing to the inadequate functional structure of the ovary or to a failure of ovarian control by higher centers. Sometimes a cycle can be established by the repeated administration of prostaglandin analogs in 10- to 14-day intervals, but it is advisable initially to use classic 'substitution' methods until cycles are achieved.

Nymphomania

Definition. Nymphomania is a syndrome caused by an abnormality of neurohormonal regulation and characterized by behavioral disorders with ovarian changes. Affected mares show long-continued, erratic signs of estrus with no regular cycle and are infertile.

Symptoms. Nymphomania is frequently evidenced by an increasing duration and intensity of estrus with progressively shorter interestrous periods, until finally estrus is constant. Affected mares are highly nervous, irritable and sometimes vicious. They kick, bite, squirt urine, and may accept the stallion but frequently refuse him. Their agitated state makes them dangerous to humans, other animals and property. Palpation demonstrates the presence of one or more follicles. The uterus and vagina show changes typical of estrus; occasionally a secretory endometritis is present. Affected mares should not be bred for the duration of their illness.

Etiology. The causes of nymphomania are not fully understood. An increased incidence sometimes can be demonstrated in certain blood lines, and severe stress factors, including psychic stresses, have been implicated. Occasionally nymphomania is associated with the improper use of estrogens or PMSG as well as with chronic uterine inflammation. The condition is due essentially to an excessive production of estrogenic hormones, with the ovarian follicles as the source. Apparently the agitated behavioral state is controlled by an increased secretion of 17-ketosteroids from the adrenal cortex in the setting of hyperestrogenism.

Differential diagnosis must be made from central nervous excitation states and masculinity of adrenal origin.

Treatment. The external signs of nymphomania can be eliminated with hormonal therapy in many cases, but a restoration of breeding soundness is often remote. Treatment consists in the injection of luteinizing hormone, chiefly chorionic gonadotropin, followed by progesterone. Ovariectomy will, of course, destroy the breeding value of the mare but will maintain her soundness for other uses.

Masculinity of Adrenal Origin (Adrenal Virilism)

Definition. Adrenal virilism refers to the development of both physical and behavioral masculine traits in the female due to an abnormality of adrenal androgen production.

Symptoms. Certain features of the syndrome are very similar to nymphomania, especially with regard to behavioral changes. However, nymphomania mainly involves an exaggeration of female sexual characteristics due to hyperestrogenism, whereas virilism involves an apparent sexual behavior change. Affected mares adopt a noticeably 'studdish' manner of behavior, will mount other mares, but will no longer accept the male. Their nervous unrest sometimes increases to the point of frenzy and destructive mania. Ovarian activity is indifferent, and the follicles that characterize nymphomania are absent. The handling of such animals is dangerous; some will permit themselves to be touched only by certain persons, or only by force. The mare may appear calm during certain periods, but it must be remembered that she is in a constant state of psychoneurotic tension, and even the slightest disturbance may be sufficient to precipitate frenzied behavior.

Etiology. Adrenal virilism is based upon a pathologic change in the adrenal cortex with an associated hypersecretion of 17-ketosteroids and androgenic substances. Higher control is effected through the increased secretion of adrenocorticotropic hormone (ACTH) by the anterior pituitary. The underlying causes are not yet known.

Treatment. Operative or conservative methods of curing or improving adrenal virilism are unknown in veterinary medicine. The confusion of this condition with nymphomania leads frequently to the inappropriate treatment of mares with adrenal virilism. The absence of response in such cases serves as a differential diagnostic criterion. Ovarion tumors (granulosa cell tumors) must be ruled out as a cause of the behavior.

2.1.11.7. Death of the Gamete, Zygote, Embryo and Fetus; Abortion

The potential causes of the death of a zygote or embryo are extremely varied. To adopt a systematic approach toward the problem of prenatal death, it appears necessary to make a general distinction between damage to the gametes occurring prior to fertilization, and abortion of the embryo or fetus occurring after fertilization.

While a classification of this type is a useful aid to diagnosis, it is still necessary to consider and evaluate other factors. These include infection, toxemia, hormonal and immune status, genetic influences, nutrition, climate, acclimatization and other stress factors.

Damage to the Gametes Prior to Fertilization

It is estimated that roughly 50 % of mares fail to conceive when first bred. This is due mainly to incorrect timing of the breeding, but other, less frequent causes include damage to the gametes resulting from inflammation in the female genital tract, and other unforeseen circumstances. Often no specific cause can be assigned. The case may involve early embryonic mortality, and although conception does occur, the mare remains barren for that breeding year (about 20 % of cases).

Embryonic and Fetal Mortality

'Embryonic mortality' is a loosely-defined term for embryonic death occurring between the early zygotic stage and the end of the 5th to 7th week, regardless of whether the embryo is resorbed or aborted. In cattle this limit is 5 weeks, inasmuch as placentation is already well established by that time. In horses, however, placental attachment of the embryo does not occur until several weeks later, accounting for the longer period during which embryonic mortality may be said to occur. This fact, plus the labile cervix of the mare, explains the relatively high incidence of embryonic abortion in this species.

The causes and prevalence of embryonic mortality are difficult to discuss in precise terms due to the variety of primary and secondary factors involved. Especially difficult to explain are the 'hidden' cases of early embryonic resorption that are apt to be mistaken for simple split estrus, cycle depression or other causes of sterility (i.e., nonconception). Often inappropriate empirical treatment is used. Moreover, if the zygote dies before about the 10th day of gestation, the next estrus can still occur on schedule, and the prenatal death will go unsuspected. In many cases too little importance is attached to minor deviations in the regularity of the estrous cycle, and to the fact that more mares in a herd conceive than remain pregnant. On the whole, continuous surveillance in a band of mares will reveal an embryonic mortality rate of about 5—10 %. This does not count the aforementioned cases that are concealed among the frequent cases of regular or irregular split estrus.

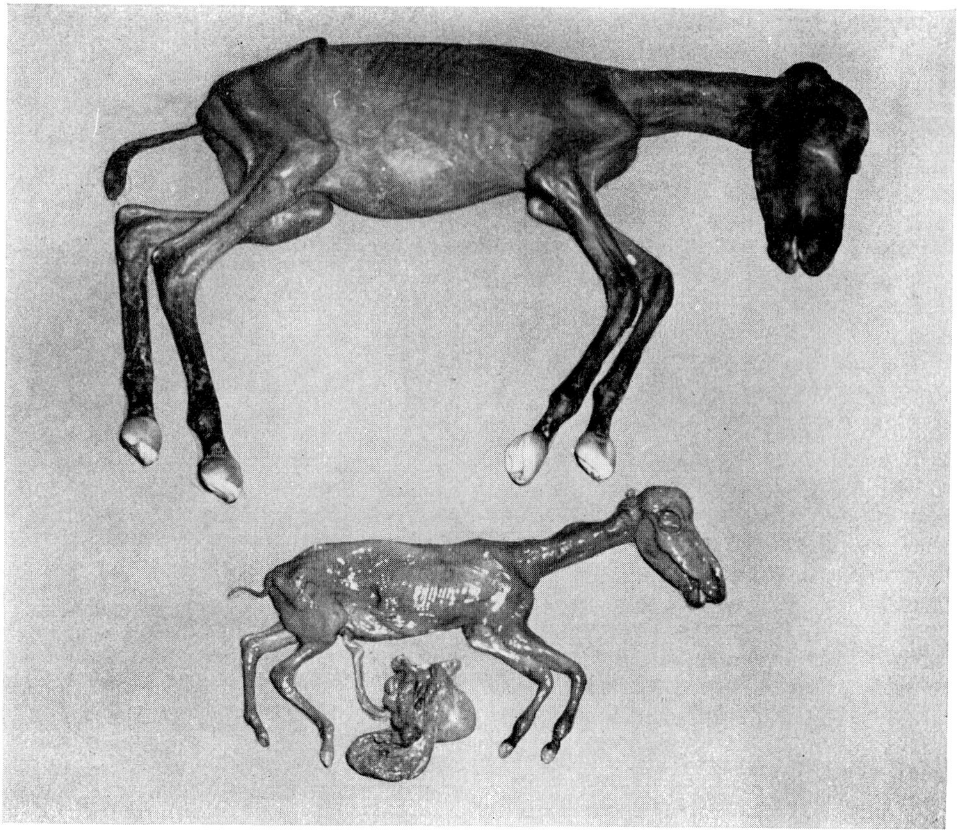

Fig. 2.1.11. — 2. Aborted fetuses.

The suspicion of an embryonic death is justified if the mare becomes estrous again more than 3 weeks after she has been bred. In most cases of early embryonic mortality, evidence is too scant to enable the cause to be specified. As gestation time increases beyond 3—4 weeks, the diagnostic prospects improve. The fundamental question for the examiner is whether the death is the result of hereditary influences, stress factors, infectious disease or a pathologic condition of the genital or other organs. Often the boundaries are indistinct, and special circumstances and processes associated with infectious or contagious abortion may be present in the late embryonic stage. More likely, the fetal stage is involved.

a) *Hereditary influences:* Certain individual animals or blood lines are relatively poor breeders. Diagnostic techniques are not yet capable of reliably differentiating stress-related factors from defects due to genetic causes. However, observations indicate that animals with roughly equivalent physiologic makeups can respond differently to the same stress factors, and that a high or even total embryonic mortality occurs with regularity in certain individuals. Often a combination of certain paternal and maternal characteristics in the embryo results in a critical incompatibility. Intrauterine isoerythrolysis (Rh disease) is unknown in horses, as the maternal antibodies cannot pass through the placental barrier. Antibodies can be transferred to the foal only post partum via the colostrum, causing neonatal isoerythrolysis. Whether genetically determined or the result of a random combination during mating, severe defects often can occur. Such mares often are simply classified as 'poor breeders' and are excluded from breeding use. Of particular interest is the high incidence of embryonic resorption in Thoroughbred mares that conceive from a '9-day breeding'. One must also consider resorption and abortion associated with twin pregnancies in mares of all breeds.

b) *Stress-related causes:* Zygotic and embryonic deaths are more the result of stress effects than of diseases affecting the reproductive organs. When excessive demands are placed on the body's capacity to deal with a stress, it responds by deactivating the 'nonvital' reproductive functions. This often occurs during extreme physical exertion or when the body is subjected to varying forms of unaccustomed stress. Because this effect on reproductive events stems from such nonspecific factors as heat, cold, hunger, thirst, deficiencies, exertion, food lesions, poisonings, diseases, etc., identification of the active stress factor is often a difficult task. It is important to note that these processes mainly represent a regulatory mechanism that is acting between the organism and its environment. Hence, any corrective measures that are undertaken should be aimed at the cause and not directed at treating the symptoms.

Stress-related reproductive disorders in the mare cover a relatively broad spectrum. A common stress that may arise at any time during the pregnancy is food poisoning from the yew tree *(Taxus baccata)*, juniper *(Juniperus sabina)* and other plants that have a contractile effect on the uterus. Besides harmful feed mixtures, abortion is also associated with the feeding of massive amounts of turnips as well as fungus-infested feeds (see Sec. 2.5.1.3.).

Drugs that stimulate peristalsis (e.g., parasympathicomimetics) and corticosteroids should be used with extreme caution in pregnant mares. Sudden cooling (e.g., from rain or drafts) as well as the rapid consumption of large amounts of cold water can also have harmful effects.

c) *Traumatic factors:* The pregnant mare is highly sensitive to kicks, blows, falls, jumps, slips, overexertion, casting for surgery, confined transport, etc. Occasionally, artificially-induced abortions result from an inept or overvigorous rectal or vaginal examination. Psychic stresses associated with fright or physical abuse are also of significance, for they often elicit abrupt responses with compression of the gravid uterus by the abdominal muscles.

d) *Other causes of abortion:* Severe systemic diseases can lead to fetal death in all stages of pregnancy (fig. 2.1.11. — 2). These include parasitic and febrile diseases as well as gastrointestinal (colic) and urinary tract disorders.

In the majority of twin pregnancies, the fetuses are either resorbed in the embryonic stage, aborted, or are expelled, together or separately, during the course of fetal development. It is rare for a twin pregnancy to reach full term, and it is equally rare for the twins to survive. Attempts have been made to control events, and thus avoid the uncertain process of self-selection (resorption of one embryo or the death of both embryos followed by a new estrus and breeding), either by inducing a complete abortion or by crushing one embryo at about the 30th day of gestation, with the object of enabling the surviving twin to continue development as a solitary fetus. The results of this procedure are not good, the incidence of abortion being about 90 %. However, even if the mare aborts, she will come into estrus several days later and will again be able to conceive.

The issue of abortion in mares raises the question of whether the laxity and distensibility of the cervix during pregnancy and the relatively late completion of placentation at about 12—14 weeks leads to a higher prevalence of non-infectious embryonic losses in the mare than in the cow. Careful estimates point to a slightly but significantly higher rate of embryonic loss in the mare.

Infectious or Contagious Abortion

The majority of infectious abortions occur in the second half of pregnancy. They are usually signaled 1 to 2 days previously by the development of edema cranial to the udder or a swelling of the udder and the area surrounding the vulva. The pelvic ligaments sink inward slightly, until finally labor commences and the embryo, usually dead, is prematurely expelled.

Abortions may be characterized according to their occurrence as symptomatic (occurring as a manifestation of infection), sporadic, enzootic or epizootic. These terms do not necessarily denote the number of animals affected, and even solitary abortions may be epizootic in origin. Thus, any premature expulsion of the embryo or fetus may be a sign that a disease is present. Both the mare and the aborted fetus should be carefully examined until the presence of an epizootic can be excluded or confirmed. It is important to realize that the organisms of infectious abortion can also be responsible for septicemia in foals as well as endometritis and resultant sterility.

Salmonella abortus equi

Definition. The disease, also known as equine paratyphoid, was widespread. It can be acutely transmitted to nearly all mares, a large percentage of which will then abort or bear a dead or nonviable foal. Afterwards the mare will have difficulty conceiving or will be infertile.

Symptoms. Ingestion is the principal mode of infection. It is unclear whether the disease can be transmitted through copulation. The incubation period is about 30 days. Abortion usually occurs between the 6th and 10th months of pregnancy, though it may occur earlier or later, and the aborting mare shows no particular signs of illness. Live foals may be born from infected mares, but most die a short time after birth. The causal organism can be demonstrated by serologic and culture methods in the mare and foal.

Control and Prevention. Control centers on the practice of organized hygienic measures. Besides strict general stable hygiene, this includes the observance of special precautions during abortions, premature births and stillbirths and in the handling of sick or dead foals. In addition, all affected mares should be subjected to close serologic and clinical surveillance and should be allowed 3 months of convalescence and sexual rest before being bred again. On the herd scale, prophylactic vaccinations with a specific bacterin was recommended. Vaccination reactions could not always be avoided in such circumstances, however, and vaccinational titers often persist for a long time. Whenever individual cases of abortion due to Salmonella are detected, the affected animals should be isolated, and the vaccination of healthy animals should be avoided so that eradication can be more easily monitored and confirmed. The continual testing of all mares between 1 and 2 years old is strongly advised, however. If the extent of an outbreak is unclear, then the best means of preventing spread is to prohibit the exchange of mares among breeding farms or across national boundaries. In any event, it is a good rule to breed only quarantined, tested animals that have checked out healthy in every respect.

Comments. The eradication of abortion due to Salmonella is possible but requires time (2—4 years) and strict adherence to a carefully designed eradication program.

Streptococcus zooepidemicus

Symptoms. This ubiquitous organism is transmitted mainly during breeding. Abortion most commonly occurs between the 4th and 7th months of pregnancy, or a weak foal is born shortly before term. While infection with *Str. zooepidemicus* does not always appear in epizootic form, the disease is considered dangerous because of the variety of its forms and manifestations and its frequently poor prognosis. It often plays a significant role as a sexually-transmitted, sterility-causing infection. Stallions can be chronic shedders of the bacteria, and large numbers of mares contract catarrhal and purulent endometritis and pyometra from which they may not recover. The organism is also important in the etiology of foal septicemia, requiring close supervision in all crops of foals that are threatened by infection.

Treatment. The abortion, which rarely is complicated, is followed by a mucopurulent discharge without particular systemic signs. It is treated locally with the usual medications and methods. The aborting mare may be bred again only after treatment is concluded and swabs are negative, i.e., subsequent to clinical and bacteriologic recovery.

Prevention and Comments. The eradication of genital streptococcal infections in horse populations is possible but requires very close supervision of breeding procedures, suitable surveillance of breeding stock and preventive medicine practices. The culling of incurable individuals is sometimes unavoidable and is even advisable in terms of preventing spread among stabled animals.

Brucella abortus

Reports to date on abortions due to brucellosis have been infrequent but are deserving of attention. At one time it was thought that it was safe for infected cattle herds to graze the same pastures used by horses. However, several abortion 'storms' on stud farms have proven that brucellosis can be transmitted to horses from aborting heifers and cows in cases where both species are grazing the same pasture.

As in cattle, the diagnosis is made on the basis of a serologic examination. Brucellosis in horses is prevented by prohibiting the grazing of cattle on studs, especially in infected regions.

Fungi

Increasingly, a connection is being observed between fungal infection and abortion in mares. *Aspergillus fumigatus* is most commonly implicated. Apparently it is possible for fungal hyphae to be introduced into the placenta from the bowel under certain circumstances. Metastasis from the lungs is also possible when fungus-laden dust is inhaled. Abortions due to fungal infection seldom occur in large numbers of animals. Diagnosis is relatively easy owing to the characteristic plaque like-lesions on the fetal membranes and the presence of well-defined fungal elements under magnification.

Viral Abortion (Equine Herpesvirus 1, EHV 1)

Definition. The incidence of abortion in mares due to EHV 1, the rhinopneumonitis virus, is increasing in almost all countries and is a particular problem in Thoroughbred breeding. Often many recently-infected mares on a farm will abort within a period of a few weeks. Viral arteritis can produce similar outbreaks but is a less frequent cause. The influenza virus usually does not cause abortion.

Symptoms. The infection is generally contracted from the inhalation of viruses shed by infected mares. After an incubation time of 3—7 days, the infection appears as a self-limiting, mildly febrile disease that runs a course of 8—10 days. Signs of upper respiratory tract disease are evident in young horses, and the temperature varies from 39 to 40 °C. Pregnant mares experience only mild symptoms with a slight temperature elevation. Abortion occurs from 3 weeks to 4 months after infection of the mare, and thus after clinical recovery, and generally between the 7th and 10th months. Abortions after the 3rd month are known. The abortions tend to occur in outbreaks. Recovery is followed by an immunity lasting for 1—3 additional foaling periods, and successive abortions are rare. An infection contracted before or at the start of pregnancy could conceivably produce immunity without abortion.

The abortion is sudden and without premonitory signs. Usually the fetus is still in fresh condition and the fetal membranes intact. Breeding may be resumed during the next breeding season, assuming there have been no postpartum complications.

Diagnosis. In aborted or stillborn fetuses, the liver shows grayish-white areas of focal necrosis. Specific inclusion bodies are found in hepatic cells bordering on the necrotic foci and in the bronchiolar epithelium. Other gross organic lesions are non-specific.

For diagnostic purposes, aborted fetuses should be promptly examined or the lung, liver, spleen and kidneys deep-frozen and submitted for analysis. Isolation of the virus in guinea pigs can confirm the histologic diagnosis.

Prevention and Control. Medical treatment is useless for preventing abortion in virus-infected animals, and the infectious process cannot be interrupted. However, prior inoculation with virus vaccine may be an effective preventive measure in endangered populations.

When viral abortion occurs, immediate control rests on management. Because fever develops 36—72 hours after the initial infection, it is necessary when abortions occur to perform immediate and continued temperature checks of all pregnant mares on the stud once or twice daily while submitting blood samples for analysis. Because antibodies are already present 10 days after infection, and the mares do not abort earlier than 18 days after infection, it is possible to isolate mares in which EHV 1 is suspected on the basis of fever. It may be diagnosed on the basis of serum titers before abortion occurs, and thus before virus is shed. When the last mare has foaled, the infection may be considered eradicated. A reinfection of nonimmunized mares during the next pregnancy period generally can be traced to new arrivals at the stud. Weanlings and yearlings pose a particular danger in this regard, for the fall 'colds' that occur in these animals can be caused by the rhinopneumonitis virus. For this reason it is a good precaution to keep pregnant mares separated from younger animals. When the occurrence of a viral abortion is confirmed on the stud, no mares should be allowed to enter or leave it until after the foaling period.

Abortions due to viral arteritis are infrequent on the European continent but are more common in the U.S., for example, where such abortions are enzootic. In contrast to the rhinopneumonitis virus, the arteritis virus produces marked clinical symptoms in infected mares, most notably a high fever, swelling of the limbs and edema of the ventral abdomen.

Other Infectious Abortions

Occasionally abortions occur in mares that have contracted an infectious disease, yet the morbidity is not of epizootic proportions and the abortion is not considered to be of the classic contagious variety. The causative organisms include staphylococci, *Actinobacillus equuli*, *Corynebacterium equi*, *Pseudomonas aeruginosa*, *Proteus vulgaris*, enteritic bacteria, etc. In addition, 'symptomatic' abortions are seen in infectious anemia, pleuritis and pneumonia, bacterial inflammation of the upper respiratory tract, and other febrile infections. In each case the course should be watched closely, for significant outbreaks, though rare, can occur if conditions are favorable.

The prevention of abortion outbreaks in horse populations is governed in each country by veterinary health regulations pertaining to the isolation of sick animals; the disinfection of stable areas, pastures and utensils; the disposal of dead fetuses and fetal membranes; procedures for surveillance and vaccination; the imposing and lifting of quarantines; convalescence prior to resumption of breeding; and precautionary measures in breeding operations.

References

Allen, W. R.; Rowson, L. E. A.: Einleitung und Synchronisation des Östrus bei Rind, Schaf und Pferd unter Verwendung von Prostaglandinen. Prakt. Tierarzt *16:* 515 (1975).

Benten, C. von; Petzoldt, K.; Sonnenschein, B.; Benten, K. von: Abortursachen in der Warmblutzucht. Dtsch. Tierärztl. Wschr. *84:* 453 (1977).

Ginther, O. J.: Occurrence of anestrus, estrus, diestrus and ovulation over a 12-month period in mares. Amer. J. Vet. Res. *35:* 1173 (1974).

Greenhoff, G. R.; Kenney, R. M.: Evaluation of reproductive status of nonpregnant mares. J. Amer. vet. med. Assoc. *167:* 419 (1975).

Knowles, R. C.; Hendricks, J. B.; King, D. D.; Hourrigan, J. L.: CEM; Contagious equine metritis. A transmissible disease with international implications. Mod. vet. Pract. *59:* 819 (1978).

Kooistra, L. H.; Ginther, O. J.: Effect of photoperiod on reproductive activity and hair in mares. Amer. J. Vet. Res. *36:* 1413 (1975).

Kuhns, B.: The effect of artificial lighting on the estrus cycle of the mare. Iowa State Univ. Vet. *3:* 85 (1975).

Küst, D.; Schaetz, F.: Fortpflanzungsstörungen bei den Haustieren, 5. Aufl. (VEB Gustav Fischer Verlag Jena und Ferdinand Enke Verlag, Stuttgart 1977).

Lieux, P.: Reproduction and genital diseases. In Catcott, E. J.; Smithcors, J. F.: Equine Medicine and Surgery, 2nd ed. (Amer. Vet. Publ. Inc. 1972).

Merkt, K.: Die Zyklusdiagnose beim landwirtschaftlichen Nutztier. Pferd. Tierzüchter *22:* 220 (1970).

Roberts, S. J.: Veterinary obstetrics and genital diseases. New York 1971 (published by the author).

Rolle, M.; Mayr, A.: Mikrobiologie, Infektions- und Seuchenlehre, 4. Aufl. (Enke, Stuttgart 1978).

Stabenfeldt, H. G.; Hughes, J. P.; Evans, J. W.: Ovarian activity during the estrus cycle of the mare. Endocrinology *90:* 1379 (1972).

Tainturier, D.; Ferney, J.; Royal, L.: La metrite contagieuse de la jument. Revue Méd. vét. *130:* 497 (1979).

Thibault, C.: Regulation of breeding season and oestrus cycles by light and external stimuli in some mammals. J. Animal Sci., suppl. 25, p. 119 (1966).

Vandeplassche, M.; Spincemaille, J.; Bonte, P.; Bouters, R.; Tijskens, R.: Aktuelle Probleme der Stutensterilität. Prakt. Tierarzt *13:* 494 (1972).

2.1.12. Breeding Practices

With the increasing concentration of breeding stock on stud farms and other establishments where horses are bred, the problem of fertility and conception rates has become a matter of great concern. In response to this challenge, breeding practices have become more sophisticated, and reproductive efficiency is improved through the control of factors that are detrimental to fertility and breeding health.

While diseases of the genital tract and abnormalities of the estrous cycle take their toll, faulty breeding practices still represent a *major* cause of poor reproductive performance. By this we mean human errors committed in the organization and conduct of breeding procedures, such as failure to recognize estrus or errors in the timing of breeding. Often these errors are the product of ignorance concerning the physiology of the estrous cycle in the mare. In other cases stallion overuse is to blame. These problems usually pose no serious difficulties in breeding operations that are run by

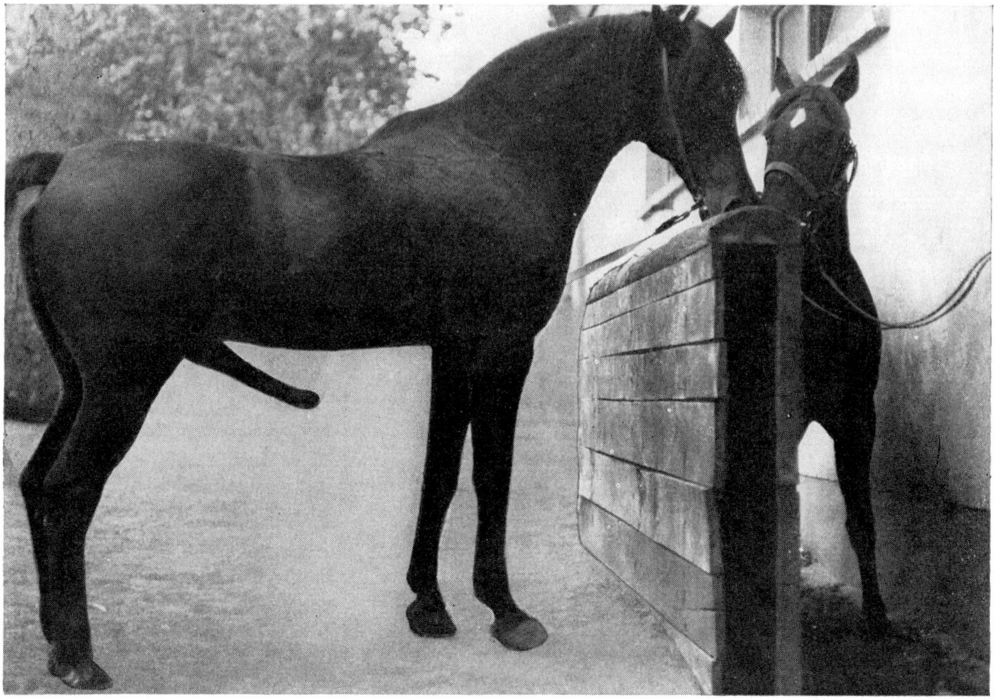

Fig. 2.1.12. — 1. Teasing the mare behind a teasing wall.

qualified and experienced personnel. However, the problems inherent in breeding management are highly complex, and years of experience are needed in order to recognize and deal with them as they arise. It is important that faulty breeding practices be considered in the diagnosis of infertility. Treatment of the cause is always the goal whenever infertility is detected; a haphazard diagnosis followed by symptomatic treatment usually does more harm than good.

Another factor detrimental to reproductive efficiency in breeding operations is the narrow limits that are assigned to the length of the breeding season. Aside from a few larger breeding establishments in which sires are available throughout the year, stallions usually are used from about February to July (in the Northern Hemisphere). In breeding farms for Thoroughbreds and Standardbreds, the breeding season starts on February 15 and ends on June 15. Restrictions of this kind preclude the breeding of many mares in which estrus is delayed or is missed for other reasons. Moreover, there is little chance that mares contracting genital infections after the first breeding will be able to be bred again in the same season.

The fewest problems arise in herds in which a single stallion has more or less constant exposure to a mare. A natural selection is operative in such situations, and a conception rate of nearly 100 % can be expected among animals in good breeding condition. For many reasons, however, this ideal situation cannot be achieved in breeding operations.

2.1.12.1. Teasing

Each phase of the estrous cycle is characterized by certain physiologic and behavioral peculiarities. Important for breeding purposes are the typical estrous behavior of the mare, by which she demonstrates a readiness to receive the stallion, and physiologic estrus with development of the follicle and ovulation. The signs of estrus can vary greatly in degree from one animal to the next. Very strong estrous symptoms are not difficult to recognize. In many mares, however, the manifestations of estrus are less obvious and may be difficult to discern. For this reason broodmares are systematically 'teased' at 1- to 2-day intervals, in this way testing them for the presence or absence of estrus.

For the safety of the animals as well as of persons standing nearby, many breeders use a teasing wall to separate the stallion and mare (fig. 2.1.12. — 1) or place the mare in a special teasing stand. The teasing wall or stand must be of a sturdy construction. Some mares will reject the teaser at the wall, yet will show definite signs of estrus while in a stall or paddock. This is especially common in Thoroughbred mares and other purebreds. One solution in such cases is to tease the mare elsewhere, having first restrained her with a sideline or hobbles; another is to try teasing her with a different stallion.

In larger breeding establishments a special teaser is used so that the breeding stallions will be spared unnecessary work.

A group of mares in a paddock can be teased by leading a quiet stallion up to the side of the paddock. Estrous mares in the band generally will approach the stallion and display an obvious readiness to breed; these animals are then removed from the paddock and prepared for breeding. In a herd, estrous mares can be identified by a use of a 'searcher'. This is a stallion whose penis has been surgically transposed in such a way that the penis is diverted caudad on erection. This will enable the stallion to mount the mare yet will prevent intromission as well as the possible transmission of infection (fig. 2.1.12. — 2). The use of these animals tends to have a stimulating effect on the mares but is possible only in herds where the mares are without foals.

2.1.12.2. Breeding and Rebreeding

Breeding should be timed such that it coincides as closely as possible with the time of ovulation. Experience has shown that breeding is best done 4/5 of the way through estrus, and thus near the end of the estrous period. In about 75 % of mares, the strongest overt signs of estrus ('peak' of estrus) approximately coincide with ovulation. Estrous signs generally disappear within 24 hours after ovulation.

NISHIKAWA [1959] reports the following statistical distribution for ovulation in mares with respect to the end of estrus:

0.9 % ovulate 3 days before the end of estrus
25.3 % ovulate 2 days before the end of estrus
64.5 % ovulate 1 day before the end of estrus
8.4 % ovulate on the last day of estrus
0.9 % ovulate 1 day after the end of estrus.

Systematic studies have shown that in 72 % of mares, ovulation occurs between 11 : 00 p.m. and 7 : 00 a.m. On the strength of these findings, it is clear that a mare should not be bred too early in the estrous period. This not only leads to avoidable overuse of stallions but also increases the risk of introducing infection into the uterus.

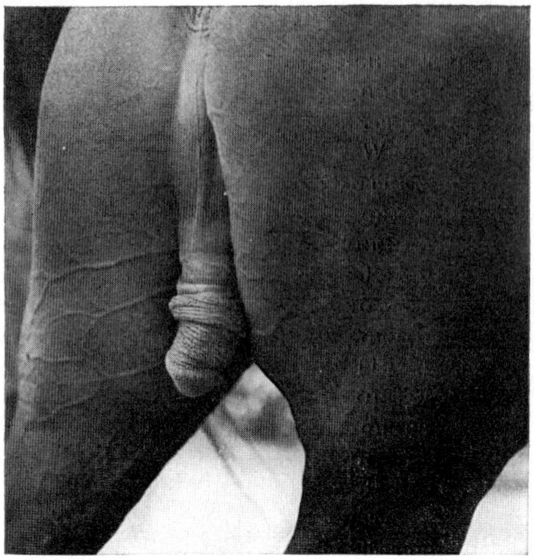

Fig. 2.1.12. — 2. 'Searcher' whose penis has been surgically transposed in a caudal direction to permit mounting without intromission.

An excellent method of timing in breeding operations is to keep an estrus chart for each broodmare, from which the length of the estrous periods, and thus the optimum breeding time, can be ascertained. These can vary greatly from one mare to the next, although the length of estrus is fairly consistent for each animal. It must be realized, however, that the cycles tend to be weak and irregular during the winter months, especially in younger animals. The cycles normalize as the season progresses, the estrous periods becoming shorter and the likelihood of conception greater.

Following a natural breeding, the spermatozoa remain active in the mare's genital tract for an average of 25—48 hours, though this will vary somewhat with the individual stallion. The ovum, on the other hand, is capable of being fertilized for only about 8—12 hours after its release. Therefore, to ensure that fertile spermatozoa will be present in the uterus or tube at the time of ovulation, the mare should be rebred about 36—48 hours after the initial breeding, and this regimen should be continued until the stallion is refused or ovulation has been confirmed by rectal examination.

Recent information indicates that artificial insemination of the mare is successful only if done no later than 8 hours after rupture of the follicle.

Due to the limited length of the breeding season, it is not uncommon for stallions to be heavily used during the spring months. Breeding operations should be organized so as to avoid stallion overuse. Development of the spermatozoa, including maturation in the epididymis, is a process that takes about 9 weeks and is fairly constant throughout the year. Frequent use of the stallion leads only to an excessive production of seminal fluid and thus to a potentially significant dilution of the semen in terms of sperm count. In the normally fertile stallion, semen production is linked to demand and is sufficient for about 1.5 ejaculations per day. Overuse is possible for brief periods, but in the long run it decreases the chance of fertilization. Individual differences among stallions also must be taken into account when breeding schedules are assigned.

Rectal palpation of the ovaries by a veterinarian provides a reliable means of monitoring follicular development and estimating the time of an impending ovulation.

Alternate-day examinations are adequate at the start of estrus, but daily examinations become necessary as the follicle matures. In this way the most favorable breeding time can be established and the number of covers substantially reduced. This measure is especially recommended for 'problem mares'.

It is possible to shift the estrous cycles, and thus achieve a more reasonable distribution of stallion service, by treating broodmares with prostaglandin $F_{2\alpha}$ or its analogs. In this way estrous periods can be skipped and the next cycle shifted ahead by 10 days.

During the actual breeding, an attendant should help guide the stallion's penis into the vagina. Ejaculation will follow after about 5—10 pelvic thrusts. During ejaculation the cranial end of the penis is pressed toward the open cervix, so that the semen is ejected into the uterus. The sperm will reach the fallopian tube in a matter of minutes, and it is there that fertilization takes place. One way to confirm the occurrence of ejaculation is to place the hand onto the exposed part of the underside of the penis; ejaculation will be evidenced by a series of palpable peristaltic waves. After breeding is completed, the mare should be walked for a few minutes to keep her from expressing the semen.

2.1.12.3. Breeding Hygiene

Breeding hygiene is of critical importance in the avoidance of sexually-transmitted infection. The regular examination of all broodmares and stallions is a highly effective preventive measure. Most sexually-transmitted infections in the horse are produced by nonspecific organisms, and such infections are relatively uncommon as long as a balance is maintained between the genital flora and the defense mechanisms of the genital mucosae, and hygienic rules are followed in breeding procedures. According to Tilmann [1975], a nonspecific, resident organism will produce infection only if:

1. the resistance and defense mechanisms of the genital mucosae are impaired;
2. the organisms are present in great numbers;
3. the organisms are highly infective.

The main natural barriers against genital tract infection in the mare are:

1. labial closure
2. vestibulo-vaginal closure
3. cervical closure
4. the antimicrobial properties of the mucosae.

These antimicrobial properties are strongest during estrus, at which time the estrogen-primed genital tract is highly resistant to bacteria introduced during coitus. However, circumstances may overtax the antimicrobial capacity of the genital mucosae to the extent that invading organisms can no longer be resisted. The stallion often acts as a carrier of infectious organisms and can transmit these organisms sexually without showing any symptoms.

A number of special precautionary measures have proved indispensible in breeding practice. To keep the stallion from being kicked during breeding, restraint of the mare is desirable. Breeding hobbles should be applied in such a way that they effectively restrain the mare, yet can be easily and quickly released if the need arises (fig. 2.1.12. — 3).

The breeding site must meet all hygienic requirements. It should be roofed and provide a quiet setting. A closed breeding shed is best. The floor should be neither dusty nor muddy but must offer traction. Fine, moist gravel and firm, nonslippery

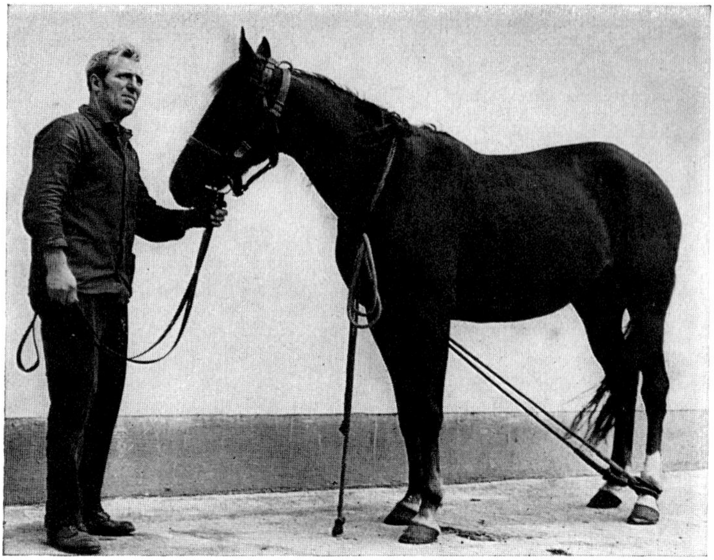

Fig. 2.1.12. — 3. Mare restrained for breeding.

surfaces such as asphalt or rubber tiles make excellent flooring. The breeding and teasing facilities should be kept as clean and germ-free as the stables, and they should not be used for any other purposes (treating sick horses, irrigating mares, etc.).

The mare is prepared for breeding by rolling a clean bandage around the upper third of the tail (fig. 2.1.12. — 4). The vulva and surrounding area are cleaned thoroughly and washed with a mild, weak scented antiseptic, taking care that no solution enters the vulvar fissure.

After breeding, the stallion's penis is rinsed with warm physiologic saline solution (9 g salt in 1 liter boiled water) or a mild antiseptic solution (e.g., acridine dye solution 1 : 1,000). The application of a thin film of a non-irritating bovoflavin ointment is also beneficial. For this purpose a gob of ointment is applied to the proximal part of the flaccid penis immediately after the stallion dismounts. As the penis retracts, the ointment will automatically become spread over the mucosa. At no time should antibiotic rinses, sprays or ointments be used. Neither is it advisable to place antiseptic ointments into the vestibule of the vagina immediately after breeding, as this might harm the sperm.

Only healthy, fully estrous mares should be presented to the stallion. The following mares should not be bred:

1. mares that are obviously sick and show signs of systemic illness;
2. mares that show outward signs of genital tract disease (purulent or pus-containing discharge);
3. mares that have aborted within the past 3 months or whose foals have died or suffered recurrent illness, unless the mares have been examined by a veterinarian and declared fit for breeding;
4. mares that have been covered or inseminated during the past 2 years and produced no live foal, unless they have been examined by a veterinarian and declared fit for breeding;

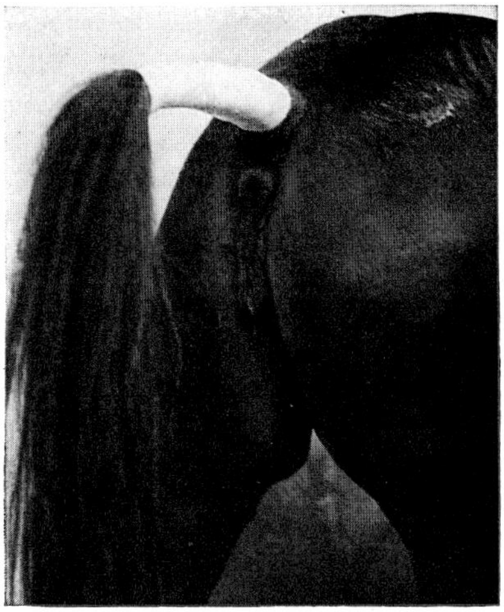

Fig. 2.1.12. — 4. The upper part of the tail is bandaged in preparation for breeding.

5. mares that have been unsuccessfully covered or inseminated in 3 consecutive estruses during the current breeding season and have not been examined by a veterinarian and declared fit for breeding or insemination.

2.1.12.4. Organization of Fertility Management and Sterility Control Practices

The control of fertility disturbances in horse breeding is essentially an organizational problem that can be solved only through a systematic, organized program of preventive medicine. This applies to stallions as well as broodmares. The examinations must be performed by veterinarians who are specialists in the field and should be patterned along the lines of an animal health service. The program is most efficient if controlled by a central agency. In the German Democratic Republic, for example, a 'Stallion Health Service' and 'Breeding Hygiene Service for Mares' have been established by the state to provide ongoing hygienic surveillance and health care for horses on stud-farms and other breeding establishments. These services adhere to a system of guidelines, or standards, that enable chronically sick, incurable or unsound animals to be promptly excluded from breeding. Curably sick animals can be identified as such and their breeding value preserved by prompt referral for veterinary examination, treatment and further supervision.

The multiplicity and variety of reproductive disorders that can arise in horse breeding are related to such factors as local conditions, nutrition, care and maintenance, breed, usage, local epizootiologic conditions, age and hereditary disposition. It is little wonder that the sterility factors at work in any given case are frequently difficult to identify.

When a mare is suspected of being infertile, the first step is to take a detailed history. The examiner must learn all he can not just about the individual animal, but also about the breeding operation and its practices. Only after these questions have been clarified should he proceed with the clinical examination. Once a diagnosis has been reached, the necessary measures and treatments can be instituted. If the etiology of the fertility disturbance is known, much can be accomplished through preventive measures.

Stallions. All breeding stallions should be examined at least once a year. These routine examinations are best conducted after the end of the breeding season, so that the animal's reproductive performance and sexual behavior can be evaluated for that season.

If reproductive performance has been poor or other problems are noted, further investigations are indicated, including a general clinical examination and special examination of the genital tract.

Semen examinations are routine for stallions that are to be used for artificial insemination. In the breeding stallion, a semen examination is indicated if:

— reproductive performance is poor,

— there is disease or any clinical change in the genital organs, or

— there is any other disease or deficiency that could adversely affect semen quality.

In some instances a bacteriologic or virologic examination of the semen or pre-ejaculate will be necessary. However, it is a sound precaution to subject the pre-ejaculate of all breeding stallions to a microbiologic analysis prior to the start of each breeding season.

All findings should be accurately recorded. They provide the basis upon which veterinary medical authorities will evaluate the soundness of the stallion for breeding or for artificial insemination and declare it to be 'sound', 'sound with reservations' or 'unsound'. The examination results are discussed with the farm management, and necessary measures are implemented.

Mares. The reproductive status of the mare should be monitored continually during the breeding season. All bred mares should be examined early for pregnancy so that they can be rebred without delay if they fail to conceive at first breeding. Due to the danger of embryonic and fetal resorption, pregnant mares should be reexamined around mid-May to verify that the pregnancy is proceeding normally, or the final pregnancy determination may be deferred until the 3rd month, by which time the danger of embryonic resorption and mortality will have passed.

In addition, a prebreeding examination by a veterinarian is indicated in all mares that:

— are barren or have been acquired with an uncertain history,

— have aborted,

— have experienced dystocia, retention of fetal membranes and/or postpartum difficulties,

— have abnormal discharge from the genital organs,

— show abnormal estrous cycles,

— have had split estruses more than twice,

— are scheduled for a follow-up examination following therapy.

Between September and December, but no later than 2 months before the start of the new breeding season, an end-of-the-year examination should be performed on all nonpregnant broodmares. This consists of a general clinical examination as well as a special breeding soundness evaluation. The latter may include a microbial examination of cervical swabs and uterine washings, serologic, parasitologic and other examinations. This should provide a clear picture of the fertility status of the individual animal and of the herd as a whole. If genital tract pathology is detected (e.g., genital infections, perineal lacerations, faulty vulvar closure, ovarian lesions), prompt medical and surgical therapy can be recommended and instituted so that the mares can be returned to breeding soundness by the start of the new season. Animals that are still anestrous at this time may or may not require special therapy later on, for experience has shown that estrous cycles often take time to become established, especially in younger mares, and that it will probably be spring before a meaningful clinical assessment can be made.

Mares with chronic, incurable diseases of the genital tract should be excluded from breeding at the earliest opportunity. The decision as to when a mare should be declared unfit for breeding is often a difficult one, and some mares may appear unsound at the moment, yet have curable diseases that do not preclude their eventual return to breeding use.

Routine breeding soundness examinations in the mare should be done early enough that the necessary treatment can be administered and concluded by the start of the new breeding season, and the mare can be allowed a sufficient period of sexual rest following treatment. It is known that even when a mare has been cured of a disease, and the cure has been confirmed on the basis of bacteriologic tests, the genital system often is still not functioning at a normal level. Experience shows time and again that a period of several weeks' or even several months' sexual rest is extremely important if conception is to occur. In severe cases, in fact, it is not unusual for an entire breeding season to pass before full breeding condition is regained.

A fertility examination should always be preceded by a thorough pregnancy examination. In doubtful cases a wait-and-see approach is recommended. In all examinations, the accurate documentation of findings will facilitate immediate prognostic evaluation and will provide a valuable reference during future examinations and analyses.

The mares can be assigned to the following 'fertility categories' based on the results of the examinations:

Fertility category	Findings	Chance of conception in %
I	Pregnant mares and maiden mares with no abnormal clinical or bacteriologic findings	70—100
II	Mares with no abnormal clinical or bacteriologic findings that have been barren for 1 year	50—70
III	Mares with no abnormal clinical or bacteriologic findings that have been barren for longer than 1 year, and recovered mares in category IV	25—50
IV	Mares with abnormal findings in the genital tract or other diseases or deficiencies that hamper fertility	0—25
V	Mares that show severe signs of genital tract disease or for other reasons have little if any chance of regaining their fertility	0

The findings of the various examinations should be discussed with the farm management, and necessary measures should be adopted. Given sufficient understanding and cooperation on the part of the farm management, a fertility surveillance program of this kind can do much to improve conception and birth rates in breeding operations.

2.1.12.5. Peculiar Breeding Habits in the Stallion

Not infrequently, stallions will display peculiar behavior toward mares that are presented to them. Some will refuse to breed mares that are in 'foal heat' or any mare that is accompanied by a foal. Others are reluctant to cover maiden mares. Sometimes it appears as if the odor of the mare plays some role in stimulating the stallion. It is known, however, that the *color* of the mare is an important factor. Many stallions prefer mares of a certain color, white and gray being the colors most preferred.

It is often reported that stallions are attracted more to outside mares than to home-owned mares to which they are continually exposed.

Sexual response varies greatly from one stallion to the next, usually without apparent reason. Most stallions will copulate rapidly. However, there are some stallions that require a prolonged period of 'foreplay' before they will cover a mare. Certain stallions have to cover the mare several times before ejaculating. Others are easily distracted from their cover by noise, movement, unfamiliar objects, etc. No generally valid rules can be applied to sexual response in the stallion.

Many young stallions require time to become accustomed to the breeding routine. In difficult cases the young stallion may benefit from witnessing older, experienced stallions engaged in copulation. It is important to be patient and avoid making snap judgments. Breeders also have frequent difficulties with imported stallions, for example, or stallions that are new arrivals on the farm. The problem in such cases is essentially one of acclimatization. Experience has shown that such problems are more common in certain breeds. For this reason it is unwise to delay scheduled transfers of breeding stock for too long.

Poor breeding habits in the stallion often prove difficult to correct. The line between physiologic and pathologic sexual behavior is difficult to draw, for training, temperament, stress and age play a major role. Often certain behavioral peculiarities must be tolerated if the stallion is to continue to do breeding service.

2.1.12.6. Incidents during Breeding

It is customary to restrain the mare for breeding by means of two ropes extending from the neck to the pasterns of the hind legs. These hobbles will prevent her from kicking the stallion during breeding. Sometimes the stallion receives deep injuries to the penile mucosa from sharp tail hairs of the mare (cf. Sec. 2.1.8.10.1.) or, less frequently, an angulation or 'rupture' of the penis occurs as a result of violent breeding. Conversely, the stallion may injure the mare severely during breeding by biting her on the crest or withers.

Superficial or deep injuries of the vagina, including perforations, can occur if there is a size disproportion between the partners, the stallion mounts obliquely, intromission of the penis is too vigorous, or there is excessive swelling of the glans. Stallions with excessive glans swelling should not breed very small mares or maiden mares. Affected mares strain heavily after copulation, show evidence of pain, and varying degrees of vaginal bleeding may be observed. If the injury is severe, cellulitis of the pelvic area with systemic signs may develop. These mares should be given immediate sexual rest and their condition promptly treated. In cases of total, extensive vaginal perforation, it is not uncommon for loops of intestine to prolapse through the vulva immediately following coitus.

Bone fractures and other limb injuries can occur if one of the animals loses its footing. The majority of these injuries can be prevented through sound, attentive breeding practices.

References

BLOBEL, K.; KLUG, E.: Tiefgefriersamen — Übertragung beim Pferd. Ein Versuch unter praktischen Gestütsbedingungen. Berliner Münchener Tierärztl. Wschr. *24:* 465 (1975).

FLÜGE, E.: Massnahmen zur Fruchtbarkeitsförderung in der Pferdezucht am Beispiel der Landespferdezucht. 4. Arbeitstagung der Fachgruppe Pferdekrankheiten der DGV, München 1975.

KLUG, E.; TOLKSDORF, E.; KOLM, H.: Zyklussteuerung im Puerperium der Stute mit Prostaglandinen analog. 4. Arbeitstagung der Fachgruppe Pferdekrankheiten der DGV, München 1975.

MERKT, H.: Maßnahmen zur Fruchtbarkeitsförderung in der Pferdezucht am Beispiel der Vollblutzucht. 4. Arbeitstagung der Fachgruppe Pferdekrankheiten der DGV, München 1975.

NISCHIKAWA, Y.: Studies in reproduction in horses. Tokyo 1959.

PARKER, W. G.; SULLIVAN, J. J.; FIRST, N. L.: Sperm transport and distribution in the mare. J. Reproduct. Fertility, suppl. 23, p. 63 (1975).

ROSSDALE, P. D.: Das Pferd — Fortpflanzung und Entwicklung (Karger, Basel 1975).

TILLMANN, H.: Paarungsinfektionen beim Pferd. 4. Arbeitstagung der Fachgruppe Pferdekrankheiten der DGV, München 1975.

VANDEPLASSCHE, M.: Die puerperale Metritis. 4. Arbeitstagung der Fachgruppe Pferdekrankheiten der DGV, München 1975.

2.1.13. Diseases of the Endocrine System

2.1.13.1. The Pituitary Gland

The pituitary gland, or hypophysis, consists of two parts which have different embryologic, morphologic and functional characteristics: the *adenohypophysis*, consisting of the pars tuberalis, pars intermedia (intermediate lobe) and pars distalis (anterior lobe), and the *neurohypophysis* (posterior lobe).

The *adenohypophysis* is composed of epithelial cells which differ in their staining properties and in which a number of hormones are synthesized. These hormones either act directly on the body (growth hormone, lipotropic hormone, prolactin, melanocyte-stimulating hormone) or regulate the development and function of other, peripheral endocrine glands (adrenocorticotropin, thyrotropin, gonadotropin) and thus exert an indirect effect on body functions. The secretion of all adenohypophyseal hormones is controlled by specific CNS hormones that are produced mainly in the hypothalamus. These hormones reach the pituitary gland via the humoral pathway, where they exert a stimulating (releasing hormones, RH) or inhibitory effect (inhibiting hormones, IH). Thus, a direct functional relationship exists between the central nervous system and the adenohypophysis. There is much evidence to indicate that an excessive or deficient secretion of RH and IH is a common primary cause of functional derangements of the adenohypophysis.

Hypofunction of the adenohypophysis (panhypopituitarism) is of no clinical importance in the horse. It is true that regressive processes occur in the adenohypophysis with advancing age [COHRS, 1970], but these are not reflected in definite clinical symptoms.

2.1.13.1.1. Tumors of the Adenohypophysis

Occurrence. Tumors of the adenohypophysis are not rare and are particularly common in older horses [Brandt, 1940; Seiferle, 1948; Tasker et al., 1966]. They must be differentiated from nodular hyperplasias, which also are fairly common. The tumors, usually benign, develop most frequently in the pars intermedia and rarely in the anterior lobe. Females are affected about twice as often as males.

Symptoms. Gribble [1972] observed the following clinical signs in 33 horses with an adenoma of the pars intermedia: muscle wasting, polydipsia, polyuria, hyperglycemia, glucosuria, hirsutism, delayed wound healing, and bilateral enlargement of the adrenal glands. A real or relative neutrophilia, lymphopenia and eosinopenia were also frequently observed. Alopecia, hyperhidrosis, blindness and locomotor disturbances were occasionally present. The clinical picture closely resembles that of Cushing's disease, suggesting that the adenomas mainly produce adrenocorticotropic hormone. Gribble [1972] also measured consistently elevated plasma levels of melanocyte-stimulating hormone, whose site of production is the pars intermedia.

The diagnosis and treatment of this disease are the same as for Cushing's syndrome and are discussed under that heading (see Sec. 2.1.13.4.3.). The prognosis for animals with hyperglycemia is poor. Horses without hyperglycemia may live for several years and do limited work when maintained on a nutritious diet and complications are controlled.

The *neurohypophysis* secretes two hormones: vasopressin, called also adiuretin or antidiuretic hormone, and oxytocin. These hormones are not produced in the neurohypophysis itself, but in the neurons of certain hypothalamic nuclei, whose axons pass via the supraoptic-neurohypophyseal tract to the neurohypophysis and terminate there. The hormones are conveyed to the neurohypophysis via these nerve fibers, stored there and released into the bloodstream as needed. The principal effect of oxytocin is on the female genital tract and the mammary gland, where contractility and milk ejection are stimulated. The main physiologic effect of vasopressin is on the kidneys. It limits water loss from the body by increasing as needed the reabsorption of water in the distal tubules, thereby inhibiting diuresis. Accordingly, the principal triggers for vasopressin release are a rise in the osmotic pressure of the blood and a fall in the blood volume. The vasopressor effect of the hormone, which is exerted on various but not all vascular regions, is evident only when relatively large doses are administered. It probably is of no importance in physiologic blood pressure regulation.

2.1.13.1.2. Diabetes insipidus

Definition. Diabetes insipidus is the term applied to a disease that is caused by a disturbance in the production or release of vasopressin and is characterized by an inability to concentrate the urine. It is rare in horses [Leemann, 1971]. The major causes of diabetes insipidus are neoplasms, inflammation, and degenerative and traumatic lesions of the hypothalamic-neurohypophyseal system. In man, moreover, there are hereditary forms based either on a congenital hypofunction of the hypothalamic-neurohypophyseal system or on a failure of renal response to vasopressin (nephrogenic diabetes insipidus). Clinical symptoms do not appear until more than 85 % of the neurons of the hypothalamic-neurohypophyseal system are lost, at which time disturbances in the regulation of diuresis become apparent. If lesions are confined to the neurohypophysis, some urine-concentrating ability will be preserved. It is likely in such cases that vasopressin enters the blood directly from the nerve fibers of the supraoptic-hypophyseal tract.

Symptoms. The cardinal symptoms of diabetes insipidus are polyuria and polydipsia. The onset may be sudden or gradual. Thirst is both excessive and compulsive. Affected animals drink up to 120 liters of water per day and will drink their own urine if water is unavailable. The urine is light-colored, contains no sugar or protein, has a low specific gravity (usually less than 1,005) and is passed in large amounts. Because the water losses cannot always be replenished right away, the mucous membranes are often dry, constipation develops, and sweat secretion is reduced. No signs of oxytocin loss are apparent, and mares with diabetes insipidus can foal normally.

Diagnosis. The diagnosis is based mainly on the history and urinanalysis. The low specific gravity and absence of sugar in the urine distinguish diabetes insipidus from diabetes mellitus, in which polyuria and polydipsia are also present. Further verification can be obtained by witholding water for 12 to 24 hours while making continual checks of urine specific gravity and, if possible, osmolarity. The resultant release of vasopressin will lead to a significant reduction in urine volume with a rise in specific gravity and osmolarity. In diabetes mellitus, these changes are absent or not as noticeable. Another method of confirming diabetes insipidus is to administer a single diagnostic injection of 10 I.U. vasopressin, and then watch for a fall of urine volume and a rise in specific gravity and osmolarity.

Treatment. Treatment consists in the daily i.m. injection of 5—10 I.U. synthetic vasopressin or a posterior pituitary extract, preferably distributed in 2 doses. For long-term treatment, long-acting preparations such as Pitressin tannate (active for 1—3 days) are recommended. The dosage should be individualized, taking into account the fact that full response is not immediate. In case of overdosage, signs of hyperhydration will appear. Water should be offered ad libitum.

Prognosis. The progress of the disease is irreversible, although affected animals can be restored to usefulness by replacement therapy.

2.1.13.2. The Thyroid Gland

The thyroid gland secretes two hormones: triiodothyronine (T_3) and tetraiodothyronine or thyroxine (T_4). They are synthesized as follows: Iodide ingested with the feed is extracted from the blood, oxidized in the thyroid to elemental iodine and incorporated into the amino acid tyrosine. The thyroid hormones then form through a condensation process and are stored in the colloid of the thyroid follicles. When released to the bloodstream, 99.95 % of T_4 and 99.85 % of T_3 are bound to proteins, leaving only a very small percentage in free, biologically active form. T_3 has a biologic half-life of 19 hours, and T_4 about 190 hours. The thyroid hormones are carried by the bloodstream to the cells of the body, where they stimulate carbohydrate metabolism, growth and maturation of the CNS, bones and muscles, heat production, oxygen consumption, cholesterol metabolism and cardiac work. T_3 is about 5 times more potent than T_4. Though the thyroid gland is not necessary for life, normal thyroid function is essential for normal somatic growth and development.

Thyroid secretion is regulated on the one hand by the iodine level of the blood, both a rise or fall causing an inhibition of thyroid function. The second major regulating factor is the thyroid-stimulating hormone (TSH) of the adenohypophysis. Its secretion is stimulated by the hypothalamic hormone TRH. A fall in the thyroid hormone level of the blood stimulates the secretion of TRH and thus of TSH, while an elevated level of T_3 and T_4 blocks the pituitary response to TRH, thereby inhibiting TSH secretion.

2.1.13.2.1. Hypothyroidism

Definition. Hypothyroidism refers to a hypofunction of the thyroid gland with a deficient secretion of triiodothyronine and thyroxine. This insufficiency may result from chromosomal abnormalities or may be acquired *in utero* or after birth. A distinction is made between primary hypothyroidism, whose cause lies in the thyroid gland, and the secondary form, in which thyroid function is impaired due to a deficient secretion of TSH. The term 'tertiary' hypothyroidism is applied if utilization of the thyroid hormones in the body periphery is impaired.

Etiology. Primary congenital hypothyroidism can occur sporadically or endemically and has its cause in developmental anomalies (hypo- or aplasia), genetically-based disturbances of enzymatic hormone synthesis, or exposure to exogenous insults during intrauterine growth (e.g., iodine deficiency or excess).

Primary postnatal hypothyroidism can result from inflammation or neoplastic disease, an iodine excess or deficiency, or the ingestion of 'goitrogenic' substances, which are especially common in plants of the cabbage and turnip families [Greer et al., 1964] and act at various sites to inhibit hormones biosynthesis. Hypothyroidism can also develop following removal of the thyroid glands.

In the absence of congenital hypoplasia of the thyroid gland, primary hypothyroidism will be associated with the development of a goiter. This occurs when the pituitary release of TSH is increased due to a reduced concentration of thyroid hormones in the blood. When the large amounts of TSH encounter reactive thyroid tissue, this tissue undergoes either a diffuse or nodular proliferation, the latter being most common in aged horses. Hypothyroid goiter in horses is most frequently observed in regions that are deficient of iodine (endemic goiter), in animals that ingest goitrogenic substances, and in coastal regions where there is an excessive amount of iodine in the environment. It is important to note that iodine becomes concentrated in the milk, and so foals may receive excessive iodine even if corresponding changes are absent in the dam.

Euthyroid or 'bland' goiter represents a compensated state in which there is a primary disturbance of hormone production. The associated increase in TSH secretion is however sufficient to keep T_3 and T_4 secretion within normal limits through the proliferation of hormone-forming thyroid tissue. In secondary hypothyroidism, which is very rare in horses, the secretion of TSH is significantly reduced due to a partial or complete failure of pituitary function. The cause may lie in the pituitary itself (inflammation, necrosis, space-occupying lesions) or in the central nervous system, involving a reduction in TRH release. This can occur, for example, during prolonged exposure to high temperatures, when TRH release is inhibited via a temperature center in the hypothalamus.

Symptoms. The symptoms of hypothyroidism are most striking when the deficiency coincides with periods of rapid growth, as in fetuses and foals. If the condition develops in utero, the foal is frequently stillborn or, if alive, is weak, may have contracted tendons and usually is unable to stand and nurse. Lowe et al. [1974] removed the thyroid gland from yearling foals and observed the following changes: absence of longitudinal growth, sensitivity to cold, a dull, scruffy haircoat and prolonged retention of winter coat, general lethargy, edema of the hind legs, low rectal temperature (especially in colts), and a reduced phosphorus level in the blood. Because ossification of the skeleton is delayed in these animals, they are prone to pathological fractures.

In older horses, the symptoms of hypothyroidism are often so vague that they go unrecognized. Frequently an enlarged thyroid gland is the only primary sign [Baker and Lindsay, 1968]. Further signs have also been reported: general lethargy; unthriftiness; bilateral, symmetric hair loss; myxedema, in which the skin is dry, cracked, spongy and thickened from mucoid deposits. In addition, there may be bradycardia due to tone loss, dilatation and in severe cases myxedematous infiltration of the myocardium; failure to express estrus; mild to moderate normochromic and normocytic anemia; and pneumonia and arthritis due to the lowered resistance to infection.

A diagnosis based on clinical findings alone is usually possible only if the goiter coexists with several of the above-mentioned symptoms; this is especially true in mature horses. The diagnosis can be confirmed by laboratory tests of thyroid function, the most important being the demonstration of a reduced T_4 or T_3 level in the plasma or serum utilizing the competitive protein-binding or radioimmunoassay technique. Kallfelz and Lowe [1970] report a normal T_4 level of $20.6 \pm 0.72\,\mu g/100$ ml, while Hightower et al. [1971] state a value of 2.57 ± 0.71. The reliability of the determination can be further enhanced by the subcutaneous injection of 15 I.U. TSH, which in healthy horses produces a 2- to 4-fold rise in the thyroxine level after 24 hours. This increase is smaller in primary hypothyroidism, and absent in secondary hypothyroidism.

Other laboratory tests involve determining the secretory rate of the thyroid hormones. Irvine [1967] measured a normal value of 1.078 mg T_4/100 kg BW/day, the level of protein-bound iodine (PBI), which ranges from 1.5—2 μg/100 ml serum [Kallfelz and Lowe, 1970], and T_3 uptake by the thyroid gland [Kallfelz and Lowe, 1970]. All these values are lowered in hypothyroidism. However, each of these investigations requires special laboratory facilities and is either less specific or involves more possible sources of error than the direct determination of hormone levels. A simpler method is to determine the serum cholesterol concentration [Kaneko and Cornelius, 1970], which is elevated in a hypothyroid metabolic state.

Differential Diagnosis. Whenever goiter is present, thyroid adenoma as well as hyperthyroidism should be considered. In foals, bone problems as well as marked systemic signs of varying etiology can produce a clinical picture similar to that of hypothyroidism. One must rely on the foregoing laboratory tests of thyroid function if goiter is absent.

Treatment. In hypothyroidism due to exogenous causes, treatment is aimed at eliminating the cause. For iodine deficiency in regions endemic for goiter, or for animals that have ingested goitrogenic substances with the feed, iodized salt may be given (1 part KI or NaI per 10,000 to 100,000 parts salt). It is better to use potassium iodate, however, owing to its greater stability. For more rapid treatment of individual animals, tincture of iodine or Lugol's solution can be applied to the skin in amounts of 2—4 ml at weekly intervals. In most cases these measures are effective in normalizing thyroid function.

If the seat of the disease is in the thyroid itself, replacement therapy is indicated. It is best to use modern combination products that contain both T_3 and T_4 and are supplemented, for example, with potassium iodide. They are active on oral dosing. The dosage must be individualized according to the severity of the condition, and this is most easily done by monitoring response and measuring the serum cholesterol. If a secondary hypothyroidism has been diagnosed from the administration of TSH, the same product may be used for replacement therapy.

Hypothyroidism contracted in adulthood has a favorable prognosis with proper treatment. In foals it is important that the disease be recognized early, before irreversible developmental defects have occurred.

2.1.13.2.2. Hyperthyroidism (Thyrotoxicosis, Basedow's Disease)

Definition. Hyperthyroidism or thyrotoxicosis denotes a condition of excessive thyroid gland activity associated with an increased secretion of T_3 and T_4.

Etiology. Even today the etiology of this disease is not fully understood. It is known that emotional disturbances (fear, fright) and stress situations are precipitating factors, but the true cause probably lies in an autoimmune response. In man, much pathogenetic importance is attached to long-acting thyroid stimulator (LATS), which has a more prolonged thyroid-stimulating action than TSH. LATS is an antibody that is formed in the mast cells and lymphocytes and directed against decomposition products of the thyroid gland [McKenzie, 1968]. It has also been suggested that the thyroid cells are directly stimulated by 'T lymphocytes' in the thyroid gland itself [Volpe et al., 1970], rather than by LATS, which has not yet been demonstrated in the horse.

The assumption of an immunologic etiology for hyperthyroidism is consistent with the fact that no elevation of TSH levels can be demonstrated. This level is, in fact, reduced, for the excessive secretion of thyroid hormones leads to an inhibition of TSH release. This is also the case with toxic adenoma, in which one or more adenomatous areas independent of pituitary control produce excessive thyroid hormone, while the remaining thyroid tissue is subject to pituitary influence and is insufficient owing to the deficiency of TSH.

Symptoms. Hyperthyroidism is frequently but not always manifested by an enlargement of the thyroid gland that is either diffuse (Basedow's goiter) or nodular (nodular goiter; fig. 2.1.13. — 1). Additional signs are tachycardia and arrhythmias, emaciation despite a good or increased appetite, restlessless, and excitement with sweating at the least provocation. In Standardbreds and Thoroughbreds, the slightest stimulus is sufficient to provoke tachycardia, arrhythmias and nervousness, often in the absence of visible thyroid enlargement, thus enabling subclinical cases to be diagnosed [Dietz, 1981]. In addition, disturbances of the creatine metabolism can lead to a myopathy whose clinical signs are muscular weakness and rapid fatigability. Exophthalmos is rarely observed in horses.

Diagnosis. If symptoms are severe, a diagnosis can be made on the basis of clinical signs. However, the subclinical forms are more frequent and require the additional use of laboratory methods discussed under Hypothyroidism. Of greatest value is the determination of an elevated serum level of T_4 or T_3. In human medicine a radiolabeled indicator (^{131}I) is injected and its uptake in the thyroid gland is measured, thereby demonstrating the presence of hyperactive regions in the gland (thyroid scintigraphy). If clinical signs point to hyperthyroidism, however, the demonstration of a reduced serum cholesterol level is often sufficient to establish the diagnosis.

Differential Diagnosis. The aforementioned methods for the study of thyroid function are used to exclude autonomic nervous system disturbances, encephalitis and non-thyroid diseases that cause emaciation through increased metabolic demands (tumors, sustained fever).

Treatment. The treatment of hyperthyroidism is aimed at inhibiting hormone synthesis in the thyroid gland. The substances known as 'thyrostatics' belong to a variety of chemical classes. Good results have been obtained with iodine or iodine

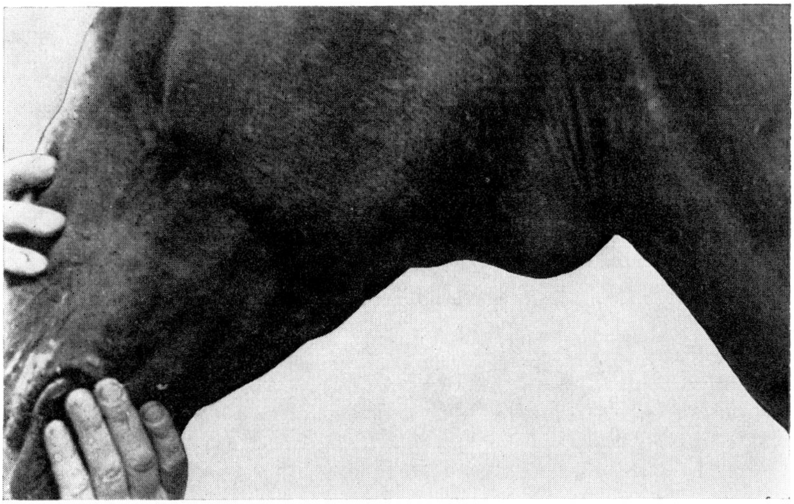

Fig. 2.1.13. — 1. Goiter.

salts (Plummer effect), radioiodine as well as thiocyanate and perchlorate, which block iodine uptake by the thyroid. Drugs of the thiouracil class (thiouracil, methylthiouracil, methimazole, etc.) interfere with the incorporation of iodine into tyrosine, thereby inhibiting hormone synthesis. Iodine salts are administered with the feed in the form of Lugol's solution or Plummer's solution; this can be augmented by applying iodine to the shaved skin over the thyroid gland or goiter at weekly intervals. According to Dietz [1981], it has proved beneficial, especially in younger horses, to administer by i.v. injection 15—20 ml of an iodine stock solution prepared by the method of Götze (pure iodine 1.0, potassium iodate 15.0, sodium iodate 15.0, distilled water to 100.0) diluted with 100 ml of distilled water, this being done on the 1st, 7th and 14th days of treatment. If nervousness is severe, sedation can be obtained with bromides, barbiturates or phenothiazine derivatives. It is important that the medical treatment of hyperthyroidism be continued only until clinical symptoms regress or the goiter disappears; otherwise hypothyroidism, iodine cachexia or iodism is a danger. Hyperthyroidism, which is rarely fatal if untreated, typically takes an intermittent course, i.e., it may revert to euthyroidism at any time, only to recur. In other cases a hyperthyroid metabolic state may persist for years without remission. Spontaneous long-term recoveries are rarely seen.

2.1.13.3. The Parathyroid Gland

In the horse the parathyroid gland is comprised of four separate bodies located in close proximity to the thyroid. The parathyroid secretes parathormone, a peptide hormone which acts with thyrocalcitonin, a hormone produced by specialized cells in the thyroid (C cells), and vitamin D to regulate the calcium and phosphate balance. In the presence of vitamin D, parathormone promotes the absorption of calcium and phosphates from the intestine. It also effects the release of calcium and phosphates from bone through the activation of osteoclasts and inhibition of osteoblasts. In addition, parathormone exerts a calcium-retaining and a phosphaturic action on the renal tubules. The net effect, therefore, is an elevation of the serum calcium level and a reduction of bone calcium. The phosphate level in the blood is increased temporarily, but then falls below normal. Thyrocalcitonin serves as the antagonist of parathormone, lowering the calcium level of the blood by inhibiting bone resorption.

The release of parathormone is increased when the calcium level of the blood falls below the normal range. High calcium levels inhibit parathormone release while increasing the secretion of thyrocalcitonin.

Primary disease of the parathyroid gland with either an excess or deficit of parathormone has not been described in the horse. Hyperparathyroidism secondary to renal disease is also uncommon in this species [Gribble, 1972].

Nutritional Secondary Hyperparathyroidism

Secondary hyperfunction of the parathyroid gland can result from a dietary excess of phosphorus relative to calcium, which is especially common in horses fed very high-grain rations without adequate calcium supplementation [Krook and Lowe, 1964; Joyce et al., 1971]. Krook [1968] states that the optimum calcium : phosphorus ratio for the horse is 1.2 : 1.

Etiology. The etiology of nutritional secondary hyperparathyroidism is not fully understood. It is assumed that a dietary phosphate excess inhibits calcium absorption from the intestine, and that a high phosphate level in the serum reduces calcium resorption from bone. Both effects reduce plasma calcium levels, which in turn stimulates secretion by the parathyroid. While the increased parathormone secretion is capable of maintaining blood calcium levels at near normal, this occurs at the expense of bone demineralization, which is associated with a proliferation of fibrous connective tissue, i.e., fibrous osteodystrophy (similar to Recklinghausen's disease of bone in man).

Symptoms. Secondary hyperparathyroidism is manifested clinically by lameness, enlargements of the maxilla and mandible, loosening of the teeth, spontaneous fractures and generalized bony atrophy. In severe cases the cortical bone is thinned.

Plasma calcium levels are normal or in the low-normal range (10—14 mg/100 ml), while plasma phosphate levels may be high normal (normal: 2.5—5.5 mg/100 ml). The calcium level in the urine is low (normal: $>$ 20 mg/100 ml), and the urinary phosphate is greatly elevated (normal: 4—18 mg/100 ml). The alkaline phosphatase activity in the blood is increased. According to Joyce et al. [1971], the *urinary* calcium and phosphate levels are more useful diagnostically than the plasma levels. Today it is possible to determine parathormone directly in the blood by radioimmunoassay and thus detect elevated levels.

Differential Diagnosis must be made from osteoporosis, in which the cortical bone is always well preserved; osteomalacia with a reduced blood phosphate level; hyperthyroidism, which is associated with hypercalciuria as well as other characteristic symptoms (see Sec. 2.1.13.2.2.); and hypervitaminosis D, which is frequently accompanied by hypercalcemia. The latter should be suspected if vitamin D has previously been administered.

Treatment. Treatment of nutritional secondary hyperparathyroidism consists of correcting the calcium : phosphorus imbalance by changing the diet (feeding clover or alfalfa) and supplementing with calcium, making sure that the phosphorus intake is not simultaneously increased.

Prognosis. The prognosis is favorable, in that recalcification of the bone can be achieved by ensuring an adequate calcium intake, though this process may require several months.

2.1.13.4. The Adrenal Cortex

The adrenal cortex is comprised of three zones in which various hormones (corticoids) are produced. The outer zona glomerulosa is the site of aldosterone formation, a mineralocorticoid of vital importance for maintaining the sodium, potassium and water balance. Its main action is on the kidneys, but it also acts on the mucous membrane of the colon and on the salivary and sweat glands. It promotes the retention of sodium ions and water while increasing the release of potassium. Aldosterone secretion is little affected by the adrenocorticotropic hormone of the pituitary; the major mechanisms for its regulation operate through the renin-angiotensin system of the kidney.

The two inner zones of the adrenal cortex are the zona fasciculata and the innermost zona reticularis, which lies adjacent to the adrenal medulla. Two further hormone groups are synthesized in these zones: the glucocorticoids (most notably cortisol and corticosterone) and the adrenal sex hormones (progesterone, estrogens and androgens).

The principal effect of the glucocorticoids is on the intermediary metabolism, where they exert primarily a catabolic effect. Through their gluconeogenic effect, i.e., the formation of carbohydrates in the liver by the mobilization and breakdown of protein and triglycerides, the glucocorticoids create an ergotropic metabolic situation in which rapidly-utilizable energy sources (glucose, free fatty acids) are made available while anabolism is inhibited. In addition, the glucocorticoids exert a 'permissive action' with regard to the metabolic and vascular effects of growth hormone, glucagon, epinephrine and norepinephrine. They also play a part in regulating the water balance by increasing glomerular filtration in the kidneys. In the blood they cause a decrease in the number of circulating eosinophils and lymphocytes while producing a real or relative increase in neutrophilic granulocytes.

Glucocorticoids are also an essential factor in the body's ability to resist stresses of many kinds. Adrenalectomized animals die from peripheral circulatory collapse when exposed even to minor stresses, and they can be saved only by the rapid administration of glucocorticoids.

Besides these physiologic effects, the glucocorticoids also exert pharmacologic actions that, today, are widely utilized therapeutically. Specifically, the glucocorticoids have an anti-inflammatory and antiallergic property which inhibits proliferative and exudative inflammatory processes and tissue antibody formation. At the same time, however, these substances retard healing processes and lower defenses to infection. Antibiotics and sulfonamides may have to be administered to counter these effects. Due to their gluconeogenic effect, the administration of high glucocorticoid doses over prolonged periods can lead to steroid diabetes, but this passes quickly when treatment is discontinued. See Dietz [1981] for further details on the potential benefits and risks of the local and systemic use of glucocorticoids in equine medicine.

The sex hormones of the adrenal cortex are probably of minor importance in the horse under normal circumstances. In mares, androgens may become important in terms of their protein-anabolic action, and they may have causal significance in nymphomania. In addition, the adrenal sex hormones supply precursors for hormone synthesis in the gonads of both sexes.

The secretion of glucocorticoids and adrenal sex hormones is stimulated by adrenocorticotropic hormone (ACTH), whose release is effected by an unidentified hormone from the hypothalamus (CRF). The physiologic inhibitor of ACTH secretion is cortisol, which halts the release of CRF when the plasma concentration of ACTH is elevated, and disinhibits CRF release when plasma levels are low. When glucocorticoids are used therapeutically, it must be understood that the long-term administration of high doses can inhibit ACTH secretion to such a degree that adrenal atrophy develops. To prevent adrenal insufficiency, the withdrawal of glucocorticoid therapy should be preceded by a gradual reduction of dosage. This is the best means of reestablishing endogenous ACTH production and restoring a normal adrenocortical response to ACTH.

2.1.13.4.1. Adrenocortical Hypofunction

Acute Adrenocortical Insufficiency

Every stress (infection, overexertion, surgery, etc.) increases the body's demand for glucocorticoids. If the function of the hypothalamic-pituitary-adrenocortical system is already marginal, the adrenal cortex will lack the functional reserves necessary to withstand the stress. Acute failure of the adrenal cortex can also be precipitated by a hemorrhagic infarction of the gland, especially when combined with septicemia. The associated clinical signs are a precipitous fall of blood pressure, cyanosis, muscle weakness, subnormal temperature, colicky episodes, and finally prostration and coma. The sodium-potassium ratio in the blood is reduced below the normal value of 40, and, in contrast to other forms of shock, the eosinophils in the blood tend to be increased rather than reduced.

Treatment must not be delayed and so must be based entirely upon clinical findings. It consists in the i.v. administration of 500—1,000 mg cortisol hemisuccinate or prednisolone hemisuccinate, the infusion of glucose solution, and the injection of norepinephrine; antibiotics are also given if septicemia is present. During subsequent days the cortisol or prednisolone should be maintained orally or intramuscularly in decreasing doses, even if acute symptoms regress.

Primary Chronic Adrenocortical Insufficiency (Addison's Disease)

Definition. Addison's disease is due to hypofunction of the adrenal cortex. Symptoms appear when approximately nine-tenths of the adrenal cortex is unresponsive.

Etiology. The disease, which is not uncommon in horses [Solomon, 1963; O'Connor, 1968], can be caused by chronic inflammatory processes, ischemia or amyloidosis of the adrenal glands, and possibly by disuse atrophy secondary to prolonged treatment with glucocorticoids. In man, circulating, organ-specific antibodies toward microsomes and mitochondria of the adrenocortical cells are found in more than 50 % of patients with primary adrenal atrophy. The disease probably has an autoimmune basis, therefore. Corresponding studies have not yet been conducted in horses.

Symptoms. The onset of the disease is usually gradual, although sudden outbreaks have been observed in connection with stressful situations. The symptoms in horses are reportedly similar to those in man [Solomon, 1963; O'Connor, 1968]: fatigue, anorexia, weight loss, alternating bouts of diarrhea and constipation, hypotension and hypoglycemia. The characteristic hyperpigmentation of the skin due to an increased secretion of melanocyte-stimulating hormone is not demonstrable in the horse. Thus, the clinical signs are relatively nonspecific, and the diagnosis should be confirmed by laboratory tests.

The cortisol level in the blood, which may be determined by competitive protein binding or radioimmunoassay, is low or low-normal and in itself is not diagnostic. A more definitive test is the response to ACTH. In normal horses the plasma cortisol and corticosterone levels (normally about 0.5 μg/100 ml) will increase 2- to 3-fold 2 and 8 hours, respectively, following the i.v. or i.m. injection of 1 I.U. ACTH/kg BW [Hoffsis and Murdick, 1970; James et al., 1970]. The absence of this increase is a sure sign of primary adrenocortical insufficiency. Additional laboratory findings are a relative lymphocytosis and increase in eosinophils, a reduction of the sodium-potassium ratio below 40, and an increased excretion of sodium. If the i.m. injection of an ACTH depot is not followed within 8—10 hours by a significant decrease of eosinophils in the blood, it may again be inferred that the function of the adrenal cortex is deficient (Thorn test).

Treatment. The treatment of Addison's disease consists of an individualized regimen of adrenocortical hormone replacement. If no serious disturbances of the mineral balance are observed, the daily administration of 60—150 mg cortisone acetate orally is sufficient; it is best to divide the dose between morning and afternoon. In place of cortisone acetate, dexamethasone may also be given in a daily dose of 2—5 mg. A mineralocorticoid deficiency is corrected by replacement with desoxycorticosterone acetate (DOCA) or fluorocortisol. Again, the dosage should be individualized. Overdosing leads to edema, while underdosing results in continued weight loss and hypotension. In many cases salt supplementation of the feed is sufficient to normalize the mineral balance. If the adrenocortical insufficiency is attributable to long-term glucocorticoid therapy, treatment is by the daily injection of 50—100 I.U. depot ACTH.

Untreated, Addison's disease is usually fatal. With appropriate replacement therapy, on the other hand, it is possible to maintain the animals at full working capacity.

2.1.13.4.2. Adrenocortical Hyperfunction (Cushing's Syndrome)

Definition. Cushing's syndrome is a condition resulting from an excess of endogenous cortisol or the excessive administration of exogenous glucocorticoids. It has been described with some frequency in the horse [Kral, 1951; Raker and Fegley, 1965; Loeb et al., 1966; Evans et al., 1968; Gribble, 1972].

Etiology. The elevated glucocorticoid level can have various causes: adrenocortical adenomas and carcinomas (primary hyperfunction), adrenocortical hyperplasia due to excessive ACTH secretion by the pituitary or ACTH-producing tumors, or the administration of high doses of ACTH (secondary hyperfunction) or glucocorticoids.

Tumors of the adrenal cortex are usually unilateral and secrete large amounts of glucocorticoid, independent of ACTH stimulation, which in turn inhibit the production of ACTH. The result is atrophy of the contralateral, unaffected adrenal gland.

Adenomas are the most common source of excessive pituitary ACTH. Most of these neoplasms develop in the pars intermedia, especially in older horses, and are composed of multiple nodules. Recent evidence suggests that these are probably not autonomous tumors subject to the laws of tumor growth, but are, rather, due to hyperplastic changes. In man, it has been shown that these tumors are particularly frequent after total adrenalectomies. This occurs at a time when there is no inhibition of hypothalamic CRF release by cortisol and there is a constant hypersecretion of ACTH. Moreover, clinical studies have shown that in patients with adrenocortical hyperplasia due to endogenous causes, the responsiveness of the hypothalamic-pituitary system to the ACTH-inhibiting effect of cortisol is markedly reduced.

Thus, whether a pituitary adenoma is absent or present, it appears that the primary cause of adrenocortical hyperplasia lies in a derangement of central nervous regulation.

In man, the bronchial carcinoma and its metastases represent the main source of ectopic ACTH production, though carcinomas of the thymus, pancreas and other organs can also produce ACTH. In all forms of secondary hypofunction, including iatrogenic Cushing's syndrome through excessive administration of ACTH, both adrenal glands are hyperplastic. By contrast, high glucocorticoid doses lead to adrenal atrophy by inhibiting endogenous ACTH secretion.

Symptoms. According to Gribble [1972], the major symptoms of Cushing's syndrome in the horse are weight loss with muscle wasting producing a swayed back and pendulous abdomen, a long, unkemp haircoat that is not shed in the spring, proneness to infectious diseases, and impaired wound healing. These are often accompanied by polyuria and consequent polydipsia, especially in the presence of pituitary neoplasms.

Cushing's syndrome can generally be diagnosed from the history and clinical signs. The diagnosis is confirmed by laboratory studies. These show a hyperglycemia with very high glucose levels (150—200 mg/100 ml) that are not significantly influenced by insulin. In addition there is glucosuria, ketonuria (if weight loss is rapid), lymphopenia, a marked eosinopenia, and a relative or absolute neutrophilia. Plasma cortisol levels may be normal or elevated, but the normal diurnal rhythm of cortisol secretion, characterized by a rise in the morning and a fall at night [James et al., 1970], is absent. Studies in adrenalectomized human patients have shown that Cushing's syndrome can be induced simply by maintaining the normal, high morning glucocorticoid levels throughout the night. When blood is drawn for laboratory tests, which should be done both morning and evening, care should be taken to avoid exciting the animal, for this can cause a transient rise in the cortisol level.

Further confirmation of the diagnosis can be obtained by the dexamethasone inhibition test. It is based on the principle that in low doses, the synthetic glucocorticoid dexamethasone strongly inhibits ACTH secretion in normal animals without significantly influencing levels of cortisol and corticosterone assayed in the blood or urine. The dexamethasone is injected i.m. in a dose of 40 μg/kg BW, and the plasma levels of cortisol or cortisol + corticosterone are determined before and 12 hours after the injection. In the normal horse these will fall to about $^1/_3$ the initial value [Hoffsis and Murdick, 1970; James et al., 1970; Gribble, 1972]. Little or no decrease will be observed in horses with Cushing's syndrome.

Differential Diagnosis. Malnutrition, masticatory difficulties or parasitisms can produce outward signs that resemble Cushing's syndrome. However, the long summer haircoat, polydipsia, and the obvious hematologic changes are indicative of adrenocortical hypofunction. Diabetes mellitus on the basis of hypoinsulinism, in which hyperglycemia, polyuria, polydipsia and emaciation are observed, can be excluded by administering insulin. In Cushing's syndrome this will produce no significant fall in the blood glucose level.

Treatment. The only sure treatment of Cushing's syndrome due to noniatrogenic causes is unilateral adrenalectomy in the case of an adrenocortical tumor, and total adrenalectomy or hypophysectomy in the case of bilateral adrenocortical hyperplasia. These operations are scarcely practical in the horse, however, and they usually require replacement therapy for life. In man, good results have been achieved with x-irradiation of the pituitary and with the intrapituitary implantation of ^{90}yttrium or ^{198}gold, either alone or in conjunction with ^{192}iridium. Use has also been made of 'adrenostatics' such as amphenone B, metyrapone, op'-DDD, which was developed from the insecticide DDT, and aminogluthetamide, all of which inhibit adrenal steroid production by various means. However, all these drugs have toxic side-effects and have not yet been used in the horse.

Prognosis. The prognosis of Cushing's syndrome is unfavorable, especially in animals with hyperglycemia. Horses without hyperglycemia may live for several years if maintained on a nutritious diet and complications are controlled.

2.1.13.5. The Adrenal Medulla

The adrenal medulla produces two hormones: epinephrine and norepinephrine. These catecholamines are synthesized in the chromaffin cells from the amino acid tyrosine. The ratio of epinephrine to norepinephrine in the horse is approximately 4 : 1. A constant stream of impulses is transmitted from the centers of the midbrain and from the medulla oblongata via splanchnic nerve fibers to the adrenal medulla, maintaining a continuous, low-level hormone secretion of about 20 ng/kg/min. However, a great variety of psychic, physical and metabolic stimuli can precipitate a sharp, sudden rise in catecholamine secretion. Epinephrine and norepinephrine are highly labile substances that disappear rapidly from the blood and are excreted in the urine mainly as metanephrine, normetanephrine and vanillylmandelic acid. The actions of epinephrine and norepinephrine are similar to those of adrenergic nervous system stimulation: increased heart rate and and blood pressure, reduced gastrointestinal motility, bronchodilation, increased sweat secretion, increased glycogenolysis and lipolysis, and an increase in the basal metabolic rate and oxygen consumption. Epinephrine is considerably more potent in its metabolic effects than norepinephrine.

The loss of adrenal medullary function produces no immediate clinical signs. This is due on the one hand to continued adrenergic nervous activity, and on the other to the fact that a portion of the medullary hormone production is probably assumed by paraganglia and groups of chromaffin cells located elsewhere in the body.

Adrenal Medullary Hyperfunction (Pheochromocytoma)

Definition. Pheochromocytomas are functioning, usually benign tumors of the adrenal medulla. They may reach the size of a hen's egg and are usually unilateral. According to Gribble [1972], they are uncommon but by no means rare in the horse. They are composed chiefly of chromaffin cells and may also develop in paraganglia. Most pheochromocytomas secrete large amounts of catecholamines, usually at a rate between 300 and 5,000 g/day in man.

Symptoms. The symptoms are referable to a catecholamine excess and may be paroxysmal or sustained [Evans et al., 1971]. The main symptoms are hypertension, tachycardia and sweating. During paroxysmal attacks, these may be accompanied by unrest, mydriasis, hyperthermia, profuse sweating and tremor. Severe cases may culminate in circulatory failure with pulmonary edema, progressive cyanosis and collapse. Attacks often end with profuse urination.

Diagnosis. The diagnosis can sometimes be made from clinical symptoms alone, but additional laboratory tests are usually required. If the disease is taking an intermittent course, these tests are useful only during periods when the tumor is active and clinical signs are present. Hyperglycemia, reduced glucose tolerance, glucosuria and neutrophilia are characteristic. Today it is possible to assay the catecholamines or their breakdown products in the urine. The values will be elevated relative to normal animals, which should be included in the study for comparison. A predominance of epinephrine production signifies a tumor of the adrenal medulla, while excess norepinephrine secretion is frequently associated with extraadrenal neoplasms.

Drug tests are useful for differentiating pheochromocytoma from other diseases with similar symptom complexes (diabetes mellitus, thyrotoxicosis, Cushing's syndrome, intoxication with lead or sympathomimetic agents). Phentolamine blocks the α-adrenergic receptors, making them inaccessible to circulating catecholamines, and thus causes a rapid fall in blood pressure and a regression of clinical symptoms. So far the phentolamine test has been used only in human patients. The dose must be selected with care, for overdosing can lead to hypotension and shock.

Treatment. Treating a pheochromocytoma by surgical excision is extremely difficult in the horse due to the problem of separating the adrenal glands from the caudal vena cava. Moreover, it is possible that the tumor may not be located in the adrenals at all. The best treatment in severe cases, therefore, is to administer α-blocking drugs (phenoxybenzamine) or drugs that block catecholamine synthesis (α-methyl-para-tyrosine). Animals with mild symptoms may live for years without treatment if strenuous work is avoided and complications are controlled.

2.1.13.6. The Endocrine Pancreas

The hormones insulin and glucagon are secreted by the islets of Langerhans in the pancreas. Gastrin is also produced in the pancreas, but its physiologic importance remains unknown. Glucagon and insulin are polypeptide hormones that are formed in the A and B cells, respectively, of the islets. The ratio of A to B cells in the horse is approximately 1 : 1.2. A glucagon-like substance (enteroglucagon) is also produced by cells of the gastrointestinal mucosa. Radioimmunoassay demonstrates an insulin level of 10—20 μU/ml in the peripheral blood of fasted horses [Argenzio and Hintz, 1971]. The glucagon level in agricultural work horses is 50—250 pg/ml [Fischer and Hommel, 1980].

Insulin is the only hormone in the body that lowers the blood glucose level while promoting energy storage in the form of carbohydrates, protein and fat. Insulin accomplishes these anabolic effects mainly by accelerating the transport of sugars and other substances into the tissues, with a subsequent increase in glycogen, fat and protein synthesis. A number of hormones act as antagonists to insulin by inhibiting the cellular uptake or intracellular utilization of glucose. These include glucagon, the glucocorticoids, growth hormone, epinephrine and the thyroid hormones, all of which have some degree of diabetogenic action when present in excess or when insulin secretion is impaired.

Insulin release is stimulated by a variety of substances (monosaccharides, amino acids, fatty acids and ketone bodies, gastrointestinal hormones, adrenocorticotropic hormone, growth hormone, cholinergics). The monosaccharides that are most effective in other species are weak stimulators of insulin secretion in the horse [Kuzuya et al., 1971]. In the glucose tolerance test, a period of 1.5 to 3.5 hours elapses between glucose loading and the return to the baseline blood glucose level [Mehring and Tyznik, 1970]. On the other hand, the short-chain fatty acids have practically no stimulative effect in the horse [Argenzio and Hintz, 1971].

The most effective stimulus for glucagon release is a fall in the blood glucose level. For this reason glucagon is also called the 'hunger hormone'. Additional stimuli are a fall in the fatty acid level and a rise in the free amino acid content of the blood.

As in man, disturbances of glucagon secretion are probably of only minor importance in the horse. Hyperinsulinism, i.e. excessive insulin production by a pancreatic tumor, has been described in dogs but apparently does not occur in horses.

Diabetes mellitus

Etiology. Diabetes mellitus is invariably based upon an absolute or relative deficiency of insulin. Hyperglycemia and glucosuria are the characteristic features of the disease. The cause may involve a disturbance of B-cell insulin biosynthesis, insulin secretion, protein binding of the hormone in the blood, the responsiveness of the target cells, or the breakdown of the hormone. Disturbances at the first two sites may be associated with morphologic changes in the pancreas (pancreatitis; JEFFREY [1968]) or an autoimmune response. In the remaining disturbances, chronic excessive demands are placed on the B cells. High blood levels of insulin antagonists can have a similar effect, and most reports of diabetes mellitus in horses have associated the condition with Cushing's syndrome [KING et al., 1962; LOEB et al., 1966; TASKER et al., 1966]. However, lesions of the B cells themselves, with a consequent inability to meet the increased insulin demand, is assumed to be present even in the secondary insufficiencies [FROESCH, 1971]. As yet there is no firm evidence of an inherited disposition to diabetes mellitus in the horse.

Symptoms. The most common symptoms of diabetes mellitus are polydipsia and polyuria, rapid fatigability, emaciation (which may lead to cachexia despite a voracious appetite), proneness to infection, rapid pulse and dyspnea. Abnormalities of the haircoat, cataracts, pain in the joints and feet, gangrene of the foot due to vascular sclerosis, and delayed wound healing may also be observed.

Diagnosis. Permanent hyperglycemia is always present in diabetes mellitus. The blood glucose level may far exceed the normal value in the fasted horse, which according to KANEKO and CORNELIUS [1970] ranges from 75 to 115 mg/100 ml. The blood glucose falls precipitously in response to insulin administration if a primary insufficiency of the islet system is involved. The plasma insulin level as determined by radioimmunoassay is also lowered in such cases. On the other hand, the glucose tolerance time in the fasted horse is always prolonged. Ketoacidosis is present in severe cases.

Ordinarily a diagnosis can be made simply by demonstrating glucose in the urine by means of reagent strips or Benedict's solution. Quantitative glucose determinations indicate a urinary excretion of up to 8 g/100 ml. This glucose increases the specific gravity of the urine to 1,040—1,060.

Differential Diagnosis. It is necessary to differentiate between diabetes due to disease of the pancreas itself, and extrainsulary forms of diabetes in which hyperglycemia and glucosuria result from the antagonizing effect of diabetogenic hormones. Most important in this regard is Cushing's syndrome due to endogenous causes or to the prolonged administration of high glucocorticoid doses, producing clinical symptoms similar to hypoinsulinism. The diagnosis of Cushing's syndrome is confirmed by the demonstration of eosinopenia and lymphopenia, a negative dexamethasone inhibition test, and by the presence of elevated or uniform glucocorticoid levels and a normal or relatively increased plasma insulin level. Also, the administration of insulin in this disease causes no significant reduction of hyperglycemia and glucosuria. In pheochromocytoma, which is also characterized by glucosuria, the paroxysmal or sustained hypertension and signs of unrest with tachycardia serve to distinguish this condition from pancreatic diabetes. Polyuria is also present in diabetes insipidus, but glucosuria is absent, and the urinary specific gravity is well below the normal value of 1,020—1,050.

Treatment. The administration of insulin forms the basis of treatment. A low-carbohydrate diet like that prescribed for human diabetics is difficult to achieve in the horse. In addition, the diabetic animal is already in a state of permanent starvation due to impaired glucose utilization, and this would contraindicate any significant degree of feed rationing.

Treatment is started with low insulin doses to avoid precipitating hypoglycemic shock. The recommended initial dose is 0.1—0.3 units/kg/day, and this can be gradually increased in accordance with the results of insulin tolerance tests. Hypoglycemic shock is characterized by muscle tremors, sweating, rapid pulse and respiration, hyperirritability, nystagmus, collapse, spasms and finally loss of consciousness. During this time the plasma glucose level falls below 20 mg/100 ml. Emergency treatment consists in the i.v. infusion of large amounts of glucose.

For long-term therapy, it is best to use depot insulin preparations that contain protamine and/or zinc and have a prolonged duration of action so that 1 or 2 injections per day will suffice. If 2 daily injections are given, it is customary to give 3/5 of the dose in the morning and 2/5 in the evening. The chosen regimen should be strictly adhered to, although it is usually possible to reduce the dose after a prolonged period of treatment. Ketoacidosis is controlled by the additional administration of sodium bicarbonate, fluids and electrolytes. Response is monitored by checking urinary glucose excretion with reagent strips; initially this should be done 2 or 3 times daily.

Prognosis. Diabetes mellitus generally carries an unfavorable prognosis. Death can result from diabetic coma due to severe ketoacidosis as well as from renal, cardiac or circulatory failure. Infections also pose a serious risk to the diabetic horse.

References

Argenzio, R. A.; Hintz, H. F.: Volatile fatty acid tolerance and effect of glucose and VFA on plasma insulin levels in ponies. J. Nutrition *101:* 723 (1971).

Baker, H. J.; Lindsey, J. R.: Equine goiter due to excess dietary iodide. J. Amer. vet. med. Assoc. *153:* 1618 (1968).

Bolz, W.; Dietz, O.: Lehrbuch der Allgemeinen Chirurgie für Tierärzte, 4. Aufl. (VEB Gustav Fischer Verlag, Jena 1970).

Brandt, A. J.: Über Hypophysenadenome bei Hund und Pferd. Skand. Vet. Tidskrift *30:* 875 (1940).

Cohrs, P.: Lehrbuch der speziellen pathologischen Anatomie der Haustiere, Teil II, 5. Aufl. (VEB Gustav Fischer Verlag, Jena 1970).

Dietz, O.: Anwendung von Hormonen in der Chirurgie und Inneren Veterinärmedizin. In: Döcke, F.: Veterinärmedizinische Endokrinologie, 2. Aufl. (VEB Gustav Fischer Verlag, Jena 1981).

Evans, L. H.; Hubben, K.; Siegel, E. T.: Adrenal cortical adenoma in a horse. J. Amer. vet. med. Assoc. *152:* 1778 (1968).

Evans, L. H.; Stewart, J.; Dodd, D. C.: Pheochromocytoma in a mare. J. Amer. vet. med. Assoc. *159:* 209 (1971).

Fischer, U.; Hommel, H.: Pankreas. In: Döcke, F.: Veterinärmedizinische Endokrinologie, 2. Aufl. (VEB Gustav Fischer Verlag, Jena 1981).

Froesch, E. R.: Pathogenese und Ätiologie des Diabetes mellitus. In: A. Labhart: Klinik der inneren Sekretion, 2. Aufl., p. 786 (Springer, Berlin 1971).

Greer, M. A.; Kendall, J. W.; Smith, M.: Antithyroid compounds. In: R. Pitt-Rivers; W. R. Trotter: The thyroid gland, vol. 1., p. 357 (Butterworths, London 1964).

Gribble, D. H.: The endocrine system. In: E. J. Catcott; Smithcors, J. F.: Equine medicine and surgery, 2nd ed., p. 433 (Amer. Vet. Public., Wheaton/Ill. 1972).

Hightower, D.; Miller, L.; Kyzar, J. R.: Comparison of serum and plasma thyroxine determinations in horses. J. Amer. vet. med. Assoc. *159:* 449 (1971).

Hoffsis, G. F.; Murdick, P. W.: The plasma concentrations of corticosteroids in normal and diseased horses. J. Amer. vet. med. Assoc. *157:* 1590 (1970).

IRVINE, C. H. G.: Thyroxine secretion rate in the horse in various physiological states. J. Endocrinology *39:* 313 (1967).
JAMES, V. H. T.; HORNER, M. W.; MOSS, M. S.; RIPPON, A. E.: Adrenocortical function in the horse. J. Endocrinology *48:* 319 (1970).
JEFFREY, J. R.: Diabetes mellitus secondary to chronic pancreatitis in a pony. J. Amer. vet. med. Assoc. *153:* 1168 (1968).
JOYCE, J. R.; PIERCE, K. R.; ROMANE, W. P.; BAKER, J. M.: Clinical study of nutritional secondary hyperparathyroidism in horses. J. Amer. vet. med. Assoc. *158:* 2033 (1971).
KALLFELZ, F. A.; LOWE, J. E.: Some normal values of thyroid function in horses. J. Amer. vet. med. Assoc. *156:* 1888 (1970).
KANEKO, J. J.; CORNELIUS, C. E. (Ed.): Clinical biochemistry of domestic animals (Academic Press, New York 1970).
KING, J. M.; KAVANAUGH, J. F.; BENTNICK-SMITH, J.: Diabetes mellitus with pituitary neoplasms in a horse and a dog. Cornell Vet. *52:* 133 (1962).
KRAL, F.: Epileptiform manifestations of endocrine disturbances associated with adrenal tumors. J. Amer. vet. med. Assoc. *118:* 235 (1951).
KROOK, L.: Dietary calcium-phosphorus and lameness in the horse. Cornell Vet. *58:* 59 (1968).
KROOK, L., and LOWE, J. E.: Nutritional secondary hyperparathyroidism in the horse. Pathol. Vet. *1:* 1 (1964).
KUZUYA, T.; KANAZAWA, Y.; HAYASHI, M.; KIKUCHI, M.; IDE, T.: Species difference in plasma insulin responses to intravenous xylitol in man and several mammals. Endocrinology (Japan) *18:* 309 (1971).
LEEMANN, W.: Diabetes insipidus. In: K. WAMBERG: Handlexikon der tierärztlichen Praxis (Med. Book Co., Copenhagen 1971).
LOEB, W. F.; CAPEN, C. C.; JOHNSON, L. E.: Adenomas of the pars intermedia associated with hyperglycemia and glycosuria in two horses. Cornell Vet. *56:* 623 (1966).
LOWE, J. E.; BALDWIN, B. H.; FOOTE, R. H.; HILLMANN, R. B.; KALLFELZ, F. A.: Equine hypothyroidism: the long term effects of thyroidectomy on metabolism and growth in mares and stallions. Cornell Vet. *64:* 276 (1974).
MCKENZIE, J. M.: Humoral factors in the pathogenesis of Grave's disease. Physiol. Rev. *48:* 252 (1968).
MEHRING, J. S.; TYZNIK, W. J.: Equine glucose tolerance. J. Animal Sci. *30:* 764 (1970).
O'CONNOR, J. T., jr.: The untoward effects of the corticosteroids in equine practice. J. Amer. vet. med. Assoc. *153:* 1614 (1968).
PFANNENSTIEL, P.: Therapie von Schilddrüsenerkrankungen (Henning, Berlin 1975).
RAKER, C. W.; FEGLEY, H.: Adrenal cortical adenocarcinoma with metastases in a mare. J. Amer. vet. med. Assoc. *147:* 848 (1965).
SEIFERLE, E.: Über Gehirnkrankheiten des Pferdes und einen Versuch zu ihrer neurologisch-psychologischen Auswertung. Schweiz. Arch. Tierheilk. *90:* 615 (1948).
SOLOMON, J. A.: The 'turning out' syndrome — a hypothesis. Blood Horse *85:* 714 (1963).
TASKER, J. B.; WHITEMAN, C. E.; MARTIN, B. R.: Diabetes mellitus in the horse. J. Amer. vet. med. Assoc. *149:* 393 (1966).
VOLPÉ, R.; EDMONDS, M. W.; CLARKE, P. V.; ROW, R. R.: A viewpoint regarding the nature of the emergence of long-acting thyroid stimulator of Grave's disease. Acta Endocrinol. Panam. *1:* 155 (1970).

2.1.14. Diseases of the Nervous System

2.1.14.1. Diseases of the Central Nervous System

2.1.14.1.1. Trauma to the Brain

Definition. A blow to the head can result in functional disturbances even in the absence of macroscopic lesions. A *concussion of the brain* is said to be present in such cases. If the trauma results in damage to brain tissue, then a *contusion of the brain* exists. Finally, trauma can cause intracranial hemorrhage with a consequent pressure increase, leading to *compression of the brain*.

Symptoms. Regardless of the severity of the trauma, clinical manifestations appear immediately after the event. In less severe cases the horse will suddenly collapse after colliding with an obstacle, or the animal will remain recumbent after the head is struck in a fall. There will be a general weakness of the muscles, and unconsciousness will be more or less complete. In mild concussions, the pulse and respiration are normal and the horse will recover within a few minutes but may continue to have an unsteady gait for up to 30 minutes. With more severe trauma, the comatose state persists for a longer time. The cutaneous and tendon reflexes are abolished. The pupils are dilated, the pupillary reflex is absent, and nystagmus may be present. In cases of moderate to severe injury, unconsciousness may last from several hours to 2 days. When the animal recovers, it generally will exhibit disturbances of consciousness such as poor balance, ataxia, incoordinated gait, compulsive movements or compulsive posturing (especially, abnormal carriage of the head), as well as paralysis of one or more cranial nerves. These defects usually persist for several days. The course depends on the severity of the trauma and especially on the degree of intracranial hemorrhage. In some cases the animal may appear to recover completely after a few hours, but the neurologic deficits become worse as time progresses. This is a sign that intracranial pressure is increasing as a result of hematoma or brain edema. Bradycardia will develop, and signs of unrest may appear. The development of fever after several days of normal body temperature may be an early sign of suppurative meningoencephalitis. This condition is especially common following skull fractures. The prognosis depends greatly on the presence or absence of a cranial fracture. Palpation may reveal a depressed fracture or crepitation. If palpation is negative, both lateral and dorsoventral radiographs of the skull should be made in severe cases. In addition, cisternal puncture is recommended to check for blood in the cerebrospinal fluid.

Etiology. Cerebral traumata are most commonly caused by collision with obstacles, falls on slippery floors, kicks to the head, and bad falls during riding. Other causes include collision between the maxilla and mandible, and striking the head while attempting to stand up. The latter can occur in animals that have been prostrate from colic, myoglobinuria, tetanus or other diseases.

Pathogenesis. In any head injury, the force of the blow is transmitted to the brain tissue. Movement of the brain within the confining space of the skull can lead to injuries of the brain substance and especially of fine capillaries on the side opposite the blow — a 'contrecoup' lesion [Palmer, 1979]. The initial reaction to the trauma is a circulatory shock which causes a transitory decrease in the blood flow to the brain. Because the brain is highly sensitive to an oxygen deficit, edema is quick to develop in the hypoxic brain. If vascular injury is present, a cerebral hemorrhage or hematoma may develop depending on the site of the lesion. Hematomas in animals are almost always of the subarachnoid type; subdural hematomas, though common in man, are rare or nonexistent in animals.

While subdural hemorrhages and cerebral edema cause compression of the brain, a subarachnoid hemorrhage can diffuse with the cerebrospinal fluid, and no symptoms of brain compression are produced.

The course depends both on the severity of the hemorrhage and on the site of the lesion. Extensive damage to the brain stem causes severe injury to the vital autonomic centers, often with a fatal outcome. Even small hemorrhages can lead secondarily to nonseptic encephalitis [Holliday, 1972]. Injuries of the cerebral cortex, such as those associated with fractures, do not necessarily lead to a fatal termination. On the other hand, basal skull fractures like those caused by mandibular violence are usually fatal, because the hematoma involves the base of the brain.

Diagnosis. A history of trauma can usually be elicited. Also, skin abrasions or injuries are likely to be found on examination of the head.

Differential Diagnosis. If an adequate history is unavailable, the following diseases should be considered: In *rabies*, the animal goes down and is unable to rise again, and death follows within 24 hours. The brain should be removed and examined if the animal has been taken from a rabies area (personal observations). *Botulism* is distinguished by a rapidly progressive paralysis, and the brain is free of gross or histologic lesions. *Trauma to the spinal cord* may be associated with tetraplegia, but the comatose state that is characteristic of brain lesions is absent, and there is little or no disturbance of sensation about the head.

Treatment. If significant improvement is not seen within a few minutes, plasma expanders should be given to correct hypovolemic shock. If symptoms of brain compression are evident as a consequence of cerebral edema or intracranial hemorrhage, fluid reduction should be attempted by the intravenous injection of 20 % mannitol (3 kg/kg BW) or 30 % urea (1—2 g/kg BW) in 10 % invertose. This may be repeated 4—6 hours later if there is no response. Urea should be used only if kidney function is still intact. If there is no visible improvement after 2 days, the further administration of hypertonic solutions is usually fruitless.

It is useful to follow dehydrative therapy with the administration of a glucocorticoid (e.g., dexamethasone). The initial dose of 500 mg is given intravenously, and subsequent doses of 100—200 mg are given intramuscularly for 3—4 days.

If water uptake is impaired, hemoconcentration should be monitored. This is achieved by continuous intravenous electrolyte solutions.

References

Holliday, T. A.: The nervous system. In: Equine medicine and surgery, 2nd ed., p. 459 (Amer. Vet. Public. Wheaton/Ill. 1972).

Palmer, A. C.: Hirn- und Rückenmarktraumata. Referat: Schweiz. Vereinigung für Kleintiermed. 8. Juni 1979.

2.1.14.1.2. Ataxia

Definition. Ataxia refers to a lack of coordination in limb movements.

The following forms of ataxia are distinguished according to the site of the lesion: cortical, subcortical, bulbar, cerebellar and spinal.

Symptoms. Cortical and subcortical ataxia are rare in the horse. They may arise during the course of other brain diseases. A cortical or subcortical ataxia should be suspected if the patient exhibits a clumsy gait and is unable to make fine adjustments during motor sequences. The animal walks with a stumbling gait and is apt to slip on smooth flooring.

Cerebellar ataxia is also rare in the horse. It is characterized by an inability to perform purposeful movements. Thus, a foal with the condition will have difficulty finding the udder, and mature animals will be unable to drink water from a pail. Some movements are hurried while others are slowed. Movements directed toward a specific target tend to 'overshoot' their mark. The sequence of limb movements is also uncoordinated. Horizontal nystagmus is frequently present. Disturbances of equilibrium become evident when the animal is blindfolded.

Spinal ataxia may be congenital ('wobbles', ataxia of foals; cf. Sec. 2.8.5.1.) or acquired. In congenital spinal ataxia, the disease symptoms appear before the second year of life. Acquired ataxia can develop at any age.

Affected foals typically show an increasing unsteadiness of gait, the hindlimbs being the more seriously affected. In other cases the onset is sudden. Signs usually are exaggerated when the horse is turned. The ataxia is manifested by crossing of the hindlimbs and by a jerky action of leg movements. A marked swaying of the hindquarters is also characteristic. Often no locomotor disturbance is apparent when the horse is walked straight ahead or when it is trotted or galloped. However, difficulties will appear when the animal is pulled up sharply, whereupon a marked sagging and swaying of the hindquarters will be noted. Backing is usually quite difficult. Often there is excessive angulation in the joints of the hind legs, even to the point of collapse. It is not unusual for affected animals to fall as a consequence of turning the head too far to one side. Pain sensation and the tendon reflexes are generally unimpaired. Involvement of the forelimbs may become apparent as the disease progresses. The animal usually has no difficulty in getting up and down until the terminal stages.

Etiology. Cortical and subcortical ataxia can develop secondarily to trauma or an infection of the CNS. In both cases the manifestations of the primary disease will be predominant. Cerebellar ataxias are the result of developmental defects during prenatal life. The cause of the defect remains unknown, however.

Signs of spinal ataxia may be delayed until the horse is 2 years or older, or may develop after the age of 4. Recent studies point to malformation of the intervertebral joints as the probable cause of the disease. The most severe changes have been found at the junction of C3 and C4, C4 and C5, and C5 and C6. Excessive mobility in one or more of these articulations apparently results in cervical subluxation and pressure on the white matter of the cord when the head is flexed forward. Eventually this leads to the degeneration of spinal cord tracts. Osteoarthritic changes in the vertebrae further exacerbate the condition.

In mature horses, trauma can cause vertebral displacement, or fissure fractures can lead to excessive callus formation. In either case there will be damage to the white matter of the cord.

Pathogenesis. The dislocation of one or more vertebrae can cause a direct contusion of the cord or cause pressure to be exerted on blood vessels, generally veins. In either case a localized edema develops that ultimately leads to a more or less circumscribed demyelination in the gray matter. The pathways that control motor coordination are the most seriously affected. Generally the condition is progressive.

Prognosis. Ataxias of long standing have an unfavorable prognosis; complete recovery is improbable.

Differential Diagnosis. Infectious diseases must be excluded. The symptoms of the primary disease will be predominant in such cases, however. Lamenesses can mimic ataxia but are distinguished by the restriction of the motor impairment to one limb. Fractures of the cervical, thoracic and lumbar vertebrae lead to paralyses or pareses of the limbs. The onset is sudden in such cases, and an immediate history of trauma will be in evidence.

Treatment. Regardless of whether the ataxia is cortical, cerebellar or spinal, treatment is unlikely to be of value. Corticosteroids or mannitol may relieve edema in very early cases of spinal ataxia. However, this does not affect the primary disease, and so a recurrence is likely.

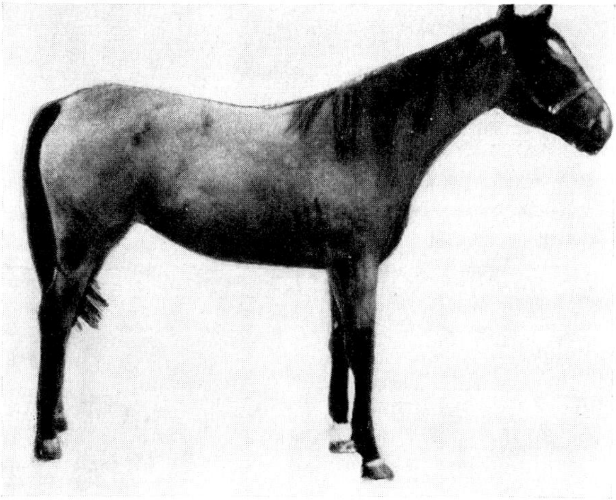

1

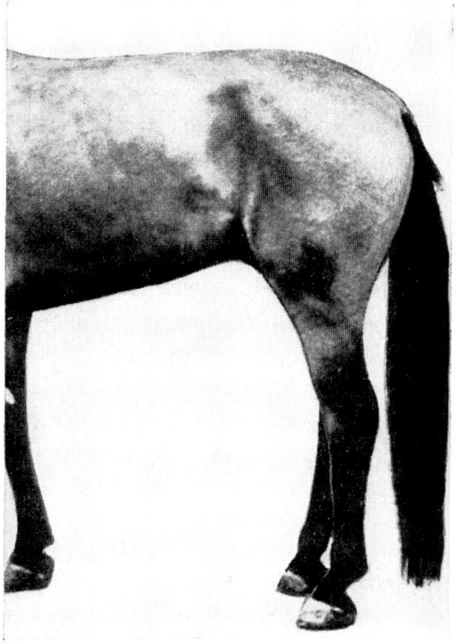

2

Fig. 2.1.14. — 1–2. Neuritis of the cauda equina.

2.1.14.1.3. Neuritis of the Cauda Equina

Definition. The disease is based on a chronic inflammation of the extradural nerve cords of the cauda equina. The term 'combined tail-sphincter paralysis' has also been applied to the disease [DEXLER, 1897].

Symptoms. In general, the onset of the disease is gradual, and the earliest symptoms are largely nonspecific. On close observation, it will be noticed that tail movements are becoming less active, and that the tail is not raised to a normal degree during movement (figs. 1.2.14. — 1 and — 2). Occasionally the tail will be held at an odd angle relative to the body. As the disease progresses, the tail loses most if not all of its muscular tone. Insects can no longer be swatted from the trunk and ventral abdomen, and the tail flails about freely during movement. On closer examination, a marked paresis or paralysis can be demonstrated. In typical cases defecation is hampered, the tail is no longer raised during defecation, and the tail hairs become soiled with feces and urine. Often the anus is open, and fecal balls drop from it during movement.

Rectal examination reveals a loss of anal sphincter tone and an accumulation of feces in the rectal ampulla. When the rectal ampulla is evacuated, urine can be readily expressed from the full, atonic bladder. In addition, spontaneous dribbling occurs, especially when the animal moves or stands up. Sensitivity tests will demonstrate a zone of complete anesthesia in the tail area that may extend to the skin around the tuber ischii. An asymmetric area of hyperesthesia is usually present cranial to this zone. The anal reflex is absent, the anus is frequently flaccid, and in mares dermatitis often develops on the inner thigh due to the dribbling of urine. Cystitis may also develop as a result of the bladder paralysis and associated retention of urine.

Atrophy of the hindquarter muscles near the tail may be present in advanced cases. Locomotor disturbances may appear in the form of hindquarter weakness or ataxia, sagging of the hindquarters under a rider, and ataxia on turning [HUTYRA et al., 1945; FANKHAUSER et al., 1975].

Laboratory Findings. Urinalysis will show proteinuria and hemoglobinuria if cystitis has developed, but other tests such as blood status, enzyme levels and serum electrophoresis are of no value.

Etiology. Opinions vary with regard to the etiology of cauda equina neuritis. Mechanical insults from traction on the tail, blows to the tail root in horse trailers, kicks, etc. [VON HUTYRA], as well as migrating parasitic larvae have all been cited as causative factors [VON HUTYRA et al., 1945; STÜNZI, 1974]. Because definitive evidence for a traumatic or parasitic etiology is lacking, however, a viral etiology appears to be the most plausible. A particularly likely candidate is the equine Herpesvirus I (rhinopneumonitis), especially since infections with this virus have been shown to be associated with CNS lesions [JACKSON].

However, there are several discrepancies that cast doubt on the herpesvirus as the sole causative factor. First, herpes infections are relatively common while the classic cauda equina neuritis is rare. Second, the disease is not observed in foals or aged horses, while herpes infections can occur at any age. Finally, the disease is more prevalent among mares than geldings [FANKHAUSER et al., 1975]. These facts make it likely that additional factors are involved in the etiology of the disease. FANKHAUSER et al. [1975] suggest that an individual predisposition to allergy may be an important factor. While this has not yet been proven, it seems a valid possibility.

Pathogenesis. If we accept the virus etiology, then the infectious agent produces an inflammation with epi- and perineural fibrosis. These changes cause damage to the nerve fibers themselves, which results in the characteristic sensory and motor losses. Because herpesvirus apparently can survive for months in the tissues, yet is included in the category of 'slow viruses' [JACK, 1974], it is possible that an allergic action of the virus is a factor in producing the lesions.

Differential Diagnosis. Fractures of the first coccygeal vertebra can cause tail paralysis. In such cases crepitation and pain will be evident during passive movement of the tail, and anal and bladder paralysis will be absent. In infections of the CNS such as Borna disease and dourine, the deficits are not restricted to the cauda equina.

Prognosis. With extensive paralysis of the tail, anus and bladder, the prognosis is unfavorable. The animal is probably still fit for light work, but it will remain susceptible to chronic cystitis as well as inflammation of the rectal mucosa with possible perforation.

Necropsy Findings. In advanced cases a firm cord of fibrous tissue will completely fill the spinal canal in the area of the filum terminale. In early cases the nerves are enmeshed in a gelatinous, blood-streaked tissue. It is possible for both recent and old lesions to coexist in the same animal.

Histologically, inflammatory reactions are considerably less common in the extradural root segments than in the intradural segments. Lymphocytic and histiomonocytic infiltration is the predominant finding; plasma cells, eosinophilic and neutrophilic granulocytes are also observed. The myelin sheaths are fragmented, and some necrosis is seen in the spinal ganglia. A marked fibrosis of the fiber bundles is invariably present [FANKHAUSER et al., 1975].

Treatment. No specific treatment is available. While glucocorticoids may relieve inflammation and reduce the allergic response, this therapy might also *activate* a herpesvirus infection.

In well-developed cases, measures are limited to manual evacuation of the rectal ampulla and emtying of the bladder.

References

Dexler, H.: Die kombinierte Schweiflähmung und Sphincterenparalyse des Pferdes (Hammelschwanz). Zschr. Thiermed. (Jena) *1:* 279 (1897).

Fankhauser, R.; Gerber, H.; Cravero, G. C.; Straub, R.: Klinik und Pathologie der Neuritis caudae equinae des Pferdes. Schweiz. Arch. Tierheilk. *117:* 675 (1975).

Hutyra, F. v.; Marek, J.; Manninger, R.; Mócsy, J.: Spezielle Pathologie und Therapie der Haustiere, 9. Aufl., Bd. 2 (Gustav Fischer Verlag, Jena 1945).

Jack, J.: Persistent infections with herpesviruses. Progr. med. Virol., vol. 18, p. 160 (Karger, Basel 1974).

Stünzi, H.; Pohlenz, J.: Zur Pathologie der Neuritis caudae equinae beim Pferd. Schweiz. Arch. Tierheilk. *116:* 533 (1974).

2.1.14.2. Paralysis of the Peripheral Nerves

2.1.14.2.1. Paralysis of the Facial Nerve

Definition. The loss of function may affect the auricular muscles, the orbicularis oculi muscle, the buccal muscles, or the muscles of the upper lip, nostrils, lower lip or chin, depending on the location of the injury.

According to Marolt, Bego and Maticic [1970], two forms can be distinguished according to the course of the nerve and the localization of the lesion: central or intracranial paralysis, and peripheral or extracranial paralysis. The intracranial form is a consequence of damage to the facial nucleus in the brain.

Extracranial facial paralysis is the more common form. It includes paralysis occurring from the site of emergence of the nerve to its ramifications.

A further distinction is made between unilateral and bilateral paralysis, and between partial paralysis (paresis) and complete paralysis.

Anatomy. The facial nerve is the 7th cranial nerve. It leaves the cranial cavity in the pons area through the stylomastoid foramen, courses along the facial canal at the inner ear, passes beneath the parotid gland, and emerges at the border of the mandible below the articular process. On the surface of the masseter muscle it ramifies into the two facial branches.

Symptoms. Unilateral paralysis is evidenced by a sagging of the upper and lower lip on the affected side. The cheek on the affected side is lax. The mouth and lips appear deviated and drawn upward toward the *normal* side (fig. 2.1.14. — 3). The nostrils on the affected side cannot dilate normally, and the nasal opening has an elongated oval ('bean') shape. This may cause respiratory difficulties during exertion. During forced respiration the nostrils tend to flutter on expiration and fall inward on inspiration.

If the nerve damage is located in the facial canal or in proximity to the middle ear, there will be concomitant injury of the auriculopalpebral nerve. Clinically this is manifested by lagophthalmos with a severe loss of tone in the orbicularis oculi muscle. The corneal reflex is slowed; the eye and nictating membrane have normal motility.

Finally, the facial paralysis may involve the caudal and internal auricular nerves. This results in paralysis of the ear, which hangs laterally and obliquely outward.

Paralysis of the lips creates difficulties with food prehension. Much time is needed for mastication, and there is a tendency for food to collect between the cheek and teeth on the affected side. Swallowing is also difficult, because the bolus cannot be easily conveyed past the tongue. Masticated food and saliva drool from the mouth

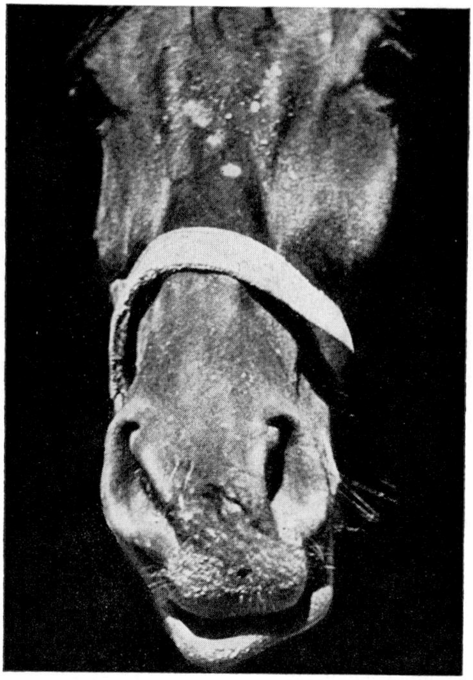

Fig. 2.1.14. — 3. Paralysis of the facial nerve.

and can be found in the feed trough. The animal drinks slowly. During this time the horse may immerse part of its nostrils in the water due to the difficulty of creating an effective sucking action with the mouth.

In bilateral facial nerve paralysis, the upper and lower lips sag symmetrically and both nostrils are constricted. A snorting or rattling sound is heard during respiration. During heavy exertion, dyspnea may become extremely severe due to the collapse of the nostrils on inspiration. Food prehension with the lips is no longer possible, and the horse must bite into the roughage or granular feed with its incisors. Even then, a portion of the food is dropped from the mouth. Drinking is very difficult. Because the lips do not close, the corners of the mouth have to be immersed before the water can be swallowed.

Etiology. Peripheral, extracranial facial nerve paralysis is caused by damage to the nerve in its anatomic course, due for example to inflammation in the middle ear region, or by contusion or rupture at points where the nerve or its branches run subcutaneously over bone.

The most frequent cause is contusion of the nerve below the temporomandibular joint at the upper, external border of the masseter muscle. Here the nerve is easily crushed by pressure from the buckle of a halter (left side) or from the buckle of the cheekpiece of a snaffle. A peripheral facial nerve paralysis of this type can occur without involvement of the auricular and palpebral muscles as a result of head trauma inflicted as the horse attempts to stand after a bout of colic, other recumbency, or during recovery from anesthesia. Central facial paralysis can be caused by encephalitis, space-occupying intracranial lesions (tumors, hematomas, leukosis [Pick and Püschner, 1970], abscesses), and by basal skull fractures.

Prognosis. Peripheral facial paralyses caused by short-term nerve compression have a good prognosis. If the nerve has been severed, the prognosis is poor. Recovery is unlikely in cases of central facial paralysis, because even if the primary disease is cured, it is improbable that the facial nucleus will regenerate. Atrophy of the masseter can seriously interfere with food ingestion. In many cases weeks or even months are required for nerve regeneration to occur. Recovery is signaled by a gradual improvement in the animal's ability to feed.

Treatment. The first step in the treatment of peripheral facial paralysis is to eliminate its cause. The horse should be placed in a well-bedded stall and the halter removed. Because feeding is a laborious and continuous process, a soft, easily masticated ration should be available at all times. A temporary tracheotomy is indicated only in cases of bilateral paralysis when the animal is in imminent danger of suffocation.

The goal of treatment is to hasten regeneration of the damaged nerve. Concentrated glucose, sorbitol and fructose solutions are given intravenously, and 10—15 ml of a vitamin B-complex solution is injected at 4- to 5-day intervals. For the first few days cutaneous massage, liniments and heat (microwave, infrared) are applied to the affected side of the face, especially over the course of the nerve and in the masseter area. Good results are obtained with stellate ganglion blockade and prednisolone injections, which may be repeated after 3—4 days in acute cases.

Comments. If the facial paralysis does not improve within 4 weeks, then recovery usually will require 3 to 4 months. The animal may be kept alive this long in unilateral cases.

In bilateral cases, starvation is always a possibility, and slaughter may have to be considered after 14 days.

2.1.14.2.2. Paralysis of the Trigeminal Nerve or its Mandibular Branch

Definition. Paralysis of the motor branches of the trigeminal nerve or of its third main division, the mandibular nerve, results in loss of function of the muscles of mastication: the masseter, temporal and pterygoid. The paralysis also affects the mylohyoid muscles, portions of the biventer muscle, and the tensor tympani muscle.

Etiology. The trigeminal nerve is the 5th cranial nerve. It lies in the trigeminal incisure of the sphenoid and petrous bone. From the semilunar (gasserian) ganglion arise the three main divisions of the trigeminal nerve: the ophthalmic and the maxillary, which are mainly sensory, and the mandibular, which is chiefly motor.

Forms and Occurrence. Central trigeminal paralysis is associated with intracranial lesions. Peripheral trigeminal paralysis is usually traumatic in origin and affects only the mandibular branch.

Symptoms. Peripheral trigeminal paralysis cannot be clinically distinguished from central paralysis. In rare cases a strangulation or contusion can be demonstrated in the cheek area. In bilateral paralysis the mouth hangs open, and the tip of the tongue protrudes between the incisors and saliva drips from the mouth. The jaws can be passively closed without difficulty. The swallowing reflex is preserved. Within a few days the breath becomes fetid. With unilateral paralysis, food can still be ingested but tends to accumulate between the cheek and teeth on the unaffected side. With bilateral paralysis there is a complete inability to eat or drink. Marked atrophy of the masseter muscle and temporal muscles is evident only 8—10 days after onset. Gradual starvation is inevitable even if the animal is fed by stomach tube.

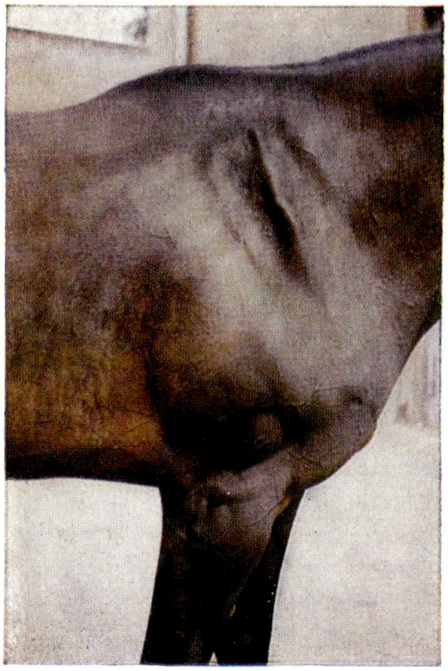

Fig. 2.1.14. — 4. Paralysis of the suprascapular nerve with atrophy of the supraspinatus and infraspinatus muscles.

Etiology. Central trigeminal paralysis can be a symptom of many brain diseases, including rabies. It can also result from brain abscesses, tumors and other lesions that are associated with a rise in intracranial pressure. Peripheral trigeminal paralysis due to strangulation is rare in horses.

Differential Diagnosis. Dislocation of the mandible is very rare in the horse and is distinguished by resistance to passive closure of the mouth.

Prognosis. The prognosis is good in paralysis due to traumatic causes; otherwise it is poor.

Treatment. It may become necessary to feed the animal by stomach tube. Alcohol-base liniments should be applied to the affected cheek. In other respects, treatment is the same as that for facial nerve paralysis.

Comments. In central paralysis, the primary disorder should be corrected if possible. Otherwise treatment is continued for 8—10 days, at which time slaughter should be considered if no improvement is seen.

2.1.14.2.3. Paralysis of the Hypoglossal Nerve

Definition. The hypoglossal nerve (12th cranial) is the motor nerve of the tongue. Its paralysis involves a uni- or bilateral neurogenic loss of function of the lingual muscles. The motor cells of the hypoglossal nerve lie in the caudal part of the medulla oblongata. The nerve leaves the skull through the hypoglossal foramen and passes oroventrally, crossing the origin of the lateral maxillary artery and accompanying its inferior border.

Symptoms. Because hypoglossal nerve paralysis is very rare and, when it occurs, tends to be unilateral, the protruding tongue generally deviates toward the right or left side. It is always held toward the unaffected side. Saliva is drooled. The tongue itself shows no changes at the onset of the disease. Later, mucosal lesions can develop with all their attendant complications. The animal is unable to eat or does so with great difficulty, and a large portion of the food is dropped from the mouth.

Etiology. The most frequent cause of hypoglossal paralysis is contusion of the nerve at the origin of the external maxillary artery or elsewhere in its course. This can occur as a result of strangulation, mandibular fracture, when the head becomes lodged between two posts, etc. Lingual paralysis of myogenic and neurogenic origin also has been observed following forcible withdrawal of the tongue. Hypoglossal paralysis of central origin can occur secondarily to rabies, botulism and other infectious brain diseases.

Differential diagnosis must be made from fractures of the hyoid bone.

Treatment and Prognosis. The prognosis is good for unilateral, peripheral hypoglossal nerve paralysis due to contusion. Prednisolone is administered in a dose of 200 mg/day for 3 to 4 days, and large doses of B-complex vitamins are given. In some cases a stellate ganglion blockade is indicated at the onset of the disease; this is done with about 100 ml of a 0.5 % procaine solution. Massaging the contused site with camphor spirit is beneficial. In paralysis due to central lesions, the prognosis is poor and treatment is generally of no value.

2.1.14.2.4. Paralysis of the Suprascapular Nerve

Definition. Suprascapular nerve paralysis is characterized by a loss of function in the motor nerves that supply the supraspinatus and infraspinatus muscles, which serve as lateral collateral ligaments for the shoulder joint.

The suprascapular nerve arises from the ventral branches of the 6th, 7th and 8th cervical components of the brachial plexus. It passes along the inner side of the scapula to the neck, where it winds around the cranial border of the scapula and passes to its outer surface.

Occurrence. The nerve is exposed to trauma as it passes around the scapula at the point of the shoulder. As as result, contusion of the nerve with consequent paralysis is not uncommon in the horse.

Symptoms. Injury to the nerve results in paralysis of the muscles that it supplies. As a result, a mild to moderate supporting-leg lameness is evident when the animal is walking. This is accompanied by a sudden lateral movement of the shoulder joint and scapula when the affected limb is bearing weight. The shoulder and elbow joints are slightly abducted when the animal is standing. The abduction of the shoulder is most easily seen when the animal is walked toward the examiner. This specific functional disturbance is not so apparent at the trot. After 8—10 days, atrophy of the spinatus muscles will cause the scapular spine to appear unusually prominent (fig. 2.1.14. — 4; Stanić and Palić [1960]). This atrophy is termed 'sweeny' by horsemen.

Sometimes soft-tissue injuries and closed or open fractures are also observed at the anterior border of the scapula.

Etiology. A single blunt trauma to the neck of the scapula is the most common cause of this paralysis. This leads to contusion, stretching or even tearing of the suprascapular nerve on the sparsely-padded bone of the scapula neck. Most cases occur when the horse jumps or runs into an obstacle. However, the paralysis has also been observed in jumping and three-day-event horses whose injuries were sustained during jumps over ditches.

Differential Diagnosis. Chronic omarthritis with associated joint deformation should be considered in chronic cases. A swinging-leg lameness distinguishes this condition from suprascapular paralysis.

Diagnosis. The lameness is characterized by lateral deviation of the shoulder joint and scapula when weight is placed on the affected limb. In many cases it appears as if a flat hand could be inserted between the scapula and thorax.

Atrophy of the affected muscles is a sign that the disease has been present for more than 8—10 days.

Prognosis. A definite prognosis cannot be given early in the disease. Contusions of the nerve may heal in a few days with or without treatment. If the nerve is stretched or torn, recovery may require 3—4 months or may never occur. If the paralysis has already existed for several weeks and muscular atrophy is complete, it is very unlikely that much improvement will be seen.

Treatment. Treatment should be immediate, and all possibilities should be exhausted. The site of the contusion can be treated with massage, moist or dry heat applications or mild rubefacient ointments. Stimulative therapy with microwaves or electric current may also be tried. B-complex vitamins, vitamin E-selenium preparations, hypertonic glucose solutions and possibly strychnine (0.1 mg/kg BW) are administered parenterally. Symptoms associated with nerve contusion are usually quickly relieved by single or repeated blockade of the stellate ganglion (approx. 100 ml of a 0.5% local anesthetic or epinephrine). Repeated prednisolone injections are helpful in promoting functional recovery [Lewandowski et al., 1969]. The horse should be allowed to exercise in a large box stall until recovery is complete.

Reversal of muscular atrophy may be hastened by administering anabolic steroids.

Comments. The function of the nerve and the muscles it supplies will return if nerve continuity has been preserved. If no improvement is seen after 4 months, it may be necessary to restrict the animal to breeding use.

2.1.14.2.5. Paralysis of the Radial Nerve

Definition. Radial nerve paralysis is characterized by a loss of function in the extensor muscles of the elbow, carpal and digital joints.

Anatomy. The radial nerve arises from the posterior part of the brachial plexus. It runs distally along the inner side of the scapula and ramifies at the level of the shoulder joint, sending motor branches to the extensor of the elbow joint, the triceps muscle. Above the humeral condyles the nerve winds laterally around the humerus and at the level of the elbow ramifies into the branches that supply the extensors of the carpal and digital joints. A sensory branch innervates the skin of the forearm.

Forms. Rooney [1963] identifies three forms of radial nerve paralysis in the horse: (1) The loss is restricted to the extensors of the elbow joint. Only the branch supplying the triceps muscle is damaged. (2) The extensors of the carpus and digit are affected. In such cases the nerve has usually been injured at the point where it winds around the humerus. (3) Both muscle groups are paralyzed (the most common form); this condition is called complete radial nerve paralysis.

Symptoms. In complete ('proximal') radial nerve paralysis, the affected limb has a characteristic appearance when the animal is standing: the shoulder joint is extended, the elbow is dropped, the carpal joint is in slight flexion and the fetlock joint in extreme flexion. This gives the limb an elongated appearance. If the horse is forced to walk, it is unable to advance the limb to place weight on the foot, and the anterior surface of the hoof drags on the ground. The animal may bear weight on the fetlock for brief periods until the carpus and elbow joints give way. If a horse with complete radial nerve paralysis lies down, it usually can get up again only if it is lying on the unaffected side. The animal can walk normally if a rope is attached around the fetlock and the affected limb is pulled forward during each swinging-leg phase. The fetlock will knuckle with each stride, but weight will be supported by the affected leg. Atrophy of the extensors of the elbow, carpal and digital joints develops within 8—10 days.

If the paralysis involves only the carpal and digital extensors, it will not be difficult to recognize this partial ('distal') radial nerve paralysis by the milder clinical signs. When the animal is standing, the elbow joint of the affected limb is not dropped relative to the normal side. Thus, the affected leg does not appear elongated. The carpal and fetlock joints are only slightly flexed. The horse can perform the swinging-leg phase without assistance. It moves in short lunges supporting itself on the healthy leg while swinging the affected leg forward. There is wear to the toe of the anterior hoof wall.

In complete (proximal) as well as partial (distal) radial nerve paralysis, there is a partial or complete anesthesia of the skin on the forearm.

Paralysis affecting only the branch supplying the triceps brachii muscle is rare. During standing the elbow joint is flexed, while the carpal and digital joints are extended and can support weight.

Etiology. Complete radial paralysis in the horse is rarely caused by direct violence. According to Rooney [1963] and based upon many years of our own experience, the most frequent cause is hyperextension of the whole limb. At one time this was a relatively common occurrence in horses that were cast onto the Vinsot-type surgery table, on which the body was drawn upward with a belly band while the limbs were pulled downward and tied. The same clinical picture can occur in horses that are inadequately anesthetized and struggle against restraint. In this case a complete radial nerve paralysis develops that affects the uppermost limb as well. The cause is a tear of the nerve in the upper portion of the limb on the medial side of the humerus.

Direct trauma, especially contusions, at the site where the nerve winds laterally around the humerus produce the clinical picture of partial (distal) radial paralysis. This can be caused by lying on a hard surface, collisions during running or jumping, a kick from another horse, etc. In rare cases distal radial paralysis is seen following deep surgical anesthesia. This is attributed to a complete relaxation of the muscles that normally cushion the nerve.

Sole paralysis of the branch supplying the triceps brachii muscle is usually caused by wounds along the medial aspect of the humerus that traumatize or tear the nerve.

As early as 1962, Marolt and colleagues suggested that transitory symptoms of radial paralysis were due not to a primary lesion of the nerve itself, but to an interruption of the blood supply from compression of the vessels, especially the axillary artery, when the horse is placed in lateral recumbency on a hard surface and the lowermost forelimb is pulled backward.

Differential Diagnosis. Fractures of the ulna produce a similar carriage of the limb while the horse is standing. The same applies to traumatic cubital (elbow) arthritis. Both conditions are characterized by local tenderness and inflammatory swelling. An ulnar fracture can be excluded by radiographs if necessary.

Diagnosis. The typical flexed positions of the elbow, carpal and digital joints are the only signs that are apparent in the limbs, although wounds may be present in characteristic locations. Abrasions may be found on the fetlock or anterior surface of the digit. Cutaneous analgesia may be demonstrated on the forearm. The presence of muscular atrophy signifies that the condition has existed for at least 8—14 days.

Prognosis. It is favorable if improvement is noted a few hours after onset of the paralysis; circulatory impairment is the probable cause in such cases. If no improvement is seen by the 3rd or 4th day, the prognosis is unfavorable, although recovery is still possible even in cases that are weeks or months old.

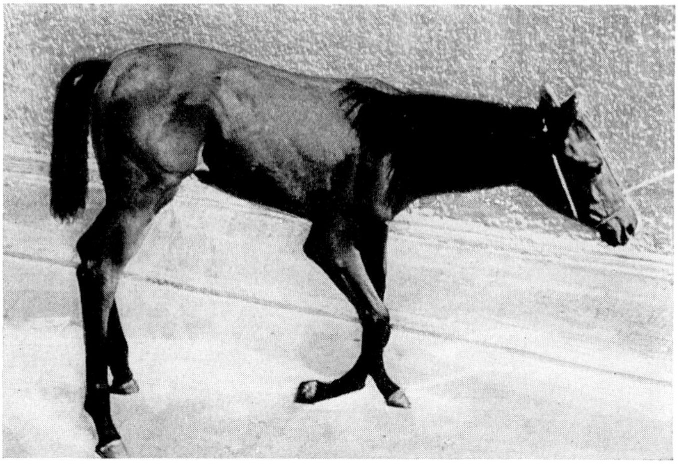

Fig. 2.1.14. — 5. Paralysis of the brachial plexus.

Treatment. Treatment is similar to that for suprascapular nerve paralysis and should not be delayed. Massage, local hyperemia, microwave and electrotherapy are worthwhile only if the radial nerve has been contused at the site where it winds around the humerus. Injections are administered as in other types of peripheral nerve paralysis. The affected horse should be allowed free mobility in a large box stall. The digital joints should be bandaged to prevent skin abrasions.

Comments. Following recovery, stumbling can still occur at fast gaits. If no improvement whatsoever is seen within 6—8 weeks, destruction of the animal should be considered.

2.1.14.2.6. Paralysis of the Brachial Plexus

Definition. This paralysis involves a loss of sensory and motor function in all peripheral nerves that supply the front limb. Anatomically the brachial plexus is formed by the ventral branches of the 6th, 7th and 8th cervical nerves and the first 2 to 3 thoracic nerves. A peripheral paralysis occurs when these branches become injured outside the spinal canal or there is injury to the plexus as a whole. A 'central' brachial plexus paralysis is present when the aforementioned ventral branches are damaged by disease of the vertebrae or lesions within the spinal canal.

Symptoms. The affected limb hangs limp from the shoulder downward. The shoulder and elbow are severely dropped, and the digital joints are flexed. If the horse is able to hobble on the remaining three legs, the paralyzed limb dangles freely, dragging the ground or striking against the healthy limb. When passively moved, the elbow joint appears to have an excessive range of motion. The animal offers no resistance to such manipulation. Skin sensation is abolished from the coronet to well above the elbow. If the digit is extended while the horse is standing and weight is placed on it, the scapula and shoulder joint will deviate laterally (fig. 2.1.14. — 5).

In addition to these symptoms, there is frequently a comminuted fracture of the scapula. There may also be tears or contusions of the muscles that insert on the scapula.

Complete, bilateral paralysis of the forequarters occurs when that portion of the cervical or thoracic cord becomes contused or compressed by a fracture of the vertebral body or vertebral arch or a dislocation of the last cervical and/or first thoracic vertebra.

Etiology. Brachial plexus paralysis is apt to occur when the horse steps into a hole, trap, etc. and then tries forcibly to free the trapped forelimb. This can result in stretching of the plexus or even avulsion of the ventral nerve branches from the spinal canal. Similar injuries can occur when a heavy frontal blow is delivered between the scapula and thorax, or when objects are thrust under the scapula. Lateral blows that produce communited or depressed fractures of the scapula can cause plexus lacerations. Brachial plexus paralysis of gradual onset is the result of abscesses, lymph node swelling, neoplasms, or heavy callus formation on the scapula or ribs.

Differential Diagnosis must be made from radial nerve paralysis, ulnar fractures, cubital (elbow) arthritis, omarthritis and dislocation of the humerus. This is done on the basis of clinical signs and, if necessary, by radiographic examination.

Diagnosis. The diagnosis is based upon a complete loss of sensation and motor function in the forelimb.

Prognosis. In paralysis associated with scapular fracture, the prognosis is poor. The same applies to paralysis of gradual onset due to subscapular neoplasms, abscesses, lymph node swelling and callus formation.

If a stretch injury of the plexus is suspected, treatment may be attempted. Avulsions of the ventral nerve roots cannot be ruled out, however. In 'central' brachial plexus paralysis there is little or no chance of recovery.

Treatment. Treatment corresponds to that for other peripheral nerve paralyses, especially those of the forelimbs. Local treatment is useless, however, owing to the anatomic position of the plexus.

Comments. If no signs of improvement are seen in 8—10 days, destruction is recommended.

2.1.14.2.7. Paralysis of the Sacral Plexus

Definition. Paralysis of the sacral plexus is characterized by a loss of sensory and motor function that simultaneously affects the tibial and peroneal components of the sciatic nerve.

The three roots of the sacral plexus (sciatic nerve) arise from the lumbosacral trunk, and its ventral rami from the last lumbar and first sacral segments. The plexus (nerve) leaves the pelvis through the greater sciatic foramen and passes downward in the angle between the femur and ischium. At the origin of the gastrocnemius muscle it divides into its two components, the tibial nerve and the peroneal nerve.

Symptoms. The limbs cannot be actively raised or adequately advanced. If a rope is attached around the fetlock and used to pull the limb forward, weight can be supported for a short time owing to preserved function in the quadriceps femoris muscle. But after a moment the limb will give way at the hock, frequently accompanied by a knuckling of the fetlock. There is usually anesthesia of the skin on the lateral and medial aspects of the limb from the stifle joint downward.

Etiology. Paralysis of the sacral plexus or sciatic nerve in the horse is almost always associated with a deep muscular wound in the region of the hip, thigh or croup. Deep abscesses can also be a cause of plexus damage. The plexus is so well protected by muscles that it is seldom damaged by blunt trauma.

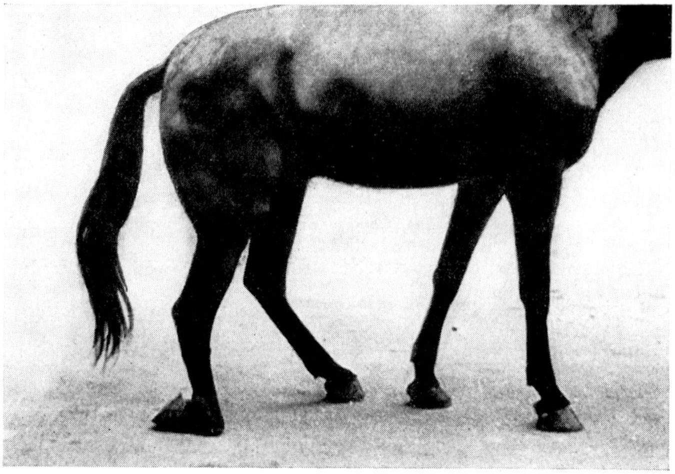

Fig. 2.1.14. — 6. Paralysis of the peroneal nerve.

Differential Diagnosis. Differentiation from peroneal nerve paralysis may be difficult unless a fresh wound or abscess-forming cellulitis can be demonstrated.

Diagnosis. The diagnosis is based on a concomitant loss of sensory and motor function in the nerves arising from the plexus.

Prognosis. The prognosis in sciatic paralysis is poor, for wounds and abscesses usually entail the destruction of nerve tissue.

Treatment. Fresh wounds that extend to the sacral plexus are managed according to the principles of general surgery. Anastomosis of the nerve with a suture is rarely successful. Abscessed cellulitis is incised and drained. Full regeneration of the damaged nerve tissue is unlikely under the best of circumstances.

2.1.14.2.8. Paralysis of the Peroneal Nerve

Definition. Peroneal paralysis is characterized by a loss of function in the flexors of the hock and extensors of the digit.

Symptoms. When the horse is standing, the hock joint of the affected limb shows almost no angulation. The digit is in extreme flexion, and weight is supported on the fetlock. This situation is quite painful and can be maintained for only a short time (fig. 2.1.14. — 6). If the animal is forced to walk, the affected limb moves forward in an outward arc, with the anterior surface of the hoof dragging on the ground. If it is necessary for the horse to walk long distances, a rope can be placed around the fetlock to pull the digit forward during the swinging-leg phase; this will enable the foot to make flat contact with the ground during each stride. No swelling, tenderness or increased warmth is noted in the affected limb, although abrasions or decubitus sores may be present on the anterior surface of the foot.

Etiology. Unilateral or bilateral peroneal paralysis is observed with some frequency when the horse is cast into dorsal recumbency with the Stuttgart casting harness, put into a shallow plane of general anesthesia, and ropes or bands are attached above the hock to obtain further abduction of the hindlimbs.

Less frequently, unilateral peroneal paralysis is caused by direct violence, such as a kick to the gaskin from another horse.

Differential Diagnosis. When peroneal paralysis is observed in the standing horse, it is apt to be confused at first sight with upward fixation of the patella. However, whereas the stifle and hock cannot be passively flexed in upward fixation of the patella, this can be done without difficulty in peroneal paralysis. Vertebral abscesses, osteomyelitic foci, and neoplasms in the lumbosacral region of the spinal column can produce similar neurologic deficits. In such cases the signs usually are limited to one side initially and spread to the opposite side within 3—4 weeks; associated paralysis of the tibial and obturator nerves may also be present.

Central paralysis of this type may appear as a symptom of vertebral luxation or subluxation, a vertebral fracture, a hematoma of the spinal canal, or a luxation in the iliosacral articulation. A history of trauma to the lumbosacral region can be elicited in such cases.

Diagnosis. The loss of angulation in the hock joint and the bearing of weight on the fetlock are characteristic. Anesthesia is sometimes present in the area supplied by the superfical peroneal nerve. If it is suspected that the paralysis is of central origin, a rectal examination can provide further diagnostic clues.

Prognosis and Treatment. The prognosis is very good for paralysis developing during general anesthesia. If standing on the fetlock is observed following recovery from anesthesia, a uni- or bilateral lumbar sympathetic blockade is performed using at least 100 ml of a 0.5 % procaine solution without epinephrine. The paralytic symptoms should regress within 24—48 hours. In paralysis of traumatic origin, the above treatment is supplemented by giving large doses of B-complex vitamins at 2- to 3-day intervals combined with the i.v. infusion of hypertonic glucose or fructose solution. Electrotherapy, vitamin E-selenium, and anabolic injections may be conducive to healing. Recovery generally follows in 2—4 weeks.

Comments. If no improvement occurs within 14 days, or if the paralysis is known to be central, it is recommended that the animal be euthanized.

2.1.14.2.9. Paralysis of the Obturator Nerve

Definition. This condition involves loss of function in the muscles that adduct the leg, especially the gracilis, pectineus, adductor and obturator externus muscles.

Symptoms. The affected leg is held in abduction while the horse is standing. During walking the affected limb is moved forward with an outward sweep of the femur. Marked atrophy of the adductor muscles develops within 8—10 days. Horses with bilateral obturator paralysis are unable to stand up, and the hindlimbs tend to straddle when the animal is lying down. No swelling or tenderness is present.

Etiology. Unilateral or bilateral obturator paralysis can develop when excessive traction is exerted during the delivery of an oversize fetus, causing the nerve to become crushed or torn within the pelvis. The most common cause is trauma to the nerve associated with pelvic fractures.

Differential Diagnosis. The history provides adequate grounds for distinguishing myositis, myoglobinemia, tying-up syndrome, and thrombosis of the terminal bifurcation of the aorta.

Diagnosis. The diagnosis is established by the characteristic symptoms and by the rectal or vaginal examination. This is necessary to exclude hematomas and pelvic fractures.

Prognosis. The prognosis is unfavorable to poor, especially with bilateral paralysis. Recovery is possible only in unilateral paralysis occurring as a sequel to dystocia.

Treatment corresponds to that for peroneal paralysis.

Comments. Horses with bilateral obturator paralysis get pressure sores and soon die from pneumonia and decubitus. Hence, euthanasia should be considered without delay.

2.1.14.2.10. Paralysis of the Tibial Nerve

Definition. There is loss of function in the extensors of the hock joint and flexors of the digit.

Symptoms. When weight is placed on the affected limb during standing or walking, excessive angulation (dropping) of the hock is evident. There is knuckling of the fetlock, the digit does not flex completely during walking, and the limb makes an outward arcing movement when it is advanced. Complete collapse of the hock joint is prevented by the action of the gastrocnemius and digital flexor muscles in the Achilles tendon complex. Neurogenic atrophy of the muscles supplied by the motor branches of the tibial nerve develops in 8—10 days. No other changes are evident in the affected limb.

Etiology. Paralysis of the motor branches of the tibial nerve is rarely the result of contusion. Transection of the nerve associated with accidents and wounds is a more frequent cause.

Differential Diagnosis. Tibial nerve paralysis may be confused with partial rupture of the Achilles tendon when the animal is standing. Wounds or avulsion fractures of the calcaneus are not difficult to exclude. A tendovaginitis of the common deep flexor tendon sheath can be excluded by palpation or radiographic examination.

Diagnosis. The diagnosis is based on characteristic signs — dropping of the hock and knuckling of the fetlock — with otherwise negative clinical findings.

Prognosis and Treatment. The prognosis is good for nerve contusions but poor if the nerve has been severed. Treatment corresponds to that for peroneal paralysis.

Comments. See Peroneal Paralysis.

References

Cox, V. S.; Martin, C. E.: Lähmung des N. peronaeus bei einer Färse. J. Amer. vet. med. Assoc. *167:* 142 (1975).

Lewandowski, M.; Kostyra, J.; Koper, St.; Lipinska, M.: Posttraumatische Nervenparese der Extremitäten von Pferden und ihre Behandlung mit Prednisolon. Med. weteryn. *25: 18* (1969).

Marolt, J.; Bego, U.; Maticić: Beitrag zur Fazialislähmung bei Pferd und Hund. Dtsch. tierärztl. Wschr. *77:* 463, 469 (1970).

Marolt, J.; Bego, U.; Vucelić, E.; Sankocie, F.; Zeskow, B.: Untersuchungen über Funktionsstörungen des Nervus radialis und des Kreislaufes in der Arteria axillaris beim Pferd. Dtsch. tierärztl. Wschr. *69:* 181 (1962).

Marolt, J.; Peitel, M.; Somek, I.: Paralysis N. radialis bei einer Kuh. Dtsch. tierärztl. Wschr. *79:* 555 (1972).

Pick, M.; Püschner, H.: Zentrale Fazialislähmung durch Leukose beim Pferd. Berliner Münchener tierärztl. Wschr. *83:* 249 (1970).

Rooney, J. R.: Radial paralysis in the horse. Cornell Vet. *53:* 328 (1963).

Stanić, M. N.; Palić, D. T.: Experimentelle Untersuchungen der Dysfunktion der motorischen Nerven der Gliedmassen bei Pferden und Rindern. I. Nervus suprascapularis. Wien. tierärztl. Wschr. *47:* 688 (1960).

Stanić, M. N.; Palić, D. T.: Experimentelle Untersuchungen der Dysfunktion der motorischen Nerven der Gliedmassen bei Pferden und Rindern. II. Nervus radialis. Wien. tierärztl. Wschr. *49:* 360 (1962).

2.1.15. Diseases of the Eye

2.1.15.1. The Eye as an Optical System

The eye consists of a neural component and its accessory structures. The neural component is represented by the visual receptors (rods and cones) located in the retina and the conduction pathways that arise from them. This component performs the true function of the eye as an organ of light perception: the reception of light stimuli and their conversion to nervous impulses that can be transmitted to the brain.

The accessory structures of the eye can be divided into external structures, consisting of the eyelids, nictating membrane, lacrimal glands and eye muscles, and internal structures, consisting of the cornea (with its precorneal tear film), the aqueous humor, the iris, the lens and the vitreous body. The latter structures are also collectively termed the dioptric apparatus. The function of this compound refractive system is to ensure that light rays entering the eye are brought to a focus exactly on the retina (emmetropia). The pigmented iris ensures the creation of an optic axis by adjusting the pupillary width to allow only a portion of incident light rays to enter the eye. The ability of the eye to adjust to objects at various distances so that a sharp, inverted retinal image is always produced is called accommodation. It is achieved mainly through changes in the thickness of the crystalline lens. The total accomodating power of the eye is called the range of accommodation. This is the distance between the near point of vision and the far point, measured in meters and expressed in diopters (D). This range varies individually and with age. In the horse the range of accommodation is only 1—2 D, compared, for example, to 2—4 in the cat and 10 in diurnal birds.

Errors of refraction are relatively common. They are dependent on a number of factors including breed, age and care. It is reported that up to 40 % of horses are myopic (myopia = nearsightedness: light rays are focused in front of the retina), the highest prevalence being reported in cold-blooded breeds. Myopia is considered to be a result of domestication and inbreeding. It can occur as axial myopia (lengthening of the visual axis due to an elongated anteroposterior diameter of the eyeball) or as refractive myopia (convergence of rays traversing the refractive media due, for example, to reduced elasticity or swelling of the lens). A myopia of no more than 3—4 D in the horse is not considered significant and should not impair the animal's usefulness. Myopias in excess of 4 D, on the other hand, can cause behavioral disturbances, such as shying, when the animal is in unfamiliar terrain or doing unaccustomed work.

Hyperopia (hypermetropia), or farsightedness, is less frequent in the horse (2—3 %). Like myopia, it may be axial (e.g., abnormal shortness of the eyeball) or refractive (flattening of the cornea due to ulcerous or inflammatory changes, aphakia). Again, deviations up to 4 D are considered to be acceptable, while hyperopia of 10—16 D like that associated with aphakia causes severe vision impairment.

Vision relies on the coordinated interaction of the neural and optical components of the eye. When considering the visual apparatus of the horse, it must be borne in mind that, aside from the various ocular diseases, there are certain breed peculiarities that can have important bearing on the care and its utilization for sport or pleasure.

The horse, being a diurnal animal, has a smaller proportion of rods (night-vision receptors) than do humans or nocturnal species, and consequently its dark adaptation is poorer than in the cat, for example. On the other hand, the presence of a 'central striate area' (collection of receptors in the form of a stripe above the optic disk) enables the horse to detect extremely small movements, especially those occurring at the periphery of the visual fields. Initially these moving objects are located outside the range of visual acuity, but despite this fact, or perhaps because of it, they are capable of triggering exaggerated reactions on the part of the animal. It is estimated that the 'blind spot' on the equine retina is relatively large. As a result of this, when the horse is looking at objects located at various distances but situated along more or less the same line of sight, it must move its head, eye or both in order to focus on the objects.

Owing to the relatively lateral placement of the eyes on the head, the visual axes of the horse are divergent, i.e., the common visual field is comparatively small, despite the compensating effect of the horizontally-shaped pupil. The horse has limited depth perception, therefore. On the other hand, the lateral placement of the eyes extends the temporal boundaries of the visual field, providing the horse with panoramic vision. Moreover, lateral head movements can compensate for the poor coordination of the eye muscles in focusing both eyes on a single object.

The horse is able to perceive colors, with the probable exception of red.

The reflex sign of retinal activity is the pupillary response to light stimuli. It is important to note that this response takes place via a reflex arc (retina — optic nerve — optic chiasm — optic tract — quadrigeminal body — interneuronal center — ciliary ganglion — iris) that bypasses the visual center. Thus, while the pupillary reflex is useful in assessing the functional status of the retinal receptors, reflex arc and oculomotor nerve pathway, it does not reflect the presence or absence of vision.

2.1.15.2. Examination of Visual Function

The functional examination tests the ability of the visual organ to receive a light stimulus, the transformation and processing of the stimulus in the brain, and the associated responses of the animal. Except for the detection and grading of abnormalities in the performance of the dioptric apparatus, the examination requires no specialized knowledge or equipment and can be done under ordinary conditions. It essentially involves testing the horse's vision while noting the direction of gaze and assessing the pupillary reflex.

Vision should be tested only in animals that have a serious vision impairment (amblyopia) or are blind in one or both eyes (amaurosis). The tests do not enable a grading of the abnormality, nor can they reveal mild vision impairments (asthenopia) or refractive errors.

Before any special tests are done, the examiner should take the necessary time to observe the overall behavior of the animal, both in daylight and at dusk, in relation to:

— familiar and unfamiliar stimuli;

— familiar and unfamiliar surroundings (in the stable, in the paddock, in the herd, at the feed trough, in a closed room, etc.) while the horse is moving freely, longed or performing work. Special note should be taken of:

— the gait (free, surefooted, hesitating, groping, stumbling, etc.);

— limb action at slow and fast gaits;

— carriage of the head (oblique, extended);

— ear play, nostrils, nasal speculum.

Having gained an impression of the animal's overall behavior, the examiner proceeds with the actual vision testing. This consists essentially of leading the animal through or over obstacles of varying size, shape and arrangement, such as elevations or depressions in the ground, or posts, boards, ladders, hurdles, walls, ropes, etc. that have been laid or stretched across the animal's path.

The eyes can be tested separately by covering each eye alternately with a hood, blinder or bandage.

Head and eye movements as well as changes in the direction of gaze in one or both eyes when following a moving object can also be of diagnostic importance. On the other hand, a rapid hand movement made in front of the eye can set up air currents that are sufficient to elicit eyelid closure and simulate a light reflex (horse-traders' trick).

The pupillary reflex has limited bearing on the quality of the animal's vision. If included in the functional examination, its main purpose is to aid in assessing the functional status of the retina. Assuming that pupillary action is not restricted by synechiae, drugs or an increased sympathetic tone, then a prompt, full reflex accompanied by a consensual reflex in the other eye enables the following conclusions to be drawn:

- sufficient light is striking the retina,
- the retina is light-sensitive,
- there is conduction in the visual pathway up to the reflex arc,
- the reflex arc and oculomotor nerve pathway are intact.

2.1.15.3. Shying

In the care and utilization of horses, shying is an undesired characteristic that all too often is attributed to inadequacies of vision and too seldom is viewed in relation to the natural flight response of the horse. Thus, the causes of shying relate mainly to the historical aspects of equine behavior in the wild that have persisted despite domestication and breeding. These essentially involve the natural protective and flight reflexes of this species in response to unfamiliar stimuli in general. But while this reaction is based upon an interplay of all sensory modalities, the fact remains that shying can be caused by ophthalmic disorders. These include the presence of floating corpuscular elements in the eyeball, opacities of the transparent ocular media, or severe refractive errors.

2.1.15.4. Diseases of the Eye

Ophthalmic diseases in the horse can seriously reduce the value of the animal, especially if it must rely on vision in the performance of its work. In this section we shall discuss diseases and lesions that are relatively frequent in the horse compared to other domestic species.

2.1.15.4.1. Diseases of the Eyelids

Examination: When examining the eyelids, attention is given to their form, position and mobility. The eyelid of the horse is covered with a fine, thin skin. Eversion of the eyelid folds, tenseness of the eyelid skin and swelling of the eyelids may signify an inflammation, effusion, neoplasm or other disease. Abnormalities of eyelid position are recognized by the shape and arrangement of the eyelid margin ('third canthus', inversion or eversion) and by the angle of the eyelashes in relation to the globe ($< 45°$ = entropion; $> 45°$ = ectropion).

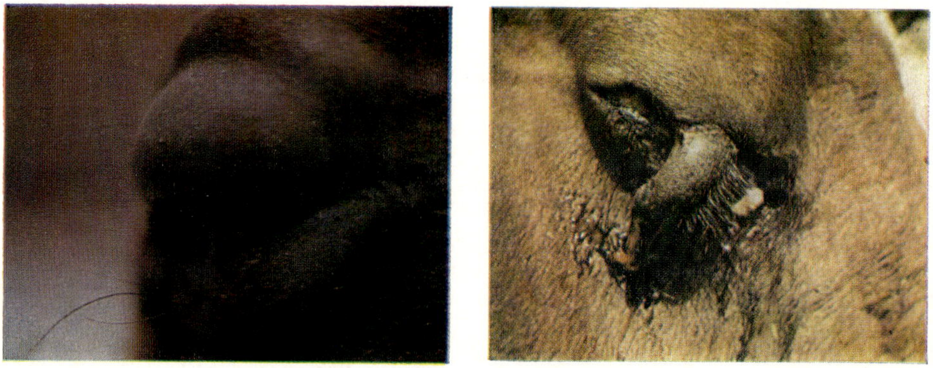

1 2

Fig. 2.1.15. — 1. Edema of the upper and lower eyelids.
Fig. 2.1.15. — 2. Full-thickness laceration of the eyelid parallel to the lid margin.

Eyelid movements are influenced by adhesions (symblepharon, ankyloblepharon), spasmodic conditions (blepharospasm), paralytic conditions (ptosis), mechanical obstructions (neoplasms, edema) and inflammation.

Changes in the palpebral fissure mainly relate to its size. The palpebral fissure is narrow or closed if the eyeball is abnormally small or retracted into the orbit (microphthalmos, enophthalmos), in the presence of adhesions (ankyloblepharon), abnormalities of eyelid position (entropion), and in inflammatory states. Widening of the palpebral fissure may be associated with enlargement or anterior displacement of the eyeball (glaucoma, macrophthalmos, exophthalmos) or with abnormalities of eyelid movement or position (lagophthalmos, ectropion).

Eyelid edema: Eyelid edema is characterized by a pathologic accumulation of fluid in the loose connective tissue of the eyelid. It is caused by local or systemic conditions that lead to an alteration in the permeability of the vessel walls (e.g., inflammation, infections, toxemia, deficiency states, organic diseases).

The characteristic symptom is swelling of the eyelid (fig. 2.1.15. — 1). Swelling of the upper eyelid may be so severe that the orbital cavity is covered and the palpebral aperture is closed (pseudoptosis). The eyelid skin is tense, and the palpebral folds are everted. In the presence of stasis edema, the skin feels cooler than normal and is nontender. If the edema is inflammatory in origin, the eyelid will be tender to palpation. The skin feels warm and is reddened in nonpigmented areas.

Treatment is directed toward the primary disorder. Supportive measures include the application of cold compresses or anti-inflammatory ointments. Cellulitis responds favorably to local hyperemia (40—45 °C compresses for 20 minutes several times daily, infrared light, heating pad). In cases of insect bites or allergy, antihistamines and antiallergic drugs may be used locally and systemically.

Eyelid injuries: The horse is prone to eye injuries and is relatively sensitive to their effects.

Eyelid contusions are caused by blunt trauma and can result from blows or bumps of the head (colic), prolonged recumbency or scraping of the eyelid on the floor while attempting to stand up. They occur mainly in the area of the superior orbital arch and quickly lead to edematous swelling of the eyelids, especially the upper lid.

Treatment is limited to applying cold compresses. In the presence of excoriations or decubitus ulcers, cooling, protective ointments (zinc, boric acid, bismuth) are

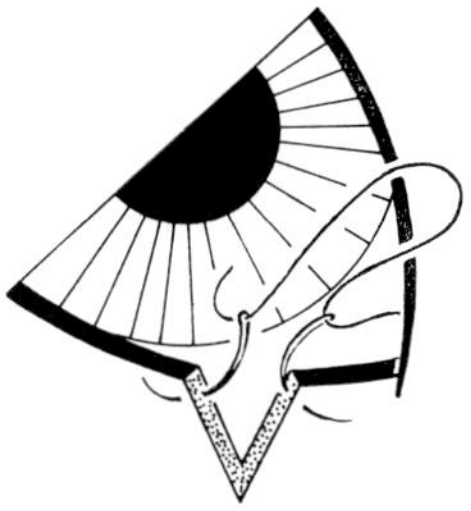

Fig. 2.1.15. — 3. Technique of the intermarginal suture.

beneficial. An antibiotic-containing ophthalmic ointment should be instilled into the conjunctival sac for prophylaxis.

Wounds affect mainly the delicate skin of the eyelids. They often present as lacerations caused by projecting, sharp or pointed objects. These wounds are characterized by a disruption of continuity in the skin of the eyelid or even in the palpebral muscles and palpebral conjunctiva, the lid being torn parallel or at right angles to the eyelid margin. With full-thickness lacerations that create a discontinuity in all eyelid layers, large pieces of lid become torn from surrounding tissues and hang loosely from the eye (fig. 2.1.15. — 2). In less favorable cases the piece of eyelid is completely torn free. The immediate reaction is a collateral edema of the eyelid that narrows or closes the palpebral fissure, and heavy lacrimation develops mixed with a seromucoid exudate.

Treatment centers on prompt surgical repair to restore tissue continuity or, if too much tissue has been lost, on blepharoplastic procedures (sliding skin flap) to obtain satisfactory eyelid closure and ensure the preservation or restoration of the precorneal tear film. Partially avulsed eyelid tissue should never be removed. Even older wounds should be surgically managed, in which case treatment consists of a careful wound excision that spares uninvolved tissues. The suturing of skin wounds is best done with synthetic material or silk (closely-spaced simple interrupted sutures of Dexon 1/0). Extensive conjunctival wounds should also be united with sutures, as they are prone to edematous swelling. This is done with absorbable material. Postoperative care includes the use of topical antibiotics and immobilization of the operative field by cross-tying the head, applying a cap bandage, or similar measures.

Neoplasms: Papillomas are the most common benign tumors in older horses, while melanomas are observed more frequently in old gray horses. The principal malignant tumors of the eyelid are the melanosarcoma, hemangiosarcoma and carcinoma. Very often it is difficult to identify visually the portion of the eyelid (skin or conjunctiva) from which the neoplasm has arisen.

Treatment. Benign tumors are excised from the eyelid in V-shaped fashion, the wound edges are carefully apposed with an intermarginal suture (fig. 2.1.15. — 3), and the wound is protected from injury. For large eyelid defects, various blepharoplastic procedures are suitable, depending on the situation.

Malignant tumors are radically excised on account of their infiltrative and destructive growth. This may necessitate removal of the globe and orbital contents in some instances (see Enucleation), and postoperative treatment with radioisotopes or cytostatics may be warranted.

Disturbances of eyelid movement: Spastic eyelid closure (blepharospasm) is a reflex phenomenon associated with irritation of the conjunctiva, cornea, uvea or retina, or it may be a symptom of degenerative neurologic disease (e.g., Borna disease). The orbicularis oculi muscle is powerfully contracted, and tight closure of the palpebral fissure is maintained for varying lengths of time.

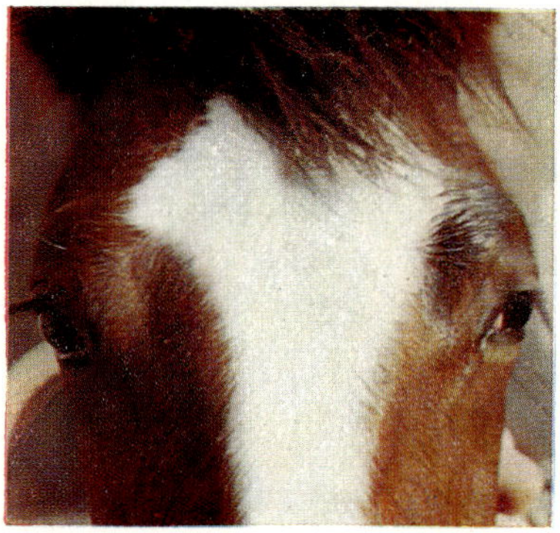

4

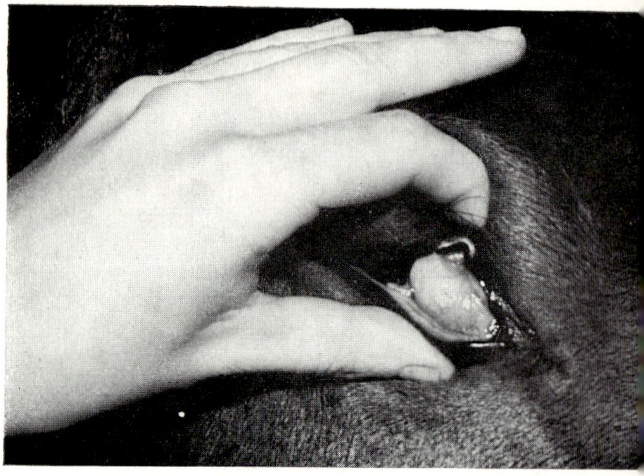

5

Fig. 2.1.15. — 4. Ptosis in a case of Horner's syndrome. (Note smaller palpebral aperture and lower angle of lashes.)

Fig. 2.1.15. — 5. Technique for visualizing the conjunctiva and especially the nictating membrane (photo courtesy of Veterinary Surgical Clinic, Leipzig).

The major goal of treatment is to relieve both the symptoms and the cause and break the vicious cycle of 'irritation, reflex inversion, irritation'. The spasm can be relieved temporarily by applying a topical anesthetic to the conjunctiva and cornea (e.g., pantocaine). Heat application has a spasmolytic effect. Finally, temporary relief can be achieved by blocking the auricular nerve (subfascial injection of 5—6 ml anesthetic into the zygomatic arch region). If the blepharospasm is symptomatic, only causal treatment is effective.

A drooping, normally developed upper eyelid in the horse is most commonly due to an edema or hematoma of the eyelid, in which case the cause is mechanical. This condition is also called false ptosis or pseudoptosis.

True ptosis is due to paralysis of the oculomotor nerve, facial nerve or frontal nerve. In the horse, temporary or sustained ptosis may be caused by contusions of the facial nerve (central portion proximal to the anatomic bend) or may be a sign of Horner's syndrome resulting from paralysis of the cervical sympathetic nerves (fig. 2.1.15. — 4). Treatment is directed toward the primary disease, i.e., swelling of the eyelids is alleviated, neoplasms are removed, and spasmodic conditions are relieved. In cases of nerve paralysis, the administration of vitamin B, glucose and local heat applications are beneficial; strychnine may also be indicated. For systemic diseases that are accompanied by ptosis, such as dourine and botulism, specific therapy is indicated.

An *abnormality of eyelid position* that is commonly observed in the horse is the 'third canthus'. This condition is present when an extraneous, canthus-like notch develops in the upper eyelid. It is associated with abnormal smallness and/or retraction of the eyeball (atrophia bulbi, phthisis bulbi, enophthalmos, etc.) and results from a constant voluntary contraction of the levator palpebrae muscle by the animal in an effort to keep the palpebral aperture open.

Therapy is directed toward the primary disorder. Treatment is useless in the case of atrophia bulbi.

2.1.15.4.2. Diseases of the Conjunctiva

Examination of the conjunctiva is done mainly by inspection. A large area can be inspected by placing the thumb and index finger onto the approximate midpoints of the upper and lower eyelids from the temporal side and then spreading the lids by pressing gently into the orbital cavity along the globe. This will evert the eyelids somewhat, causing the nictating membrane to protrude. It is now possible to inspect portions of the bulbar conjunctiva, palpebral conjunctiva and outer surface of the nictating membrane (fig. 2.1.15. — 5).

To inspect the fornix, a topical anesthetic is applied and special instruments are used to immobilize and evert the eyelid (e.g., palpebral forceps or lid retractors).

Special attention should be given to the nictating membrane, the cartilage-supported conjunctival duplication that presents in the medial canthus.

Conjunctivitis. General remarks on symptoms and etiology: An inflammation of the conjunctiva may be primary (from physical, chemical or infectious causes), secondary (from the spread of inflammatory processes) or associated with influenza, rhinopneumonitis or other diseases.

The normal conjunctiva is pale red in color, smooth and glistening. The initial symptom of conjunctivitis is hyperemia. The differentiation of conjunctivitis from other diseases of the anterior segment of the eye relies mainly on the nature of the vascular filling (vascular congestion), which may be conjunctival or ciliary. Conjunctival congestion as a sign of conjunctivitis is due to active hyperemia of the vascular system located within the conjunctiva. The engorged, brick-red vessels follow a tortuous course that is most prominent in the palpebral conjunctiva and fornix. The vessels constrict and the redness disappears when a 0.1 % Suprarenin solution is topically applied.

Ciliary congestion as a symptom of inflammation of the anterior eye segments (cornea and iris) is characterized by hyperemia of the subconjunctival network of blood vessels. The very thin, bluish-red vessels are difficult to distinguish individually. The topical application of 0.1 % Suprarenin produces no change, and the redness persists.

The serous infiltration that invariably accompanies a severe conjunctivitis leads to chemosis, or excessive edema of the conjunctiva. This can also occur as a symptom of inflammatory changes in the tissues surrounding the eye, in which case the term ‘collateral edema’ is applied. With the increased congestion comes exudation from the conjunctival vessels. The exudation may be serous, mucoid, fibrinous or purulent (fig. 2.1.15. — 6). Increased lacrimation frequently accompanies the inflammatory exudation. The exudate is washed over the lid margin by the lacrimal fluid, causing tracks to form at the medial canthus.

In longstanding cases the acute conjunctivitis passes into a chronic stage. The conjunctiva gradually loses its smooth texture; often it is only moderately reddened and may appear greatly thickened. The depths of the fornices are filled with a mucoid, fibrinous or purulent exudate or membranous coatings. Marked dilatation may be evident in some blood vessels.

Treatment is initially directed toward the cause. Afterward, cleansing, soothing, anti-inflammatory therapy is indicated. The rule is to treat uncomplicated inflammation with mild-acting astringents and antiseptics, if possible. In longer-standing cases, a change in the selection of medications is recommended. For the first few days the conjunctival sac and nasolacrimal duct are irrigated repeatedly with warm solutions of borated water (2 %), oxycyanated mercury (1 : 4,000), potassium permanganate (1 : 10,000), physiologic saline, etc. A mild compacting and drying effect

6 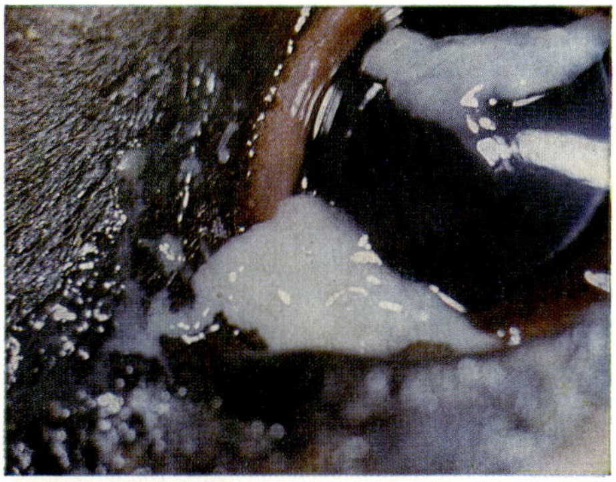

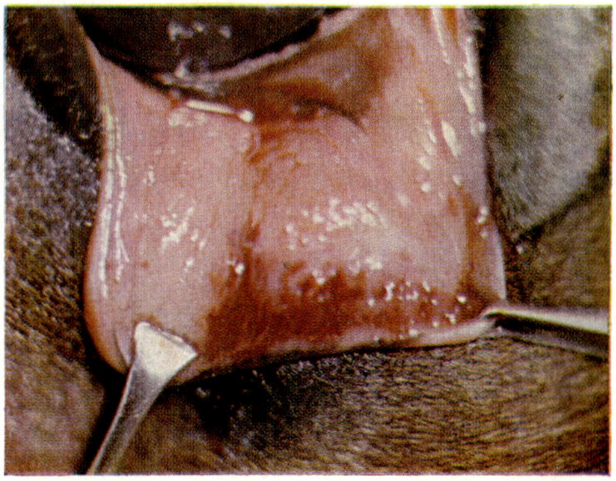 7

8 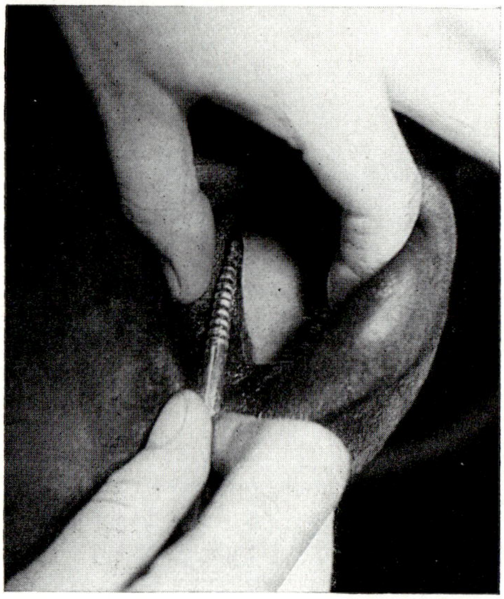

Fig. 2.1.15. — *6.* Flocculent, purulent discharge due to conjunctivitis.

Fig. 2.1.15. — *7.* Bulbar surface of the nictating membrane in follicular conjunctivitis.

Fig. 2.1.15. — *8.* Cannulating the nasolacrimal duct.

on the conjunctival tissue can be obtained with 1 % tannic acid, 0.5—1 % zinc sulfate, 0.5 % zinc chlorate, or 1 % salicylic acid or resorcinol in ointment form.

The colloidal silver compounds Targesin 3 %, Protargol 3 %, as well as 0.25—0.5 % silver nitrate solutions may be beneficial. In many cases vigorous treatment by direct application of 2 % silver nitrate or crystalline copper sulfate is successful (caution: follow by neutralizing with saline!). In cases where there is spasm, topical anesthetics are effective in temporarily relieving pain (caution: these agents have epitheliolytic and allergenic properties).

The following have proved useful in the treatment of purulent inflammation:

— Penicillin in the form of sodium penicillin G. It is highly effective against hemolytic streptococci and is active against certain staphylococci. The 1.5 % ointment is applied at least every 2 hrs, or the 0.15 % aqueous solution every 30 minutes, to achieve a therapeutic level. Efficacy is prolonged with subconjunctival application. For this an aqueous solution of at least 50,000 I.U./ml should be prepared, and applications should be repeated every 6 hrs.

— Tetracyclines (chlortetracycline, oxytetracycline) with a broad activity spectrum against all gram-positive and gram-negative bacteria, many rickettsia species, several large viruses, certain spirochetes and leptospirae, but not against certain *Pseudomonas* strains, *Proteus* and staphylococci. They are suitable for topical use in the ointment or drop form (0.5—1 %). They are applied hourly for the first 6 hours, and then once every 3 hours thereafter.

Follicular conjunctivitis is relatively common in the horse. It occurs as a sequel to chronic conjunctivitis and is characterized by the appearance of pinhead-size, glassy, hard, firmly-embedded subepithelial nodules. On the medial surface of the nictating membrane, a great number of these nodules are arranged into a flat packet with an irregular, granular, bright-red surface (fig. 2.1.15. — 7).

Treatment is essentially the same as for chronic conjunctivitis. Following topical anesthesia and eversion of the nictating membrane, the 'follicular packet' on the bulbar surface of the membrane is curetted toward the cornea with a sharp ophthalmic curet, preferably with the aid of a loupe, treated topically with 2 % $AgNO_3$ solution, then neutralized with 1 % NaCl. Surgery is followed by a 3-day course of topical antibiotics. Vitamin A supplementation will aid in promoting epithelialization. Treatment is continued with zinc sulfate drops. The treatment is repeated after 8—10 days if necessary.

Prolapse of the nictating membrane: When the nictating membrane protrudes, it covers part if not most of the cornea. The possible causes are numerous:

— mechanical prolapse due to microphthalmia or spasm of the retractor oculi muscle (tetanus symptom!);

— prolapse from enlargement of the nictating membrane due to inflammatory or neoplastic swelling;

— prolapse resulting from central or peripheral paralytic conditions (administration of hypnotics, neuroplegics, sign of Horner's syndrome).

Treatment is directed toward the primary disease. No treatment is given for microphthalmos or enophthalmos. If the nictating membrane is involved in neoplasia, excision of the membrane is indicated. The standing animal is given a narcotic or sedative, and local anesthesia is administered (topical, infiltration or nerve block). The nictating membrane is grasped with forceps, exteriorized, and sectioned at its base with a curved scissors. Bleeding is controlled by direct pressure.

2.1.15.4.3. Diseases of the Lacrimal Apparatus

Examination. When examining the lacrimal apparatus of the horse, the main point to consider besides the functional status of the secretory organs (lacrimal gland, nictitans gland, accessory glandular tissues in the conjunctiva) is the patency of the tear-conveying structures, especially the nasolacrimal duct. This is tested by introducing a special cannula (nasolacrimal duct cannula) or flexible catheter into the distal orifice of the nasolacrimal duct at the mucocutaneous junction on the nasal floor (fig. 2.1.15. — 8). A fluid that has been warmed to body temperature (physiologic saline, potassium permanganate solution, etc.) is then injected into the nasolacrimal duct through flexible tubing connected to the cannula. If the duct is patent, a fine stream of the solution will flow from the lacrimal puncta of the cannulated side.

Stenoses of the nasolacrimal duct are manifested clinically by persistent lacrimation from the medial canthus, conjunctivitis, and, if the tear flow is prolonged, hair loss and dermatitis along the track of the discharge. The nasolacrimal duct can become

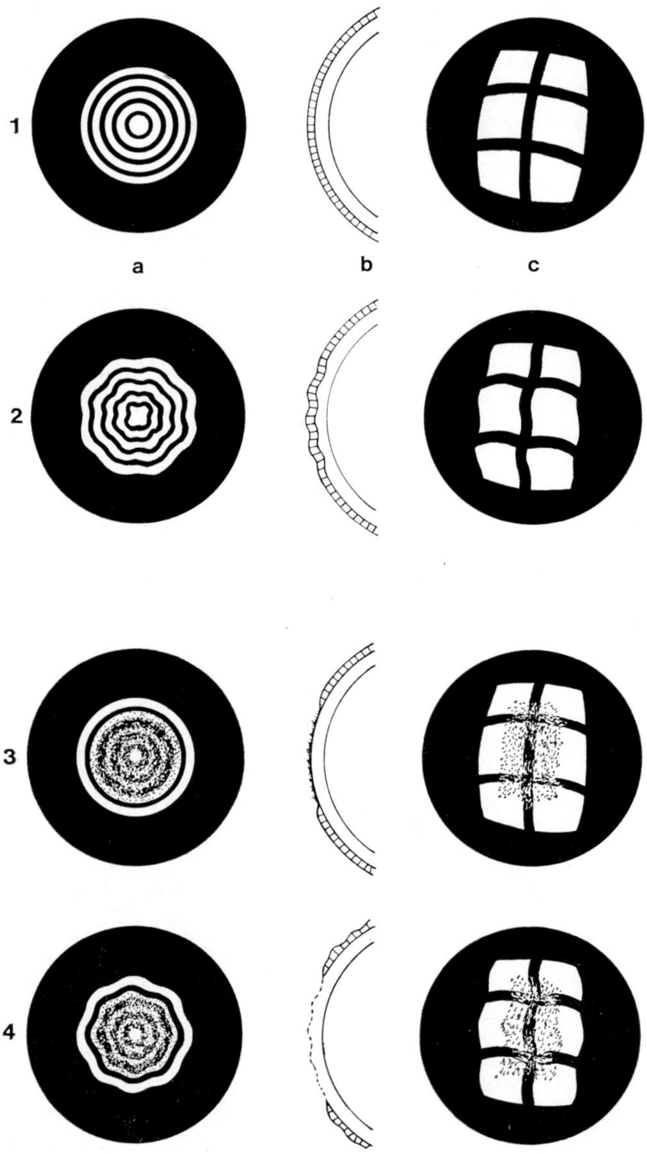

Fig. 2.1.15. — 9. Assessment of the corneal surface with the aid of reflected images. 1—4 see explanations in text; a = keratoscope; b = cross-section of cornea; c = window bars.

stenosed due to compression from enlargements or swellings of the maxilla or nasal bone. Very often the duct becomes obstructed by inflammatory products, foreign bodies or parasites.

Treatment. Obstructions of the nasolacrimal duct can usually be relieved by single or repeated flushing of the duct. Aqueous antibiotic solutions are administered if necessary.

In compression of the nasolacrimal duct, treatment is directed toward the primary disorder.

Atresia of the excretory papilla of the nasolacrimal duct is characterized clinically by a round, fluctuant swelling of the nasal mucous membrane at the opening of the nasolacrimal duct. The swelling spreads in a proximal direction and causes bulging of the skin above the nostrils on the affected side.

Treatment is surgical. With the animal recumbent, a piece of mucosa is excised through the nasal opening, and an artificial orifice is created for the nasolacrimal duct. Multiple flushings through this orifice on subsequent days maintain patency of the fistula while cleansing the nasolacrimal duct of residual secretions.

2.1.15.4.4. Diseases of the Cornea

Examination. The cornea is examined for surface irregularities, opacities and abnormalities of curvature. The normal corneal surface is smooth, even and shiny, and reflected images (contours of light source, window bars, keratoscope) are sharp, regular and have smooth edges (fig. 2.1.15. — 9, 1). Reflections with wavy edges on a shiny surface are a result of scar indentations or cellular infiltrations that do not disrupt the epithelial layer (fig. 2.1.15. — 9, 2). A distorted reflection combined with localized dullness signifies irregularities due to disruptions of the epithelial layer (lesions, wounds), cellular infiltrations or liquefactive processes (ulcers) (fig. 2.1.15. — 9, 3). Dull reflections with unsharp boundaries signify edema of the corneal epithelium (fig. 2.1.15. — 9, 4). Epithelial lesions can be clearly demonstrated by applying a drop of 2 % fluorescin solution and then rinsing off the excess dye with physiologic saline.

The cornea is transparent when the deeper parts of the anterior eye segment (anterior chamber, iris and pupil) can be inspected without difficulty. Corneal opacities may be smoky, milky, porcellan-white or brown in appearance; they may be spotty, flakey, plexus-like, diffuse or circumscribed. Yellowish-gray opacities are associated with heavy leukocyte and lymphocyte infiltration, bluish-white or white opacities with scarring, and brown opacities with pigmentary deposits or infiltration. Transparency is also affected by vascularization.

A distinction is made between superficial and deep vascularization, as this is important in determining whether pathologic changes are localized in the cornea, or there is involvement of the uvea in the disease process.

Keratitis: Superficial keratitis is caused mainly by physical trauma, which is especially common in racing animals. The injury involves the corneal epithelium and superficial parenchymal layers. Most injuries of this type go unrecognized until subjective symptoms appear: photophobia in the affected eye, narrowing or spastic closure of the palpebral fissure, retraction of the globe, abnormal lacrimation, restrained or shy behavior. A mucoid or mucopurulent conjunctival discharge is not uncommon. There is diffuse or circumscribed opacification of the cornea, and the fluorescin test is positive. Edematous loosening of the corneal ground substance quickly develops, starting at the edge of the defect and progressing toward the periphery. The end-result is profound and extensive corneal change and a generalized, milky opacification of the cornea. This is prone to purulent liquefaction and even perforation as a result of secondary infection. In the horse in particular, the reaction to deeper corneal lesions and inflammation is swift and severe. The reaction is sometimes dramatic, and consists in inflammatory involvement of the uvea with consequent miosis, hypopyon or hyphema, and synechiae.

The following principles are important in the *treatment* of keratitis, even when the deeper corneal layers are involved:

— prevention of infection or spread by secondary pathogens, which are ubiquitous in the conjunctival sac;
— immobilization of the iris of the ciliary body;
— prevention of synechiae;
— reduction of pain;
— promotion of corneal regeneration and healing.

Secondary infections are most effectively controlled with broad-spectrum antibiotics. Combination products containing corticosteroids inhibit regeneration of the corneal epithelium, hamper the desired restoration of epithelial continuity, prolong healing, and predispose to complications. If a corneal perforation is present, local treatment should be supplemented with systemic antibiotics due to the breach of the blood-aqueous barrier. The remaining requirements (relaxation of the iris and ciliary body, pharmacologic immobilization of the inner eye, prevention of synechiae, pain relief) are best answered with the topical administration of atropine. By blocking the cholinergic sphincter pupillae muscle, atropine leads to a passive mydriasis. At the same time, the radially-oriented ciliary muscle relaxes due to a predominance of sympathetic outflow, and cycloplegia develops. With relaxation of the ciliary spasm, pain is reduced. Atropine also blunts impulses from the sensory nerve endings of the cornea, which further contributes to pain relief.

Atropine sulfate is used in the form of a 1 % ointment or 0.5—1 % aqueous solution. Mydriasis begins within 15—20 minutes; the effect is maximal in about 2 hours and persists for up to 8 days.

Warm, moist compresses (40—50 °C) applied to the closed eyelids for 20—30 minutes several times daily are helpful in relieving pain and promoting absorption. After initial resistance, the horse should submit to this treatment. The compress is wetted with boiled water to which antiseptics may be added if desired. Atropine and heat applications also are extremely beneficial in promoting regeneration of the corneal epithelium.

In cases of *deep keratitis* (parenchymatous keratitis, keratitis profunda punctata) that have not developed from a superficial keratitis or been caused by the direct action of inflammatory agents (bacterial invasion, damage by toxins), an allergic reaction to infectious or toxic processes in the body should also be considered as a possible cause. Reactions of this type are common in the equine eye (cf. pathogenesis of 'moonblindness'). A diffuse, milky opacification of the cornea, possibly accompanied by stipple-like areas of increased opacity, is characteristic of corneal edema. Conjunctival and scleral vascular congestion appear a short time later as a sign of inflammation. The dense corneal opacities in such cases reflect a cellular infiltration in the form of fibroblasts (keratoblasts) and especially macrophages, which are responsible for eliminating some of the antigen (or toxic/infectious agent) that is present in the cornea.

The *course* varies with the cause. Inflammation that develops from chronic, superficial processes generally takes a refractory, usually chronic course that is characterized by vascularization and opacification. Not infrequently, infiltrates remain in the cornea causing dense, permanent opacities. Keratitis due to endogenous causes either regresses very quickly with a restoration of corneal transparency, or takes a more serious course characterized by purulent liquefaction due to invasion by secondary pathogens.

Treatment is always directed toward the primary disease.

In keratitis that is caused or perpetuated by exogenous influences, the primary concern, besides antibiotic coverage, is the restoration of epithelial continuity. All measures that enhance the regenerative capacity of the epithelium are beneficial in this regard (cf. treatment of superficial keratitis). Once epithelial continuity has been restored, exudative and infiltrative processes in the corneal tissue are inhibited by vigorous local treatment with glucocorticoids. Various preparations may be administered conjunctivally for this purpose: cortisone (1—2 % ointment or drops q. 3—4 h), hydrocortisone (0.5—1 % drop or ointment q. 3—4 h), and prednisone or prednisolone (0.25 % drop or 0.5—1.5 % ointment q. 6—8 h); 100 mg of a 1 % aqueous solution of cortisone or 50 mg hydrocortisone are suitable for subconjunctival use.

Chronic inflammation with associated dense infiltration is often highly refractory to treatment. The recommended procedure in such cases is first to convert the process to an acute condition by means of measures that promote hyperemia and lymph flow. These measures may be physical (heat) or pharmacologic (iodine in the form of tincture of iodine or 6—10 % aqueous potassium iodine solution, iodoform powder or 10 % iodoform ophthalmic ointment; hydrargyrum precipitatum in the form of 1 % white precipitate ointment and mercurous chloride (calomel), ethylmorphine hydrochloride (dionin), in ointment or drop form in increasing concentration from 1 to 10 %, ammonium sulfobituminosum contained in 2—5 % ichthyol ophthalmic ointment). Then, in a second treatment phase, it will be easier to remove the infiltrates by the local use of glucocorticoids.

Nonspecific protein therapy and antihistamines may be beneficial. Atropine is indicated to prevent the complications of an accompanying iritis and reduce pain.

In the event of purulent liquefaction, the conjunctival, subconjunctival and systemic administration of antibiotics is of prime concern (cf. treatment of conjunctivitis). Irrigation with mild antiseptics is done to remove pathogenic organisms and autolytic exudate. Hyperemia with physical (irrigations, compresses) and pharmacologic methods (white precipitate ointment, collargol, dionin = ethylmorphine hydrochloride) is recommended to aid absorption and regeneration.

With horses that resist repeated conjunctival medication, subpalpebral instillation is recommended. In this method the medicament is instilled through a length of soft plastic tubing that is inserted into the conjunctival sac, brought out through the upper eyelid via an artificial tissue channel, and fastened to the skin at some distance from the eye. The palpebral fissure is closed by suture after the tubing is inserted (fig. 2.1.15. — 10).

2.1.15.4.5. Diseases of the Uveal Tract

Examination. The uveal tract (vascular tunic) consists of the iris, ciliary body and choroid. Only the iris is completely accessible to direct examination. Points to be evaluated are the color of the iris, the relief of its surface features, and the pupil. Color deviations may be associated with congenital pigmentary abnormalities or inflammatory changes. The 'relief' of the iris (represented by the lattice structure of the iridal tissue and by muscular and vascular folds) is velvety or effaced when the iris is edematous, and inflammatory exudate may be present in the folds. Contour is lost in iridal atrophy. With respect to the pupil, points to note are its shape, margin, size and responsiveness. Deviations or irregularities of pupillary shape are a sign of lens-iris or cornea-iris adhesions. The pupillary margin should be freely mobile and show no discontinuities. The pupillary response to light is tested by interrupted light

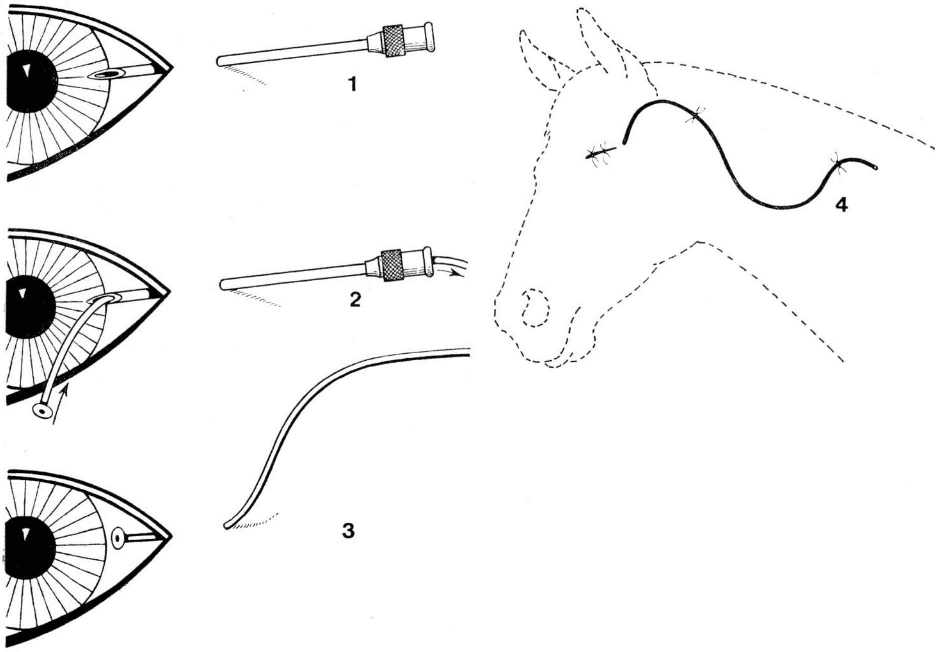

Fig. 2.1.15. — 10. Subpalpebral medication. *1* Creating a tissue channel with a large-gauge cannula; *2* Introducing a plastic tube through the cannula; *3* The plastic tube terminates in the conjunctival sac; *4* Situation following placement of the plastic tube.

stimuli that elicit a pupillary reflex (note that this reflex in itself is not proof of vision!).

A pathologic constriction of the pupil (miosis) may be spastic in nature [irritation of the pupillary sphincter due to inflammation of the uvea, trauma to the iris, cerebral disease, intoxication (morphine, urea), infection, or the administration of parasympathomimetics (eserine = physostigmine, pilocarpine)]. A paralytic miosis can be caused by paralysis of the pupillary dilator muscle, whose innervation is chiefly sympathetic. It is a sign of various conditions, including Horner's syndrome.

A pathologic dilatation of the pupil (mydriasis) may be spastic, due to irritation of the pupillary dilator (sympathetic nervous system irritation in epilepsy), or paralytic, due to paralysis of the pupillary sphincter associated with intoxication (e.g., solanine), inflammation of the retina or optic nerve, infections (e.g., tetanus, anthrax) or the use of parasympatholytic drugs (atropine, homatropine, scopolamine).

Disturbances of the pupillary reflex become evident only when there is a loss of function in the sphincter, which is more powerful than the dilator. The main sign of such disturbances is a dilated or fixed pupil, and the principal causes are damage to the retina and/or optic nerve, interruption of the reflex arc (reflex mydriasis), and insufficiency of the oculomotor nerve pathway (paralytic mydriasis).

As for the examination of the other two parts of the uveal tract, the ciliary body cannot be examined in life, and the retina-covered choroid can only be partially visualized during examination of the ocular fundus. Particular note should be taken

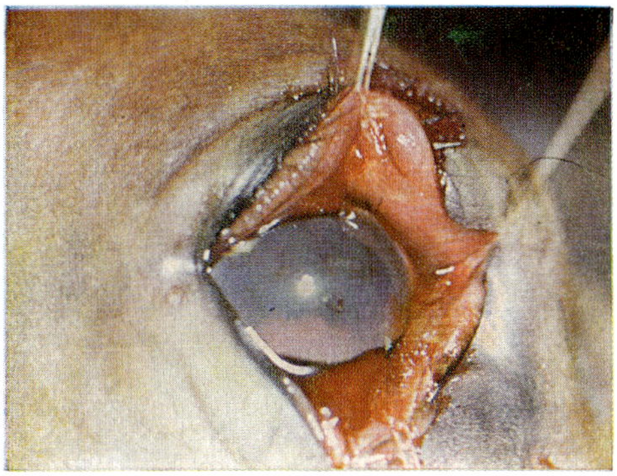

11

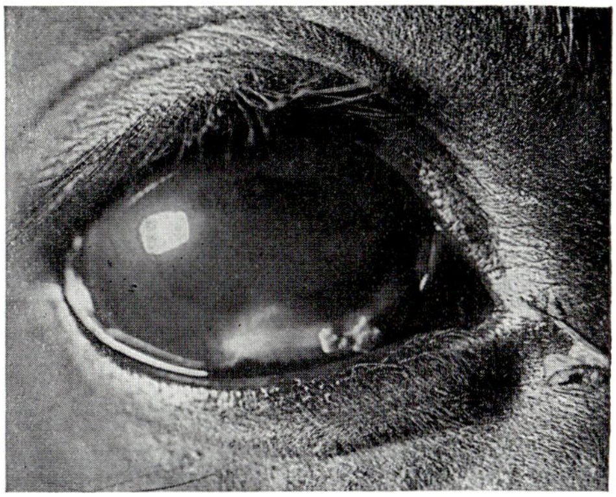

12

Fig. 2.1.15. — 11. Hemorrhagic iritis in foal septicemia.
Fig. 2.1.15. — 12. Acute periodic ophthalmia with exudate in the anterior chamber (pupil dilated by medication).

of color anomalies of the tapeta that may signify inflammatory, degenerative or atrophic processes or congenital pigmentary abnormalities.

Pigmentary abnormalities: Deficiencies of pigmentation are the most common pigment irregularities in the horse. Those involving the iris are the most easily recognized. The stroma is chiefly affected, displaying a bluish-gray to grayish-white color (the pigmented pars iridis of the retina is still present and creates a bluish sheen that is visible through the nonpigmented stroma). In some cases the entire iridal stroma is devoid of pigment ('glass eye', cf. Sec. 2.8.3.4.), but circumscribed depigmented areas are more commonly seen. In rare cases there is a difference of color in the two irides (heterochromia iridis). Depigmentation of the choroid appears to be more common than iridal depigmentation in the horse. If the entire choroid is involved, the nonpigmented fundus appears red when viewed through the pupil. Often, however, the depigmentation is partial and presents during the ophthalmoscopic examination as a focal depigmentation or 'tapetal island' confined mainly to the tapetum nigrum. Congenital depigmentation of the uveal tract is of no clinical importance.

Inflammatory changes: The three parts of the uvea (iris, ciliary body and choroid) are derived from the same germ layer and form a continuous structure. As a result, they can undergo very similar reactions, mainly inflammatory, those of endogenous origin being the most important in the horse. Involvement of the uvea is not uncommon in infectious diseases. For example, the hemorrhagic iritis that accompanies foal septicemia (fig. 2.1.15. — 11) is a consequence of the special vascular affinity of the organism and the rich vascularity of the uveal tract.

Periodic ophthalmia, known also by such names as recurrent uveitis, recurrent ophthalmia, recurrent lymphocytic iridocyclitis and 'moonblindness', is, as its name implies, an inflammatory condition of the middle tunic of the eye whose classic feature is the periodic recurrence of symptoms.

Periodic ophthalmia is a devastating disease in horses due to its effect on the animal's performance. It is regarded as a specific ophthalmic disease of equidae, although it is known that an endogenous, recurrent uveitis with similar symptoms also occurs in cattle.

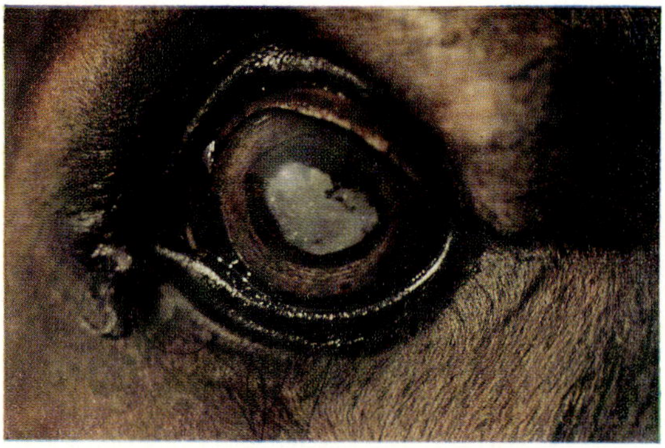

13

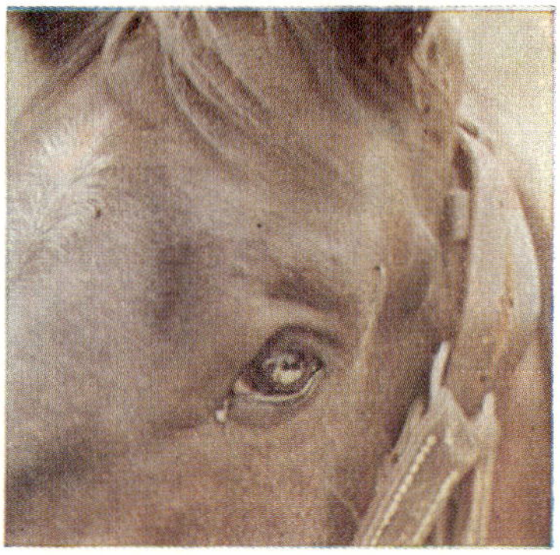

14

Fig. 2.1.15. — 13. Chronic periodic ophthalmia: adhesive iritis, secondary cataract.

Fig. 2.1.15. — 14. Late stage of chronic recurrent panuveitis: microphthalmia, prolapse of nictating membrane, third canthus, adhesive iritis, cataract.

Although the disease has been known and scientifically studied for many decades, its *etiology* remains something of a mystery. Besides hereditary, climatic and geographic factors, the following causes have been postulated:

— Autointoxication from the absorption of histamines or partially-degraded proteins as a consequence of digestive disturbances and/or the ingestion of spoiled feed or harmful food contaminants (mold, putrifaction and fermentation products);

— parasitic invasion (*Onchocerca cervicalis* microfilariae);

— leptospirosis *(L. grippotyphosa, L. pomona, L. icterohemorrhagiae);*

— viral infections, especially of the upper respiratory tract;

— bacterial infection.

Infectious organisms or parasites exert a direct pathogenic effect on the vascular tunic of the eye (strangles, foal septicemia), especially during an initial infection. However, much attention has been given recently to the possibility that the symptoms of recurrent endogenous uveitis in horses are based upon an anaphylactic reaction of the body and ocular tissues to the repeated and latent presence of certain substances, metabolic or degradation products, pathogenic organisms or their toxins. This would mean that all the factors mentioned above are of potential causal significance in the disease. Apparently, periodic ophthalmia is a symptomatic panuveitis which, as a result of inflammatory reactions in the uvea — an organ that responds exquisitely to immunologic processes — leads to general inflammation of the globe, i.e., to ophthalmia.

Symptoms and Course. The clinical picture is characterized by a paroxysmal, serofibrinous irodocyclochoroiditis with associated severe pain, sometimes accompanied by a mild conjunctivitis and keratitis. The course may be acute, subacute or chronic.

Acute attacks are manifested by a sudden photophobia, blepharospasm, increased warmth of the eyelids, heavy lacrimation, ciliary congestion, and possibly conjunctivitis and keratitis. As a rule, however, the symptoms become more severe during subsequent days and then show all the features of an iritis (fig. 2.1.15. — 12) such as loss of iridal contour, miosis, sluggish pupillary reflex, and fibrino-hemorrhagic exudation, first in the anterior uvea and shortly therafter in the choroid (floating vitreous opacities). There may be a mild systemic reaction with a 1 °C rise of body temperature. After a peak is reached on about day 5, the inflammatory symptoms gradually regress, and the attack is over by about day 14. At that time the eye appears healthy, and only ophthalmoscopic examination will disclose residual signs of inflammation (loss of iridal relief, sluggish pupillary reflex, vitreous opacity, focal infiltration of the choroid).

In exceptional cases the attacks are of longer duration, sometimes lasting 6 to 8 weeks (subacute form). The clinical picture in such cases is dominated by exudative inflammation of the iris without further local or systemic signs. Subacute, protracted cases characterized by an exudative iritis lasting for up to 2 months are very rare.

If acute symptoms regress quickly, the next attack will probably occur in 4—6 weeks and may in turn be followed by subsequent attacks that initially occur at approximately equal intervals but later tend to become less frequent.

The reactive changes in such cases progressively assume a chronic character and present as an adhesive iritis with the development of lens-iris adhesions. The iris loses contour and becomes atrophic, the pupil becomes distorted and irregular, and the pupillary margin acquires a frayed appearance (fig. 2.1.15. — 13). Irregular, brown shreds of lenticular tissue can be seen on the lens surface. A diffuse opacity of the lens develops with accompanying points or streaks of increased opacity. Dislocation of the lens sometimes occurs. The choroid, retina and optic nerve progressively undergo first inflammatory, then degenerative changes that ultimately lead to blindness. In the final stage the globe softens and becomes atrophic (fig. 2.1.15. — 14).

Initially, disease symptoms are usually limited to one eye. The other eye may become involved during the course of subsequent attacks. The course described is a common one, although it is possible for severe, chronic changes to develop after only the first attack. The disease apparently has its highest incidence in animals less than 7 years old.

Even with clinical recovery, the *prognosis* is guarded due to the likelihood of a recurrence. The more severe the inflammatory symptoms, the less favorable the prognosis in terms of preservation of vision.

Treatment. Treatment encompasses both local and systemic measures. Local measures include:

— heat in the form of warm dressings or compresses (for 30 min several times daily) to relieve pain and promote absorption;

— atropine (1 % solution, 2 drops twice daily) to induce mydriasis and prevent synechiae;

— glucocorticoids, initially combined with antibiotics, to reduce inflammation (applied conjunctivally several times daily, later applied subconjunctivally).

Systemic treatment consists in the administration of antihistamines and glucocorticoids to minimize the allergic response. Nonspecific protein therapy is also recommended. Antibiotics are administered parenterally to control infection. Absorption is enhanced by systemic osmotherapy, i.e., the administration of concentrated solutions (40 % glucose, 10 % calcium chloride), diuretics and potassium iodate (8 g/d for 5 days).

Prophylactic measures are dictated by the suspected cause. The feeding of moldy or spoiled feeds should be avoided. Leptospiral infections can be controlled by eradicating the intermediate hosts (mice, rats) or by avoiding contact with infected wild and domestic animal species. Allergenic foci of infection in the body should be cured by local or systemic measures. Riboflavin (40 mg/d given with the feed) is reportedly effective in preventing new outbreaks. General measures include the elimination of resistance-lowering factors (poor care, poor nutrition, overexertion, parasitism, etc.) and adherence to hygienic practices.

2.1.15.4.6. Diseases of the Lens

Examination. Pathologic conditions of the lens affect mainly its transparency and position. The lens is examined in incident light and by transillumination using daylight, a lamp with focused light or an ophthalmoscope with the pupil widely dilated. A transparent or nearly transparent lens can be examined with the aid of Purkinje-Sanson mirror images (principle: formation of reflected images at optical interfaces). Besides the clear and well-defined corneal image, a virtual, noninverted image is visible on the anterior lens surface, and a real, inverted image is visible on the posterior lens surface in the normal eye.

Sometimes fissures develop between the cortex and nucleus of the lens, causing double lenticular images to be produced (= presence of additional optical interfaces).

In aphakia (absence of the lens), no lenticular images are formed. A second mirror image, if present, represents the anterior border of the vitreous body. In this case details of the ocular fundus are visible in incident light without the aid of an ophthalmoscope, and they do not appear magnified.

The lens can be examined for opacities using incident light. True cataracts are grayish-white in color, while false cataracts appear brown or black. Lens opacities are always rigid and immobile. Dislocation of the lens leads to alterations of refraction and reflection. A lens that has luxated into the anterior chamber magnifies the portion of the iris that it covers when direct illumination is applied (assuming a transparent cornea).

With luxation of the lens into the vitreous body, a crescent-shaped area of lens-free pupil appears over the sharply-defined lens equator. The ocular fundus is clearly visible through this area without an ophthalmoscope, and its features do not appear magnified (absence of lenticular magnification).

Cataracts. Congenital cataracts in the horse may be based upon abnormalites of the germ layer itself or upon secondary damage to the lens. Because congenital cataracts often show a breed and familial predilection, a genetic influence is presumed. The cataracts present as bluish-white or milky opacities of variable shape that arise in the central embryonic nucleus or cortex. In cataracts of the central embryonic nucleus, the lens remains soft and contains circumscribed areas of compaction in addition to liquified material. 'Sutural cataracts' (cortical cataracts) present clinically as sharply-circumscribed, regular, white opacities located in the pole of the lens. Frequently the opacities assume a Y-shape in accordance with the triradiate sutural lines of the lens. They are found in the cortex or beneath the capsule and sometimes are composed of minute punctate or vesicular opacities. They remain visible on transillumination and differ in this respect from the 'sutural reflex', an apparent opacity produced by a change of refraction under incident light. Sharply-circumscribed sutural cataracts apparently do not have a serious effect on vision. Nuclear cataracts, on the other hand, can cause significant visual impairment. Vision can be improved in such cases by aspirating the cataractous material. For this purpose the bulbar conjunctiva is dissected free, an incision is made through the sclera adjacent to the limbus at the 12 o'clock position, a large-gauge cannula is inserted through this incision into the globe and into the lens, and the cataractous lens material is aspirated. Then the small incisional wound is closed by attaching the prepared conjunctival flap to its edges. The lens capsule remaining in the eye will undergo imbibition and eventual absorption. A lens-induced uveitis resulting from the release of lens proteins (which act as foreign proteins) is prevented by local and systemic corticosteroid therapy.

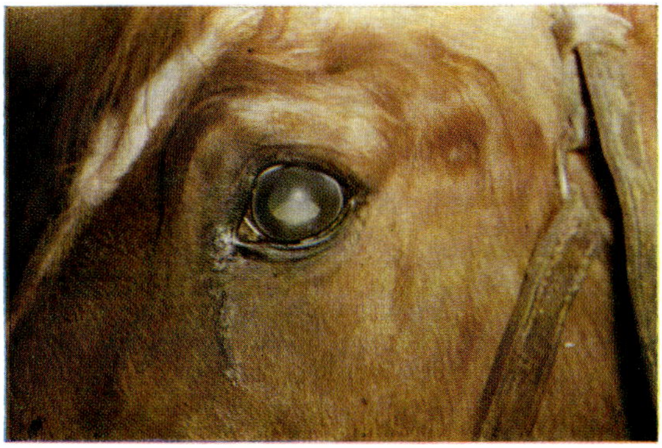

Fig. 2.1.15. — 15. Posterior luxation of the lens.

Acquired cataracts in the horse most frequently develop secondarily to periodic ophthalmia and may be associated with lens luxation (fig. 2.1.15. — 15). The lens opacity and luxation in such cases are symptoms of profound, irreversible, pathologic ocular changes. No special lenticular therapy is indicated.

2.1.15.4.7. Diseases of the Vitreous Body

Examination. The recognition of vitreous changes depends both on the experience of the examiner and, to a large degree, on the examination technique and apparatus used. Useful results are obtained when the vitreous body is transilluminated with a focal light source (Zeiss penlight, otoscope, etc.) by holding the light source between the animal's nostril and the examiner's temple and pointing it in a rostrodorsal direction. The physiologic transparency of the vitreous can be altered by the presence of cholesterol crystals (synchysis scintillans), which sometimes is congenital, as well as by pathologic conditions that are associated with exudative inflammation and affect mainly the choroid or retina. In this case the vitreous substance, which is liquefied or altered in its consistency, contains exudates (blood, fibrin, pus) in the form of very small conglomerates which swirl when the head is moved rapidly (main criterion for differentiation from fixed lens opacities), mobile or oscillating intravitreal strands or membranes, or a diffuse collection of exudate that renders the vitreous nontransparent. In some circumstances the entire vitreous body may appear red as a result of extravasation or vascular congestion. The presence of grayish-yellow strands or filaments coursing between the lens and optic papilla in the mature horse may be indicative of a persistent hyaloid artery. On the other hand, in 70 % of all newborn foals these membranes simply represent a regressing hyaloid vessel and so are not considered abnormal.

Pathologic vitreous inclusions: Perforating injuries of the eye can allow foreign bodies to enter the vitreous. Depending on their chemical properties, these bodies may cause no reaction (glass, stone), or they may evoke an inflammatory response (wood), undergo a reaction with the moist environment (metals), or lead to infection and suppurative inflammation through the introduction of pathogenic organisms. Foreign bodies that cause no immediate reaction remain embedded in the eye until reactive changes occur. Infections are difficult to control and are an indication for vigorous local and systemic therapy. If treatment is unsuccessful, enucleation is indicated.

Intravitreal hemorrhages occur as a result of traumatic vascular lesions associated with violence to the eye or surgical procedures in or around the eye, or may be a symptom of inflammatory diseases of the ocular tissue based on infectious or toxic processes. Sometimes the entire vitreous body is suffused with blood (hemophthalmos) and appears bright red, reddish-brown or dark and opaque, depending on when the extravasation occurred. The pupillary orifice is red, and vision is seriously impaired or abolished. As the condition progresses, there may be destruction of the fibrillary framework of the vitreous, liquefaction of the vitreous, or the formation of dense vitreous opacities with subsequent retinal detachment or degeneration. If massive extravasations are absorbed, indurated membranes may remain which traverse the vitreous body, abut against the posterior lens surface and cause considerable vision impairment.

Besides therapy directed at the cause, there are various primary measures that can reduce extravasation in cases of acute intravitreal hemorrhage: the application of cold dressings or compresses, the administration of substances that reduce vascular permeability and promote coagulation (ascorvit, calcium, vitamin K, rutabion, etc.), and immobilization of the eye. Once the hemorrhage is controlled, measures are taken to promote its absorption. This can be done with warm compresses, irradiation (shortwave, ultrasound), subconjunctival injections of hypertonic saline, retrobulbar injections of streptokinase or hyaluronidase preparations, or the conjunctival administration of 2% potassium iodide or diethylmorphine-containing ophthalmic ointments or drops.

Liquefaction of the vitreous body: Liquefaction of the vitreous body (synchysis corporis vitrei) is mainly observed in animals with periodic ophthalmia. It has been found that the liquefaction originates in the nasodorsal region in such cases. The exudative products of uveal inflammation appear as opaque points, specks or filaments that swirl gently within the vitreous. Initially, foci of liquefaction form in the nuclear region of the vitreous body and spread outward, but they do not involve the more dense cortical zone. This is accompanied by a concomitant degeneration of the fibrillary framework, which then forms a free-floating opacity in the fluid. The liquefaction reduces the intraocular pressure and predisposes to luxation of the lens as well as to partial or nearly complete detachment of the retina (affecting all but the papillary region). The consequences are vision impairment and bulbar atrophy.

Age-dependent liquefaction of the vitreous body occurring in horses more than 10 years of age takes a gradual course and causes minimal vision impairment. Liquefaction of the vitreous does not respond to therapy.

2.1.15.4.8. Diseases of the Retina and Optic Nerve

Examination. Examination of the ocular fundus (portions of the retina, choroid and optic disc) serves to disclose grossly visible changes of the choroid and retina and is done exclusively by ophthalmoscopy. The prior induction of mydriasis is recommended.

Three parts can be distinguished in the ocular fundus (eyeground) of the horse:

— The triangular or hemispheric tapetum lucidum; this structure is located in the upper half of the fundus, is pale yellow-green to light blue in color and presents numerous violet-red dots representing vascular rami of the choriocapillary layer.

— The optic disc (optic papilla), which represents the entrance of the optic nerve; it is located in the tapetum-free area near the margin of the tapetum lucidum, has a transverse oval shape, is orange-red in color with a dark-shaded center, and has a light ring-shaped border (representing the nerve sheath).

Vessels: peripheral, radial arrangement of thin papillary vessels which extend past the disc margin and are lost in the periphery.

— The nontapetal area making up the remaining portion of the fundus; it is brownish with red, olive-green or black hues.

Points to be noted in particular are color anomalies of the tapetal and nontapetal portion of the fundus and optic disc, as well as abnormalities of disc shape, vascular course and vascular filling. These may denote pathologic states which affect the retina and/or choroid and account for specific functional losses.

Retinitis: Inflammation of the retina is rarely confined to the retina alone, but usually is associated with inflammatory changes of the uveal tract or optic nerve (chorioretinitis, papilloretinitis).

The etiology may be unknown, or the inflammation may develop either from the extension of pathologic processes affecting neighboring ocular structures (retinitis per continuitatem) or from encephalotropic viral infections (Borna disease).

Symptoms. In acute cases there is marked irritation manifested by photophobia, conjunctival and episcleral vascular congestion, and lacrimation. On ophthalmoscopy, fundus details appear hazy (due to exudation or hemorrhage), the vitreous body is clouded, and the pupil is narrow. The arteries and veins of the fundus are tortuous and distended. Irreparable inflammatory states lead to the degeneration of portions of the retina and are characterized by depigmented spots or areas of varying size with an indistinct vascular pattern. The pupil in this case is fixed and dilated, and there are varying degrees of vision impairment depending on the extent of the inflammatory changes.

Treatment. The subjective symptoms of acute retinitis can be relieved by shielding the eye from light, preferably by placing the horse in a darkened room. The absorption of exudates is promoted by local subconjunctival injections of hypertonic saline, heat application with compresses, systemic osmotherapy, and salicylic acid preparations. A short time later, retrobulbar and subconjunctival injections are highly effective, and soluble glucocorticoids are indicated. Vascular permeability can be reduced by giving vitamin C and calcium preparations systemically, and the administration of vitamin K may aid cases of hemorrhagic exudation. Vitamin A and B preparations can be given to enhance retinal function. Metastatic infections and retinal involvement in systemic diseases require appropriate systemic therapy.

Retinal hemorrhage: Retinal hemorrhages most commonly result from contusions of the globe due to trauma but may also occur in connection with inflammation of the choroid (periodic ophthalmia) and systemic diseases that increase hemorrhagic tendency (foal septicemia).

Ophthalmoscopy reveals striate or spotty fundus discoloration that is irregular in outline. Initially it is reddish in color, later becoming brownish-yellow and finally gray-white. Smaller extravasations are eventually absorbed without visible clinical consequences, while larger extravasations can lead to retinal detachment, vitreous opacities and vision impairment.

Treatment is analogous to the absorption-promoting regimen used in retinitis, and also includes primary measures to control bleeding.

Retinal detachment is caused mainly by choroid exudation or hemorrhage but may also result from intraocular tensile forces (contraction of the vitreous body, lens luxation or extraction, atrophy of the ciliary body, fibrous organization of intraocular inflammatory products or blood clots, proliferative retinal-vitreous changes, fall of intraocular pressure) (cf. Sec. 2.8.3.3.).

Treatment is at present limited almost exclusively to conservative measures aimed at promoting the absorption of exudates and immobilizing the eye for the purpose of avoiding further detachment. The primary disease is also treated.

Atrophy of the optic nerve and optic disc in the horse represents the final stage of destructive processes involving the globe, retina, choroid and optic nerve. Objective and subjective symptoms of a mild or severe vision impairment or blindness are present, depending on the extent and duration of the atrophy. The pupillary reflex is sluggish or absent. Atrophy of the optic disc can be detected by ophthalmoscopy only in the advanced stage, at which point the disc appears pale, yellowish-white, gray-white or stark white. Its size is diminished, and its margins are partially indrawn or have a ragged appearance. Treatment is futile if the atrophy is complete.

2.1.15.4.9. Diseases of the Globe and Orbit

Examination. Examination of the globe as a whole includes a careful evaluation of the area surrounding the eye, and of the entire side of the head if possible. This will disclose any asymmetry of the head or bony orbit in the form of protrusion, enlargement or indentation. Note should be taken of skin changes in the form of excoriations, scars, discharge tracks, etc.

The globe is assessed with regard to its size (microphthalmos, macrophthalmos), mobility (nystagmus) and the position of the ocular axis (strabism), taking into account species peculiarities.

Inflammatory conditions of the orbit: Inflammation of the bony orbit (orbital periostitis and ostitis) usually results from the spread of inflammatory or suppurative processes from adjacent areas, especially inflammation of the nasal cavities and the maxillary and frontal sinuses, strangles, etc. This spread of inflammation is promoted by the venous plexus of the basal orbital region, which communicates with the veins of the nose, paranasal sinuses and cerebral network (sinus cavernosus). The main clinical feature is tenderness of the orbital region to pressure. Swelling of the eyelids (collateral edema) and chemosis are sometimes observed.

Treatment is directed toward the precipitating cause. Diseased teeth are extracted, sinus empyema is drained, abscesses are incised, and necrotic portions of the bony orbit are removed.

Local and systemic antibiotics are administered.

Injuries of the orbit are caused mainly by direct or indirect trauma, such as kicks or blows. They create disruption in the continuity of tissues of the orbital cavity and of the orbital contents, very often associated with wounds of the eyelids and orbital skin. An accurate diagnosis is crucial if a specific *treatment* is to be rendered. Radiographic examination is of much help in this regard.

Treatment follows the general surgical principles. Foreign bodies should always be removed if possible, as they may lead to orbital tissue irritation and fistulization. Eyelid wounds should always be sutured in the interest of preserving lid function. Open treatment is indicated for all other deep wounds of the immediate orbital region.

Orbital cellulitis is a complication of injuries to periocular tissues and the ocular appendages. It involves an inflammation of the orbital tissue with infiltration and purulent liquefaction of retrobulbar tissues, sometimes with extension to the cavernous sinus and meninges (owing to the common venous network).

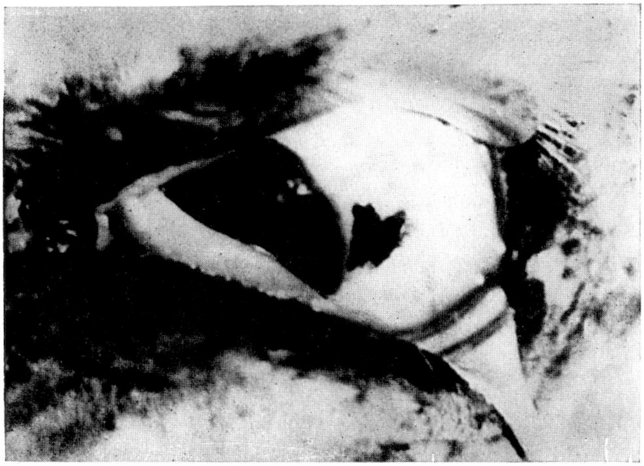

Fig. 2.1.15. — 16. Enophthalmos in tetanus, with prolapsed nictating membrane.

Clinically, orbital cellulitis is marked by extensive swelling of the tissues surrounding the eye, especially the lids. There is marked heat and tenderness to pressure in the orbital region. Very often feed is refused on account of pain associated with mastication. A general temperature elevation is sometimes present. The eyeball protrudes and is reduced in its mobility. Vision may be impaired due to compression of the optic nerve, circulatory disturbances or neuritis. The vessels of the fundus and optic disc appear congested on ophthalmoscopic inspection. In unfavorable cases the causal organisms may gain entry to the globe and cause a panophthalmitis. Involvement of the basal venous network leads to orbital thrombophlebitis.

The *prognosis* is guarded to poor due to the variety of complications that may arise.

Treatment must be prompt, vigorous, and aimed at eliminating or localizing the purulent liquefactive process. This can be achieved by stimulating local hyperemia (using physical or pharmacologic means) and by the topical and systemic use of antibiotics and sulfonamides. Open treatment is indicated for infected wounds. Abscesses should be incised after the acute inflammatory swelling has passed, and managed by open treatment according to general surgical principles.

Exophthalmos: Protrusion of the globe (exophthalmos) is either the result of space-occupying lesions of the orbital cavity or an enlargement of the globe itself. Not infrequently, protrusion of the globe is combined with lateral deviation and a reduction of ocular mobility.

Besides inflammatory conditions of the orbit (orbital cellulitis) and injuries with retrobulbar hemorrhage, the major causes of exophthalmos in the horse are neoplasms that displace the eye either through retrobulbar extension from a paranasal sinus or through enlargement of a carcinoma or sarcoma of the eyelid or nictating membrane.

The *prognosis* is favorable in terms of eye preservation only if the tumor is readily accessible to surgery and can be extirpated in its entirety. In all other cases the eye will eventually be lost as a result of tumor invasion.

The *treatment* for accessible, early-stage tumors consists of total removal by surgical excision or cryosurgery. Tumors that have spread to involve the globe or are situated behind the globe will necessitate enucleation. Tumors of the bony orbit or paranasal sinuses are inoperable as a rule.

Enophthalmos (recession of the globe) is based upon either a real increase in the volume of the orbital cavity due to fractures of the orbital bone, a reduction in the volume of retrobulbar tissues (as in cachexia), or spastic contraction of the retractor bulbi muscle associated with painful conditions of the eye or tetanus (fig. 2.1.15. — 16). It is also seen in cases of congenital or acquired small globe (fig. 2.1.15. — 14), paralysis of the cervical motor sympathetic chain (including ptosis and miosis = Horner's syndrome) as a result of trauma, destructive neoplasms in the region of the neck and thoracic inlet, or a stellate ganglion blockade done for the purpose of inducing hyperemia (fig. 2.1.15. — 4).

Symptoms. The globe is deeply recessed in the orbital cavity. Eversion of the lower eyelid (ectropion) and drooping of the upper eyelid (ptosis) are sometimes present. The animal tries to keep the eye open through sustained contraction of the levator palpebrae muscle, which eventually leads to the formation of a 'third canthus' (fig. 2.1.15. — 14).

The prognosis and treatment are determined by the primary disease.

References

Ammann, K.; Müller, A.: Das Bild des normalen Augenhintergrundes beim Pferd. Berliner Münchener Tierärztl. Wschr. *81:* 370 (1968).

Barron, C. N.; Saunders, L. Z.: Intraocular tumors in animals. II. Primary non-pigmented intraocular tumors. Cancer Res. *19:* 1171 (1959).

Barron, C. N.; Saunders, L. Z.; Jubb, K. V.: Intraocular tumors in animals. III. Secondary intraocular tumors. Amer. J. vet. Res. *24:* 835 (1963).

Bayer, J.: Tierärztliche Augenheilkunde (Braumüller, Wien 1914).

Bentz, H.; Klaus, H.; Richter, J.; Münchow, P.: Rezeptformeln für die Veterinärmedizin (VEB Gustav Fischer Verlag, Jena 1966).

Bistner, S.; Wiebe, E.: Traumatic panophthalmitis in a horse. Cornell Vet. *61:* 415 (1971).

Böke, W.: Der Einfluss der Nebennieren-Corticoide auf die entzündlichen Reaktionen des Auges (VEB Georg Thieme, Leipzig 1960).

Bruce, D. F. M.: The use of the ophthalmoscope in veterinary practice. Vet. Med. *50:* 599 (1955).

Cohen, Ch. M.; Reinke, D. A.: Equine tonometry. J. Amer. vet. med. Assoc. *156:* 1884 (1970).

Eichholtz, F.: Lehrbuch der Pharmakologie (Springer, Berlin 1957).

Eriksson, K.: Hereditary aniridia with secondary cataract in horses. Nord. Vet.-Med. *7* (1955).

Farris, H. E.; Fraunfelder, F. T.; Mason, C. T.: Cryotherapy of equine sarcoid and other lesions. Vet. Med. and Small Animal Clinician *71:* 325 (1976).

Formston, C.: Examination of the eye with special reference to the horse and dog. Vet. Rec. *68:* 984 (1956).

Formston, C.: Keratitis in animals. In: Aspects of Comparative Ophthalmology. Proc. of a Symposium org. by the Brit. Small Animal. Vet. Assoc. (Pergamon Press, Oxford 1965).

Frank, A.; Marolt, J.: Mikroskopische Veränderungen am Auge bei der symptomatischen periodischen Augenentzündung der Pferde und Rinder. Dtsch. Tierärztl. Wschr. *77:* 207 (1970).

Friedenwald, J. S.; Buschke, W.: Mitotic and wound healing activities of the corneal epithelium. Arch. Ophthalmol. *32:* 410 (1944).

Fröhner, E.; Neumann-Kleinpaul, K.; Dobberstein, J.: Lehrbuch der Gerichtlichen Tierheilkunde, 11. Aufl., S. 70 (Parey, Berlin 1955).

Gelatt, K. N.: Blepharoplastic procedures in horses. J. Amer. vet. med. Assoc. *151:* 27 (1967).

Gelatt, K. N.: Postoperative subpalpebral medications in horses and dogs. Vet. Med. and Small Animal Clinician *62:* 1165 (1967).

Gelatt, K. N.: Veterinary ophthalmic pharmacology and therapeutics. 1. Introduction. Vet. Med. and Small Animal Clinician *63:* 547 (1968).

Gelatt, K. N.: Veterinary ophthalmic pharmacology and therapeutics. 2. Topical anesthetics. Vet. Med. and Small Animal Clinician *63:* 751 (1968).

GELATT, K. N.: Veterinary ophthalmic pharmacology and therapeutics. 3. Antimicrobial agents. Vet. Med. and Small Animal Clinician *63:* 892 (1968).

GELATT, K. N.: Pseudomonas ulcerative keratitis and abscess in a horse. Vet. Med. and Small Animal Clinician *69:* 1309 (1974).

GELATT, K. N.: Corneolimbal squamous cell carcinoma in a horse. Vet. Med. and Small Animal Clinician *70:* 53 (1975).

GELATT, K. N.; FINOCCHIO, E. J.: Variations on the normal equine eye. Vet. Med. and Small Animal Clinician *65:* 569 (1970).

GELATT, K. N.; KRAFT, W. E.: A technic for aspiration of cataracts in young horses. Vet. Med. and Small Animal Clinician *64:* 415 (1969).

GELATT, K. N.; MYERS jr., V. S.; MCCLURE jr., J. R.: Aspiration of congenital and soft cataracts in foals and young horses. J. Amer. vet. med. Assoc. *165:* 611 (1974).

GORDON, D. M.: The clinical use of corticotropin, cortisone and hydrocortisone in eye disease (Charles C. Thomas, Springfield 1954).

GUNDERSON, TH.: Vascular obliteration for various types epithelium. Arch. Ophthalmol. *21:* 76 (1939); ref. Zbl. ges. Ophthalmol. *43:* 502 (1939).

HAMM, K.: Neurofibrome der Retina an beiden Augen eines Pferdes. Wien. tierärztl. Mschr. *46:* 117 (1959).

HATZIOLOS, B. C.; SASS, B.; ALBERT, TH. F.; STEVENSON, M. C.: Ocular changes in a horse with gutturomycosis. J. Amer. vet. med. Assoc. *167:* 51 (1975).

HEUSSER, H.: Über Flecken und Vaskularisation der Hornhaut des Pferdes. Vet.-med. Habil.-Schrift, Zürich (1921).

HILBERT, B. J.; FARRELL, R. K.; GRANT, B. D.: Cryotherapy of periocular squamous cell carcinoma in the horse. J. Amer. vet. med. Assoc. *170:* 1305 (1977).

HURTIENNE, H.: Klinische Diagnostik bei Glaskörperveränderungen des Pferdes. Dtsch. Tierärztl. Wschr. *79:* 537 (1972).

JONES, T. C.: Riboflavin and the control of periodic ophthalmia. J. Amer. vet. med. Assoc. *114:* 326 (1949).

KAMER, O.: Über Farbanomalien im Augenhintergrund von Haustieren. Schweiz. Arch. Tierheilk. *102:* 501 (1960).

KAMPEN, K. R. VAN; JAMES, L. F.: Ophthalmic lesions in locoweed poisoning of cattle, sheep and horses. Amer. J. Vet. Res. *32:* 1293 (1971).

KNILL, L. M.; EAGLETON, R. D.; HARVER, E.: Physical optics of the equine eye. Amer. J. Vet. Res. *38:* 735 (1977).

KOLB, E.: Lehrbuch der Physiologie der Haustiere, 2. Aufl. (VEB Gustav Fischer Verlag, Jena 1967).

KOMAR, G.; SZUTTER, L.: Tierärztliche Augenheilkunde (Akadémiai Kiadó, Budapest 1968).

KRAWITZ, L.: Clinical examination of the canine and feline eye. J. Amer. vet. med. Assoc. *147:* 33 (1965).

KRUININGEN, J. H. VAN: Intracapsular cataract in the horse. J. Amer. vet. med. Assoc. *145:* 773 (1964).

LAHUNTA, A. DE: CUMMINGS, J. F.: Neuro-ophthalmologic lesions as a cause of visual deficit in dogs and horses. J. Amer. vet. med. Assoc. *150:* 994 (1967).

LEOPOLD, J. H.; KROMAN, H. S.; GREEN, H.: Intraocular penetration of prednisone and prednisolone. Transact. Amer. Acad. Ophthalmol. Otolaryng. *59:* 771 (1955).

MAGRANE, W. G.: Cortisone in ophthalmology. Amer. Vet. *32:* 763 (1951).

MAGRANE, W. G.: Periodic ophthalmia. Progress in Equine Practice *328* (Amer. Public. Inc., Wheaton/Ill. 1966).

MAKSIMOVIĆ, B.: Akinesie des M. orbicularis oculi bei Rind, Pferd und Hund. Vet.-med. Diss., Belgrad (1953).

MAROLT, J.: Die periodische Ophthalmie als ein Symptom von Viruskrankheiten bei Pferd und Rind. Ein Vorschlag für entsprechende forensische Beurteilung und eine Namensänderung. Dtsch. Tierärztl. Wschr. *75:* 189 (1968).

MAROLT, J.; BEGO, U.; FRANK, A.; MATICIK, Z.: Beitrag zur Ptose und Akinesie des M. orbicularis oculi beim Pferd. Dtsch. Tierärztl. Wschr. *78:* 378 (1971).

MITCHELL, J. S.; ATTLEBERGER, M. H.: Fusarium keratomycosis in the horse. Vet. Med. and Small Animal Clinician *68:* 1257 (1973).

MORGAN, J.: Ocular tumours in animals. J. small Anim. Pract. *10:* 563 (1969).

MUSSCHE, A.; VANDERVELDE, A.: Atresie van de onderste afvoeropening van het traankanaal bij een paard. Vlaams Diergeneeskd. Tidskr. *30:* 302 (1963).

OHMS, K.-D.: Der Hornhautastigmatismus und sein Vorkommen bei den Haustieren unter besonderer Berücksichtigung des Pferdeauges. Vet.-med. Diss., Leipzig (1950).

OKSALA, A.: Das Echogramm in der Diagnostik von Augenkrankheiten. Klin. Zbl. Augenhk. *137:* 72 (1960).

PRINCE, J. H.; DIESEM, C. D.; EGLITIS, I.; RUSKELL, G. L.: Anatomy and histology of the eye and orbit in domestic animals (Thomas, Springfield/Ill. 1960).

RIESE, K.: Veränderungen des Glaskörpers beim Pferd. Literatur, klinische und biochemische Untersuchungen. Vet.-med. Diss., Hannover (1974).

ROBERTS, E. J.: Some modern surgical operations applicable to the horse. Vet. Rec. *76:* 137 (1964).

ROBERTS, S. R.: Animal vision. J. Amer. vet. med. Assoc. *127:* 236 (1955).

ROBERTS, S. R.: A system of testing vision in animals. J. Amer. vet. med. Assoc. *128:* 544 (1956).

ROHEN, J. W.: Das Auge und seine Hilfsorgane; in MÖLLENDORF; BARGMANN, Handbuch der mikroskopischen Anatomie des Menschen (Springer, Berlin 1964).

ROESTI, W.: Über Drusenbildung am Sehnervenkopf des Pferdes — Neuritis exsudativa nervi optici. Arch. Tierheilk. *77:* 81 (1941).

RUBIN, L. F.: Indirect ophthalmoscopy in veterinary medicine. J. Amer. vet. med. Assoc. *137:* 648 (1960).

SAUNDERS, L. Z.: Pathology of the eye of domestic animals (Parey, Berlin 1968).

SCHLEITER, H.; DIETZ, O.: Antibiose am und im Bulbus unter besonderer Berücksichtigung der Blut-Kammerwasser-Schranke. Wien. tierärztl. Mschr. *44:* 641 (1957).

SCHMIDT, TH.: Über fixe und flotierende Membranen im Glaskörperraum des Pferdeauges. Mh. prakt. Tierhk. *17:* 166 (1905).

SMYTHE, R. H.: Veterinary ophthalmology (Baillière, Tindall and Cox, London 1958).

STEHLE, O.: Histopathologische Untersuchungen der Sehbahn bei Erblindungen ohne äusserlich erkennbare Ursache (Amaurose). Vet.-med. Diss., München (1939).

STRUBE, G.: Literaturstudie über Ätiologie, Diagnostik und Therapie der ‚Periodischen Augenentzündung der Pferde'. Vet.-med. Diss., Hannover (1971).

SZÚTTER, L.: Die bläschen- und sternförmigen Linsenstare des Pferdeauges. Vet.-med. Diss., Budapest (1924).

SZÚTTER, L.: Untersuchungen über die Pigmentmangelflecke im Augenhintergrund der Pferde. Acta vet. Acad. Sci. Hung. *7:* 329 (1957).

SZÚTTER, L.: Ophthalmoskopische und Lupenspiegeluntersuchungen an neugeborenen Haustieren. Acta Veterin. Acad. Sci. Hung. *10:* 45 (1961).

SZÚTTER, L.: Ophthalmoskopische und Lupenspiegeluntersuchungen an neugeborenen Haustieren, I—II. Acta. Vet. Acad. Sci. Hung. *11:* 183 (1961).

ÜBERREITER, O.: Die Mikroskopie am lebenden Tierauge mit einer Spezialspaltlampe. XV. Internat. Tierärztekongr., Stockholm 1953, Teil II, S. 366.

ÜBERREITER, O.; DREIER, H.: Der Y-Star (Embryonalstar) beim Pferde. Wien. tierärztl. Mschr. *27:* 1 (1940).

ÜBERREITER, O.; KÖHLER, H.: Primäre Tumoren der Cornea. Wien. tierärztl. Mschr. *50:* 70 (1963).

UVAROV, O.: Corticosteroids in veterinary medicine. Vet. Rec. *71:* 335 (1959).

VIERHELLER, R.: Clinical experiences with indirect ophthalmoscopy. Mod. vet. Pract. *47:* 41 (1966).

WEBER, W.: Angeborener Star, eine rezessive Mutation beim Pferd. Schweiz. Arch. Tierhk. *89:* 397 (1947).

WIESNER, E.; WILLER, S.: Veterinärmedizinische Pathogenetik (VEB Gustav Fischer Verlag, Jena 1974).

WILDI, G.: Vergleichend-anatomische Untersuchungen am Spaltlampenmikroskop über die Persistenz des Canalis hyaloideus mit besonderer Berücksichtigung der sogenannten Bogenlinien und der Linsennähte. Vet.-med. Diss., Zürich (1924).

WOODS, A. C.: Endogenous inflammations of the uveal tract (Williams and Wilkins, Baltimore 1961).
WYMAN, M.: Surgery of the cornea and anterior segment of the horse's eye. J. Amer. vet. med. Assoc. *153:* 1703 (1968).
ZIMMERMANN, L. E.: Lens-induced inflammation in human eyes; in MAUMENSEE; SILVERSTEIN, Immunopathology of uveitis (Williams and Wilkins, Baltimore 1964).

2.1.16. Diseases of the Ear

2.1.16.1. Diseases of the Earflap

2.1.16.1.1. Othematoma (Hematoma of the Ear)

Definition. Othematoma, or hematoma auris, is a subcutaneous hematoma of the inner or outer surface of the earflap resulting from a prior contusion. It is relatively rare in the horse but is occasionally seen in ponies.

Symptoms. The head is carried at an angle with the affected side lowermost. Head shaking is frequent due to the weight of the hematoma. In most cases a round to oval subcutaneous swelling will be evident on the inner surface of the earflap near the apex. The outer surface of the earflap is seldom affected. The swelling is not warm and causes little pain. The affected ear can no longer be brought to an upright position as a sign of attentiveness. Fluctuation is present in recent cases.

Etiology. A frequent cause of aural hematoma in ponies is playful bites from dogs in situations where both are kept in the same yard or turned out on the same field.

Prognosis. It is more favorable in the horse than in the dog, because the auricular cartilage is relatively strong, and the ear can be held erect even if some residual fibrous thickening is present. In ponies, moreover, the inner surface of the earflap usually has a thick hair covering that minimizes the importance of cosmetic defects.

Treatment. A small, fresh hematoma is treated topically with ointments that promote dispersion and absorption. If the hematoma is approximately plum-size and the ear cannot be held erect, the procedure is similar to that for small animals, i.e., the hematoma is evacuated about 8—10 days after the injury, by which time the ruptured vessel will have been clotted. Then a bandage is applied to ensure that the skin is closely applied to the underlying tissue, and that dead space is eliminated. The hematoma can be evacuated by aspiration in some cases, but it is usually necessary to make 2 or 3 parallel incisions over the hematoma to ensure a complete evacuation.

2.1.16.1.2. Wounds of the Earflap

Definition. By far the most common ear wounds in the horse are lacerations and bite wounds. With lacerations, the ear generally is split inward from its periphery so that individual flaps are formed. Dog bites in ponies cause tissue loss from the earflap or create perforations in the ear. A bite on the ear from another horse leaves an ugly, infected, contused wound that may involve considerable tissue loss.

Symptoms. Generally the earflap is split inward from its border. In acute cases there is usually heavy bleeding that is further exacerbated by constant head shaking. The majority of ear wounds are assumed to be heavily contaminated with bacteria, and this must be given due consideration with regard to the prophylaxis of infection. Cellulitis will develop in ear wounds that are several days old. The ear droops to one side on account of its weight, and its abnormal size and position have a generally disfiguring effect.

Prognosis. If a portion of the tip of the earflap has been avulsed, it is seldom possible to restore a normal appearance to the ear. An ear that is split or punctured should be surgically repaired without delay in order to achieve a good cosmetic result.

Treatment. Treatment follows the rules of general surgery. In acute cases hemostasis has first priority. Next the wound edges are excised, including the cartilage if necessary. Divided cartilage is not sutured; the skin is merely closed over the cartilage on the inner and outer surfaces of the ear. It has proved advantageous to stitch a thin, light plastic disk to the inner or outer surface for 8—10 days to provide support for the healing earflap. This will ensure complete immobilization of the wound edges and a good cosmetic result. The horse is cross-tied so that it cannot rub the injured ear against a wall or other object. Tetanus antitoxin or toxoid is administered postoperatively. The administration of a polyvalent clostridial anti-serum may be beneficial following surgery. An antibiotic spray is applied daily to the ear wound to promote primary healing.

Comments. A cosmetic restoration of the earflap is important in riding horses and especially in show horses. Hence, surgical intervention should not be deferred if optimum results are to be achieved.

2.1.16.1.3. Auricular Cellulitis

Definition. Auricular cellulitis is an inflammatory condition of the earflap resulting from the pyogenic infection of ear wounds.

Symptoms. The earflap is swollen to a thickness of 1—2 cm, is warm and painful. The increased weight of the earflap causes it to droop to one side, and it cannot be raised to an erect position. Serous fluid exudes from the swollen skin and dries to form crusts on the inner and outer ear surfaces.

Treatment. An attempt is made to bandage the ear, having first packed the external auditory meatus with cotton. The bandage is moistened with warm Burow's solution every 2 hours. Large antibiotic doses are given concurrently for 5—7 days. Either resorption will occur, or small abscesses will form over the earflap within 6—7 days. These abscesses are managed according to general surgical principles, taking care not to split the cartilage when the abscesses are incised. If cartilage necrosis has developed, a partial amputation of the earflap is necessary.

Prognosis. It is unfavorable in terms of the cosmetic result.

2.1.16.1.4. Ear Fistula (Ear Cyst, Fistula auris congenita)

Definition. An ear fistula is a unilateral or bilateral dentigerous cyst with a fistulous opening located on the anterior edge of the ear. A purulent or milky-white fluid is discharged from it (fig. 2.1.16. — 1).

Symptoms. Mainly young horses and foals are affected. An approximately pea-size opening is found on the anterior edge of the ear 1, 2 or 3 cm from its base. It exudes a gray mucoid or purulent fluid that runs down the temporal and buccal regions and gradually dries. The fistulous opening is always indrawn and covered with epithelium. The fistulous tract can be followed along the edge of the ear to the

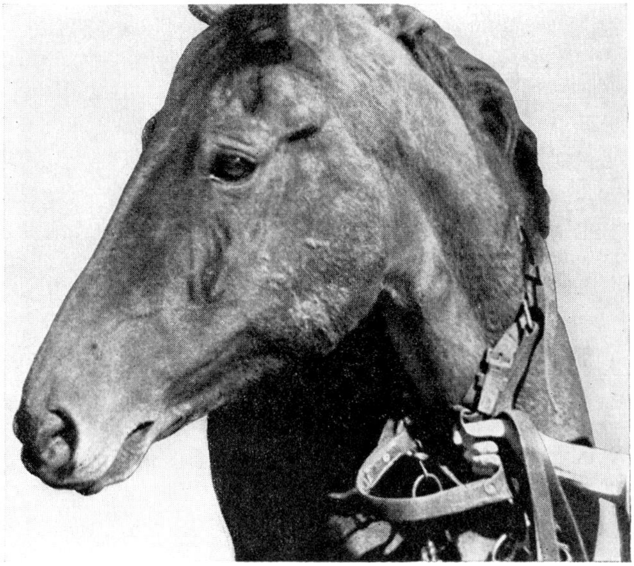

Fig. 2.1.16. — 1. Ear fistula.

fistular base by external palpation or by introducing a probe. Anterior to or below the external auditory meatus, this fistulous tract communicates with a nodular or tooth-like structure of variable size. This structure usually represents an aberrant, stunted tooth. It tends to have a firm attachment with the temporal bone, although sometimes it can be moved a millimeter or so. If a metal probe can be passed all the way through the fistulous tract, this structure will be encountered. The aberrant tooth is usually surrounded by a cyst wall. If pressure is applied to the cyst and tooth, a large amount of mucopurulent fluid usually will drain from the fistulous opening. There may be excoriation of the skin surrounding this opening.

Etiology. The cause of the cyst is an embryonic malformation arising from the first branchial pouch at the base of the ear. This malformation contains tooth germ, which grows into molar-like structures. However, the ear cyst can also result from the splitting-off of embryonic tissues having odontogenic properties. The origin of this tissue is the first branchial arch, from which the mandible develops.

Prognosis. The prognosis is excellent following surgical excision of the fistulous tract and of the cyst located at its base.

Treatment. Under general anesthesia, an elliptical incision is made completely around the fistulous opening on the anterior edge of the ear. A probe is inserted into the fistulous tract, and the tract is split on the probe. Then the wall of the tract is shelled out. The fistulous tract dilates in funnel-like fashion toward the cystic sac. This sac is extirpated together with all its contents. Any remnants of the tract likewise are removed. The tooth-like teratoma usually lies within the cyst sac. An attempt is now made to grasp this aberrant tooth bud with a strong forceps and move it slightly laterally or rotate it somewhat in order to loosen it from its bed. If this is not possible, dental forceps are used. If this also fails, a chisel may be used to separate the tooth from its bony attachment with the temporal bone, taking great care not to damage the skull. Once the chisel is in place, however, it is nearly always

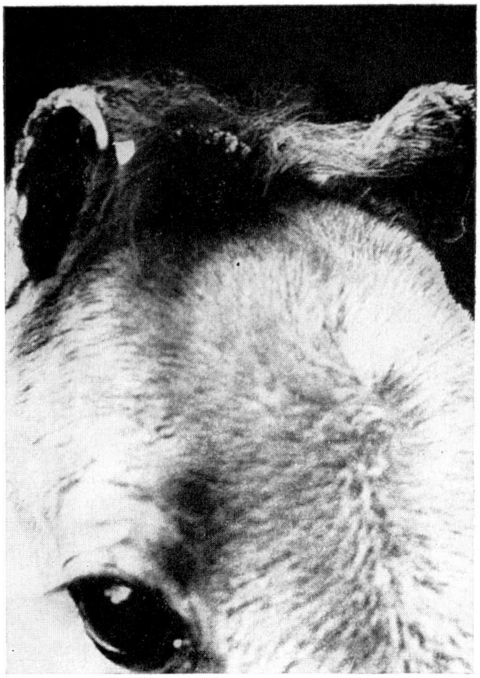

Fig. 2.1.16. — 2. Stubby ears secondary to poisoning with *Secale cornutum.*

possible to loosen the aberrant tooth with a simple prying motion. After the tooth has been removed, hemostasis is obtained. The skin is then closed with simple interrupted sutures. Good granulation healing should ensue within 2—3 weeks.

2.1.16.1.5. Neoplasms of the External Ear

Occurrence. Papillomas or warts occur on the edge of the ear and sometimes on the inner and outer auricular surfaces. They are essentially cosmetic defects, but they may grow so large that they hamper ear movements or create unsightly blemishes on riding stock. 'Papillary acanthomas' occur on the inner auricular surface. These are tumors of epithelial origin that later spread to involve the corium. They appear as flat, dry, pale or pigmented warts. It is possible for the entire inner surface of the earflap to become covered with acanthomas of this type. The surface of these tumors may be rough or covered with crusts or scales.

Deeper auricular tissues may be affected by adenomas, atheromas, dermoid cysts, chondrosarcomas, and rarely squamous-cell carcinomas. These neoplasms may completely obstruct the inlet to the external auditory meatus.

Large, spheroidal neoplasms of a reddish color that produce an oily, seropurulent, foul-smelling discharge are sometimes encountered on the edge of the ear, where they are adherent to the cartilage. Nearly all of these tumors are fibromas.

Prognosis. The prognosis depends on the nature of the tumor.

Treatment. Neoplasms on the edge of the earflap and its inner and outer surfaces are surgically removed. In the case of fibromas, it is necessary to include a piece of cartilage in the resection. Some disfigurement of the earflap is unavoidable in such cases.

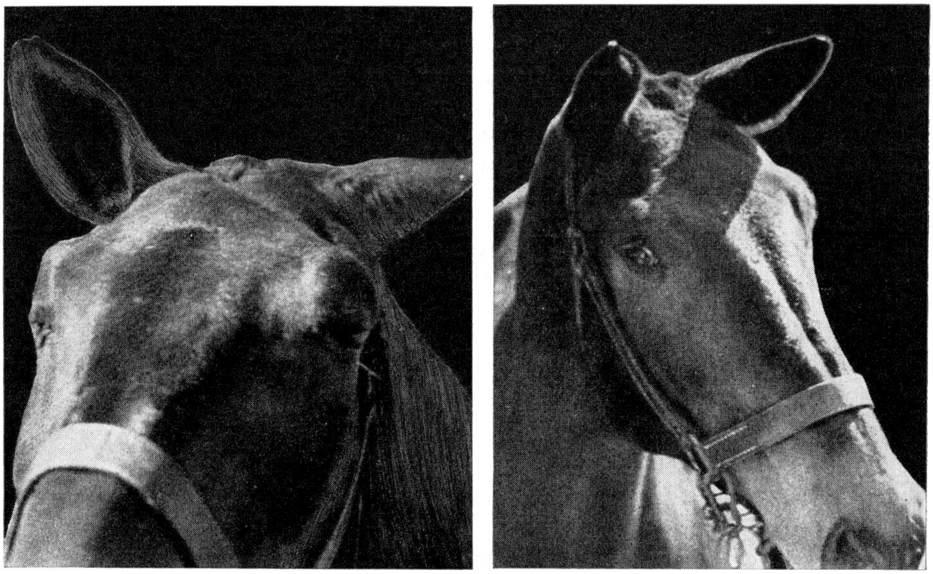

3 4

Fig. 2.1.16. — 3–4. Floppy ears.

2.1.16.1.6. Deformities of the External Ear and Abnormalities of Ear Carriage

Stubby ears: This is a condition in which the earflaps are abnormally small and short. It may be congenital, especially in Shetland ponies.

An acquired form can occur unilaterally or bilaterally following accidents, ear tip avulsions, damage from frostbite, amputations, and poisoning by *Secale cornutum* (fig. 2.1.16. — 2). No treatment is indicated for either the congenital or acquired form.

Floppy ears: In this condition the ears are disproportionately large. As a result, ear movements become irregular, the ears cannot be brought fully to the erect position, and the concave surface of the auricle cannot be directed forward with accuracy. The ears tend to flop about during walking and at faster gaits — a hightly undesirable trait in show and jumping horses (figs. 2.1.16. — 3 and — 4).

Treatment. Surgical size reduction of the earflap is sufficient in many cases to correct the abnormal ear carriage. In other cases it may prove necessary to shorten the adductor muscles of the ear to restore the earflap to an upright position. Technique: A skin incision is made at the base of the ear toward the dorsal midline of the neck, the muscles are exposed, and a 1- to 2-cm segment of muscle is resected.

2.1.16.1.7. Diseases of the External Auditory Meatus

The external auditory meatus is a cartilaginous tube that runs downward as a continuation of the funnel-shaped apex of the earflap. The terminal segment of the cartilaginous meatus makes an approximately 90° bend in the direction of the petrous bone, at which point it becomes encased in bone. This external meatus then tapers in conical fashion until it terminates at the eardrum, which marks the start of the middle ear.

Foreign Bodies in the External Auditory Meatus

Occurrence. Foreign bodies are rare in the external auditory meatus. They are occasionally found in smaller horses. The objects most commonly found are pebbles, small pieces of wood, and fir and pine needles (in hunting and eventing horses).

Symptoms. Foreign bodies in the external auditory meatus may produce no symptoms for some time. In the case of larger foreign bodies, there may be itching that causes the horse to shake its head constantly or hold the head with the affected side down. If the foreign body is firmly lodged in the external auditory meatus, a suppurative inflammation of the meatus will gradually develop over a period of days or weeks. Examination will reveal a purulent, foul-smelling exudate pooling within the ear or draining from it.

Treatment. The hairs in the external auditory meatus are clipped, and the meatus is cleansed by irrigating with 3 % hydrogen peroxide solution. Then the interior of the earflap is well illuminated, and a search is made for the foreign body. Once located, it is extracted with forceps. Inflammation of the meatus regresses spontaneously following the instillation of an antibiotic ointment, the application of zinc oil, or the application of a glucocorticoid-containing ointment.

The *prognosis* is favorable.

Otitis externa

Definition. Otitis externa is an inflammation of the cutaneous lining of the external auditory meatus. In horses, the disease is generally caused by the presence of foreign bodies in the external acoustic meatus. In all other cases, there will be a purulent discharge from the meatus signifying disease of the middle ear.

2.1.16.1.8. Diseases of the Middle and Inner Ear

Otitis media, Otitis interna

Definition. Otitis media is an inflammation of the tympanic cavity. In otitis interna, the inflammation has spread to involve the cavity system of the petrous bone; this results in disease of the balance organs (vestibule, semicircular canals). The tympanic cavity, or middle ear, communicates with the pharynx via the eustachian tube, and thus via the gutteral pouch.

Symptoms. Inflammation of the middle and internal ear is invariably associated with systemic signs (fever, anorexia, possible emaciation). Facial paralysis is also present. The head is largely immobile and is rotated with the affected side down. A foul-smelling pus drains from the external ear, soiling the hairs below it. When the earflap is touched or the external auditory meatus is palpated externally, the horse will show resentment and back away from the examiner or fall while attempting to do so. The most common cause of otitis media and internal in the horse, besides foreign bodies and eardrum perforations, is ascending inflammation of the pharynx. Purulent infection of the upper respiratory tract can lead to involvement of the eustachian tube. This in turn leads to inflammation and empyema of the tympanic cavity, with erosion of the tympanic membrane from within. Coexisting disease of the guttural pouch is always present in such cases. Involvement of the internal ear leads to marked disturbances of equilibrium, swaying, walking in circles, and nystagmus. The animal has a tendency to fall if handled or exercised.

Prognosis and Treatment. The prognosis is guarded to poor. Antiseptic irrigations of the external auditory meatus may be tried, followed by topical antibiotic therapy. Large antibiotic doses should also be given systemically. Medical treatment is successful in only a small percentage of cases, however.

Reference

BARNETT, R. E.: Wiederherstellung eines verletzten Ohres bei einem Hengstfohlen. Mod. vet. Pract. *55:* 799 (1974).

2.1.17. Diseases of the Skull, Spine and Pelvis

Function. The spine, or vertebral column, is an organ of support and movement which represents the central pillar of the animal skeleton. Like the limbs and limb muscles, the spine forms one component of the integrated locomotor system. Both these components are closely interconnected in the horse, and each influences the other. Nevertheless, the spine has certain characteristics that distinguish it from the rest of the skeletal system from both a morphologic and functional standpoint. These peculiarities, and the functional role they play in biodynamics and locomotion, have an important bearing on the origin and development of pathologic processes on the vertebral column as well as the extremities. Age-related changes in the equine skeleton also have pathogenic significance.

The *skull* of the horse has the shape of a four-sided pyramid whose base faces the cervical vertebrae. It is made up of the cranial bones and the mandible, which are joined at the temporomandibular articulation.

The bones of the skull are divided into those of the cerebral cranium and those of the visceral, or facial, cranium. The cranial bones enclose the cranial cavity, the space occupied by the cerebrum and cerebellum. The visceral part of the cranium consists of the maxillary and nasal bones and the mandible. These bones form the oral and nasal cavities as well as the maxillary and frontal sinuses.

In the posterior intermandibular area lies the hyoid bone, which supports the root of the tongue, pharynx and larynx.

The *vertebral column* of the horse is a skeletal organ of support and movement. It is made up of individual vertebrae that are interconnected by intervertebral discs, articulations and ligaments. The total number of vertebrae in the horse, including the coccygeal, varies between 50 and 55. These consist of 7 cervical vertebrae, 18 (rarely 17 or 19) thoracic vertebrae, 6 lumbar vertebrae, 5 sacral vertebrae (which join to form the sacrum), and 15—19 coccygeal vertebrae.

All the vertebrae resemble each other in certain structural features and differ in others. All vertebrae with the exception of the 1st cervical and last coccygeal have a vertebral body, situated ventrally, and a dorsally-situated vertebral arch (neural arch), whose pedicles connect it with the body. The body and arch enclose an opening called the vertebral foramen. All the vertebral foramina collectively form the vertebral canal. Projecting upward from the vertebral arch is the spinous process. These processes are arranged longitudinally along the dorsal midline, flanked by paired transverse processes. The articular processes of the vertebrae project craniad and caudad. The latter form the dorsal boundaries of the cranial and caudal vertebral notches, which together define the borders of the intervertebral foramen. From these openings emerge the spinal nerves that form the sympathetic chain, nerve plexuses and individual nerves.

The *pelvic girdle* is comprised of the pelvic bones: the ilium, pubic bone and ischium. The pelvis is joined to the spine at the sacroiliac joint. This relationship is important in the function of the pelvic limbs — the forward shift of the torso during forward progression by the animal. The pelvic girdle possesses powerful muscles which give the horse its extraordinary running and jumping abilities and, with suitable training, enable the horse to stand and even move on its hind limbs alone.

2.1.17.1. Injuries of the Skull

Classification. Head injuries in the horse occur in varying forms and degrees. They may be associated with hematoma formation, lymph extravasation, complete or incomplete bone fractures, dental fractures, and dislocation of the temporomandibular joint. Open injuries (wounds) can occur anywhere on the head and may be complicated by infection.

2.1.17.1.1. Skull Fractures

General. Skull fractures can result from extreme violence to the head during accidents, kicks, malicious blows, or falls. Skull injuries in newborn foals may be caused by careless obstetrical practice such as the use of obstetric hooks for delivering the fetus or the placement of a loop around the fetal mandible. The inept cutting or extraction of teeth can similarly lead to fractures of the mandible.

Occurrence and General Symptoms. Skull fractures in horses may involve the cerebral cranium (occiput, sphenoid, temporal, parietal, frontal, lacrimal, zygoma) as well as the visceral cranium (mandible, maxilla, premaxilla, palatine, sphenoid, nasal, ethmoid, hyoid). The fractures most commonly seen in practice involve the nasal bones and premaxilla, the maxilla and mandible at the level of the dental roots, transverse fractures through the pars incisiva of the mandible (uni- or bilateral), mandibular symphysis fractures, and chip fractures of the mandibular angle, condyloid process or coronoid process.

General symptoms of open skull fractures are hemorrhage and deformity of the affected region. Food ingestion is impaired in all forms of mandibular fracture.

Besides general clinical signs there are certain special symptoms that are characteristic of specific cranial bone fractures. For example, in fractures of the nasal bone, especially depressed fractures, there may be damage to the nasal conchae with associated profuse hemorrhage. Depressed fractures of bony processes, on the other hand, can cause severe respiratory impairment. In fractures of the mandibular symphysis, abnormal mobility of the right and left mandibular rami will be noted on each side of the fracture line. Bilateral transverse fractures through the interdental space are marked by a dropping of the pars incisiva. Bone splinters in mandibular fractures may cause injury to the tongue, gingiva or soft palate, causing profuse bleeding from the oral cavity.

Fractures of the cerebral cranium are usually accompanied by direct cerebral trauma from indriven bone fragments. Cerebral compression due to intracranial hemorrhage is not unusual. Most fractures of this type have a fatal outcome.

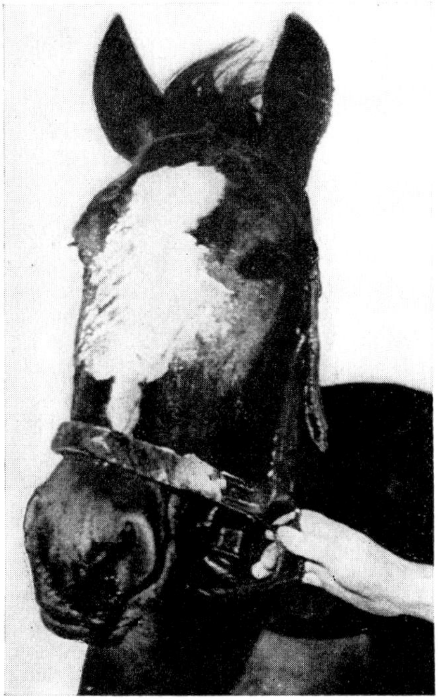
1

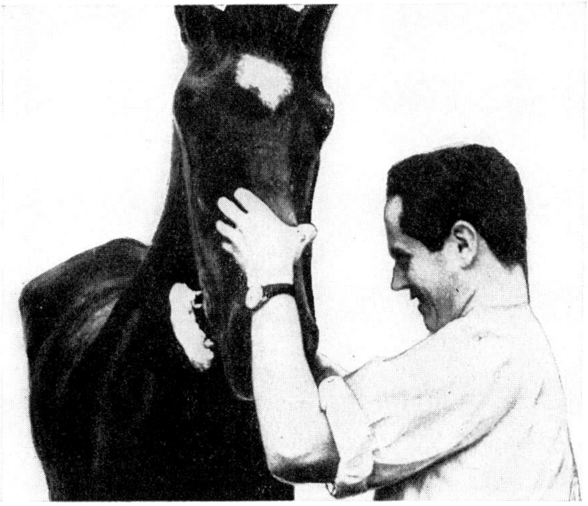
2

Fig. 2.1.17. — 1. Bilateral, closed, depressed fracture of the nasal bone.
Fig. 2.1.17. — 2. Fracture of the pars incisiva of the maxillary bone.

Prognosis. Nasal bone fractures, chip fractures of the outer mandibular border, and fractures of the premaxilla and mandibular symphysis have a favorable prognosis. Extensive, compound skull fractures, fractures of the mandibular body and intra-articular fractures have an unfavorable prognosis.

Fractures of the Nasal Bone

Occurrence. Fractures of the nasal bone are not at all uncommon in racing horses. The fracture may be unilateral or bilateral, closed or open, simple or comminuted, and may take various forms (longitudinal, transverse, depressed, infraction, fissure).

Symptoms. The main symptom is a swelling about the dorsum of the nose that greatly alters the normal nasal contour. Abrasions and skin lacerations may also be present. The area is tender to palpation. With injury to the nasal mucosa, profuse hemorrhage is observed. Air may periodically enter the subcutaneous connective tissue during expiration, producing a diffuse subcutaneous emphysema of the head.

Depressed fractures cause an indriving of bone fragments (fig. 2.1.17. — 1) whose sharp edges damage the nasal conchae or septum, leading to epistaxis. There is swelling of the nasal mucosa with a narrowing of the nasal passages. This causes respiratory difficulties that can be life-threatening in severe cases. The dyspnea usually persists for 5 to 7 days. Loss of patency in the nasolacrimal duct is manifested by blood-tinged lacrimation.

Complicated fractures can lead to purulent exudate of the frontal and sometimes the maxillary sinus. The defects in the nasal bones and in other flat cranial bones initially undergo fibrous-tissue cicatrization.

The nasal cavity and paranasal sinuses may have to be opened if trephination cannot allow adequate pus drainage and bone fragment removal, in which case fistulization must be expected.

Etiology. Kicks, collisions with obstacles, falls, gunshot wounds.

The *prognosis* is favorable for closed fractures. Complicated cases are marked by necrosis of the nasal bone and conchae or by empyema of the paranasal sinuses.

Treatment. With closed fractures, a wait-and-see approach is recommended. Cold compresses may be applied for the first few days.

In depressed fractures complicated by life-threatening respiratory distress, a tracheotomy must be performed before any other aid is rendered. Once the horse is breathing well, surgical reduction of the bone fragments may be undertaken.

Primary surgical wound care is necessary in complicated fractures: loose bone fragments are extracted, sharp bony points and edges denuded of periosteum are smoothed, and mild antiseptic lavage is carried out, followed by routine wound care measures. Treatment also involves prophylactic antibiotics and sulfonamides.

Fractures of the Maxilla and Premaxilla

Occurrence. Fractures of these bones are frequently accompanied by damage to the nasal conchae. The fractures may be unilateral or bilateral, simple or comminuted.

Symptoms. In fractures of the palatine process, there is bleeding from the oral cavity, and food cannot be chewed. Examination of the mouth reveals wounds of the gingiva and palate and the loosening or loss of one or more teeth (fig. 2.1.17. — 2).

Closed fractures of the maxilla are manifested initially by an indentation ('dimple') and later by swelling, heat and tenderness. In complicated fractures the skin is disrupted and the maxillary sinus is breached, allowing a fistula to develop (fig. 2.1.17. — 3). Emphysema of the head can develop if air from the maxillary sinus collects subcutaneously. Injury to the inner lining of the maxillary sinus by bone splinters is evidenced by hemorrhage. Infection results in the development of a purulent sinusitis.

The *prognosis* is favorable for closed fractures but is guarded in open fractures due to the risk of suppurative maxillary sinusitis, suppurative periodontitis or dental fistulization.

Treatment. In acute cases, hemorrhage is controlled and loose bone fragments are removed. If no dental roots are exposed and the gingiva is intact, there is no need to extract loose teeth. Clinical observations show that such teeth can contribute to stable occlusion if left in place. Extraction is unavoidable, however, if the root is exposed. Thorough disinfection of the wound is necessary following the extraction.

Reduction of depression fractures must be carried out if displacement is present. If there is significant depression in the fracture area, treatment is as follows: A burr hole is placed near the edge of the bone that is large enough to accomodate a finger or curved metal probe. The finger or probe is used to push the depressed area outward until the normal contour is restored. The surgical wound is closed by routine suture techniques. Liquid nutrition, preferably administered by nasogastric tube, is given for several days postoperatively.

2.1.17.1.2. Osteodystrophia Fibrosa

Definition, Pathogenesis and Etiology. Osteodystrophia fibrosa is a disease of bone that is based upon a derangement of bone metabolism. It is characterized by fibrous tissue growth in the medullary cavities and vascular channels of the cortical bone, replacing the yellow and red marrow.

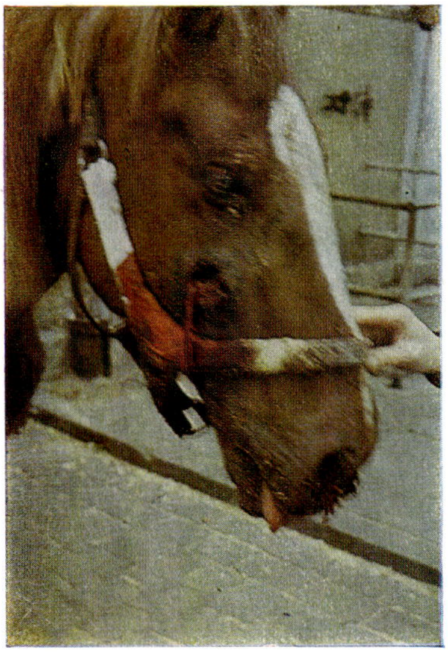

3

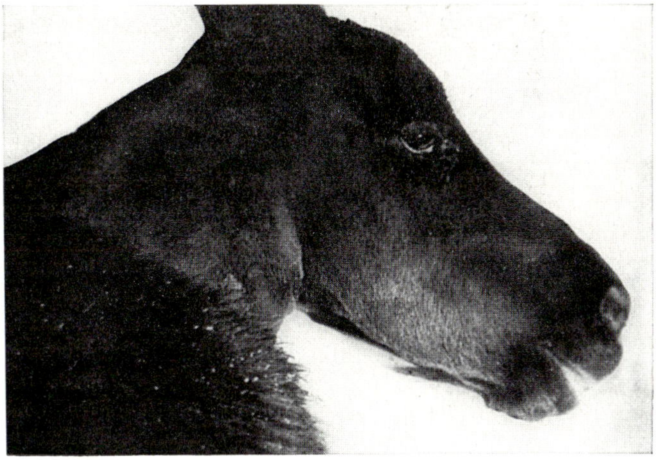

4

Fig. 2.1.17. — *3.* Open fracture of the maxillary bone.
Fig. 2.1.17. — *4.* Osteodystrophia fibrosa.

Osteodystrophia fibrosa is characterized morphologically by a preponderance of bone resorption over bone formation, osteoporotic processes, and occasionally by the formation of pathologic osteoid tissue like that seen in ricketts. In some cases only primitive structures are formed during osteogenesis. These structures may be laid down in entirely random aggregations like those seen in osteodystrophy due to parathyroid disease. Less frequently, and especially in osteodystrophy due to nephrogenic causes, there is an increase in bone-forming processes resulting in osteosclerosis.

Thus, the changes in osteodystrophia fibrosa relate mainly to structural alterations in the bony tissue. These occur essentially by way of resorption and replacement, rather than by a degeneration of preexisting bone.

In domestic animals the facial bones and the subepiphyseal zones of the long bones, especially the femur, are most commonly affected.

The causes of osteodystrophia fibrosa in horses is due to excessive dietary phosphorus. The disease mainly affects young animals, and it is based upon a dysfunction of the endocrine system, most notably the parathyroid gland.

Often the condition is accompanied by hypertrophy of the parathyroid. A low serum calcium level may be observed in affected animals.

Symptoms. Few systemic signs are present. Affected bones show marked enlargement. Clinical changes are most apparent in the facial bones. The increased mass of the mandible frequently causes the teeth to separate and loosen. Mastication may be seriously hampered. Respiration is stertorous. A mucoid nasal discharge is present, and the retropharyngeal lymph nodes may be enlarged and indurated. Compression of the nasolacrimal duct results in continuous lacrimation. Fibrous tissue proliferation appears on the periosteum, and the mandibles and paranasal sinuses contain large amounts of fibrous tissue in which cysts may form. If the mandible is affected, the process can easily spread to involve the region of the tooth roots. The mandible has an enlarged cross-section, and its inferior border is rounded. The cortical layer of the

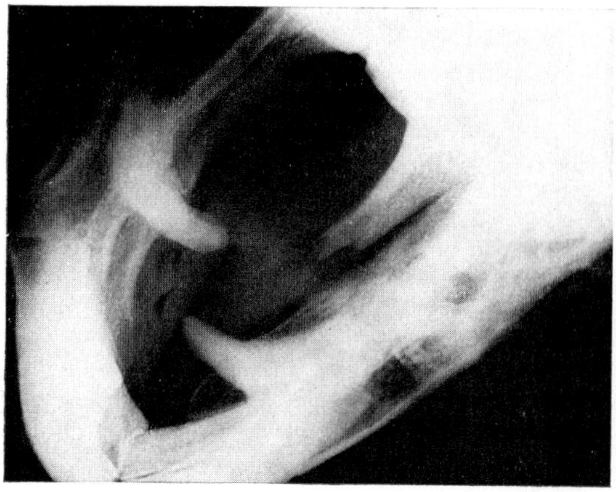

5

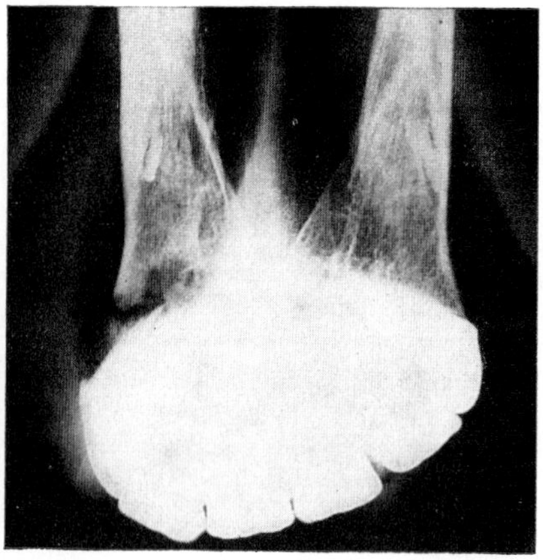

6

Fig. 2.1.17. — 5. Open fracture of the mandible.
Fig. 2.1.17. — 6. Bilateral fracture of the mandible, reduced by percutaneous fixation.

bone is replaced with fibrous tissue. As a result, the long bones are greatly weakened and fracture easily. Lameness is sometimes evident. The bones are enlarged in the region of the epiphysis, and their periosteum is thickened and spongy.

In young horses the osteodystrophic process is usually confined to the maxilla and mandible, including the teeth (fig. 2.1.17. — 4). This can lead to cement hypoplasia, caries of the premolars, enamel hypoplasia of the incisors, shortening of the roots, and abnormalities of occlusion.

The periosteum of the enlarged maxilla and mandible tends to be thickened, while the underlying cortex is thinned. The cysts that form may reach several inches in diameter. Often they are loculated by fibrous septae or by porous bony or fibrous tissue. There may be continuous or intermittent lameness. Emaciation and an unkempt haircoat are seen in the late stages.

Radiography confirms the extreme calcium depletion of the bones. Localized areas of lucency are observed. The cortical layer is thinned and bowed. Fibrous septae and cysts of varying size are seen in the cancellous bone. No cysts are observed in the flat bones of the skull. Deposits are visible on the periosteum of the long bones.

The *prognosis* of osteodystrophia fibrosa is unfavorable when clinical signs are marked.

Treatment. Treatment is ineffectual in most cases. Supplementation of the diet with calcium can effect some improvement in the animal's condition while arresting or at least slowing the progression of symptoms. Surgical procedures, such as resection of the nasal conchae or the removal of altered cancellous tissue through burr holes in the mandible, are of no value.

2.1.17.1.3. Diseases of the Mandible

Fractures of the Mandible

Definition, Forms. Mandibular fractures may be open or closed, uni- or bilateral, comminuted or simple, and may be characterized as transverse, longitudinal, oblique, intra-articular, or involving the coronoid process or posterior angle.

Symptoms. Bilateral fractures through the mandibular body result in a downward displacement of the pars incisiva. Fractures that open into the oral cavity are accompanied by injuries of the mucosa with associated hemorrhage. Eating is extremely difficult. Palpation reveals tenderness along the fracture line and crepitation. In closed fractures of the symphysis, the mandibular halves can be moved relative to each other, and a gap is formed between the first two incisors. A unilateral oblique fracture of the mandibular body causes the lower incisors to deviate toward the affected side, producing a change in occlusion.

With a closed fracture of the coronoid process, the contours in the temporomandibular joint region are altered as in open fractures (fig. 2.1.17. — 5). Contraction of the temporalis muscle pulls the coronoid process upward, and so crepitation usually cannot be detected. However, palpation reveals mobility of the process and tenderness. Food generally is masticated only on the unaffected side.

With an intra-articular fracture of the condyloid process, food is refused for several days after the injury. The animal will take food after the pain has abated, but will chew it only on the healthy side. Secondary arthritic changes may develop leading to deformity and ankylosis of the temporomandibular joint. Fractures may be complicated by facial or trigeminal nerve paralysis, injuries to the salivary gland and its ducts, or by damage to the teeth, oral mucosa and skin.

Etiology. Severe trauma, gunshot wounds, careless tooth extraction. Faulty obstetric practices are also responsible in some instances in the neonate. Predisposing factors may include 'ricketts' (epiphysitis), osteomyelitis and tumors.

The *prognosis* depends on the nature of the fracture. It is favorable in the case of closed, simple fractures. Comminuted and intra-articular fractures have a favorable prognosis in terms of functional recovery. Separations at the symphysis associated with pars incisiva fractures always have a favorable prognosis.

Treatment. The reduction and fixation of symphyseal or pars incisiva fractures may be carried out under local or general anesthesia depending on how extensive the repair will have to be. Fixation can be achieved with intraoral wire splints, metal plates or metal pins applied in accordance with AO/ASIF principles (fig. 2.1.17. — 6).

Comminuted fractures are managed in the same way, except that general anesthesia is almost always required.

Pars incisiva fractures often run transversely through the interdental space or cause a separation at the symphysis. Closed symphysis fractures usually show little displacement, whereas open symphysis fractures are susceptible to much greater displacement. Fixation is achieved by wiring the incisors together, thereby stabilizing the fragments.

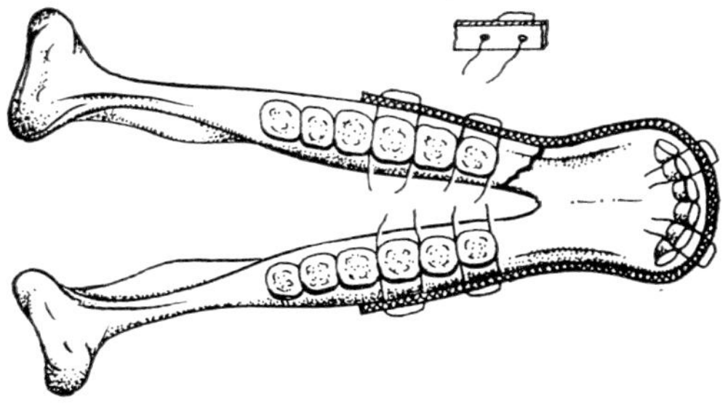

7

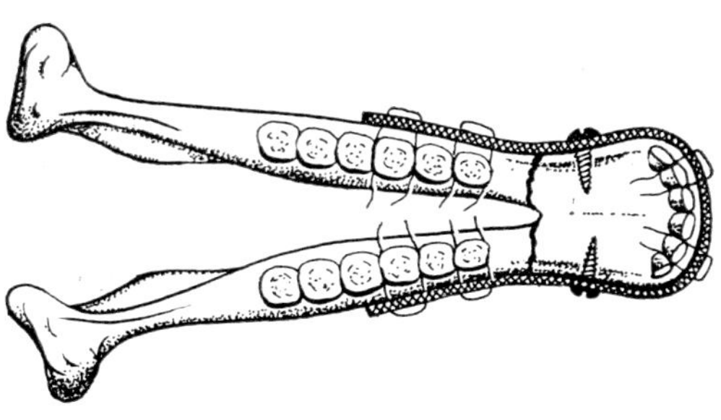

8

Fig. 2.1.17. — 7. Fixation of a mandibular fracture with the U-bar technique of GABEL [1959].
Fig. 2.1.17. — 8. Use of GABEL's [1959] U-bar technique for a transverse mandibular fracture.

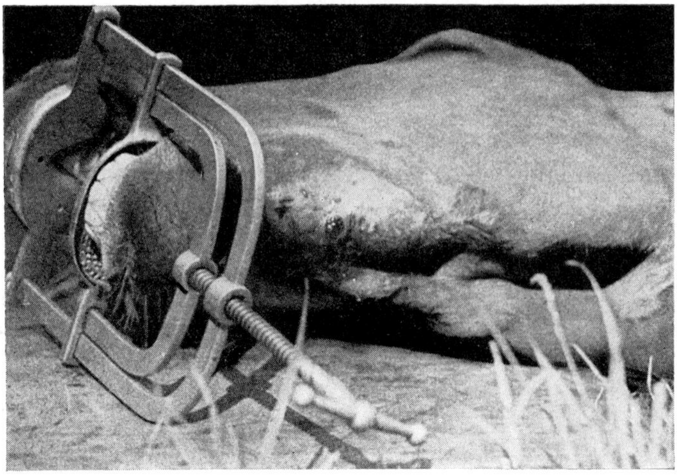

Fig. 2.1.17. — 9. Osteomyelitis of the mandible with fistulization secondary to alveolar periostitis.

Transverse fractures through the pars incisiva result in a dropping of the lower incisors, making eating extremely difficult. Following reduction, the fracture is immobilized with a wire placed around the corner incisors and canines or the first premolars on both the right and left sides. This is augmented by circumferential wiring (cerclage) from the inferior surface of the mandible or by applying a small compression plate to each side of the jaw.

Techniques of intraoral splinting have been proposed for the bony fixation of mandibular fractures [Smith and Michols, 1957; Gabel, 1959; figs. 2.1.17. — 7 and — 8]. These techniques are advocated on the assumption that wire fixation is unsatisfactory for oblique fractures, because tightening of the wire causes a shortening of the fractured bone, leading to a change of occlusion in cases where the fracture is unilateral. This problem is solved by the use of metal plates. The technique of Gabel [1959], in which an U-shaped rod is anchored with wire to the incisors and premolars, has proved particularly useful in longitudinal fractures of the pars incisiva and in unilateral oblique fractures of a mandibular ramus. However, this fixation technique is not entirely suitable for bilateral fractures of the interdental region. This has led us to develop a modification of the technique in which the splint is additionally anchored by means of screws inserted into the bone fragment distal to the fracture line. Fractures of the mandibular body are best immobilized by compression plating.

Full recovery of function may be expected in 8—12 weeks. Systemic antibiotics are administered for 8—10 days. In the case of open comminuted fractures, removal of the fragments is usually indicated. This is necessary to prevent fistulization and osteomyelitis with sequestra formation.

Comments. In the case of open mandibular fractures complicated by purulent osteomyelitis, recovery is unlikely, and euthanasia may be neccessary.

Osteomyelitis of the Mandible

Etiology, Pathogenesis. Mandibular osteomyelitis can occur in connection with open fractures, complicated cases of acute, diffuse, purulent alveolar periostitis or pulpitis of the cheek teeth (fig. 2.1.17. — 9).

In purulent osteomyelitis there is primary damage to the cancellous bone with eventual involvement of all bony tissue elements.

When an infectious agent (staphylococcus, streptococcus) invades the bone marrow, the initial reaction is an inflammation characterized by vasodilation and hyperemia of the cancellous bone and an inflammatory edema. This is followed by the development of blood vessel thrombosis as well as a fibrinous swelling of the vessel walls and necrosis. The bone marrow becomes permeated with a serofibrinous and later purulent exudate. The suppurative, necrotizing process may spread to involve the cortex, periosteum and soft tissues.

Symptoms. The clinical course of mandibular osteomyelitis is highly variable. Acute cases manifest symptoms of a severe infectious process. The body temperature is elevated, as are the pulse and respiratory rate, a leukocytosis develops. Depression and anorexia are present. Pain is elicited by palpation and percussion of the affected side. In later stages, diffuse swelling appears due to the development of an ossifying periostitis and collateral edema. Abscesses form in adjacent soft tissues, and these rupture to form fistulas that communicate with the medullary cavity. A purulent, putrid-smelling exudate is discharged from the fistulous openings. This discharge usually contains fat droplets from the marrow and small fragments of devitalized bone.

Chronic osteomyelitis leads to excessive periosteal bone formation, rarefaction of the cortical bone and necrosis. The formation of sequestra and accumulation of pus in the cancellous bone leads to enlargement of the bone, and proliferative processes develop in surrounding tissues. Externally the skin is swollen, firm and non-tender and feels abnormally tense and immobile.

Treatment. In acute cases of purulent osteomyelitis, general nursing care (rest, good nutrition) in conjunction with antibiotic and sulfonamide therapy to prevent septicemia, may limit the infectious process and help natural defenses. Local anesthesia of the cranial sympathetic ganglion may also be used. Acute cases respond favorably to the local injection of antibiotics and local anesthetic into the infected area. In cases that are associated with progressive changes in the bone or severe toxemia, it is wise to intervene surgically at the earliest opportunity. The object of the surgery is to remove the suppurative, necrotizing focus by opening the pus-filled abscess cavity and resecting all affected bone until healthy tissue is reached. Afterward the cavity is flushed with alcohol or acridine dye solution and packed with gauze soaked in a sulfonamide solution which has osmotic activity. The packing is changed at 2- or 3-day intervals. A streptomycin emulsion may also be used.

Comments. Recovery depends on removal of the primary cause of the osteomyelitis.

Neoplasms of the Mandible

Neoplasms of the mandible are not uncommon in horses. Osteomas, osteosarcoma-like tumors and fibrosarcomas are most commonly observed (fig. 2.1.17. — 10 to — 12). The majority of these tumors are primary, although metastatic tumors are not unusual. Adamantinomas are rarely seen. One such tumor was described by Hanselka et al. [1974] in an 11-year-old horse. In most cases the tumor arises from the periosteum. The tumor grows slowly and may spread to adjacent soft tissues. Mandibular neoplasms may grow large enough to interfere with mastication. Such tumors are constantly susceptible to trauma, leading to secondary infection and the formation of necrotic foci. Osteosarcoma-like tumors are occasionally accompanied by mandibular fractures.

The *prognosis* is unfavorable in malignant cases. Osteomas are amenable to surgical removal.

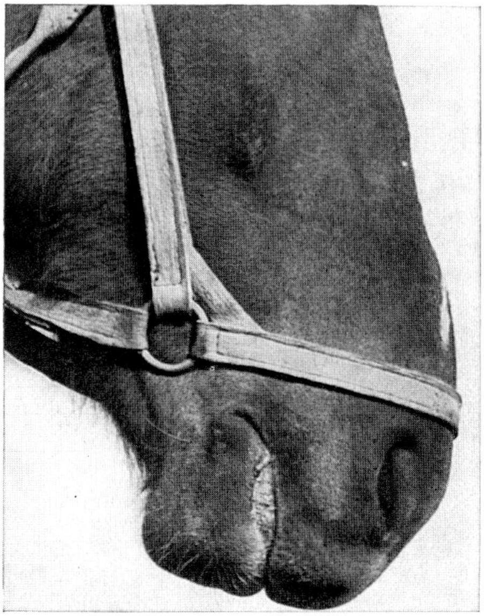
10

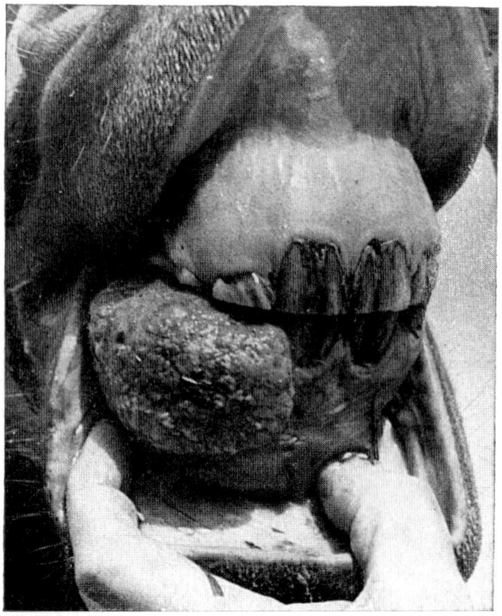
11

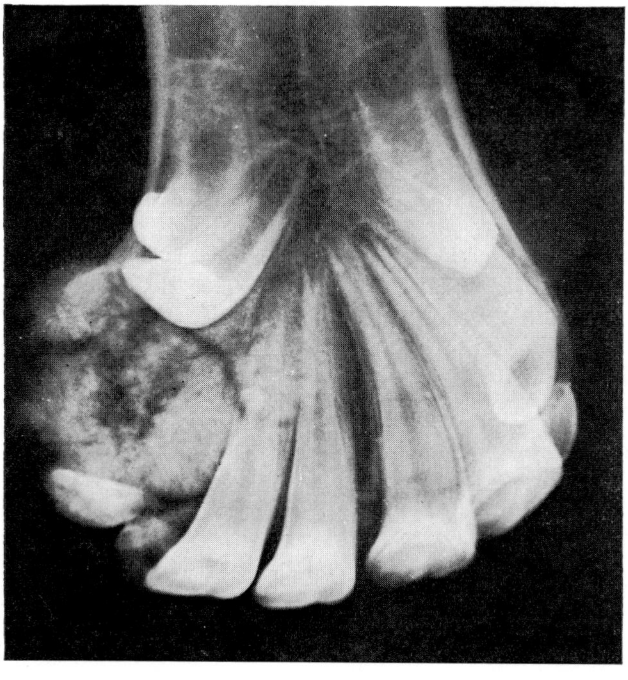
12

Fig. 2.1.17. — *10–11.* Fibrosarcoma of the mandible.

Fig. 2.1.17. — *12.* Osteosarcoma-like lesion of the pars incisiva of the mandible with impaired dentition.

2.1.17.2. Diseases of the Cervical, Thoracic and Lumbar Spine

Injuries

Closed injuries of the vertebral column (involving the bone and overlying soft tissue) can occur as a result of direct or indirect violence of varying force and duration. The most frequent causes of spinal injuries are falls at high speed or jumps, traffic accidents, blows against low-hanging crossbeams during standing, falls from a height, etc.

The spine can suffer various morphologic changes depending on the magnitude, direction and localization of the traumatizing force. Contusions, ligament ruptures, dislocations and vertebral fractures are possible in a great variety of combinations.

A spinal injury may be characterized as 'complete', and thus affecting an entire transverse plane of the spine, or 'partial', with damage limited to one process or vertebral arch. Complete injuries include:

1. vertebral fractures with associated tears of the ligaments and surrounding soft tissues;
2. complete transverse ruptures of all the spinal ligaments, without an associated vertebral fracture.

Ligament ruptures with vertebral displacement are called dislocations (or luxations). Complete injuries of the spine are associated with varying degrees of functional disability and impairment of general health. The degree of the disturbance depends on the character of the spinal injury and its location, and especially on whether injury to the spinal cord is involved.

Thus, a distinction must be made between uncomplicated spinal injuries involving no damage to the spinal cord or its meninges, and complicated injuries with associated cord lesions. In injuries of the latter variety, paralysis of the limbs is instantaneous. If a hematoma forms within the vertebral canal or edema develops, paralysis gradually develops.

Contusions of the spine are caused by direct violence and are usually limited to injuries of the soft tissues or bone surface without involvement of the cord. The resulting pain, which restricts mobility, is transitory and less severe than in the case of vertebral fractures. Associated symptoms tend to increase in severity for several days after the injury and then regress, disappearing in 9—12 days. Injuries of this type are treated with anti-inflammatory drugs.

Fractures and Dislocations of the Cervical Vertebrae

Occurrence. Fractures and dislocations of the cervical vertebrae are more common in the horse than in other animal species.

Symptoms. Symptoms depend on the location and character of the fracture or dislocation. For example, a fracture or dislocation that is accompanied by spinal cord lesions usually terminates fatally within a few hours. If a vertebral body or neural arch is fractured and there is no displacement of the processes or direct involvement of the cord, paralytic symptoms may worsen during subsequent days as a result of spinal meningitis and the accumulation of exudate in the vertebral canal. In the case of comminuted fractures, several days may pass before bone fragments work their way into the vertebral canal, causing paraplegia or even death.

In all fractures and dislocations of the cervical vertebrae, the most prominent clinical signs are limited cervical mobility and obvious pain when the head is forcibly pushed downward or turned to the side. Occasionally a painful swelling may be present at the fracture site due to a hematoma or collection of purulent exudate in the soft tissue. The head is held in a lowered position with the neck turned slightly

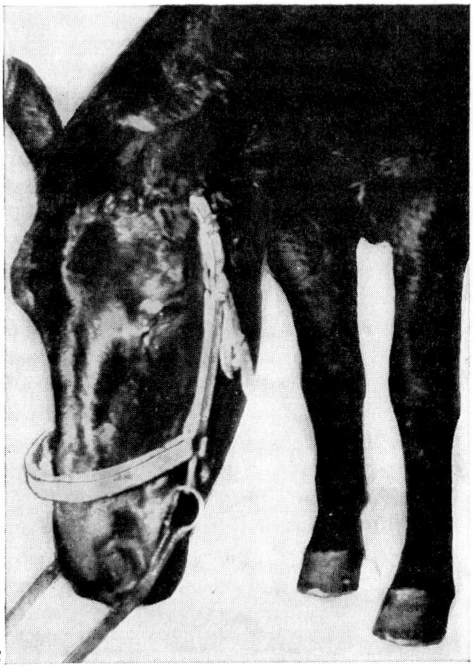

13

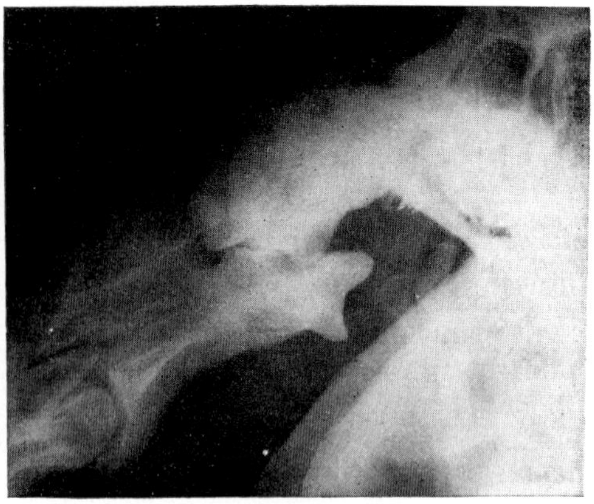

14

Fig. 2.1.17. — 13. Fracture of the cervical vertebrae: torticollis.
Fig. 2.1.17. — 14. Dislocation of the axis.

to one side. Congestive or dependent edema may develop in the head region (fig. 2.1.17. — 13).

Etiology. Most injuries and displacements of the cervical vertebrae in horses result from falls at high speed, falls onto the head during jumps, gunshot wounds, and other violent trauma. Predisposing factors include bony changes associated with osteoporosis-like conditions, osteochondrosis, epiphysitis, tumors, etc.

Diagnosis. With fractures of the 1st and 2nd cervical vertebrae, palpation reveals changes in the normal position of the vertebrae and in some cases crepitation. Determining the nature and exact location of the fracture or dislocation by clinical methods is difficult. Radiographic examination is necessary to arrive at an accurate diagnosis (fig. 2.1.17. — 14). In addition, puncture of the spinal canal through the foramen magnum can be performed to obtain cerebrospinal fluid for evaluation. The presence of blood in the fluid is sufficient to suspect a vertebral fracture.

Prognosis. Fractures of the vertebral body or neural arch and dislocations of the cervical vertebrae have an unfavorable prognosis. The outlook is favorable for closed fractures of the longitudinal or transverse processes if they are chipped. In open fractures, and especially in fractures complicated by infection, the prognosis is guarded or unfavorable.

Treatment. We do not believe that treatment is indicated in vertebral body or neural arch fractures or in dislocations where marked paraplegic symptoms are exhibited. In fractures where spinal cord functions are not impaired, measures should be taken to immobilize the head and neck.

Epidural Hematoma

Occurrence. Epidural hematomas and hemorrhage within the spinal cord sometimes occur as a sequel to trauma. The hematoma may or may not be associated with damage to the vertebrae or intervertebral ligaments. Hematomas are most common in the region of the cervical spine [Bolz, 1966].

Wehnert [1920] found a hemorrhagic effusion into the epidural space with subsequent hematoma formation in T_{17-18} of a horse. The blood entering the fatty epidural tissue can spread freely along the epidural space, causing compression of several cord segments. Nevertheless, the pressure of the epidural hematoma rarely leads to complete compressive paralysis of the cord, for the bleeding from small-caliber vessels and especially from thin-walled veins stops spontaneously. But even partial disruptions of the conduction pathways in the cord can result in severe loss of function in the locomotor organs. Symptoms can be exacerbated by fibrous scar-tissue formation at the site of the effusion.

Symptoms. Epidural hematoma is manifested by progressive paralysis due to cord compression. When the hematoma is located in the cervical region, paraplegia of the forelimbs soon develops. Apathy or stupor is usually present.

The pulse rate is elevated initially but later falls to a normal or even subnormal level. Respiration is calm, deep and predominantly costal. Berge and Müller [1965] observed severe respiratory distress due to diaphragmatic paralysis associated with fractures of C4 through C7. Dietz et al. [1965] reported no such clinical signs in horses with epidural hematomas.

The internal body temperature is usually normal. In isolated cases it may rise to 39.5—40.1 °C, returning to normal over the next 2—3 days. An improvement of general condition is also noted at this time. The appetite returns, but food prehension and mastication are still difficult.

Initially the head is moved as little as possible, and nuchal rigidity is present. During subsequent days the head is held progressively lower until it is only 20—30 cm from the ground. Thus, the horse stands quietly, but unsteadily, without turning its neck to the side or rotating it about the long axis. The limbs are usually held in a straddled position. The horse refuses to lie down for the first several days or does so only with extreme caution. It avoids any unnecessary movement and is especially reluctant to move the neck laterally. This makes eating and drinking difficult. Cutaneous sensation is not affected. On the other hand, edema of the head is fairly common. Palpation of the neck reveals only those changes associated with trauma to the vertebrae or soft tissues.

Radiographic examination of the cervical vertebrae is an important aid to differential diagnosis. It is useful in excluding vertebral fractures and dislocations. With an epidural hematoma in the thoracic or lumbar region, clinical signs generally do not appear for several hours. Only after this time do neurologic symptoms appear in the form of paresis of the hindquarters and pelvic organs (impaired micturition and defecation) and sensory loss in the associated cutaneous zones.

Etiology. Epidural hematomas most commonly result from a severe blow to the side of the head (collision with trees, walls or fences) or from extreme lateral flexion of the vertebral column without cord involvement or vertebral deformation. Epidural hematomas can also be caused by a severe spinal shock and by contusions and dislocations of intervertebral joints due to sudden violence.

The *diagnosis* is based upon the history, course, typical head carriage with consequent edema, inability to rotate the neck, the characteristic reaction to forcible raising of the head, negative radiographic findings, and the occurrence of ataxia, paresis and paralysis. An epidural hematoma of the thoracic and lumbar spine and of the sacrum is recognized from the clinical symptoms described above.

Differential Diagnosis. In edema of the head due to other causes, passive movements of the neck do not produce pain.

Contusions and sprains of the intervertebral joints are usually distinguished by marked local swelling and tenderness. These signs are not pronounced in subluxations and incomplete fractures of the vertebrae. When these lesions involve the cervical vertebrae, they can be demonstrated by radiography. Epidural hematoma may also be present in such cases.

Dislocations and fractures of the cervical vertebrae are distinguished by such local findings as deformity, swelling, crepitation, and marked disturbances of cord function (paraparesis, dyspnea). Radiographic examination can establish the diagnosis. Dislocations and fractures of the thoracic and lumbar vertebrae are easily recognized, especially if there is a complete disruption of spinal cord pathways causing a total, instantaneous loss of function in the hind limbs and pelvic organs.

In the presence of torticollis, the dorsal and ventral midlines are no longer parallel, and there is a twisting of the neck that may be combined with lateral, upward or downward deviation.

Tumors of the spine develop gradually and are slow to produce changes in the posture of the neck. They can be excluded by radiographic examination [Bolz]. Lesions due to fungal infection of the thoracic, lumbar and sacral vertebrae are relatively uncommon in the horse and, when they occur, are difficult to diagnose.

Open injuries of the vertebral column are rarely accompanied by epidural hematoma.

Prognosis. The prognosis is favorable if the right balance is achieved between pressure and counterpressure in the area of the hematoma when the animal is standing quietly. As the extravasation is absorbed, the pressure will gradually lessen, the animal's condition will improve, and clinical symptoms referable to the hematoma will disappear. However, if the trauma recurs or the process is reactivated, there will be renewed hemorrhage leading to progressive paresis and paralysis or even to death from respiratory arrest.

Treatment. The goal of treatment is the reduction and elimination of cord compression caused by the extravasation. The main emphasis is not on the use of drugs, but on the careful management of the patient, including the provision of complete rest. The horse is confined in a large box stall. Food should be placed on the floor. Any lifting of the head or turning of the neck to one side (e.g., by leading on a halter) is dangerous. This also contraindicates tying the animal on a short rope.

If the horse is lying quietly, it should not be disturbed or made to stand. Calm animals may be placed in a sling. In most cases the horse will refuse to lie down or will do so only with great caution.

Edema of the head usually requires no special treatment and will regress spontaneously when circulatory conditions are improved. As the edema fluid is absorbed, the head will be held more upright.

Vasotonic agents, local irritants and heat applications are contraindicated.

Very light exercise may be started after 14 days. Ataxic signs should disappear in 2—3 weeks. Recovery may be complete as early as the 5th week, although it is wise to limit exertion for several weeks thereafter.

Absorption of the edema may be hastened by administering hypertonic glucose, fructose or sorbitol solutions. Large doses of B-complex vitamins are given simultaneously.

Torticollis (Wryneck) (cf. Sec. 2.8.6.1.)

Definition and Etiology. This relatively rare condition is occasionally seen in racing horses. It can have various causes: fractures of the articular processes of the cervical vertebrae, strains and ruptures of tendons and muscles, neurogenic paralyses of the cervical muscles, joint contracture of the cervical spine. Sometimes torticollis occurs as a result of local toxicity from tetanus toxoid following inoculations. In cases of unilateral muscular tears, contraction of the contralateral muscles can produce a myogenic torticollis.

Symptoms. The head is usually lowered. The neck is twisted and drawn to one side, so that one side of the neck is convex and the other concave. Acute cases and those due to muscular disease may be marked by tenderness, local heat and a firm, boardlike swelling. It may be possible to extend the neck by applying pressure to the swelling with one hand while turning the head toward the side of the lesion, but the torticollis will return when the hand is removed. In long-standing cases passive congestion occurs, and the head becomes edematous. In cases due to vertebral lesions, the neck generally cannot be straightened by passive manipulation.

Prognosis. If inflammatory muscle changes are responsible for the torticollis, the prognosis is favorable. With disease of the articular processes, the prognosis is poor. The same applies to joint contractures, neurogenic muscular paralyses and dislocations.

Treatment. If inflammatory symptoms are present, treatment follows general surgical rules: immediate application of cold, later of heat; moist, drying alcohol dressings; paraffin fomentations; shortwave; massage; systemic and topical glucocorticoids.

Sprains of the Vertebral Column

Sprains of the vertebral column involve incomplete lesions of the spinal ligaments or intervertebral discs. They can result from sudden, uncoordinated movements, sharp turns or falls.

Sprains are accompanied by minor dislocations of the vertebrae and by more or less permanent functional disability of the vertebral column. The major symptoms are severe pain in the area of the trauma and restricted movement, especially during turns. A diagnosis of 'sprain' or 'strain' can be made only on the basis of a thorough clinical examination (including neurologic tests and a radiographic evaluation if possible), once a vertebral fracture or dislocation has been excluded. No differentiation need be made between a sprain and strain.

Treatment. Rest, heat application with paraffin, microwave therapy, glucocorticoids, phenylbutazone.

Fractures of the Thoracic and Lumbar Vertebrae

Classification. Fractures are a common form of injury sustained by the thoracic and lumbar spine. Two basic types are recognized:

— isolated fractures of one part of the vertebra (spinous, transverse or articular process, neural arch or body);

— combined fractures of the body, neural arch and processes.

Symptoms and Treatment. Isolated fractures of the spinous processes are mainly caused by direct trauma from above and by falls onto the back. A sharply-circumscribed area of tenderness, swelling and possible crepitation is detected following the injury. The horse stands with its back slightly arched.

Treatment is conservative and consists of rest and the application of anti-inflammatory ointments, followed by massage.

Neural arch fractures result from violence to the spinous processes. Displacement of the bone fragments with impingement on the cord is possible in severe cases.

The degree of cord involvement is determined from the clinical examination, during which the nature of the functional disturbances is also ascertained. It is useful to gain some idea of the degree of vertebral damage that has occurred. In the case of the spinous processes, this is best done by radiography.

If there is evidence of cord damage associated with a neural arch fracture, surgery is indicated. This consists in a laminectomy for the purpose of removing bone fragments.

Fractures of the vertebral bodies are caused by extreme violence associated with falls, blows to the back from low overhead beams or partitions, or sudden flexion of the spine caused by extreme force (falling trees, rocks). In contrast to dislocations, which tend to occur in the most mobile segments of the spine (e.g., the cervical vertebrae), fractures of the vertebral body tend to occur at junctions between mobile and immobile segments. The lumbar vertebrae are predisposed. Excessive bending of the spine causes compression of the intervertebral cartilage and exerts extreme pressure on the adjacent vertebrae. The result of this is a 'wedge fracture', i.e., a compression fracture in which the vertebra is crushed and assumes the shape of a wedge.

If unusually large forces are involved, two adjacent vertebral bodies may be crushed, both becoming impacted to form a single wedge-shaped mass. In very severe cases the vertebral injury is accompanied by ligamentous ruptures, vertebral dislocations and cord lesions.

Depending on the elasticity of the bony tissue and on the magnitude and degree of the compression, the damage to the vertebral body may take the form of a weakening, fissure fracture, wedge fracture, transverse fracture, oblique fracture, or complete destruction of the vertebral body.

The *clinical diagnosis* of a vertebral body fracture is based on the history, the mechanism of the injury and the clinical symptoms. The latter consist of tenderness to palpation at the fracture site, restricted motion, depression, a defect in the normal contour of the backline, and signs of impaired cord function. Percussion causes obvious pain in the area of the associated spinous process and is a valuable diagnostic aid. Sweating localized to zones and hindquarter paralysis point to a vertebral body or neural arch fracture with cord compression.

The *prognosis* of vertebral fractures is unfavorable in racing animals, especially with cord involvement. Euthanasia is the recommended action in such cases. In vertebral fractures without associated cord injury, recovery is possible. The animal will be unsound for future athletic use because ataxic symptoms tend to persist.

Puncture wounds and incised wounds of the spine may be associated with cord injury if the sharp object penetrates the vertebral canal. Paralysis of the limbs and pelvic organs may develop, depending on the level of the injury. Occasionally only a hemiplegia occurs, and sometimes spinal fluid is discharged from the wound. The injury may introduce pathogenic organisms into the depths of the wound, leading to the development of a purulent meningitis or myelitis. Sometimes a foreign body is left within the vertebral canal.

Puncture and incised wounds of the back and lumbar region may be associated with damage to the pleura or peritoneum in addition to the spinal injury. The neurologic deficits caused by direct damage to the cord are irreversible and make the horse unsound for further use. Puncture wounds of the back that do not penetrate the vertebral canal, leave no residual foreign bodies, and do not invole the cord usually have a favorable prognosis. Vertebral injuries that impinge on the spinal canal are an

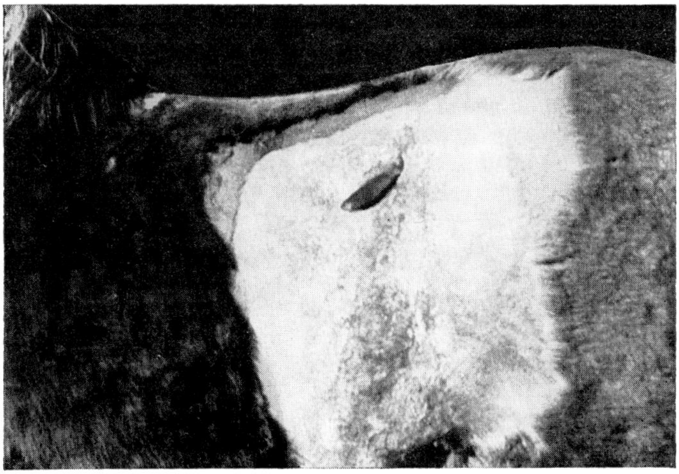

Fig. 2.1.17. — 15. Fistula of the lumbar spine following a fracture of the transverse process.

indication for surgery. Bone splinters and foreign bodies must be removed. Injuries in proximity to the vertebral column will lead to abscessation in the psoas muscles and to fistulization, possibly accompanied by hemiplegia, unless wound care is immediate and thorough (fig. 2.1.17. — 15).

Gunshot wounds of the spine are grave injuries that are fraught with potential complications. They are commonly associated with severe cord damage.

A distinction is made between perforating and nonperforating injuries of the spine. In perforating injuries, there is a breach in the bony wall of the canal system (arch, body, spinous or transverse process, upper surface of vertebral body). Nonperforating injuries are characterized by damage to parts of the vertebra that do not form a portion of the vertebral canal (inferior and central portions of the vertebral body, tips of the spinous and transverse processes). While the dura mater is not damaged, some contusion of the cord is generally present.

Gunshot injuries of the vertebral column in which the missile track runs dorsoventrally may be associated with perforating abdominal wounds, damage to the abdominal organs, or, if the thoracic spine is involved, damage to the pleural cavity and lung.

It is not always easy to recognize combined injuries of this type, because the deficits caused by the spinal cord trauma (urine retention, bowel paresis, sensory disturbances) may be masked by symptoms referable to the abdominal injury.

Systemic Diseases of the Vertebral Column

Generalized Osteodystrophia fibrosa

In the generalized form of osteodystrophia fibrosa, the vertebral column undergoes changes analogous to those seen in other skeletal regions. In the early stage of the disease, signs of osteoporosis appear in the vertebral bodies. The intervertebral discs are not affected. The disease is gradually progressive in character, and the prognosis is poor.

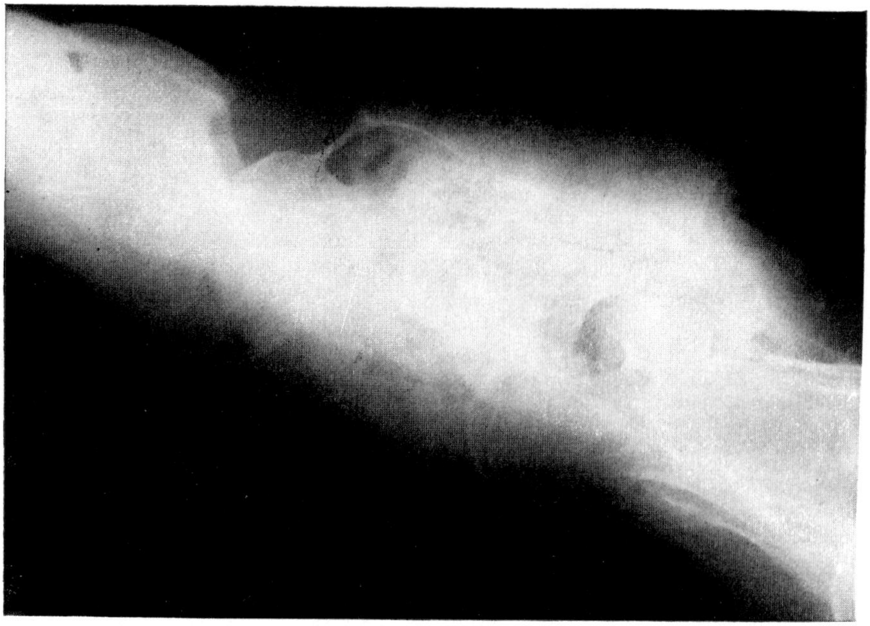

Fig. 2.1.17. — 16. Tuberculous osteomyelitis of the axis.

Vertebral Osteomyelitis

Osteomyelitis develops mainly as a complication of open fractures that have become contaminated with bacteria. In some cases osteomyelitis develops by the hematogenous route in connection with infected cutaneous wounds, skin diseases and other purulent processes (fig. 2.1.17. — 16). Acute, suppurative osteomyelitis takes a fulminating course and terminates fatally within a short time, the inflammation spreading rapidly from the neural arch to the cord.

Chronic osteomyelitis is less common than the acute form. It may result from the progression of an acute osteomyelitis or may show chronic features from the outset. The etiology is the same as in the acute form. Systemic signs need not be present. In chronic cases the suppurative focus in the vertebral body spreads to involve the intervertebral discs. The patient is depressed and shows signs of pain during movement, especially when turning. If the osteomyelitic process has its seat in the cervical vertebrae, the mobility of the neck will be limited. Slightly elevated temperatures are occasionally seen.

The prognosis is unfavorable with regard to a complete restoration of soundness. A spondylitis or spondylosis usually develops.

Treatment is conservative but is of little benefit.

Spondylosis

Definition. Spondylosis is a chronic degenerative disease of the vertebral column. The lesions in spondylosis are located in those parts of the spine that are subject to the greatest mechanical stresses, i.e., the lumbar region. Morphologically, spondylosis is characterized by changes in the ventral longitudinal ligament, the intervertebral discs and the vertebral bodies. Degenerative spondylosis is extremely rare in racehorses.

Symptoms. Affected horses are reluctant to lie down or have difficulty standing up. The animal resists being saddled and mounted by a rider, is reluctant to jump, and may refuse many gaits.

In work horses, the development of kyphosis is a frequent symptom of spondylosis.

Etiology and Pathogenesis. The etiologic factors in spondylosis relate to trauma, excessive and prolonged stress, and primary degenerative changes in the annulus fibrosus of the intervertebral disc cartilage. Abnormal use can also contribute to the progression of spondylosis. Stretch injuries of the spinal ligament, especially the longitudinal ligaments, produce lesions of the fibrous tissue. Degenerative changes of the spinal ligaments are demonstrable in such cases. The longitudinal ligaments respond to the inflammatory process with calcification, the formation of periosteal deposits and subsequent ossification. Thus, spondylosis always involves secondary changes in the spinal ligament system. The deformities that develop in the vertebrae essentially represent late manifestations of spinal disease and usually are present morphologically long before they produce clinical signs. The degenerative changes in the vertebral bodies progress very slowly and only to a certain point.

Diagnosis. Radiographic changes can be demonstrated in some cases.

The *prognosis* is unfavorable due to the lack of an effective therapy. Horses with spondylosis are considered to be unsound.

Overlapping of Thoracic and Lumbar Spinous Processes ('Kissing' Spines)

Definition. Two or more spinous processes of the thoracic and lumbar vertebrae are in contact or overlap as a result of extreme enlargement. The condition was first described in 1968 by Roberts, who discussed its symptoms and surgical treatment.

Symptoms. Faults of gait in the hindquarters of trotting horses, or repeated breaks from the trot, may be symptomatic of overlapping spinous processes in the thoracic-lumbar region. Affected riding horses frequently exhibit classic symptoms of 'saddle shyness', and will buck or lie down when the cinch is tightened. Some horses will show signs of pain when standing up, or will groan or show other signs of discomfort when saddled or when landing after a jump. Other horses will resist being mounted by a rider or will refuse to jump altogether. Local examination reveals marked tenderness over the affected spinous processes. Many horses will lie down during this palpation or swing the hindquarters away from the examiner.

Etiology. Often a history of trauma to the spine can be elicited, possibly caused by a fall onto the back. In other cases no obvious cause can be demonstrated. Following a blunt trauma to the spinous process of the thoracic and lumbar vertebrae, the horse may remain asymptomatic for months or even years, until overlapping of the spinous processes develops following a prolonged inflammation of the cartilaginous caps of the spines.

Diagnosis. Palpation of the spinous processes should begin at the withers and work backward. In many cases this will reveal a widening and hardening of the cartilaginous caps of the spinous processes. In extreme cases an interspace can no longer be felt between two adjacent spines. A local examination of this type yields better and more accurate results if the animal is cast under light general anesthesia supplemented with muscle-relaxing drugs. While local tenderness cannot be demonstrated in such circumstances, the relaxed back muscles will allow a 'deep' palpation of the spinous processes in the thoracic and lumbar region. Overlapping of the spinous processes is evidenced not only by an absence of interspace between adjacent spines, but also by an extreme ossification and rigidity of the cartilaginous caps. A positive diagnosis can be established by radiography. Again, visualization of the overlap is enhanced if the animal is cast for the examination.

Differential Diagnosis. Similar symptoms exist in the tying-up syndrome, degenerative spondylosis and spondylarthritis, but these conditions mainly affect older draft horses. Subluxations of the sacroiliac joint can also mimic overlapping spines. Differentiation is made by palpation and radiographic evaluation.

Treatment. Surgical treatment may produce consistently good results. The horse is cast under general anesthesia and positioned in lateral recumbency. A skin incision is made about 2 cm from and parallel to the dorsal midline on each side. The touching or overlapping spinous processes are exposed from both sides by carefully dissecting away the attached back muscles. The resection is performed with the aid of a wire saw. The sharp edges of the spinous stumps are rounded, and the muscles and skin are reapproximated and sutured. Roberts [1968] recommends 2 months of stall rest postoperatively, after which time the animal may be exercised on a lead for 1 month.

Prognosis. The majority of patients are free of pain postoperatively and can be returned to work.

Neoplasms

Both benign and malignant tumors of the vertebral column are uncommon in the horse. A primary osteosarcoma has been described by Bolz [1965]. Metastases from malignant neoplasms, especially melanomas, are occasionally reported.

Treatment is useless, and the prognosis is unfavorable.

2.1.17.3. Diseases of the Sacrum and Pelvis

Fractures of the Sacrum

Occurrence and Etiology. Fractures of the sacrum are relatively uncommon. They result from direct trauma associated with falls, blows or collisions with vehicles.

Symptoms. Palpation of the sacrum may reveal an indentation or protrusion. Fractures of the sacrum may be accompanied by injuries of the lumbosacral plexus, in which case symptoms of sciatic paralysis will be evident. In fractures of the lateral parts of the sacrum with concomitant damage to the tubera sacralia of the ilium, the horse will have difficulty standing up. It is reluctant to lie down, and lameness is apparent on walking. Fractures of the sacrum always produce an asymmetry about the hip that is obvious on inspection. The fracture of a vertebral segment is palpable during rectal examination. Crepitus can sometimes be detected by placing one hand on the sacral region and 'pumping' the tail with the other.

With paraplegias and paralyses of the urinary bladder, rectum and tail, the prognosis is unfavorable and slaughter should be considered.

Treatment. Rest for 5—7 weeks, local heat applications, anti-inflammatory drugs (where required).

Fractures of the Pelvis

Occurrence and Classification. Fractures of the pelvic bones are more frequent than those of the vertebrae. The fracture may be transverse or oblique, the latter being associated with displacement of the fragments as a result of muscle contractions. Pelvic fractures can be classified into two groups. The first group includes fractures that involve separation of the pelvic girdle (pelvic ring fractures). These are parallel fractures of the ascending pubic ramus, the acetabulum and iliac shaft, or the medial iliac spine. The second group includes fractures of the pelvic brim. These are chip fractures of the tuber coxae, tuber ischii or symphyseal ramus of the ischium.

Symptoms. The symptoms vary with the nature of the fracture. Fractures of the iliac shaft and tuber coxae result in asymmetry of the croup. The avulsed tuber coxae is pulled downward by contraction of the tensor fasciae latae and internal abdominal oblique muscles. Initially there is a severe swinging-leg lameness that passes in 2—3 weeks. Fractures of the iliac shaft produce severe lameness or recumbency. The avulsed tuber coxae can be detected by palpation. One can also measure the distance from the tuber sacrale to the superior angle of the tuber coxae on the affected and unaffected sides. If the two distances are equal, absence of a fracture of the iliac shaft must be assumed. If the distance is longer on the affected side, however, a fracture of the tuber coxae is indicated. On rectal examination in the standing or recumbent position, the fracture line in the iliac shaft, pubic ramus, ischial ramus or pelvic symphysis can be palpated during passive movement of the limb. Fractures of the iliac shaft may be complicated by ruptures of the external iliac artery and vein. When the artery is ruptured, a rapidly progressive and often fatal blood loss will develop as a result of intra-abdominal hemorrhage.

Often crepitation can be detected by placing the free hand over the tuber coxae or tuber ischii while the rectum is being explored. Transrectal or transvaginal radiography may be attempted.

The *prognosis* for closed, uncomplicated fractures of the tuber coxae, tuber ischii and iliac shaft is favorable in terms of survival but unfavorable in terms of restoring the animal to working or racing soundness. The formation of a large callus, especially in a displaced fracture of the iliac shaft, leads to a narrowing of the pelvic ring that could cause dystocia in mares.

Treatment. In closed fractures of the tuber coxae or tuber ischii, reduction is extremely difficult due to the considerable downward displacement of the fragment. Attempts at internal fixation are not successful. But because the use of the limb is not impaired in this type of fracture, no treatment is indicated in closed fractures. A racing animal can easily be rendered unsound by such an injury.

Open fractures are managed surgically, with removal of the displaced fragment.

With a fracture of the iliac shaft, reduction and fixation are virtually impossible. However, because such fractures show minimal displacement, the fracture is able to heal without treatment. In the case of symphyseal fractures, euthanasia should be considered.

Subluxation of the Sacroiliac Joint

Definition. The sacroiliac joint in the horse is a diarthrosis formed by the articular surfaces of the sacrum and the ilium. In the mature horse, little or no movement is possible in this diarthrosis due to the bony fusion that has occurred between the cartilage layers. The entire diarthrosis is surrounded by a strong ligament system. The ventral sacroiliac ligament reinforces the lower portion of the joint. In addition, a strong ligament system is present between the angle of the ilium and the sacrum or its spinous processes. Because the sacroiliac joint is not meant to be mobile in the adult, violence to this region can cause a loosening of the diarthrosis or even a partial or complete rupture of its ligament system, resulting in subluxation. As long as mobility exists in the sacroiliac joint, chronic pain is present.

Symptoms. The most common symptom is evidence of pain when the animal stands up. The horse may emit painful grunts during this time. Some stiffness of the hindquarters is apparent during movement. Pain may be elicited by pressing on the tuber coxae or tuber sacrale, due to the associated rotation of the pelvis. In normal horses, the right and left tubera sacralia can be felt on deep palpation, and the sacrum can be palpated in a depression between the tuber coxae. When the sacroiliac joint is subluxated, this deep palpation produces pain. Inequalities in the distance between the sacrum and tuber sacrale may be palpable in some cases. The muscles overlying the sacral region may be painful. If the subluxation is of chronic duration, an asymmetry of the tuber sacrale will be evident when the animal is viewed from the side or from behind. This unevenness is considered a reliable sign of sacroiliac subluxation. In acute cases, it is reported that crepitation can be elicited by applying digital pressure over the sacroiliac joint. Many horses with chronic subluxation refuse to jump or perform any kind of rapid gait. Symptoms in chronic cases can sometimes mimic a unilateral or bilateral hip lameness. The rectal examination can be useful. This is especially true in cases with marked ventral displacement of the sacrum which narrows the palpable space between the sacrum and tuber sacrale. In chronic cases the rectal examination is of limited value. ADAMS [1969] recommends that the rectal examination be done while the horse is walking slowly. While one hand is inserted in the rectum, the other hand is placed over the tuber sacrale. A mobility, and sometimes even a kind of crepitation, can be detected under these conditions. In some cases sacroiliac joint mobility can also be detected by backing the horse for one or two steps and then having it walk forward a step or two.

Etiology. Subluxation of the sacroiliac joint can result from falls, slips and any other trauma causing stress to the sacroiliac region.

Diagnosis. The demonstration of loosening and movement of the tubera sacralia during walking confirms the diagnosis. Asymmetry of the tubera sacralia is also an important sign. In addition, there must be some degree of stiffness in the movement of the hindquarters. ADAMS [1969] states that when evidence of pain is present, the injection of a local anesthetic and steroids could be a useful aid to differential diagnosis (similar injections are used to relieve the pain of sacroiliac subluxation in humans). If pain were relieved by such injections, then the diagnosis would be established. As ADAMS points out, the injections would have to be extensive to cover the ligamentous attachments and the joint.

Differential Diagnosis. Thrombosis of the terminal aorta or its bifurcation is excluded by rectal exploration. Stiffness occurring as a sequel to tying-up syndrome can be excluded by the history. Overlapping of the lumbar spinous processes is excluded by palpation. According to ROBERTS [1968], a hormone-related loosening of the sacroiliac ligaments should be considered in older horses.

Treatment. If a trauma has been identified as the cause of the subluxation, sufficient time must be allowed for ligamentous healing to occur. This means complete rest for at least 2 months. Injections of sclerosing agents are recommended to enhance stability in the lax sacroiliac joint. The injection of glucocorticoids prevents or delays stabilization.

The *prognosis* is always guarded, especially in cases where adequate rest cannot be enforced. Experience shows that if the joint is adequately stabilized, a recurrence is unlikely.

2.1.17.4. Diseases of the Tail

Fractures of the Coccygeal Vertebrae

In fractures of the 1st coccygeal vertebra with associated injury to the cauda equina, paralysis of the tail results. The tail hangs limp, and crepitation is detected on palpation. All cutaneous sensation is lost, and the root of the tail is no longer raised during defecation.

In injuries of the last coccygeal vertebrae, no signs of tail paralysis are present. The only visible change is an abnormal mobility at the fracture site that is easily detected. Radiographs in two planes provide the best means of localizing and evaluating the fracture.

With paralysis of the tail that is unresponsive to treatment, amputation is indicated.

Open fractures of the coccygeal vertebrae may be complicated by suppurative, necrotizing processes that lead to fistulization. Hence, primary surgical wound care for the prophylaxis of infection is of special importance in this type of fracture. All loose bone fragments are removed, and the wound is closed by suture or a bandage is applied. In complicated fractures, gangrene of the tail is a great danger and, when present, necessitates amputation.

Tail Muscle Contracture, Crooked Tail

A crooked tail represents a significant handicap for show horses and jumpers. A myotomy or myectomy of the contracted tail muscles is curative.

References

Adams, O. R.: Subluxation of the sacroiliac joint in horses. Proc. Amer. Assoc. Equine Pract., p. 191 (1969).

Auge, G.; Casieux, A.: Elements de diagnostic radiologique des lesions rachidiennes. Rev. Méd. Vét. *122:* 2 (1971).

Bolz, W.: Das klinische Bild nach einem Fibromyxoosteosarkom der Halswirbel beim Pferd. Tierärztl. Umschau *20:* 10 (1965).

Bolz, W.: Epidurales Hämatom der Halswirbelsäule beim Pferd. Dtsch. Tierärztl. Wschr. *73:* 23 (1966).

Buscher, D.: Operative Behandlung einer Unterkieferfraktur bei einem Warmblutfohlen. Prakt. Tierarzt *54:* 12 (1973).

Gabel, A. A.: A method of surgical repair of the fractured mandible in the horse. J. Amer. vet. med. Assoc. *128:* 155 (1959).

Göbel, P.: Eine Schläfenbeinfraktur beim Pferd. Mh. Vet.-Med. *19:* 503 (1956).

Hanselka, D. V., et al.: Adamantioma of the equine mandible. Vet. Med. and Small Animal Clinician *69:* 2 (1974).

Hustienne, H.; Wissdorf, H.: Beitrag zur Behandlung von Frakturen am Kopf des Pferdes. Dtsch. tierärztl. Wschr. *72:* 23 (1972).

Laefler, K.: Die Wirbelsäule und ihre Erkrankungen beim Haustiere. Prakt. Tierarzt *48:* 6 (1967).

Marcenac, L.: La Pathologie du cheval de selle. Rév. Elevage *20:* II (1965).

Matthias, D.; Dietz, O.; Rechenberg, S.: Zur Klinik und Pathologie der spinalen Ataxie der Fohlen. Arch. exp. Vet.-Med. Sonderheft, S. 19 (1965).

Muzafarow, K. F.: Röntgenologische Untersuchungen bei Pferden. Vet.-med. Diss., Moskau (1971).

Roberts, E. J.: Resection of thoracic or lumbar spinous processes for the relief of pain responsible for lameness and some other locomotor disorders of horses. Proc. Amer. Assoc. Equine Pract., p. 13 (1968).

Roberts, E. J.: Amputation of a lumbar spinous process in the horse. Proc. Amer. Assoc. Equine Pract., p. 115 (1968).

Rooney, J. R.: Biomechanics of lameness in horses (Williams and Wilkins, Baltimore 1969).

Rooney, J. R., et al.: Sacroiliac luxation in the horse. Proc. Amer. Assoc. Equine Pract., p. 193 (1969).

Rooney, J. R., et al.: Sacroiliac luxation in the horse. Equine Vet. J. *1:* 287 (1969).

Rooney, J. R.: Etiology of the Wobbler syndrome. Mod. Vet. Pract. *53:* 9 (1972).

POMMER, A.: Röntgenologische Darstellung der Kiefergelenke beim Pferd. Wien. tierärztl. Mschr. *36:* 5 (1949).

SMITH, W. B.; MICHOLS, M. D.: External fixation of a compound fracture of the equine mandible. West. Vet., p. 4 (1957).

STIHL, H. G.: Frakturen als orthopädisches Problem beim Sportpferd. Schweiz. Arch. Tierhk. *110:* 309 (1968).

DUCHARME

Diseases of the Horse

A Handbook for Science and Practice

Part 1

Edited by

Prof. Dr. sc. med. vet. Olof Dietz, Berlin

Prof. Dr. sc. med. vet. Ekkehard Wiesner, Berlin

English translation edited by

Dr. A. S. Turner, Fort Collins, Colo.

73 figures (partly in color), 31 tables, 1984

KARGER

S. Karger · Basel · München · Paris · London · New York · Tokyo · Sydney

Translated from the original German edition by TERRY C. TELGER, Marina, Calif.

National Library of Medicine. Cataloging in Publication

Handbuch der Pferdekrankheiten für Wissenschaft und Praxis. English.
Diseases of the horse: a handbook for science and practice / edited by Olof Dietz, Ekkehard Wiesner; English translation edited by A. S. Turner. Basel; New York: Karger, 1984. Translation of: Handbuch der Pferdekrankheiten für Wissenschaft und Praxis.
1. Horse Diseases I. Dietz, Olof II. Turner, A. Simon III. Wiesner, Ekkehard
ISBN 3-8055-3497-3
SF 951 H 236

Printed in the German Democratic Republic
ISBN 3-8055-3497-3

Contents of the Present Volume

Contents of the Complete Work

Part 2/II Special Part (Continuation)

Contributors

Friedrich Berschneider, D. Sc., Food Chemist and Senior Assistant, Division of Nutritional and Hereditary Diseases, Section of Animal Production and Veterinary Medicine, Humboldt University, Berlin, GDR

Walter Busch, D. V. M. Sc., Veterinary Consultant, Professor and Head, Division of Reproductive Physiology and Pathology and Head of Obstetric Clinic, Section of Animal Production and Veterinary Medicine, Humboldt University, Berlin, GDR

Hedwig Daniels, D. V. M., Specialist in Internal Medicine, Hochmoor Veterinary Clinic, FRG

Olof Dietz, D. V. M. Sc., Professor and Head, Division of Surgery and Radiology, Veterinary Surgical Clinic, Hoppegarten Veterinary Clinic, and Head of Central Radiology Department, Section of Animal Production and Veterinary Medicine, Humboldt University, Berlin, GDR

Friedemann Döcke, D. V. M., Lecturer, Institute for Experimental Endocrinology, Humboldt University, Berlin, GDR

Karl Elze, D. V. M. Sc., Ph. D., Veterinary Consultant, Division of Reproductive Physiology and Pathology, Section of Animal Production and Veterinary Medicine, Karl Marx University, Leipzig, GDR

Horst Gängel, D. V. M., Lecturer and Physician-in-Chief, Division of Surgery and Radiology, Veterinary Surgical Clinic, Hoppegarten Veterinary Clinic and Central Radiology Department, Section of Animal Production and Veterinary Medicine, Humboldt University, Berlin, GDR

Johannes Gruner, D. V. M., Senior Veterinary Consultant and Head, Lutherstadt-Wittenberg Veterinary Clinic, Institute of Veterinary Science, Halle, GDR

Klaus Hartung, D. V. M., Ph. D., Clinic for Equine Diseases and General Surgery, Free University of Berlin, West Berlin

Theodor Hiepe, D. V. M. Sc., Senior Veterinary Consultant, Professor and Head, Division of Parasitology, Section of Animal Production and Veterinary Medicine, Humboldt University, Berlin, GDR

Friedhelm Horsch, D. V. M. Sc., Veterinary Consultant, Professor and Head, Division of Microbiology and Epizootiology, Section of Animal Production and Veterinary Medicine, Humboldt University, Berlin, GDR

Bernhard Huskamp, D. V. M., Specialist in Veterinary Surgery, Head of the Hochmoor Veterinary Clinic, FRG

Tadeusz Janiak, D. V. M., Professor and Director, Veterinary Medical Clinic, School of Veterinary Medicine, Wrocław Agricultural College, Poland

Klaus-Dieter Jentzsch, D. V. M., Ph. D., Lecturer, Institute for Pharmaceutical Research, Department of Pharmacology II, Academy of Sciences of the GDR, Berlin

Peter Knezevic, D. V. M., Professor and Head, Animal Orthopedic Clinic and Department of Animal Orthopedics, Veterinary Medical University of Vienna, Austria

Norbert Kopf, D. V. M., Surgical and Ophthalmic Clinic, Veterinary Medical University of Vienna, Austria

Hans-Joachim Kuller, D. V. M., Veterinary Consultant, Head of the Center for Equine Health, Dahlwitz-Hoppegarten, GDR

Werner Leemann, D. V. M., Professor and Director, Veterinary Medical Clinic, College of Veterinary Medicine, University of Zurich, Switzerland

Jürgen Mill, D. V. M., Senior Physician, Division of Surgery and Radiology, Hoppegarten Veterinary Clinic, Section of Animal Production and Veterinary Medicine, Humboldt University, Berlin, GDR

Antoine de Moor, D. V. M., Professor and Director, Veterinary Surgical Clinic, University of Ghent, Belgium

GERHARD PRIETZ, D. V. M. Sc., Veterinary Consultant and Senior Physician, Division of Surgery and Radiology, Section of Animal Production and Veterinary Medicine, Humboldt University, Berlin, GDR

WILFRIED RICHTER, D. V. M. Sc., Veterinary Consultant and Physician-in-Chief, Hoppegarten Veterinary Clinic, Section of Animal Production and Veterinary Medicine, Humboldt University, Berlin, GDR

FRANZ SCHAETZ, D. V. M. Sc., D. M. V. h. c., Senior Veterinary Consultant, Professor Emeritus, Section of Animal Production and Veterinary Medicine, Humboldt University, Berlin, GDR

MAGNUS SCHÄFER, D. V. M. Sc., Professor and Head, Division of Veterinary Internal Medicine and Pathologic Physiology, Section of Animal Production and Veterinary Medicine, Karl Marx University, Leipzig, GDR

HANS SCHLEITER, D. V. M. Sc., Senior Veterinary Consultant, Professor and Head of the Veterinary Surgical Clinic and Division of Surgery and Radiology, Section of Animal Production and Veterinary Medicine, Karl Marx University, Leipzig, GDR

VERA SCHMIDT, D. V. M. Sc., Veterinary Consultant, Professor and Head of the Small-Animal Division and Small-Animal Clinic, Section of Animal Production and Veterinary Medicine, Karl Marx University, Leipzig, GDR

HANS-JOACHIM SCHNEIDER, D. V. M., Veterinary Consultant and Physician-in-Chief, Division of Surgery and Radiology and Veterinary Surgical Clinic, Section of Animal Production and Veterinary Medicine, Karl Marx University, Leipzig, GDR

NIKOLAI ALEXANDROWITSCH SUDAKOV, D. V. M. Sc., Ph. D., Head, Department of Therapeutics and Clinical Diagnosis, College of Veterinary Medicine, Ukranian Agricultural Academy, Kiev, USSR

PJOTR TERECHOV, D. V. M. Sc., Ph. D., Veterinary Surgical Clinic, Veterinary Medical Academy of Moscow, USSR

ROLF TEUSCHER, D. V. M. Sc., Senior Veterinary Consultant, Naumburg/Saale, GDR

EKKEHARD WIESNER, D. V. M. Sc., Professor and formerly Head, Division of Nutritional and Hereditary Diseases, Section of Animal Production and Veterinary Medicine, Humboldt University, Berlin, GDR

SIEGFRIED WILLER, D. V. M., Lecturer and Senior Assistant, Division of Nutritional and Hereditary Diseases, Section of Animal Production and Veterinary Medicine, Humboldt University, Berlin, GDR

Foreword

I first learned about the three-volume German publication *Diseases of the Horse: A Handbook for Science and Practice* while visiting Dr. BERNARD HUSKAMP of the Animal Clinic, Hochmoor, West Germany in 1981. During this visit I began to appreciate the enormous communication gap that exists between European countries and English-speaking countries especially in the field of veterinary medicine.

Because of my personal inability to efficiently read scientific German literature, I heretofore failed to recognize their contributions to our scientific discipline. I felt that some of their many techniques and ideas could possibly remain unknown to virtually all veterinarians of the English-speaking world. For this reason, I was most interested to see this 'handbook' for horse diseases translated into English.

Mr. TERRY C. TELGER accomplished the monumental translation effort with recognizable professional skill. Some German terms in veterinary medicine are difficult to translate and if left unaltered could confuse the reader familiar with other standard English word usage. I therefore carefully read the translation and in many instances made these appropriate changes, and in some instances I took some small liberties to alter the text, primarily to improve the handbook's overall appeal to the English-speaking reader.

I certainly do not want to give readers the impression that I endorse or recommend everything in this book. Most diseases or conditions are handled in an identical manner to the way they would be in our clinics but some are handled differently. Certain medications and drugs cited in the handbook are unavailable, at least in North America. However, I do not feel that this is a major drawback since, in most cases, products with similar modes of action are available. The conditions of husbandry and feeding may vary a little from North American methods, but this should not be a problem for either the veterinarian or horse owner reading this book.

The handbook is a very comprehensive one with a wide variety of topics covered. It will be particularly useful for those in institutions faced with unearthing literature that has been published in Europe on some of the more uncommon conditions seen in the horse. I stumbled across some diseases that are either non-existent or extremely rare in North America. However, if an animal presents with such a disease, this book will be a useful source of information. *Diseases of the Horse* should be of value to veterinarians in specialty practice, horse owners, trainers, or anyone associated with the industry.

Fort Collins, Colorado, USA, 1983 — A. S. TURNER

Preface to the German Edition

The world horse population declined greatly in the first decades after World War II, almost to the point where extinction of the species was feared. Since then, however, the horse population not only has become reestablished, but actually has displayed a continuing upward trend. With this has come a resurgence of interest in the care, breeding and use of horses, particularly the athletic and pleasure breeds. Horses have also gained increasing practical value, whether as suppliers of serum for the manufacture of vaccines, or as beasts of burden in timber-cutting regions.

As a result, equine medicine has emerged in many countries as a veterinary specialty in its own right. This is made necessary not only by the growing numbers of horses, but also by the substantial economic investment that many horses represent. A top-notch performance horse may sell for several hundred thousand dollars, while top breeding stallions may be valued in the millions.

Because no textbooks or handbooks on equine medicine had been published in the German-speaking world since the 1930s, there was a pressing need to produce a standard, up-to-date reference work for equine specialists, practicing veterinarians, and students of veterinary medicine. *Diseases of the Horse* draws upon the combined experience of thirty-two authorities from eight countries in an effort to meet this need. Given the volume of material at hand, it was necessary to make two major subdivisions in the text. Thus, the book is divided into a general part presenting basic information on the diagnosis and treatment of diseases, and a more specialized part dealing with specific diseases.

The editors and authors hope that they have provided the reader with a reference of the highest scientific value that incorporates the most recent findings in all areas of equine research. The combined textbook and handbook format of the work, though difficult to achieve editorially, was designed to serve the broadest possible readership. It is hoped that this book succeeds in its goal fo reviewing, supplementing and updating our knowledge of equine diseases.

We express our appreciation to the publishers for recognizing the necessity of such a voluminous text and for their usual excellent production work and advice, and we convey special thanks to Dr. ITTERHEIM for his meticulous editing of manuscript.

Berlin, summer 1981 E. WIESNER and O. DIETZ

1. General Considerations

1.1. Examination of the Horse

1.1.1. Clinical Examination

The systematic application of clinical methods enables the veterinarian to differentiate between normal and diseased animals on the basis of comprehensive knowledge in anatomy, physiology, pathology and behavioral research [KELLY, 1971]. Often it is impossible to render an exact diagnosis, i.e., to specify the organ as well as the nature and etiology of the pathologic process. Moreover, it is seldom possible to make a diagnosis on the basis of a single presenting sign.

Methods of Symptom Recognition

In examining the animal, the veterinarian utilizes his senses: sight, touch, hearing and smell. The interiors of the hollow organs are not visible externally although they may be examined by endoscopic means. The basic techniques of the physical examination are: palpation; percussion; auscultation.

Modern diagnostic procedures such as pulmonary function tests, blood gas analyses, electrocardiography, phonocardiography, cardiac catheterization, radiography and ultrasound (for further detail the reader is referred to the work of VASALL; SASSE; MEISTER; SPÖRRI; HAHN; BARNER; PIPERS; HAMLIN) can provide a clearer picture of the nature and severity of the disease process than clinical examination. Nevertheless, clinical examination, especially involving the processes of auscultation and percussion, remains an indispensible part of the diagnostic program, despite their frequent subjectivity. As in the past, a thorough clinical examination forms the cornerstone for diagnosis, prognosis and therapy. As for specialized examinations, one must always weigh the risks and costs against the potential gain of information and correlate the results with the clinical picture.

There is no question that the various laboratory and technical aids have enriched diagnosis and therapy to an extraordinary degree. The result is a growing and sometimes bewildering flood of information. Such information not only exceeds the capacity of diagnostic departments, but also threatens to overtax the interpretive ability of the diagnosing physician [NILIUS and NEEF, 1979].

1.1.1.1. Examination of the Head (Oral Cavity, Nose, Paranasal Sinuses)

When inspecting the head, attention must be given to the facial expression, which reflects the mental state of the animal. A horse in good health has a bright appearance and responds to stimuli in a physiologic manner. Central nervous disorders (states of depression and excitation) are accompanied by changes in expression and behavior. Symmetrical as well as asymmetrical enlargements of the maxilla or mandible are indicative of disease in this region. Alterations in the contour of the soft tissues may denote tumors or lymph node enlargements. Other soft-tissue changes include the increased muscle tone of tetanus, which produces dilatation of the nostrils, rigidity of the ears and prolapse of the nictitating membrane. In examining the nasal region, attention is given to the area around the nasal opening, movements of the nostril, respiratory sounds, expiratory air, nasal discharge, the color of the mucous membranes, and the paranasal sinuses. The large, flexible nostrils of the horse give them a mobility that is distinctive compared to other species.

In inspiratory dyspnea there is a forced dilation of the nostrils during inhalation; with expiration the nostrils return to their normal position. The nasal mucosa is accessible to direct visual inspection in the lower third of the nasal cavity. At the junction of the skin and mucosa, the openings of the nasolacrimal canals are clearly seen on the arch of the nasal fossa. Whenever nasal discharge is present, it should be determined whether it originates entirely or in part from the conjunctival sac, escaping from the nostrils via the nasolacrimal canals. The principal changes of the nasal mucosa include pallor, congestion, petechiae, erosions and ulcerations. A rhinolaryngoscope is also useful for examining the nasal passages and mucous membranes in the horse.

Examination of the Nasal Cavity and Paranasal Sinuses

External inspection will disclose thickenings and swellings of the skin in the area of the nasal inlet. Visible swellings in the area of the nasal bones, frontal bones, maxillary bones and zygomata may be caused by cellulitis, fractures, empyemas or neoplasms of the nasal, frontal and maxillary sinuses.

Chronic unilateral nasal catarrh is of considerable clinical importance. It may denote various pathologic states, depending on the quantity, color, consistency and odor of the discharge [DEEGEN, 1973]. A unilateral, purulent, fetid, and discolored discharge which empties rapidly when the head is lowered is characteristic of empyemas of the maxillary sinus or guttural pouch.

Palpation of the outer wall of the maxillary and frontal sinus is usually done to ascertained localized temperature elevation, tenderness, and the consistency of the various swellings.

Percussion with the fingers or percussion hammer elicits sounds that can be useful diagnostically. In healthy animals, the percussion sound is clear and loud. If the maxillary sinus is filled with exudate, tissue or a cyst, a dull sound is elicited. It is important to note, however, that percussion sounds vary even under normal circumstances depending on the age of the animal, the thickness of the skin and the momentary jaw position. Since small collections of fluid are often insufficient to muffle the sound, negative percussion findings do not necessarily mean that the sinuses are healthy. In percussion studies of the maxillary sinuses, the findings on one side must be compared with those on the other. The findings are diagnostically significant only if marked disparities are present.

The examination of the nasal cavity and paranasal sinuses is generally combined with examination of the lymph nodes of the throat region. Their form, size, consistency and tenderness are noted, as well as their resistance to passive movement.

Examination of the Oral Cavity

A mouth speculum should be used when examining the oral cavity. Occasionally the animal must be sedated before the examination. Inflammation of the oral mucosa may be caused by infectious, chemical or physical irritants. Color changes of the oral mucosa may be associated with jaundice or vascular changes (hyperemia, hemorrhage). Excessive salivation sometimes occurs in painful inflammatory states.

The presence of pus or blood in the saliva is a sign of purulent or hemorrhagic inflammation or injuries of the oral or pharyngeal mucous membranes. The tongue should be examined for injuries, swelling due to cellulitis and neoplasms. Prolapse and paralysis of the tongue may be caused by paralysis of the hypoglossal nerve as well as central paralysis. Myogenic paralysis may follow tongue injuries, hyoid bone fractures or glossitis. Extension of the tongue is an idiosyncrasy of horses (play instinct) that is not necessarily abnormal, but may also be prompted by dental defects or glossal paralysis.

When inspecting the teeth, the examiner should note overall abnormalities of dentition (shear mouth, step mouth, wave mouth, parrot mouth, crossbite) as well as disorders of individual teeth, such as missing teeth, entrapped food material, tooth length irregularities, chipped and fractured teeth, lateral deviations, and the presence of pits and cavities (caries, excavations). Enlargements or tumors on the palpable portion of the jaw should also be noted. The lower jaw is examined for injuries, contusions, as well as bony swelling. Deformities of the jaw can occur as a result of fractures and neoplasms. Swellings in the mandibular area, combined with mastication abnormalities and atrophy of the masseter muscle, are symptomatic of a chronic inflammation of the temporomandibular joint. Examination of the oral cavity should include assessment of the mouth odor. A characteristic carious smell is noted in the presence of entrapped food, dental caries and necrosis of the bone. An acrid, sweet or putrid odor is a sign of pharyngitis or the presence of food matter lodged between the teeth and check.

Often in the horse, the upper molars will have sharp edges on the buccal side, while the lower molars will be sharp on the lingual side, as a result of the natural disparity in jaw width. This can result in mucous membrane injury and ulceration which likewise produces a sweetly stale odor.

Internal Palpation of the Pharynx

The entire pharynx can be examined in the sedated horse with the aid of a mouth speculum. This examination is useful for revealing foreign bodies and neoplasms as well as for ascertaining the size of pharyngeal lymph nodes. In the healthy animal, insertion of the hand into the pharynx will evoke a strong swallowing reflex (contraction of the pharynx followed by swallowing movements). This reaction is weak or absent in pharyngeal paralysis, compressive lesions, local suppuration, and in botulism. The parotid salivary gland is located subcutaneously in the upper cervical region and is also palpable during examination of the pharynx.

Examination of the Guttural Pouch

Diseases of this organ (usually inflammatory or purulent in nature), can cause swelling of the upper cervical region in the area of the parotid gland. Severe swelling of both guttural pouches can cause respiratory distress and difficulties in swallowing. The swelling, which is often unilateral, is soft and cushion-like to the touch; sometimes a splashing sound is heard on palpation. With the aid of a rhinolaryngoscope, the opening of the guttural pouch can be directly observed. An endoscope with an angled tip can be passed into the guttural pouch cavity [Breuer, 1978; Boening, 1978].

Radiographic examination can also provide useful information on the condition of the guttural pouches.

Examination of the Larynx

During the external examination, the laryngeal area is palpated to check for circumferential enlargement, tenderness, and the ease with which a cough is elicited.

In healthy animals, auscultation of the larynx discloses sounds that are similar to those heard over the bronchial regions. In animals with laryngitis or with tumors are laryngeal paralysis (hemiplegia), there are extraneous inspiratory sounds that may be characterized as whistling, roaring, hissing or wheezing. In glottic stenosis the laryngeal sounds are whistling (stenotic) in character. In such cases a vibration (laryngeal fremitus) can be felt by pressing on the skin over the larynx.

Constriction of the lumen of the larynx may be edematous or allergic in origin, or may be caused by acute inflammatory disease. In the clinical examination for laryngeal paralysis, the open hand is placed onto one side of the larynx, while the fingertips of the other hand press inward on the larynx on the opposite side. If laryngeal paralysis is present, this will elicit an abnormal inspiratory sound caused by narrowing of the reina glottis. Stenotic sounds from laryngeal paralysis occur only during inspration, because only in this phase, does the paralyzed arytenoid cartilage and vocal cord prolapse into the laryngeal lumen to produce the narrowing.

Laryngoscopy

The laryngoscope [Cook, 1970; Gratzl, 1964] consists of a tube about 76 cm long which is equipped with an optical system and a light source. The laryngoscope is inserted through the ventral nasal passage of the immobilized horse. The examiner holds the protruding portion of the instrument firmly in his hand while simultaneously grasping the medial nasal wing. With this instrument it is possible to examine the nasal mucosa thoroughly. Portions of the nasal concha, larynx, guttural pouch openings and soft palate can also be viewed. The larynx is visible at the base of the pharyngeal cavity; the epiglottis, arytenoid cartilages, vocal cords, lateral ventricles and parts of the trachea can be visualized. In laryngeal hemiplegia (roaring) the vocal folds (cords) and larynx appear asymmetrical, and the mobility of one or both vocal folds (cords) is lost. In catarrhal laryngitis the mucous membrane is reddish-gray in color and has a heavy mucous coating. Edema in this region is characterized by indistinctness of the laryngeal contours. With the tip of the laryngoscope positioned above the larynx, the instrument can be rotated 45° to the right or left to view the entrance of the guttural pouch (eustachian tube) lying as a vertical fold in the pharyngeal wall. In suppurative diseases of the guttural pouch, there may be a purulent discharge from the ventral commissure of the orifice.

1.1.1.2. Examination of the Respiratory System

Much information can be gained on the conditions of the respiratory system from a physical examination of the lung region [Cook, 1965], using the techniques of palpation, percussion and auscultation

The value of the results varies with the method and experience of the examiner as well as the physical condition of the animal.

Percussion of the chest wall makes it possible to define the position of the normal lung and detect abnormalities by eliciting various percussion sounds (resonance). Percussion of the lung is generally done by the hammer-pleximeter method [Steck, 1969], but finger percussion may also be used [Miklaušic and Dolinar, 1966]. A narrow, spatula-like instrument with a contact width of 8—10 mm makes an excellent pleximeter. The percussion hammer should have a weight of 50—70 g and be fitted with a soft rubber cap. The following guidelines are recommended for the examination technique:

— Very gentle tapping, or 'treshold percussion', induces vibration of the lung tissue below the chest wall, while more forceful percussion essentially sets the chest wall itself in vibration.
— Percussion should keep strictly within the intercostal spaces.
— The contact pressure of the pleximeter should be as high as possible.
— Strictly intercostal percussion can be achieved only with a correspondingly narrow pleximeter ($\leq$ 10 mm) or by finger percussion [Deegen and Zichner, 1970].

Owing to variations of percussion technique, varying topographic results are reported in the literature, such as those relating to the course of the caudoventral boundary of the lung. As mentioned, intercostal percussion with very gentle tapping is the recommended technique. The pleximeter is applied to the intercostal space and is pressed firmly against the chest wall. It is struck in a quiet area with just enough force to elicit an audible sound.

If pulmonary percussion in the healthy animal is begun in the dorsal region of the thorax in the manner described, the first sound to be heard is a characteristic *loud, full pulmonary sound*. A *dull sound* is obtained when air spaces are displaced by tissue or fluid, while the presence of excessive air gives an *overloud* or *tympanitic sound*. When percussion is carried out in the ventral region of the thorax, a point is reached where the sound quality changes, becoming higher, softer and shorter. This point forms a portion of the caudoventral lung boundary. As percussion is carried farther ventrally, a zone of increasing dullness about 3—5 cm wide is demonstrated. This 'zone of relative dullness' is bounded ventrally by a point beyond which the dullness is absolute. If points of similar sound quality are connected along the individual intercostal spaces, the following *boundary lines* are obtained: An upper line, which is straight for three quarters of its length and turns dorsally in its final quarter, forming an obtuse angle with the straight portion; and a lower line, which is curved for its full extent. The upper, angled line, is useful diagnostically. For example, with the elasticity loss that occurs in moderate cases of chronic obstructive pulmonary disease (COPD) the obtuse angle becomes smaller, so that the angled limb approaches a perpendicular. In more advanced cases of COPD the angled boundary line is replaced by a deformed line that is curved throughout.

The anatomical reference points used in the literature for defining the lung borders (tuber coxae, tuber ischii, point of shoulder) relate to the aforementioned boundary level for absolute dullness. Due to the individual variability of the reference points, however, this level is no longer recommended for diagnostic purposes.

Another phenomenon that has diagnostic applications is the zone of hyperresonance. In work horses and in athletic horses, this zone occupies an area of 3—4 fingers' breadth at the edge of the lung field, dorsal to the caudoventral lung boundary. It expresses the increased air content of the alveoli at the pulmonary border. In low-to moderate-grade COPD, the zone is 1—2 hands wide. In high-grade COPD, it can extend some distance dorsally from the caudoventral lung boundary, occupying up to two-thirds of the total lung field. Finally, zones of dullness can occur in the lung field either alone or combined with symptoms of elasticity loss. These may denote areas of infectious pneumonia, acute pleuritis or chronic pleuritis with adhesions. Percussion may be supplemented by auscultation for the detection of infiltrative lesions at deeper levels. A suitable stethoscope is essential for obtaining optimum, clinically useful auscultatory findings. The stethoscope tubing should be 30 to 50 cm long, with an inside diameter of 3—6 mm and a fairly rigid lumen. The inside diameter of the endpiece should not exceed 30 mm, or else the soft, higher-frequency vibrations will not be audible. In the normal horse the soft, gentle *vesicular sound* is audible at rest only during the inspiratory phase.

Expiration is physiologically silent in the adult horse. If the sharper, harsher *bronchial sound* is heard over the chest wall during inspiration and especially during expiration, abnormal conditions are assumed to exist in the lung area. This sound, which occurs in the larynx, trachea and main stem bronchi during each respiratory movement, becomes audible on chest wall auscultation only when sound conduction in the lung is accentuated due to pathologic congestion of the alveoli with secretions, as in pneumonia or edema. Intermediate between the vesicular and bronchial breath sounds is the *increased vesicular sound*, which is especially pronounced in chronic bronchitis. It is about as sharp as the bronchial tone, but is heard only during inspiration. Louder râles and rhonchi are caused by secretion accumulations in the bronchial space (bronchitis, bronchopneumonia, allergies). Soft crackling heard during inspiration is indicative of heavy secretions in the alveoli (especially in edema!), while loud crackling is symptomatic of interstitial emphysema.

1.1.1.3. Examination of the Cardiovascular System

The cardiovascular system is composed of two main functional units: the heart and the blood vessels. Both maintain the circulation of blood and ensure a normal exchange of gases, electrolytes and fluids. The autonomic nervous system controls both components.

Anatomic Relationships. In the horse the heart occupies an asymmetrical position; a little more than half the organ lies to the left of the median plane, the base extending from the 2nd to the 6th intercostal space. The cardiac apex is situated centrally about 1.3 cm above the last sternal segment. The posterior border is nearly vertical and lies at the level of the 6th rib. The right atrioventricular orifice (tricuspid valve) lies opposite the 4th intercostal space, about 7.5 cm above the lower end of the 4th rib. The pulmonary orifice (pulmonary semilunar valve) lies opposite the 3rd intercostal space just above the plane of the atrioventricular orifice. The left atrioventricular orifice (bicuspid valve) is located opposite the 5th intercostal space, about 10 cm above the sternal end of the 5th rib. The aortic orifice (aortic semilunar valve) lies opposite the 4th intercostal space, level with the point of the shoulder [Marek and Mócsy, 1956; Kelly, 1971].

Examination of the Pulse

Along with examination of the cardiac cycle and the subcutaneous veins, an assessment of the pulse can provide information on the state of the circulatory system. When the pulse is taken, its rate, rhythm and quality are noted. An elevation of the *pulse rate* is present in painful disorders and many diseases that do not primarily involve the heart and circulatory system. It is also a principal feature of the fever. The *pulse rhythm* is determined by estimating the time intervals between successive pulse waves. The sequence may be regular or irregular. Abnormalities of rhythm may themselves occur at regular or irregular intervals. The irregular dropping of a pulse wave occurs without obvious cause and is usually associated with irregularities of the pulse volume resulting from variations in the cardiac stroke volume. The most frequent causes of irregular pulse irregularities are extrasystolic arrhythmia and atrial fibrillation. Most of these irregularities are accentuated by movement. The *pulse quality* depends chiefly on the amplitude of the pulse waves, which can vary because the degree of diastolic filling influences the stroke volume. The pulse quality is estimated from the degree of digital pressure required to obliterate the pulse wave in the artery. Changes in the pulse character may be caused by organic and functional cardiac diseases. In assessing the pulse, it must always be borne in mind that a number of pulse abnormalities reflect the functional state of the heart, which is influenced in a variety of ways.

Abnormalities of Pulse Rate. A strongly elevated pulse rate is called *tachycardia*. In sinus tachycardia, the impulse has its origin in the sinus node. Paroxysmal tachycardia is the sudden occurrence of periods of tachycardia of relatively short duration. Sinus tachycardia occurs in febrile diseases, in shock, and in circulatory failure. In simple tachycardia the pulse rate rises with exercise and falls during rest.

Bradycardia (slow pulse) represents a decline in the rate of the sinoatrial impulse. It is important to distinguish between sinus bradycardia and the form that occurs with atrioventricular block. In the first case there is the usual rise of pulse rate in response to movement and excitement. Opinions vary as to the origin of bradycardia in horses that have undergone high-performance training [LUTZ et al., 1976].

Abnormalities of Rhythm. In the irregular pulse the intervals between successive pulse waves are of varying length. These abnormalities of rhythm are always associated with a change in the pulse amplitude such as occurs in atrial fibrillation, atrial flutter or generalized myocarditis. In serious febrile and toxic states with increased cardiac activity, an irregular pulse may be a transitory phenomenon. An intermittent pulse is one where individual pulse waves are lost in an otherwise regular sequence. If there is a corresponding interruption of the heart beat, the pulse is said to be absent. If a heart beat occurs, but is too weak to generate a palpable pulse wave, the pulse is described as intermittent. An intermittent pulse may be found in horses in a high peak of training (sinus arrhythmia). Irregularities and interruptions can be triggered by irregular stimulation in the atria (atrial flutter and fibrillation) as well as in the overall cardiac muscle (extrasystole).

Abnormalities of Quality. These are the result of variations in the stroke volume and vasomotor effects. A distinction is made between the full and strong pulse, the small and weak pulse, the soft pulse, the irregular pulse, and the alternating pulse.

Jugular Pulse. The jugular pulse may be observed subcutaneously in the jugular furrow. A negative jugular pulse is normal. A strong pulsation may be seen in tricuspid valve stenosis as well as in heart block and pericarditis. The positive jugular pulse consists of true pulse waves which pass from the thoracic inlet to the mandibular arch. It occurs in tricuspid valve insufficiency.

Dilatation of the Veins. A continuous dilatation of superficial veins is observed in all conditions in which there is an obstruction to the venous blood flow (myocardial diseases, heart block, endocarditis). In the short-winded horse, for example, venous dilatation appears rapidly with exercise and persists much longer than in healthy fit individuals.

Examination of the Heart

Inspection. The visible expression of the cardiac action is the movement of the chest wall during systole by the 'apex beat'. This beat is also observed in healthy animals, but it is more pronounced when cardiac activity is increased (overexertion, anemia).

Palpation. The strength and size of the cardiac impulse can be estimated by placing the palm of the hand onto the cardiac area. The apex beat is felt with the tip of one finger. The heart beat is not palpable if the heart has been forced away from the chest wall such as would occur in pericarditis, pleuritis or hydrothorax).

Percussion. This is done in the same way as described for the lung; usually the heart and lung are percussed at the same time. Percussion is always carried from areas of increased resonance to areas of dullness. The area of absolute cardiac dullness in the horse covers an approximately palm-size area on the left chest wall and lies behind the shoulder, above the line of the elbow, in the area of the 3rd and 5th intercostal space.

On the right side of the chest, the area of cardiac dullness is considerably smaller than on the left. The area of cardiac dullness is extended in cardiac enlargement, fluid distension of the pericardial sac, and lateral displacement of the heart (unilateral pneumothorax). This area is reduced in chronic obstructive pulmonary disease, when more than the usual amount of lung is interposed between the heart and chest wall.

Auscultation. By careful auscultation, useful information can be gained on the functional state of the heart. The auscultation is carried out with the aid of a phonendoscope. The aim is to determine the character of the heart sounds and to detect the presence of abnormal sounds. Points to be noted are the number, rhythm, intensity and quality of the heart sounds; abnormal sounds must be related to the functional activity of the heart. The first heart sound is dull, loud and prolonged. It is immediately followed by the second heart sound, which is shorter and higher-pitched. In the horse a third heart sound, which is short and quite soft, is audible at the start of diastole; the mechanism of this sound remains unclear. Unnaturally loud heart sounds are associated with cardiac hypertrophy and anemia. The intensity of the heart sounds is diminished when cardiac performance is impaired (advanced cardiac insufficiency). An accentuated second heart sound is generally the result of increased blood reflux against the closed valves. The second sound is weakened when the arterial pressure is low.

Splitting of the first and second heart sounds can occur in normal horses as well as in animals with elevated blood pressure. Splitting of the second heart sound results from asynchronous closure of the semilunar valves. A further goal of auscultation is to evaluate the cardiac rhythm, which has a regular, cyclic form in most normal horses. The rhythm is influenced to a slight degree by respiration (sinus arrhythmia). Full-blown cardiac arrhythmias are attributable to conduction disturbances in the bundle of His. The importance of cardiac arrhythmias can be ascertained and diagnostically evaluated by means of electrocardiography. Auscultation of the heart before and after exercise provides the clearest indication of arrhythmias, which become more clearly audible after exertion.

Extraneous Heart Sounds. Abnormal sounds may replace or accompany one or both of the normal sounds. The extraneous sounds that originate within the heart itself are caused by valvular lesions (vegetative endocarditis or valvular adhesions), valvular insufficiency and abnormal orifices (ventricular septal defect, patent ductus arteriosus). These murmurs may be described by terms such as hissing, humming buzzing or vibrating. Thus, the murmur of stenosis is harsh and buzzing, while that associated with valvular insufficiency has a softer, hissing quality. Endocardial murmurs are caused by chronic valvular endocarditis, cardiac dilatation, acute endocarditis and neoplasms. Endocardial murmurs may be systolic as well as diastolic. Systolic murmurs indicate either stenosis of the semilunar valves of insufficiency of the atrioventricular valves.

Diastolic murmurs are caused either by stenosis of the atrioventricular valves or by semilunar insufficiency. Mitral murmurs in the horse are heard in the 5th intercostal space on the left side, level with the point of the shoulder, and pulmonic murmurs in the 3rd intercostal space on the left side, level with the olecranon. In advanced pulmonary diseases, a marked accentuation of the second heart sound over the middle valvular field or even a reversal of the normal heart sound intensity can be found. The second sound may become louder than the first. A louder second heart sound is also characteristic of certain acute pulmonary diseases.

Blood Pressure. Blood pressure measurement has not become a routine procedure in the clinical examinaton of the horse. The blood pressure can be measured indirectly by applying a cuff to the root of the tail. Direct and indirect blood pressure measurements can be carried out using a variety of techniques [Eberly et al., 1964; Bayer, 1967; Förster, 1976; Hahn and Garner, 1977].

Electrocardiography. While the ECG cannot replace the clinical examination, it can nevertheless enhance the diagnosis of certain functional cardiac diseases. ECG studies permit an accurate determination of the heart rate and cardiac rhythm, while providing a record that may demonstrate the need for further investigations. It is important to note that deviations in the ECG are not necessarily indicative of disease.

Phonocardiography. This is a technique for the graphic recording of heart sounds. The apparatus includes a timing system for recording a pulse curve and electrocardiogram [Spörri, 1975; Spörri and Leemann, 1972].

1.1.1.4. Examination of the Digestive System

Inspection of the abdomen will reveal distension in cases of primary tympany. External palpation is of limited value. Auscultation of the abdomen is useful because the functional activity of the intestines can be assessed on the basis of the peristaltic sounds.

Rectal Examination. After insertion of the hand into the rectum, the amount of feces present and the rectal muscle tone are evaluated. The condition of the pelvis and sacrum should be assessed. Under normal circumstances only a few sections of bowel are palpable on rectal examination. The segments can be readily identified if a portion is distended with gas, obstructed or displaced. The small colon lies in irregular loops in the posterior part of the abdominal cavity and is accessible in the pelvic cavity. In obstructions of the small colon, the fecal balls may range from fist- to coconut-size. In many normal horses, portions of the dorsal and ventral loops of the large colon and the pelvic flexure are palpable. It is important to note that the left loops of the large colon may be located at the midline or even to the right of it. The ventral segment of the large colon is 12—30 cm in diameter, and its surface is marked by longitudinal, band-like thickenings (teniae) as well as circumferential constrictions and sacculations (haustra).

The pelvic flexure of the large colon is about 7—10 cm in diameter. Its surface is smooth and possesses only one longitudinal tenia near the attachment of the mesentery along its concave face. The diaphragmatic and sternal flexure of the large colon are out of reach. The stomach-like dilatation of the right dorsal colon is occasionally palpable in small to medium-size horses. The most frequent disorder of the large colon is impaction of the left ventral colon. Such impactions are most pronounced in the pelvic flexure. On the right side in the upper cranial portion of the abdominal cavity, the round, immobile base of the cecum can be reached with the fingertips. In most cases, however, the cecum can be easily identified only if it is enlarged by solid or gaseous contents. Cecal enlargements may occur as the result of impaction or tympany. The terminal ileum of the small intestine, whose thick muscular wall distinguishes it anatomically from the remaining thin-walled segments, can occasionally be palpated. It lies in the upper cranial region of the abdominal cavity and can normally be identified as a tubular structure 5—8 cm in diameter running horizontally or obliquely from left to right to the base of the cecum. Its left portion is somewhat mobile, while the right portion is fixed at its entry into the cecum. Impactions of the jejunum are recognized by the empty, contracted state of the large intestines and the marked gas or fluid distension of small-intestine loops. The duodenum cannot be identified by rectal examination.

Normally the stomach cannot be palpated unless it is acutely enlarged. The spleen often can be felt only with the fingertips at its caudal border. The posterior border of the spleen is located near the left costal arch. The position of the spleen is influenced by the degree of distention of the stomach. With gastric distention, the spleen is displaced caudally and medially. Intestinal loops may come between the spleen and abdominal wall, either from below or from above, across the renosplenic (nephrosplenic) ligament. Splenic enlargements may be palpable in congestive heart failure, portal obstruction or neoplastic disease. Nodular enlargements occur in tuberculosis. The left kidney lies somewhat cranially against the dorsal chest wall below the last rib and adjacent to the transverse processes of the first 2—3 lumbar vertebrae. Only the caudal pole of the kidney can be palpated; the right kidney is out of reach. The ureter is identified only if it is dilated or thickened. The abdominal aorta is felt as a strongly pulsating tube below the lumbar spine. The bifurcation of the left and right iliac arteries is palpable below the sixth lumbar vertebra. Thickenings and irregularities of the arterial wall are indicative of thrombosis, or arteritis. The anterior mesenteric artery and several of its branches can be palpated by following the abdominal aorta forward. A pulsating vessel running vertically downward can be felt at the level of the first lumbar vertebra. In verminous arteritis, the vessels are thickened at their origin and have a rough, knobby surface. If a thrill is noted on palpation of the anterior mesenteric artery (root of mesentery) instead of individual pulse beats, the presence of a thrombus should be suspected.

The urinary bladder is palpated below the rectum on the pelvic floor. It is about the diameter of a coconut when empty. When filled, it is felt as a solid structure whose cranial end extends over the pelvic brim to the abdominal floor. Palpation can disclose bladder stones or thickenings of the bladder wall. The urethra in the male horse is felt as a cylindrical structure running forward on the pelvic floor. The inguinal rings should be examined in the stallion. When the abdominal wall is palpated to the right or left of the midline, the split-like apertures of the inguinal rings are felt and generally are large enough to accommodate three fingertips. The spermatic duct is also felt as a pencil-thick structure running downwards through the inguinal canal. If a portion of the bowel has been displaced into the inguinal canal and has become incarcerated there, a thick cord will be felt entering the inguinal ring. In the mare, the uterus is palpable as a short structure interposed between the rectum and bladder. Its horns curve somewhat dorsally. The uterus is located by first finding an ovary and following the horn to the uterus, which then is palpated in a systematic fashion. The ovaries are located bilaterlly in the lumbar region, ventral to the fourth or fifth lumbar vertebra in close proximity to the abdominal wall.

The visceral and parietal peritoneum can be felt only in caudal aspect of the abdominal cavity. In cases of gastric or intestinal rupture, the peritoneal surface is roughened by food particles.

Special Examination of the Abdomen. Direct inspection of the abdominal viscera is possible by means of a laparotomy or with a laparoscope. To establish the nature of the abdominal fluid (useful in the diagnosis of colic), abdominal paracentesis with subsequent analysis of the fluid can provide useful information. Radiographic examination of the abdomen is informative only in small horses, unless higher power radiographic equipment is available.

1.1.1.5. Examination of the Urinary and Genital System

Signs indicating disease of the urinary organs are often subtle. They include: the duration of the urination act, the volume of urine passed, the color of the urine, and evidence of pain on urination. Abnormally frequent urination may or may not be accompanied by an increased urinary volume. Polyuria is most often seen in chronic interstitial nephritis and after the administration of diuretics. Frequent urination with no increase in urine volume is observed in irritation to the bladder or urethra (acute nephritis, cystitis). Bladder stones may provoke frequent voiding. Oliguria and anuria are often the result of renal disease. Diseases of the urinary tract can cause acute abdominal pain. The kidneys and urinary organs are not accessible to external palpation. During the rectal examination (see 1.1.1.4.), only the caudal portion of the left kidney can be felt in large horses. Points to be noted are the relative size of the kidney, its consistency and surface contour as well as tenderness to pressure. Examination of the bladder is done by rectal palpation (bladder neoplasms, bladder stones). The patency of the urethra can be assessed by catheterization. The preputial area should also be examined in male animals (obstruction of urethral process, inflammatory swelling of prepuce).

Special Examination of the Urinary Organs
Urine samples are obtained by collecting spontaneously voided urine or by catheterization. Mares can be easily catheterized (sterile metal catheter and mare speculum). In the male horse the penis must be withdrawn from the prepuce; the prior administration of an ataractic type tranquilizer makes this easier. The catheter for the male horse must be strong but sufficiently elastic to pass around the ischial arch. Urinalysis is useful for demonstrating the presence of renal or bladder disease. Renal function tests and pyelography are occasionally indicated.

Examination of the Male Genital Organs
External inspection and palpation are used to examine the skin of the prepuce and scrotum, the inner surface of the preputial cavity, the glans penis, as well as the distal portion of the penis. Sedation of the horse is usually required. In both the stallion and gelding, the penis can be withdrawn by inserting the hand into the preputial space and grasping the penis. In pudendal nerve paralysis and paraphimosis, the penis will hang from the sheath. It may swell in this condition due to the increase of hydrostatic pressure caused by venous constriction. Hardened concretions of smegma (preputial stones) are occasionally found in the preputial cavity and urethral sinus and may interfere with the passage of urine. Examination of the inguinal region is especially important in colts and stallions in cases of incarcerated or strangulated inguinal hernia.

The inguinal hernia is accompanied by a unilateral hot, painful swelling of the testis. Changes in the testis and scrotum (neoplasms, acute inflammatory processes) are evident on palpation. The internal male genital organs are accessible during the rectal examination (see 1.1.1.4.). The prostate is composed of two lateral lobes that are directed cranially. The seminal vesicles are paired blind sacs about 15—20 cm long and 2.5 cm wide and can be felt on both sides of the pelvic portion of the urethra. The sexual drive may be heightened or diminished. Not infrequently, an abnormal libido is the result of gonadal disease but may also be caused by other genital abnormalities including psychological disorders. Occasionally a bacteriologic examination of the preputial secretion is indicated. A semen analysis is warranted if a stallion's fertility is in question.

Examination of the Female Genital Organs
The clinical examination is done by direct inspection. The vaginal depths are examined with the aid of a speculum, which also allows the cervix to be viewed. The position of the internal genital organs is assessed during the rectal examination. The rectal pregnancy determination can be supplemented by laboratory tests (Friedman test, Cuboni test) [Walker, 1977].

1.1.1.6. Examination of the Central Nervous System

Deviations in the mode of behavior of an animal can be manifested in various ways. They include dullness and apathy, the degree of which can be estimated from the animal's response, or lack of response, to normal stimuli. The 'dummy' syndrome is the advanced stage. The terminal stage of apathy is coma, in which the animal no longer responds to painful stimuli. The neurological examination includes an assessment of locomotor function. For evaluation the animal is allowed to move freely or is led through various gaits and observed for motor disturbances (stumbling, swaying, hindquarter weakness, compulsive movements). These disturbances may be continuous or transient. Diseases must be differentiated from faults and vices such as balking on leading or riding, resistance to saddling, head sensitivity, shying from certain objects, viciousness and possessiveness toward food, and weaving.

Diseases of the nervous system may occur as the result of certain infectious diseases, including listeriosis, tetanus, rabies, toxoplasmosis, Borna disease, and herpesvirus infections [Dinter and Klingborn, 1976; Little and Thorsen, 1976; Charlton et al., 1976].

Developmental defects of the central nervous system, such as congenital hydrocephalus, can occur. Secondary diseases of the nervous system may be caused by infectious or toxic processes associated with other organic diseases [Fankhauser, 1968; Binkhorst, 1976; Mayhew et al., 1978; Wiese, 1976].

Due to the limited responsiveness of certain parts of the nervous system, it is not always possible to deduce the nature of the disease from clinical signs alone. Diseases in which there is impairment of nervous function with corresponding symptoms, but there is no demonstrable lesion, are called functional disorders. They are seen in metabolic diseases, biochemical abnormalities, and various other conditions.

The clinical neurological examination is confined to a few areas. The history will assist the examiner in narrowing the scope of his investigation. In all clinical examinations of the nervous system, the observation of the animal's interactions with its environment and response to stimuli is of paramount importance. The systematic examination begins with inspection and palpation of the cranium. The spinal column is examined for deformities (kyphosis, lordosis and scoliosis). Nervous disorders are localized as central, peripheral or autonomic, depending on whether the disease has its seat in the brain or spinal cord or in the sympathetic and parasympathetic nervous system. Motor or sensory disturbances may be predominate, depending on the nervous component involved. An exaggeration of motor nerve activity produces the clinical picture of spasm. When motor nerve function is depressed, the result is partial paralysis or paresis. When loss of function is complete, the result is paralysis. Sensory nerve activity may also be heightened or diminished, giving rise to corresponding increases or decreases of sensitivity. Paralyses are classified as central or peripheral, depending on the anatomic location of the lesion. The central paralyses may be spinal or cerebral in origin. Peripheral paralyses affect only the region supplied by one or more nerves. The paralysis may be of the flaccid type, with an absence of muscle tension. Spinal paralyses are generally bilateral (paraplegia), their extent varying with the site and severity of the spinal cord damage.

Serious injuries of the spinal cord cause immediate flaccid paralysis. Cerebral dysfunction is often accompanied by a loss of consciousness. The loss of function is confined to one side of the body. In cases of muscular atrophy or muscle wasting, a distinction is made between atrophy of disuse and the degenerative atrophy that occurs in the various paralyses. Muscle spasms are classified as tonic or clonic. A tonic spasm is one in which there is sustained muscular rigidity; it is characteristic of trismus (in cases of hypocalcemia) and tetanus. A clonic spasm is one in which the muscular contraction is followed by immediate relaxation. Tetany is marked by tonic muscle spasm, excitation and labored breathing. Tremor is a rapid succession of limited clonic muscular contractions (trembling). Abnormal movements of the eyeball (horizontal, vertical or rotatory) are termed nystagmus and may accompany meningitis and cerebellar disease. Ataxia denotes a failure of functional coordination between different parts of the muscular system. Compulsive movements are defined as coordinated muscular movements performed in response to excitation of the motor centers (cerebral hemorrhage, intracerebral parasites, generalized brain disease). Abnormal movements or modes of behavior can be caused not only by the paralysis or spasm of individual muscle groups, but also by injuries to the muscles, tendons or bones (q.v.). Sensory disturbances may affect the senses of touch, vision, smell, taste or hearing. Abnormalities of this type are difficult to demonstrate due to the absence of subjective symptoms.

The functional state of the nervous system is assessed by determining the integrity of certain reflexes. A reflex may be absent, depressed or exaggerated. When the *cornea* is touched, the horse should respond by blinking. Touching the *palpebral conjunctiva* evokes a similar response. The *pupillary reflex* is tested by covering both eyes and then shining a flashlight into one eye. Normally the pupil dilates in darkness and contracts rapidly on exposure to light. The pupil is fixed and contracted with increased intracranial pressure, cervical cord disease and cranial injury. The pupil is fixed and dilated in conditions such as retinal detachment and intoxications (atropine, botulism). A fixed pupil (after exclusion of internal ocular diseases) is a common symptom of brain disease. Cutaneous reflexes are tested by touching or gentle stabbing with a pin. The *pedal reflex* can be examined by stabbing the coronet. The *anal or perineal reflex* is tested by touching the anus. In the recumbent horse the absence of this reflex denotes a profound impairment of nervous function. *Tendon reflexes:* see lameness examination.

Psychic disturbances (neuroses) are not uncommon in the horse. The vices, such as wind-sucking and weaving, are included in this category. Special examinations are done to ascertain the cerebrospinal fluid pressure and composition. Radiographic examinations (cerebral angiography, pneumoencephalography and ventriculography) may also be performed. Electroencephalography is used as an adjunctive method to assess the function of the nervous system for experimental studies.

References

Bayer, A.: Unblutige Messung des systolischen Blutdruckes mit einem neuartigen Pulsfühler beim Pferd. Berliner Münchener tierärztl. Wschr. *80:* 84 (1967).

Binkhorst, G. J.: Ataxie-Syndrom bei jungen Pferden. Vet.-med. Diss. Utrecht 1976.

BOENING, K. J.: Klinische und endoskopische Beobachtungen beim „Follikelkatarrh" der Pferde. Prakt. Tierarzt *59:* 300 (1978).

BREUER, D.: Diagnose und Therapie der Luftsackerkrankungen des Pferdes. Prakt. Tierarzt *59:* 295, 299 (1978).

CHARLTON, K. M.; MITCHELL, D.; GIRARD, A.; CORNER, A. H.: Meningoenzephalomyelitis bei Pferden mit Herpes-Virus-1-Infektion. Vet. Pathol. *13:* 59 (1976).

COOK, W. R.: Die Diagnose von Erkrankungen der Atmungswege beim Pferd. Vet. Rec. *77:* 516 (1965).

COOK, W. R.: Instrumentenspezifikation für die Endoskopie des oberen Luftweges und des Luftsackes beim Pferd. Vet. Rec. *87:* 429 (1970).

DEEGEN, E.: Ursachen des Nasenausflusses beim Pferd. Tierärztl. Praxis *1:* 169 (1973).

DEEGEN, E.; ZICHNER, M.: Zur klinischen Diagnostik chronischer Lungenerkrankungen des Pferdes. Dtsch. tierärztl. Wschr. *77:* 601 (1970).

DINTER, Z.; KLINGBORN, B.: Serologische Untersuchung über den Ausbruch einer Parese, hervorgerufen durch bei Pferden auftretenden Herpes-Virus-1 (EHV-1). Vet. Rec. *99:* 10 (1976).

EBERLY, V. E.; GILLESPIE, J. R.; TYLER, W. S.: Herzkreislaufbefunde beim Pferd. Amer. J. vet. Res. *25:* 109 (1964).

FANKHAUSER, R.: Entzündliche Gefäßveränderungen als Grundlage von Rückenmarkläsionen beim Pferd. Schweiz. Arch. Tierheilk. *110:* 171 (1968).

FISCHER, J.; DEEGEN, E.: Bronchoskopische Untersuchung bei Pferden mit chronisch obstruktiver Bronchitis. 7. Arbeitstag. Fachgr. Pferdekrankh. der Dtsch. Vet.-Med. Ges., Hamburg, Okt. 1980.

FÖRSTER, W.: Eine Methode zur indirekten Blutdruckbestimmung bei Kalb und Rind mit Hilfe des Ultraschall-Doppler-Effekts. Dtsch. tierärztl. Wschr. *83:* 64 (1976).

GRATZL, E.: Instrumentarium zur Rhinoskopie und Laryngoskopie an Pferden. Wiener tierärztl. Mschr. *51:* 203 (1964).

HAHN, A. W.; GARNER, H. E.: Indirekte Blutdruckmessung bei Tieren. Advances vet. Sci. comp. Med. *21:* (1977).

KELLY, W. R.: Tierärztliche klinische Diagnostik (VEB Gustav Fischer Verlag, Jena 1971).

LITTLE, P. B.; THORSEN, J.: Disseminierte nekrotisierende Myeloenzephalitis. Eine neurologische Erkrankung der Pferde durch Herpes-Infektion. Vet. Pathol. *13:* 161 (1976).

LUTZ, G.; SCHNEIDER, J.; PANNDORF, H.; PREUSSE, C.; GRÜN, E.: Das Verhalten der Ruheherzfrequenz beim trainierten Galopprennpferd. Mh. Vet.-Med. *31:* 134 (1976).

MAREK, J.; MÓCSY, J.: Lehrbuch der klinischen Diagnostik der inneren Krankheiten der Haustiere; 5. Aufl. (VEB Gustav Fischer Verlag, Jena 1956).

MAYHEW, I. G.; LAHUNTA, A.; ROBER, H.; KROOK, L.; TASKER, J. B.: Rückenmarkerkrankung (CSM) beim Pferd. Cornell Vet. Suppl. *68:* 207 (1978).

MEISTER, U.; GERBER, H.; TSCHUDI, P.: Die arterielle Blutgasanalyse in der Diagnostik und Überwachung chronisch lungenkranker Pferde. Schweiz. Arch. Tierheilk. *118:* 99 (1976).

MIKLAUSIC, B.; DOLINAR, Z.: Die digito-digitale Perkussion und topographische Grenzbestimmung der Herzdämpfung beim Pferd. Vet. Arh. (Zagreb) *36:* 284 (1966).

NILIUS, R.; NEEF, L.: Über Beurteilungskriterien diagnostischer Methoden, zugleich ein Beitrag zur rationalen Anwendung von klinisch-chemischen Tests in der Labordiagnostik. Dtsch. Gesundh.-Wesen *34:* 577 (1979).

PIPERS, F. S.; HAMLIN, R. L.: Echokardiographie beim Pferd. J. Amer. vet. med. Assoc. *170:* 815 (1977).

SASSE, H.: Lungenfunktionsprüfung beim Pferd. Tierärztl. Praxis *1:* 49 (1973).

SPÖRRI, H.: Pathophysiologie des Blutkreislaufes. Pathophysiologie der Haustiere. (Hrsgb. H. SPÖRRI und H. STÜNZI). Verlag Paul Parey, Berlin (West) und Hamburg 1969.

SPÖRRI, H.: Elektrokardiographie: Grundlagen der Elektrokardiographie. 1.—3. Mitt. Tierärztl. Praxis *3:* 1; 139; 263 (1975).

SPÖRRI, H.; LEEMANN, W.: Zur Pathophysiologie der Aortenklappeninsuffizienz des Pferdes. Berliner Münchener tierärztl. Wschr. *85:* 441 (1972).

STECK, W.: Mechanik, Technik und Ergebnis der perkutorischen Feststellung thorakaler Schallgrenzen beim Pferd. Schweiz. Arch. Tierheilkunde *111:* 1 (1969).

VASALL, H.: Beitrag zur klinischen Untersuchung von Sportpferden. Vet.-med. Diss., Berlin-Dahlem (1968).

Walker, D.: Labormethoden der Trächtigkeitsdiagnose beim Pferd. Vet. Rec. *100:* 396 (1977).
Wiese, A.: Literaturstudie über die „Spinale Ataxie des Pferdes". Vet.-med. Diss., Hannover (1976).

1.1.1.7. Examination for Locomotor Disturbances and/or Lameness

Definition. A *locomotor disturbance* is present if both forelimbs, both hind limbs or all four limbs show abnormalities of movement. Three grades of locomotor disturbance are recognized — mild, moderate and severe — and the associated symptoms are described in more or less exhaustive detail.

For the detection of locomotor disturbances (table 1.1. — 1), the horse is closely observed in various gaits (walk, trot, gallop) on hard and soft ground, on a lead, uphill and downhill, over jumps, unsaddled and under saddle (with various riders), hitched to a cart, and with various bits. The breed, sex, age and use of the animal must also be taken into account.

The *lameness diagnosis* must be based upon a thorough examination of the *entire locomotor system.* Due to the varied etiology of motor disturbances, such as colic, diseases of internal organs, nervous disorders, metabolic diseases, intoxications, as well as diseases of the postural and locomotor apparatus, it is necessary to examine the entire animal. The horse is repeatedly led and ridden for the examiner (on different days if neccessary) and is observed during backing, changing from one gait to another, pivoting, etc. Finally, various *provocative tests* can be administered by flexing or extending joints for several minutes to increase the stress on these regions and thereby localize the causes of locomotor disturbances or lameness.

The *wedge test* and *board test* are included among the provocative tests (see below).

The term *lameness* is applied to a disturbance in the use of one limb, two diagonally opposed limbs, or two limbs on the same side. Thus, there can be no lameness of the left *and* right forelimbs or hindlimbs; this technically would be classified as a *locomotor disturbance.*

There are three types of lameness, depending on the phase of the stride in which the lameness appears: *supporting and swinging leg lameness,* in which the stride is disturbed in the supporting and swinging phase, respectively, and *mixed lameness,* in which the disturbance extends over both phases or parts of them.

Degree of Lameness

Supporting leg lameness (table 1.1. — 2) has four degrees, or grades, of severity:

Grade 1: audible; the healthy adjacent foot strikes the ground with a louder sound owing to its greater load. (This can be mistaken for the lame foot by an inexperienced observer.)

Grade 2: audible and visible; the horse drops its head when the healthy forelimb bears weight or drops the croup in lameness of a hind limb.

Grade 3: The foot of the lame limb bears weight only on the toe of the shoe; dorsiflexion or striding through in the fetlock joint is absent or incomplete.

Grade 4: The foot of the lame leg does not bear weight or does so only with great hesitancy; the horse hobbles on three legs.

In '*swinging leg lameness*' (table 1.1. — 3) and '*mixed lameness*' (table 1.1. — 4), the severity is described as mild, moderate or severe.

Many severe lamenesses can be seen while walking. Often, however, lameness first becomes apparent while trotting. Lameness cannot be detected in the galloping horse, a fact exploited by deceptive dealers!

Most cases of lameness are of the supporting leg type. Swinging leg lameness is less common. Mild mixed lameness may be quite difficult to detect.

Variable lameness is one in which the degree of severity fluctuates (mild to moderate-grade, grade 1 to grade 2); it is frequently seen in arthrosis.

In *paroxysmal* or *intermittent lameness*, the disturbance 'comes and goes'. Paroxysmal lameness includes the syndrome of *intermittent claudication*, which encompasses lamenesses associated with thrombosis of the external iliac, hypogastric or femoral arteries and, less frequently, of the caudal aorta, the latter producing a locomotor disturbance. Rarely is the brachial artery involved.

Table 1.1. — 1. Types and causes of some common locomotor disturbances

Type of disturbance	Possible cause(s)
a) Forelimbs	
Constrained or choppy gait	1. Bilateral contracted heels 2. Bilateral metacarpal periostitis ('bucked shins') 3. Tendinitis of superficial flexor tendon and/or interosseous muscle (suspensory desmitis) 4. Bilateral deep digital flexor tendon contraction 5. Bilateral superficial digital flexor contraction 6. Bilateral sidebones 7. Bilateral corns
Shuffling, plodding gait	1. Bilateral navicular disease 2. Bilateral degenerative joint disease of the proximal and distal interphalangeal joints
b) Hindlimbs	
Exaggerated hip action 'Stabbing' movement of leg	Bilateral spavin/bone spavin
Bilateral loss of flexion in hock joint	Bilateral osteochondritis dissecans/osteochondrosis of hock joint
Waddling, staggering gait	Bilateral spavin and/or myopathy of back muscles, mainly in trotting horses; CNS disturbances that make up 'wobbler syndrome'.
c) All four limbs	
'Refusal to move'	Acute laminitis of all 4 feet
Stiff, stilted gait	1. First, improper shoeing of a (too) young, immature horse 2. Degenerative joint disease of numerous joints including the spinal column (e.g., old riding-school horse) 3. Fatigue, poor training, unfit horse. 4. Chronic coronary band inflammation in all 4 feet
'Tying up' mainly of both hindlimbs	Myoglobinuria, 'Monday morning disease', myositis of back muscles
Waddling, unsteady gait	Cervical instability, cervical stenotic myelopathy, equine degenerative myeloencephalopathy, Herpes I myelitis.

A *shifting of the lameness* is observed in some circumstances, such as would occur following nerve block of the palmar digital nerves in navicular disease. Navicular disease (podotrochleosis) develops insidiously, usually in *both* thoracic limbs, in horses that are in use. It leads to a bilateral lameness (motor disturbance) that often goes unrecognized until *supporting leg lameness* arises from a predominance of pain in one foot. If the pain in the lame limb is temporarily alleviated by a nerve block, thus eliminating the cause of the lameness, the supporting leg lameness will 'shift' to the foreleg that previously appeared sound.

Table 1.1. — 2. Supporting leg lameness, common causes and grades of severity

Supporting leg lameness in a forelimb		Supporting leg lameness in a hindlimb	
grade	cause(s)	grade	cause(s)
1—2	Navicular disease (process is *bilateral* but one limb is more severely affected) Degenerative joint disease of proximal and distal interphalangeal joints (high and low ringbone)	1—3	Spavin Gonitis (usually in older horses) Osteochondrosis (usually in younger horses)
1—3	1. Fresh hoof wall crack 2. Hollow wall	2—4	Stepping on a nail, puncture wounds in the hoof
1—4	Improper shoeing: nail compression nail prick following shoeing ('quicked')		
2—4	Coronary band injury due to interfering		

Table 1.1. — 3. Swinging leg lameness, common causes and grades of severity

Swinging leg lameness in a forelimb		Swinging leg lameness in a hindlimb	
grade	cause(s)	grade	cause(s)
low to high	1. omarthritis or 2. myositis of shoulder muscles (biceps brachii) or 3. radial nerve paralysis	low to high	1. gonitis or 2. coxitis or 3. femoral nerve paralysis

Table 1.1. — 4. Mixed lameness, common causes and grades of severity

Mixed lameness in a forelimb		Mixed lameness in a hindlimb	
grade	cause(s)	grade	cause(s)
low to high	navicular disease and podarthrosis omarthritis	low to high	spavin and coxitis

A horse with a *'cold' lameness* will show a marked degree of lameness when first saddled or hitched but then warms out of the lameness after a short time. The lameness of low-grade spavin lameness can often be 'ridden away'. Warmup pain is typical of early degenerative joint disease.

Causes of Locomotor Disturbances and Lameness

Experience has demonstrated that most cases of locomotor disturbance and/or lameness have not just one cause but a number of causes that may involve virtually the entire locomotor system. This accounts in part for the extreme difficulty of localizing *all* the causes (table 1.1. — 5). Having performed a relatively simple examination of the distal parts of the limb and obtained a positive nerve block with radiographic change, the inexperienced examiner may conclude that he has identified all the causes. However, residual locomotor disturbances that have their seat in the proximal portion of the musculoskeletal system (spinal column, back muscles, large proximal joints, etc.) are likely to be overlooked. Here the examination becomes particularly difficult, especially in the adult horse, and a diagnosis by a process of elimination may be the only recourse. In many cases, it is necessary despite great advances, to rely on response to therapy. The proximal portions of the locomotor system still represent something of a void that can be illuminated only by repeated careful examinations and the exhaustion of *all* available resources, as well as by the increasing experience of the examiner.

The indiscriminate use of potentially harmful drugs such as corticosteroids to 'see if the lameness goes away' is to be condemned.

The numerous causes of locomotor disturbances and/or lamenesses can be divided into three broad groups:

1. Pain: *'pain lameness'*
2. Limitations of joint motion with little or no pain: *'mechanical lameness'* (ankyloses, contractures, etc.).
3. Nervous disorders: *'neurogenic lameness'* (paralysis, paresis).

The boundaries between these groups are indistinct (see also table 1.1. — 6).

Chronic, longstanding lamenesses, such as those associated with spavin, disrupts the statics and dynamics of the affected limb as well as other parts of the locomotor system, producing various symptoms:

Table 1.1. — 5. Causes of locomotor disturbances or lameness

Painful		Nonpainful
podo-dermatogenic	originating in the hoof matrix	youth lack of training
dermatogenic	originating in the skin (e.g., of the fetlock)	excess fatigue absent or restricted movement in one or more joints: 'mechanical lameness'
arthrogenic tendogenic osteogenic neurogenic myogenic angiogenic	(Note: Boundaries are indistinct!)	

Table 1.1. — 6. Terminology occasionally used for describing lamenesses by the localization of their causes

Term	Localization of cause
Hoof lameness	The horny wall and the structures it encloses (matrix, coffin joint, lateral cartilages, coffin bone, etc.)
Joint lameness	One or more joints of the limbs
Tendon lameness	Flexor tendons and suspensory ligament (interosseous muscle)
Bone lameness	Bone (usually several) or periosteum
Nerve lameness	Peripheral or central nervous system
Muscle lameness	Muscle (myopathy, myositis, muscle degeneration)
Vascular lameness	Blood vessels (thrombosis, intermittent claudication) or lymph vessels (lymphangitis)

1. In the limb affected with spavin lameness: bony swelling on the medial side of the hock, atrophy of gluteal muscles, excessive toe wear, etc.

2. In the rest of the locomotor system: favoring of entire croup and lumbar region, hypertrophy of muscles of sound (or more sound) adjacent limb, increased weight bearing by forelimbs, possible spinal deformity, etc.

According to their *course*, locomotor disturbances and lamenesses may be classified as *acute* or *chronic*.

In all disturbances of gait it is necessary to conduct a careful, systematic examination of the entire locomotor system, beginning with the foot.

In many cases, such as prepurchase exams, full examination of the locomotor system is indicated, even in the absence of obvious abnormalities. Here one must be guided by the shape and condition of the feet, the quality of the shoeing, etc., and make a prognosis accordingly.

Disorders of the equine locomotor system are among the most difficult to diagnose in veterinary medicine. In part, this is due to the great diversity of causes that may result in similar lameness symptoms. In examining the locomotor system, the veterinarian should be systematic in his efforts by adhering closely to an *examination routine* (table 1.1. — 7).

1. Careful *history-taking* must include the time of onset of the lameness or locomotor disturbance, the animal's appearance at the onset, previous diagnoses or treatments by a veterinarian or layman, and the course of the symptoms. Care is taken to obtain an accurate accounting, since information given by owners, attendants or agents may be intentionally or unintentionally misleading.

Of particular importance in hoof lameness is the time of the last shoeing and whether the shoe has been reset. The possibility of tetanus must not be overlooked in certain foot conditions.

Due to the scarcity of competent farriers, horses often go too long between shoeings, and the quality of the shoeing as well as the shoe itself is apt to be poor. Often the history must be obtained by telephone because the rider, driver or owner are unable to be present at the time of examination.

2. *Recording of patient data* (table 1.1. — 8). Already the examiner gains an appreciation of the animal's general appearance (atrophied muscles, exostoses, soft tissue, swellings, etc.), as well as its behavior, temperament, character, general care, etc., thus expediting the inspecion that follows.

3. *Inspection.* The horse should be made to stand on a level floor for inspection. With damage to the locomotor system, the animal may not be able to distribute its weight evenly on all four legs and feet. The animal's behavior, the position it assumes, and the manner in which weight is borne by the feet, provide important diagnostic clues. The examiner also assesses the general condition of the feet and type of shoeing, checking for ring formation, separation of the hoof wall, injuries or fistulas at the coronary band, soft tissue, swellings, etc.

Table 1.1. — 7. Routine for the orthopedic examination of the horse

1. History	
2. Patient data	
3. Inspection: general appearance (head, neck, torso, spine, limbs)	
leg position	
pastern and foot axes	
hoof shape	
animal is viewed from the front, from both sides and from behind	
4. Examination of gait (at walk, trot, and perhaps gallop)	
5. Check for pulsation (in palmar or plantar digital arteries)	
6. Reaction to hoof tester	
7. Percussion of hoof	
8. Palpation of the entire limb with both hands	
9. Check for localized temperature increases	
10. Flexion tests	
11. Wedge test	
12. Board tests	
13. Nerve blocks	
14. Radiography	
15. Rectal examination	
16. Test of skin sensitivity (if paralysis is suspected)	
17. Laboratory tests	
18. Further investigations	
a) Electrical stimulation	e) Arthroscopy
b) Oscillometry	f) Ungulography with DMS
c) Angiography	g) Electromyography
d) Scintigraphy	h) Thermography (etc.)

Table 1.1. — 8. Relevant patient data

1. Color
2. Sex
3. Markings: congenital and acquired, starting with head and proceeding to neck and limbs
4. Age
5. Height at withers: linear rule and tape measure
6. Breed
7. Use
8. Name of horse
9. Blood type (if necessary) for identification and verification of parentage
10. Pedigree papers present and consistent?
11. Body weight in kg or lb. (weighed or estimated)

4. *Examination of gait.* With a halter or bridle on the horse, it is first led in a straight line at a walk, on even ground, on both hard and soft surfaces, without a rider. The patient is observed from the front, rear and both sides. The path traveled by the feet during each stride is recorded, be it a straight line, an inward semicircle (brushing) or an outward semicircle (circumduction). The examiner also notes whether the feet meet the ground flat or on the toe, heel or edge, as well as the length of the stride, the height of the step, and any other noticeable variations from 'normal'. Next the horse is trotted. The object of this examination is:

a) to identify the lame limb(s),
b) to ascertain the type of lameness (supporting leg, swinging leg or mixed),
c) to obtain evidence of the causes of the lameness.

The four points of the examination routine listed thus far are usually sufficient to identify the lame limb(s). In many cases the experienced examiner already has formed an opinion as to the seat of the lameness (usually there are several) and perhaps even the causes of the lameness.

Some examples: Lameness from ringbone or navicular disease improves to a varying degree with exercise. Sometimes the lameness is exacerbated *on turning.* Other diseases may lead to intermittent lameness such as intermittent claudication of iliac thrombosis, from verminous arteritis or joint mice that very occasionally become incarcerated between the weight bearing surfaces of articular cartilage.

The remaining points in the examination routine are as follows:

5. *Check for pulsation* in the palmar or plantar digital arteries. This can give evidence of inflammatory processes in the distal part of the limb. Strong pulsation of the arteries with an increase of caliber compared to the healthy adjacent foot is termed 'increased digital pulse'.

6. *The use of the hoof tester* provides important information on painful lesions of structures enclosed in the hoof wall.

7. *Percussion of the hoof* is done with a closed hoof tester or with hoof percussion hammers.

8. *Palpation* is done proximal to the hoof and should be continued up the entire limb as well as to the back and remaining parts of the locomotor system.

9. The local *temperature* of the hoof wall is checked as well as other regions of the locomotor system that may be involved in inflammation.

10. The *flexion tests* represent the provocative tests that can be performed on the various joints.

11. *Wedge test.* This is also classified as a provocative test. This test is positive in the presence of chronic degenerative joint disease.

12. The *board test* also gives similar results in the presence of arthritic conditions.

13. *Nerve blocks* are among the most important clinical tests and should always be done prior to radiographic examination (point 14). They also form an important part of the clinical training of students and veterinarians.

Points 5 through 14 of the examination routine, serve to localize the causes of the lameness and help establish the cause(s) of lameness in the limb(s).

The following examinations are done for lamenesses or locomotor disturbances involving the hindlimbs:

15. *Rectal examination.*

16. *Test of skin sensitivity if paralysis is suspected.*

17. *Laboratory tests* relating to blood status, muscle enzymes, urinary findings, etc.

Points 15—17 are supplementary examinations for differential diagnosis in cases not involving hoof lameness.

18. Further investigations of the locomotor apparatus that may be done in suitable equipped clinics include: (a) electrical stimulation; (b) oscillometry; (c) angiography; (d) scintigraphy; (e) arthroscopy; (f) ungulography with DMS; (g) electromyography; (h) thermography.

If uncertainty persists as to the seat or cause of the lameness, it is often useful to (a) repeat the examination in one or two days, or (b) conduct the examination under conditions of natural weight-bearing, or (c) examine the horse under a rider or under various riders, or hitched to a cart, or (d) examine the horse exercising on a track or in pasture. The latter is particularly indicated for lameness having its seat in the proximal portions of the limbs, the spinal column or the CNS.

Arthroscopy, with Guidelines for Intra-articular Operative Technique under Arthroscopic Control

Introduction. Increasingly, veterinarians are relying upon the direct technique of arthroscopy in the diagnosis of joint disease. A number of reasons are responsible for this: (1) improved aseptic and atraumatic techniques in veterinary surgery; (2) modern, small-caliber telescopes with bright, 'cold' illumination from an external source; (3) the necessity, especially in large animals, of subjecting the proximal joints to meticulous inspection with minimal trauma. In addition, the arthroscope provides a means of performing intra-articular operations under visual control. Modern devices also enable findings to be documented by photography.

We shall relate briefly our experience with arthroscopy during the past six years, placing special emphasis on the examination technique in the horse.

Problems of Arthroscopy. A prerequisite for the endoscopic examination of a joint is the presence of a sufficiently large space to accommodate the telescope. The large proximal joints, i.e., the hip and shoulder joints and especially the stifle joint, are important in this regard. The possibilities of examining these joints are limited. As is known, it is difficult to obtain good radiographs of the stifle or shoulder joint in the standing horse. The double-contrast films of the knee joint commonly taken in human patients are much more problematic in large animals and are seldom obtained. Films of the hip joint in large animals require particularly costly x-ray apparatus and a recumbent patient. One can appreciate the need for casting the horse in order to conduct a thorough examination of these large proximal joints. To avoid repeated casting, diagnosis is often followed by treatment (e.g., arthrotomy) in the same sitting. One should always endeavor to reach the desired goal with an absolute minimum amount of trauma. For this reason arthroscopy is the method of choice. Cartilage injuries, for example, can be diagnosed only by means or arthroscopy or arthrotomy.

Instruments. We first used the arthroscope developed by Wruhs [1969] for humans, which allows simultaneous photodocumentation. Lumina optics with a forward (180°) and lateral view angle (100°) are used, to which the fiberoptic cable is rigidly attached. The light source is a triple-intensity projection lamp. The arthroscope is available in two models: a diagnostic instrument with a trocar sheath 3 mm in diameter, and an 'operative arthroscope' with a larger 5-mm trocar sheath through which grasping forceps, diathermy loops, scissors, and similar instruments can be introduced into the joint. Recently we have also used a large-caliber arthroscope with an 8-mm diameter. For smaller animals we use finer instruments. The aforementioned instruments are equipped with insulated shafts and thus can be safely used for electrocoagulation. A side attachment with a two-way stopcock can be fitted to the arthroscope sheath for flushing the joint space after the drainage of effusions and for the insufflation of gas. We use sterile filtered air. Thermal damage to the joint is prevented by the cold-light optics. To protect the delicate optics, the instruments are sterilized with ethylene oxide in a sterilization box at room temperature. It should be remembered that the small-caliber arthroscopes are highly sensitive to all mechanical stresses such as bending or pressure and should be handled appropriately.

Practice on cadaveric joints will aid the operator in correct approaches, improving instrument handling, and indicating the limits of vision into articular spaces.

Viewing conditions in the joint space are greatly enhanced by the insufflation of sterile air. With expansion of the synovial lining, the joint can be systematically inspected. Ballottement of the patella when the stifle joint is being examined can also obtained with this method, enabling the arthroscope to be slipped beneath the patella without trauma. The viewable joint area can be increased by careful angling of the scope, using both the forward-view and angled optics, and by moving the joint itself.

Strict asepsis is essential. As mentioned, the optics and light cable are sterilized in a gas sterilizer with ethylene oxide, and everything else is autoclaved. The hair is clipped and then the are around the joint to be examined is shaved (unfortunately this is often possible only under general anesthesia). After the skin is defatted, it is scrubbed several times with a suitable surgical soap or disinfectant and prepared for a septic surgery in a routine manner. Then the area is draped with large split towels and a commercially available self-adhering incise drape. The limbs and hooves are cleaned prior to the surgical scrub and the distal parts of the limbs covered with a sterile stocking. This enables the surgeon to move the joint intraoperatively without a break in aseptic technique (fig. 1.1. — 1).

As a general rule, the *indication* for arthroscopy is present if a definitive diagnosis cannot be made by any other examination method. This applies especially to the stifle joint as well as to the hip and shoulder. In addition, there are certain sesamoid fractures that can be assessed more accurately by arthroscopy than by radiographic means. It may also be indicated for monitoring the progress of a disease once the diagnosis is made.

Arthroscopy is *contraindicated* in severe general illnesses that would carry a high anesthetic risk, as well as in the presence of overlying skin changes that would contraindicate joint puncture.

Examination Technique. Arthroscopy in the horse is carried out under general anesthesia (for example using halothane administered by endotracheal tube). A pneumatic tourniquet is applied for arthroscopy of the distal limb but is unsuitable for the stifle, hip, shoulder and elbow joints. Frequently the arthroscopy is followed by an arthrotomy, and so all necessary preparations should be made beforehand. The animal is examined and operated on in lateral recumbency. The surgery table described by Knezevic [1971] is useful for positioning a horse for arthroscopy (fig. 1.1. — 1).

The *approaches to the joints* are selected according to the diagnostic goal and anatomic constraints (fig. 1.1. — 2). In the horse we use the dorsal approach to the superior recess for arthroscopy of the femoropatellar joint, and approach the femorotibial joint from the cranial, medial and lateral directions, as is done in human arthroscopy.

For *photography*, an assistant attaches the sterile phototube with camera to the arthroscope, always observing strict aseptic technique. On completion of the examination the unsufflated air is expressed through the trocar sheath after removal of the telescope. If this is not done, subcutaneous emphysema can be felt for several

1 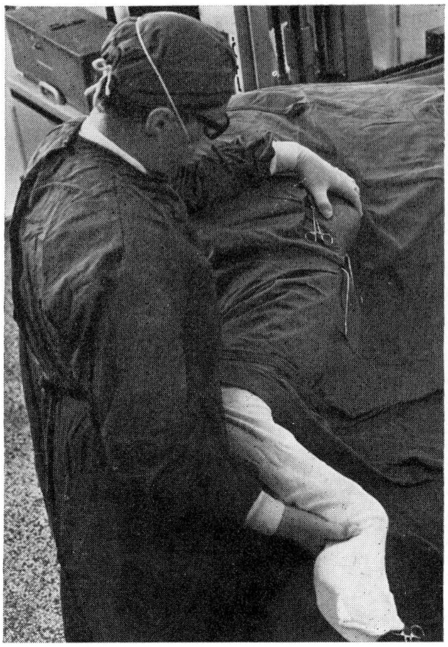 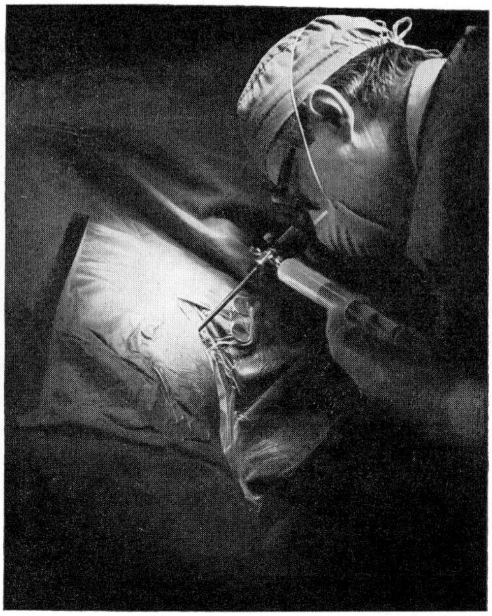 2

Fig. 1.1. — 1. Arthroscopy. Horse in left lateral recumbent position, right stifle joint prepared for arthroscopic examination. The hindlimb is covered with a sterile stocking. The sterile draping is done such that the limb can be flexed or extended as needed during the examination.

Fig. 1.1. — 2. Arthroscopy of right femoropatellar joint. The operative field is additionally draped with a self-adhesive film. Sterile filtered air is insufflated to expand the synovial membrane.

days postoperatively. The skin incision is closed with a temporary suture. Antibiotics are administered for a period of several days.

In all animals we have noticed a more or less pronounced joint distention after arthroscopy including some swelling of the adjacent soft tissues. This usually disappears after a few days of box stall confinement. If the swelling persists, elastic pressure bandages are applied and anti-inflammatory drugs administered. No case of post-arthroscopic infection was observed.

Results. The hip, shoulder, stifle, elbow, tarsal and fetlock joints have all been arthroscopically examined in the horse. The principal endoscopic findings were cartilage damage, meniscal injuries, and the presence of loose or foreign bodies in the joint (fig. 1.1. — 3 to 1.1. — 6). Changes in the synovial membrane have also been observed. Various sesamoid fractures, that are difficult or impossible to demonstrate radiographically, can be verified by arthroscopy. Arthroscopy can provide a guideline whether the operative removal of the osteochondral fragments is indicated.

Arthroscopy is of unquestionable value in the diagnosis of severe cartilage erosion not demonstrable by x-ray. Despite various radiographic techniques carried out at the various institutions, it has never been possible to demonstrate cartilage damage by indirect methods prior to the development of obvious secondary bony change. With arthroscopy, a rapid, definitive diagnosis is possible. Formerly these changes could be detected only by an exploratory arthrotomy.

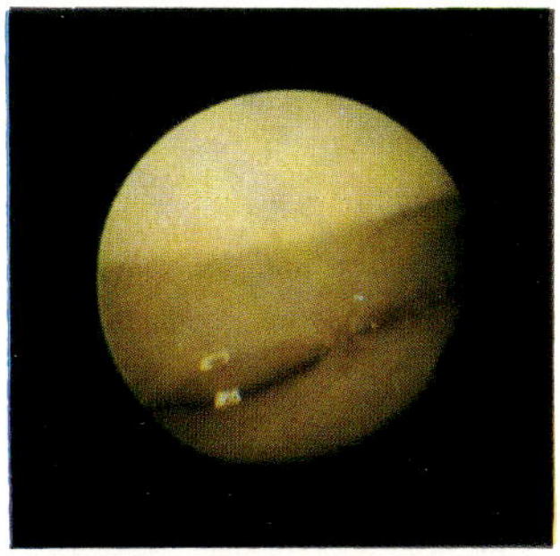

3

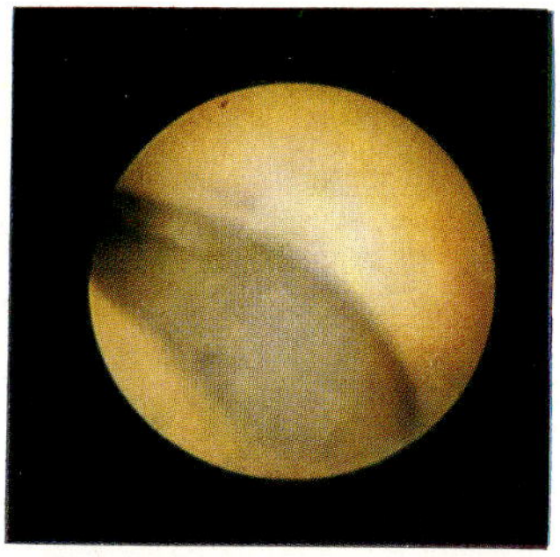

4

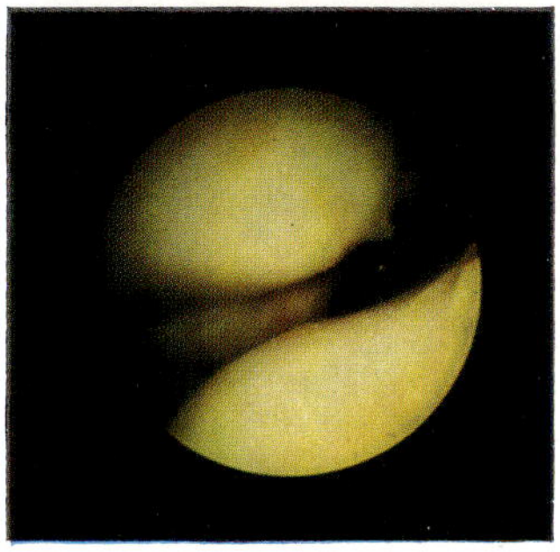

5

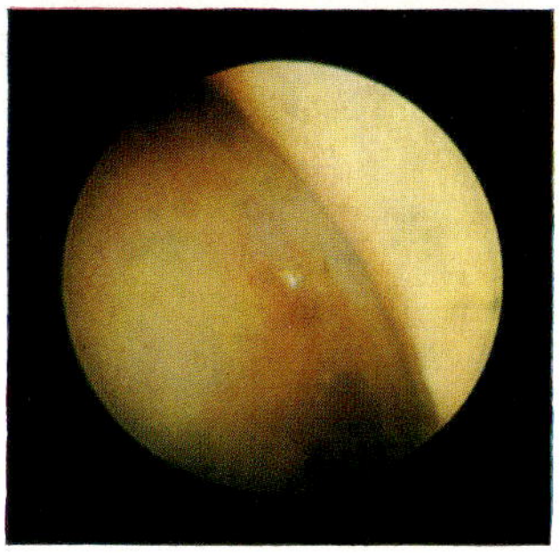

6

Fig. 1.1. — 3. Femoropatellar joint. Wavy joint contour line denoting cartilage ulceration. Isolated air bubbles are visible in the synovial fluid.

Fig. 1.1. — 4. View into the femoropatellar joint from the superior recess. Three joint mice can be discerned.

Fig. 1.1. — 5. Femorotibial joint: Portions of the medial meniscus are torn.

Fig. 1.1. — 6. Metacarpophalangeal joint of a jumper; several cartilage lesions are evident.

Risks and Complications. The risks of arthroscopy include infection, joint effusion, and injuries that may result from insertion of the trocar or manipulation of the arthroscope in the joint space. Damage to the endoscope itself is often first manifested by distortion of the photographs, rather than by direct viewing through the instrument. Besides minor damage to the optics, no complications have yet been observed.

Summary. Our six years' experience with arthroscopy of the hip, shoulder, stifle, elbow, tarsal and fetlock joints in the horse is briefly reviewed. Arthroscopy represents a valuable contribution to the diagnosis of equine joint disease. It provides an atraumatic means of gathering information that formerly could be obtained only by arthrotomy. Lesions of the articular cartilage, capsular tissue and menisci can be demonstrated by the systematic inspection of all joint compartments and can be documented with photographs. The arthroscope also permits intra-articular surgery under visual control with minimal trauma. Following the arthroscopic diagnosis, the necessary arthrotomy, if indicated, can be undertaken at the most favorable site, and can thus be kept as atraumatic as possible. In addition osteochondral fragments can be moved about within the joint and removed under optimum conditions.

References

KNEZEVIC, P.: Ein fahrender Grosstier-Operationstisch. Wiener Tierärztl. Mschr. *58:* 173 (1971).

KNEZEVIC, P.: Zur Endoskopie des Kniegelenkes beim Pferd. XI. Congr. European Soc. of Veterin. Surgery, Copenhagen 1975, p. 57.

KNEZEVIC, P.: Zur Geschichte der Gelenkendoskopie in der Veterinärmedizin. Historia Med. Veterin. *1:* 19 (1976).

KNEZEVIC, P.; WRUHS, O.: Endoskopische Gelenkdiagnostik bei Pferd und Rind. XX. Welttierärztekongress, Thessaloniki 1975, p. 707.

KNEZEVIC, P.; WRUHS, O.: Möglichkeiten der Arthroskopie bei Pferd und Rind. Wien. Tierärztl. Mschr. *62:* 300 (1975).

KNEZEVIC, P.; WRUHS, O.: Die Arthroskopie bei Pferd, Rind, Schwein und Hund. Vet.-med. Nachr. *1:* 53 (1977).

WRUHS, O.: Die Arthroskopie und Endophotographie zur Diagnostik und Dokumentation von Kniegelenkverletzungen. Wien. Med. Wschr. *120:* 126 (1970).

WRUHS, O.: Indikationen, Technik und Ergebnisse der Arthroskopie des Kniegelenkes. Sandorama II, 1971, p. 4.

WRUHS, O.: Die Arthroskopie. Langenbeck's Arch. Klin. Chir. (1972), 332, Kongreßbericht.

WRUHS, O.: Die Endoskopie des Kniegelenkes zur Diagnostik und Dokumentation von Binnenschäden und Erkrankungen. Fortschr. der Endoskopie *4:* 225 (1973a).

WRUHS, O.: Die Arthroskopie des Kniegelenkes. Z. Orthopädie *111:* 525 (1973b).

WRUHS, O.: Die Arthroskopie des Kniegelenkes. Z. Orthopädie *111:* 664 (1973c).

WRUHS, O.: Die Arthroskopie. Orthopäd. Praxis *9:* 75 (1973d).

WRUHS, O.: Der Informationswert der Endoskopie des Kniegelenkes (Verlag Brüder Hollinek, Wien 1974).

1.1.2. Hematology and Biochemistry of the Normal Horse and the Significance of Pathologic Variation

The use of laboratory tests and the analysis of the composition of various body fluids have become an established part of veterinary diagnostics. The need for an accurate diagnosis reflects the growing demand for specificity of treatment, which is why laboratory tests of specific parameters are often essential for supplementing clinical findings, confirming the diagnosis or refining the differential diagnosis. Such tests are also indispensable for making a prognosis and assessing the results of therapy. In addition, many hematologic and biochemical values are highly useful from the standpoint of early detection of various disease states. They also provide a means of evaluating responses to training in the case of the athletic horse.

In the horse, diagnosis is basically concerned with the individual animal. Methods of herd diagnosis are applied only when dealing with special problems. Since the information derived from each parameter varies, the usual practice is to measure several parameters which are mutually supplementary, for each particular organ system (panel).

Every effort must be made to minimize the sources of error in the determination of individual values. Thus, some parameters may be influenced by the time of day, food consumption, stress or concurrent medication. Blood samples should be drawn at a standardized time such as before the morning feeding. For comparative purposes, ideally it is essential that the samples be stored in clean containers and that anticoagulants or preservatives be added, depending on the nature of the test to be performed. The storage must conform to the particular character of the sample and parameter of interest. It is important that all rules be adhered to, otherwise the sample may be useless for the particular test and the results may lead to false conclusions.

Even with complete standardization of the examination methods and the assurance of optimum conditions of sample taking, transport and storage, minor variations are unavoidable. It is important to note that age, sex and breed can be a source of variations.

Normal values are always average values. For this reason the normal range, usually defined as the mean $\pm$ 2 standard deviations, is of greater importance for clinical purposes.

Ideally it would be desirable to refine the data for the horse with consideration for the various influencing factors, and establish normal and borderline values for the principal breeds, types and age groups.

1.1.2.1. Blood

Blood samples are drawn from the jugular vein in the horse. Heparin, EDTA or some other anticoagulant is added to the collecting tubes if the test is to be performed on whole blood or plasma. If the tests are to be done on serum, nothing is added to the sample. Hemolytic serum or plasma is unsuitable for most determinations. Yellow staining by bile pigments or milky turbidity caused by lipids can also distort the various tests. The blood samples are used in the clinical laboratory for the determination of hematologic or biochemical values.

1.1.2.1.1. Hematologic Examinations

The hematologic analysis includes an assessment of the cellular elements of the blood, specifically the determination of the hematocrit, hemoglobin concentration, erythrocyte count, leukocyte count, and the red and white blood cell morphology (table 1.1. — 9). The parameters of blood coagulation may be included among the hematologic values together with the erythrocyte sedimentation rate (ESR).

Changes in erythrocytic parameters that are manifested by an increase in the hematocrit, hemoglobin concentration and erythrocyte count are termed polycythemia. Most important clinically is the reason why the blood becomes concentrated. This may be a result of fluid loss or, as in the case of anemia, a decrease in the proportion of corpuscular elements per unit blood volume. Regardless of the various precipitating causes, anemia always results when the breakdown of erythrocytes exceeds the maximum capacity for their production, or there is a primary impairment of erythropoesis. The determination or calculation of the parameters as well as the examination of the blood smear are sufficient in most cases to identify the form of anemia present. Acute posthemorrhagic anemias are rarely observed in the horse, because even extensive blood losses are overcome with amazing rapidity and without pronounced regenerative changes. Hemolytic anemias are observed in infectious anemia, leptospirosis, and as a result of various immune responses. These forms of anemia are typically accompanied by icterus, bilirubinemia, and hemoglobinuria. With impaired hematopoiesis, the anemia usually has a hypochromic character, and altered cell forms are observed.

Changes in the leukocyte count may be nonspecific. Leukocytosis is a feature of many infectious or inflammatory diseases. It can be interpreted as the result of an injurious agent and the animal's response to that agent. Conversely, leukopenia

Table 1.1. — 9. Normal range of hematologic values in the adult horse (except Thoroughbreds)

Parameter	SI units		Old system	
	units of measure	quantity	units of measure	quantity
Hematocrit	'one'	0.32···0.45	Vol.-%	32···45
Hemoglobin	g/dl	10···14	g/100 ml	10···14
Erythrocytes	10^{12}/l	6···9	$10^6/\mu l$	6···9
MCV	$10^{-9}\,\mu l$ = fl	34···58	μm^3	34···58
MCHC	mmol/l (Hb/4)	19.24···22.96	9 %	31···37
Leukocytes	10^9/l	6···10	$10^3/\mu l$	6···10
Basophils	%	0···2	%	0···2
	abs/μl	0···90	abs/μl	0···90
Eosinophils	%	2···6	%	2···6
	abs/μl	100···700	abs/μl	100···700
Nonsegmented neutrophils	%	2···5	%	2···5
	abs/μl	120···500	abs/μl	120···500
Segmented neutrophils	%	35···65	%	35···65
	10^9/l	2.5···6.5	$10^3/\mu l$	2.5···6.5
Lymphocytes	%	20···45	%	20···45
	10^9/l	1.5···4.5	$10^3/\mu l$	1.5···4.5
Monocytes	%	1···6	%	1···6
	abs/μl	100···600	abs/μl	100···600
Platelets	10^9/l	200···500	$10^3/\mu l$	200···500

signals a failure of the body's defense mechanisms. Severe viral infection, endotoxic shock, intoxication or radiation injury may be responsible. The changes in leukocyte count do not affect the different types of white blood cells equally. Eosinophilia may indicate parasitic infestation or allergic diseases, while eosinopenia is associated with an increase of glucocorticoid excretion. The neutrophilic granulocytes determine the white blood picture in the horse and are the principal agents of cellular defense. Their quantitative behavior as well as the predominance of younger or older cell forms (called a left and right shift, respectively) mainly reflect the stage of the disease. Marked lymphocytosis in the horse occurs in chronic infections such as infectious anemia or the rarely seen case of tuberculosis or lymphatic leukosis. It may also accompany the healing phase of inflammatory diseases but is then only a transient phenomenon. Very low platelet counts are found in hemorrhagic diathesis and disseminated intravascular coagulation (DIC) syndrome.

A further blood study is the determination of the erythrocyte sedimentation rate (ESR). It is performed by various methods using a vertical or slanted tube. Citrate solution is used as the anticoagulant, in accordance with prevailing rules. The results are nonspecific, providing information that is more prognostic than diagnostic. An accelerated ESR is seen in anemias, febrile diseases and local suppurative processes, and a decreased ESR in states of hemoconcentration, and in an agonal situation.

Table 1.1. — 10. Normal range of biochemical blood values in the adult horse (except Thoroughbreds)

Parameter	SI units		Old system	
	units of measure	quantity	units of measure	quantity
Total bilirubin	μmol/l	···34.2	mg/100 ml	···2.0
Glucose	mmol/l	2.8···5.0	mg/100 ml	50···90
Lactate	mmol/l	0.33···1.78	mg/100 ml	3···16
Total lipids	g/l	3.7···6.7	mg/100 ml	370···670
Total cholesterol	mmol/l	1.8···3.1	mg/100 ml	70···120
Urea	mmol/l	3.3···6.7	mg/100 ml	20···40
Total protein	g/l	60···78	g/100 ml	6.0···7.8
Albumin	%	32···49	%	32···49
α-Globulin	%	7···23	%	7···23
β-Globulin	%	11···33	%	11···33
γ-Globulin	%	10···32	%	10···32
Sodium	mmol/l	126···157	mg/100 ml	290···360
Potassium	mmol/l	3.3···5.6	mg/100 ml	13···22
Calcium	mmol/l	2.0···3.3	mg/100 ml	8···13
Magnesium	mmol/l	0.5···1.0	mg/100 ml	1.3···2.5
Inorg. phosphate	mmol/l	0.6···1.8	mg/100 ml	2.0···5.5
pH		7.35···7.42		
pCO_2	kPa	4.7···6.7	mm Hg	35···50
Base excess	mmol/l	0···3.0	mval/l	0···3.0
AspAT (GOT)	μkat/l	1.33···2.33	E/l (U/l)	80···140
AlAT (GPT)	μkat/l	···0.38	E/l (U/l)	···23
CPK	μkat/l	···0.67	E/l (U/l)	···40
SDH	μkat/l	···0.02	E/l (U/l)	···1.3
ALD	μkat/l	···0.11	E/l (U/l)	···6.5
AP	μkat/l	···3.67	E/l (U/l)	···220

1.1.2.1.2. Biochemical Examinations

Determinations of the levels of blood constituents have become increasingly important, and the number of assayable metabolites is steadily increasing. At present, however, only a limited number have attained recognized diagnostic value. What is more, the time and apparatus required for some determinations still represent a limiting factor in many cases. The principal metabolites and enzymes that are routinely determined in the blood are listed in table 1.1. — 10 together with their normal ranges of variation, without specification of the methods used. Almost all these constituents are determined in the serum or plasma. In whole blood, most of the parameters undergo rapid change despite refrigeration. Serum samples, on the other hand, can be refrigerated for several days or frozen for weeks and even months without significant change. Determinations of the acid-base status are more demanding. They are done on whole blood collected in evacuated tubes and must be performed without delay.

In most cases several parameters are determined simultaneously so that a comprehensive evaluation can be made. A number of metabolites are useful indicators of the intermediary metabolism as well as the functional state of organs such as the liver and kidneys.

A very important parameter in the horse is the serum bilirubin, which is elevated in liver parenchymal disease, hemolysis and biliary obstruction. The simultaneous determination of the direct bilirubin combined with determinations of the urinary bilirubin and urobilin enable an accurate differentiation of the various forms of icterus. An elevated serum urea level is indicative of uremia due to renal, prerenal (shock) or postrenal causes (outflow obstruction).

The enzymatically determined plasma glucose level is of less importance in the horse than in other domestic animals. Hyperglycemia is occasionally seen in diseases of the central nervous system, though it may also be caused by extreme excitement. The lactate and pyruvate concentrations show a particularly marked increase in paralytic myoglobinuria (tying-up syndromes); strenuous exertion and respiratory distress can also provoke a lactic acid increase. The lipid status (total lipids, free fatty acids, cholesterol) is of interest in ponies with suspected hyperlipemia.

Changes in the total serum protein are often the result of hemoconcentration or hemodilution. True decreases affect mainly the albumin fraction. Digestive disorders, chronic liver damage and endoparasites are the principal causes. Hyperproteinemia is the result of increased globulin formation. The individual protein fractions may also be elevated with no corresponding effect on the total serum protein. The α-globulins (α_2 fraction) are increased in febrile states, viral infections and inflammatory reactions of the bones and joints. A rise of the β-globulin fraction is often associated with chronic foci of inflammation or chronic infections such as mesenteric abscessation. Hypergammaglobulinemia may be demonstrated in cirrhosis of the liver or after immunizations. Mares sometime display a marked rise of gamma globulin levels in late pregnancy.

Electrolyte determinations in the horse are mainly of value in assessing disturbances of the water, electrolyte and acid-base balance. The results may indicate a need for supplementing intravenous therapy. In choosing the proper intravenous solution, it is extremely important to know whether an existing state of dehydration is hypertonic, hypotonic or isotonic in character. The principal cations to be determined are sodium, potassium, calcium and magnesium; the most important anions are bicarbonate, chloride and phosphate.

Of equal importance is the acid-base balance of the blood. By performing a blood gas analysis with a suitable instrument setup, the pH, pCO_2 and standard bicarbonate or base excess can be ascertained. The results of the urinalysis may be included in the evaluation (table 1.1 — 11).

Of the various respiratory disturbances, acidosis is the most important with respect to its occurrence in diseases such as pneumonia and chronic obstructive pulmonary disease (COPD). Metabolic acidosis may be seen in cases of acute diarrhea. It is also seen in cases of paralytic myoglobinuria (tying-up syndrome) or organic acid buildups from other causes, such as endotoxic shock in intestinal obstruction. Starvation or renal insufficiency can also cause acidosis in rare instances. Metabolic alkalosis seldom occurs in horses.

Enzyme determinations center on the group of intracellular enzymes. The demonstration of increased enzyme activities in the serum is a reliable indicator of cellular damage. Some enzymes are particularly abundant in certain organs, although no enzyme can be said to be completely organ-specific. Thus, it is best to determine the activities of a spectrum or panel that includes such enzymes as glutamic oxaloacetic transaminase (GOT) (aspartate aminotransferase), glutamic pyruvic transaminase (GPT) (alanine aminotransferase), creatine phosphokinase (CPK), aldolase (ALD) and akaline phosphatase (AP). These tests are sufficient to demonstrate as well as differentiate muscular lesions and liver diseases. Sorbitol dehydrogenase

Table 1.1. — 11. Disturbances of the acid-base balance

Disturbance	Blood gas analysis			Urinalysis		Compensation by
	pH	pCO_2	BÜ	pH	NSBA	
Metabolic acidosis						Hyperventilation
decompensated	↓	→	↓	↓	↓	
compensated	→	↓	↓	↓	↓	
Metabolic alkalosis						Hypoventilation
decompensated	↑	→	↑	↑	↑	
compensated	↗	↗	↑	↑	↑	
Respiratory acidosis						Renal excretion of H^+ and Cl^-
decompensated	↓	↑	→	↓	↓	
compensated	→	↑	↑	↓	↓	
Respiratory alkalosis						Renal excretion of HCO_3
decompensated	↑	↓	→	↑	↑	
compensated	→	↓	↓	↑	↑	

(SDH) has also proved useful in the diagnosis of liver damage. Along with glutamate dehydrogenase (GDH), it is practically liver-specific, although its sensitivity is poor and its activity changes are demonstrable for only a short time.

1.1.2.2. Urine

The urinalysis is an essential part of the diagnostic workup of diseases of the kidneys and urinary organs. Because the kidneys play a critical role in the maintenance of homeostasis, analysis of the urine also gives valuable information on renal disease as well as disturbances of other organs.

In the mare, urine is best obtained by catheterization of the urinary bladder. In the male catheterization is possible only after the penis has been prolapsed manually or by medication, and precautionary measures are necessary during catheter insertion.

In most cases the objective of the urinalysis is to confirm clinical suspicions or shed light on known metabolic disorders or impairments of organ function. In either case it is important to obtain a result as quickly as possible, even at the cost of greater accuracy, so that further diagnostic or therapeutic measures can be instituted without delay. Hence, the urinalysis is limited in most cases to a physical examination of the fresh urine and the application of qualitative or semiquantitative methods of analysis. These quick methods can be followed if need be by accurate chemical determinations, microscopic examination of the urinary sediment, as well as microbiological studies if inflammatory changes are apparent.

If the analysis cannot be done right away, the urine specimen should be stored in the refrigerator. Formalin, boric acid or chloroform may be added as preservatives.

During the physical examination of the urine, the volume, color, odor, transparency and viscosity are noted. Normal horses excrete 3—6 l per day, and perhaps as much as 10 l. Equine urine is a viscous, mucus like, stringy fluid. It may be light yellow to light brown or even yellow-red in color. The odor is species-specific and is often compared to that of beef broth or rotting hay. A large amount of sediment forms within a short time; this consists mainly of calcium carbonate and smaller amounts of calcium oxalate, calcium sulfate and hippuric acid. In an uncapped container the superficial layer of urine soon takes on a darker color, which intensifies and spreads to deeper layers.

The properties of equine urine make assessment difficult, for they may mask turbidity resulting from inflammatory urinary tract disease. Slight color changes, such as those associated with hematuria or the reddish-brown discoloration following the administration of the anthraquinone laxative Istizin[1] may also escape notice. However, hemoglobinuria and especially myoglobinuria may be so intense that they cause the urine to take on a reddish-brown to dark brown color, perhaps even turning it inky black.

Equine urine has a density of 1.025—1.060 and is usually alkaline (pH 8). Values in the acidic range reflect renal compensation in response to an acidotic insult. In such cases the urine becomes clear and watery.

The chemical examination of the urine is ordinarily limited to the demonstration of protein, bilirubin and urobilinogen, hemoglobin and glucose. This can be done in a matter of minutes by the use of the commercially available reagent strips. If renal or urinary tract disease is suspected, the protein test is of primary interest. If proteinuria is demonstrated, microscopic examination of the urinary sediment should follow without delay. Glucosuria is uncommon in horses but may occur in conjunction with certain diseases of the central nervous system (Borna disease).

Tests for bilirubin and urobilinogen in the urine are important in the diagnosis of icterus. Bilirubinuria occurs only in parenchymatous and obstructive jaundice; urobilinogenuria is characteristic of liver parenchymal damage and hemolytic icterus.

Hemolytic diseases are also typically accompanied by hemoglobinuria. Its differentiation from myoglobinuria is best accomplished by observing the clinical picture, which is one of anemia in the case of hemoglobinuria and signs of acute muscular disease in the case of myoglobinuria. If redness of the urine and hemoglobinuria are the result of hematuria, this can be readily determined by letting the urine stand. All doubts are finally resolved by microscopic examination of the sediment. Isolated red cells may be observed despite a negative hemoglobin test. Besides primary renal damage or urinary tract disease, hematuria is a consistent feature of all hemorrhagic diatheses.

The quantitative urinalysis is a special examination done to resolve a specific question. Such tests can be very useful in providing more precise information on certain metabolic disorders. The following substances are most commonly determined:

Substance	Urine concentration in the normal horse	
Urea	333—666 mmol/l	(20—40 g/l)
Phosphate	0.16—0.65 mmol/l	(0.5—2.0 mg/ml)
Indican		(12—300 mg/100 ml)

The urea content of the urine, together with the urea level in the blood, can serve as a useful index of the protein supply. Marked phosphaturia always signifies an acidotic stress on the organism. High urinary indican levels are particularly common in intestinal diseases.

[1] Danthron Winthrop (Sterlin Drug Co., New York, N.Y.).

The microscopic examination should be carried out promptly after sedimentation or centrifugation of the sample.

Of the inorganic constituents, the crystals of calcium carbonate and calcium oxalate are of no diagnostic importance, although the absence of the former is considered a pathologic finding. Triple phosphate crystals in the fresh urine are a sign of urinary tract infection.

Other formed elements that may occur in the sediment are red cells, white cells, epithelial cells from the kidneys and urinary tract, as well as various types of casts. The latter in particular, underscore the presence of renal disease. Most chronic forms of renal damage are distinguished by unremarkable urinary findings, however. Large amounts of epithelial cells and triple phosphate are indicative of cystitis and pyelitis. Isolated epithelial and white blood cells may also be found in normal animals.

1.1.2.3. Cerebrospinal Fluid

Examination of the cerebrospinal fluid (CSF) is useful in the diagnosis or differential diagnosis of central nervous disorders. The fluid is collected by cisternal puncture in the anesthetized horse or lumbosacral puncture in the standing sedate horse. After successful puncture, the CSF escapes in drops or in a thin stream; about 40 to 100 ml can be collected. The CSF pressure in the normal horse is 270—490 mm H_2O. It is markedly elevated in chronic internal hydrocephalus.

The normal CSF is clear and colorless, like water, and has the following characteristics:

Cell content	0/3—8/3 per microliter
Cell differentiation	lymphocytic, up to 20% neutrophils
Protein content	0.29—0.72 g/l (29—72 mg/100 ml)
Albumin	0.27—0.68 g/l (27—68 mg/100 ml)
Globulin	0.02—0.25 g/l (2—25 mg/ml)
Pandy reaction	—/+
Nonne-Apelt reaction	—/+
Glucose	2.22—4.33 mmol/l (40—78 mg/100 ml)

Abnormal values are most commonly seen in Borna disease (which is seldom observed in the United States). Usually a slight to moderate xanthochromia is apparent at the time of collection. The qualitative protein reactions are positive, and the total protein content is markedly increased. There is a moderate pleocytosis (20—200/3 cells) which is almost entirely lymphocytic.

In cases of purulent meningitis, the cell content is greatly increased (200—1000/3 cells), often causing clouding of the fluid. In the various hepatic encephalopathies, which are important in terms of differential diagnosis, the CSF examination often shows no abnormalities.

1.1.2.4. Peritoneal Fluid

Abdominal paracentesis with subsequent examination of the peritoneal fluid has attained much diagnostic and prognostic importance in the various forms of equine colic. It is done if abnormal fluid in the abdominal cavity is suspected.

The fluid is drawn with the animal standing. The recommended site is on the midline between the sternum and umbilicus, about a hand's width caudal to the xiphoid process. Some authors recommend puncture somewhat left of the linea alba. The risk of bowel perforation is usually low but may be higher in cases of gaseous distention of the bowel. In cases of bowel distension and depressed peristalsis, paracentesis may be contraindicated. This also applies to mares in late pregnancy.

The volume of fluid obtained can vary greatly. Usually only 2—3 ml of a clear, pale-yellow to amber-colored fluid is collected.

The sample should be examined grossly, noting its color and transparency. It is further useful to centrifuge the fluid and examine the sediment. Small amounts are collected at once on a glass slide.

A layering of cells can be observed in the sediment. There is often an erythrocyte layer at the top, below which are further cellular elements that are gray in color. Food particles, if present, are found at the bottom. Microscopic examination can provide further clarification.

The presence of blood in the fluid is easily recognized, provided the lumen of the needle is not blocked. In cases where there has been rupture of an organ (liver, spleen) or arterial aneurysm, death from intra-abdominal hemorrhage can occur rapidly. Blunt abdominal trauma or prior castration can lead to similar results. Paracentesis findings should always be interpreted within the context of the clinical picture.

Blood-tinged transudate is yellow-red in color. It is commonly associated with displacements and incarceration of bowel. The volume of fluid collected varies with the degree and extent of strangulation and the amount of necrotic bowel, as does the thickness of the erythrocyte and leukocyte layer following centrifugation. In thromboembolic colic, the fluid is also blood-tinged and highly turbid.

Gastric or intestinal contents mixed with blood indicate bowel rupture. Intestinal contents withdrawn inadvertently by puncture of the bowel are usually not mixed with blood unless a hemorrhagic enteritis is present. In bowel rupture, the fluid has a 'dirty' appearance, is gray-red or green in color, and is usually voluminous. Food particles can usually be recognized. More detailed information is provided by the sediment. Microscopic examination can usually distinguish between gastric and intestinal contents, because undigested starch granules and micrococci occur only in the stomach. In rare cases the contents of a ruptured stomach may become trapped in the omentum, resulting in a negative abdominal paracentesis.

Exudates signify peritonitis but may also be associated with neoplastic diseases. The fluid is highly turbid and is yellow-gray to green in color. It contains abundant sediment that consists mainly of leukocytes and epithelial cells. Its density is high (above 1.018). The protein content is well above 2.5 g/100 ml. If it exceeds 4.0 to 4.5 g/100 ml and if the gamma-globulin content is above 3.0 g/100 ml, the sample will give a clearly positive Rivalta test, making it still easier to distinguish the fluid from transudate (the latter test is seldom used in the United States).

In ascites, copious amounts of transudate escape from the peritoneal cavity on paracentesis. The fluid is light and clear, contains very few cells, and has a low density.

References

Blackmore, D. J.; Kent, J. E.: Serum enzyme and protein concentration in English shire horses. Vet. Rec. *100:* 91 (1977).

Bokori, J.; Csek, J.; Tölgyesi, G.: Über die Intraabdominalflüssigkeit des Pferdes und den diagnostischen Wert der mit ihr vorgenommenen Rivaltaschen Probe. Acta vet. hung. *10:* 431 (1960).

Bokori, J.; Tölgyesi, G.: Über die Untersuchung der pathologischen Körperhöhlenflüssigkeiten von Haustieren. Acta vet. hung. *11:* 79 (1961).

CHRISTOPH, H.-J.; MEYER, H.: Klinisches Laboratorium (S. Hirzel Verlag, Leipzig 1971).

DANIELS, HEDWIG: Die Bauchhöhlenpunktion beim Pferd — Technik und Interpretation. Prakt. Tierarzt *59:* 268 (1978).

Deutsche Veterinärmedizinische Gesellschaft: Arbeitswerte in der Laboratoriumsdiagnostik. Kalender für tierärztliche Praxis 1977, Beilage zu Tierärztl. Praxis *4* (1976).

GERBER, H.: Enzymdiagnostik bei inneren Krankheiten des Pferdes. Zbl. Vet.-Med. R. A *11:* 135 (1964).

GERBER, H.; MARTIG, J.; STRAUB, R.: Enzymuntersuchungen im Serum von Großtieren im Hinblick auf Diagnose und Prognose. Tierärztl. Praxis *1:* 5 (1973).

GLASENAPP, H. v.: Über die Brauchbarkeit der Aktivitätsbestimmung spezifischer Serumenzyme für die Diagnostik von muskelbedingten Bewegungsstörungen bei Pferden — insbesondere bei Trabrennpferden. Vet.-med. Diss., Berlin (West) 1972.

HEJLASZ, Z.: Rownowaga kwasowo-zasadowa jako wykladnik wydolnosci oddechowej u koni z pecherzykowa rozedma pluc. Med. weterin. (Warszawa) *32:* 108 (1976).

HIEPE, TH.: Die Bornasche Krankheit. Wiss. Zschr. Karl-Marx-Univ. Leipzig, Math.-nat. R. *8:* 263 (1958).

KOMAREK, J.; STROS, K.; SYKORA, J.; KYNCLOVA, J.; JADRNY, L.; SELINGER, P.: Hodnoty acidobazicke rovnovahy krve nekterych druhu domacich zvirat. Vet. Med. (Praha) *21 (49):* 51 (1976).

KUDRJAVCEV, A. A.; KUDRJAVCEVA, L. A.; PRIVOL'NEV, T. I.: Gematologija životnych i ryb. (Izdat. Kolos, Moskva 1969).

LIPPMANN, R.: Vorkommen und Nachweis von Bilirubin im Liquor cerebrospinalis bei Pferd, Schaf und Rind. Arch. exp. Vet.-Med. *23:* 279 (1969).

LIPPMANN, R.: Kolloidreaktionen im Liquor cerebrospinalis des Pferdes. Acta vet. hung. *19:* 229 (1969).

MEMEDEJKIN, V. G.: Koncentracija močeviny v krovi u lošadej v zavisimosti ot razlicnych faktorov. Naučni tr. VNII konevodstva *25:* 183 (1971).

NIKOV, S.: Vyrchu normalnata kryvna kartina pri našite kone. Naučni tr. Vet.-med. Inst. ,,Prof. Dr. G. Pavlov" Sofia *9:* 115 (1961).

NIKOV, S.; GABRASCHANSKI, P.: Propedevtika na vytrešnite bolesti na domašnite zivotni (Zemizdat, Sofija 1977).

PINKIEWICZ, E.: Podstawowe badania laboratoryjne w chorobach zwierzat. Panstwowe wydawnictwo rolnicze i leśne, Warszawa 1971.

SCHMIDL, M.: Laboruntersuchungen für die Diagnose und Verlaufskontrolle. Boehringer Mannheim GmbH, 1978.

SCHOTMAN, A. J. H.; WAGENAAR, G.: Hyperlipemia in ponies. Zbl. Vet.-Med. R. A. *16:* 1 (1969).

SEDLAK, TH.: Erythrozytäre Messwerte beim Pferd unter Berücksichtigung des Alters, der Rasse und des Geschlechts. Vet.-med. Diss., Leipzig (1972).

SOMMER, H.; BEST, J.; GÖRNER, M.: Untersuchungen über die Aktivität von Enzymen im Blutserum bei Galoppern unter besonderer Berücksichtigung ihrer Rennleistung. Berliner Münchner Tierärztl. Wschr. *91:* 433 (1978).

STRAUB, R.; PETITJEAN, J.; TSCHUDI, P.: Serumlipide und -lipoproteide bei gesunden Equiden. Schweiz. Arch. Tierheilk. *119:* 93 (1977).

ZAJCEV, V. J.; SINEV, A. V.; JONOV, P. S.; VASIL'EV, A. V.; ŠARABRIN, I. G.: Kliničeskaja diagnostika vnutrennich boleznej selsko-chozjajstvennych životnych. 3rd ed. (Izdat. Kolos, Moskva 1971).

1.1.2.5. Synovial Fluid

The fluid from a diseased synovial space (joint, tendon sheath, bursa) reflects the changes occurring in that space in a highly specific manner. Such changes enable us to make a diagnosis and prognosis from the synovial fluid sample and thereby effectively supplement clinical and radiographic examination. Synovial fluid is readily obtained during intrasynovial anesthesia and therapy, thus requiring no additional traumatization of the synovial space. Owing to the dynamics of inflammation, the values obtained are strongly dependent on the stage and severity of the synovitis, and the examination of the fluid represents its condition at one point in time.

The often small volume of fluid present in certain synovial spaces limits the number of examinations that can be made. This makes it necessary to follow a sequence: (1) Gross examination such as overall appearance, turbidity and visual estimation of viscosity; (2) cell count; (3) differential cell count. These values are most useful to the clinician and results are obtainable within a short time thereby markedly influencing treatment. An assessment of clotting ability and a bacteriologic examination are also done if possible. All further tests, such as enzyme determination, provide additional useful information and are indicated in certain situations.

Appearance. Normal synovial fluid is yellow to colorless and contains no grossly visable particulate matter. The presence of red streaks indicates fresh intrasynovial bleeding caused by the tap, while a homogenous red tinge signifies a prior trauma to the synovial space associated with a contusion, intra-articular fracture, etc. A dark-yellow to pale-brown color is caused by free bilirubin from the breakdowns of erythrocytes and indicates that a more chronic injury to the synovial space has occurred. Pyogenic synovitis is characterized by a gray-white to yellow exudate. When the synovial fluid loses its viscosity in cases of sepsis, the exudate is commonly reddish brown.

Turbidity. Normal synovial fluid is clear. Turbidity occurs when there is an increase in colloidal and formed substances. An erythrocyte count up to 2,500/mm^3 after traumatization of the synovial space does not alter clarity. Counts up to 10,000/mm^3 cause slight turbidity, and counts over 10,000/mm^3 produce heavier turbidity. The increase in white blood cells in response to inflammation causes a very slight clouding in subacute aseptic synovitis. This clouding increases in the acute and peracute synovitis forms and eventually becomes quite marked in purulent and putrid synovitis. The presence of flakes signifies a serofibrinous inflammation. In chronic aseptic synovitis the fluid may be clear, slightly turbid or turbid.

Viscosity. The viscosity of the normal synovial fluid varies. This applies to all types of synovial spaces regardless of their anatomy. The values stated in the literature often cannot be compared due to variations of analytical method. Generally speaking the average relative viscosity is inversely proportional to the size of the joint and the average volume of synovial fluid. Thus, for example, the hock joint contains about 10 ml of synovial fluid with a relative viscosity of 4.43, while the fetlock joint contains about 4.5 ml with a relative viscosity of 46.68 [van Pelt, 1962].

The viscosity of the synovial fluid is a reflection of its hyaluronic acid content. The viscosity also serves as a measure of quantity, quality and degree of polymerization of hyaluronic acid. All three factors can change in diseases of the synovial space. To date, no objective data on pathologic equine synovial fluid have been obtained with the aid of viscosimeters. The clinician makes a gross assessment of the viscosity by rubbing the fluid between two fingers or by the length of the thread formed by a falling drop of synovial fluid. Fluid from hygromas usually shows a markedly decreased viscosity and may even have a watery consistency. In acute synovitis the viscosity varies. Viscosity is generally increased in chronic arthritis deformans.

Cytologic Examination. Normal synovial fluid contains *no erythrocytes*. Their presence is generally the result of a traumatic tap, even in pathologic specimens. In these cases the fluid has a blood-streaked appearance.

Nucleated cells in the form of synoviocytes and neutrophilic granulocytes occur in a specific number and specific ratio to each other in the fluid of normal as well as diseased synovial spaces.

The quantitative cell determination is performed using a hemacytometer or a Coulter counter. For extremely high cell counts the sample can be diluted.

The qualitative cell determination is done using Wrights or Wright-Giemsa stains or any Romanowski type of stain.

The average nucleated cell count and percentage of neutrophilic granulocytes are indicated below for fluid from normal and diseased synovial spaces:

	Nucleated cells/mm³ (mean value)	% Neutrophilic granulocytes (mean value)
1. Normal synovial spaces:		
Small joints	209.8	5.3
Large joints	301.9	5.9
Tendon sheaths	189.5	2.3
2. Hygromas have the lowest cell count and highest percentage of neutrophilis granulocytes:		
Small joints	241.2	2.0
Large joints	296.0	1.4
Tendon sheaths	181.1	2.6
Bursae	81.7	1.0
3. The cell counts in joints with chronic arthritis deformans and periarthritis correspond to those in hygromas: 199.4 and 152.9, respectively. The average percentage of neutrophilic granulocytes is higher, however, with respective values of 6 and 3.		
4. In chronic aseptic serous synovitis both the cell count and % neutrophilic granulocytes are markedly increased in the synovial fluid:		
Small joints	649.4	9.1
Large joints	1,023.5	12.7
Tendon sheaths	957.4	10.3
Bursae	670.7	7.7
5. In acute aseptic serous synovitis there is a further increase in both values:		
Small joints	1,179.0	11.5
Large joints	4,035.1	30.4
Tendon sheaths	17,683.0	63.3
6. The highest values occur in septic or purulent synovitis:		
Small joints	118,195.0	82.3
Large joints	45,134.0	73.4
Tendon sheaths	161,553.7	84.2
Bursae	105,158.6	83.7

The cell count and percentage of neutrophils are considerably lower in the stage of pyogenic synovitis and higher in purulent panarthritis.

Clotting Ability. Normal synovial fluid does not clot. The selective permeability of the synovial membrane prevents the passage of all clot-promoting substances. Occasionally the fluid becomes viscid, but it regains its normal consistency on shaking. The fluid from hygromas rarely clots. In chronic aseptic serous synovitis the fluid either fails to clot or does so after 48 h; in chronic deforming arthritis it clots in 15 to 125 minutes; in acute aseptic and purulent synovitis it clots within an hour.

Bacteriologic Examination. In suspected joint infections the synovial fluid should be subjected to a bacteriologic examination if the volume of fluid obtained permits. In suppurative arthritis, only about 20% of the specimens will show a positive result on routine microbiologic examination. Despite the presence of infection, the various causative organisms often cannot be demonstrated in the synovial fluid even after a short period of time. The few positive findings in spontaneous joint infections are commonly streptococci, making the choice of a suitable antibiotic for intraarticular or parenteral administration relatively simple.

Protein Content. The total protein content of normal synovial fluid is relatively low: 0.5—1.9 g/dl, with a mean value of 1.1 g/dl. It is determined by the biuret method. The albumin fraction accounts for 42.9% of the total protein and is thus higher than in the serum (37.0%); the albumin: globulin ratio is 1.108 in the synovial fluid compared to 0.754 in the serum. The average globulin values are as follows: α-globulin 14.9%; β-globulin 24.1%; γ-globulin 18.1%.

Thus, the α- and γ-globulin content of the synovial fluid is lower than that of the serum. The protein fractions are determined by electrophoretic methods.

Diseases of the synovial spaces lead to changes in the total protein content of the synovial fluid and its fractions:

Serous, aseptic arthritis:	Total protein 1.0—4.8 g/dl Mean value 2.9 g/dl
Arthritis deformans:	Total protein 2.0—5.1 g/dl Mean value 3.2 g/dl
Septic, infectious arthritis:	Total protein 3.3—6.6 g/dl Mean value 4.8 g/dl

In the first two types of arthritis there is no significant shift of the *protein fractions*, whereas in septic arthritis there is a fall of albumin and an increase of globulin.

Glucose. Normally the serum and synovial fluid glucose levels are approximately equal in the horse. Both levels are determined simultaneously in order to provide a useful, individualized reference quantity for the synovial fluid glucose level in the diseased joint.

The normal synovial fluid values are 5.08 to 5.75 mmol/l with an average of 5.41 ± 0.22 mmol/l. The corresponding serum glucose values range from 4.52 to 5.48 mmol/l.

In degenerative joint diseases the synovial fluid glucose is 1.55 mmol/l *higher* on the average than the serum level. In all the other joint diseases mentioned, the synovial fluid glucose is below that of the serum by the following values (in mmol/l):

Hydrarthrosis	0.0555
Suppurative arthritis with no demonstrable organism	1.39
Infectious arthritis with demonstrable organism	1.94

[VAN PELT, 1962, 1974].

Hyaluronic Acid. The quantity and degree of polymerization of the hyaluronic acid determines the viscosity of the synovial fluid. In synovitis both factors are subject to characteristic changes. The hyaluronic acid content can be determined indirectly by determination of the glycosaminoglycan (GAG) level [SUNDBLAD, 1953]. For purposes of clinical diagnosis, the mucin clot test of VAN PELT [1962] is more practical. The reaction is divided into four grades:

1. compact flake in a clear solution;
2. soft mass in a turbid, pale yellow or pale brown solution;
3. small, crumbly masses in a solution of grade-2 turbidity;
4. several clumps in a very turbid, pale yellow to dark brown solution.

The precipitate contains the hyaluronic acid and about 75% of the protein in a normal sample.

The quality of the mucin precipitate (MPQ) is usually normal (= grade 1 or 2) in degenerative joint diseases, osteochondritis dissecans, osteochondromatosis, chronic traumatic arthritis and in hygromas of the tarsal joint. In hygromas, however, the size of the precipitate is smaller due to the smaller amount of hyaluronic acid. In suppurative and infectious arthritis the MPQ corresponds to grades 3 and 4.

Enzyme Activities. In diseases of synovial structures, enzyme levels in the synovial fluid are altered as a result of (a) permeability changes in the synovial membrane and (b) tissue destruction, allowing the entry of these enzymes into the synovial fluid. Their quantitative demonstration can be useful diagnostically. Enzymes include lactate dehydrogenase (LDH), alkaline phosphatase (AP) and glutamic oxaloacetic transaminase (GOT), (aspartate aminotransferase). The importance of enzyme analysis lies in the possible differentiation of various forms of arthritis. Blood-tinged synovial fluid samples are unsuitable for enzyme analysis.

Lactate Dehydrogenase (LDH). Colorimetric studies indicate the following mean values (in Berger-Broida units):

Normal joints	108
Hydrarthrosis	100
Degenerative arthritis (arthrosis)	211
Suppurative arthritis	262
Infectious arthritis with demonstrable organism	1197

[VAN PELT, 1974]

The values are broken down as follows with the aid of agar gel electrophoresis (in U/l):

Normal joints	88	
Serous arthritis	292	
Osteochondrosis dissecans	291	(with simultaneous elevation of the isoenzyme LDH_5)
Arthrosis	739	(with simultaneous elevation of the isoenzyme $LDH_{4/5}$)

[REJNO, 1976].

Alkaline Phosphatase (AP). The alkaline phosphatase activity in synovial fluid is identical to that of the cartilage. As with lactate dehydrogenase, the activity is increased in joint lesions that are accompanied by cartilage destruction and allow release of the enzyme into the synovial fluid. The mean values are as follows (in Sigma units/ml):

Normal joints	1.02
Hydrarthrosis	1.24
Degenerative joint disease	1.35
Suppurative arthritis without demonstrable organism	2.72
Infectious arthritis with demonstrable organism	23.20

Glutamic Oxaloacetic Transaminase (GOT, Aspartate Aminotransferase). The measurement of this enzyme activity is also a useful diagnostic aid according to VAN PELT [1974]. The values are as follows (in Sigma Frankel units/ml):

Normal joint	53
Hydrarthrosis	50
Degenerative joint disease	70
Suppurative arthritis without demonstrable organism	128
Infectious arthritis with demonstrable organism	118

References

CABAUD, P. A.; WRÖBLEWSKI, F.: Colorimetric measurement of lactic dehydrogenase activity of body fluids. Amer. J. Clin. Pathol. *30:* 234 (1958).

DABICH, D.; NEUHAUS, O. W.: Proc. Soc. Exp. Biol. Med. *123:* 584 (1966); cit. PANNDORF, H.; GRÜN, E. (1978).

EISENMENGER, E.: Gelenkpunktionen für Diagnostik und Therapie. Tierärztl. Praxis *2:* 401 (1974).

FOLIN, O.: Two revised copper methods for blood sugar determination. J. Biol. Chem. *82:* 83 (1929).

FOLIN, O.; WU, H.: A system of blood analysis. A simplified and improved method for determination of sugar. J. Biol. Chem. *41:* 367 (1920).

GÄNGEL, H.: Diagnostische Aspekte der Synoviazytologie bei Pferd und Rind. Arch. exp. Vet.-Med. *25:* 65 (1971).

KERSJES, A. W.: Over synovia en synovitis. Vet.-med. Diss., Utrecht (1963).

LANGE, W.: Zur klinischen Verwertbarkeit zytologischer Synoviauntersuchungen beim Rind. Arch. exp. Vet.-Med. *15:* 993 (1961).

MATRENIN, A. N.: O metodach podstachota eritrozitow i lejkozitow pri issledowanii krowi selskochosjajstwennych shiwotnych. Trudy Burjat — Mongolskogo Zoo — Veterinarnowo Instituta (russ.) *7:* 100 (1951); cit. LANGE, W. (1961).

MICHELETTO, B.: Annali Fac. Med. vet. Torino *101:* 541 (1957); cit. PERSSON (1971).

PANNDORF, H.; GRÜN, E.: Zum Verhalten einiger Enzymaktivitäten in der Synovia erkrankter Gelenke und Sehnenscheiden des Pferdes. Mh. Vet.-Med. *12:* 449 (1978).

PELT, R. W. VAN: Properties of equine synovial fluid. J. Amer. Vet. Med. Assoc. *141:* 1051 (1962).

PELT, R. W. VAN: Interpretation of synovial fluid findings in the horse. J. Amer. Vet. Med. Assoc. *165:* 91 (1974).

PERSSON, L.: On the synovia in horses. Acta vet. scand., Suppl. *12:* 35 (1971).

REJNO, S.: LDH and LDH isoenzymes of synovial fluid in the horse. Acta vet. scand. *17:* 178 (1976).

SEYFARTH, H.: Gelenkergüsse und Gelenkresorption (Johann Ambrosius Barth, Leipzig 1956).

SUNDBLAD, L.: Studies on hyaluronic acid in synovial fluids. Acta Soc. Med. Upsal. *58:* 3, 113 (1953).

1.1.2.6. Feces

Macroscopic Examination. The sample is grossly examined for the presence of adult ascarids, strongyles, oxyurids and tapeworm segments. Technique: If no parasites are visible on the surface of the fecal sample, specimens are taken from various sires, liquefied with water and strained through a sieve. The sieved material is then examined macroscopically.

Microscopic Examination (fig. 1.1. — 7). *Flotation method:* For the demonstration of nematode and cestode eggs. Principle: The parasitic structures rise to the surface of a solution of higher specific gravity. Technique: A certain quantity of feces (e.g., 10 g) is ground in a mortar or glass beaker, flotation solution is added (generally saturated saline solution, density 1.18), and the mixture is strained through a sieve (250—300 μm mesh) into a beaker (150—200 ml). Then enough flotation solution is added through the sieve to fill the beaker 3/4 full. The liquid is allowed to stand for 20 min. Then, with a right-angled wire loop (5 mm diameter), 5 drops are collected from the surface of the liquid column (1 from the center, 4 from the zone between the edge and center) and mounted on a glass slide for microscopic examination.

Sedimentation method: For the demonstration of trematode eggs and Eimeria oocysts. Principle: The parasitic structures sink in water owing to their higher specific gravity. Technique: A certain quantity of feces (10 g) is mixed with tapwater and strained through a sieve into a beaker (150—200 ml). The beaker is filled close to

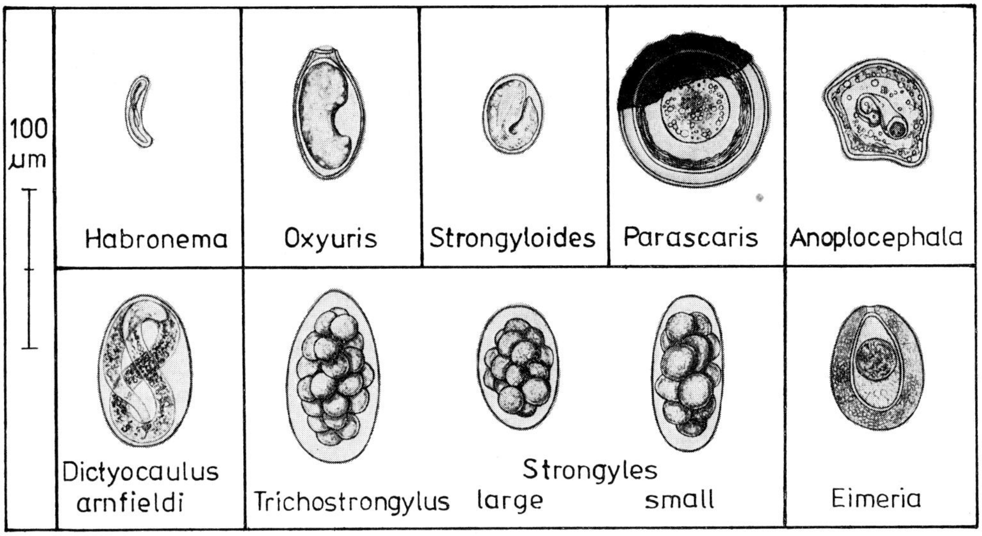

Fig. 1.1. — 7. Helminth eggs and coccidian oocysts demonstrable in the stool.

the top with water and allowed to stand for 2 min. Then the water with the suspended fecal particles is decanted from the sediment and the beaker refilled with water. This is done 3 times. The sediment is transferred to a flat Petri dish and examined microscopically.

Migration method: For the demonstration of lungworm larvae (at least 7 h after collection) and other nematode larvae from 'old' fecal specimens, e.g., Strongyloides and strongyle larvae. Principle: Worm larvae migrate from the stool into the water; unable to swim, they sink to the bottom. Technique: A certain quantity of feces (10 g) enclosed in a gauze bag is introduced into a funnel glass filled with lukewarm water such that about half the fecal sample is immersed. The sample is allowed to stand for at least 8 h. Then about 2 ml of liquid is collected from the bottom of the funnel with a pipette and examined microscopically in a small dish.

1.1.3. Radiographic Examination

1.1.3.1. Radiographic Technique

1.1.3.1.1. Apparatus

One of the most difficult tasks for the equine practitioner is the selection of a suitable x-ray machine. A great variety of machines are available, but many are developed for human medicine and have certain deficiencies when applied to animals. No machine is ideal, and a unit must be selected that conforms most closely to the demands of equine radiography.

There are several basic requirements that all x-ray machines must satisfy:

1. The output of the machine must be adequate for the intended range of application. In animals, it is essential that the exposure time be kept to an absolute mini-

mum in order to prevent motion. The exposure time is a function of the tube current (mA). The machine may have an output from 10 to 1,000 mA, depending on its design. The quantity of the radiation is directly dependent on the exposure time and the tube current. The product of exposure time and tube current, expressed in milliampere seconds (mAs), is an accurate measure of the degree of exposure of a radiograph. This means that the higher the output of the machine in mA, the shorter the exposure times can be.

The output that is adequate for a particular case depends on the type of object to be radiographed, i.e., whether the digits are to be examined or more proximal thicker parts as well. An x-ray machine for equine practice should have a minimum output of 40 mA.

The quality of the radiation (kilovoltage) is adequate in all modern x-ray machines. Even small units have means for adjusting the kilovoltage between 50 and 90 kV. This range is entirely adequate for diagnostic purposes.

2. The x-ray tube and housing must be freely mobile. In particular, it must be possible to lower the tube close to the floor so that foot films can be made in the standing horse. The upper limit of tube mobility depends if head films are to be taken.

3. The cost of the machine must be within acceptable limits. The higher the output of the machine, the more complex its construction and the higher the cost. One must decide what requirements the unit must meet in order to strike a proper balance between economy and machine performance.

Additional features that are desirable include stability, as well as easy mobility to allow response to sudden movements by the horse. The machine should also be quiet so it will not startle a nervous animal. A unit intended for field use must be easy to load and unload or dismantle and must be of a sturdy construction.

Every x-ray machine must have adequate radiation safety features. Besides the tube shielding, devices which confine the primary beam to the object (diaphragms, cylinders) and project a light beam showing the exact configuration of the selected field, should be included.

1.1.3.1.2. Accessory Equipment

As important as the selection of the x-ray machine itself is the availability of adequate accessory equipment.

Intensifying Screens. A considerable amount of x-ray exposure is needed to form an image on a film. While such films have a very high intrinsic definition, they are often unsharp due to the length of time needed to expose the film. Films can be exposed more quickly by visible light (low-energy electromagnetic wave radiation). In radiography this light is derived from fluorescence, the ability of certain crystalline salts (called phosphors) to emit light when excited by x-rays. Intensifying screens consist of a thin layer of phosphor applied to a radiolucent base. The screens are inserted into the front and back of the x-ray cassette. When the cassette is closed, the screens come in contact with the x-ray film, which has photosensitive emulsion on both sides. On irradiation, the screens fluoresce and expose both sides of the film. Calcium tungstate has been used as a phosphor since the early days of radiography. In recent years new screens have been introduced which contain rare earths such as lanthanum or gadolinium oxysulfide as phosphors. These screens have a higher light output than calcium tungstate screens.

Table 1.1. — 12. Intensification factors for conventional screen types

Screen type	Intensification factor compared to nonscreen film	Phosphor
Detail	10	$CaWo_4$
Par	20	$CaWo_4$
High-speed	40	$CaWo_4$
Rare earth	40—60	Rare earths

The intensification factors for the conventional screen types are given in table 1.1. — 12.

As a general rule, screens with higher intensification factors accentuate any technical unsharpness that may be present.

When intensifying screens are used, the exposure time can be reduced by a factor of up to 1/50 compared to nonscreen film. This is particularly advantageous in the case of relatively low-output x-ray machines, where the exposure times can be sufficiently reduced to eliminate motion.

Intensifying screens must be handled with care. Scratches or spots on the screens lead to a loss of light output at that site, leading to local image flaws (artifacts).

Grids. In every x-ray film a portion of the radiation is absorbed, a portion passes straight through the object, and a portion is deflected or 'scattered'. This scatter radiation is a source of blurring. The thicker the object and the stronger the radiation (high kV), the greater the amount of scatter radiation, and the less sharp the final radiograph. This radiation can be largely eliminated by placing grids between the object and the film. Grids consist of a parallel series of thin lead strips embedded in plastic which are oriented at right angles to the path of the primary beam. All x-rays that do not travel in the direction of the primary radiation are absorbed by the lead strips.

Since the scatter radiation also contributes to the total exposure of the film, the exposure time must be *increased* by a factor of 2 to 3 when a grid is used. This limits the use of grids, especially with small x-ray machines, since in some cases, exposure times may be so prolonged that motion becomes a problem.

Opinions vary as to the types of radiograph for which a grid should be used. In some clinics, films of the fetlock joint are made with grids, while elsewhere grids are not used, even for films of the stifle joint. Their use in a given case will depend essentially on the overall equipment. In any event, they are a necessary adjunct for x-ray studies of thick objects with much soft tissue.

Filming Aids, Cassette Holders. Only a few aids are needed for making radiographs of the limbs in equine practice, but they are indispensable.

Films of the digits require positioning blocks of various sizes on which the foot can be rested. If the horse stands directly on the floor, the coffin and pastern joints become distorted, since the central beam cannot be directed exactly horizontally that close to the floor. Blocks of varying thickness may be used, depending upon whether the limb is to be radiographed in a stressed or unstressed position.

For radiographs of the distal (3rd) phalanx and distal sesamoid (navicular) bone in the AP projection, special blocks are used. These place the anterior hoof wall in a vertical position, providing a better overview of the entire distal phalanx. In this position the distal sesamoid or navicular bone is also projected for its full width over the middle (2nd) phalanx and is therefore more easily identified (see also p. 54).

Since most radiographs of the limbs are made in the standing horse, it is imperative for safety reasons that cassette holders be used. The cassette should be held directly in the lead-gloved hand only in exceptional cases. As a general rule, it must be held by means of an extension device to ensure that the assistant holding the cassette will remain clear of the primary beam and will remain an adequate distance from the scattering object. This will also reduce the danger of the assistant being kicked by a fractious patient.

The design of the cassette holder is limited only by the ingenuity the veterinarian. Care should be taken, however, not to make the apparatus too heavy or complex. It is often sufficient to clamp the cassette in a simple frame which itself is attached to a bent rod made of lightweight aluminium.

Film Identification. Accurate marking of all radiographs is essential. The marking must identify the animal to which the film belongs, as well as the particular object that is visualized. The latter is particularly important when many films are taken so there will be no confusion between right, left, thoracic and pelvic limbs.

All markings should be affixed directly to the film itself in an unmistakable, tamper-proof fashion. There are various means of marking patient data; the simplest is to write the information on the developed and dried film. This is not recommended. The chance of a mixup is too great. It is far better to use markings that are projected onto the film at the time of exposure, such as lead letters or lead-containing screens that are attached to the cassette during the exposure. These procedures are mandatory for films made outside the office or clinic that are developed later in a darkroom. Of course, all markings should be kept to a minimum so as not to mask portions of the image. In some cases it is sufficient to mark the film with a serial number which corresponds to a more detailed entry in a log-book. For films that are developed at once, it is possible to mask a narrow strip of the screen in the cassette to keep that portion of the film from being exposed. Then, in the darkroom, a device can be used to print the desired patient data onto the unexposed strip of film.

Marking of the limb must be done during the initial exposure. This is best accomplished with lead letters or letter combinations which briefly identify both the limb and the projection.

1.1.3.1.3. Preparation of the Horse

The main purpose behind preparation of the horse for radiographs is to eliminate external objects that could cause artifactual shadows on the radiograph. This means that any shoes, plates, halters, snaffles, bandages and dressings should be removed, if at all possible. If this is not possible, such as the radiographic examination of a fracture beneath a cast or dressing, this additional material must be taken into account when setting the exposure.

Equally important, but easily overlooked, is debris on the skin in the form of sand, dirt, liniments or medications. A number of externally applied medications are strong x-ray absorbers, and even wet hair left by washing can make a distinct shadow. Highly absorptive medications may even mask the object and render it invisible. Less absorptive medications can be an even greater problem. They can make shadows (densities) on the developed film that mimic periostitis, or conversely, a periostitis may be overlooked because it is taken for a shadow caused by such medications. Meticulous cleansing of the patient is therefore essential if the examiner is to be able to recognize and interpret subtle changes on the radiograph.

1.1.3.1.4. Radiation Protection

Protection in the radiographic examination of animals is somewhat simpler than in human medicine, in that only the protection of the attending personnel need be considered. Protection of the patient, from a genetic standpoint, is usually ignored in domestic animals. Accordingly, national radiation protection standards pertain only to the safety of personnel.

Protection against exposure to ionizing radiation is regulated by law in all countries. The regulations may vary slightly from one country to the next, but all conform in essence to the recommendations of the ICRP (International Commission on Radiological Protection). Owing to the variations in legal standards, the regularions will not be discussed further here. Instead, the important general principles of radiation protection in the radiographic examination of horses will be focussed on.

Only essential personnel should be present during the examination. All other persons must leave the examination room or, in outdoor examinations, must stand far enough away to preclude exposure. Persons under 18 years of age and pregnant women should not take part in the examination under any circumstances.

The examination itself must be conducted in such a way that personnel exposure is minimized. With proper awareness of radiation safety, this should pose no difficulty. All rules are based upon simple principles. Personnel must keep out of the primary beam at all times, even if protective clothing is worn. Conventional lead-lined clothing is designed only for scatter radiation, not for primary radiation. This clothing must be worn by all persons who are assisting.

The precaution of leaving the room, as commonly practiced in human medicine, is generally impractical in veterinary medicine. In most cases it is necessary to maintain contact with the animal, which may not cooperate with the examiner and many times tends to resist the procedure. There are some clinics in which it is mandatory to leave the room during every radiographic examination. In some countries, this precautionary measure is a binding rule. This means that the animal must at least be sedated, if not anesthetized, for every examination. We feel that such precautions are exaggerated, considering the doses.

The examination should be conducted in a calm, unhurried manner. There is little point in quickly making a film that later is difficult to interpret because of poor technique or faulty projection. Every repeat examination means increased x-ray exposure for personnel. Another important safety measure is dose monitoring, which is prescribed by law in most countries. The measurement of a single increased dose should prompt a reappraisal of one's entire radiographic routine.

1.1.3.2. General Radiography

1.1.3.2.1. Epiphyseal Closure

The bones of vertebrates are not yet fully developed at birth. In some species only centers of ossification can be seen in some bones. In others, the epiphysis and diaphysis are ossified and separated only by an epiphyseal plate, also called the growth plate. Man and the dog, for example, belong to the former group, while the horse is representative of the latter. During the course of further growth, ossification progresses until epiphyseal closure occurs. Equine bones are largely ossified at birth, more so than in other animal species. In some bones an epiphyseal plate can no longer be

Table 1.1. — 13. Times of radiographic closure of various epiphyseal and apophyseal plates in the horse (months after birth)

Part		Adams	Schmidt	Myers/Emmerson
Forelimb	Scapula: distal	—	18	—
	proximal	9—12	—	27
	Humerus: distal	14—18	14	14—15
	proximal	15—18	14	14
	Radius: distal	24—30	24	24
	Ulna: proximal	24—30	18	27—30
	Metacarpus	9—12	6	7
	1st phalanx: proximal	6—9	6	8
	2nd phalanx: proximal	6—9	6	8
Hindlimb	Femur: distal	24—30	24	22
	proximal	30—36	—	36
	Tibia: distal	22—26	—	17
	Calcaneus	—	—	20
	1st phalanx: proximal	6—9	6	8
	2nd phalanx: proximal	6—9	6	8
	Metatarsus	9—12	6	7

The mean closure times were determined in horses of the following breeds:
Adams: Thoroughbreds, quarterhorse
Schmidt: various breeds
Myers/Emmerson: Arabians.

demonstrated radiographically at birth (e.g., 3rd phalanx, distal epiphyseal plate of 2nd phalanx, proximal epiphyseal plate of metatarsal and metacarpal bones).

Other epiphyseal plates are evident at the time of birth as non-ossified zones of varying width between the epiphysis and diaphysis. At this stage the bony components appear rounded at the plate; later they join even at the edges, and only a very fine line remains. Radiographically, the remodeling of the plate proceeds from the center. Shortly before final closure a small notch can still be seen at the margins.

On completion of radiographic closure, a zone of increased density is apparent at the site of the former epiphyseal plate. This can still be observed in later life. If epiphyses or apophyses (traction epiphyses) are visible in the radiographs of young horses, a film of the contralateral limb should be made for comparison. This can be a useful aid in recognizing lesions of the epiphysis. For every epiphysis there is a normal time of anatomic closure, which varies somewhat with breed and sex. It is important to know the time of epiphyseal closure in order to recognize any delays of closure or premature closure. The approximate times of epiphyseal closure in the horse are reviewed in table 1.1. — 13. These investivations were carried out in various equine breeds, and so the times may vary. All times indicated correspond to radiographic closure; anatomic and histologic closure occurs several months later.

1.1.3.2.2. Radiography of Degenerative Joint Disease (DJD)

Joint diseases are the most frequent indication for radiographic examinations in equine practice. Nevertheless, the quality of radiograph and subsequent evaluation are often less than satisfactory. This is often due to the highly varied radiographic manifestations of DJD. A diagnosis of DJD alone is of little use to the clinician, who requires information as to the duration and activity of the process. Radiography not only discloses the extent of the changes, but in some cases permits an understanding of the pathologic process; for example whether the DJD is primary or secondary. Secondary DJD can occur as a result of an intraarticular fracture. Primary DJD, on the other hand, is initiated by cartilage or synovial membrane changes. Nevertheless, it is often impossible to distinguish between primary or secondary DJD on either clinical or radiologic grounds. When we consider that primary DJD has its origin in disease of the cartilage or synovial membrane it becomes clear why the radiographic finding of DJD is usually a late diagnosis. Cartilaginous erosion and synovial membrane changes are invisible in the radiograph. Occasionally cartilage damage can be inferred from a narrowing of the joint space and changes in the joint position. Generally speaking, however, radiographic demonstration is successful only in the stage of DJD, when there is bony involvement. Radiographic diagnosis is further hampered by the fact that many cases of DJD have not produced external changes to the bones. Cartilage changes may be the only pathologic finding in such cases. Nevertheless, with sophisticated radiographic technics and accurate film interpretation, it is still possible to detect early radiographic changes. Weiss [1968] has made a systematic search for the radiographic signs of DJD and has succeeded in finding several that are indicative of the disease in its early stages.

Cartilage changes that determine the pathologic picture of incipient DJD are not demonstrable, since the uncalcified cartilage cannot be visualized radiographically. The area generally termed the 'joint space' in the radiograph is in reality the space occupied by the radiolucent cartilage of the bones that make up the joint. This space is bounded on both sides by calcifying cartilage and subchondral bone. If the cartilage loses elasticity, this bone-cartilage boundary is subjected to abnormally high stresses. In response, the calcified cartilage layer and bony boundary layer thicken. This process is evidenced radiographically by increased density (subchondral sclerosis).

An associated 'narrowing' of the joint space is frequently observed. It must be understood that this does not involve the loss of free space, but rather an erosion of the radiolucent cartilage (and thinning) coupled with a thickening in the subchondral region. This 'narrowing' of the visible joint space is of limited diagnostic value, however, because the width of the space varies with age. Moreover, the width can be assessed only if the central beam strikes the joint space at precisely a horizontal angle.

An important radiographic sign of the presence of DJD is subchondral remodeling including subchondral sclerosis. This remodeling may be a response to excessive stress on the bone and can in some circumstances lead to extensive deformity of the particular joint. Cystic changes in the subchondral area may also be visable radiographically. These are visible only after attaining a certain size. In time a bony margin forms around these cysts which is visible on the radiograph. Such cysts tend to be relatively small in the tarsal joint but can reach a considerable size in other joints. These lesions may be static or may enlarge under sustained functional loading. Complete or partial regression of the lesions is also known.

If such cystic changes are numerous, necrosis of the bone may result. Initially the necrotic bone cannot be distinguished from normal, healthy bone on radiograph. Because the mechanical quality of this bone is poor, defects at the bone-cartilage boundary soon result.

A similar picture develops if the articular cartilage is completely destroyed during the course of the disease, and ulcerations form on the bone itself. These changes are particularly evident in the distal joints of the tarsus. If bony ulceration or necrosis are present, there is almost always a severe lameness. Ankylosis of the distal tarsal joints is quite common in advanced stages of the DJD of the hock. If, with loss of cartilage, the underlying bony end plate is exposed, it becomes covered with pannus. If the opposing bony end plates are congruent, the fibrous tissue on both sides can bridge the joint space, and an internal ankylosis results. This union may be formed by bone or connective tissue. A fibrous ankylosis is difficult to demonstrate radiographically, while a bony ankylosis is easily recognized because the joint space will be obliterated in all projections. A common feature of DJD is spur formation or lipping at the joint margins. This is a most characteristic sign of DJD but need not always be present.

The changes that appear during the course of the disease are often dependent on the localization of the primary cartilage lesion. The first cartilage changes are often observed at the periphery of the joint. Benninghoff [1970] attributes this to the especially high tensile stresses that act on the peripherally located cartilage. The bone then reacts to any erosions or losses of substance that may occur, and these reactions produce the radiographic picture of spur formation. Spurs are most frequently observed on the outer bone margin. They develop from subchondral cancellous bone and are quickly covered with cartilage. Periosteal bone proliferation may also occur, however. Just as spurs form at the outer joint margins, spurs can form within the joint at the insertion sites of intra-articular ligaments.

An important component of the joint is the joint capsule, which, being a soft tissue, is not demonstrable by radiograph. One can only infer a thickening or distension of the capsule by fluid accumulation based on external contour. Pathologic conditions of the capsule may be accompanied by radiographic bone changes at the site where the fibrous capsule inserts on the periosteum. As the disease progresses a circumscribed osteoporosis may develop which can result in a circumscribed loss of bone. This is demonstrable as a more or less deep notch or depression on the radiograph. If the defects extend close to the cartilage-covered joint surface, spur formation will also occur in that area. The cartilage-covered joint surface is undermined, provoking subchondral ossification at the cartilage border. The marginal spur becomes especially prominent due to the underlying bony substance. These changes, too, become apparent only after a latent period.

The proliferation of fibrous tissue in the capsule can impair joint mobility, creating a fibrous ankylosis that may eventually ossify. It is important to note that inflammatory capsular lesions in the development of DJD are often accompanied by cartilage and bone formation in the joint capsule itself. If such cartilaginous bodies are formed in synovial villi, they may lose their pedicles and become free bodies or joint mice. Joint mice may also form by other mechanisms during the course of DJD. For example, cartilaginous fragments may detach in the area of circumscribed cartilage damage and then enter the joint cavity. Joint mice can also result from the avulsion of large osteophytes on the joint margins by the action of shearing forces. The best example of this is an avulsion at the extensor process of the distal phalanx. Such fragments are demonstrated radiographically if they are calcified or ossified. Then they make shadows of varying density, depending on their degree of calcification. If they become lodged between the joint surfaces, they can produce severe lameness as well as erosive or abrasive lesions.

In some circumstances free bodies or joint mice may be the only sign of DJD. It may then be impossible to distinguish DJD from OCD even by arthrotomy or radiography [Weiss, 1968].

1.1.3.2.3. Radiography of Bone Fractures and Fracture Healing

Radiographic examinations should not only demonstrate or exclude the presence of discontinuity of bone such as occurs in a fracture but demonstrate the number of fragments and the degree of their displacement. It may also be necessary to assess the quality of the bone (e.g., in osteoporosis, pathologic fractures) as well as the duration of the changes.

Fractures are always obvious on radiograph if the fragments are separated, the gap being filled by soft tissue, blood and serum. If there is no gap between the fragments, either because of impaction or close apposition of the fragments, the fracture line may be difficult to demonstrate radiographically. In the relatively dense bones of the horse, such fractures may be demonstrable only if the path of the central beam coincides precisely with that of the fracture line. In this case the radiograph will show an extremely fine line or perhaps only an irregularity of the adjacent cancellous bone. Sometimes a fresh fracture cannot be visualized at all.

A complete fracture is present if the discontinuity extends across the entire bone. In a fissure fracture, there is a hairline crack in the cortex that does not extend completely through the bone.

It is important, particularly from a prognostic standpoint, to ascertain the configuration of the fracture, i.e., whether it is transverse, oblique, comminuted, a Y-fracture, etc. Young animals may sustain epiphyseal injuries, the most common type being an epiphyseal separation in which part of the fracture line is in the epiphyseal plate and part is in the metaphysis (Type II Salter fracture).

Radiographs in two planes are mandatory in every fracture. An undisplaced fracture with few fragments is often demonstrable in one plane only. Moreover, the two-dimensional radiograph often fails to reflect the degree of displacement, which can be assessed only by viewing two films taken perpendicular to each other.

The demonstration of a fracture and the analysis of its configuration, to determine the method of treatment, are only part of the task of radiography in fracture management. Equally important is the monitoring of the healing process. To assess this correctly, a knowledge of the reparative processes of bone healing is imperative. Essentially bone healing takes place under the same conditions as other types of healing, i.e., the picture is one of an aseptic inflammatory process.

Bone healing, like that of the soft tissues, may be primary or secondary. For primary healing to occur, the bone ends must be held rigidly in perfect approximation throughout the healing period. This prevents the formation of a fracture gap into which vessels or other tissue elements can interpose. Osteons form 'cones' that grow directly into the opposing fracture surface during the course of healing. Thus, the fracture is bridged at once by bone, these processes occurring almost entirely within the cortex. Since the fracture site is bridged directly by bone with no callus formation, the fracture fragments undergo little or no resorption. The radiographs show only a transitory widening of the fracture defect followed by its gradual disappearance.

Because optimum fixation and rigid immobilization of the fracture fragments are difficult in adult horses with longbone fractures, primary bone healing is rarely achieved. Most fractures in the adult horse and even foals undergo secondary-type healing.

Secondary bone healing is characterized by the following stages:

1. Clotting of the hematoma formed at fracture.
2. Organization of the clot.
3. Formation of fibrous callus.
4. Formation of woven bone.

5. Replacement with lamellar bone.
6. Functional reconstruction, and remodelling.

Bone at the immediate edge of the fracture site is always damaged and becomes necrotic. Although the degree of necrosis may vary according to the configuration of the fracture and degree of trauma, it must be assumed that some bone will succumb to necrosis. These processes are accompanied by the necrosis of tissue debris in the fracture site. Osteoclasts and phagocytes are mobilized to absorb the dead bone and tissue debris. There is an overall widening of the fracture gap, and the fracture site becomes osteoporotic, because of the pronounced hyperemia in the fracture site.

Blood clot becomes infiltrated by fibroblasts and this granulation tissue develops into the fibrous callus which unites the bone ends. At the same time, collagen fibrils and hyaline ground substance are secreted between the ends of the fragments.

At sites subjected to mechanical loads, there is an early formation of woven bone in the fibrous callus. This forms a trabecular network whose orientation at this point bears no apparent relation to the lines of tension and compression. This woven bone may form between the bone ends or may form a rounded collar-like structure that spans the fracture site (periosteal callus). The periosteal callus approaches the fracture site beginning from the angles formed by the bone and the periosteum. The callus then unites with callus of the other side. This collar of woven bone is usually separated from the fracture by cartilaginous callus, which is gradually replaced with osseous callus. Finally the callus unites with the fracture margins to form a rigid bony meshwork. At this stage the woven bone is gradually converted to lamellar bone and the outer surface becomes remodeled by removal of excess bone. In the last stage of healing the callus adapts to mechanical loads, and a cuff of solid cortical bone is formed.

The various stages of fracture healing are well demonstrated radiographically. First a marked widening of the fracture defect is observed. Though present in every case, this phase may not always occur. This apparent widening of the fracture gap is particularly evident in fractures in which little or no primary defect can be recognized. In these fractures a widening of the defect by even a few millimeters will be more noticeable than in fractures with greater displacement.

In the horse, this widening is especially common in fissure fractures of the proximal phalanx (P1). The clinical diagnosis of fissure fracture of P1 cannot be confirmed radiographically until follow-up films are made at two or three weeks, by which time the defect will have widened. This widening of the fracture defect must not be confused with displacement resulting from inadequate immobilization. The widened fracture line is less sharply defined at this stage, and the adjacent bone appears less dense radiographically. Resorption is also evidenced by a rounding-off of fragments that were sharp at the time of injury.

A failure of resorption occurs in comminuted fractures in which some fragments have been separated from their blood supply. These fragments make a dense shadow for a longer period compared with other parts of the bone.

As bone healing progresses, the fracture defect gradually becomes less distinct. After about three weeks the first signs of a periosteal bridging callus can be seen on the periphery of the bone in underexposed films. This callus formation intensifies during the weeks that follow, becoming radiographically more distinct. As long as this tissue is active, it has a rough surface and a cloudy appearance.

When healing is virtually complete, i.e., the fragments are firmly united, the external callus becomes smoother and its structure becomes more dense and homogenous. The callus also decreases markedly in size. At this stage the fracture line itself can scarcely be discerned. In its place is a zone of dense bone. This bone does not yet have the structure of normal bone, but presents as a dense, unorganized mass. Only during the stage of functional adaptation, or remodeling, does this mass become less dense and more organized, although a zone of densification often persists in the area of the healed fracture.

Any movement between the fragments during healing seriously disrupts the repair process, especially the formation of the callus. More hyaline cartilage is formed in such cases, and the more hyaline cartilage is present, the longer the formation of lamellar bone is delayed. If movement in the fracture area is prolonged and excessive, a complete failure of bone formation can occur. Fracture healing is arrested in the fibrous callus stage leading to pseudarthrosis formation [Preiss, 1952].

Such a situation is frequently observed in horses with small metacarpal or metatarsal (splint) bone fractures that have not been treated surgically. A large callus may form, or a cartilaginous union may result, depending on the mobility of the fragments.

1.1.3.2.4. Contrast Studies

Radiographic examinations with the aid of contrast media are not as important in equine practice as in small-animal practice. This is due to the fact that the internal organs of the horse are poorly accessible to radiographic study owing to the animal's body mass. Nevertheless, there are some contrast studies that have been used clinically and can be performed, with some limitations, on an outpatient basis. These methods will be described or simply mentioned in accordance with their importance for the equine practitioner.

As a rule, one or more scout films should be made before the contrast study in order to demonstrate shadows that could be masked by the contrast medium.

Esophagography. Radiographic contrast studies of the esophagus can generally be performed in the standing horse without difficulty.

Indication: To establish the diagnosis of esophageal obstruction or its displacement due to periesophageal diseases, esophageal necrosis or strictures (e.g., cicatricial strictures) or to investigate other causes of recurrent dysphagia.

Contrast Medium: Positive contrast medium: $BaSO_4$ solution; negative contrast medium: air.

Hertzsch [1978] stresses the advantage of negative contrast media due to the danger of aspiration pneumonia when solutions are used.

Technique: The contrast medium is introduced into the esophagus through a stomach tube in the standing, sedated animal. Lateral (or latero-lateral) films are made at varying intervals after introduction of the contrast medium.

Even with smaller x-ray machines, good views of the cervical portion of the esophagus can be obtained even in large horses. The thoracic portion of the esophagus can be demonstrated with high-output units.

Arteriography. The visualization of blood vessels by contrast filling, while routine in human medicine and small-animal clinics, is still somewhat uncommon in equine clinics. Arteriograms in the horse are limited almost exclusively to the distal portions of the limbs. They can be very useful in the diagnosis of all diseases that are accompanied by an alteration of blood flow. Experimentally, arteriography has been important in identifying the causes of certain syndromes, such as laminitis [Benninghoff et al., 1970] or navicular disease [Colles and Hickmann, 1977].

Indication: Angiograms have been performed in acute and chronic laminitis [Ackermann et al., 1975; Scott et al., 1978], in flexor tendon diseases [Norberg et al.,

1968], and in blood flow disturbances of varying etiology such as luminal changes, wall changes and obliterations [SCHMIDT and JENNY, 1976; SCOTT et al., 1978; HERTZSCH, 1978].

Contrast Medium: Triiodinated water-soluble contrast medium.

Technique: The examination should be performed under deep general anesthesia, since the contrast medium has an irritating action on the vessel wall and may trigger movements in the unanesthetized animal.

A suitable artery proximal to the site of the presumed blood flow disturbance is punctured with a cannula, and the contrast medium is rapidly injected under pressure. Because the contrast medium is removed very quickly by the bloodstream, it is necessary to take the first film during the injection itself. To demonstrate the functional state of the vessels, including the venous phase if possible, several films should be made in rapid sequence. Automatic cassette changers are very useful for this purpose, but even home-made cassette changers that are hand-operated are satisfactory.

Myelography. In studies of the vertebral column, the visualization of the spinal canal can be a useful adjunct to the clinical and radiographic examination.

Indication: In disturbances of coordination as well as some forms of paralysis, the radiographic examination is often conclusive. A contrast study may demonstrate a spinal cord compression in such cases. The suspected diagnosis can be confirmed, especially in the 'wobbler' syndrome.

Contrast Medium: Water-soluble iodinated contrast material.

Oil contrast media are poorly absorbed from the lumbar canal. Most water-soluble contrast media cause meningeal irritation. At present only Metrazamid (170 mg/ml) can be recommended for cervical myelography.

Technique: The examination is conducted under deep general anesthesia. A short-bevel stylet-armed needle is inserted into the spinal canal at the anterior border of the atlas. After 20 ml of spinal fluid is withdrawn, an equal volume of contrast medium is instilled. The head and neck of the animal should be kept elevated for several more minutes.

Lateral (or latero-lateral) films of the cervical spine are taken at intervals of several minutes until the entire spinal canal is well visualized.

Tendography. Negative contrast media can be administered to delineate certain portions of the tendons and tendon sheaths, especially in the area of the flexor tendons.

Indication: To assess the severity of tendonitis, adhesions, swellings and ruptures of the flexor tendons.

Contrast Medium: Air.

Technique: The examination can be done in the standing horse under mild sedation. A total of 200—300 ml air is injected in 2 or 3 depots subcutaneously between the flexor tendons and into the flexor tendon sheath.

Slightly underexposed films are taken in various projections after the injection is completed.

1.1.3.3. Radiographic Technique

In this section we shall present some guidelines for obtaining radiographs in the horse. Space is limited to give detailed instructions for all structures of potential interest; for this the reader should consult various texts that deal exclusively with diagnostic radiography (e.g., SCHEBITZ and WILKENS [1978]; DOUGLAS and WILLIAMSON [1977]). We must limit our discussion to some basic, general rules. In addition, we shall explain the techniques of radiographing certain special objects that cannot be demonstrated by the basic techniques (e.g., the distal sesamoid [navicular] bone) or which, for various reasons, are difficult to visualize (e.g., the stifle).

All the techniques describes are for the standing horse, for in our opinion it is rarely necessary to anesthetize a horse for radiographic examination. The technique recommended here have stood the test of time in our clinic. We acknowledge that other techniques may be equally useful, however.

Nomenclature of Radiographic Views of the Limbs. Radiographs should be made using standardized techniques. Standardized examination techniques such as those described in the literature may be modified in practice, however it is important to adopt a correct and uniform nomenclature for designating radiographic views.

We favor the nomenclature advocated by ZELLER et al. [1975], which is very similar to that recommended by the American Association of Equine Practitioners.

The terms anteroposterior (AP) and posteroanterior (PA), drawn from human medicine, are obsolete. According to the most recent anatomic nomenclature (NAV, 1971), they should be replaced by the following terms:

AP	by dorso-palmar	for the distal portion of the forelimbs up to and including the carpus
AP	by dorso-plantar	for the distal portion of the hindlimbs up to and including the tarsus
AP	by cranio-caudal	for the areas proximal to the carpus and tarsus.

Analogous terms apply to the opposite projections.

For lateral views the terms latero-medial, medio-lateral and latero-lateral are used.

Oblique projections are required for many special films. These should be designated in degrees, 0° being the dorsal or cranial aspect, 360° the palmar or caudal aspect, 90° the lateral aspect, and 270° the medial aspect. In this way any oblique projection can be accurately defined by its corresponding angle. This system has the advantage of permitting the same parts (e.g., the lateral sesamoid of the right and left limb) to be x-rayed at equal angles (in the example, about 50°).

1.1.3.3.1. General Radiographic Technique for Limb Films

Whenever possible, films of the limbs should be made in two planes. In dense equine bone, such features as bony deposits and osteochondral fragments may go unrecognized if they are superimposed on the parent bone. Thus, horizontal films in the latero-medial and dorso-palmar or dorso-plantar projection (standard views) are indicated in routine examinations of the bones and joints. In doubtful cases additional films, especially oblique views, may be needed.

In examinations of the joints, it must be understood that only one joint can be accurately demonstrated on any one x-ray film. If the central beam is at the level of the pastern joint (proximal interphalangeal), the neighboring coffin (distal interphalangeal) and fetlock (metacarpophalangeal) joints will be more or less distorted owing to the divergence of the beam. In joints that are more closely adjacent, this distortion is relatively unimportant. However, when the localization of the disease is uncertain, it is better to make several films of the various joints than try to demonstrate all the joints between the distal phalanx and distal radius with a single long cassette. There is little chance that any of the joints would be well demonstrated with such a technique, and an accurate interpretation would be impossible.

Different radiographic techniques may be needed to demonstrate different lesions, even in the same bone. 'Soft' films (low exposure settings) are excellent for defining the outer contours of bones; fine bony deposits and increased soft-tissue densities are especially well demonstrated. They provide little osseous structural detail, however. 'Harder' films (higher exposure settings) bring out detail of the bone structure and joint surfaces, although fine calcifications (e.g., in early exostoses) as well as weakly calcified osteochondral fragments tend to be 'burnt out'. With an uncertain clinical diagnosis, it would of course be optimal to obtain two films for each bone or joint — one a little underexposed and the other a little overexposed. In some clinics this is done by attaching a nonscreen film to the cassette. A medium (hard) exposure then produces an underexposed image on the nonscreen film for contour detail, and a more fully exposed image on the screen film for structural detail.

However, we believe that it is neither necessary nor economically feasible to make two films in every case. One should first obtain a film which provides relatively good contour and structural detail. If further changes are suspected, then an additional overexposed or underexposed film may be taken.

1.1.3.3.2. Special Radiographic Techniques

Forelimb

Navicular (Distal Sesamoid) Bone. Navicular bone examinations pose special difficulties for the radiologist. The narrow bone can seldom be adequately assessed in lateral views. In a simple dorso-palmar film, the navicular bone is superimposed on the articular surfaces of the proximal and middle phalanges, so that the navicular itself is difficult to assess owing to the structures in this region. For this reason special projections have been devised. In all cases careful preparation of the sole is necessary in order to eliminate shadows from the sulci of the frog, air in spaces in the sole, and dirt, which will make it difficult or impossible to assess the navicular bone. Sometimes, the hoof must be carefully trimmed before each examination. In addition, the median and lateral sulci must be packed with a material that is similar in density to the horny wall (e.g., a soft soap).

Radiographic Technique

1. Standing limb (high coronary view). In this technique the foot is placed onto the cassette, and the central beam is directed obliquely from the dorsal aspect onto the coronary band at varying angles to the floor (45—80°).

2. Upright pedal view. The upright pedal view is one of the most commonly used. The foot is placed onto an angled hardwood or plexiglas positioning block such that the anterior hoof wall is nearly vertical. The central beam is then directed horizontally at the coronary band. In this view the entire navicular bone is superimposed on the homogenous middle phalanx (P_2) permitting an assessment of both its contour and structure.

3. Proximo-distal projection (palmar-dorsal skyline view). The leg is placed somewhat back on the cassette. The x-ray tube is behind the leg to be examined, at the level of the proximal third metacarpal bone. The central beam is directed obliquely from above (about 30° craniad) toward the bulb of the heel so that the navicular bone is visualized without superimposing the proximal sesamoid bone. The navicular bone is well demonstrated by this view, and the flexor surface can also be assessed [O'Brien et al., 1975].

Proximal Sesamoid Bones. The proximal sesamoid bones cannot be adequately assessed in the standard projections. The distal third metacarpal bone is superimposed in the dorso-palmar view, and both proximal sesamoids are superimposed over each other in the latero-medial view.

Radiographic technique for demonstrating a specific sesamoid bone:
approx. 50° oblique for the lateral sesamoid,
approx. 310° oblique for the medial sesamoid.

Small Metacarpal (Splint) Bones. The third metacarpal bone is superimposed in the standard projections.

Radiographic technique for demonstrating a specific splint bone:
approx. 70° oblique for the lateral splint bone,
approx. 290° oblique for the medial splint bone.

Carpal Joint. Chip fractures of the carpal bones are often difficult to recognize, and their size and location are often difficult to determine.

Radiographic Technique

1. Flexed latero-medial. The carpal joint is held in full flexion, and the cassette is placed on the medial aspect of the joint. In this view the joint is opened, and fracture lines can often be clearly demonstrated.
2. Skyline or tangential view. The carpus is fully flexed, and the cassette is placed on the dorsal aspect of the third metacarpal bone. The central beam is directed obliquely from the front and above toward the dorsal border of the carpus at an angle of about 30° to the cassette. Slab fractures (in a frontal and sagittal plane) of the third carpal bone as well as chip fractures of the other bones can be demonstrated with this view.

Scapulo-humeral (Shoulder) Joint. In the standing animal the shoulder joint is located behind the large shoulder muscles and thoracic cavity. Thus, the joint cannot be well demonstrated without a special technique.

Radiographic Technique

An assistant grasps the limb to be examined in the area of the proximal interphalangeal (pastern) joint and slowly and carefully pulls it forward as far as possible. The head of the animal should be moderately elevated.

The cassette is placed on the outer aspect of the shoulder. The central beam is directed obliquely (about 285°) and laterally through the scapulo-humeral joint.

Hindlimb

Proximal Sesamoid Bones see Forelimb.

Small Metatarsal (Splint) Bones see Forelimb.

Tarsal (Hock) Joint. Standard radiographs of the tarsus should always include oblique views, which should demonstrate changes affecting the dorsal and dorso-medial surfaces of the central and third tarsal bones. Often the first radiographic signs of spavin are noted in this region. Osteochondral fragments in the tibial tarsal joint are also well demonstrated by the oblique views.

Radiographic Technique

The central beam is directed obliquely from the dorsal through the center of the tarsal joint at an angle of 45° (Zeller) or 70° (Schebitz).

Stifle Joint. The stifle joint is a relatively difficult joint for radiographic examination. The lateral view must be taken at the level of the abdominal cavity, while in the cranio-caudal or caudo-cranial view there is a relatively large amount of intervening soft tissue.

Radiographic Technique

Medio-lateral view: The tube is on the side opposite that being examined, with the central beam directed below the abdomen toward the medial aspect of the stifle joint. The limb should be slightly abducted. In some circumstances the central beam must be directed obliquely downward. The cassette is placed on the lateral side of the joint.

Caudo-cranial view: The central beam is directed obliquely downward from behind at an approximately 30° angle about a hand's width above the bend between the ischial muscles and tarsus. The cassette is held against the cranial side of the patella.

Pelvis and Hip Joints. The equine pelvis and hip joints are radiographed only in the recumbent animal and, owing to the large mass of the subject, only with high-output units.

Radiographic Technique

The anesthetized animal is placed in dorsal recumbency, in a 'frog leg' position with the hindlimbs abducted slightly. The central beam is directed vertically downward through the pelvic region; the cassette is beneath the animal.

The transrectal technique of visualizing the hip joint in the standing horse can be practiced by the method described by Paesch and Nagel [1968].

Spinal Column

The equine spinal column can be radiographed in the latero-lateral projection, or dorso-ventral projection.

The cervical spine can be well demonstrated in its entirety. The dorsal processes in particular are easily visualized in the thoracic spine, while in the lumbar region they are usually demonstrable only in rather thinly muscled animals. The posterior coccygeal vertebrae can be demonstrated in the latero-lateral and dorso-ventral views.

Films of the spinal column in flexion are necessary to demonstrate the vertebral changes in spinal ataxis ('wobbler syndrome'). Because the spinal flexion must be maximal, these films can be made only in the recumbent, anesthetized animal.

Head

Radiographic Technique

1. Latero-lateral view: This view is useful for visualizing changes in the region of the nasal cavities, maxillary sinuses, cranium and facial bones.

2. Dorso-ventral views: Radiographs in the dorso-ventral projection are useful for delineating lesions of the nasal cavities and nasal septum. The posterior portions of the head, especially the cranium, are not well demonstrated in dorso-ventral views. To visualize the individual upper incisors, a dorso-ventral film is made with the cassette placed in the oral cavity. The lower incisors are radiographed in the dorso-ventral projection, also with an intraoral cassette.

3. Oblique views: Two rows of teeth are superimposed in each of the latero-lateral and dorso-ventral views. This makes it impossible to assess such features as individual dental roots or alveoli. To visualize a single row of teeth, oblique views of the jaws are needed.

Maxilla. The central beam is directed obliquely downward from the opposite side through the dorsum of the nose. The cassette is placed on the outer aspect of the jaw to be examined.

Mandible. The central beam is directed obliquely upward from the opposite side through the midline between the mandibular rami. The cassette is placed on the outer aspect of the jaw to be examined.

References

Ackermann, N.; Garner, H. E.; Coffman, J. R.; Clement, J. W.: Angiographic appearance of the normal equine foot and alterations in chronic laminitis. J. Amer. vet. med. Assoc. *166:* 58 (1975).

Adams, O. R.: Lamenesses in Horses (Lea & Febiger, Philadelphia 1972).

Benninghoff, G.; Coffman, J. R.; Johnson, J. H.; Guffy, M. M.; Finocchio, E. J.: cited in K. Weiss (1968), Hoofcirculation in equine laminitis. J. Amer. vet. med. Assoc. *156:* 76 (1970).

Colles, C. M.; Hickman, J.: The arterial supply of the navicular bone and its variations in navicular disease. Equine Vet. J. *9:* 150 (1977).

Douglas, S. W.; Williamson, H. D.: Grundlagen der Röntgenologie in der Veterinärmedizin (Verlag Paul Parey, Berlin (West) und Hamburg 1977).

Hertzsch, B.: Spezielle Röntgenuntersuchungsverfahren beim Pferd. Vortrag, gehalten auf der 1. Fortbildungstagung der ATF, 1978.

Myers, V. S.; Emmerson, M. A.: The age and manner of epiphyseal closure in the foreleg of two Arabian foals. J. Amer. vet. Rad. Assoc. *7:* 39 (1966).

Nagel, E.: Zur Röntgenologie der Speiseröhre beim Pferd und Rind. Schweiz. Arch. Tierheilk. *110:* 320 (1968).

Norberg, A. L.; Raker, C. W.; Dodd, D.: Equine tendinitis — an angiographic and histologic study. Proc. 13th Annual Conv. Equine Pract. *13:* 243 (1968).

O'Brien, T. R.; Millman, T. M.; Pool, R. R.; Suter, P. F.: Navicular disease in the thouroughbred horse: A morphologic investigation relative to a new radiographic projection. J. Amer. Vet. Rad. Assoc. *14:* 39 (1975).

Paesch, R.; Nagel, E.: Zur Röntgendiagnostik des Beckens erwachsener Rinder. Medizin. Versorgung *4, 5:* 230 (1968).

Preiss, G. A.: Knochenbruch und Knochenbruchheilung. Lehrbuch der Röntgendiagnostik, vol. 1, p. 238 (Verlag Thieme, Stuttgart 1952).

Schebitz, H.; Wilkens, H.: Atlas der Röntgenanatomie vom Pferd (Verlag Paul Parey, Berlin (West) und Hamburg 1978).

Schmidt, G.: Epiphysen und Apophysen in der röntgenologischen Darstellung der Vorder- und Hinterextremitäten der Fohlen. Vet.-med. Diss., Hannover (1960).

Schmidt, S.; Jenny, U.: Zur Angiographie beim Pferd — zwei Anwendungsbeispiele. Schweiz. Arch. Tierheilk. *118:* 257 (1976).

Scott, E. A.; Sandler, G. A.; Shires, M. H.: Angiography as a diagnostic technique in the equine. J. Equine Med. Surg. *2:* 270 (1978).

Stowater, J. L.; Kneller, S. K.; Froehlich, P. S.: Metrizamide myelography in two horses. Vet. Med. Small Animal Clinician 177 (1978).

Verschooten, F.; de Moor, A.: Tendinitis in the horse: Its radiographic diagnosis with air-tendograms. J. Amer. Vet. Rad. Assoc. *19:* 23 (1978).

Weiss, K.: Degenerative Gelenkerkrankungen. Handbuch der Medizin, Radiologie Bd. V/3, 543 (1968).

Zeller, R.: Der Spat des Pferdes. Vet.-med. Habil.-Schrift, Berlin-Dahlem (1969).

Zeller, R.; Hertzsch, B.; Wilkens, H.; Neurand, K.; Hartung, K.: Die Bezeichnung der Aufnahmerichtungen bei der Röntgenuntersuchung in der Veterinärmedizin. Dtsch. Tierärztl. Wschr. *82:* 22 (1975).

1.1.4. Age Determination

The approximate age of a horse can be determined by examining the teeth. This is the most reliable method of age estimation.

Designation of Teeth. Incisors (I), canines (C), premolars (P), molars (M). Deciduous (milk) teeth are indicated by the prefix D.

Foals. 24 deciduous teeth.

Incisors (DI)	12
Premolars (DP)	12

DP	DI	DI	DP	
3	3	3	3	Upper
3	3	3	3	Lower

The very short deciduous canine teeth (DC) (3—5 mm long) do not generally erupt in stallions and geldings.

Mare. 36 permanent teeth (without counting the wolf teeth).

Incisors (I) 12
Premolars (P) 12
Molars (M) 12

M	P	I	I	P	M	
3	3	3	3	3	3	Upper
3	3	3	3	3	3	Lower

In the mare the canine teeth are usually very small or do not erupt.

Stallion and Gelding. 40 permanent teeth (without counting the wolf teeth).

Incisors (I) 12
Canines (C) 4
Premolars (P) 12
Molars (M) 12

M	P	C	I	I	C	P	M	
3	3	1	3	3	1	3	3	Upper
3	3	1	3	3	1	3	3	Lower

The wolf tooth (P 1) often found in the upper jaw is not shed.
The permanent teeth are divided into two sets:
Successional Permanent Teeth. 12 incisors, 12 premolars.
The successional permanent teeth erupt to replace corresponding milk teeth.
Superadded Permanent Teeth. 12 molars.
The superadded permanent teeth have no deciduous predecessors.

Age Determination. Dental age determination is based on three factors:

1. Eruption of the deciduous teeth.
2. Eruption of the permanent teeth.
3. Wear of the cups, or inner enamel rings of the incisors.

1. Eruption of the deciduous teeth. *Foals* are born with 12 premolars (DP 2, DP 3, DP 4). The *nippers* (central or first incisors) are usually present at birth; otherwise they erupt no later than 8—10 days after birth. The *middles* (middle or second incisors) erupt within 4—6 weeks. The *corners* (outer or third incisors) erupt when the animal is 6—9 months old. As a rule, the upper nippers appear somewhat earlier than the lower ones. In shape the temporary incisors resemble a shovel (crown) with a narrow shaft (root). *Temporary incisors also have cups,* which are 3—4 mm deep. The cups disappear on the *nippers* at about 1 year of age, on the *intermediates* at 1—$1^{1}/_{2}$ years, and on the *corners* at 2 years. Once the cups are worn away, the deciduous teeth cease to grow. They are then shed, or pushed out by the erupting permanent teeth below.

2. Eruption of the permanent teeth. The temporary incisors are replaced with permanent teeth in the order of their appearance, the *nippers* being replaced at $2^{1}/_{3}$ to 3 years, the *intermediates* at $3^{1}/_{2}$ to 4 years, and the *corners* at $4^{1}/_{2}$ to 5 years. At 5 years, replacement of the incisors is complete.

Premolars: The wolf teeth are without deciduous counterparts. They are not always present as permanent teeth and are sometimes counted among the premolars and are designated P 1.

The second premolar is replaced at $2^{1}/_{2}$ years of age, the third premolar at 3 years, and the fourth premolar at $3^{1}/_{2}$ to 4 years.

Inadequate mastication in horses that are $2^{1}/_{2}$ to $3^{1}/_{2}$ years old may be caused by eruption of the permanent premolars. Removal of the deciduous caps is beneficial in such cases.

Molars: The first molar appears at 1 to $1^{1}/_{2}$ years of age, the second molar at 2 to $2^{1}/_{2}$ years, the third molar at 4 to 5 years, and the permanent *canines* at 4 to 5 years. At 6 years, eruption of the canines and molars is complete.

3. Wear of the cups. Beyond age 5, the age of the horse is determined by the degree of cup wear. The cups are 6 mm deep in the lower incisors and 12 mm deep in the upper incisors. Accordingly, the cups of the lower incisors are worn away more rapidly. Cup wear begins in the month when the corresponding upper and lower incisors come into occlusion. With normal dentition, about 2 mm of wear will occur each year.

In accordance with their order of eruption, the nippers come into wear first, followed by the intermediates and then the corners.

Age (in years) at which the incisor cups are completely worn away:

	Corners	Middles	Nippers	Nippers	Middles	Corners
Maxilla	11	10	9	9	10	11
Mandible	8	7	6	6	7	8

When the animal is 7 years old, the mandible begins to grow forward. As a result, only half the lower corner incisor comes in contact with the upper corner. By age 9 or 10 this produces an indentation ('dovetail') in the upper corner. This notch disappears by age 11 or 12.

Contour of the Incisor Tables. This feature provides a rough guideline for age estimation. The tables of the lower incisors have a transverse-oval contour at 6—12 years, a rounded contour at 13—18 years, a triangular contour at 18—23 years, and a somewhat rectangular contour in horses older than 23 years.

Contour of the Lower Incisor Tables at Various Ages (in Years)

	Nippers	Middles	Corners
Transverse oval	6—11	7—12	8—13
Rounded	12—17	13—18	14—19
Triangular	18—23	19—24	20—25
Rectangular	over 23	over 24	over 25

This method is of limited use in wind-suckers or crib-biters, as these animals subject the cups and dental tissue to abnormal wear.

Cup Remnants on the Lower Incisors. The cups start to disappear on the nippers, middles and corners at age 6, 7 and 8, respectively. By 13, 14 and 15 years, respectively, the cups have entirely disappeared from these teeth. At age 8 the dental star appears in front of the cup remnant and persists even after the cup remnant has disappeared. The cup remnant is always elevated slightly above the level of the table surface.

Changes in the Incisor Arch. Up to age 11 the dental arch is crescent-shaped. From age 11 to 17 the arch becomes flatter, and from age 17 to 23 it is nearly linear. After age 23 it forms a straight line through the nippers and middles.

Changes in the Direction of the Incisors. Up to age 8 the incisors are oriented in a nearly perpendicular direction. From age 8 to 15 the lower incisors are elongated and directed more obliquely. After age 15 both the upper and lower incisors are elongated and angled outward.

Groove on the Upper Corner Incisors (Galvaynes Groove). This groove is in the upper third of the labial surface at 10 years of age, the upper half at age 15, the lower half at age 25, and is present only in the lower third at age 30.

Age Characteristics of the Cheek Teeth

		Eruption	Replacement
Temporary premolars (DP)	PD 2	present at birth	$2^1/_2$ years
	PD 3		3 years
	PD 4		$3^1/_2$ to 4 years
Premolars (P)	P 2	$2^1/_2$ to 3 years	
	P 3	3 to $3^1/_2$ years	
	P 4	$3^1/_2$ to 4 years	
Molars (M)	M 1	1 to $1^1/_2$ years	
	M 2	2 to $2^1/_2$ years	
	M 3	3 to 4 years	

Age Determination by Radiographic Visualization of the Cheek Teeth

Mandible. All 3 temporary premolars are radiographically demonstrable at birth as hard structures at equal stages of development. At age 2 only deciduous premolar 4 has a clearly discernible root, because this tooth lags behind the other temporary premolars in its development. Deciduous premolar 2 and 3 no longer have demonstrable roots. Their disappearance begins at 10—12 months. The calcified rudiments of premolar 2 and 3 are evident at 20 months, and that of premolar 4 at 26 months. In the 3-year-old horse the premolars have developed into elongated columns.

The calcified rudiment of the first molar is already demonstrable at birth. The second molar rudiment is visible at 8—10 months, and the third molar rudiment at 26 months.

Maxilla. As in the lower jaw, the structures of the upper temporary premolars (except the roots) are already demonstrable at birth. The gradual disappearance of the roots begins when the horse is 10—12 months old.

The first structures of the second premolar are apparent at 14 months. At 20 months, the third and fourth premolar are also clearly demonstrable.

The rudiment of the first molar is visible at birth. Structures of the second molar are found at 8—10 months, and of third molar at 20—24 months.

Length Increase of the Roots of the Lower Cheek Teeth and their Increasing Distance from the Mandibular Border (Distance from Cortex) after Westhues [1942]

	Second premolar (P 2)	Third premolar (P 3)	Fourth premolar (P 4)	First molar (M 1)
8 years	Root 10 to 15 mm long, 15—30 mm from cortex	Root 20 mm long, 20—30 mm from cortex		Root 30—40 mm long, 40—50 mm from cortex
10 years	Root 30 to 40 mm long, 30—40 mm from cortex	Root 30 to 35 mm long, 40 mm from cortex	Root 20 to 25 mm long, 50 mm from cortex	Root 30 mm long, 50—55 mm from cortex

12 to 14 years	Roots 30 to 50 mm long, 20 and 40 mm from cortex	Root 40 to 50 mm long, 40—50 mm from cortex	Roots 50 and 60 mm from cortex	Roots 30 and 40 mm long, 60 and 70 mm from cortex
15 to 20 years	Root tips are sharper and even more distant from the cortical bone; their low mineral content makes them difficult to demonstrate radiographically			

Age Determination in the Horse

1st week	Eruption of temporary nippers (DI 1)
4 to 6 weeks	Eruption of temporary middles (DI 2)
6 to 9 months	Eruption of temporary corners (DI 3)
12 months	Disappearance of cups in lower DI 1 Eruption of M 1
18 months	Disappearance of cups in lower DI 2
2 years	Disappearance of cups in lower DI 3 Eruption of M 2
$2^1/_2$ to 3 years	Replacement of nippers and both anterior premolars (P 2, P 3)
$3^1/_2$ to 4 years	Replacement of middles and both posterior premolars (P 4)
4 to 5 years	Eruption of canines (C) and M 3
$4^1/_2$ to 5 years	Replacement of corners
6 years	Disappearance of cups in lower nippers (I 1)
7 years	Disappearance of cups in lower middles (I 2)
8 years	Disappearance of cups in lower corners (I 3)
9 years	Disappearance of cups in upper nippers (I 1)
10 years	Disappearance of cups in upper middles (I 2)
11 years	Disappearance of cups in upper corners (I 3)
12 years	Table of lower nippers has rounded contour
13 years	Table of lower middles has rounded contour
14 years	Table of lower corners has rounded contour
15 years	Cup remnants gone, dental arch flattened, table rounded, Galvaynes groove in upper half of corner incisors
18 to 20 years	Incisors angled outward, dental arch almost straight, tables triangular
20 years	Galvaynes groove extends full length of corner incisors
25 years	Table of lower incisors rectangular, sharp outward angulation of all incisors, groove in lower half of upper corner incisors, teeth very long
30 years	Galvaynes groove in lower third of corner incisors

Age Determination in the Pony

1 to 4 weeks	Eruption of temporary nippers (DI 1)
3 to 4 months	Eruption of temporary middles (DI 2)
7 to 11 months	Eruption of temporary corners (DI 3)
18 to 23 months	Disappearance of cups in lower incisors
21 to 27 months	Disappearance of cups in upper incisors
$2^1/_2$ to 3 years	Replacement of nippers
$3^1/_2$ to 4 years	Replacement of middles
$4^1/_2$ to 5 years	Replacement of corners
$4^1/_2$ to 10 years	Incisor tables have transverse-oval contour

$6^1/_2$ years	Disappearance of cups in lower nippers (I 1)
8 years	Disappearance of cups in lower middles (I 2)
$9^1/_2$ years	Disappearance of cups in lower corners (I 3)
up to 11 years	Incisors nearly vertical
11 years	Disappearance of cups in upper nippers (I 1)
11 to 17 years	Incisor tables rounded
15 years	Disappearance of cups in upper middles (I 2)
17 to 18 years	Disappearance of cups in upper corners (I 3)
over 18 years	Incisors angled outward
over 22 years	Incisor tables triangular

Age Changes in the Skeleton

The time of ossification of the epiphyseal plates can also serve as a basis for age determination in the horse.

Epiphyseal closure occurs at the following ages for various bones:

8 days	10—12 months	12—15 months	15—18 months
Distal proximal and middle phalanges	Proximal middle phalanx, ilium-pubis-ischium, scapula-coracoid	Distal third metatarsal and metacarpal bone, proximal phalanx	Distal [sic.] third metatarsus and metacarpus proximal radius

2 years	3 years	$3^1/_2$ years	4—5 years	5 years
Distal tibia and fibula	Tuber calcis	Proximal humerus proximal and distal femur, proximal ulna, tibia, distal radius	Vertebrae	Iliac angle and tuber ischii

References

Brömler, K.: Die Altersbestimmung beim Kleinpferd auf Grund der Zahnentwicklung und -abnutzung. Vet.-med. Diss., München (1954).

Butz, H.; Böttger, Th.: Das Zahnalter des Pferdes (Verlag Schaper, Hannover 1946).

Habermann, U.: Zur röntgenologischen Darstellung der maxillaren Backenzähne des Pferdes. Vet.-med. Diss., Hannover (1963).

Habermehl, H. K.: Altersbestimmung bei Haustieren, Pelztieren und beim jagdbaren Wild. 2. Aufl. (Verlag Paul Parey, Berlin (West) und Hamburg 1975).

Henricson, B.: Altersbestimmung von Pferden. Medlemsbl. Sveriges Vet.-Förb. *10:* 369 (1958).

Jahn, W.: Die röntgenologisch nachweisbaren Veränderungen im Bereich der maxillaren Backenzähne des Pferdes in den verschiedenen Altersstufen. Vet.-med. Diss., Hannover (1966).

Knezevic, P.: Ein Beitrag zur Persistenz der Milchzähne bei Pferden. Mh. Vet.-Med. *12:* 19 (1957).

Krüger, G.: Der Zahnbogen der Traber als Hilfsmittel zur Altersfeststellung. Mh. Vet.-Med. *7:* 51 (1952).

Küpfer, M.: Backenzahnstruktur und Molarenentwicklung bei Esel und Pferd (Gustav Fischer Verlag, Jena 1937).

Leue, P.: Einbiss oder Einschliff. Tierärztl. Rundsch. *45:* 150 (1939).

Pörschmann, F.: Zur röntgenologischen Darstellung der mandibularen Backenzähne des Pferdes unter Berücksichtigung verschiedener Altersstufen bis zum 3. Lebensjahr. Vet.-med. Diss., Hannover (1966).

ROSENBERGER, F.: Irregularistüten im Zahnwechsel bei spätreifen Pferderassen. Wien. Tierärztl. Mschr. *42:* 549 (1955).

SANNEMANN, H.: Grundlagen der Altersbestimmung des Pferdes. Eine Literaturstudie. Vet.-med. Diss., Hannover (1949).

SASSEN, W.: Beitrag zur Beurteilung der Furche und des Einbisses an den Eckzähnen des Pferdes für dessen Altersbestimmung. Vet.-med. Diss., Hannover (1950).

SAUER, R.: Untersuchungen über die Anwendbarkeit der Röntgenkontrastaufnahmen zu Zahn- und Kieferaufnahmen beim Pferd. Vet.-med. Diss., Berlin (1950).

SCHÖNHERR, H.: Die Darstellung der Zähne des Pferdes im Röntgenbild. Vet.-med. Diss., Leipzig (1959).

WESTHUES, M.: Die Altersschätzung des Pferdes durch das Röntgenbild der Backenzähne. Tierärztl. Rdsch. *48:* 232 (1942).

1.2. Anesthesiology

1.2.1. General

General anesthesia in the horse can pose special problems due to the temperament and physical size of the animal as well as peculiarities of its circulatory and respiratory system. Even the casting of an adult horse, especially the Thoroughbred, presents a difficult problem. It is however manageable with well trained, experienced help. Animals who struggle or fall violently during casting can suffer serious injuries to the head, vertebral column and limbs. Excitement associated with anesthesia induction or recovery can be physically difficult to manage. Postoperative excitement can be prevented or minimized by safeguarding against triceps rhabdomyolysis or so-called 'radial nerve paralysis', and hindquarter muscle ischemia in dorsal recumbency by careful positioning and padding. Adminstering oxygen postoperatively, and by placing the animal into a padded recovery stall will also help prevent these problems.

If the anesthesia is too light, serious injury can occur to the spine and limbs, particularly if the animal is not well restrained. In addition, some Thoroughbreds become extremely tense during light anesthesia, even to the point of causing rectal prolapse.

Besides the complications cited above, which can be avoided to some degree with suitable drugs and anesthetic techniques, several other problems must be considered. For example, the horse with intestinal obstruction is at risk from the standpoint of developing endotoxic shock. The large pulmonary dead space (V_D/V_T) in the horse must be taken into account, especially when an anesthetic machine is used. The horse is also subject to marked ventilation-perfusion disturbances of the lungs and a large right-to-left shunt. The latter may result from occlusion of the terminal bronchioles, possibly accompanied by severe hypotension in the pulmonary circulation. As a result it may be difficult or even impossible to achieve adequate oxygen delivery to the tissues especially in old and heavy animals in the dorsal recumbent position.

1.2.1.1. Premedication

Premedication is the administration of certain agents which reduce the risk of anesthesia, surgery and recovery to the patient as well as facilitate the induction of anesthesia. All these requirements cannot be satisfied in every case, however. Some drugs have a strong sedating effect and thus facilitate anesthesia induction, yet have unfavorable or even dangerous side-effects.

Atropine[1]. Opinions differ as to the value of administering the anticholinergic drug atropine. We recommend it in the horse for preventing excessive fluid loss from sweat-

[1] Atropine sulfate. Burns Biotec, Omaha, NE 68103 (USA).

ing and protecting against cardiac arrhythmias associated with the use of succinylcholine or analgesics. The 2nd-degree heart block that occurs after the i.v. injection of Rompun[1] can be prevented with atropine. Atropine is also beneficial in animals with chronic obstructive pulmonary disease (COPD). It is highly doubtful whether atropine protects against the cardiac and respiratory effects of vagal reflexes in its normal dose of 5—20 mg s.c. or i.m. (or 1 mg/kg bw i.v.). Since halothane[2], the most widely used inhalation anesthetic, does not irritate the air passages and does not increase salivary and respiratory secretions, the routine use of atropine prior to halothane anesthesia appears to be unnecessary. Atropine depresses gastrointestinal motility which is a distinct disadvantage particularly in gastrointestinal surgery. As well, atropine causes mydriasis, which makes it difficult or impossible to assess the pupillary size as a criterion for the depth of anesthesia.

Atropine also causes a slight decrease in the arterial oxygen pressure (PaO_2), but this has practically no effect on arterial oxygen saturation [DeMoor, 1968a]. The fall of the PaO_2 may result from the increase in the pulmonary dead space. Atropine decreases ciliary activity, thus hampering the transport of mucus to the larynx. This can be disadvantageous in chronic bronchitis with retention of secretions [Annis et al., 1976].

1.2.1.2. Sedation

Sedation is used either for premedication before general anesthesia or as a means of quieting temperamental or difficult horses before examination or treatment. Phenothiazine derivatives such as Promazine[3] and Acepromazine[4] are the most widely used agents. The use of sedatives and tranquilizers prior to general anesthesia can facilitate induction as well as reduce the necessary dose or concentration of the hypnotic or anesthetic agents. Moreover, the recovery phase after barbiturate anesthesia is quieter than when no premedication is given. Phenothiazine derivatives also have certain side-effects, however, which require that their dose be kept to a minimum. In some situations they are contraindicated. Higher doses do not seem to improve their tranquilizing properties. In very difficult or refractory animals, moreover, tranquilizers appear to be of limited value. Phenothiazine derivatives have an α-adrenergic blocking effect, i.e., they abolish the compensatory vasoconstriction produced by tissue α-receptors in response to hemorrhage, for example. This can be very dangerous unless the circulating blood volume is maintained by the infusion of blood, plasma, plasma expanders or electrolytes. On the other hand, this α-adrenergic blocking effect can be advantageous in terms of preventing shock or in the treatment of shock due to blood loss, but only if the circulating blood volume is sufficiently large. If the circulating volume is small, as frequently occurs in shock, marked peripheral pooling of blood can occur especially in the splanchnic area, with an inadequate venous return. The α-blocking effect also causes a marked pooling of erythrocytes in the spleen, which is not influenced by the administration of atropine. After the i.v. injection of the phenothiazine tranquilizers propionylpromazine and promethazine in a dose of 8 mg/100 kg, 1,423 ml of O_2-transporting erythrocytes/100 kg

[1] Xylazine. Haver-Lockhart, Shawnee, KS 66201 (USA).
[2] Fluothane. Ayerst Laboratories (American Horse Products Corp.), New York, NY 10017 (USA).
[3] Promazine hydrochloride. Fort Dodge Laboratories, Inc., Fort Dodge, IA 50501 (USA).
[4] Acepromazine maleate. Ayerst Laboratories (American Horse Products Corp.), New York, NY 10017 (USA).

were removed from the circulation over a period of several hours [DEMOOR et al., 1975]. This means that more than one-third and in some cases more than one-half of the circulating erythrocytes were sequestered in the spleen. This effect is also observed with promazine [DEMOOR et al., 1972b]. Hence, phenothiazine tranquilizers are contraindicated in acute or chronic anemia, in circulatory disturbances, and as premedication for surgery involving a potentially large blood loss. Tranquilizers prolong the recovery phase of anesthesia and cause hypothermia, which can be particularly disadvantageous during protracted recovery at a low ambient temperature.

High doses of phenothiazine tranquilizers can cause incoordination, which may be a problem if the animal is to be treated or operated in the standing position. Some tranquilizers, such as chlorpromazine and propionylpromazine, occasionally cause paradoxical reactions when injected intravenously. The horse may become violent, sinking down on its haunches only to plunge forward suddenly. The combination of a tranquilizer with promethazine can prevent this paradoxical reaction with almost 100% certainty. In the stallion and gelding phenothiazine derivatives cause a slight to moderate prolapse of the penis that persists for several hours. In stallions and geldings under testosterone therapy, there is a danger of penile paralysis if an erection occurs shortly before or after the injection of propionylpromazine or acepromazine. The most widely used phenothiazine derivatives are promazine hydrochloride, and acepromazine.

Promazine hydrochloride is generally administered by the i.v. route in a dose of 50 mg/100 kg. It produces moderate sedation.

Propionylpromazine is usually combined with promethazine and administered i.v. in a dose of 5—6 mg/100 kg. This relatively small dose produces good sedation in most cases. The dose for intramuscular injection is 0.25 mg/kg. Proprionylpromazine may also be combined with the analgesic methadone. The doses are 10 mg/100 kg each of proprionylpromazine and methadone and 1 mg/100 kg atropine, with a maximum dose of 50 mg propionylpromazine and 50 mg methadone per animal. Very good sedation and analgesia are obtained with this combination.

The sedative effect of *acepromazine* is superior to that of promazine. It is administered i.v. or i.m. in a dose of 5—10 mg/100 kg. It may also be combined with methadone in the following dose: 5—10 mg/100 kg acepromazine + 10—15 mg/100 kg methadone + 1 mg/100 mg atropine i.v.

Stresnil[1], a butyrophenone derivative, is a neuroleptic agent commonly used in swine. It produces good sedation in a dose of 0.5—0.8 mg/kg i.m., achieving maximum effect after 20—60 min. The effect persists for 2—6 h. There is a 30—40% decrease in the arterial blood pressure, an effect which lasts longer than the actual sedation. According to Serrano and Lees, side-effects can occur (perspiration, muscle tremor, salivation). Azaperone probably increases the secretion of ACTH, with a rise of the plasma 11-hydroxycorticoid concentration [MACKENZIE and SNOW, 1977]. Azaperone should not be given intravenously, because it tends to cause excitement, ataxia and in some cases collapse [DODMAN and WATERMAN, 1979].

Rompun[2], a thiazine derivative, is a sedative and muscle relaxant with analgesic properties. The dose is 0.4—0.8 mg/kg i.v. or 1.5—2 mg/kg i.m. It is an excellent sedative. Its onset of effect is rapid even on intramuscular injection, but it does not cause the animal to fall. Its duration of action is shorter than that of the phenothiazine derivatives. It causes no penile paralysis and does not depress respiration [KERR

[1] Azaperone. Pitman Moore Inc., Washington Crossing, NJ 08560 (USA).

[2] Xylazine. Haver-Lockhart, Shawnee, KS 66201 (USA).

et al., 1972 b]. It significantly increases the resistance of the nasal passages as well as the respiratory laryngeal resistance [ROBINSON et al., 1975]. Intravenous injection is followed by an immediate rise of blood pressure, followed by a fall of pressure 2 min later. Xylazine decreases the left ventricular contractile force and cardiac activity and (unlike the phenothiazine derivatives) increases the peripheral resistance [McCASHIN and GABEL, 1975]. The blood pressure remains fairly stable following i.m. injection. Intravenous injections nearly always cause cardiac arrhythmias with a 2nd-degree AV block. These side-effects can be avoided by the i.v. injection of 1 mg/100 kg atropine immediately before the xylazine is given. Cardiac arrest has been observed after the i.v. injection of xylazine alone [NDRITO and ENOS, 1977]. Excitement has also occurred in isolated cases. Xylazine may be administered in conjunction with methadone and atropine. Seemingly better results are achieved if it is given several minutes before the methadone. The combination of xylazine, proprionylpromazine and methadone can sometimes cause very violent paradoxical reactions [FRITSCH, 1975]. According to KERR et al. [1972 a], xylazine is an excellent preanesthetic prior to thiobarbiturate anesthesia or thiobarbiturate and halothane anesthesia; it causes only slight respiratory depression and provides greater cardiovascular stability than acetylpromazine. In addition, the animal is quiet during recovery and does not attempt to rise before it is able.

1.2.1.3. Analgesia

Narcotic analgesics may be indicated for pain relief (e.g., in the postoperative period) or may be used in combination with a tranquilizer for premedication.

Morphine[1] should be administered only in small doses in the horse. Pain sensation is diminished, motor activity is decreased, and mild sedation is obtained. Doses greater than 200 mg should be avoided, for they usually cause psychic and motor unrest or even excitement [LAGERWEIJ, 1975). The danger of excitement is much smaller when the animal is in pain. Good sedation and analgesia can be obtained by the i.v. injection of xylazine in a dose of 1.1 mg/kg, followed by a morphine dose of 0.6 mg/kg i.v. after 2—5 min [HUSKA, 1977]. Many horses exhibit head-shaking, however, and excitement with diminution of the sedative effect of the xylazine is sometimes observed. Xylazine and morphine are of clinical value however because they stabilize the circulation and respiratory center [MUIR et al., 1979]. The drug is not commonly used in North America.

Demerol[2]. Meperidine hydrochloride (Demerol) is a less potent analgesic than morphine but exerts a strong spasmolytic effect. The dose is 0.5—1.5 mg/kg i.m. It is used for premedication as well as for postoperative pain relief. Intravenous injections may cause mild excitement or incoordination in some cases.

In the pony its half-life is 66 $\pm$ 8.7 min [ALEXANDER and COLLETT, 1975]. It produces excitement when administered by nasogastric tube.

Methadone[3]. Dolophine hydrochloride (methadone) is a more powerful analgesic than morphine. It is a less potent sedative, however, so it is often combined with a tranquilizer. The dose is 10—15 mg/100 kg i.v. It is usually administered in conjunction with an atropine-like substance such as Polamivet. The narcotics of the analgesic group cause negligible respiratory depression in and of themselves. Morphine, me-

[1] Morphine sulfate. Eli Lilly, Indianapolis, IN 46206 (USA).

[2] Meperidine hydrochloride. Winthrop Laboratories (Sterling Drug Inc.), New York, NY 10016 (USA).

[3] Dolophine hydrochloride. Eli Lilly, Indianapolis, IN 46206 (USA).

perdine and methadone do not alter the PaO_2, $PaCO_2$ or pH_3 [Muir et al., 1978a]. They can, however, potentiate the respiratory depression caused by barbiturate or halothane anesthesia.

A great advantage is the availability of an antidote, nalorphine, which acts as a morphine antagonist. The drug, like morphine, is not commonly used in North America.

Talwin-V[1]. Pentazocine (Talwin) can be administered for pain in a dose of 0.3 to 0.6 mg/kg by the s.c., i.m. or i.v. route. It is a potent, fast-acting analgesic, though it can cause mild ataxia in some cases. If respiratory depression occurs as the result of an overdose or hypersensitivity reaction, naloxine hydrochloride can be given as an antidote. Nalorphine is less effective.

M99. M99 (Etorphine hydrochloride) is a very potent analgesic that can be used intravenously or intramuscularly together with acepromazine under the name of Immobilon. The animal collapses and exhibits a very strong analgesia. Violent side-effects such as sweating, excitement and severe dyspnea are fairly common, especially in the large breeds. Other frequent effects are a fall of the PaO_2 [Hillidge et al.; Lees, 1975b], tachycardia, and a marked decrease in the stroke volume [Lees et al., 1971]. Despite the lowered PaO_2, the oxygen saturation remains adequate, probably by virtue of the cardiac output and PCV [Hillidge, 1976]. Reversible myocardial hypoxia resulting from coronary insufficiency is a possibility, however [Hillidge, 1978]. If etorphine and acetylpromazine are given after glyceryl guaiacolate, the circulatory effects are less severe [Schatzmann and Held, 1975]. Diprenorphine hydrochloride or nalorphine can be given as antagonists. Some fatalities have been observed after use of the antidote, however [Hillidge and Lees, 1974]. Etorphine alone is used in zoo animals but the etorphine/acepromazine combination is presently unavailable for use in horses in North America.

1.2.1.4. Preanesthetic Examination and Preparation

After taking the history a brief clinical examination must be made before premedicating for general anesthesia. Points to be noted are the animal's temperature, the quality and rate of the pulse, the peripheral perfusion of the mucous membranes (anemia, congestion, slow capillary filling, icterus), the presence or absence of venous congestion, the state of hydration (eyes, skin), the respiratory rate, as well as the type and quality of the respiration. Pulmonary auscultation is indicated. The status of the CNS (depression, excitement) should be noted. If the animal can be exercised without difficulty, then accessory heart sounds that were noted during auscultation may vanish. These may not neccessarily signify an anesthetic risk. Murmurs in the chest wall at the level of the heart are usually pathologic, however. Such animals require particularly close observation during anesthesia.

This basic examination routine can be completed in a matter of minutes. In certain cases additional examinations such as blood and urine studies, EKG or chest radiographs may be warranted. If an abnormality is noted during the preoperative examination, the owner must be warned of this as objectively as possible. In some cases, such as when an obvious infection of the respiratory system is present and the operation is not urgent, it is prudent to postpone the procedure.

The animal should be fasted prior to the induction of general anesthesia. Water may usually be given until 2—4 h before anesthesia. Food should be withheld for

[1] Pentazocine. Winthrop Laboratories (Sterling Drug Inc.), New York, NY 10016 (USA).

8—12 h preoperatively. The duration of fasting depends on the nature of the procedure; intra-abdominal surgery requires longer fasting than other operations. The ingestion of bedding material must also be prevented by muzzling the animal if necessary. Roughage should be reduced for several days prior to major intra-abdominal surgery. Withholding food and especially water for too long a period can have adverse effects. For example, the reduction of circulating blood volume that occurs with dehydration can be a problem, particularly with anesthetics that cause cardiovascular depression (e.g., halothane). Moreover, dehydration or Na^+ deficits reduce the influx of extracellular water into the blood vessels following a bleeding episode. Fasting for too long a period may impair the ability of the liver to detoxify certain anesthetic agents, presumably by exhausting its protein and glycogen stores.

If gastric dilation is present as a result of intestinal obstruction, some fluid must be siphoned off by means of a stomach tube to avoid gastric rupture when the animal is cast. Animals that show signs of 'shock' or marked dehydration and require immediate surgery must be treated appropriately before the induction of anesthesia, and their dehydration corrected to the extent that time allows.

1.2.1.5. Casting with Chemical Agents and Induction of Anesthesia

The technique of casting a horse with chemical agents, the induction of anesthesia and the agents to be used are dependent upon various factors. These include the experience of the assistants, the size and temperament of the animal, the type of surgery table available, and the nature and duration of the operation.

Chloral hydrate is a safe, practical basal hypnotic that is still widely used in equine surgery. The dose is 8—10 g/100 kg i.v. of a 10—20% solution. It is essential that this solution be given intravenously due to the danger of thrombophlebitis and periphlebitis (at 20% pH 2.9). Because the animal may struggle during restraint, the use of restraining ropes is advised. The solution is infused in the standing animal, the ropes are applied, and at the onset of hypnosis and ataxia the animal is cast. If restrained too soon, the animal may struggle violently. Chloral hydrate produces a shallow narcosis but not true anesthesia. The animal is still sensitive to pain and can make sudden violent movements. Therefore, supplementary local or regional anesthesia and suitable physical restraint are usually necessary prior to commencing surgery. A standard dose rarely causes cardiovascular or respiratory depression, and so monitoring should pose no difficulties. The recovery time is short. If a recovery stall is not available, the animal may be kept under physical restraint until able to rise after 45 min to 1 h. Chloral hydrate is not suitable for high-risk procedures. It is useful as a basal hypnotic and may be combined with other agents such as thiopental, pentobarbital[1] (1—2 g) or halothane to deepen the level of anesthesia. A muscle relaxant, such as glyceryl guaiacolate (see below) can be given to prevent struggling after the horse has been restrained with chloral hydrate. For an operation of approximately 30 min duration we infuse 10—15 g/100 kg glyceryl guaiacolate (GG), in which is dissolved 1 g thiopental/100 kg. An alternative and perhaps better method is to give chloral hydrate after casting the horse with glyceryl guaiacolate.

Pentothal. Pentothal (Thiopental sodium[2]) is a short-acting thiobarbiturate that can be administered in various ways. Premedication with a tranquilizer or xylazine (Rompun) is advised [Skarda et al., 1970]. This simplifies the injection while pre-

[1] Chlorpent. Fort Dodge Laboratories, Inc., Fort Dodge, IA 50501 (USA).

[2] Thiopental sodium. CEVA Laboratories, Overland Park, KS 66212 (USA).

venting the postoperative excitement that often follows thiobarbiturates. Thiopental is chiefly administered by *rapid i.v. injection in the standing animal.* The rapid injection of 1 g/100 kg causes the horse to fall in 20—40 s. According to Langley, the excitement that sometimes results from a rapid injection can be avoided by extending the injection over a period of 15—25 s. After premedication with xylazine, the induction time for lateral recumbency after thiopental is much longer than after premedication with acetylpromazine [Frankland and Camburn, 1977]. On very slow injection, however, the horse is apt to become highly excited. No restraining ropes are necessary when casting the animal. It is well to have an experienced assistant standing at the horse's head. His task is to ease the animal's fall and prevent it from striking the side of the head violently on the floor.

Apnea often occurs during rapid induction. This is usually of short duration and is seldom dangerous, and affects mainly the expiratory phase. Spontaneous breathing can generally be restored by firm compression of the thorax. Moderate tachycardia and a slight fall of mean arterial pressure may also be noted. Serious arrhythmias do not occur, however [Tavernor and Lees, 1970]. Despite a decreased stroke volume, there is a moderate increase in cardiac output as a result of the tachycardia. The increase in coronary blood flow does not appear adequate for the increased myocardial metabolism, however [Patschke, 1976]. Thiopental is contraindicated in the presence of cardiovascular abnormalities. The duration of surgical anesthesia is 5—15 min, the recovery period 30—45 min. The duration of anesthesia should not be prolonged by repeated thiopental injections. This significantly increases the recovery time, because thiopental is short-acting only with single use.

The animal's fall can be made quicker and more gentle by the rapid i.v. injection of 0.08—0.1 mg/kg suxamethonium immediately after the thiopental injection. Thiopental can also be used to deepen the level of chloral hydrate anesthesia. The animal cast with chloral hydrate is given a rapid injection of one-third the calculated dose. After 1 min the injection is slowly continued 'to effect' while monitoring the animal's reflexes, breathing and pulse. A period of apnea will follow. This method is useful for avoiding a relative overdose, while prolonging somewhat the duration of surgical anesthesia. A smaller dose is sufficient following a large blood or fluid loss. Excited animals require a larger dose, since the injected thiopental is more rapidly eliminated from the brain and carried to the well-perfused muscles. Thiopental can also be administered prior to casting with glyceryl guaiacolate. If the animal begins to show ataxia during the infusion of glyceryl guaiacolate, a rapid i.v. injection of 0.5—0.75 g/100 kg thiopental is given. This is usually sufficient to produce a gentle fall. When a thiobarbiturate is combined with glyceryl guaiacolate, a somewhat longer period of apnea usually results [Schatzmann, 1975].

Pentobarbital. Pentobarbital is unsuitable for general anesthesia in adult horses, except when used in certain cases to increase the depth of chloral hydrate anesthesia. The recovery period is long and is marked by struggling. Pentobarbital may be used in foals in cases where thiopental anesthesia is too brief and inhalation anesthesia is not available.

Metomidate. Metomidate, a hypnotic commonly used in swine, can also be used in the horse after premedication with azaperone. Metomidate is injected intravenously in a dose of 3.5 mg/kg bw. Induction is quiet, muscle relaxation is good, and no respiratory or circulatory problems arise. The duration of anesthesia is 5—10 min. Recovery usually takes 30—60 min, though it may vary between 14 and 120 min [Hillidge et al., 1973]. The following side-effects can occur during emergence: sweating, tremor of the limbs and neck, and excitement, particularly after premedication with a small dose of azaperone [Hillidge and Lees, 1972]. Metomidate causes a mild hemolysis [Serrano et al., 1976]. The drug is not available for use in the horse in North America.

Ketamine[1]. Ketamine (Ketamine hydrochloride) is a dissociative anesthetic; it produces a dose-dependent increase in the cardiac output, blood pressure and heart rate in various animal species. It is considered a good, safe, short-acting agent with a good sedative effect *after satisfactory premedication with xylazine* (Rompun). Xylazine is given in a dose of 1.1 mg/kg i.v. Prior medication with atropine is sometimes performed as well. Ketamine is given i.v. in a dose of 2.2 mg/kg several minutes after the administration of xylazine. The horse will generally down quietly into lateral recumbency within 30—60 min after the i.v. injection of ketamine. It produces excellent analgesia and mild anesthesia, but the sensitivity to metallic noise is heightened in horses premedicated with promazine [Fuentes, 1978]. If promazine and ketamine are given together intravenously, the result is a mild muscle tremor, limb rigidity and unrest. The combination of xylazine and ketamine is easy to administer but expensive [Ellis et al., 1977]. Circulatory function remains within normal limits with a rise of the mean arterial pressure and fall of cardiac output. The duration of anesthesia is about 15 min. The recovery period is free of struggling. Higher ketamine doses (6.6 mg/kg) cause serious side-effects, such as muscle tremor, rigidity, mydriasis, sweating, hypertension, tachycardia and hyperthermia during recovery [Muir et al., 1979]. Continuous infusion or repeated i.v. injection is not advised, as this lengthens the duration of anesthesia and prolongs recovery time [Kaka et al., 1979]. Ketamine can also be given i.v. in a dose of 1.7 mg/kg after premedication with xylazine at the conclusion of glyceryl guaiacolate infusion. The animal goes rapidly and safely into lateral recumbency, with very good muscular relaxation and analgesia. Recovery is quiet and rapid. After this combination, halothane anesthesia can be induced with a relatively low, safe concentration [Muir et al., n.d.]. Glyceryl guaiacolate and ketamine provide stable cardiovascular function in the laterally recumbent horse, although a fall of the PaO_2 sometimes occur in spontaneously breathing animals [Muir et al., 1978 b].

Quelicin[2] *(Suxamethonium)* Sucostrin. Succinylcholine is a muscle relaxant which causes depolarization at the level of the motor end-plate. It may be given either prior to casting with chemical agents or during general anesthesia to achieve strong muscular relaxation. The dose is 0.08—0.1 mg/kg i.v. A possibly painful muscular twitching develops a few seconds after the injection is given. The horse goes down in 30—40 s and remains in a relaxed state for several minutes. An apneic spell lasting from 30 s to 3 min can occur after the animal falls. In some cases it is advisable to administer oxygen and apply artificial respiration. Succinylcholine also produces marked tachycardia (3 to 6 times the normal rate) and may raise the blood pressure to 400 mm Hg or more. Premedication with a tranquilizer greatly reduces this hypertension and improves hypoxemia [Zinn et al., 1970]. Arrhythmias are common but can be prevented with atropine premedication. The PaO_2 can fall significantly. To prevent the tachycardia and avoid arrhythmias, a dose of 0.1 mg/kg propanol hydrochloride can be given before the succinylcholine injection. Propanol hydrochloride is a β-receptor blocking agent that inhibits sympathetic effects on the heart [Tavernor and Lees, 1970]. During halothane anesthesia, the tachycardia and hypertension are much less severe than in the conscious animal, and a regular cardiac rhythm is maintained. Halothane anesthesia and artificial respiration prevent arrhythmias and blood pres-

[1] Ketamine hydrochloride. Parke Davis (Warner Lambert Corp.), Morris Plains, NJ 07950 (USA).
[2] Succinylcholine chloride, Sucostrin. E.R. Squibb & Sons, Princeton, N.J. (USA).

sure elevations and significantly decrease the tachycardia caused by succinylcholine [BENSON et al., 1979].

These cardiovascular effects may be dependent on two mechanisms: (1) a β-stimulating action on the heart resulting from respiratory depression and anxiety in the conscious animal, and (2) a direct stimulatory effect on the peripheral autonomic ganglia [LEES and TAVERNOR, 1969]. During halothane anesthesia succinylcholine can also be slowly infused at a rate of 0.03 mg/min/kg bw [HALL]. If succinylcholine is given during general anesthesia, artificial respiration is essential. The relaxation produced by succinylcholine allows a more effective artificial respiration to be applied [BENSON et al., 1976].

Succinylcholine is superior to glyceryl guaiacolate in that only a very small volume need be injected — a particular advantage in difficult and temperamental horses. The anxiety and possible pain caused by the drug in the conscious animal are best alleviated by premedication with a tranquilizer and by the injection of 0.75 g/100 kg thiopental i.v. just before the succinylcholine is given. Atropine is always given during premedication as a precaution against cardiac arrhythmias.

There are various contraindications to the use of succinylcholine. Large verminous aneurysms, for example, are susceptible to rupture from the strong hypertensive action of the drug. Organophosphates suppress the plasma cholinesterase concentrations (an enzyme which breaks down succinylcholine into choline and succinic acid) for a period of at least 14 days. It sometimes takes 7—8 weeks for initial values to be restored [BELLO et al., 1974]. Applications of organophosphates increase the danger of respiratory arrest and serious cardiac arrhythmias after the administration of succinylcholine, and there is a stronger decline in the PaO_2 and pH [SHORT et al., 1971]. Organophosphates can be dangerous if administered within 8 days *prior* to the injection of suxamethonium due to the prolonged apnea that occurs with induction [KELLER and MÜLLER, 1979].

Various antibiotics, such as streptomycin, neomycin, polymyxin, colistin and possibly even tetracycline and kanamycin, have a neuromuscular-blocking action that can accentuate the effect of succinylcholine. If a serious hepatocellular dysfunction is present, the plasma cholinesterase level may not be high enough to degrade succinylcholine. It is still unclear whether it causes a dangerous hyperkalemia in horses after severe muscle trauma and tetanus, as it does in humans and dogs. EISENMENGER reports on the occurrence of only a single death in conjunction with 800 administered doses (= 0.125%); that death was the result of an aneurysmal rupture. The American Association of Equine Practitioners recorded a somewhat higher mortality: 300 deaths out of 160,000 administered doses (0.188%; TIEGLAND [1969]). If anesthesia is induced directly with high doses of halothane after casting the animal with succinylcholine, there is a danger of fatal cardiac arrhythmias resulting from a halothane-induced sensitization of the myocardium toward catecholamines released by succinylcholine [HEATH and GABEL, 1970].

Glycodex[1]. Guaifenesin (Glyceryl guaiacolate) acts at the level of the internuncial neurons rather than the level of the motor end-plate. It has the useful property of paralyzing the skeletal muscles without affecting the respiratory muscles when administered in suitable concentration. Unlike succinylcholine, however, a rather large volume of the drug must be infused which can be a disadvantage in the casting of difficult horses. Only a 10—15% solution is used, as more concentrated solutions can cause hemolysis. A 20% solution can cause thrombophlebitis. The occurrence

[1] Guaifenesin. Burns-Biotec Laboratories (Chromalloy Pharmaceuticals, Inc.), Omaha, NE 68103 (USA).

and degree of relaxation depend on the rate of infusion. If the dose is infused under pressure in 30—60 s, the horse goes down quickly and quietly. Slow infusion can produce an ataxic state in which the animal can barely stand but is not relaxed enough to go down [Schatzmann et al., 1978]. Guaifenesin also has a weak sedative and analgesic effect. Recumbency is produced by the infusion of 10 g/100 kg of a 10—15% solution. The animal usually falls quietly before the total dose is infused. The infusion is then completed in the recumbent animal. Overdose leads to extensor rigidity and labored breathing. For short-lasting operations, thiopental, ketamine or chloral hydrate can be given after the infusion. For longer operations, inhalation anesthesia with halothane is preferred. In ponies, the recovery time after guaifenesin is more prolonged in males than in females, this due to the slower elimination of the drug from the plasma [Davis and Wolf, 1970]. This difference has not been confirmed in other studies, however [Ketelaars et al., 1979]. The arterial oxygen pressure (PaO_2) is higher after guaifenesin than after succinylcholine [Yoshida et al., 1975].

1.2.2. Fundamentals of General Anesthesia

1.2.2.1. Components of General Anesthesia

General anesthesia is characterized by a sequence of varying states: narcosis (unconsciousness), analgesia (loss of pain sensation), and muscular relaxation. Some protection is advisable to protect the patient from exaggerated sympathetic or parasympathetic reactions. Some agents used in the horse do not produce complete anesthesia. For example, while chloral hydrate produces a loss of consciousness, it does not provide suitable analgesia or muscle relaxation. Succinylcholine, on the other hand, is a good muscle relaxant but does not reduce pain sensation or level of consciousness. Complete anesthesia can be obtained in two ways: The first method is to induce complete anesthesia with a single drug, such as thiopental, pentobarbital or halothane. In order to achieve adequate narcosis, analgesia and muscle relaxation with a single agent, it must be administered in large doses at high concentrations. This can cause metabolic disturbances by having adverse effects on the cardiovascular and respiratory system, the kidneys and the liver. The second method is to obtain the various components of general anesthesia by means of a combination of different drugs, each with a more or less specific action. For example, a tranquilizer, perhaps combined with atropine, and a narcotic analgesic may be used for premedication; a short-acting barbiturate and short-acting muscle relaxant for induction of anesthesia; and halothane, nitrous oxide and perhaps a muscle relaxant for maintenance of anesthesia. The advantage of such a combination technique is that the drugs need be given only in small doses or low concentrations, thus minimizing any toxic effects that may occur. However, the anesthetist must be familiar with the properties, side-effects and possible interactions of the agents used. When complications arise, it is sometimes difficult to know exactly which drug is responsible, and what treatment is indicated.

1.2.2.2. Depth and Stages of Anesthesia

For the safe administration of the anesthetic it is extremely important to be able to assess accurately the depth of anesthesia. To estimate the depth of anesthesia in man, Guedel divided anesthesia into four stages. This empirical division holds mainly for drugs which have a long induction time, such as diethyl ether and methoxyflurane, but these agents are very seldom used in the horse. The Guedel stages are less satisfactory for drugs which have a short induction time, such as barbiturates, or agents characterized by rapid changes in depth of anesthesia, such as halothane. Moreover, individual differences must be taken into account, as well as the type of induction and premedication. When atropine is used, for example, the pupil size can no longer serve as a criterion for the depth of anesthesia. After a strong muscle relaxant is given, moreover, certain movements and reflexes can no longer be monitored. Thus, while these stages are of only relative value and are much less objective than measurements of the agents in the blood or end expiratory gas concentrations, they nevertheless provide a simple, useful means for anesthetic monitoring in the horse.

Stage I, or the *analgesic stage*, is important only in man. Stage II is characterized by *unconscious excitement*. This excitement depends on the agent used: It is seldom seen with chloral hydrate or halothane and is more frequent with barbiturates. The temperament of the animal and its environment may also play a role such as loud noises. During the excitement stage the breathing is deep and irregular, while the heart rate and arterial blood pressure are elevated. Mydriasis and a rapid nystagmus are present. The swallowing reflex is usually preserved. Muscle tone is increased, and involuntary muscle contractions and struggling movements occur that usually are accompanied by apnea. The oxygen demand is greatly increased by the muscular contractions, which can be quite dangerous if the PaO_2 is lowered as a result of induction with thiobarbiturates. The barbiturates are eliminated from the brain more rapidly by the increased muscular perfusion, requiring that a greater dose be given. Sensitivity to pain is also heightened during the excitement stage. The onset of this stage is sometimes marked by *conscious excitement*, the animal showing resistance to restraining measures or i.v. injection. The excitement stage can usually be prevented by suitable premedication and proper induction. Stage III is the *surgical stage*, which currently is divided into three substages. Stage III_4 of the original Guedel classification is no longer considered part of the surgical stage, but is the result of anesthetic overdose. The transition between these three substages is not always clearly defined. The *first substage* (*III_1*) *is marked by superficial anesthesia*. The breathing is regular, and the nystagmus slows and finally disappears between III_1 and III_2 or at the beginning of III_2. Muscle relaxation is not very pronounced. The swallowing reflex is slowly lost. The palpebral reflex (closure of eyelid in response to tapping of the lid or lashes) becomes less intense. The pupil is constricted. There may still be some pain response in this stage. In some cases, e.g., in high-risk patients, it may be prudent to perform the operation in this stage (III_1), perhaps supplementing the general anesthesia with a local or regional anesthetic. The *second substage* (*III_2*) *is distinguished by a moderate surgical anesthesia*. Eye movements are absent. The corneal reflex (closure of the eyelid when the cornea is touched) weakens and is gradually lost. Lacrimation is decreased, giving the conjunctivae and cornea a dry appearance. Miosis is still present, and the pupillary reflex is weak. Muscle relaxation becomes more pronounced in this stage, but the abdominal muscles are not yet fully relaxed. Cardiovascular depression slowly develops, especially with halothane or barbiturates. *Substage III_3 is marked by deep anesthesia*. All ocular reflexes are absent, and the pupils slowly begin to dilate. The muscles, including the abdominal muscles, are well relaxed. Respiration is for the most part abdominal because the intercostal muscles are paralyzed. Respiratory acidosis and hypoxemia (low PaO_2) develop unless an oxygen-rich mixture is administered. Surgical operations should be minimal during this stage, and artificial respiration should always be given. If good muscular relaxation is desired, it is better to administer a muscle relaxant. Cardiovascular depression is very pronounced. Practically all reflexes are absent. Only the vagal reflexes can still be elicited by tension on abdominal or thoracic structures. *Stage IV* is reached by a *large overdose* and is marked by asphyxia. There is complete paralysis of the abdominal and intercostal muscles. Diaphragmatic activity is preserved initially, but this cannot prevent the extreme respiratory acidosis and hypoxemia that may occur. The pupils are widely dilated and do not respond to light. The arterial blood pressure plummets and respiration ceases. The heartbeat continues for a time until cardiac arrest supervenes.

1.2.2.3. Inhalation Anesthesia

Inhalation anesthesia is recommended for prolonged operations or procedures that require complete unconsciousness. The principal agent for inhalation anesthesia in horses is halothane, possibly combined with nitrous oxide. This form of anesthesia is advantageous, for the depth of anesthesia can be rapidly controlled and adapted to the demands of the procedure. Recovery is rapid, even after prolonged anesthesia. Because the anesthetic agent is delivered in oxygen, there is little danger of hypoxemia with its attendant complications even with pronounced respiratory depression. The main disadvantage is the need for continuous delivery under careful control. For this, an anesthetic machine is required.

1.2.2.3.1. Inhalation Equipment and Techniques

The simple Ayre T-piece is suitable for spontaneous as well as artificial respiration in foals. This is the simplest anesthetic unit, consisting of a rubber tube about 1 m long and 2.5 cm in diameter connected to an endotracheal catheter. The gases to be administered (halothane in O_2 or in O_2/N_2O) are delivered at the junction between the endotrachial catheter and rubber tube (fig. 1.2. — 1). The apparatus is based on the following principle: The exhaled gases are driven out by the inflowing stream of fresh gases. Just after the completion of expiration, the tube is completely filled with

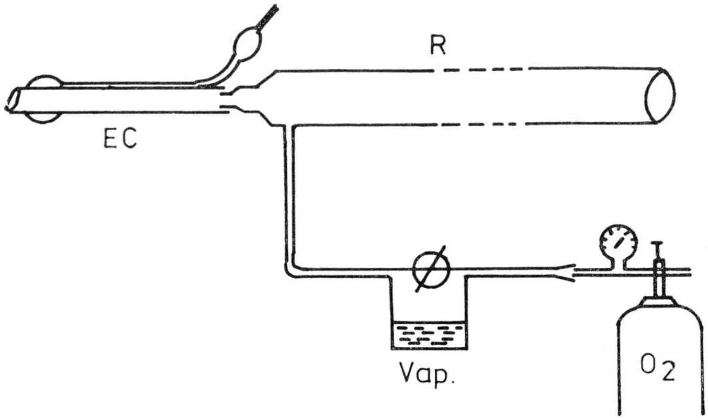

Fig. 1.2. — 1. Ayre T-piece for foals. EC = endotracheal catheter; R = rubber tube (~ 1 m); Vap. = vaporizer.

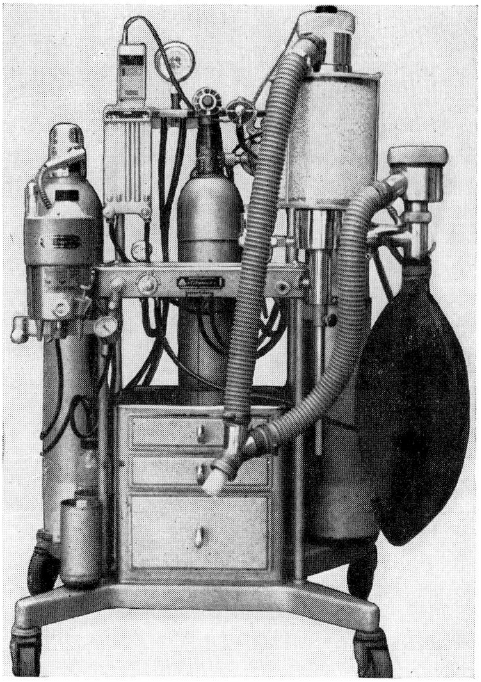

2

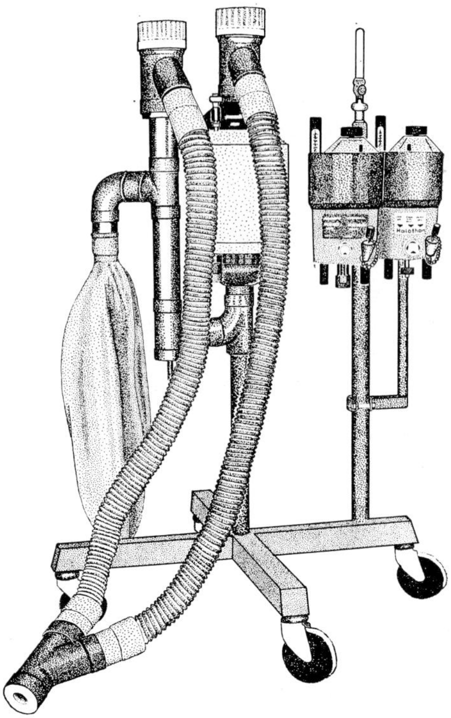

3

Fig. 1.2. — 2. Circle respiration system for horses.

Fig. 1.2. — 3. Circle respiration system (Narkovet-E, Dräger) with absorbers for halothane and methoxyflurane.

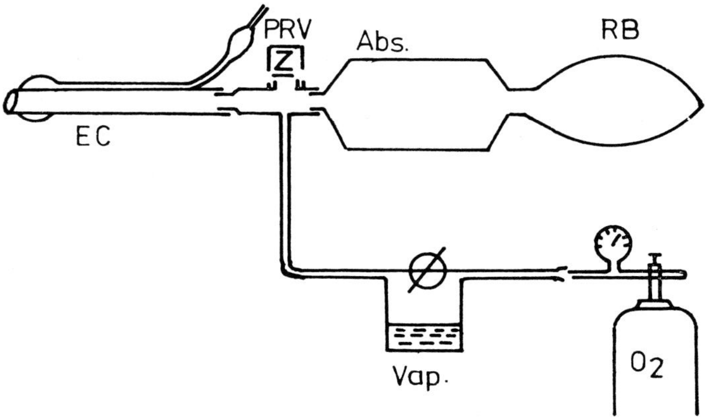

Fig. 1.2. — 4. Schematic diagram of the to-and-fro system. EC = endotracheal catheter; PRV = pressure-relief valve; Abs. = absorber; RB = reservoir bag; Vap. = vaporizer.

fresh gases, which are then inhaled during the next inspiration. The advantages of this system are that it is simple and safe, has no dead space, and offers little resistance to respiration. Its disadvantage is that a large gas flow must be maintained to prevent the rebreathing of CO_2. Other disadvantages are the very high consumption of anesthetic agent and carrier gas, and the discharge of the gases into the environment. The tube length must be in proper relation to the size of the animal. If the tube is too short, air will be inhaled during the inspiratory phase. If it is too long, CO_2 rebreathing will occur unless the fresh gas flow is very high and is at least 3 times the respiratory minute volume, or there is a long pause after exhalation. Most suitable is a tube whose volume is somewhat greater than the tidal volume. Artificial respiration can also be applied with this simple apparatus: If the tube opening is held shut, the stream of fresh gases will enter the lungs. The thorax having been adequately inflated, the tube is reopened, and passive expiration follows. Artificial respiration can also be applied by attaching a reservoir bag with side outlet to the end of the exhalation tube. The systems that exhaust all expiratory gases to the outside are safe but are not very economical.

Open or semiopen systems like the once-popular chloroform masks have become largely obsolete due to their various disadvantages.

Closed and semiclosed systems are most widely used in equine practice. These systems may be of the 'circle' or 'to-and-fro' type. The circle system contains two valves with minimal flow resistance to ensure a one-way flow of gas. The diameters of the horses, the connections to the endotracheal catheter, reservoir bag and CO_2 absorbers, and the valve apertures must be sufficiently large to minimize resistance during inspiration and expiration. A high resistance prevents good ventilation, which in turn can have adverse and even dangerous cardiovascular effects. Although Short [1970] reports no difference between a circle system with a large diameter and one with a small diameter (2.25 cm) in terms of ventilation during one hour of anesthesia, it is, nonetheless, generally agreed that the diameter in such a system must be at least 5 cm (fig. 1.2. — 2 and — 3). In a circle semiclosed system, the exhaust valve of the expiratory hose is mounted in front of the CO_2 absorber. The escaping expiratory gases no longer pass through the CO_2 absorber, which will therefore retain its absorbency for a longer period [Thurmon, 1972]. In a to-and-fro system, which contains no valves and is simpler in design, the gases pass back and forth through a CO_2 absorber between the animal and the reservoir bag (fig. 1.2. — 4).

A horizontal or vertical absorber can be used in the to-and-fro system (fig. 1.2. — 5). Although the respiratory gases in this system pass through the absorber during both inspiration and expiration, the resistance is usually low in a well designed system. The disadvantages of the system are as follows: The absorber, which is located close to the animal, is rapidly exhausted, resulting in a gradual increase in the dead space. In addition, the inspiratory gases are heated by the chemical reaction in the CO_2 absorber. If a horizontal absorber is used, it must be filled completely with granules, for otherwise the air will follow the path of least resistance, and CO_2 absorption will be incomplete. There is also a danger that the horse will inhale irritant material from the lime absorbent during induction.

In the semiclosed system the anesthetic agent can be delivered in O_2 or in a mixture of O_2 and N_2O. The flow rate of the carrier gas is less than the minute volume but greater than the volume consumed by the animal and the absorber. Excess gas is vented to the outside or, for safety reasons, should be scavenged. The rest passes through the absorber. A semiclosed system is safer than a closed system, in which the volume of oxygen supplied corresponds to that consumed by the animal and the absorber. In a completely closed system the gas delivery must be in perfect equili-

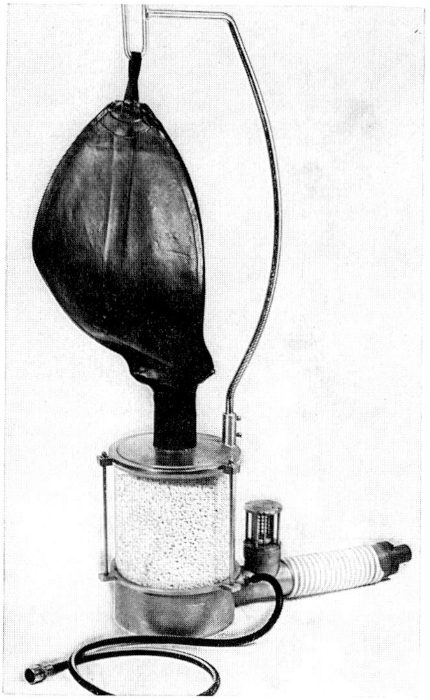

Fig. 1.2. — 5. To-and-fro system with vertical absorber.

brium with the gas consumption. Closed systems are chiefly used in horses, though in reality most of these systems are not completely closed. A closed system is very economical in its consumption, since no oxygen or anesthetic agent is lost. Owing to the smaller gas flow, the absorption of CO_2 is improved. The inspired gases are humidified, which is beneficial in terms of ciliary function in the airways, and the exothermic reaction in the absorber warms the inspiratory gases, thus protecting against hypothermia. The closed system also eliminates the possible escape of anesthetic gases into the environment. On the other hand, the less efficient semiclosed system is advantageous in that the anesthetic can be delivered in a mixture of oxygen and nitrous oxide in a 1: 1 to 1: 3 ratio. Owing to the analgesic effect of the nitrous oxide, smaller concentrations of halothane may be used, thereby reducing the adverse cardiovascular side-effects of this agent (see below). Without control of the inspiratory oxygen concentration, nitrous oxide is safe to use only in the semiclosed system, in which the excess can escape, thereby eliminating the danger of hypoxemia. The smaller the gas flow, the higher the O_2: N_2O ratio must be in order to achieve an adequate O_2 concentration [Schilling and Weis, 1973a]. The highest inspiratory O_2 concentration is obtained with systems in which the fresh gas is delivered in close proximity to the inspiratory valve. The differences are particularly marked at small gas flows and low O_2 concentrations [Schillig and Weis, 1973b]. If means are available for monitoring the inspiratory O_2 concentration or the arterial O_2 pressure (PaO_2), then nitrous oxide can be used even in closed systems [Skarda, 1974].

'Diffusion hyperoxia' can develop during the induction of nitrous oxide anesthesia. This involves an increase in the alveolar O_2 concentration brought on by the rapid diffusion of nitrous oxide from the pulmonary tissues into the blood.

In both the closed and semiclosed systems, it is preferable to use a transparent absorption canister. This contains granules composed chiefly of $Ca(OH)_2$, which absorb the expired CO_2 to form $CaCO_3$ and H_2O. The reaction is exothermic. An indicator is added to the $Ca(OH)_2$ that will cause it to change color when saturated, thus indicating that the absorber is exhausted; in addition, no further heat is generated. The more free water is present in the absorber, the more pronounced the color change. The color indicator is not completely reliable, and marked differences exist between the different absorbent granules available. The air space between the granules should at least equal the animal's tidal volume. When completely filled, about 50% of the volume of the absorber is occupied by granules. When respiration is monitored with a capnograph, it can be seen that the absorber usually retains its absorbency much longer than its color index would suggest. An absorber with a volume of 7—10 l should be satisfactory. Two absorbers, one on top of the other, can be used to reduce consumption of the lime absorbent. When the first absorber is completely exhausted, it is filled with fresh lime, and the second absorber is mounted in its place. 'Canalization', or the flow of gas through areas of least resistance, and the associated loss of absorber efficiency can be prevented by packing the granules densely and uniformly in the canister or by arranging them in concentric lamellae [Zetner, 1973]. The lime absorbent is less rapidly consumed in a semiclosed system, because a portion of the expired CO_2, together with excess gases, escapes through the exhaust valve ahead of the absorber.

The reservoir bag must be able to expand during expiration without offering too much resistance and must have an adequate reserve volume. The reservoir bag is usually kept $^2/_3$ to $^3/_4$ full during anesthesia. If the reserve volume is too small, the animal may inhale air during a deep inspiration; if the bag is overfilled, the expiratory resistance becomes too high. A volume of 20—30 l is necessary in horses. The gas volume within the system and reservoir bag dilutes the inflowing anesthetic gases, however, thereby prolonging the time needed to establish equilibrium between the expired and inspired anesthetic gases. The volume of the circle system and reservoir bag should not be too large [Steffey and Howland, 1977]. The reservoir bag in the circle system may be on the inspiratory or expiratory side of the circuit. If attached on the expiratory side, the expiratory resistance is low; if on the inspiratory side, the inspiratory resistance is low [Schreiber, 1972].

In both the circle and to-and-fro systems, a suitable vaporizer must be present for the anesthetic agent. In the to-and-fro system the vaporizer is always placed outside the system (out of circuit) in the fresh gas stream. In the circle system the vaporizer may be mounted in-circuit or out-of-circuit. An in-circuit vaporizer is preferred for substances that do not vaporize readily, such as methoxyflurane, or for substances administered in high concentrations, such as diethyl ether. To avoid overdosing, the vaporizer for halothane anesthesia is usually mounted *out-of-circuit*. Overdose is a particular danger when switching from spontaneous breathing to artificial respiration. In hypoventilation, for example, little halothane is inhaled. When artificial ventilation is started, a large dose of the anesthetic is suddenly delivered to the lungs. During artificial ventilation, then, it is best to use an out-of-circuit vaporizer. One difficulty with in-circuit vaporizers is the condensation of water in the vaporizer. Vaporizers that are designed for out-of-circuit use should not be installed in-circuit due, among other things, to their high resistance.

Halothane vaporizers that are to be operated in the fresh gas stream (that is, outside the circuit) are available in both a simple (fig. 1.2. — 6) and a high-precision design. The Vapor® precision vaporizer, for example (fig. 1.2. — 7), differs from the simple model in that it indicates the exact concentrations of the anesthetic regardless

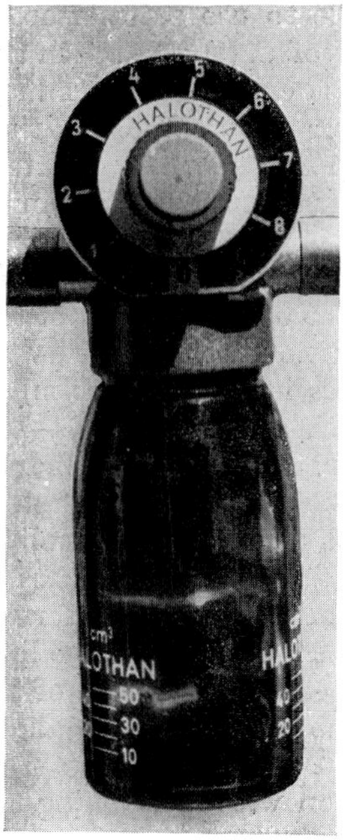

6

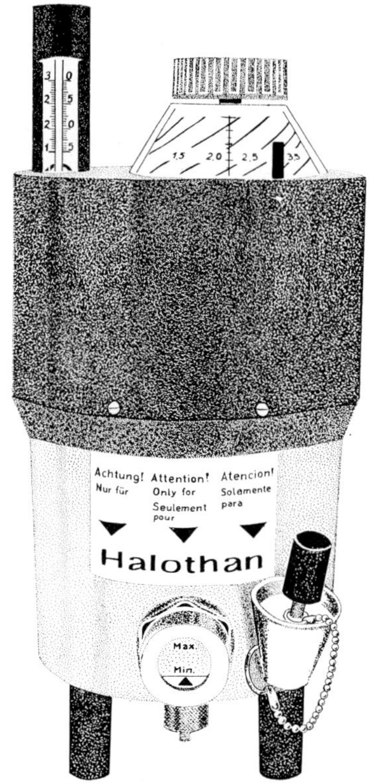

7

Fig. 1.2. — 6. Halothane vaporizer.
Fig. 1.2. — 7. Vapor® high-precision vaporizer.

of temperature and at flow rates between 300 ml and 10 l/min. Pressure variations that can arise during artificial respiration also have no effect on the concentration. It should be noted, however, that the inspired concentration does not coincide with the vaporizer concentration outside the circuit. Owing to the diluting effect of the expired gases, the inspired concentration is usually lower.

The horse should be connected to the anesthesia machine via a mask or endotracheal tube. With a mask it is more difficult to obtain an airtight seal. An advantage of the endotracheal tube is that the upper airways remain free at all times, and saliva, gastric contents, blood or pus cannot be aspirated. Moreover, the dead space is smaller with the endotracheal tube.

Intubation is a relatively simple procedure in the horse and can practically always be done 'blindly'. The largest sized tube that can be easily passed should be used (i.e., at least 30 mm for mature horses) in order to minimize airflow resistance. The curved endotracheal tubes are more easily passed than straight ones. For intubation the animal is placed in lateral recumbency, the head is held in moderate extension, a mouth speculum is inserted, and the tongue is pulled forward. The tube, which is lubricated with a suitable jelly, can then be pushed through the larynx without difficulty in most cases. The curved tube is best introduced into the mouth with its concave side toward the hard palate. With its tip in the pharynx, the tube is rotated 180°, and with the tip centered, the tube is advanced through the larynx into the trachea during the next inspiration [HALL, 1971 b]. The cuff should be inflated, but not overinflated (see below), to obtain an airtight seal. The adapters for connecting the tube to the anesthesia machine should not be smaller in diameter than the endotracheal tube.

1.2.2.3.2. Inhalation Anesthetic Agents

Chloroform. Chloroform, which was formerly administered to horses by mask, is now obsolete. It was used in semiopen systems with a mask or in closed or semiclosed systems following induction with chloral hydrate, glyceryl guaiacolate or a barbiturate. Though potent and inexpensive, chloroform is hepatotoxic, and an overdose can cause severe cardiovascular depression. With close cardiovascular and respiratory monitoring, chloroform anesthesia would presumably be less dangerous than in earlier years when this agent was used in semiopen systems, without oxygen, and with minimal monitoring of cardiovascular and respiratory functions.

Diethyl Ether. Diethyl ether is less toxic, produces good muscle relaxation, causes no respiratory depression, and is inexpensive. Its great disadvantage is that it is flammable and explosive in both oxygen and air. Due to its slow induction, ether should be given only after induction with another drug. The high concentrations necessary for anesthesia can generally be attained only with the aid of an in-circuit vaporizer. Ether vapors cause mild irritation of the respiratory passages. It is not used for general anesthesia in horses in North America.

Metofane[1]. Methoxyflurane is not widely used in horses. Induction is slow, recovery is prolonged, and respiratory depression is marked. Cardiovascular depression is less pronounced than with halothane. Methoxyflurane should be administered with an in-circuit vaporizer. No studies are available in the horse relating to a possible nephrotoxic effect of methoxyflurane, like that occurring in humans. The fluorine released by the metabolic breakdown of methoxyflurane is responsible for this effect.

Fluothane. Fluothane (Halothane) is neither flammable nor explosive. It is a very potent anesthetic that is widely used in horses in both closed and semiclosed systems; it is often combined with nitrous oxide. Induction is best obtained with guaifenesin, followed by a low dose of thiopental thiamylal or ketamine. Induction with thiopental sometimes causes severe hypoventilation or induction apnea, with the result that too little halothane is inspired. The horse is connected to the anesthesia machine by endotracheal tube. Normal halothane anesthesia provides moderate muscle relaxation; however, high concentrations can have dangerous cardiovascular effects and cause extreme muscular relaxation. Halothane causes moderate to strong respiratory depression [Müller, 1967]. The depressive effect of halothane on respiration diminishes during anesthesia of several hours' duration, although prolonged halothane anesthesia can have an adverse effect on the surfactant in the lungs — an effect that may be accentuated by artificial respiration. Halothane causes a marked, dosedependent hypotension, mainly during the first 15 min of anesthesia. The systolic and diastolic pressures then rise again but do not attain their initial values [Lees et al., 1971]. The partial reversal that follows the initial depression of cardiac function may be the result of respiratory acidosis [Hillidge and Lees, 1977b]. It may also reflect the end-point of cardiovascular depression by the inducing agent such as thiopental [Hillidge and Lees, 1977c]. The cardiodepressive effects of low halothane concentrations are probably reversible to some degree by surgical stimulation. Completely divergent effects of halothane on the total peripheral resistance have been reported by various authors [Hillidge and Lees, 1977a; Steffey and Howland, 1978]. The

[1] Methoxyflurane. Pitman Moore, Washington Crossing, NJ 08560 (USA).

hypotension caused by halothane is not ordinarily dangerous at the usual concentrations [NEUMANN and WINTZER, 1975]. Like most anesthetic agents, halothane causes a concentration-dependent decrease in myocardial contractile force with a fall of the stroke volume and heart rate, i.e., a decline of the cardiac output.

The depression of myocardial contractility is probably not a product of metabolism. Halothane may decrease the amount of Ca^{++} available for the contractile proteins and inhibit the reaction between Ca^{++} and these proteins [PRICE, 1974]. This is manifested by a blood pressure drop, since halothane also exerts a direct relaxing effect on the vascular smooth muscle. Because halothane also has an inhibitory effect on the sympathetic nervous system, the depression of the myocardium and peripheral blood vessels cannot be compensated for by an increase in the heart rate or by peripheral vasoconstriction. A rise of the hematocrit occurs with increasing concentration [STEFFEY et al., 1977b]. Recovery is rapid but is sometimes marked by muscular tremor and impaired coordination on rising.

Nitrous Oxide. Nitrous oxide (N_2O) is a gas with a weak anesthetic action. Its use in horses is principally in combination with another anesthetic agent, such as halothane. It is generally assumed that N_2O has no adverse effects on the myocardium (see Oxygen Supply). The best means of obtaining an N_2O concentration that is as high as possible but not hypoxic, is to completely eliminate nitrogen as much as possible. This can be done by emptying the reservoir bag several times via the pressure relief valve, especially during induction of anesthesia, and then partially refilling it with O_2 and N_2O. To avoid diffusion hypoxia when turning off the machine, the administration of N_2O should be discontinued 15 min before the end of anesthesia.

Nitrous oxide is contraindicated if a closed, air-filled space is present in the animal, such as might occur in pneumothorax or intestinal obstruction. This is because the diffusion of N_2O into these spaces is 35 times greater than its diffusion from them. This can lead to a critical pressure of volume increase, especially during prolonged anesthesia with high nitrous oxide concentrations (SCHUH [1975]; fig. 1.2. — 8). Animals that have not been fasted are highly prone to tympany caused by accumulation of the gas in the digestive tract.

Isoflurane. (Compound 469, or Forane)[1]. Induction and recovery are rapid, and coordination on rising is good [AUER et al., 1978]. Isoflurane causes a halothane-like hypoventilation.

Enflurane. (Ethrane)[2] Enflurane, like isoflurane, is chemically similar to methoxyflurane. Its properties are similar to those of halothane. Enflurane causes greater cardiovascular depression than isoflurane, deeper hypotension, and in some cases abnormal muscular contractions or epileptoid movements, especially at high concentrations. The flow rate is very high, requiring a reservoir bag of at least 20-liters capacity. The margin of safety for producing respiratory and circulatory arrest is smaller than with most inhalation anesthetics. Enflurane is, therefore, less safe [STEFFEY, 1978].

1.2.2.3.3. Artificial Respiration

Artificial respiration is indicated in cases of marked hypoventilation or respiratory failure. It is also indicated during prolonged halothane anesthesia or operations on animals in 'shock' that show a fall of pH from an inadequate CO_2 excretion that is

[1] Compound 469 (or Forane). Ohio Medical Products, Madison, Wisc. (USA).
[2] Ethraine. Ohio Medical Products, Madison, Wisc. (USA).

accentuated by lactic acid accumulation. Respiratory failure resulting from induction of anesthesia with thiobarbiturates can be treated by extending the head and applying rhythmic pressure on the thorax. The animal usually responds to each compression of the thorax with a spontaneous inspiration. If spontaneous inspiration fails to occur, one can try pulling the uppermost foreleg upward and craniad, especially in young animals. This will stretch the thorax somewhat. At the same time, oxygen can be administered by nasopharyngeal catheter (insufflation) or even by intubation via tracheostomy.

With normal cardiac function, it is unnecessary to support artificial respiration by drug therapy. Spontaneous respiration usually recommences after a few minutes. For the treatment of more prolonged apnea after succinylcholine and/or barbiturates,

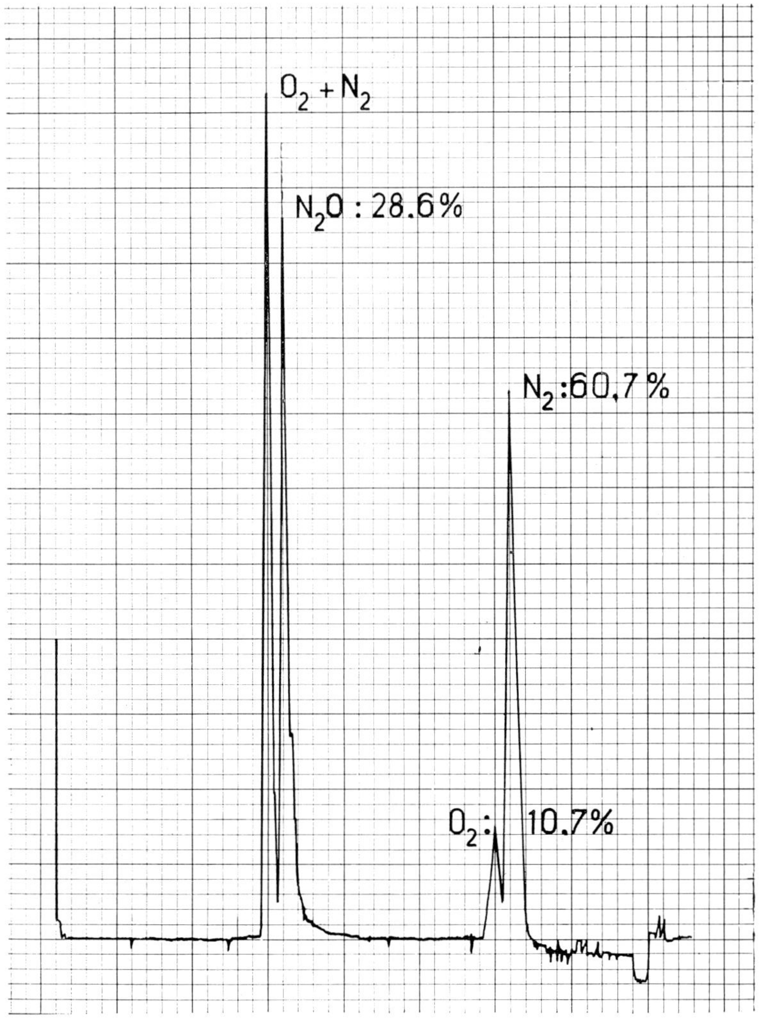

Fig. 1.2. — 8. Nitrous oxide concentration in the jejunum of a foal with volvulus of the jejunum after 1 h and 45 min of halothane/N_2O/O_2 anesthesia.

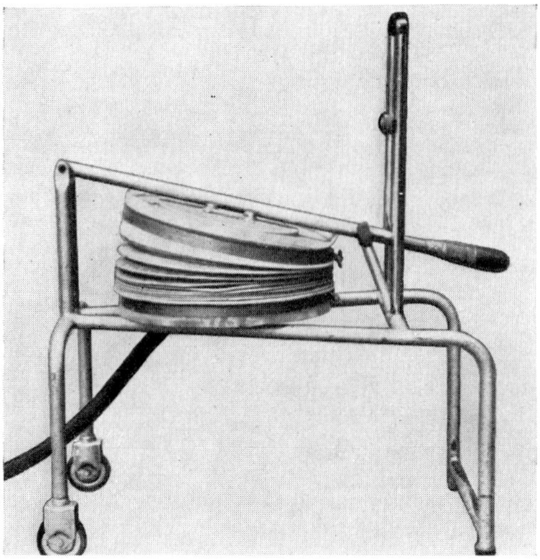
9

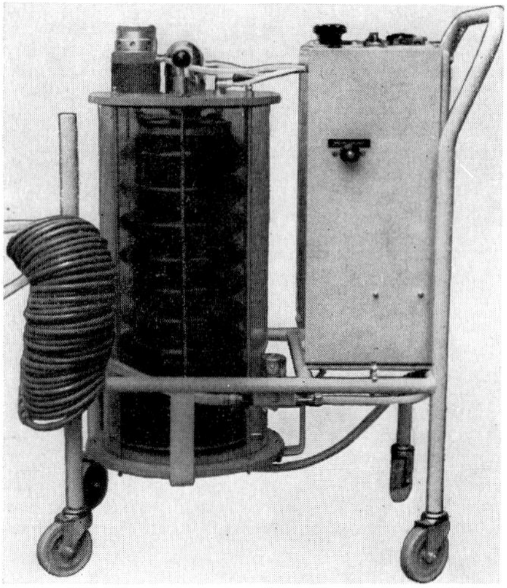
10

Fig. 1.2. — 9. Bellows for artificial respiration.
Fig. 1.2. — 10. Smith respirator.

a simple respirator has been described [SHORT et al., 1971]. If the horse is connected by endotracheal tube to a closed or semiclosed system, artificial respiration can be conducted in various ways.

Manual compression of the reservoir bag is (except in foals) effective for only a short time. Mature horses can be very effectively ventilated with a simple bellows apparatus (fig. 1.2. — 9). Both intermittent positive pressure and alternating pressure can be applied with this device. In *alternating pressure ventilation* the respiratory gases are introduced into the lungs under a positive pressure of 15—30 cm H_2O, while in the expiratory phase the gases are drawn out of the airways by a slight negative pressure. This negative pressure stimulates the venous return to the heart. Alternating pressure ventilation is undesired in open-chest operations, because the negative pressure reduces the diameter of the alveoli during the expiratory phase, predisposing to alveolar collapse and atelectasis. In *intermittent positive pressure ventilation* the respiratory gases are delivered to the lungs under a pressure of 15—30 cm H_2O, but the pressure at the end of expiration is zero. This method hampers venous return, though this can be compensated for in healthy animals by peripheral venous constriction. This technique can be dangerous in animals with hypovolemia, especially in the presence of high pressures and a too high ratio of inspiration time to expiration time. A ratio of 1 : 2 or even 1 : 3 is desirable in hypovolemia. Ventilation should be regulated such that the arterial CO_2 pressure ($PaCO_2$) is about 40 mm Hg. The minute volume should be approximately 10 l/100 kg. Artificial respiration is carried out at a rate of 5—15 excursions/min. The bellows or respirator should be adjusted to deliver 4—6.5 l per inspiration to a mature horse. In a semiclosed system, 5 l O_2 and 5 l N_2O per min should be given. Thoroughbreds seem to have a greater respiratory volume than other breeds. The tidal volume of adult Thoroughbreds is 7.5—12 l, with a minute volume of 36—96 l [PURCHASE, 1965]. With a minute volume of 7.6 l/100 kg during spontaneous respiration, a minute volume of 18.5 l/100 kg is necessary during artificial respiration in order to obtain a $PaCO_2$ of 5.33 kPa [WEAVER and WALLEY, 1975]. SCHATZMANN (1978), however, found that a minute volume of 6 to

15 l/100 kg was adequate during controlled respiration in 85 horses. The large alveolar-arterial O_2 gradient cannot be prevented by setting the end-expiratory resistance at a pressure of 10—20 cm H_2O during spontaneous respiration [HALL and TRIM, 1975].

An alternative to the simple bellows, of course, are automatic respirators. The peak inspiratory delivery rate for lightly anesthetized horses with a body weight of 350—500 kg varies between 250 and 500 l/min. Therefore, artificial respirators for horses must be capable of supplying a flow of at least 250 l/min [STEFFEY and BERRY, 1977]. The switch from the inspiratory to the expiratory phase in these machines is accomplished chiefly by three different mechanisms:

1. *Pressure-controlled respirators*, such as the Bird Respirator[1], switch from inspiration to expiration when a specific pressure is attained in the airways [SKARDA et al., 1974]. The disadvantage of these units is that they deliver an increasingly smaller volume as the airway resistance rises. Once the designated pressure is reached, the gases are not uniformly distributed in the lungs.

2. *Volume-controlled respirators* deliver a constant volume to the lungs with each inspiration, regardless of the pressure in the airways. Some of these units, such as the Smith respirator (fig. 1.2. — 10) also have an end-expiratory plateau, which provides better distribution of the gases in the lungs

3. *Time-controlled respirators* change from inspiration to expiration after a designated time. These respirators are not always efficient, however.

Artificial respiration is usually of the controlled type. That is, the animal no longer breathes spontaneously, and both the volume and rate are controlled by the anesthetist. With certain respirators, such as the Bird or Smith, assisted respiration can also be given, i.e., the animal still breathes spontaneously and determines its own respiratory rate. If the spontaneous rate is too low, a respiratory assist may not be adequate. Nevertheless, every inspiration is carried to a designated volume or airway pressure by the machine. These units can usually be adjusted to switch from assisted to controlled respiration if the delay between breaths is too long. With a bellows or well-adjusted automatic respirator, the transition from spontaneous to artificial respiration in the horse is smooth, despite the departure from the spontaneous respiratory pattern. Muscle relaxants are unnecessary during the transition to artificial respiration. If muscle relaxants are desired, however, Flaxedil (gallamine triethiodide[2]) can be given in a dose of 0.5—1.5 mg/kg i.v. or the infusion of succinylcholine at a rate of 20 μg/kg/min [MUIR and SKARDA, 1976]. At the end of the relaxation period, 30—50 mg atropine is given i.v. followed by the i.v. injection of 5—20 mg Styglin (neostigmine methylsulfate[3]). The Smith respirator can be adjusted to a tidal volume of 2—12 l. It can develop a positive pressure of 80 cm H_2O, which is ample; it can develop a pressure of —5 cm H_2O during the expiratory phase. The respirator can be operated in either the pressure-controlled or volume-controlled mode, and both controlled and assisted respiration can be given. A manual control feature is also present. Young foals can be ventilated with the anesthesic machines as well as with respirators designed for human use (fig. 1.2. — 11).

When the time comes to conclude artificial respiration, the animal is allowed to lighten as much as possible from the anesthesia, while the minute volume is reduced until the $PaCO_2$ rises sufficiently to stimulate the respiratory center. Care is taken, however, to avoid hypoxemia or excessive respiratory acidosis. As long as

[1] Bird Man 7 ventilator. Bird Corporation, Palm Springs, Calif. (USA).

[2] Flaxedil. Davis and Geck, American Cyanamid Company, Pearl River, N.Y. (USA).

[3] Styglin. Pitman Moore, Washington Crossing, N.J. (USA).

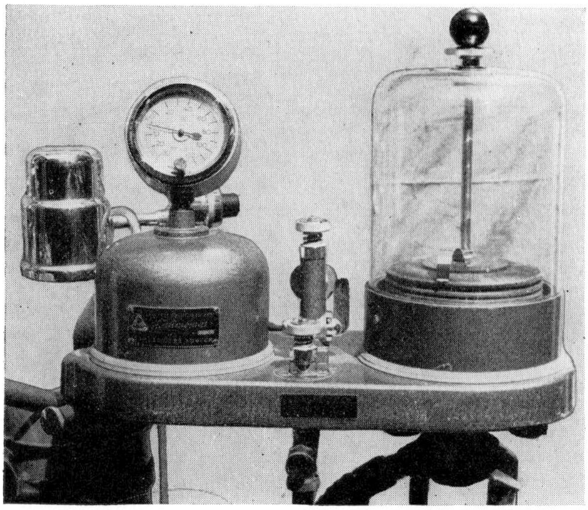

Fig. 1.2. — 11. Pulmonat respirator (Dräger).

spontaneous breathing is poor, artificial respiration must be regularly applied. Some horses resume spontaneous breathing quickly after artificial respiration, while others require several minutes. Spontaneous breathing can be established almost immediately by the intravenous injection of 0.5 mg/kg Dopram (doxapram hydrochloride)[1]. This drug does not cause muscle contraction or spasms and acts by stimulating the peripheral chemoreceptors of the carotid artery [Mitchell and Herbert, 1975]. In horses it is a safe and highly effective drug. It has no antianalgesic effect with respect to the morphine derivatives. Its duration of action is 8—12 min.

1.2.2.3.4. Oxygen Supply and Acid-Base Balance during General Anesthesia

During general anesthesia and the postanesthetic period, it is essential that an adequate tissue oxygen delivery be maintained, and the arterial CO_2 pressure ($PaCO_2$) and pH remain within normal limits. The total O_2-carrying capacity of the blood is calculated as follows:

O_2 (ml/min) = cardiac output (ml/min) × O_2 content of arterial blood
= cardiac output × arterial O_2 saturation SaO_2 (%) × hemoglobin content (g/ml) × 1.39 (where 1.39 represents the ml of O_2 that can be transported by one gram of hemoglobin).

The O_2 uptake of the tissue per minute is then given by the product of the cardiac output and arteriovenous O_2 difference (av DO_2). If the transport capacity of the blood is impaired by a decrease in the cardiac output, hemoglobin content or degree of saturation, the body can still meet the tissue oxygen demand by increased O_2 extraction from the blood. This is difficult in the myocardium, however, because its O_2 extraction is normally very high, and the O_2 content of the coronary venous blood is very low.

This formula, of course, can be applied only with a normal microcirculation. If the microcirculation is impaired, as in various forms of shock, the O_2 delivery to the tissues is always deficient. Nevertheless, this seemingly theoretical formula is still

[1] Doxapram hydrochloride. A. H. Robbins, Richmond, VA 23220 (USA).

of considerable practical importance. If any one of the three variables is decreased, there will be a proportionate decrease in the O_2-carrying capacity of the blood. For example, if the cardiac output is reduced by half, the O_2-carrying capacity will also be reduced by half. A very large fall of the cardiac output can further cause a decrease in the arterial O_2 pressure (PaO_2) and thus in the O_2 saturation (SaO_2) as well. If two of the three factors are reduced by half, the O_2-carrying capacity is reduced by three-fourths.

What changes do these three factors undergo during general halothane anesthesia in the horse?

1. Cardiac output. Halothane causes a marked, concentration-dependent decrease in the cardiac output [EBERLY et al., 1968; GILLESPIE et al., 1969].

This fall of the cardiac output is chiefly the result of a diminished stroke volume and heart rate. The decrease in the stroke volume and cardiac output are usually most pronounced during induction of anesthesia. Thereafter the stroke volume slowly increases, with an associated rise in the cardiac output. With a rise of the $PaCO_2$, the cardiac output falls sharply [HILLIDGE and LEES, 1975a]. GILLESPIE and coworkers, however, found a less pronounced depression of the cardiac output with a high $PaCO_2$. During spontaneous respiration ($PaCO_2$ of 8.64 kPa) the cardiac output is nearly twice as high as during artificial respiration ($PaCO_2$ of 4.66 kPa). This is due to the much higher ejection volume during spontaneous ventilation [STEFFY and HOWLAND, 1978a]. While respiratory acidosis has a depressive effect on myocardial contractility, it can also stimulate the heart via central sympathetic pathways, though this mechanism may be less effective during general anesthesia. The cardiac output of the horse in dorsal recumbency is less than in lateral recumbency. In addition, ventilation-perfusion disturbances and shunting in combination with a low cardiac output can account for the poor arterial oxygen supply and unfavourable cardiovascular state in old and heavy horses in dorsal recumbency. In view of the fact that the depression of the cardiac output is concentration-dependent, halothane anesthesia in the horse should be kept as shallow as possible. The palpebral reflex should almost always remain, and a slow nystagmus may even be present in some horses. This is a good method of avoiding hypotension and severe depressions of the cardiac output. Another method of minimizing cardiac output depression is to deliver the anesthetic agent in an N_2O/O_2 mixture instead of pure oxygen; nitrous oxide causes virtually no myocardial depression [GOLDBERG et al., 1972; STOELTING et al., 1972]. If halothane is used with 70—75% N_2O, the peripheral vascular resistance and cardiac output may even increase in the dog: These differences are particularly evident during spontaneous respiration [STEFFEY et al., 1975]. In spontaneous respiration the combination of halothane, nitrous oxide and oxygen causes less cardiovascular depression than halothane with oxygen alone. During artificial respiration, the difference between the two combinations (halothane/N_2O/O_2 and halothane/O_2) in terms of cardiovascular depression is much less apparent or even absent [STEFFEY and HOWLAND, 1978b]. Hence, a mixture of N_2O and O_2 should be used to deliver the anesthetic agent in horses that are in poor general health (e.g., in shock).

2. Arterial O_2 saturation of the hemoglobin (SaO_2). The oxygen saturation of the hemoglobin is mainly dependent on the arterial oxygen pressure (PaO_2). This is expressed in an O_2 dissociation curve. The O_2 dissociation curve of the horse is very similar but not identical to that of man [SCHMIDT-NIELSEN and LARIMER, 1958]. This curve indicates how much O_2 is carried in the blood at a given O_2 pressure. At an O_2 pressure of 100 mm Hg, approximately 20 ml of O_2 are bound to hemoglobin and 0.3 ml dissolved in the plasma per 100 ml of blood. According to the curve, a decrease in the PaO_2 does not always result in a corresponding decrease in the O_2

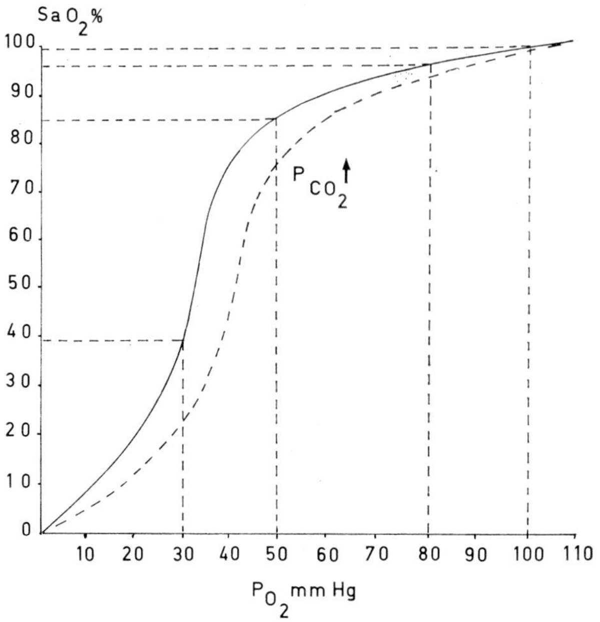

Fig. 1.2. — 12. Oxygen dissociation curve.

saturation (fig. 1.2. — 12). For example, a decrease in the PaO_2 from 100 to 80 mm Hg will cause only a slight change in saturation, while a fall of the PaO_2 from 50 to 30 mm Hg will produce an enormous change.

The O_2 dissociation curve can be shifted to the right or left by various factors. A right shift means that the saturation is lower for the same O_2 pressure, but the O_2 release to the tissues is improved. At a high arterial O_2 pressure, however, a right or left shift has practically no effect on hemoglobin saturation. A right shift of the curve can have various causes, including a rise of the $PaCO_2$, a fall of the pH, a temperature increase, and an increase in the content of 2,3-diphosphoglycerate (DPG) in the erythrocytes. In acidosis, however, a right shift is compensated for by a decrease in the 2,3-DPG content of the erythrocytes, resulting in a left shift [BELLINGHAM et al., 1971]. The right shift of the O_2 dissociation curve caused by an increased $PaCO_2$ is more pronounced in the horse than in man [RIGGS, 1960]. To maintain an adequate arterial O_2 pressure (PaO_2), an inspiratory O_2 pressure of at least 200 mm Hg is needed during general anesthesia. There is an inspiratory arterial O_2 gradient of approximately 0.87 kPa (65 mm Hg) during the inspiration of air without anesthesia (from 21.3 kPa, or 160 mm Hg, in the air to 12.7 kPa, or 95 mm Hg, in the arterial blood). The main cause of arterial hypoxemia is a) a low alveolar O_2 pressure (P_AO_2) and/or b) an increase in the alveolar arterial O_2 gradient $P(A - a)O_2$.

a) A decrease in the alveolar O_2 pressure (P_AO_2) can have the following causes:

(i) A decrease in the inspiratory O_2 concentration: This can result from an inadequate oxygen flow in the closed system, too much N_2O/O_2 in a closed or semiclosed system, or postanesthetic diffusion hypoxia. In a closed system, an oxygen flow of 2 l/min is nearly always sufficient to maintain a satisfactory inspiratory O_2 concentration. The closed system is first flushed with O_2 and then filled with 6—8 l of O_2 and perhaps two to three times as much N_2O (16—18 l). The thorax is manually compressed at the end of an expiration in order to eliminate as much N_2-containing air as possible; then the endotracheal tube is connected to the closed system. The nitrous oxide is now switched off. Oxygen concentrations of 40—50% are obtained after 5 min spontaneous respiration by this method. These concentrations gradually increase, reaching about 55% after 15 min, 60—65% after 30 min, and about 70% after 1 h [DeMoor and van den Hende, 1972]. It is unnecessary in a closed system to empty the reservoir bag at regular intervals in order to eliminate the N_2 and achieve an adequate O_2 concentration. However, more N_2O can be given after emptying the bag shortly after the induction of anesthesia.

(ii) A decrease in alveolar ventilation. Any reduction of alveolar ventilation by premedication, indication, halothane or muscle relaxants under conditions of constant CO_2 production will cause an elevated alveolar or arterial CO_2 pressure along with a decreased P_AO_2. Halothane anesthesia produces an alveolar hypoventilation that can become severe at high concentrations and during prolonged anesthesia and may be accompanied by an extreme hypercapnia and respiratory acidosis. (This is not observed at very low concentrations despite an increased production of CO_2.) Owing to the fact that the inspiratory O_2 concentrations are usually high when anesthesia machines are used, the alveolar hypoventilation often will not provoke arterial hypoxemia, unless there is a marked increase in the alveolar-arterial O_2 gradient, or if O_2 is not administered during the postanesthetic period. Hypercapnia can have various adverse consequences, such as fall of the pH, cardiac arrhythmias, and a heightened cardiac response to vagal stimulation (especially in hypoxia), as well as a posthypercapnic cardiac irritability. Unanesthetized horses respond to a rise of the $PaCO_2$ with an increase in the respiratory minute volume, caused by an increase in the tidal volume. At a low $PaCO_2$, by contrast, the respiratory minute volume is increased mainly by a rise in the respiratory rate [Muir et al., 1975a]. General anesthesia alters this stimulatory effect of a low PaO_2 and high $PaCO_2$ on the respiration, however.

In the dog, extreme hypoxemia acts to stimulate the cardiac output and ventilation at low halothane concentrations. At higher concentrations, however, respiratory or cardiac arrest develops. Thus, in severe hypoxemia it is mainly the halothane concentration that determines whether there will be a stimulation or depression of respiration and cardiac output [Cullen and Eger, 1970]. In unanesthetized dogs and at low halothane concentrations (e.g., 1% alveolar), there is an increase in ventilation with progressive hypercapnia. As the halothane concentration is increased, this response diminishes, while 2.25% halothane produces respiratory depression with a rise of the P_ACO_2 above 80 mm Hg [Brandstater et al., 1965]. The stimulatory effect of CO_2 on respiration in the dog is weakest when hypoxemia is present [Weiskopf et al., 1974].

Barbiturates, especially pentobarbital, also strongly suppress the stimulatory effects of hypoxemia and hypercapnia on respiration [Heath, 1973]. Even the administration of tranquilizers in the horse inhibits respiratory stimulation by hypoxemia or hypercapnia. The inhalation of 100% O_2, however, causes no respiratory depression, in contrast to an O_2 content of only 20% in the inspired air [Muir and Hamlin, 1975]. Thus, during prolonged halothane anesthesia and in animals in poor general health (shock, intestinal obstruction), artificial respiration by endotracheal tube is indicated, together with treatment of the cause of hypoventilation.

(iii) A mechanical obstruction of any variety. These include trauma or obstruction of the upper airways, trachea or bronchi; flexion of the head; abnormal body position; respiratory secretions; the aspiration of gastric contents, pus or blood; pneumothorax; compression of the thorax; increased resistance from the use of narrow-lumen endotracheal tubes; and an increase in the respiratory dead space. The latter cause is important in the horse, for this species has a very large respiratory dead space. The volume ratio of dead space to tidal volume is quite high during halothane anesthesia: 0.6 to 0.75 [HALL, 1971a]. This dead space can be further increased during anesthesia by the apparatus used. The respiratory dead space in the dog is also increased by emphysema or chronic bronchitis, by heavy bleeding or hypotension [SUWA et al., 1966], and during a fall of the pulmonary arterial blood pressure. Induction of anesthesia with chloral hydrate, succinylcholine or thiopental usually causes alveolar hypoventilation with a low PaO_2 and high $PaCO_2$. In some cases, however, it is difficult to determine whether arterial hypoxemia is the result of a decrease in the alveolar O_2 pressure (PaO_2) or an increase in the alveolar-arterial O_2 gradient. If the hypoxemia is the result of decreased alveolar ventilation, then there will be a simultaneous rise in the arterial CO_2 pressure ($PaCO_2$).

b) An increase in the alveolar-arterial O_2 gradient is characterized by a decreased PaO_2, a more or less normal $PaCO_2$, and a normal inspiratory O_2 pressure (P/O_2). The causes of an increased alveolar-arterial O_2 gradient ($P(A - a)O_2$) are:

(i) Diffusion loss of O_2: This diffusion gradient is very small and almost never causes hypoxemia, even in pulmonary disease.

This factor can be entirely eliminated by increasing the inspiratory O_2 concentration.

(ii) Ventilation-perfusion disturbances: These disturbances involve an imbalance between the ventilation and perfusion of various lung regions and can be an important factor in increasing the alveolar-arterial O_2 gradient. These ventilation-perfusion disturbances occur in both lateral and dorsal recumbency. During lateral recumbency, the function of the lower lung progressively deteriorates in unconscious and anesthetized horses, while in dorsal recumbency both lungs show an impairment of performance [HALL, 1979]. During chloral hydrate and halothane anesthesia, the lateral position decreases the volume of the lower lung regions, which are also poorly ventilated Turning the horse on its other side does not improve ventilation in the lung that was previously lowermost [MCDONELL et al., 1979]. In horses anesthetized in lateral recumbency, the lower lung receives only 25% of its normal blood supply, while the upper lung receives a greater-than-normal blood flow [STOLK]. These disturbances are particularly important in the horse because of its very large lungs. It is assumed that ventilation-perfusion defects in the horse are more pronounced in dorsal recumbency than in the lateral position [DE MOOR, 1968b; HALL, 1968; STEFFEY et al., 1977a].

It has been shown that the arterial oxygen pressure in the dorsally recumbent horse is lower than in lateral recumbency [MITCHELL and LITTLEJOHN, 1974]. This rise of the alveolar-arterial O_2 gradient can assume extreme proportions in dorsal recumbency, particularly in old and heavy animals [DE MOOR and VAN DEN HENDE, 1978]. However, the fact that the arterial oxygen supply sometimes cannot be improved in these cases by the inspiration of 100% O_2 demonstrates that the inadequate oxygen supply in dorsal recumbency cannot be a pure ventilation-perfusion disturbance, unless this disturbance is very severe. Because the alveolar-arterial O_2 gradient is also very large during artificial respiration, and the gases are distributed fairly evenly in the lungs during artificial respiration [BERGMAN, 1963], it is apparent that ventilation-perfusion disturbances are not the prime factor in the development of a large alveolar-arterial O_2 gradient. Ventilation-perfusion disturbances can for the most part be eliminated by the inspiration of 100% O_2.

Ventilation-perfusion disturbances in the horse increase with age. A fall of the PaO_2 can be seen in both lateral and dorsal recumbency with advancing age. The alveolar-arterial O_2 gradient develops rapidly in the horse after the induction of anesthesia and shows a further increase in open-chest procedures [GILLESPIE et al., 1969].

Ventilation-perfusion disturbances can also play a role during the postoperative period.

(iii) A third cause of a high alveolar-arterial O_2 gradient is a pathophysiologic right-to-left shunt, whereby mixed venous blood enters the pulmonary venous circulation via the pulmonary arterial circulation without coming in contact with ventilated alveoli. The anatomic shunt ($< 2\%$ of the cardiac output) is caused by the entry of venous blood from the general and pulmonary circulation into the pulmonary venous circulation. The total shunt is approximately 5% of the cardiac output in the normal standing horse, rising during halothane anesthesia to 11% [GILLESPIE et al., 1969], 20% [HALL, 1971a], or even 30% [WEAVER and WALLEY, 1975]. This shunt is most often caused by the perfusion of unventilated alveoli. The shunt effect cannot be eliminated by the administration of pure O_2.

The cause of the shunt has been the subject of much discussion. Formerly the shunt was attributed mainly to atelectasis in portions of the lung. But if this were the case, one would expect a progressive increase in this shunt during anesthesia. This does not occur in horses or humans. Atelectasis has been observed in dogs only during positive-negative pressure ventilation under open-chest conditions [ROLLY, 1971]. Besides the anatomic shunt, which remains fairly constant and is of little importance, a recent theory cites occlusion of a portion of the small terminal bronchioles and alveoli from the upper airways as being responsible for a shunt increase and the large alveolar-arterial O_2 gradient. Very small air passages decrease in size just as the pulmonary volume itself decreases during expiration. This happens mainly in the lowermost parts of the lung by virtue of its weight. If 100% O_2 is breathed, the shunt also increases; this may be due to a local pulmonary vasodilation in the non-ventilated lung regions [LAVER, 1975].

(iv) A fourth cause of the increase in the alveolar-arterial O_2 gradient is a decline of the cardiac output. Besides an increase in the respiratory dead space, a fall of the cardiac output leads to an increase in the alveolar-arterial O_2 gradient as a result of the decreased O_2 content of the mixed venous blood. This decrease in the venous O_2 content is the result of increased oxygen extraction by the tissues in response to a slowing of the blood flow. GILLESPIE and colleagues could not significantly increase the low venous oxygen pressure (PvO_2) at a low cardiac output by switching from air to 100% O_2. Thus, it is important that measures be taken to avoid an extreme fall of the cardiac output and arterial blood pressure; a fast-acting digitalis preparation, such as gitoformat (Formiloxin), in a dose of 1—3 mg i.v. is indicated. A second, equal dose may be given if need be. A fall of the mixed venous oxygen pressure and subsequent rise of the alveolar-arterial O_2 gradient also result from increased oxygen consumption, as may occur during postanesthetic unrest, fever, hemorrhage or anemia. If the horse is turned onto its other side after one hour of halothane anesthesia, no increase in the alveolar-arterial oxygen gradient is observed [DE MOOR et al., 1974]. While arterial hypoxemia does not usually develop during anesthesia, despite the large alveolar-arterial oxygen gradient because of the high alveolar oxygen pressure that is maintained, severe arterial hypoxemia very often develops during the postoperative period when the animal is returned to breathing air. Besides inadequate saturation and in some cases cellular hypoxia, this hypoxemia can also lead to cerebral hypoxia with excitement. Such excitement must be prevented in the horse if at all possible.

Most of the factors cited above contribute to the development of postoperative hypoxemia. This is not a matter of pure respiratory depression, for the hypercapnia in such cases (high $PaCO_2$) is less pronounced than the hypoxemia. The following factors promote the development of postoperative hypoxemia:

— Diffusion hypoxia after the use of N_2O/O_2;
— low inspiratory oxygen concentration;
— ventilation-perfusion disturbances that are still present but are gradually diminishing, and shunting;
— increase in oxygen consumption, especially after trembling, that regularly occurs after prolonged halothane anesthesia;
— hypoventilation following artificial respiration or muscle relaxants.

Hypoxemia is especially marked in old animals, in pulmonary disease, in pain during respiration following certain operations, and at low arterial oxygen pressures at the end of anesthesia. Oxygen toxicity to the lungs, cited by some authors as a cause of postoperative respiratory complications, could scarcely play a role after operations lasting only a few hours, even if 100% oxygen is administered [Winter and Smith, 1972]. The horse usually recovery from postanesthetic hypoxemia in 1 to 3 h [De Moor, 1968b]. This hypoxemia can be prevented by administering oxygen by endotracheal tube at a rate of 15—20 l/min. The horse is dragged into the recovery stall with the endotracheal tube still in place. The tube is removed when the animal starts to swallow. Until the horse rises to its feet, an oxygen flow of 15 to 20 l/min should be maintained via a nasopharyngeal tube. This flow rate is necessary in view of the strong dilution that occurs when oxygen is administered by nasal catheter. In man, an O_2 concentration of 25.4% has been measured in the trachea with a flow rate of 5 l O_2/min, 30.6% at a rate of 10 l/min, and 44.5% at a rate of 15 l/min [Gibson et al., 1976]. Oxygen administration during the recovery period increases the PaO_2 to a much smaller degree than in the unanesthetized horse [Garner et al., 1977]. The hazardous postoperative hypoxemic phase can be eliminated this method [De Moor et al., 1974].

3. Hemoglobin level. A low hemoglobin level is unfavorable for good tissue oxygenation. Marked anemia must always be corrected by a blood transfusion before or during anesthesia. The splenic storage of erythrocytes that occurs after the use of α-adrenergic blocking agents such as phenothiazine tranquilizers and pentobarbital must be taken into account. This storage effect is very pronounced in the horse and is not affected by the simultaneous administration of atropine [De Moor and van den Hende, 1978].

1.2.2.3.5. Patient Monitoring during General Anesthesia

Respiration, cardiac function, and anesthetic depth must be monitored regularly during general anesthesia. The depth of anesthesia is usually regulated such that the palpebral reflex is maintained. To monitor the end-expiratory halothane concentration a Hook and Tucker meter is used. However this device is extremely complex, and difficult to control (fig. 1.2. — 13). Although EEG pattern changes can be monitored, depending on the depth of anesthesia, this technique is too complicated for clinical use [Auer et al., 1979].

Cardiac function is best monitored by taking the pulse with the fingers, with a pulse monitor, or by direct of indirect measurement of the arterial blood pressure. In lateral recumbency, the arterial blood pressure can be measured in the dorsal metatarsal artery IV with a sphygnomanometer. By tightening the air-release screw, it is also possible to visually monitor the pulsations on a continuous basis (fig. 1.2. — 14). This is a reliable instrument that is advantageous in terms of motion artifacts, and with which the systolic and diastolic blood pressure can be very accurately determined [Werner et al., 1977]. The optimum cuff bladder width is 1: 4 or a little more than

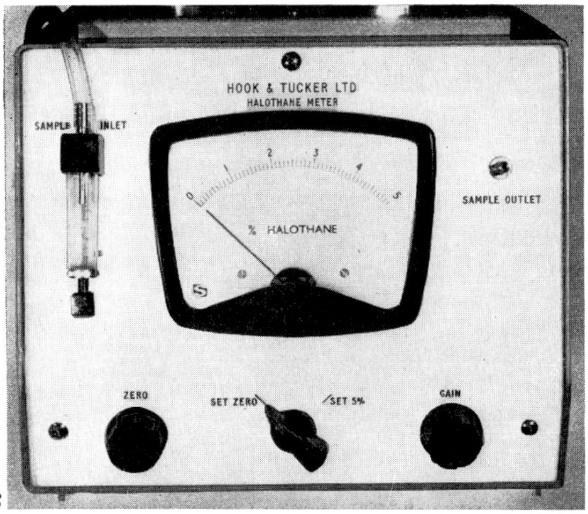

13

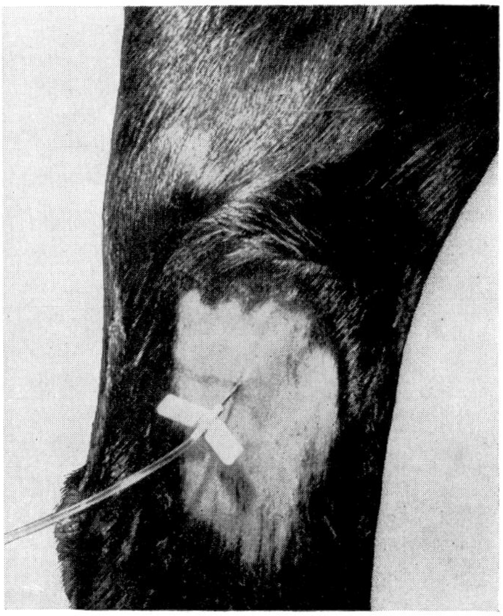
15

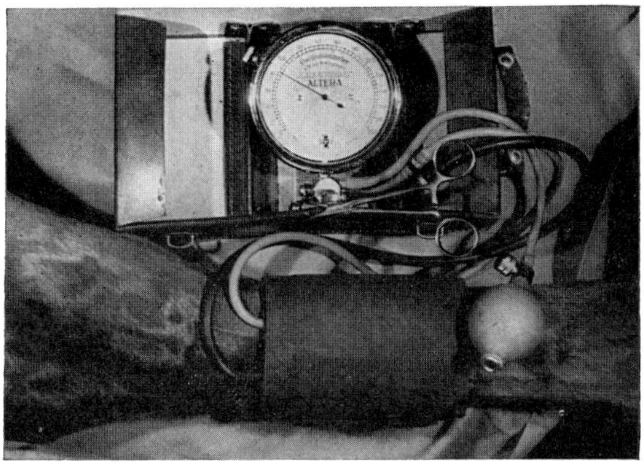
14

Fig. 1.2. — 13. Hook and Tucker apparatus.
Fig. 1.2. — 14. Oscillotonometer.
Fig. 1.2. — 15. Catheterization of the great metatarsal artery.

one-fifth the tail circumference [GEDDES et al., 1977]. The use of a cuff that is too wide underestimates the blood pressure, and if too narrow overestimates the pressure. With an optimum cuff width and good oscillometric method, a mean blood pressure could be obtained indirectly even in hypotensive horses with a mean blood pressure of 40 or even 30 mm Hg [LABHAW et al., 1979]. Although the systolic and diastolic pressure cannot be accurately measured with a sphygnomanometer, the instrument does convey a useful picture of cardiac work by relatively simple means.

The blood pressure in laterally or dorsally recumbent animals can be measured by the Doppler ultrasound technique. The systolic and diastolic values measured by this method agree well with pressure measurements made by direct arterial methods [GARNER et al., 1972], even in hypotensive horses [KVART, 1979]. An indirect pressure measurement can also be carried out by amplifying the Korotkoff sounds; again, the results correlate well with intra-arterial measurements. This method is unsuitable in shock, however, because the Korotkoff sounds are too low in frequency to be of value [ELLIS, 1975].

Monitoring of the pulse waves, which reflect the pumping activity of the heart, is much more important than the use of a cardiac monitor or oscilloscope, which indicate only the electrical activity of the heart. In many cases the heart may demonstrate a more or less normal electrical activity at a time when it is already in failure and can no longer maintain an effective circulation. The use of the oscilloscope requires considerable skill in interpretation and an understanding of the limits of the method. Measurement of the central venous pressure may also be indicated in conditions of shock or hypovolemia, mainly as a guide to therapy.

Respiratory monitoring is also of prime importance in the anesthetized horse. Often such monitoring is limited to recording the respiratory rate and the presence or absence of cyanosis. However, a rapid but shallow respiration is less effective in terms of gas exchange than a slow, deep respiration. In addition, cyanosis cannot be recognized in the presence of peripheral vasoconstriction or severe anemia. The absence of cyanosis, moreover, provides no measure of the arterial CO_2 pressure ($PaCO_2$). Accurate monitoring of ventilation can be accomplished only by studies of the arterial O_2 pressure (PaO_2) and arterial CO_2 pressure ($PaCO_2$).

In horses that are in poor general health (shock, intestinal obstruction, etc.) and during prolonged anesthesia, blood gases should be monitored by means of an indwelling intra-arterial catheter (fig. 1.2. — 15). Artificial respiration can be employed in such cases to prevent a rise of the $PaCO_2$. The elimination of CO_2 can also be determined continuously by means of an infrared absorption capnograph (fig. 1.2. — 16). During normal ventilation, the CO_2 concentration amounts to 5.6% of the total expired gas volume. Sometimes an arterial-alveolar CO_2 gradient develops that can reach extreme values of more than 50 mm Hg, especially in COPD, ventilation-perfusion disturbances and hypotension [ECKENHOFF et al., 1963]. With every fall of the cardiac output and the associated decrease in pulmonary blood flow, a smaller amount of CO_2 will enter the alveoli, and so less will be exhaled. Thus, based on the measured alveolar CO_2 pressure, one might gain the impression that a given respiratory depression is less hazardous than it actually is. When very high expiratory CO_2 values are present, artificial respiration is always indicated. In the absence of clear-cut pulmonary hypotension, the artificial respiration can be well regulated on the basis of the expiratory CO_2 level. If the artificial respiration is well regulated and the $PaCO_2$ is constant, then the infrared absorption capnograph is also a good indicator of the circulation and an excellent monitor of technical defects in the anesthesia machine. Finally, the respiratory minute volume can also be measured with a spirometer. This is not however as accurate as arterial blood-gas analysis. Either the Wright spirometer (fig. 1.2. — 17) [MITCHEL, 1972] or a dry gas meter [ADAMS et al., 1974] may be used. If N_2O, which is more dense than air, is used during anesthesia, then the measured values will be somewhat too high. The inspiratory oxygen concentration can be determined with an oxygen analyzer (fig. 1.2. — 18). The distal chamber of the analyzer can be filled with hygroscopic silica gel granules to prevent the condensation of water vapor on the sensor membrane as well as preventing failure of the instrument during prolonged, closed-system anesthesia [MOENS, 1978].

1.2.2.3.6. Complications of General Anesthesia

Various complications can arise both during and after general anesthesia. The occurrence and severity of the complications depend essentially on the nature of the anesthesia, the mode of administration of the anesthetic agent, the quality of the monitoring, the duration of the anesthesia, and the general condition of the animal. Some complications take an acute course and must be recognized at once to enhance the prospects of successful treatment, while other complications do not appear until after recovery.

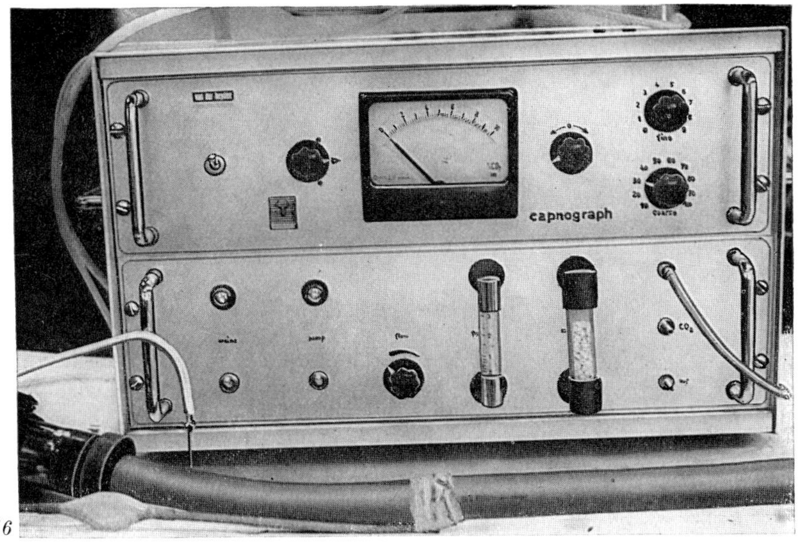

16

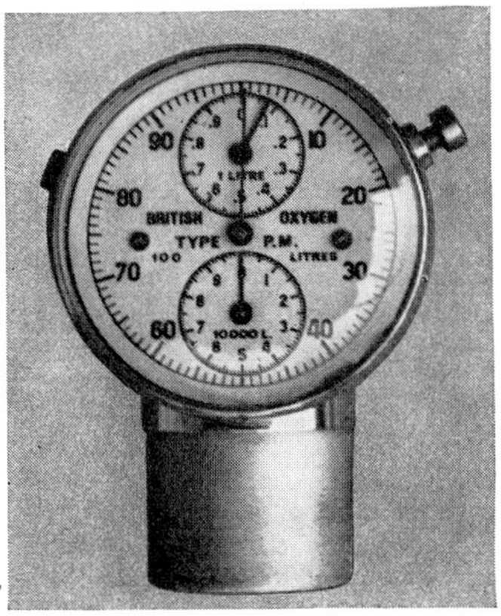

17

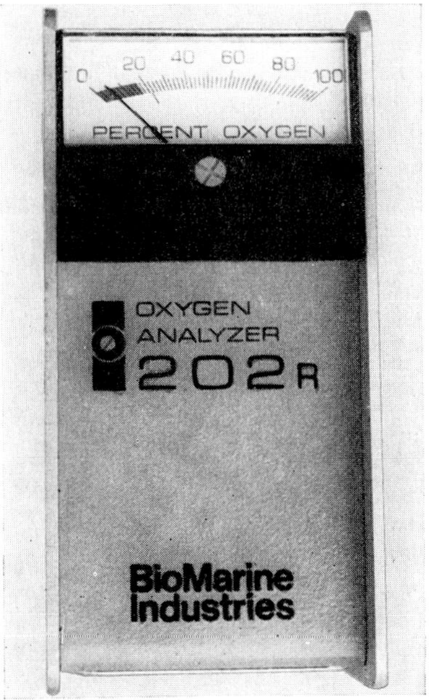

18

Fig. 1.2. — 16. Infrared absorption capnograph.
Fig. 1.2. — 17. Wright spirometer.
Fig. 1.2. — 18. Oxygen analyzer.

Complications during Anesthesia

1. Circulatory system. Practically all agents that produce general anesthesia also cause a concentration-dependent decrease in the force of myocardial contraction. The effects on cardiac output and especially the arterial blood pressure can vary greatly, however. These varying effects on the arterial blood pressure can result from a direct influence on certain hemodynamic variables, such as the stroke volume, heart rate, cardiac output, peripheral vascular resistance and central venous pressure. Cardiovascular reflexes and alterations in autonomic nervous activity can also play a role.

a) Cardiac arrest. Ventricular asystole during anesthesia is somewhat more frequent than ventricular fibrillation. The principal causes of cardiac arrest are a relative or absolute anesthetic overdose, heavy bleeding, untreated apnea, myocardial hypoxia, an acute anaphylactic reaction, or a vagal reflex, especially that resulting from strong tension on the viscera. Reflex cardiac arrest seldom occurs during well balanced anesthesia with a normal circulatory volume, a good PaO_2, and a normal pH. Irregular breathing may continue for 30—45 s after cardiac arrest (or even several minutes in very young foals) before anoxia of the respiratory center occurs.

The treatment of choice is cardiac massage. No time should be wasted on drug injections, which are rarely successful. Cardiac massage must be applied quickly, however; that is, the arrest must be quickly diagnosed, for the brain will suffer irreversible damage after a 3—5 min period of anoxia. This period is somewhat longer during general anesthesia owing to the decreased oxygen consumption of the brain and its increased glycogen content. Cardiac massage is generally successful only in cases where the arrest is sudden and the animal's general condition is good. In cases of preexisting cardiac failure or poor general health, cardiac massage is usually futile. *External cardiac massage* is chiefly indicated in young animals whose chest wall is still sufficiently compliant to allow adequate compression of the heart. It is performed by applying forceful lateral compressions of the thorax at a rate of 30—40 per min. In the foal, the thorax can be compressed with both hands with the arms outstretched, or with one or both feet. In mature horses it is very difficult if not impossible to apply effective external cardiac massage. If the heart can be compressed, an adequate circulation is obtained, especially in the brain. The extreme pupilary dilation that occurs with cardiac arrest is lost, and in favorable cases, the heart resumes beating within a few minutes. Because cardiac arrest is rapidly followed by a cessation of breathing or is the result of it, artificial respiration with 100% oxygen should always be given. Administration of the anesthetic agent is discontinued. A mixed acidosis usually develops, which can be corrected by giving an alkaline solution. If external cardiac massage proves ineffective, or the heart cannot be adequately compressed, *open cardiac massage* is indicated. After rapid disinfection with tincture of iodine or alcohol/chlorhexidine, the thorax is opened in the 5th or 6th intercostal space, preferably on the left side, with a large incision. The incision must not be carried too deeply, due to the danger of severing the internal thoracic vein and external thoracic artery and vein. A large chest-wound retractor is inserted, and the heart is compressed against the lower ribs with both hands. If cardiac arrest occurs during a laparotomy cranial to the umbilicus, the diaphragm can be divided to permit cardiac massage to be performed. If no spontaneous heartbeat appears after several minutes, then epinephrine, 5—10 ml of a 1: 10,000 dilution, can be injected into the left ventricle, supplemented if necessary by 10—20 ml of a 10% calcium gluconate solution. Calcium chloride is more strongly ionized and therefore more effective than calcium gluconate. With the resumption of cardiac activity, some bleeding will occur in the thoracic wound. The bleeding vessels are quickly ligated to prevent the entry of blood into the thoracic cavity. Having successfully resuscitated the heart, the surgeon should wait several minutes before closing [De Moor et al., 1972b]. The most favorable sign of successful cardiac resuscitation is the rapid reestablishment of spontaneous breathing. This is proof that the brain stem and medulla oblongata have suffered no serious damage. If severe convulsions occur, the prognosis is poor. Transitory neurologic deficits, such as blindness or cranial nerve paralysis, sometimes occur.

b) Acute hypotension. Acute hypotension is not uncommon, marked by the absence of a palpable peripheral pulse and by circulatory failure, even though the heart continues to show a more or less normal electrical activity. This hypotension is mainly the result of surgical stimulation of the celiac plexus, splanchnic nerve, or from tension on the viscera.

Acute hypotension is especially dangerous if the circulatory volume is low. Atropine cannot prevent such hypotension. When an episode occurs, the precipitating tension on the viscera must cease.

c) Disturbances of heart rate. *Tachycardia* is most likely to occur following the use of atropine, succinylcholine or thiobarbiturates. If muscle relaxants are used, tachycardia may be a sign of pain resulting from a too shallow level of anesthesia. Bradycardia, which can be prevented with atropine, occurs after halothane, xylazine (Rompun) or analgesics of the narcotic group.

d) Arrhythmias. Various types of cardiac arrhythmia can arise during general anesthesia. They are most commonly associated with the use of succinylcholine, thiamylal and xylazine. Although various anesthetic agents, including halothane and methoxyflurane, sensitize the heart to the arrhythmic action of catecholamines, arrhythmias seldom occur in the horse during halothane anesthesia. Most arrhythmias can be detected only on the basis of the EKG record, not by examination of the pulse. Many arrhythmias are caused by activation of the sympathetic nervous system and in some cases by a depression of the parasympathetic system with an increase in the heart rate and blood pressure, e.g., as a result of excitement during induction of anesthesia, a high $PaCO_2$ or low PaO_2, surgical stimulation during an inadequate depth of anesthesia, or a sudden blood pressure drop or abrupt fall of the $PaCO_2$. Most arrhythmias are transitory in nature and disappear once their cause is removed. Premedication with atropine and tranquilizers can prevent many arrhythmias. Propanolol, a β-blocking agent, is also effective [Lees and Tavernor, 1970]. However it is contraindicated in clinical anesthesia due to its cardiovascular effects. In rare cases severe, persistent arrhythmias develop, which can be controlled with 1 mg/kg lidocaine.

2. Respiratory system. A common respiratory complication of general anesthesia is hypoventilation. Apnea is also fairly common (see Oxygen Supply and Acid-Base Balance, Artificial Respiration). Laryngospasm and bronchospasm are virtually unheard of in the horse.

Various materials may be aspirated into the trachea and bronchi: fluid and food material during the treatment of pharyngeal obstructions, gastric contents during regurgitation secondary to abdominal surgery, and sometimes pus or blood. These complications can be prevented by the use of a cuffed endotracheal tube and, when gastric dilation is present, by siphoning the stomach contents prior to induction and during the anesthesia. If an endotracheal tube is not used, then the head must be angled downward and held in that position while the material is removed or aspirated from the pharynx as quickly as possible. The depth of anesthesia should not be increased at once, due to the resultant depression of the swallowing and cough reflexes. Material that is already in the trachea can be aspirated. This therapy should be combined with a large dose of broad spectrum antibiotics. The course of such a complication is dependent on the nature, quantity and pH value of the fluid that has entered the bronchi.

3. Complications related to injections

a) Intra-arterial injection of tranquilizers or thiopental. If the jugular vein is punctured with a fine, sharp needle and the technique is faulty, or the animal struggles during the injection, there is a danger that the needle will pass through the jugular vein and pierce the carotid artery. In some animals the injection of these agents causes no apparent harm, while in others the intra-arterial injection of tranquilizers causes unrest, head shaking, collapse and convulsions. In some cases the symptoms disappear after a few minutes and leave no neurologic deficit; in other cases death occurs within a few hours. The symptoms are caused by spasm of the cerebral arteries, swelling of the arterial endothelial cells, wall necrosis, and in some cases thrombosis with ischemic brain damage [Christian et al., 1974]. If the faulty injection is noticed, and the needle is still within the artery, 20 ml of 2% procaine of 1% lidocaine may prevent arterial spasm, together with heparin to prevent coagulation. The intra-arterial injection of a corticosteroid may also be beneficial.

b) Air embolism. Needles and catheters that are not closed can allow air to enter the vein and accumulate in the right heart and pulmonary artery, especially in the standing animal. If significant, this entry of air can assume life-threatening proportions. For example, less than 1 liter of air can cause death in the horse as a result of cardiac dysfunction. The average lethal air volume varies between 700 and 6,000 ml in experimental horses [Heath et al., 1969]. The symptoms are hypotension, tachycardia or apnea and hypoxemia. Animals that are lying down or have collapsed should be placed on their left side to facilitate outflow from the right heart. Oxygen is administered, and artificial respiration is applied if necessary. In some cases the injected air can be aspirated with the aid of a catheter. If N_2O is being used for anesthesia, it must be discontinued at once and flushed completely out of the system. This is necessary because N_2O tends to diffuse into the air bubble, greatly increasing its volume. If N_2O has already diffused into the embolism, the bubble should decrease in size after the delivery of N_2O is stopped.

c) Thrombophlebitis.

Etiology. Thrombophlebitis of the jugular vein can develop after injections of irritating substances. Agents with extremes of pH, such as chloral hydrate (pH = 3) or thiopental (pH = 11), are particularly irritating to vascular tissues. The degree of intimal damage and consequent blood coagulation with thrombosis of the vein also depends upon the concentration of the offending substance and its rate of injection. More prolonged infusions with a relatively inelastic PVC catheter often cause thrombosis from mechanical irritation of the intima. Polyethylene catheters always produce intimal irritation after about an hour, especially at the catheter tip [Schlichting and Zeller, 1971]. Foals are more susceptible to jugular thrombosis than mature horses. Catheters made of silicone rubber are less irritating but are somewhat difficult to handle. Infections can play both a primary and secondary role. Mechanical or chemical irritation of the intima can also decrease the fibrinolytic activity of the venous wall, predisposing to progressive thrombosis [Gervin et al., 1975].

Symptoms and course. An uninfected thrombophlebitis lesion feels like a firm mass or cord that is slightly to moderately painful. Sometimes mild edema develops at the level of the parotid and in the submaxillary region. This edema can be quite marked in bilateral thrombophlebitis of the jugular vein. In time, the thrombus fuses with the venous wall. Sometimes it is canalized, though valveless, while in other cases a collateral circulation develops. If the thrombus is infected or even suppurative, a painful edematous swelling develops. One or more abscesses may form in the thrombosed vein and subsequently erupt through the skin. The prognosis is guarded, especially with multiple abscess formation, and drainage is usually necessary.

Treatment. As a precaution, irritating agents should be injected in the lowest possible concentrations, and the injection should be as atraumatic and aseptic as possible. Catheters for long-term infusions should ideally be made of silicone rubber, or small amounts of heparin should be added to the infusion liquid. Uninfected thromboses can be treated by administering heparin or drugs having a fibrinolytic action.

If the thrombosis is infected, high doses of antibiotics should be given systemically, and nonirritating antibiotics may be helpful when infiltrated locally. If only one or two abscesses are present in the vein, drainage may be sufficient. With multiple abscesses it is best to resect the infected segment following proximal and distal ligation of the vessel.

d) Periphlebitis. The partial or complete perivenous injection of irritating agents can result in perivenous irritation with swelling or even necrosis, depending on the nature, concentration and volume of the product used. This process may even invade the vein wall, causing a rupture that can lead to a dangerous or even fatal hemorrhage. When periphlebitis is combined with thrombophlebitis, bleeding is absent. The skin overlying the lesion may become necrotic. The little viable tissue present is highly prone to infection. Paralysis of the recurrent laryngeal nerve, which may be involved in the inflammatory process, can lead to laryngeal hemiplegia (roaring). The best prophylaxis is adherence to meticulous injection technique and the application of adequate pressure to the puncture side after the needle is withdrawn. Intravenous solutions are best administered with a catheter that can be advanced into the vein. When using a needle, the needle placement must be checked at frequent intervals. A fall in the level of the intravenous fluid does not guarantee the fluid is within the vein.

Treatment consists of diluting the perivenously injected substance by infiltrating $^1/_2$ to 1 l of a 0.9% NaCl solution as rapidly as possible, perhaps combined with hyaluronidase and (if available) penicillin. This is followed by local heat (hydro) therapy to promote absorption. In the presence of venous wall necrosis with hemorrhage, general anesthesia should be induced as rapidly as possible, and the defect repaired or the affected segment excised.

1.2.2.3.7. Postanesthetic Complications

1. Bronchitis. Bronchitis can develop as the result of aspiration of irritating substances (see above). If a to-and-fro anesthesia system is used in which the CO_2 absorber is close to the animal, some $Ca(OH)_2$ dust may enter the air passages during induction, causing irritation. The movement of the respiratory cilia is slowed during general anesthesia, thus hampering the transport of mucus and secretions to the larynx. Various factors can contribute to this, including atropine premedication [Annis et al., 1976], the presence of the tracheal tube, poorly humidified anesthetic gases, as well as anesthesia itself.

2. Postoperative colic. Factors such as whether the animal has been fasted or not, the nature of the operation, and the primary disease, play a more important role in the origin of postoperative colic than does the anesthesia itself. The small intestine regains its activity rather rapidly, while the stomach and colon are slow to recover. Preanesthetic atropine can predispose to ileus and signs of colic. All food and water should be withheld for several hours after anesthesia. This period may be lengthened after intestinal surgery.

3. Congestion of lower lung regions. Congestion and atelectasis of the lower lung regions can occur during a prolonged and difficult recovery and after lying for too long on one side. This can be prevented by turning the animal at intervals of 1 to 2 h.

4. Liver damage. Chloroform is the only agent that has a direct hepatotoxic action and causes reproducible liver damage under experimental conditions. Halothane, by contrast, causes only mild impairments of liver function in the horse. In some

cases it produces slight to moderate histopathologic alterations of the liver tissue [De Moor et al., 1974; Norby and Link, 1970; Wolff et al., 1967]. Centrilobular necrosis with cellular infiltration has been demonstrated histologically in the horse after the oral administration of chloroform. No centrilobular necrosis was observed after halothane, although some liver cell vacuolation, cellular infiltration and glycogen loss occurred. These changes are slight but reproducible. At the same time, an increase in the serum activity of the liver-specific enzymes sorbitol dehydrogenase and glutamate dehydrogenase has been demonstrated, especially after the initial use of halothane [Jones, 1971]. The reverse effect of halothane on the liver cannot be ruled out in some horses [Wintzer et al., 1979]. Hypersensitivity reactions to halothane may occur, in which case the degree of damage usually bears no relation to the dosage or the duration of anesthesia. The danger of liver damage from halothane is apparently greater after repeated exposures to the agent and after premedication with phenobarbital. Phenobarbital is a drug that induces the release of hepatic microsomal enzymes that are active metabolically [Stenger and Johnson, 1972]. As yet, little is known concerning the metabolism of halothane in the horse and the possible toxicity of its metabolites or intermediaries. However, a rather high serum bromine concentration is found after prolonged halothane anesthesia in the horse. This ion is probably liberated during the metabolism of halothane to trifluoroacetic acid. Eighteen days after anesthesia, the plasma bromide concentration is still markedly elevated [De Moor et al., 1978]. A high plasma bromide can occur in horses that are reanesthetized with halothane a few days after prior anesthesia. Halothane is contraindicated in animals that show signs of liver damage after previous halothane anesthesia. Before attributing postanesthetic liver damage to halothane, one should note that factors other than halothane can have an adverse effect on the liver. These include fasting, severe hypotension with a marked reduction of hepatic blood flow, hypoxemia, acidosis, shock, infections, surgical trauma, and other substances administered before, during and after anesthesia.

5. Renal damage. Renal function may be impaired during general anesthesia, especially when there is a fall of blood pressure. This impairment results from a decline of the glomerular filtration rate, a decrease in the excretion of urine and Na^+, etc. Widespread ischemia and necrosis of the gluteal muscles of horses in dorsal recumbency can cause renal damage by obstruction of the tubules with myoglobin. Nephropathy after methoxyflurane as a result of fluorine metabolites has not been demonstrated in the horse.

6. Nerve paralyses

a) Facial nerve paralysis. If a horse is laterally recumbent for some time on a hard surface, the pressure from a halter strap or buckle can cause unilateral peripheral paralysis of the facial nerve. This paralysis spontaneously regresses after a few weeks or months.

b) 'Radial nerve' paralysis. After deep and prolonged anesthesia in lateral recumbency, a syndrome that resembles radial nerve paralysis can develop in the lowermost forelimb. The prognosis depends chiefly on the depth and duration of the anesthesia. In mild cases the 'paralysis' passes within minutes, but in most cases it persists for 1 to 2 days and sometimes longer. Severe 'radial nerve' paralysis can cause problems during the postoperative period, because the animal will find it difficult or impossible to get to its feet and excitement sometimes occurs. This is particularly dangerous if there is an injury such as a fracture of the other foreleg that impairs its weight-bearing ability. If the other forelimb can bear weight, it should be on the down side of the recumbent animal in order to facilitate standing. In some horses it may be beneficial to suspend the animal in a sling for one or more days. The symptoms of so called 'radial nerve' paralysis are very similar to those of ischemia of the triceps muscle group, which also occurs after lateral recumbency. This ischemia is distinguished by hard, swollen muscles and by a marked elevation of muscle-specific enzymes in the serum.

7. Muscle damage. Some large muscle groups may be subjected to considerable pressure during prolonged, deep anesthesia on a hard operating table. This produces an impairment of blood flow or even a complete loss of perfusion at low blood pressures especially in heavy animals. Commonly affected are the gluteal muscles and proximal portions of the biceps femoris and semitendinosus muscles in dorsal recumbency, and the triceps brachii muscle in lateral recumbency. Severe cell damage or ischemic necrosis can develop. As a result, the animal may be unable to bear weight on a foreleg (triceps muscle) or unable to raise its hindquarters (gluteal muscles), with potentially fatal consequences. The muscles feel hard and swollen on palpation. The SGOT and CPK activities are markedly increased [Trim and Mason, 1973]. To prevent these changes, the animal should be adequately padded during surgeries in lateral recumbency. The horse should be placed on padding such as an inflated air mattress or waterbed and positioned in such a way that the limbs are elevated. In dorsal recumbency the hindlimbs can be raised to alleviate pressure on the high and back muscles. In four horses with obvious clinical and biochemical symptoms of myositis following halothane anesthesia, an increase in muscular sensitivity to halothane and caffeine was demonstrated in vitro. The signs ranged from localized (lumbar) or generalized stiffness to generalized pain. Dantrolene Sodium was found to be of therapeutic benefit when administered sufficiently early [Waldron-Mease and Rosenberg, 1979].

8. Hypothermia. Hypothermia is common both during and after general anesthesia, especially in young and small animals. Hypothermia is particularly marked when the temperatures of the operating table and recovery stall are low. It is also seen during prolonged anesthesia with agents that cause peripheral vasodilation such as halothane or pentobarbital. During pentobarbital anesthesia, for example, the recovery period is considerably prolonged by marked hypothermia. The prolonged duration of action of pentobarbital in hypothermia is due to the slower course of the enzymatic reactions that metabolize the drug. Severe hypothermia leads to increased myocardial excitability, a fall of the cardiac output, a depression of respiration and liver function, and a decline of ACTH and the adrenal hormones. The animal usually attempts to rise during the postoperative period, thereby increasing its oxygen consumption and creating a danger of hypoxemia. Hypothermia can be prevented by providing a sufficiently high ambient temperature and by placing the animal on a warm-water mattress if necessary during the anesthesia [Heath, 1973]. A closed anesthesic system can prevent hypothermia by virtue of the exothermic reaction of CO_2 absorption and the return of the warm expiratory gases. If a tremor is present, oxygen should be administered by nasopharyngeal catheter.

9. Postanesthetic excitement. Postanesthetic excitement can occur in animals that are unable to stand because of nerve paralysis, muscular ischemia, etc. The most important causes of excitement, however, are severe hypoxemia and cerebral hypoxia. It is essential to maintain an adequate oxygen supply during the postanesthetic period. Excitement following halothane anesthesia can be almost entirely prevented by adequate oxygen administration. A quiet, padded recovery stall is very advantageous in avoiding traumatic injuries that may accompany complications during the recovery period. If a recovery stall is not available, or there is no place where the animal can recover quietly, it is left restrained in lateral recumbency until it is able to stand without danger.

10. Tracheal injury from the cuff of the tracheal tube. The cuff of the tracheal tube must be inflated so as to produce an airtight seal between the cuff and tracheal wall. In many cases, however, the cuff is overinflated. One cause of this is expansion of the cuff contents with a rise of temperature. In some cases excessive pressure in the trachea can lead to respiratory arrest. An overinflated cuff can cause damage to the tracheal mucosa, especially during prolonged anesthesia, which in turn can lead to inflammation, hyperemia, hemorrhage and even ischemic necrosis of the mucosa and submucosa. At high oxygen concentrations (75 %), small amounts of oxygen (which diffuses 3 to 4 times better than nitrogen) can diffuse into the lumen of the cuff. At oxygen concentrations of 25—50% this diffusion is negligible. Thus, it is advisable during prolonged anesthesia to reduce the cuff pressure periodically. If nitrous oxide is used to deliver the anesthetic agent, this gas, too, can diffuse into the cuff lumen and produce a pressure and volume increase. During anesthesia with N_2O, therefore, it is better to inflate the cuff with N_2O/O_2 or N_2O or else release some pressure at regular intervals [Stanley, 1975].

11. Paraplegia secondary to hematomyelia. Two cases of paraplegia caused by hemorrhage into the thoracolumbar cord have been described after 1 to 2 hours' anesthesia in the dorsally recumbent horse [Schatzmann et al., 1979]. The etiology of this rare condition is unknown.

References

Adams, A. P.; Vickers, M. D. A.; Munroe, J. P.; Parker, C. W.: Dry displacement gas meters. Brit. J. Anaesthesia *39:* 174 (1974).

Alexander, F.; Collett, R. A.: Pethidine in the horse. Res. Veterin. Sci., Oxford, *17:* 136 (1974).

Annis, P.; Landa, J.; Lichtiger, M.: Effects of atropine on velocity of tracheal mucus in anaesthetized patients. Anesthesiology *44:* 74 (1976).

Auer, J.; Amend, J.; Garner, H.; Hutcheson, D.; Salem, C.: Electroencephalographic responses during volatile anesthesia in domestic ponies: a comparative study of isoflurane, enflurane, methoxyflurane, and halothane. J. Equine Med. Surg. *3:* 130 (1979).

Auer, J.; Garner, H.; Amend, J.; Hutcheson, D.; Salem, C.: Recovery from anaesthesia in ponies: a comparative study of the effects of isoflurane, enflurane, methoxyflurane and halothane. Equine Vet. J. *10:* 18 (1978).

Bellingham, A. J.; Detter, J. C.; Lenfant, C.: Regulatory mechanism of hemoglobin oxygen affinity in acidosis and alkalosis. J. Clin. Invest. *50:* 700 (1971).

Bello, T. R.: Amborski, G. F.; Torbert, B. J.: Effects of organic phosphorus anthelmintics on blood cholinesterase values in horses and ponies. Amer. J. Vet. Res. *35:* 73 (1974).

Benson, G.; Hartsfield, S.; Smetzer, D.; Thurmon, J.: Physiologic effects of succinylcholine chloride in mechanically ventilated horses anesthetized with halothane in oxygen. Amer. J. Vet. Res. *40:* 1411 (1978).

Benson, G.; Thurmon, J.; Hartsfield, S.: Physiologic effect of succinylcholine in the anesthetized and mechanically ventilated horse. Proc. 22th Ann. Conv. Amer. Assoc. Equine Pract. 1976, 347.

Bergman, N. A.: Distribution of inspired gas during anaesthesia and artificial ventilation. J. Appl. Physiol. *18:* 1085 (1963).

Brandstater, B.; Eger, E.; Edelist, G.: Effect of halothane, ether and cyclopropane on respiration. Brit. J. Anaesthesia *37:* 890 (1965).

Christian, R. G.; Mills, J. H. L.; Kramer, L. L.: Accidental intracarotid artery injection of promazine in the horse. Canad. Vet. J. *15:* 29 (1974).

Crowhurst, R. C.; Simpson, D. J.; McEnery, R. J.; Greenwood, R. E. S.: Intestinal surgery in the foal. J. South. African Vet. Assoc. *46:* 59 (1975).

Cullen, D. J.; Eger, E. I.: The effects of halothane on respiratory and cardiovascular responses to hypoxia in dogs. A dose-response study. Anesthesiology *33:* 487 (1970).

Davis, L. E.; Wolf, W. A.: Pharmacokinetics and metabolism of glyceryl guajacolate in ponies. Amer. J. Vet. Res. *31:* 469 (1970).

De Moor, A.: Influence of atropine on arterial oxygen tension, acid-base status and tissue hypoxia in the conscious horse. Zbl. Veterinärmed., R. A. *15:* 494 (1968a).

De Moor, A.: Influence of closed circuit halothane anaesthesia on acid-base status and oxygenation in the horse. Proc. VIIIth Congr. Europ. Soc. Vet. Surg. Bologna, p. 89 (1968b).

De Moor, A.; Desmet, P.; van den Hende, C.: Influence of promazine on the equine venous haematocrit and plasma protein concentration. Proc. XI Congr. Europ. Soc. Vet. Surg. Copenhagen, p. 136 (1975).

De Moor, A.; Desmet, P.; Verschooten, F.: Influence of position change in the horse in lateral recumbency anaesthetized with halothane on arterial oxygenation and acid-base status and efficiency of post-anaesthetic oxygen administration. Zbl. Vet.-Med., R. A. *21:* 525 (1974).

De Moor, A.; van den Hende, C.: Effect of Propionylpromazine, Promethazine and Atropine on packed cell volume and circulatory red cell mass in horses and cattle. Zbl. Vet.-Med., R. A. *15:* 544 (1968).

De Moor, A.; van den Hende, C.: Inspiratory concentrations of O_2, N_2, and N_2O arterial oxygenation and acid-base status during closed system halothane anaesthesia in the horse. Zbl. Vet.-Med., R. A. *19:* 1 (1972).

De Moor, A.; van den Hende, C.; Moens, Y.; Desmet, P.: Increased plasma bronude concentration in the horse after halothane anesthesia. Amer. J. Vet. Res. *39:* 1624 (1978).

De Moor, A.; van den Hende, C.; Verschooten, P.; Desmet, P.; Watte, R.: Influence of a clinical anaesthesia-technique (Premedication with tranquilizers and atropine, induction with chloralhydrate, maintenance with halothane in a closed circle system) on liver function tests in horse. Zbl. Vet.-Med. R. A. *16:* 906 (1969).

De Moor, A.; Verschooten, F.; Desmet, P.; Muylle, E.; Steenhaut, M.: Intrathoracic cardiac resuscitation in the horse. Equine Vet. J. *4:* 31 (1972).

Dodman, N. H.; Waterman, A.: Paradoxical excitement following the intravenous administration of azoperone in the horse. Equine Vet. J. *11:* 33 (1979).

Eberly, V.; Gillespie, J.; Tyler, W.; Fowler, M.: Cardiovascular values in the horse during halothane anesthesia. Amer. J. Vet. Res. *29:* 305 (1968).

Eckenhoff, J. E.; Hale Enderby, G. E.; Larson, A.; Edridge, A.; Judevine, D. E.: Pulmonary gas exchange during deliberate hypotension. Brit. J. Anaesthesia *35:* 750 (1963).

Eisenmenger, E.: Arbeitst. Fachgr. Pferdekrankh., Wien 1974.

Ellis, P. M.: The indirect measurement of arterial blood pressure in the horse. Equine Vet. J. *7:* 22 (1975).

Ellis, R.; Lowe, J.; Schwark, W.; Taylor, J.: Intravenously administered xylazine and ketamine HCl for anesthesia in horses. J. Equine Med. Surg. *1:* 259 (1977).

Frankland, A.; Camburn, M.: Induction of anaesthesia using thiopentone sodium in the horse. Veterin. Rec. *100:* 472 (1977).

Fritsch: personal communication (1975).

Fuentes, V.: Short term immobilization in the horse with ketamine HCl and promazine HCl combinations. Equine Vet. J. *10:* 78 (1978).

Garner, H. E.; Coffman, J. R.; Hahn, A. W.; Hartley, H.: Indirect blood pressure measurement in the horse. Proc. 18th Ann. Conv. Amer. Assoc. Equine Pract. p. 343 (1972).

Garner, H.; Moore, J.; Amend, J.: Post-operative management of hypoxia in the equine abdominal crisis. Proc. 23th Ann. Conv. Amer. Assoc. Equine Pract. p. 177 (1977).

Geddes, L.; Chaffee, V.; Whistler, S.; Bourland, J.; Tacker, W.: Indirect mean blood pressure in the anesthetized pony. Amer. J. Vet. Res. *38:* 2055 (1977).

Gervin, A. S.; Mason, K. G.; Sulkin, M. D.; Hufnagel, H. V.: Drug induced hypofibrinolysis: a cause of venous thrombosis. J. Surg. Res. *19:* 233 (1975).

Gibson, R. L.; Comer, P. B.; Beckham, R. W.; McGraw, C. P.: Actual tracheal oxygen concentrations with commonly used oxygen equipment. Anesthesiology *44:* 71 (1976).

GILLESPIE, J.; TYLER, W.; HALL, L.: Cardiopulmonary dysfunction in anesthetized, laterally recumbent horses. Amer. J. Vet. Res. *30:* 61 (1969).

GOLDBERG, A.; SOHN, Y.; PHEAR, W.: Direct myocardial effects of nitrous oxide. Anesthesiology *37:* 373 (1972).

HALL, L.: Some aspects of equine anesthesia. Proc. VIIIth Congr. Europ. Soc. Vet. Surg., Bologna p. 79 (1968).

HALL, L.: Disturbances of cardiopulmonary function in anaesthetised horses. Equine Vet. J. *3:* 95 (1971a).

HALL, L. W.: Textbook of Veterinary Anaesthesia. In: SOMA, L. R. (The Williams & Wilkins Co., Baltimore 1971b).

HALL, L. W.: Oxygenation of pulmonary vein blood in conscious and anaesthetised ponies. Equine Vet. J. *11:* 71 (1979).

HALL, L. W.; TRIM, C. M.: Positive end-expiratory pressure in anaesthetized spontaneously breathing horses. Brit. J. Anaesthesiol. *47:* 819 (1975).

HEATH, R. B.: Anaesthetic management and recovery of large orthopedic patients. Vet. Clin. North. Amer. *3:* 127 (1973).

HEATH, R. B.; GABEL, A. A.: Evaluation of thiamylal sodium, succinylcholine, and glyceryl guaiacolate prior to inhalation anaesthesia in horses. J. Amer. vet. med. Assoc. *157:* 1486 (1970).

HEATH, R. B.; GABEL, A. A.; MCCASHIN, F. B.: Accidental air embolism — a cause of death in horses. Proc. 15th Amer. Conv. Assoc. Equine Pract. p. 243 (1969).

HILLIDGE, C.: Some effects of Immobilon in ponies. Proc. Assoc. Vet. Anesthesiol. Great Brit. & Ireland, *6:* 60 (1976/77).

HILLIDGE, C.: The influence of neuroleptanalgesia on the serum activity of muscle enzymes in ponies. Equine Vet. J. *10:* 60 (1978).

HILLIDGE, C.; LEES, P.: Metomidate/Azaperone anaesthesia in the horse: a clinical and pharmacological study. Proc. Assoc. Vet. Anesthesiol. Great Brit. & Ireland *3:* 84 (1972).

HILLIDGE, C.; LEES, P.: Fatility after Reviron. Vet. Rec. *94:* 476 (1974).

HILLIDGE, C. J.; LEES, P.: Cardiac output in the conscious and anaesthetised horse. Equine Vet. J. *7:* 16 (1975a).

HILLIDGE, C. J.; LEES, P.: Influence of the neuroleptanalgesic combination of etorphine and acepromazine on the horse: blood gases and acid-base balance. Equine Vet. J. *7:* 148 (1975b).

HILLIDGE, C.; LEES, P.: Influence of general anaesthesia on peripheral resistance in the horse. Brit. Vet. J. *133:* 225 (1977a).

HILLIDGE, C.; LEES, P.: Studies of left ventricular isotonic function in conscious and anaesthetized ponies. Brit. Vet. J. *133:* 446 (1977b).

HILLIDGE, C.; LEES, P.: Left ventricular systole in conscious and anaesthetized horses. Amer. J. Vet. Res. *38:* 675 (1977c).

HILLIDGE, C.; LEES, P.; SERRANO, L.: Investigations of azaperone/metomidate anaesthesia in the horse. Vet. Rec. *93:* 307 (1973).

HIRSHMAN, C. A.; MCCULLOUGH, R. E.; COHEN, P. J.; WEIL, J. V.: Hypoxic ventilatory drive in dogs during thiopental, ketamine or pentobarbital anesthesia. Anesthesiology *43:* 628 (1975).

HUSKA, G.: Xylazine-morphine sequence to obtain analgesia in the horse and dog. Canad. Vet. J. *18:* 317 (1977).

JONES, R. S.: Anaesthesia and the equine liver. Proc. Assoc. Vet. Anesthesiol. Great. Brit. & Ireland *2:* 23 (1971).

KAKA, J.; KLAVANO, P.; HAYTON, W.: Pharmacokinetics of ketamine in the horse. Amer. J. Vet. Res. *40:* 978 (1979).

KELLER, H.; MÜLLER, R.: Erhöhung des Narkoserisikos durch den Einsatz moderner Anthelminthika beim Pferd. Berliner Münchener tierärztl. Wschr. *92:* 63 (1979).

KERR, D. D.; JONES, E. W.; HOLBERT, D.; HUGGINS, K.: Comparison of the effects of xylazine and acetylpromazine maleate in the horse. Amer. J. Vet. Res. *33:* 777 (1972a).

KERR, D. D.; JONES, E. W.; HUGGINS, K.; EDWARDS, W. C.: Sedative and other effects of xylazine given intravenously to horses. Amer. J. Vet. Res. *33:* 525 (1972b).

KETELAARS, H.; VAN DIETEN, J.; LAGERWEIJ, E.: Untersuchung von Guajakolglyzerinäther bei Pferden und Ponys. Berliner Münchener tierärztl. Wschr. *92:* 211 (1979).

KVART, C.: An ultrasonic method for indirect blood pressure measurement in the horse. J. Equine Med. Surg. *3:* 16 (1979).

LABHAW, H.; FESSLER, J.; WHISTLER, S.; GEDDES, L.: Indirect measurement of mean blood pressure in the normotensive and hypotensive horse. Equine Vet. J. *11:* 191 (1979).

LAGERWEIJ, E.: Psychosedativa in de diergeneeskunde. Tijdschr. Diergeneeskunde *100:* 546 (1975).

LANGLEY, J. A.: Demonstration in the use of Thiopentone by slow injection. Proc. Assoc. Vet. Anesthesiol. Great Brit. & Ireland *3:* 8 (1972).

LAVER, M. B.: Acute respiratory failure: more questions, fewer answers. Anesthesiology *43:* 611 (1975).

LEES, P.; HILLIDGE, C. J.: Neuroleptanalgesia and cardiovascular function in the horse. Equine Vet. J. *7:* 184 (1975).

LEES, P.; TAVERNOR, W. D.: The influence of suxamethonium on cardiovascular and respiratory function in the anaesthetized horse. Brit. J. Pharmacol. *36:* 116 (1969).

LEES, P.; TAVERNOR, W. D.: Influence of halothane and catecholamines on heart rate and rhythm in the horse. Brit. J. Pharmacol. *39:* 149 (1970).

LEES, P.; TAVERNOR, W. D.; HILLIDGE, C. J.: The effects of some anaesthetics and ancillary agents on adrenoceptive receptors. Proc. Assoc. Vet. Anesthesiol. Great Brit. & Ireland *2:* 50 (1971).

LEVY, W.; GILLESPIE, J. R.: Emergency ventilator for resuscitating apnoic horses. J. Amer. veterin. med. Assoc. *161:* 57 (1972).

MACKENZIE, G.; SNOW, D.: An evaluation of chemical restraining agents in the horse. Vet. Rec. *101:* 30 (1977).

McCASHIN, F. B.; GABEL, A. A.: Evaluation of xylazine as a sedative and preanaesthetic agent in horses. Amer. J. Vet. Res. *36:* 1421 (1975).

McDONELL, W.; HALL, L.; JEFFCOTT, L.: Radiographic evidence of impaired pulmonary function in laterally recumbent anaesthetised horses. Equine Vet. J. *11:* 24 (1979).

MITCHELL, B.: Relationship between body weight and tidal volume during general anaesthesia in sheep, cattle, pigs and horses. Proc. Assoc. Vet. Anesthesiol. Great Brit. & Ireland *3:* 56 (1972).

MITCHELL, R. A.; HERBERT, D. A.: Potencies of Doxapram and Hypoxia in stimulating carotid-body chemoreceptors and ventilation in anaesthetised cats. Anesthesiology *42:* 599 (1975).

MITCHELL, B.; LITTLEJOHN, A.: The effect of anaesthesia and posture on the exchange of respiratory gases and on the heart rate. Equine Vet. J. *6:* 177 (1974).

MOENS, Y.: Eine einfache Modifikation zur Verbesserung der Genauigkeit eines Sauerstoffmessgerätes während langdauernder Anästhesien im geschlossenen System. Anaesthesist *27:* 401 (1978).

MÜLLER, W.: Halothan-Narkosezwischenfälle beim Pferd. Vet.-med. Diss., Zürich (1967).

MUIR, W. W.; HAMLIN, R. L.: Effects of acetylpromazine on ventilatory variables in the horse. Amer. J. Vet. Res. *36:* 1439 (1975).

MUIR, W. W.; MOORE, C. H.; HAMLIN, R. L.: Ventilatory alternations in normal horses in response to changes in inspired oxygen and carbon dioxide. Amer. J. Vet. Res. *36:* 155 (1975).

MUIR, W.; SKARDA, R.: Stabilization and Monitoring of the equine emergency patient. Proc. 22th Ann. Conv. Amer. Assoc. Equine Pract. (1976), 33.

MUIR, W.; SKARDA, R.; MILNE, D.: Evaluation of xylazine and ketamine hydrochloride for anaesthesia in horses. Amer. J. Vet. Res. *38:* 195 (1977).

MUIR, W.; SKARDA, R.; SHEEHAN, W.: Cardiopulmonary effects of narcotic agonists and a partial agonist in horses. Amer. J. Vet. Res. *39:* 1632 (1978a).

MUIR, W.; SKARDA, R.; SHEEHAN, W.: Evaluation of xylazine guaifenesin and ketamine hydrochloride for restraint in horses. Amer. J. Vet. Res. *39:* 1274 (1978b).

MUIR, W.; SKARDA, R.; SHEEHAN, W.: Hemodynamic and respiratory effects of Xylazine-Morphine Sulfate in horses. Amer. J. Vet. Res. *40:* 1417 (1979a).

MUIR, W.; SKARDA, R.; SHEEHAN, W.; GATES, B.: Evaluation of thiamylal, guaifenesin, and ketamine hydrochloride combinations administered prior to halothane anesthesia in horses. J. Equine Med. Surg. *3:* 178 (1979b).

NDRITU, C.; ENOS, L.: Adverse reactions to drugs in a veterinary hospital. J. Amer. vet. med. Assoc. *170:* 335 (1977).

NEUMANN, H.; WINTZER, H. J.: Das Verhalten des systolischen Blutdruckes während der Fluothan-Narkose beim Pferd. Berliner Münchener tierärztl. Wschr. *88:* 365 (1975).

NORBY, M. A.; LINK, R. P.: Effect of halothane anesthesia on liver function in the horse. Vet. Med. and Small Animal Clinician *65:* 946 (1970).

PATSCHKE, D.: Koronardurchblutung und myokardialer Sauerstoffverbrauch während der Narkoseeinleitung. Anaesthesiology and Resuscitation 96 (Springer-Verlag, Berlin (West) 1976).

PEARSON, H.; WEAVER, B.: Priapism after sedation, neuroleptanalgesia and anesthesia in the horse. Equine Vet. J. *10:* 85 (1978).

PRICE, H. L.: Calcium reserves myocardial depression caused by halothane. Site of action. Anaesthesiology *41:* 576 (1974).

PURCHASE, I. F. H.: Some respiratory parameters in horses and cattle. Vet. Rec. *77:* 859 (1965).

RIGGS, A.: The nature and significance of the Bohr effect in mammalian hemoglobins. J. General Physiol. *43:* 737 (1960).

ROBINSON, N.; SORENSON, P.; GOBLE, D.: Patterns of airflor in normal horses and horses with respiratory disease. Proc. 21th Ann. Conv. Amer. Assoc. Equine Pract. (1975), 11.

ROLLY, G.: Arterial oxygenation during anesthesia and controlled ventilation. Anaesthesist *20:* 85 (1971).

SCHATZMANN, U.: The induction of general anesthesia in the horse with glyceryl guaiacolate. Comparison when used alone and with sodium thiamylal. Equine Vet. J. *6:* 164 (1974).

SCHATZMANN, U.: Investigations of the applicability of controlled ventilation during routine anesthesia in the horse. J. Equine Med. Surg. *2:* 453 (1978).

SCHATZMANN, U.; HELD, J.: Use of Immobilon® glyceryl guaiacolate in the horse. Proc. Veterin. World Congr., Thessaloniki (1975), 1700.

SCHATZMANN, U.; MEISTER, V.; FANKHAUSER, R.: Akute Hämatomyelie nach längerer Rückenlage beim Pferd. Schweizer Arch. Tierheilk. *121:* 149 (1979).

SCHATZMANN, U.; TSCHUDI, P.; HELD, J.; MUHLEBACH, B.: An investigation of the action and haemolytic effect of glyceryl guaiacolate in the horse. Equine Vet. J. *10:* 224 (1978).

SCHILLING, R.; WEIS, K. H.: Zur Sauerstoffkonzentration im Narkosekreissystem. 1. Mitt. Abhängigkeit vom Frischgasstrom. Anaesthesist *22:* 198 (1973a).

SCHILLING, R.; WEIS, K. H.: Zur Sauerstoffkonzentration im Narkosekreissystem. 2. Mitt. Abhängigkeit vom Typ des Kreissystems. Anaesthesist *22:* 202 (1973b).

SCHLICHTING, K.; ZELLER, R.: Untersuchungen über Gefässwandschäden an der Vena jugularis externa des Pferdes bei Verwendung von Kunststoffkanülen. Berliner Münchener tierärztl. Wschr. *91:* 232 (1978).

SCHMIDT-NIELSEN, K.; LARIMER, J. L.: Oxygen dissociation curves of mammalian blood in relation to body size. Amer. J. Physiol. *195:* 424 (1958).

SCHREIBER, P.: Anaesthesia Equipment Performance, classification and safety (Springer-Verlag, Berlin (West) 1972).

SCHUH, F. F.: Nebenwirkungen von Lachgas. Anaesthesist *24:* 392 (1975).

SERRANO, L.; LEES, P.: The applied pharmacology of azaperone in ponies. Res. Vet. Sci. *20:* 316 (1976).

SERRANO, L.; LEES, P.; HILLIDGE, C.: Influence of azaperone/metomidate anesthesia on blood biochemistry in the horse. Brit. Vet. J. *132:* 405 (1976).

SHORT, C. E.: Evaluation of closed, semiclosed and nonrebreathing inhalation anesthesia systems in the horse. J. Amer. vet. med. Assoc. *157:* 1500 (1970).

SHORT, C.; CUNEIO, J.; CUPP, D.: Organophosphate-induced complications during anesthetic management in the horse. J. Amer. vet. med. Assoc. *159:* 1319 (1971).

SKARDA, R.: Intubationsnarkose bei Pferden mit Fluothan und Lachgas nach Prämedikation mit Vetranquil, Atropin und Niederlegen mit My 301 und Pentothal. Schweiz. Arch. Tierheilk. *116:* 507 (1974).

SKARDA, R.; BACKES, G.; FACKELMAN, G. E.: Improving pulmonary ventilation in anaesthetized horses with the Bird Mark 9 respirator. Vet. Med. and Small Animal Clinician *69:* 754 (1974).

SKARDA, R.; BEDLINGER, R.; MÜLLER, A.: Das Verhalten von Kreislauf und Atmung beim medikamentösen Niederlegen des Pferdes mit Rompun und Pentothal. Schweiz. Arch. Tierheilk. *112:* 458 (1970).

SMITH, M.: A respirator for large animals. Nord. Vet.-Med. *23:* 537 (1971).

STANLEY, T. H.: Nitrous oxide and pressures and volumes of high- and low-pressure endotracheal-tube cuffs in intubated patients. Anaesthesiology *42:* 637 (1975).
STEFFEY, E.: Enflurane and isoflurane anesthesia: a summary of laboratory and clinical investigations in horses. J. Amer. vet. med. Assoc. *172:* 367 (1978).
STEFFEY, E.; BERRY, J.: Flow rates from an intermittent positive pressure breathing-anesthetic delivery apparatus for horses. Amer. J. Vet. Res. *38:* 685 (1977).
STEFFEY, E. P.; GILLESPIE, J. R.; BERRY, J. D.; EGER, E. I., RHODE, E. A.: Circulatory effects of halothane and halothane-nitrous oxide anesthesia in the dog. Spontaneous ventilation. Amer. J. Vet. Res. *36:* 197 (1975).
STEFFEY, E.; HOWLAND jr., D.: Rate of change of halothane concentration in a large animal circle anesthetic system. Amer. J. Vet. Res. *38:* 1993 (1977).
STEFFEY, E.; HOWLAND, D.: Cardiovascular effects of halothane in the horse. Amer. J. Vet. Res. *39:* 611 (1978a).
STEFFEY, E.; HOWLAND, D.: Potency of halothane-N_2O in the horse. Amer. J. Vet. Res. *39:* 1141 (1978b).
STEFFEY, E.; HOWLAND, D.; GIRI, S.; EGER, E.: Enflurane, halothane, and isoflurane potency in horses. Amer. J. Vet. Res. *38:* 1037 (1977b).
STEFFEY, E.; WHEAT, J.; MEAGHER, D.; NORRIE, R.; MCKEE, J.; BROWN, M.; ARNOLD, J.: Body position and mode of ventilation influences arterial pH, oxygen, and carbon dioxide tensions in halothane-anesthetized horses. Amer. J. Vet. Res. *38:* 379 (1977a).
STENGER, R. J.; JOHNSON, E. A.: Effects of pentobarbital pretreatment on the response of rat liver to halothane administration. Proc. Soc. Exp. Biol. Med. *140:* 1319 (1972).
STOELTING, R. K.; REIS, R.; LONGNECKER, D. E.: Hemodynamic response to nitrous oxide-halothane in patients with valvular heart disease. Anaesthesiology *37:* 430 (1972).
STOLK, P.: personal communication.
SUWA, K.; HEDLEY-WHITE, J.; BENDIXEN, H.: Circulation and physiologic dead space changes on controlling the ventilation of dogs. J. Appl. Physiol. *21:* 1855 (1966).
TAVERNOR, W. D.; LEES, P.: The influence of thiopentone and suxamethonium on cardiovascular respiratory function in the horse. Res. Vet. Sci. *11:* 45 (1970).
TIEGLAND, M. B.: Drug Survey. Proc. Ann. Conv. Amer. Assoc. Equine Pract. (1969), 299.
THURMON, J. C.: Some aspects of large animal inhalation anaesthetic equipment. Proc. 18th Ann. Conv. Amer. Assoc. Equine Pract. (1972), 465.
TRIM, C. M.; MASON, J.: Post-anaesthetic forelimb lameness in horses. Equine Vet. J. *5:* 71 (1973).
WALDRON-MEASE, E.; ROSENBERG, H.: Post anesthetic myositis in the horse associated with in vitro malignant hyperthermia susceptibility. Vet. Sci. Comm. *3:* 45 (1979).
WEAVER, B. M. Q.: Mechanical control of ventilation in horses. Vet. Rec. *80:* 249 (1967).
WEAVER, B. M. Q.; WALLEY, R. V.: Ventilation and cardiovascular studies during mechanical control of ventilation in horses. Equine Vet. J. *7:* 9 (1975).
WEISKOPF, R. B.; RAYMOND, L. W.; SEVERINGHAUS, J. W.: Effects of halothane on canine respiratory responses to hypoxia with and without hypercarbia. Anesthesiology *41:* 350 (1974).
WERNER, J.; SCHÄFER, E.; TRAUTVETTER, E.: Zur unblutigen Blutdruckmessung an Haustieren. I. Methodik, Gerät, blutige Vergleichsmessungen, Manschettenbreiten und erste Messungen an Ratten und Rhesusaffen. Zbl. Vet.-Med., R. A. *24:* 229 (1977).
WINTER, P.; SMITH, G.: The toxicity of oxygen. Anaesthesiology *37:* 210 (1972).
WINTZER, H. J.; KELLER, H.; MÜLLER, R.; JAESCHKE, G.: Die Halothan-Sauerstoffnarkose beim Pferd nach Prämedikation mit Atropin/Combelen® und Chloralhydrat. Berliner Münchener tierärztl. Wschr. *92:* 81 (1979).
WOLFF, W. A.; LUMB, W. V.; RAMSAY, M. K.: Effects of halothane and chloroform anaesthesia on the equine liver. Amer. J. Vet. Res. *28:* 1363 (1967).
YOSHIDA, S.; TAKENAGA, S.; HARA, H.; OKUDA, Y.; KUMAGAYA, U.: Measuring value of blood halothane concentration, blood gas and pH in anesthetized horses. Exper. Rep. Eq. Hlth. Lab. *12:* 12 (1975).
ZETNER, K.: Konstruktion und klinische Anwendung eines Kreisatemsystems für Grosstiere. Wien. Tierärztl. Mschr. *60:* 127 (1973).
ZINN, R. S.; GABEL, A. A.; HEATH, R. B.: Effects of succinylcholine and promazine on the cardiovascular and respiratory system of horses. J. Amer. vet. med. Assoc. *157:* 1495 (1970).

1.2.3. Local Anesthesia

Advantages. In addition to its diagnostic value, local anesthesia has several other advantages in the horse:

— The drugs used are relatively inexpensive, and no special instruments or equipment are needed.
— The toxicity is low with proper dosage, and there are few complications with correct technique.
— Some operations can be performed under a lighter plane of anesthesia (e.g., chloral hydrate anesthesia).
— Certain procedures can be done with the animal standing, thus eliminating the problems of casting and postoperative recovery.
— Operations can be performed on animals that are poor risks for general anesthesia.

Disadvantages. Certain procedures performed in the standing horse are not recommended for nervous or dangerous animals, although good sedation can often solve this problem in these situations. Some procedures, such as eye operations, require absolute immobility of the patient. These operations can be done only under deep general anesthesia.

1.2.3.1. Common Local Anesthetic Agents

1. *Procaine* (Novocain) is an economical drug with low toxicity and a duration of effect from 30 min to 1 h. Its penetrating ability is relatively poor, and it causes local vasodilation. Procaine is not used for topical anesthesia. For infiltration anesthesia the strength used is 1—2%; for conduction anesthesia, 2—5%. Due to its low infiltrating ability and acidic pH (3.6—4.4), however, it is less suitable for conduction anesthesia.

2. *Tetracaine hydrochloride* (Pontocaine) is used mainly as a topical anesthetic agent in a 2% solution. The spray form is particularly suited for anesthesia of the mucous membranes.

3. *Hydroxycaine hydrochloride* (Cornecaine) is a nonirritating, potent and fast-acting topical anesthetic agent for the eye when applied in 1—3% solutions.

4. *Proxymetacaine* is a topical anesthetic agent for the eye (0.5%).

5. *Lidocaine* is about 2 times as potent as procaine, has a markedly higher penetrating ability, and is therefore suitable for infiltration anesthesia. It does not cause vasodilation. Its duration of action is 1 to $1^1/_2$ h. One-half to 1% solutions are used for infiltration anesthesia, 1—2% solutions for conduction anesthesia, and 2—6% solutions for topical anesthesia.

6. *Mepivacaine hydrochloride* (Carbocaine, Scandicaine) is somewhat less toxic than lidocaine and causes mild vasoconstriction. Its duration of effect is $1^1/_2$ to $1^3/_4$ h. Mepivacaine hydrochloride causes practically no tissue irritation.

7. *Butanilicaine* (Hostacaine) has properties similar to lidocane. However, its acidic pH (4.15) makes it less suitable for nerve blocks of the limbs; it can cause perineural irritation.

8. *Bupivacaine hydrochloride* (Marcaine) is about 4 times as potent as lidocaine. Its duration of effect is 3—5 h. It is used mainly for nerve block in solutions of 0.25—0.5%; it is usually combined with epinephrine in a concentration of 1: 200,000.

Addition of other drugs to local anesthetic agents: Other substances can be added to local anesthetics, such as epinephrine, levarterenol (norepinephrine), ornithine-vasopressin, phenylephrine, dextran and hyaluronidase.

1. Hyaluronidase greatly increases the diffusion of the anesthetic agent. It is usually combined with epinephrine to delay absorption and thus increase the duration of anesthesia. Hyaluronidase may be indicated for infiltration anesthesia of fibrous connective tissue and for the blocking of nerves that are difficult to reach.

2. Drugs used to prolong local anesthesia

a) Vasoconstricting agents: Vasoconstrictors are added mainly to delay absorption of the local anesthetic agent, prolong its duration of action, and increase the safety margin with regard to toxicity. They also reduce bleeding in the operative area during infiltration anesthesia. If large amounts of such a local anesthetic are injected, however, toxic quantities of epinephrine or levarterenol may be absorbed. Intravascular injection is a danger in extremely vascular tissues. In addition, subsequent wound healing may be delayed by the infiltration of vasoconstrictors, and persistent tissue hypoxia can lead to wound necrosis and infection. These complications can be avoided by using epinephrine or levarterenol only in very low concentrations (1: 200,000) or by using agents such as ornithine-vasopressin that are less hazardous in terms of local or systemic side-effects. The gradual breakdown of epinephrine in anesthetic solutions can be a problem during storage. In the process, hydrogen ions (H^+) are released, and the pH may fall to values as low as 2.8 resulting in possible tissue irritation [Sack, 1975]. This deterioration is accelerated by exposure to light and oxygen.

b) Dextran (6%), ammonium sulfate (20%) or oily solutions: The addition of dextran or ammonium sulfate or the use of oily solutions can also prolong the effect of local anesthetic agents.

1.2.3.2. Toxicity of Local Anesthetic Agents

Besides the toxic action of epinephrine or norepinephrine and the rare occurrence of allergic reactions, the local anesthetics themselves can exert toxic effects as the result of overdosage or intravascular injection. As well, too rapid absorption caused by hyaluronidase or injection into tissues with a rich blood supply can produce toxicity.

Intravascular injections are most common in heavily vascularized tissues. This may occur during the blocking of nerves that are closely associated with blood vessels, or during epidural anesthesia as a result of accidental puncture of a vein situated on the floor of the spinal canal. To prevent intravascular injections, repeated aspiration should be carried out before and during the injection. Toxic reactions are manifested initially by an excitatory phase with convulsions, hyperventilation and tachycardia, which is followed by a depressive phase with apnea, sphincter paralysis and coma. Sudden cardiac arrest sometimes occurs. Peripheral vasodilation with a resultant fall of blood pressure can be observed in most cases. The convulsions increase oxygen consumption, leading to hypoxemia. Lidocaine, by contrast, tends to cause depression rather than stimulation. Convulsions are treated mainly by the intravenous injection of short-acting barbiturates and, if necessary, by artificial respiration with oxygen. Analeptics are contraindicated. If the fall of blood pressure is severe, treatment with vasopressors is indicated. Cardiac massage is the treatment of choice for cardiac arrest.

1.2.3.3. Infiltration Anesthesia

The purpose of infiltration anesthesia is to deaden the nerve endings in the area of operation. The agents of choice are procaine (1—2%), lidocaine, mepivacaine hydrochloride or butanilicaine (0.5—1%). For linear incisions, the infiltration is made along the proposed line of incision. For this purpose the anesthetic agent is injected into the subcutaneous tissue as well as into deeper layers that must be incised during the operation. For a laparotomy, for example, the subcutaneous tissue and various muscle layers of the flank are infiltrated down to the peritoneum. To avoid struggling during the subcutaneous or deeper injection, some of the agent can be injected intracutaneously with a fine needle. This will desensitize the skin almost immediately, and the needle can be passed deeper through the skin wheal. To obtain good subcutaneous injection of the agent, it is advisable to grasp a fold of skin with the left hand and raise it somewhat. A good subcutaneous injection is evidenced by the presence of a visible swelling. For the suturing of skin wounds under local anesthesia, the needle can be inserted subcutaneously at the edges of the disinfected wound, rather than through the skin. This is less painful, and the animal will show only a slight reaction in most cases. In certain operations, such as the removal of tumors, the agent should be infiltrated so as to create a rhomboid or pyramid-shaped field block around the operative site. The addition of vasoconstrictors is contraindicated in such cases, due to the danger of tissue necrosis. In operations on the limbs, a 'ring block' can be done by infiltrating the soft tissues around the limb to produce anesthesia distal to the site of injection. Intravenous local anesthesia is very seldom performed in the horse. According to Arnberg and Sønnichsen [1973], the risk of a toxic reaction is greater in horses than in cattle.

1.2.3.4. Nerve Blocks (Conduction Anesthesia)

In conduction anesthesia, the nerve or nerves that innervate the operative area are blocked by the perineural injection of an anesthetic agent along their course. The advantage of this method is that a relatively large area can be desensitized with a small amount of anesthetic agent, and the agent does not interfere with wound healing. Because the agent must be injected as close to the nerves as possible, this method is suitable only for nerves with a constant anatomically accessible location. No fascia must be present between the nerve and the injected agent, because fascial layers act as barriers to the drug. Besides their use in surgery, such nerve blocks are also useful in lameness diagnosis. Nerve blocks are contraindicated in incomplete or fissure fractures (such as occurs in the proximal phalanx) because they may encourage the horse to bear full weight on the affected limb or even enable it to run, with consequent dehiscence of the fracture or fissure. Another contraindication is present in severe degenerative processes of the flexor tendon and partial divisions of this tendon, due to the danger of rupture. The animal should not be allowed to gallop or run on a hard surface following nerve block anesthesia. If the horse no longer limps, it may be assumed that the painful lesion has been localized within the densitized area. It must be noted, that occasionally some lamenesses spontaneously regress with exercise, and that this may be cause for a misdiagnosis. If the horse is still lame after nerve block anesthesia, the painful lesion must lie outside the desensitized region, usually proximal to it. The lameness may occasionally be due to mechanical reasons, such as ankylosis.

1.2.3.4.1. Nerve Blocks of the Head Region

Nerve blocks in the head region are very useful in the horse, because they permit certain operations to be performed with the animal standing.

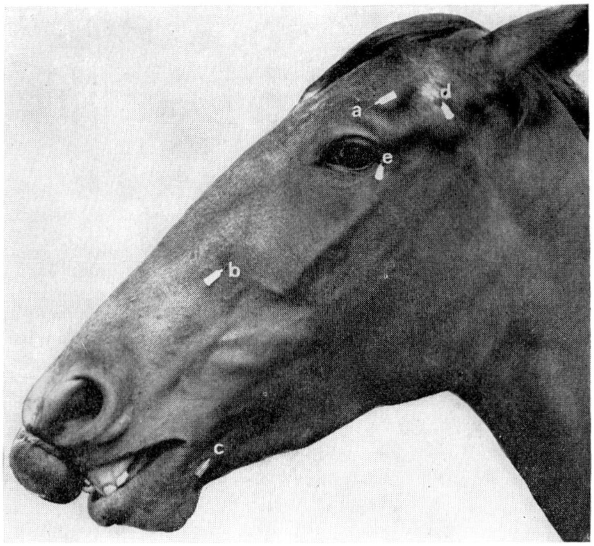

Fig. 1.2. — 19. Nerve blocks of the head region. a = frontal nerve; b = infraorbital nerve; c = mandibular alveolar nerve; d = auriculopalpebral nerve; e = ophthalmic nerve.

Supraorbital Nerve (branch of the trigeminal, fig. 1.2. — 19, a). The supraorbital nerve emerges from the orbit via the supraorbital foramen. This foramen is located slightly medial to the highest point of the supraorbital arch on a line running through the medial canthus parallel to the midline of the head. This block desensitizes (but does not paralyze) the upper eyelid, especially its medial portion, and the medial region of the forehead. The dose is 5 ml.

Infraorbital Nerve (branch of the trigeminal, fig. 1.2. — 19, b). The infraorbital nerve can be reached at the level of the infraorbital foramen or in the infraorbital canal. The infraorbital foramen is located on a line starting from the medial canthus and running parallel to the facial crest, about 1 cm anterior to the rostral end of this crest. The posterior edge of this foramen is easily palpated, especially in thin animals. For the injection, the levator labii maxillaris muscle is pushed upward, and 10 ml of anesthetic agent are injected through the thin levator nasolabialis muscle. This produces anesthesia of the upper lip and nostril. To block the nerve within the infraorbital canal, the needle is inserted about 1 cm rostral to the infraorbital foramen and advanced into the canal to a depth of 5—8 cm. A short-bevel needle that is not too sharp is preferred. A correctly placed needle should have no lateral freedom of movement. An injection of 10 ml desensitizes the upper lip and nostril for a distance of 2.3 cm rostral to the medial canthus, the incisors, the premolars and the 1st and 2nd molars together with their corresponding gingivae. If all the maxillary teeth and entire upper gum are to be anesthetized, the infraorbital nerve can be blocked at its point of entry into the upper jaw, the maxillary foramen. This technique is of less practical value, however. It is performed with a 10-cm needle inserted in a medial direction 2.5 cm ventral to the lateral canthus of the eye, precisely at the lower margin of the facial crest. The needle is advanced in a slightly dorsal direction past the maxillary tuber into the pterygopalatine fossa, and 10 ml of a suitable agent are injected. Vascular puncture must be avoided.

Mental Nerve and Mandibular Alveolar Nerve (branch of the trigeminal, fig. 1.2. — 19, c). The mental nerve is accessible at the level of the mental foramen, and the mandibular alveolar nerve in the mandibular canal. The mental foramen is located between the canine tooth and 1st premolar, 2—3 cm below the angle of the mouth. The lower lip is desensitized by an injection of 10 ml local anesthetic. By injecting the same dose through the mental foramen 3—5 cm deep in the mandibular canal, anesthesia is produced in the lower lip, a portion of the mandible, the incisors, and in some cases the 1st molar (M 1). To obtain anesthesia of the mandible, lower teeth and lower lip, the mandibular alveolar nerve is blocked at the level of the mandibular foramen. This foramen is located on the medial aspect of the mandible at the point where the continuation of the occlusal surface of the lower molars intersects a vertical line through the lateral canthus of the eye. A 15-cm needle is inserted at the ventral border of the mandible below the mandibular foramen and is advanced to the foramen. The level of the foramen should be marked on the needle in advance. From 10 to 20 ml of anesthetic are injected.

Auriculopalpebral Nerve (branch of the facial nerve, fig. 1.2. — 19, d). A block of the auriculopalpebral nerve paralyzes the orbicularis oculi muscle, thus preventing voluntary or reflex closure of the eyelids. There is no desensitization of the lid or eye, however. This block is used for surgery of the lid or eye and during subconjunctival injections in order to prevent lid movements. It is also indicated during ocular examinations or for the relief of severe blepharospasm that may cause entropion. The needle is inserted 1.5—2 cm below the highest point of the caudal part of the dorsal margin of the zygomatic arch and is advanced to the superior margin of the zygomatic arch. The anesthetic is injected subfascially in a dose of 5 ml. Absolute akinesia is not obtained in many cases, however, probably due to the presence of small accessory motor branches given off by the main branch arising from the facial nerve.

Ophthalmic Nerve Block at the Level of the Orbital Fissure (fig. 1.2. — 19, e). To produce anesthesia of the eyelids, conjunctivae and eye, a 10- to 12-cm needle is inserted through the skin or conjunctiva to puncture the orbit in the direction of the contralateral temperomandibular joint. A dose of 20—30 ml is injected at the level of the orbital fissure at a depth of 7—10 cm. This usually blocks the abducent, oculomotor and trochlear nerves as well, thus producing full ocular paralysis. Mydriasis is obtained by blocking the parasympathetic innervators of the iris sphincter. Care must be taken to avoid the puncture of blood vessels or injury to the optic nerve. Anesthesia of the eye only can be obtained by the retrobulbar injection of 20—30 ml of a suitable agent. This is done with a 10-cm needle inserted 1.5 cm behind the midpoint of the zygomatic process of the frontal bone in the direction of the last upper premolar of the contralateral side. In the process, the hard periorbita is punctured. Immobility of the eye is not usually obtained with this technique.

1.2.3.4.2. Nerve Blocks of the Limbs

a) Forelimb

Median Nerve (fig. 1.2. — 20, a). The block can be done at the level of the median nerve, or a median nerve block can be combined with a block of the ulnar and musculocutaneous nerves in some cases (e.g., carpal wounds). The median nerve innervates the radial head and medial and distal parts of the humeral head of the deep digital flexor muscle, and the flexor carpi radialis muscle. It also gives off sensory branches during its course, bifurcating proximally to the carpus to form the lateral and medial palmar nerves. The median nerve can be blocked by subfascial injection slightly below the elbow joint on the medial side. The nerve is easily palpated at this location. Puncture of the median vein and artery must be avoided. The needle is inserted obliquely in a proximal direction, and a dose of 10—20 ml is injected.

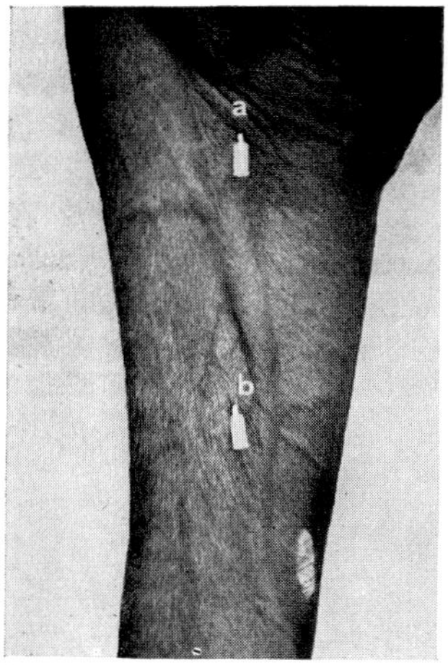

20

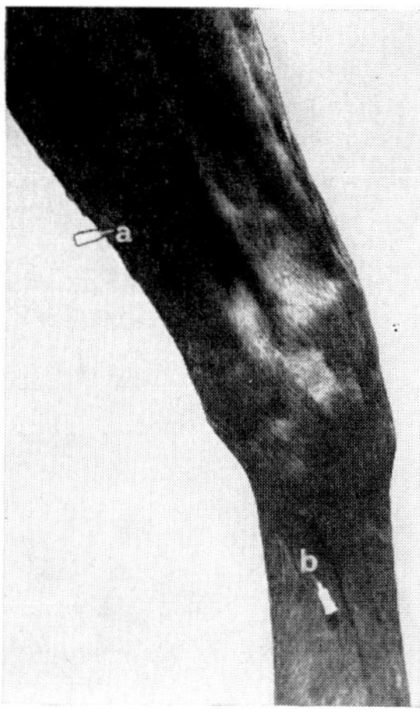

21

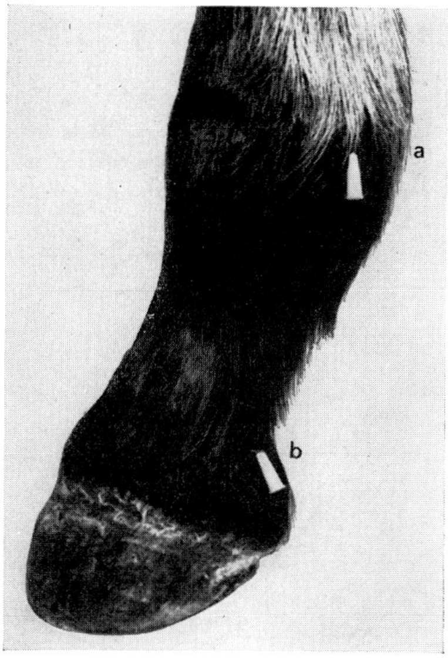

22

Fig. 1.2. — 20. Blocking the median nerve and musculocutaneous nerve. a = median nerve; b = main branch of musculocutaneous nerve.

Fig. 1.2. — 21. Blocking the ulnar nerve and palmar nerves (proximal). a = ulnar nerve; b = lateral palmar nerve.

Fig. 1.2. — 22. Blocking the palmar nerves and palmar digital nerves. a = lateral palmar nerve; b = palmar digital nerve.

Ulnar Nerve (fig. 1.2. — 21, a). An ulnar nerve block desensitizes the skin on the dorsolateral aspect of the distal forearm, carpus and metacarpus. It is also useful in the diagnosis of 'splints' or damage to the suspensory ligament and proximal portion of the sesamoids. The ulnar nerve is blocked on the lateropalmar aspect in the groove between the flexor carpi ulnaris and ulnaris lateralis muscles. The needle is inserted horizontally to a depth of 1—2 cm, and 10 ml of anesthetic are injected beneath the fascia.

Musculocutaneous Nerve (fig. 1.2. — 20, b). The musculocutaneous nerve sends branches to the biceps brachii, coracobrachialis and brachialis muscles and innervates mainly the dorsolateral skin from the lower half of the forearm down to the fetlock joint.

The main branch of the musculocutaneous nerve is blocked about a hand's breadth proximal to the chestnut, between the cephalic vein and medial border of the extensor carpi radialis muscle. At this point the nerve is subcutaneous and can usually be palpated.

Lateral and Medial Palmar Nerves. Blocks of the lateral and medial palmar nerves or their branches are often used for surgery distal to the carpus and as an aid in the diagnosis of lameness. The lateral and medial palmar nerves are subfascial at the level of the metacarpus at the border of the deep flexor tendon. The nerves are connected by a communicating branch which leaves the medial palmar nerve in the proximal third of the metacarpus and anastomoses with the lateral palmar nerve at the level of the proximal part of the distal third of the metacarpus. Proximal to the fetlock joint the palmar nerves are subcutaneous and divide into two digital branches. One of these branches, the dorsal, has a highly variable course: It usually arises proximal to the fetlock joint, but may arise at the level of this joint or somewhat distal to it. Sometimes a branch of the palmar metacarpal nerve passes dorsal to the dorsal branch on the medial side, passing to the coronet. This branch sometimes communicates with the dorsal branch. According to Sack [1975], however, these nerves simply cross without exchanging fibers. On the lateral aspect, a branch of the lateral palmar nerve arising distal to the carpus sometimes passes dorsal to the dorsal branch. The dorsal branch supplies the skin on the dorsal and lateral aspect of the fetlock joint down to the coronary band as well as the coronary band itself, the perioplic corium, parts of the laminar corium, a portion of the lateral cartilage, the dorsal part of the distal phalanx, proximal interphalangeal (pastern) joint, and distal interphalangeal (coffin) joint. Branches of the dorsal branch also supply the skin and laminar corium in the pastern region. According to Sack [1975], the distal interphalangeal joint is not supplied by the dorsal branch, because this nerve releases only a few subcutaneous twigs in a dorsal direction distal to the proximal interphalangeal (pastern) joint and thus innervates only the coronary corium but not the laminar corium.

The lateral or medial palmar digital nerve passes on the palmar side of the blood vessels at the level of the deep flexor tendon and reaches the lateral cartilage on the medial aspect. The palmar digital nerve innervates the caudal part of the hoof, the skin of the metacarpophalangeal (fetlock) joint and heel, the corium of the sole, the distal phalanx, the navicular bursa, a portion of the lateral cartilage, part of the laminar corium, the flexor tendon, the palmar part of the metacarpophalangeal (fetlock) joint, the coronet joint and the distal interphalangeal (coffin) joint.

The metacarpophalangeal (fetlock) joint is supplied by the following nerves on the palmar side: the lateral and medial palmar nerves, the lateral and medial palmar digital nerves, and the lateral and medial palmar metacarpal nerves (which arise from the deep and palmar branches of the ulnar nerve).

In some horses the dorsal pouch of the metacarpophalangeal (fetlock) joint capsule is innervated by the dorsal branch of the lateral and medial palmar digital nerves. The proximal interphalangeal (pastern) joint is supplied on its palmar surface only by branches of the lateral and medial palmar digital nerves, and on its dorsal surface by the dorsal branch of the lateral and medial palmar digital nerves.

The nerve distribution in the front digit shows a high degree of individual variation, however [Pohlmeyer and Redecker, 1974a].

Palmar Nerve Block in the Proximal Metacarpus (fig. 1.2. — 21, b). The needle is passed through the skin and fascia several centimeters to one handbreadth below the carpus at the level of the deep flexor tendon. The nerve is not palpable at this location. The injection must be made beneath the fascia, and so only a slight swelling should be visible at the injection site. A dose of 10 ml is injected, usually with the carpus in the flexed position. The needle and syringe should be directed toward the carpus, so that sudden forward movements by the limb will not cause the needle to break or penetrate deeper. Before the agent is injected, it must be certain that the needle has not entered a blood vessel. If that is the case, the needle must be repositioned before injecting. To block the more proximal, main branches of the ulnar or musculocutaneous nerve, an additional 5 ml of anesthetic can be injected subcutaneously. In this way the digit is anesthetized up to and including the metacarpophalangeal (fetlock) joint and up to the carpus on the palmar side. The medial palmar nerve, unlike the lateral palmar nerve gives off large branches only distal to the communicating branch [Sack, 1975]. The strip of skin at the level of the proximal part of the medial palmar nerve is supplied by a branch of the ulnar nerve and

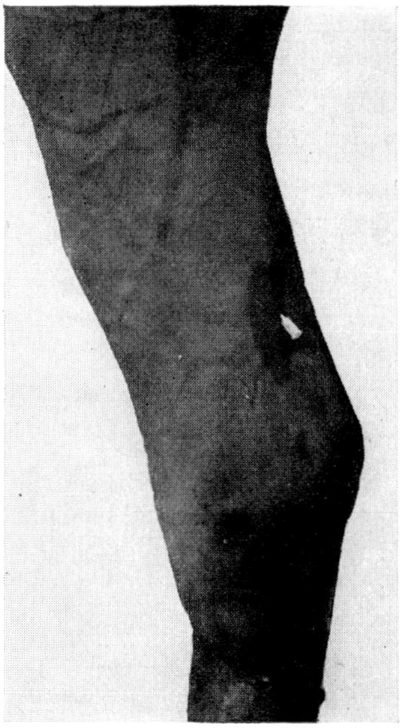

23

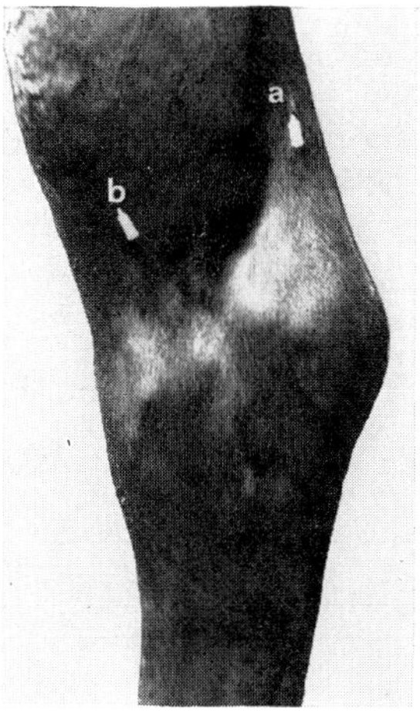

24

Fig. 1.2. — 23. Blocking the tibial nerve.

Fig. 1.2. — 24. Blocking the caudal sural cutaneous nerve and fibular nerve. a = caudal sural cutaneous nerve; b = fibular nerve.

by branches of the lateral palmar nerve. In certain diseases of the fetlock joint, lameness may persist despite a successful nerve block. Assuming the lameness is not of the 'mechanical' type, its cause can be eliminated by doing an additional ring block around the metacarpus.

Palmar Nerve Block at the Level of the Fetlock Joint (fig. 1.2. — 22, a). At the level of the proximal sesamoids, the nerve and blood vessels can be palpated on the lateropalmar and mediopalmar side, unless there is significant edema or marked subcutaneous fibrosis. The dose is 5 ml injected subcutaneously. A block at this level anesthetizes the foot up to a plane through the fetlock joint, which itself is usually only partly desensitized. Anesthesia of the digit may also be only partial if the nerve distribution is unusual. To obtain anesthesia of the small metacarpal (splint) bones, the palmar metacarpal nerves must also be blocked. This is done by injecting 3—4 ml bilaterally with a fine needle inserted to a depth of 1 cm between the suspensory ligament and the splint bone.

Palmar Digital Nerve Block (fig. 1.2. — 22, b). This is used primarily to assist in the diagnosis of navicular disease, lesions of the distal phalanx (coffin bone), and other pathologic states in the palmar region of the digit. The nerve is palpable, and it is blocked with 2 ml of anesthetic injected just proximal to the lateral cartilage. The dorsal and lateral coronary skin remains sensitive to pain. If a larger dose is injected, however, the dorsal branch is also blocked, thus negating the diagnostic value of this block for changes in the palmar region of the digit. For anesthesia of the navicular bone and navicular bursa, the posterior branch of the palmar digital nerve must be blocked. To ensure this a needle is inserted 1 to 1.5 cm deep on the medial side of the lateral cartilage near its palmar border and injecting 5 ml of anesthetic agent. The dorsal branch is not concurrently blocked by injection at this site [Zeller, 1978].

b) Hindlimb

Tibial Nerve (fig. 1.2. — 23). The anesthetic is injected on the medial side of the limb about 10 cm above the proximal part of the calcaneus, in the groove formed by the Achilles tendon and flexor digiti I longus muscle. When the joint is flexed slightly, the nerve is usually well palpable. The needle is inserted beneath the fascia, and about 15 ml of anesthetic are injected. An additional 5 ml are injected subcutaneously as the needle is withdrawn in order to block the medial tarsal cutaneous branch, which supplies the skin on the medial aspect of the hock joint and proximal third metatarsal bone. The tibial nerve block provides anesthesia of the interphalangeal joints, the skin and the deeper tissues [proximal sesamoids, digital sheath, flexor tendons and small metatarsal bones (splints)]. For the diagnosis of spavin the tibial nerve block is combined with a block of the deep fibular nerve. Another cutaneous branch of the tibial nerve, the *lateral caudal sural cutaneous nerve*, unites with a branch of the superficial fibular nerve about a handbreadth above the tuber calcis to supply the skin on the lateral surface from the level of the tarsus and metatarsus down to the fetlock. This *caudal sural cutaneous nerve* is blocked on the lateral side of the limb at the level of the proximal half of the Achilles tendon (fig. 1.2. — 24, a). The needle is inserted beneath the fascia at the lateral border of the Achilles tendon; 10 ml of anesthetic are injected subfascially, and an equal dose subcutaneously.

Fibular Nerve (fig. 1.2. — 24, b). The two branches of the common fibular nerve, namely the deep fibular nerve and the superficial nerve, can be blocked at two sites. The first site is located slightly distal to the bifurcation of the nerve at the level of the fibular head on the lateral side of the limb. The needle is inserted obliquely beneath the fascia in a proximal direction, and 10 ml of a local anesthetic are injected. Because the digital extensors are blocked, the typical picture of a knuckled fetlock develops. Sometimes the superficial fibular nerve is not blocked. Somewhat more distally, the two fibular nerve branches can either be blocked together or separately. This is done about 10 cm above the tibiotarsal joint in the groove between the long and lateral digital extensors. Here the superficial fibular nerve can be palpated beneath the skin. The deep branch is blocked by inserting the needle obliquely upward and injecting 10—15 ml of anesthetic beneath the fascia. The superficial branch is blocked with 10 ml injected subcutaneously. The superficial fibular nerve sends branches to the hock joint and supplies the skin on the dorsolateral side of the tarsus and metatarsus and on the dorsal side of the pastern down to the hoof. The deep fibular nerve supplies the digital extensors and hock joint and, in conjugation with superficial fibular nerve branches, the skin on the dorsodistal surface of the limb.

Saphenous Nerve (fig. 1.2. — 25). The saphenous nerve gives off branches to the stifle joint and innervates the skin on the medial side of the lower leg, hock joint and metatarsus down to the fetlock. The saphenous nerve can be palpated subcutaneously next to the saphenous vein on the medial side of the limb and is blocked by the subcutaneous injection of 10—15 ml at the point where the saphenous vein disappears in the femoral canal.

Plantar Nerve Block at the Level of the Fetlock Joint (fig. 1.2. — 26). The medial and lateral plantar nerves are blocked with about 10 ml of anesthetic in a manner analogous to that described for the palmar nerves of the forelimb. To obtain complete anesthesia of the digit from the fetlock down, an additional 10 ml are injected both laterally and medially just dorsal to the collateral ligaments of the fetlock joint. With this method the lateral (branch of deep fibular) and medial plantar metatarsal nerves and the medial metatarsal nerve are blocked.

Plantar Digital Nerve Block. The technique is the same used in the forelimb. The nerve distribution may show variations, however [Pohlmeyer and Redecker, 1974, b]. The lateral and medial plantar nerves, the lateral and medial plantar digital nerves, and the lateral and medial plantar metatarsal nerves supply the plantar surface of the fetlock joint. Plantar and dorsal innervation is sometimes provided by the dorsal metatarsal nerve (branch of the fibular); the dorsal surface is sometimes

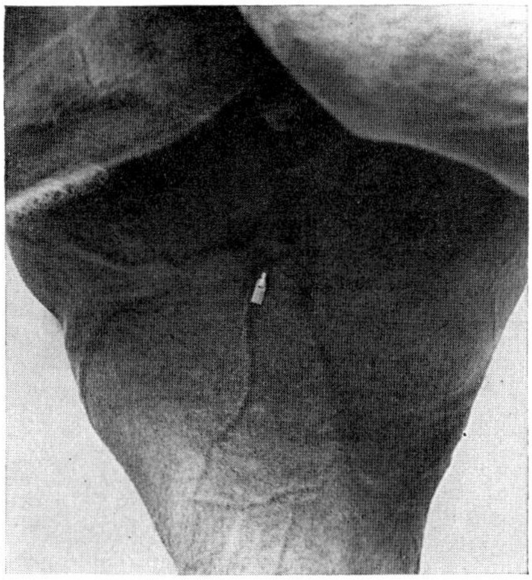
25

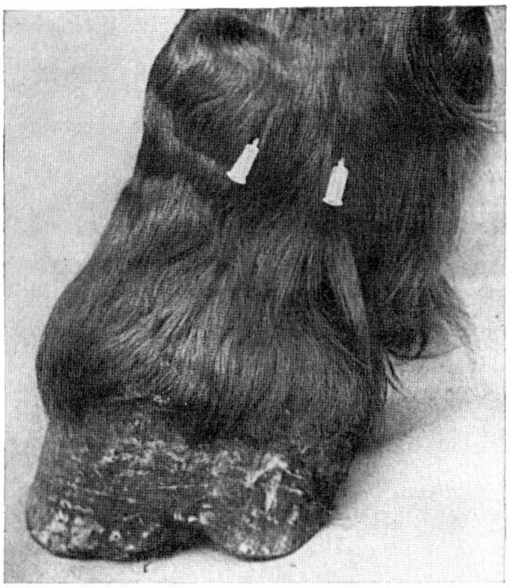
26

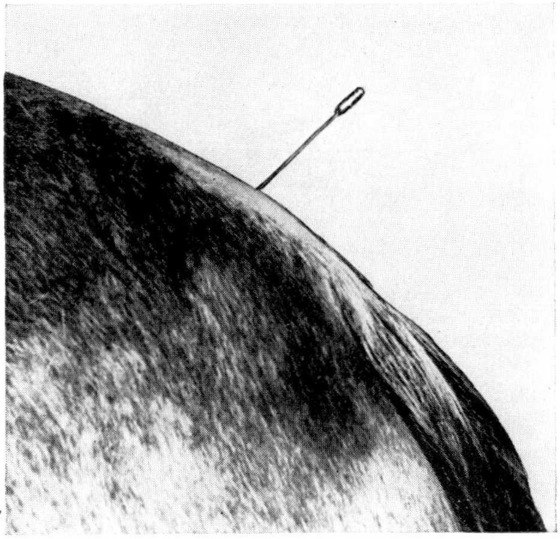
27

Fig. 1.2. — 25. Blocking the saphenous nerve.
Fig. 1.2. — 26. Distal plantar nerve block.
Fig. 1.2. — 27. Epidural anesthesia.

supplied by the dorsal branch. The pastern joint is supplied on the plantar side by the lateral and medial plantar digital nerves and the lateral and medial dorsal metatarsal nerves (branches of the fibular). It is also supplied on the dorsal side by the lateral and medial dorsal branch and by branches of the lateral and medial dorsal metatarsal nerves.

1.2.3.4.3. Epidural Anesthesia

Epidural anesthesia is generally administered in the caudal area, specifically in the first intercoccygeal space because Cy 1 is often fused with the sacrum (fig. 1.2. — 27). When the tail is moved upward and downward, a depression can be felt between Cy 1 and Cy 2 cranial to the 2nd, more mobile vertebra. It is located about 2—5 cm cranial to the first long tail hairs. This site is sometimes difficult to palpate in fat or heavy animals because of the thick soft-tissue covering. At parturition it is easier to palpate owing to the laxness of the tissues. A 10-cm needle is inserted at a 45—60° angle to a depth of 2—8 cm, taking care to keep the point on the midline. Usually the needle is directed toward the caudodorsal part of the body of the 1st coccygeal vertebra. A dose of 8—10 ml of a 2% lidocaine solution in the adult horse will desensitize the tail, anus, rectum, vulva and vagina. A test aspiration should be done before injecting as a precaution against intravascular injection. Overdosage carries a risk of incoordination and hindquarter paralysis, possibly resulting in severe injuries. Repeated puncture of the floor of the vertebral canal can cause damage to the coccygeal nerves with transitory paralysis of the tail.

Cranial epidural anesthesia is seldom if ever performed in the horse due to the danger of excitement (caused by hindquarter paralysis) and convulsions.

1.2.3.4.4. Topical Anesthesia

Skin. The intact skin will not absorb local anesthetic agents unless they are applied in very high concentrations and in a suitable solvent. The pain of excoriations and certain forms of dermatitis can be reduced or eliminated by local anesthetics, possibly applied in ointment form. The intact skin can be anesthetized for short periods by freezing or by spraying ethyl chloride onto the skin surface.

Cornea and Conjunctiva. Topical anesthesia in the eye is obtained with a 1—3% solution of hydroxycaine hydrochloride (Cornecaine), 0.5% proxymetacaine, 2—4% lidocaine, or 1—5% tetracaine hydrochloride (e.g., Pantocaine). However, the repeated or prolonged use of local anesthetics in the eye can cause epithelial damage and delay wound healing. Except with lidocaine, epithelialization is usually delayed.

Mucous Membranes. Effective topical anesthesia of the mucous membranes of the nose, pharynx, mouth, penis, prepuce and vagina is obtained by spraying with a 0.5—2% solution of tetracaine hydrochloride or a 4—10% solution of lidocaine.

Joints and Tendon Sheaths. Anesthesia of the joints and tendon sheaths plays an important role in lameness diagnosis. The local anesthetic agent produces desensitization of the synovial membrane. Lidocaine and mepivacaine hydrochloride in 2% concentration are most commonly used. The agent must be injected using strict aseptic technique. The hair is clipped and the skin is thoroughly disinfected. The presence of increased synovial fluid facilitates the injection, while injections in so called 'dry' joints may prove difficult. To prevent the animal from moving and ensure safe intra-articular needle placement, it is often prudent first to apply subcutaneous and pericapsular local anesthesia with a very fine needle. Intra-articular needle placement is confirmed by the escape of synovial fluid. Care must be taken not to confuse the joint, tendon sheath and bursa. Joints that contain little fluid may produce a 'dry' tap. The injection should be done gently, using minimal pressure. If excessive synovial secretions are present, it is best to drain the fluid to minimize dilution of the anesthetic drug and avoid an excessively high intra-articular pressure. The dose is 10—50 ml, depending on which joint is being blocked.

Shoulder Joint (fig. 1.2. — 28, a). The needle is inserted at the cranial border of the tendon of the infraspinous muscle just proximal to the point where this tendon crosses over the caudal part of the greater tubercle of the humerus. The needle is inserted horizontally in a caudal direction to a depth of 5—10 cm, and about 50 ml of anesthetic are injected.

Intertubercular Bursa of the Biceps brachii Muscle (fig. 1.2. — 38, b). This bursa is accessible on the lateral side of the limb just above the proximal end of the deltoid tuberosity, behind the biceps brachii muscle. The 10-cm needle is inserted obliquely in a proximal direction until the humerus is reached, and is advanced between the humerus and biceps brachii to deposit the anesthetic agent.

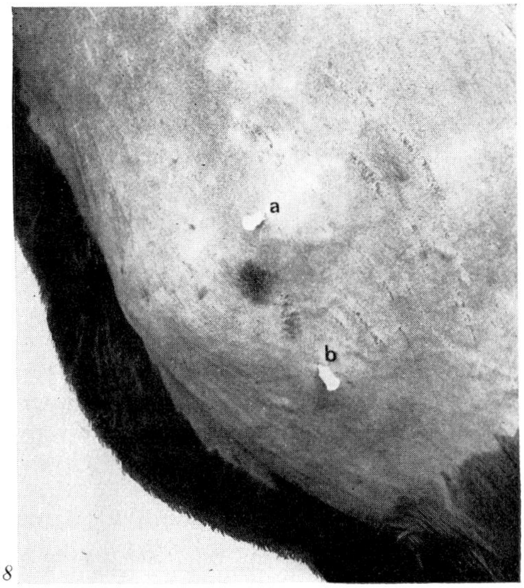

28

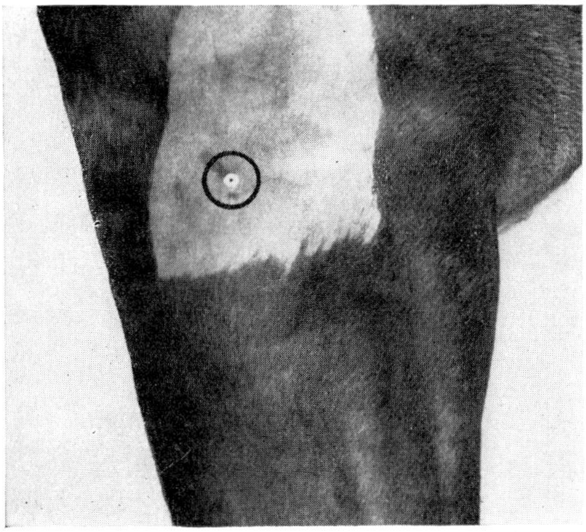

29

Fig. 1.2. — 28. a = Anesthesia of the shoulder joint; b = anesthesia of the intertubercular bursa of the biceps brachii muscle.
Fig. 1.2. — 29. Anesthesia of the elbow joint.

Elbow Joint (fig. 1.2. — 29). The needle can be passed either cranially or caudally to the lateral collateral ligament. For injection cranial to the ligament, the needle is advanced slightly obliquely along the bone and below the lateral condyle of the humerus. The lateral collateral ligament is usually palpable. The elbow joint is located about one handbreadth distal and cranial to the olecranon process of the ulna at the junction between the middle and distal third of the collateral ligament.

Carpal Joint (fig. 1.2. — 30).

a) Radiocarpal joint: This joint is easily injected on the dorsomedial side of the flexed limb between the radius and the proximal row of carpal bones. Another site is on the lateral aspect of the limb, proximal to the accessory carpal bone, between the radius and extensor carpi ulnaris muscle. The needle must be inserted distally and as close to the radius as possible to reduce the danger of piercing the carpal sheath. The radiocarpal joint does not communicate with the intercarpal joint.

b) Intercarpal joint: With the carpus in flexion, the needle is inserted between the proximal and distal row of carpal bones.

c) Carpometacarpal joint: This joint always communicates with the mediocarpal joint and so does not require a separate injection.

Carpal Sheath. The common tendon sheath of the superficial and deep flexor tendon is injected a handbreadth distal to the accessory carpal bone on the lateral surface of the limb. The needle is inserted just anterior to the flexor tendon and is kept as close to this tendon as possible. Another site for this injection is located proximal to the accessory carpal bone, caudoproximal to the injection site for the antebrachiocarpal artery, between the extensor carpi ulnaris muscle and the tendon of the extensor digitalis lateralis muscle.

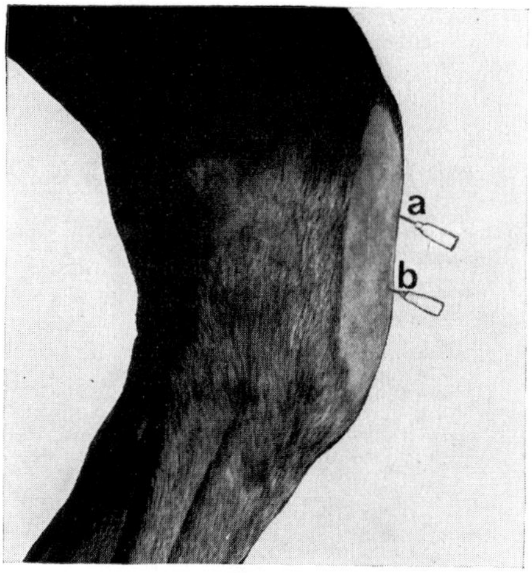

30

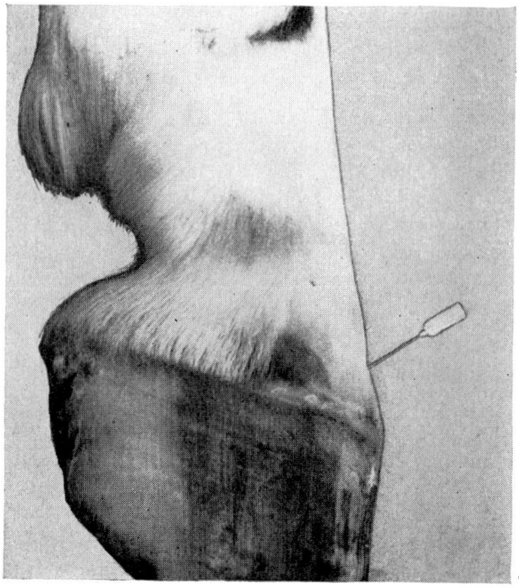
32

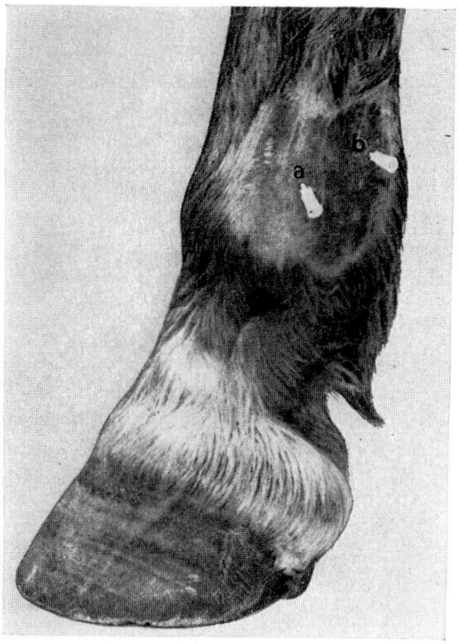

31

Fig. 1.2. — 30. Anesthesia of the carpal joint. a = radiocarpal joint; b = mediocarpal joint.

Fig. 1.2. — 31. a = Anesthesia of the fetlock joint; b = anesthesia of the digital sheath.

Fig. 1.2. — 32. Anesthesia of the coffin joint.

Metacarpophalangeal (Fetlock) Joint (fig. 1.2. — 31, a). The fetlock joint can be reached on the lateral surface of the limb at the proximal border of the lateral sesamoid between Mc III and the suspensory ligament. In quiet animals, the opposite foot should be raised during the injection to place weight on the limb being anesthetized. This will make it easier to detect any distention of the joint. The injection can also be made on the dorsal side, beside the extensor tendon, as well as distal to the abaxial border of the lateral sesamoid bone and dorsal to the superficial flexor tendon [VAN PELT, 1962].

Digital Sheath (fig. 1.2. — 31, b). The injection is made near the tendon of the deep digital flexor muscle, 3—4 cm proximal to the lateral sesamoid bone between the suspensory ligament and the deep digital flexor tendon. The dose is 20 ml.

Proximal Interphalangeal (Pastern) Joint. The sites of insertion of the collateral ligaments on the pastern bone are palpated. The pastern joint is located 1 cm below the line connecting these two points. The injection is made 1—2 cm lateral or medial to the midline, lateral to the extensor tendon at the level of the collateral ligament insertion sites; the needle is passed obliquely downward beneath the extensor tendon.

Distal Interphalangeal (Coffin) Joint (fig. 1.2. — 32). The coffin joint is easily injected from the dorsal aspect of the foot. The foot is lifted forward and held in slight flexion. After subcutaneous infiltration anesthesia on the midline, 1—1.5 cm proximal to the coronary border, the needle is inserted through the common digital extensor tendon into the dorsal pouch of the coffin joint capsule. It is then advanced obliquely in a distal and medial direction beneath the extensor tendon, and about 10 ml of anesthetic are injected. Some authors believe the anesthetic agent diffuses through the coffin bone navicular ligament and enters the navicular bursa. We have been unable to confirm this observation with contrast studies of the coffin joint, however (fig. 1.2. — 33). Following experimental determination of the concentration of a local anesthetic agent in the synovial fluid of the coffin joint and navicular bursa after intra-articular injection, the notion of an effective diffusion of anesthetic solutions from the coffin joint into the navicular bursa 'appears highly doubtful if not untenable' [Wintzer et al., 1976]. A communication between the coffin joint and digital sheath may be present in foals [Calislar and St. Clair, 1969].

Navicular Bursa. If an injection of the navicular bursa is planned, in our opinion an x-ray contrast study is mandatory (fig. 1.2. — 34). The close relations between the coffin joint and bursa make them impossible to differentiate during 'blind' in-

33
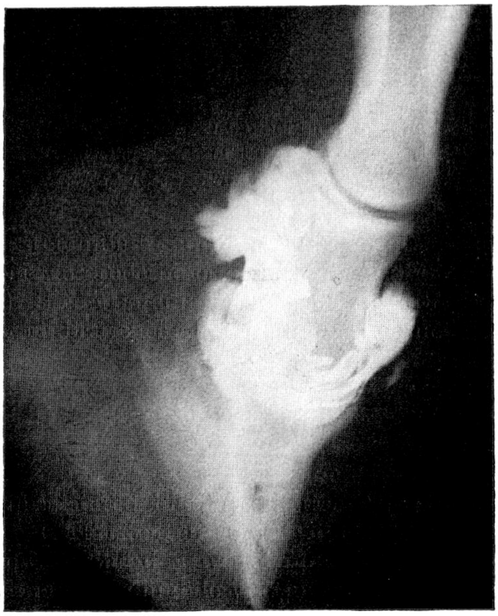

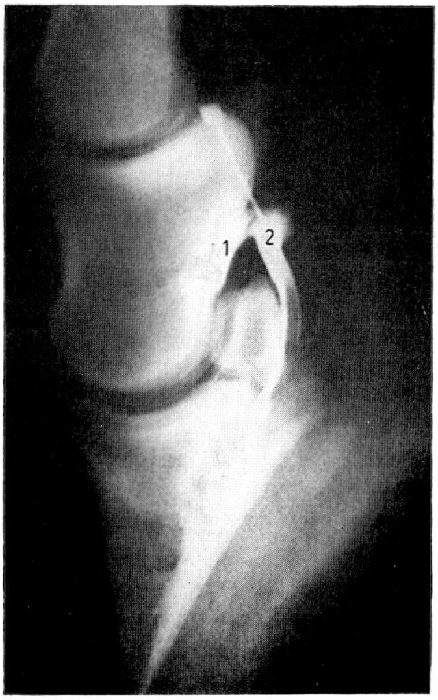

34

Fig. 1.2. — 33. Contrast material has been injected into the coffin joint, showing an absence of communication with the navicular bursa. Radiograph taken 5 min after injection.

Fig. 1.2. — 34. Anesthesia of the navicular bursa, which has been filled with contrast material. 1 = coffin joint; 2 = navicular bursa.

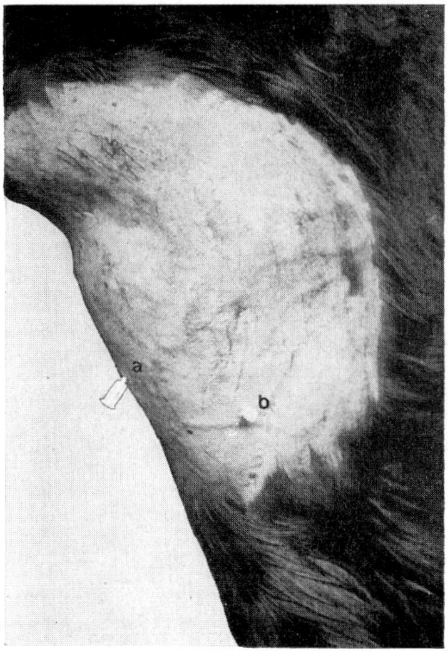

35

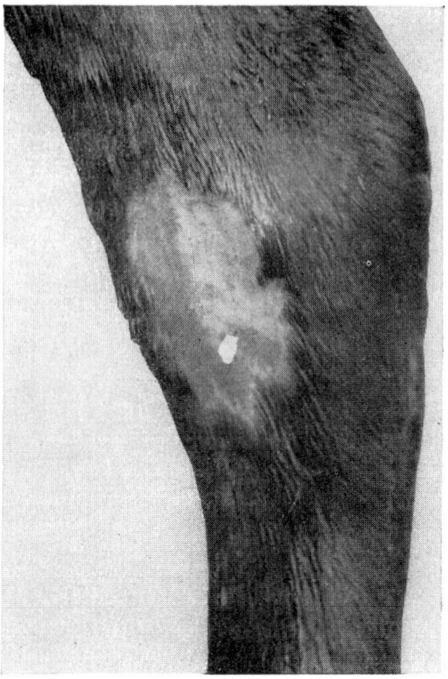

36

Fig. 1.2. — 35. a = Anesthesia of the femoropatellar joint; b = anesthesia of the femorotibial joint (lateral half).

Fig. 1.2. — 36. Anesthesia of the hock joint.

jection. The navicular bursa can be injected from the posterior side through the deep flexor tendon, as well as from the lateral side.

Local or conduction anesthesia and surgical skin preparation are necessary. For a posterior injection, a 0.9 × 55-mm needle is inserted at the midpoint of a line connecting the lateral and medial cartilages of the hoof near the deep flexor tendon. The needle is directed obliquely toward the anterior wall of the hoof.

For a lateral injection the needle is inserted above the middle of the coronary band along a line between the deep flexor tendon and palmar limit of the coffin bone at a slight angle (25—30°) to the horizontal.

Sometimes synovial fluid is obtained immediately. Then 1—2 ml of the radiopaque material are injected, and a radiograph is made. If the palmar recess of the coffin joint has been punctured, a second needle is inserted parallel to the first but 0.5—1 cm caudal to it. An additional 1—2 ml of contrast material is injected, and a new radiograph is taken. More than two injections of contrast medium are seldom necessary. When the needle is positioned within the navicular bursa, the injection may be made; in this case there is no doubt that the agent is being injected into the bursa. No communication between the bursa and coffin joint has been found.

Coxofemoral (Hip) Joint. If the production of synovial fluid is increased, injection of the hip joint is difficult, especially in heavy animals. After infiltrating the area with local anesthetic, a puncture is made with a large-gauge needle; then a smaller gauge needle at least 10 cm long is passed through the notch on the anterior side of the greater trochanter and is advanced along the femoral neck.

Stifle Joint (fig. 1.2. — 35). The stifle joint consists of three parts: the femoropatellar joint, and the lateral and medial femorotibial joints.

The femoropatellar joint communicates with the medial femorotibial joint in 75% of all horses, while it communicates with the lateral femorotibial joint in only about 5%. The two femorotibial articulations rarely communicate with each other.

Femoropatellar Joint (fig. 1.2. — 35, a). A long needle is inserted distal to the patella between the medial and middle patellar ligaments. The needle is inserted horizontally and in a caudal direction. An alternate site is between the middle and lateral patellar ligaments. This interspace tends to be smaller than between the middle and medial ligaments, although the space between these ligaments, too, may be reduced by the protruding medial ridge of the trochlea and by fatty tissue, especially that covering the tibia. The best insertion site in fat animals, therefore, is between the middle and lateral patellar ligaments.

Medial Femorotibial Joint. This joint is accessible between the medial patellar ligament and medial collateral ligament, proximal to the tibial condyle. If the needle is passed too far cranially, it may penetrate through the joint in some circumstances and enter the fatty tissue beneath the patellar ligaments. If inserted too far caudally or distally, on the other hand, the needle may cause meniscal damage. The dose is 30—50 ml.

Lateral Femorotibial Joint (fig. 1.2. — 35, b). Two routes are available for anesthetic injections: either between the lateral patellar ligament and lateral collateral ligament, above the lateral tibial condyle, or through the pouch of the joint capsule overlying the common tendon of the peroneus tertius and long digital extensor muscle. The injection is made just proximal to the lateral tibial condyle, between the common tendon of the peroneus tertius and long digital extensor and the lateral collateral ligament.

Hock Joint (fig. 1.2. — 36). The tibial tarsal joint always communicates with the proximal intertarsal joint. Injection is very simple and is carried out on the dorsomedial aspect between the long digital extensor tendon and the medial collateral ligament distal to the medial malleolus of the tibia. Care must be taken to avoid injury to the saphenous vein. If the synovial fluid is increased, then the pouches located proximoplantar to the lateral and medial malleolus may also be injected. The dose is 30—50 ml.

The distal intertarsal joint sometimes communicates with the tarsometatarsal joint. Injection of this joint is difficult due to the very narrow interarticular space.

Tendon Sheath of the Flexor Digiti I longus and Tibialis caudalis Muscles. This tendon sheath usually communicates distally with the more dorsally located sheath of the flexor digitalis longus tendon. The needle is inserted on the medial side of the tarsus, slightly proximal or distal to the chestnut at the level of the deep flexor tendon. An alternate site is the point where the flexor digiti I longus tendon is palpable; this is about one handbreadth below the tuber calcis (calcaneal tuber).

Calcaneal Bursa under the Superficial Digital Flexor Tendon. With the needle directed horizontally, the injection is made on the medial side 3—4 cm above the tuber calcis at the plantar border of the Achilles tendon.

References

Arnberg, J.; Sonnichsen, H.: Lokal intravenos analgesi. Nord. Vet.-Med. *25:* 575 (1973).

Calislar, T.; St. Clair, L.: Observations on the navicular bursa and the distal interphalangeal joint cavity of the horse. J. Amer. vet. med. Assoc. *154:* 410 (1969).

Pohlmeyer, K.; Redecker, R.: Die für die Klinik bedeutsamen Nerven an den Gliedmassen des Pferdes einschliesslich möglicher Varianten. Dtsch. Tierärztl. Wschr. *81:* 501 (1974a).

POHLMEYER, K.; REDECKER, R.: Die für die Klinik bedeutsamen Nerven an den Gliedmassen des Pferdes einschließlich möglicher Varianten. Dtsch. Tierärztl. Wschr. *81:* 537 (1974b).
SACK, W. O.: Nerve distribution in the metacarpus and front digit of the horse. J. Amer. vet. med. Assoc. *167:* 298 (1975).
SCHMIDT, K.: HELLER, W.; SCHORER, R.: Untersuchungen zur Stabilität adrenalinhaltiger Lokalanaesthetika. Anaesthesist *25:* 342 (1976).
VAN PELT, R.: Intra-articular injection of the equine carpus and fetlock. J. Amer. vet. med. Assoc. *140:* 1181 (1962).
WINTZER, H. J.; FREY, H. H.; FITZEK, A.: Untersuchungen zur Diffusion lokalanästhetischer Lösungen vom Hufgelenk in die Bursa podotrochlearis beim Pferd. Schweiz. Arch. Tierheilk. *118:* 233 (1976).
ZELLER, R.: Die Lokalanästhesie bei der Lahmheitsuntersuchung. Berliner Münchener tierärztl. Wschr. *91:* 166 (1978).

1.3. Equine Nutrition

Nutrition is an important key to the successful keeping and breeding of horses. Following the decline from World War II through the 1960's, there has been a steady rise in the world horse population since 1970. With this has come a significant shift: While the number of horses used for agriculture has steadily declined, the number used for recreation, racing and breeding has undergone both a relative and an absolute increase. In earlier years little was known about the nutrition of the horse compared to other domestic animals. Today, with the high demands placed upon many horses, a review of this species' nutritive requirements is a matter of considerable importance. Physical development and racing performance are directly related to nutrition. Next to training nutrition has the strongest influence on the animal's ability to perform.

1.3.1. Digestion

The nutrients ingested with the feed are transformed by the physical and chemical processes of digestion into a form that can be absorbed by the animal. Thus, proteins are split into amino acids, carbohydrates (crude fiber, N-free extracts [sugar, starch]) are broken down into low fatty acids or monosaccharides, and fats are split into glycerol and saturated and unsaturated fatty acids.

The digestive tract resembles a long, tube which begins at the mouth and ends at the anus. At various locations it dilates into chambers of varying size, and at many points glands secrete their product into the digestive tract. Food entering the mouth is first crushed and pulverized by mastication (this is done almost entirely with the molars in the horse) and thoroughly mixed with the secretions of the salivary glands. This not only softens the food but partially dissolves it by the action of enzymes in the saliva. The food then enters the stomach, where it is divided into horizontal layers.

The gastrointestinal tract of the horse is small and short compared to that of a cow of equal body weight (table 1.3. — 1).

The horse has a relatively small, unicameral *stomach* whose initial portion (the pars proventricularis) is lined with stratified squamous epithelium. It cannot accommodate large quantities of food at one time and must be presented with smaller rations several times a day. Horses should have three main feedings from 90 to 120 min in duration. Smaller in-between feedings may be given under conditions of extreme exertion. The evening feeding is generally the longest, for then ample time is available for the process of digestion.

The remainder of the stomach contains an abundant bacterial flora [Alexander and Davies, 1963], which breaks down a considerable portion of the soluble carbohydrates into lactic acid which, according to Alexander, is absorbed in the caudal ileum. In the fundus gland zone and pyloric gland zone, lactic acid fermentation is suppressed by the hydrochloric acid-pepsin milieu in favor of protein digestion.

Table 1.3. — 1. Relative sizes of the bovine and equine digestive tracts

Species	Length		Capacity in l		Distribution of capacity in l		
	absolute in m	ratio to body length	absolute	per 100 kg b.w.	stomach	bowel	cecum
Horse	30	20 : 1	200—230	40	10—15	190	30
Cow	50	30 : 1	310—320	50	200	110	10

Table 1.3. — 2. Digestibility of various feedstuffs in horses and cattle

Feed	Crude fiber content, %	Species	Organic matter %	Crude protein %	Crude fat %	N-free extracts %	Crude fiber %
Corn	2	Horse	89	76	61	92	40
		Cattle	90	72	89	95	58
Oats	10	Horse	69	80	71	75	29
		Cattle	70	76	80	76	28
Pasture hay, good quality	22	Horse	58	63	22	65	48
		Cattle	67	65	57	68	63
Wheat straw	41	Horse	21	28	—	28	18
		Cattle	42	4	31	37	50

Ingested material remains in the *stomach* and *duodenum* of the horse for 6—12 h. It generally takes from 12 to 24 h to traverse the remainder of the bowel, though the transit time may be as long as 5 days.

In the *small intestine*, food is broken down chiefly by the enzymes of the pancreas and intestinal juice; bacterial digestion plays a less important role.

About one-third of the digestible *crude protein* is digested in the small intestine. The *fats* are quantitatively split and absorbed in the small intestine without prior hydration, which also accounts for the high content of unsaturated fatty acids in equine fat [GEYER, 1974]. ALEXANDER and CHOWDHURY [1958] could demonstrate no lipase activity in the caudal ileum. HERTEL [1969, 1970] found the highest net absorption of crude fat in the ileum; this absorption decreases in the lower bowel as a result of bacterial fat synthesis [HOLASEK, 1954].

The soluble *carbohydrates* are broken down mostly into glucose in the small intestine and are absorbed in that form. Some 80% of the N-free extracts are digested in the small intestine [GEYER, 1974].

As a rule of thumb, GEYER states that about two-thirds of the digestible organic matter is broken down and absorbed in the small intestine of the horse.

The *crude fiber* undergoes no digestion in its passage through the small intestine to the cecum.

Due to the lack of predigestion by ruminal bacteria and the shorter transit time in the gastrointestinal tract, the utilization of foods high in crude fiber is less efficient in horses than in cattle (table 1.3. — 2).

As the table shows, the higher the crude fiber content of the feed, the lower the digestibility in all nutrient groups.

Digestion in the *large intestine* is important in the horse owing mainly to the activity of intestinal bacteria, rather than enzymatic processes. In contrast to ruminants, however, the fermentation chambers formed by the cecum and large intestine, which are analogous to the rumen, are located beyond the enzymatic digestion of the stomach and small intestine. As a result, a considerable amount of predigestion and absorptive volume reduction has already taken place by the time the chyme enters the fermentation chambers. In the cecum and large intestine, *cellulose* is broken down by cellulolytic bacteria into volatile fatty acids. According to ELSDEN et al. [1946], 67% is converted to acetic acid, 19% to propionic acid and 14% to butyric acid, which, according to BARCROFT et al. [1944], are also absorbed there. The cellulolytic activity decreases in a cranio-caudal direction from the cecum to the dorsal colon.

Protein digestion in the large intestine is determined by the type and abundance of the microorganisms that colonize its various segments. The breakdown of the cell walls (cellulose) releases the crude protein contained in the cells, which, together with the crude protein not yet digested in the small intestine, is then broken down by bacterial enzymes into CO_2 and NH_3 as well as the amino acids [DREPPER, 1976]. Quantitative data are not yet available on the extent of protein hydrolysis or extent of absorption of amino acids. The proteolytic activity in the large intestine segments is not very high [KERN et al., 1974] but does increase from the cecum to the dorsal colon.

1.3.2. Nutrient and Vitamin Requirements of the Horse

The nutrient requirement of a horse varies according to its age, breed, temperament, usage, degree of activity, etc. Thus, it is very difficult to establish general standards for nutrient requirements in the horse per unit body weight. In principle, all nutrients contained in digestible organic matter can be utilized for energy. However, the energy value of feeds is mainly dependent on their crude fiber content. Because all horses (except for foals, see below) require a certain content of structured material (crude fiber) in their diet (15—20% crude fiber, about half of which is structured), it may be quite difficult to reconcile both demands if the animal's energy requirement is high.

1.3.2.1. Energy

The energy requirement is made up of the maintenance requirement and the performance requirement (of working animals). The energy content of the feed that is capable of being utilized by the animal is called the net energy. The scientific unit of measure of a feed's energy value in use since 1970 in the German Democratic Republic is the kilocalorie of net energy for fattening (NEF). This represents the quantity of feed or nutrients that increases the body's energy by 1 kcal (approx. 4.18 kJ) during the fattening of adult animals. For practical use, the 'energy feed unit' (EF), which is a multiple of 1 kcal, was introduced to characterize the energy value of feeds and rations as well as the energy requirement of animals. For practical reasons, the energy feed unit was given different values for different domestic species, as shown below:

Cattle:	$1\ EF_c = 2.5$ kcal, or $1\ kEF_c$	$= 2{,}500$ kcal (10,450 kJ)
Swine:	$1\ EF_s = 3.5$ kcal, or $1\ kEF_s$	$= 3{,}500$ kcal (14,630 kJ)
Poultry:	$1\ EF_p = 3.5$ kcal, or $1\ kEF_p$	$= 3{,}500$ kcal (14,630 kJ).

The energy value of feed for horses is placed in the same group as that for cattle (i.e., 1 'EF_h' = 1 EF_c). Swine (including rabbits and fur-bearing animals) and poultry form separate groups (EF_s and EF_p) mainly because of their different digestive processes.

Other countries employ different feed units, although all these units are based on the energy concept. To permit comparisons of data in the international literature on the energy requirement of the horse and the energy content of the ration, it appears necessary to examine this subject in greater detail.

The establishment of feed units is based upon different precepts in different countries: raw nutrients, digestible nutrients or total energy, digestible energy or net energy. Because the use of raw nutrients or total energy does not make allowances for differences in digestion and utilization among different animal species, we do not favor evaluation systems that are based on such concepts.

KELLNER was the first to develop a feed evaluation system based on net energy, a system that is still is use today. As a reference substance he chose starch, with its energy production value of 2,356 cal/g in the fattening of adult cattle (1 *starch equivalent* [SE] = 2,356 kcal NEF), and related the energy production of the other nutrients to that substance. Thus, with the energy value of digestible starch defined as 1.00, digestible gluten protein has a relative value of 0.94, digestible fat from rapeseed 2.41, digestible fat from grain 2.12, digestible fat from roughage 1.91, digestible crude fiber 1.00, and digestible raw sugar 0.76. For each 1% crude fiber, KELLNER subtracted 136 cal (= 0.58 starch equivalent) due to the associated reduction in utilization. In cases where the calculated energy value did not correspond to the measured value, even in the case of feed concentrates, KELLNER introduced the concept of 'quality quotient':

$$\text{Quality quotient} = \frac{\text{experimentally determined net energy}}{\text{calculated net energy}} \times 100.$$

But because the starch equivalent represents such varying energy outputs in different animal species, it corresponds to entirely different values for the net energy. Thus, it cannot be transferred from one species to another, particularly from cattle to monogastric animals.

Using the same basis, the directly determined content of net calories, the U.S. researcher ARMSBY developed in 1917 the unit of the *therm* (1 therm = 1,000 kcal). This unit has not found wide acceptance, however.

The concept of digestible nutrients serves as a basis for the *total nutrient* evaluation system (for swine and poultry only) and for the *TDN* (total digestrible nutrient) system developed in the U.S. The TDN is calculated as follows: TDN = digestible (crude protein + crude fiber + N-free extracts) + 2.25 × digestible crude fat. Depending on the type and composition of the feed, the content of digestible energy in terms of TDN ranges from 3.8 to 5.5 kcal/g. Because there is no subtraction for crude fiber content in the TDN system, nor any allowance for the 'quality quotient', forages, for example, are rated more highly than in the KELLNER or EF_c system. When calculating the net energy content, 1 g TDN in feeds high in crude fiber (e.g., straw) does not even correspond to 1 kcal, while in concentrates and grain seeds it corresponds to more than 2 kcal.

The reformed *Danish feed unit* (FE, also known in France as the *unite fourragere* or U.F.) was developed on the basis of comparative barley feeding experiments in cattle. In this system the digestible nutrients are calculated in a manner similar to the KELLNER ('starch-equivalent') system, except that a utilization factor of 1.43 is assumed (but not scientifically proved) for digestible crude protein, and the subtotal is multiplied by 1.33. As a result, the FE cannot be compared with feed units based on net energy or metabolizable energy.

The *Soviet feed unit* is computed from the content of digestible nutrients, which is multiplied by the 'starch-equivalent factors' and, after allowance for the quality quotient, is divided by 0.6.

Because the *net energy* makes up about half the digestible energy (1 kg digestible fat produces 0.474—0.597 kg body fat), the energy values of the former must be approximately doubled to convert to feed units for digestible energy; thus, 1 Mcal = 200 EF_c or 212 SV, 1 EF_c = 0.005 Mcal, and 1 SV = 0.0047 Mcal.

The energy values required by the horse are very much a function of its physical condition, age, breed, type of work performed, state of training and handling, as well

Table 1.3. — 3. Energy requirement for natural movement of the horse over level ground (body wt. 500 kg)

Speed km/h		Energy requirement kJ (kcal)/km
Walk	4	624 (149)
	5.4	791 (189)
Trot	10.6—12.3	1185 (283)

Table 1.3. — 4. Energy requirements of the horse for effective work performance

Type of work	Speed km/h	Energy requirement kJ (kcal)/100 kg/draft work unit
Pulling load on level ground	4.0 (walk)	3.148 (0.752)
Pulling load on level ground	9.2 (trot)	3.148 (0.752)
Pulling load up 10% grade	4.8 (walk)	4.325 (1.033)
Carrying load on level ground	5.4 (walk)	0.980 (0.234)
Carrying load on level ground	11.5 (trot)	1.507 (0.360)
Carrying load up 10% grade	5.4 (walk)	2.868 (0.685)

as climatic conditions. They also show much variation in the international literature depending on the unit of evaluation employed. It is hardly possible to treat them dogmatically, therefore. When calculating the energy requirement, moreover, it must be considered that heavy (larger) horses have a smaller maintenance requirement per unit weight than do smaller animals. The daily maintenance requirement of a riding horse weighing 500 kg is reported to be 3,000—3,500 EF_c.

In the working (riding) horse, the energy intake beyond the maintenance requirement is utilized for natural movement and work. Even with light work, the energy requirement exceeds the maintenance value by about 50%. The galloping of Thoroughbreds during training and racing is reflected in the energy balance. Thus, an optimum energy intake is essential for maintaining condition in race horses, and the liberal feeding of easily digested carbohydrates will provide an excellent energy source during the racing period.

The studies of von Zuntz and Hagemann, as quoted by Schreiber [1965], illustrate the complexity of calculating the exact energy requirement of the working horse (table 1.3. — 3 and — 4). Certain adjustments must be made for movement over sloping terrain.

As table 1.3. — 4 shows, the energy requirement per unit draft work load is the same for both walking and trotting. It increases markedly only when the load is pulled or carried uphill, specifically by about 40% on a 10% grade.

1.3.2.2. Protein

Protein intake in the growing horse serves to replace protein losses associated with the various body functions, and above all to provide raw material for the synthesis of new protein in the body. This is why young horses have a considerably higher protein requirement per kilogram body weight than do adult animals. As the growth rate slows, the requirement for digestible crude protein decreases. In adult animals, protein intake with the ration serves only to replace protein losses. In horses doing strenuous work the intensity of protein metabolism is increased by muscular exertion, and some N-containing substances are lost in sweat. On the whole, however, physical exertion is associated with a much greater consumption of energy than of protein. Also, it is far more economical to support performance by means of carbohydrates or even fats in the diet than by feeding protein.

The figures cited by DREPPER [1976] for the daily protein requirement of the growing horse are presented in table 1.3. — 5.

According to NEISSER and VON GAGERN [1977], the daily requirement of digestible crude protein for English Thoroughbred foals between the 8th and 18th month of life is 450 to 800 g, depending on age. An average protein-energy quotient (PEQ) of up to 150 is called for.

The proportion of high-quality protein contained in the total digestible crude protein should be gradually reduced up to the age of 8 months. Young foals appear to have a particularly high requirement for lysine [HINTZ et al., 1971; BREUER and GOLDEN, 1971]. If it is true, as recently claimed, that there is no absorption of bacterially synthesized essential amino acids in the large intestine of the horse, then increased attention should be paid to the qualitative as well as quantitative protein nutrition of both young and mature horses. In that event there could be no utilization of the feed protein 'refined' in the large intestine, and the entire amount of undigested feed nitrogen that had reached the lower bowel would be excreted in the stool. It would be necessary to check digestibility values and establish the requirements for essential amino acids in the horse [DREPPER, 1977].

The daily maintenance requirement for digestible crude protein in the horse is generally assumed to be 53—68 g/100 kg body weight. As stated earlier, while the energy requirement for working horses increases considerably with the level of activity, the need for digestible crude protein shows a less dramatic rise. Thus, the daily nutrient requirement standards for a sport-horse weighing 550—600 kg and working at a moderate performance level is, on the average, 550—600 g digestible crude protein and 5.5—6.3 kEF_c. Crude protein and energy show a ratio of about 1: 10, as in the maintenance requirement. On the other hand, a 550-kg horse performing heavy work would require 650—700 g crude protein and about 7.5—8.0 kEF_c. The energy demand has increased both relatively and absolutely with the increase in work load giving a crude protein-energy ratio of approximately 1: 11.5.

1.3.2.3. Crude Fiber

Feed for horses should contain about 15—20% crude fiber, which is given in the form of bulk feeds (pasture, hay, straw, chaff). According to ZELLWEGER [1973], a sufficient crude fiber intake is essential for normal digestion in horses for several reasons:

1. to provide a feed volume sufficient to produce a feeling of fullness;
2. for mechanical stimulation of the gut wall, which promotes intestinal activity and peristalsis;
3. for expanding a too narrow nutrient range by mixing with concentrates.

Beyond this, up to one-fourth of the total absorbed energy in the horse can come from the volatile fatty acids formed by microorganisms in the large intestine. Thus, besides its stimulatory effect on digestion, crude fiber plays an important role in energy production. Even in animals which require feed with a very high energy concentration, it is not wise to meet this requirement too heavily at the expense of the structured portion of the diet. The horse, which digests crude fiber less efficiently

Table 1.3. — 5. Requirement of digestible crude protein for the growing horse

Age in months	Body wt. in % of adult weight	Body weight of adult horse in kg 300		600	
		b.w. kg	daily dig. cr. protein req. in g	b.w. kg	daily dig. cr. protein req. in g
3	30	90	300	180	500
6	45	135	340	270	580
12	64	192	370	384	680
18	77	231	310	462	570
24	85	255	250	510	460
42 (adult)	100	300	230	600	420

than ruminants, requires about 5—6 kg of bulk feed per day, which, for the reasons cited earlier, is best given during the evening feeding.

The upper limit of the crude fiber portion is about 18% for Thoroughbred foals and yearlings, and 22% for horses doing moderately heavy work.

1.3.2.4. Minerals and Trace Elements

Unlike other farm animals, the horse appears to require only relatively small amounts of these substances in its diet. On the other hand, even small concentrations of these substances seem to have very beneficial effects on health and performance, especially in Thoroughbreds.

It is believed that the following minerals in particular are essential for the horse: calcium, phosphorus, sodium, magnesium, potassium, sulfur and chlorine. Because the natural supplies of magnesium, potassium, sulfur and chlorine are abundant in the German Democratic Republic, no deficiency symptoms have yet been observed for any of these minerals, and so they need not be supplemented in the horse ration.

Besides their essential role in many other metabolic processes, certain minerals are particularly important for the development of a strong skeletal structure, and thus of a healthy, sound locomotor system. For this reason the necessary minerals and trace elements must be presented to the animal not only in adequate amounts, but also in the correct proportion to one another, especially in high-performance animals. In most cases failure to meet the mineral requirement is first noticed when marked deficiency symptoms appear.

According to Tuschy [1973], the method of choice for determining the mineral requirement is the factorial method. In this method the net requirement for endogenous losses in the urine and stool is added to the net requirement for growth, pregnancy and lactation; this total requirement is then multiplied by the absorption rate to obtain the gross requirement.

Using this method, Tuschy [1973] calculated the following gross mineral requirements for foals (warm blooded breeds) (table 1.3. — 6). It should be noted that while these values have been experimentally verified, they are for the most part slightly lower than the values calculated by other authors in recent years.

Belechov and Tschubinskaja [1960] report the following daily mineral requirements for breeding horses (table 1.3. — 7). These values should be increased by 30% during light work.

Table 1.3. — 6. Daily gross mineral requirement for hot-blood foals

Age in months	500 kg end-weight					600 kg end-weight				
	Weight kg	Ca g	P g	Na g	Mg g	Weight kg	Ca g	P g	Na g	Mg g
0···6	120	22	19	4	0.9	120	25	21	5	2
7···12	230	20	15	6	1.4	265	24	18	8	3
13···18	320	21	15	8	1.7	380	24	18	10	4
19···24	375	21	14	10	2.0	445	26	18	12	5
25···42	450	21	14	11	2.5	540	25	16	14	6

Table 1.3. — 7. Daily mineral requirement for breeding horses

		Body wt. kg	Ca g	P g	NaCl g
Pregnant broodmares	Riding and trotting horses	400	50	35	28
		450	55	40	32
		500	60	45	35
		550	65	50	38
	Heavy work horses	600	70	50	42
		650	70	50	45
		700	75	50	49
		750	80	50	52
Lactating mares	Riding and trotting horses	400	60	35	28
		450	70	40	32
		500	75	45	35
		550	80	50	38
	Heavy work horses	600	80	55	42
		650	85	60	45
		700	90	65	49
		750	100	70	52

Calcium and *phosphorus* are necessary in young horses for sound bone development. Both requirements are highest, both absolutely and relatively, during lactation and in early growth but decrease per kilogram body weight with increasing age. Nursing mares and foals generally require supplementary calcium and phosphorus beyond that supplied in mixed horse feeds. A Ca : P ratio of 1.2 to 1.5 : 1 has proved to be optimal. In calculating the necessary calcium and phosphorus content of the ration, it must be considered that the content of these elements in certain feed plants does not always correspond to standard values, but is dependent upon various external factors. Among these, BRONSCH [1963] cites the amount of precipitation and its yearly distribution, the temperature, the soil type and properties (e.g., moisture, mineral content, acidity, humus content), the stage of growth of the plant, as well as storage conditions in the case of preserved feedstuffs. Studies by HOYER [1975] have shown that while the absolute calcium and phosphorus intake may be ensured (except in nursing foals), the ratio of the two minerals to each other rarely corresponds to physiologic demands. The relative phosphorus excess is particularly great in very high-grain diets (Ca : P ratio of approx. 0.2 : 1), despite the fact that up to half the phosphorus contained in grains may be bound in compounds (e.g., inositol hexaphosphoric acid ester) that are poorly utilized by the horse. As a general rule, and especially in performance horses fed large amounts of concentrates with a P excess, calcium should be given in the form of calcium carbonate to establish a proper Ca : P ratio. For example, approximately 10 g of calcium are needed to offset the P excess in 1 kg of hay.

Sodium, as a component of salt, is especially important for horses engaged in strenuous competitive and training activity, because large amounts are lost in sweat. It may be assumed that a horse doing vigorous work will excrete about 50—60 g of salt in the sweat and another 35 g in the urine. This represents a total excretion of about 35 g of sodium. Serious sodium deficiency can develop in sport and racing horses as well as in lactating mares, with consequent adverse effects on performance and milk production. Sodium intake may be particularly jeopardized if nutrition is not based on root crops or their by-products [Anke, 1977]. Therefore, horses should be given free access to block salt to ensure the replenishment of salt losses through excretion. According to Bronsch [1963], studies in various animal species have shown that with an adequate NaCl intake, a supply-demand balance is established which will remain constant under normal circumstances. This is made possible by the body's osmoreceptors, which 'set' a constant osmotic pressure in the body fluids by regulating the craving for salt in accordance with the quantities excreted. Thus, if horses are given free access to salt in block form, it is highly unlikely that they will 'abuse the privilege'.

With regard to the *potassium* requirement of the horse, we must rely on analogy with other species, in which the optimum K : Na ratio is 5 : 1.

The *trace elements* essential for the horse include iron, manganese, zinc, copper, cobalt, selenium and iodine. Based on personal experience, we recommend the following concentrations for horse rations (table 1.3. — 8).

Generally speaking, the *iron requirement* of the horse does not exceed 50 mg/kg ration dry matter and can thus be furnished by all horse feedstuffs. No dietry supplementation is necessary. Higher concentrations can adversely affect performance, food consumption, weight gain and the utilization of manganese leading to symptoms of secondary manganese deficiency.

The *manganese requirement* of horses in all performance groups does not exceed 60 mg/kg ration dry matter with a normal iron intake. In mares, a manganese deficiency may be manifested by a weak estrus, predisposition to abortion, and a greater tendency to bear female offspring than males.

The *zinc requirement* of the horse is approximately 40 mg/kg ration dry matter but is influenced antagonistically by various factors, such as a calcium excess, phytin, or certain protein constituents. Zinc deficiency causes hair and epithelial damage and adversely affects body size and fertility. It can affect horses in certain locations.

Table 1.3. — 8. Recommended concentrations of trace elements in equine rations

Trace elements	mg/kg dry matter
Iron	50—100
Manganese	50—65
Zinc	30—50
Copper	6—8
Cobalt	0.1
Selenium	0.2—0.6
Iodine	2

Table 1.3. — 9. Daily requirement of trace elements for broodmares

	Cu, mg	Zn, mg	Mn, mg
Barren and nonpregnant mares	50	350	400
Pregnant mares	65	400	500
Lactating mares	80	500	600

The mineral mixture produced for horses in the German Democratic Republic has the following formula (g/kg): 64.00 phosphorus, 273.00 calcium, 76.00 sodium, 1.22 manganese, 0.37 copper, 0.02 cobalt, 1.23 zinc.

It is recommended that up to 100 g of this mixture be given to foals, and up to 150 g to pregnant or lactating mares and breeding stallions.

The *copper requirement* of the horse, which generally is adequately met, is about 6 mg/kg ration dry matter. Molybdenum and cadmium act as antagonists, however. Because foals obtain little copper from milk and must rely for some time on reserves stored in utero, particular care should be taken to ensure an adequate copper supply in pregnant mares so that deficiency-related skeletal and vascular abnormalities can be avoided.

The *iodine requirement* of the horse is approximately 2 mg/kg ration dry matter. In iodine-deficient areas where goiter has been observed, special attention should be given to the needs of pregnant and lactating mares, which are best met by providing iodized cattle salt (5 mg KI/kg).

Based on personal experience, we estimate the trace element requirement of broodmares as follows (table 1.3. — 9).

1.3.2.5. Vitamins

The horse, like other animals, requires vitamins to maintain its metabolism during rest and exercise and to cope with stressful situations. Although a limited microbial synthesis of B-complex vitamins occurs naturally in the large intestine of the horse, both fat- and water-soluble vitamins are given due to the uncertain conditions of absorption. Horses that are grazing on pasture or receiving green feed in the stall will receive an adequate supply of the vitamins A and D, although in winter these vitamins, too, must be supplemented. Adams [1972] describes deficiencies of folic acid, choline and biotin in racehorses fed rations containing too little protein. Niacin synthesis is also impaired by protein deficiency, especially if the tryptophan intake is poor.

Without detailing the functions of the individual vitamins, which are generally known, we shall point out only the most important functions as they relate to the horse.

Vitamin A, or carotene, is essential for the horse. In breeding practice, vitamin-A deficiency leads to fertility disturbances and predisposes to abortion and premature births. Vitamin-D deficiency becomes important only if there is a deficiency or imbalance of calcium and phosphorus in the diet. The true rachitic diseases seldom occur in horses, therefore. Vitamin E in the horse acts as a regulator of metabolic functions, most notably cell respiration; this can have a beneficial effect on the heart and muscles of performance horses [Zellweger, 1973]. Studies on the exercise physiology of horses have demonstrated that normal stress in the trained horse is accompanied by marked changes in the vitamin-C content of the blood, while horses not in training

Table 1.3. — 10. Level of daily vitamin intake in the horse (after CUNHA [1980])

	Foals				Mares			Stallions	
	Birth to 2 months	2 months to weaning	Weaning to training	during training	Pregnancy	Lactation	Barrenness	Not in breeding season	In breeding season
Vitamin A, IU	5,000	10,000	20,000	40,000	40,000	40,000	60,000	40,000	60,000
Vitamin D, IU	750	1,500	3,000	6,000	6,000	6,000	6,000	6,000	9,000
Vitamin E, IU	10	20	40	80	80	80	120	80	120
Vitamin K, mg	2.5	5	10	20	20	20	30	20	30
Thiamine, mg	3	6	12	24	24	24	36	24	36
Riboflavin, mg	5	10	60	40	40	40	60	40	60
Niacin, mg	15	30	60	120	120	120	180	120	180
Pyridoxine, mg	1.5	3	6	12	12	12	18	12	18
Pantothenic acid, mg	6	12	24	48	48	48	72	48	72
Choline, mg	75	150	300	600	600	600	900	600	900
Vitamin B_{12}, μg	15	30	60	120	120	120	180	120	180
Folic acid, mg	1.5	3	6	12	12	12	18	12	18

show little or no adaptation of their vitamin-C levels. The biochemical regulatory mechanisms that are stressed during physical exertion are to a large extent vitamin-C-dependent in the horse [ZELLWEGER, 1973]. Reportedly the seminal quality of breeding stallions is also improved by vitamin C.

The recommended daily allowances of vitamins according to CUNHA [1980] are shown in table 1.3. — 10. Somewhat higher values are cited by GIDEON [1977], who included in his list a vitamin-C requirement of 135 mg for newborn foals.

1.3.3. Special Feeds

Equine nutrition has undergone numerous changes in recent decades. In particular, it has been recognized that there are many other feedstuffs besides hay, oats and chaff that not only are highly palatable to the horse, but also make it possible to better adapt the diet to specific needs than was possible with the three 'mainstays' just mentioned. Such feeds include mixed rations, sugar beets and the various by-products of their industrial processing, silages, dry forage and mineral mixtures.

DREPPER [1974] states that the horse should consume 2 % of its live weight in the form of air-dry substances. When the horse was used chiefly as an agricultural beast of burden, a greater portion of its diet consisted, for economic reasons, of farm-produced feeds. The sport and pleasure horses of today, on the other hand, must often be given commercial feeds in order to ensure a correct supply of energy, protein, vitamins and minerals. The amounts of feed consumed increase continuously with age.

The horses of today are often fed 'complete feeds' that are supplemented with vitamins and minerals. These are mixed feeds which in themselves cover all the animal's energy, nutrient and vitamin requirements. According to GÜTTE [1973], complete feeds for horses usually contain 40—60% concentrates combined with a roughage portion in the form of dried forage. In stalls without straw bedding, however, it is recommended that feed straw also be given in order to satisfy the animal's natural chewing urge and thus help to prevent cribbing and other vices. Complete feeds can be granulated or pelletized. Numerous formulas are known and proved.

Horses should be well supplied with drinking water, especially if complete feeds are given. Automatic waterers are best for this purpose. The level of water intake depends on many factors, such as the dry matter content of the ration, the protein and energy metabolism, the mineral intake, the animal's size and body surface area, its degree of activity, the ambient temperature, etc. The average daily requirement is 30 to 50 l. Because thirsty horses eat poorly, they should be watered just before feeding. Horses that have been worked strenuously, however, should be given some hay before they are allowed to drink. Free access to water should also be withheld before racing.

1.3.3.1. Nutrition of Broodmares

If broodmares are used for regular work, they can be given the same feed as work horses for most of the year. Again, nutrition should be adjusted primarily to maintain the animal at a constant body weight while preventing emaciation or obesity. Special supplements have no effect on the pregnancy rate [Voss and Pickett, 1974]. On the other hand, an energy deficiency can lead to fetal resorption in some circumstances. The requirements of the fetus, which acquires some 80% of its birthweight during the last 4 months of intrauterine development, need be considered only in the last months of pregnancy. Later on, during lactation, the level of milk production must also be considered. Thus, broodmares are fed essentially the same diet as other working horses during the first 6—7 months of pregnancy, especially since they generally perform the same type of work as these horses during that time. If the hay rations are small, pregnant mares in the 5th and 6th month can be fed an extra ration of good-quality hay to provide protein and minerals needed for sound fetal development. If abundant hay rations are already being fed, it is well to supplement the rations with small amounts of concentrates. Then, in the last third of pregnancy, all bulk feeds should be strongly limited. The feeding of large amounts of root crops, which have traditionally served as an energy source for agricultural work horses, appears to have an adverse effect on fertility in breeding stock.

A mare weighing 550 kg and doing light work receives up to the 7th month of pregnancy about 480 g of digestible protein in about 4.5 kEF_c, which could be provided, for example, by 25 kg of green feed, 2 kg of mixed horse feed, and 2 kg of chaff. In the 8th through 11th months of pregnancy, the protein requirement gradually increases to 630 g, and the energy requirement to about 5.5 kEF_c.

Minerals that promote fetal bone development must not be neglected during pregnancy. The mineral intake should be increased to 100 g in the 10th month and later to 150 g (cf. tables 1.3. — 7 and — 9). The vitamin requirement is shown in table 1.3. — 10. In addition, recent evidence indicates that deworming the pregnant mare 4—6 weeks before foaling time is a wise precaution. Because the pregnant mare seems to be more susceptible to colic than other horses, special care should be taken to provide a clean, palatable, digestible feed. The feeding of unusally cold liquids or solids should also be avoided, as this could potentially harm the fetus. Frozen feeds should never be given. Moreover, no major dietary adjustments should be made during the final weeks of pregnancy. Special feeding rules are necessary only around foaling time. Shortly before foaling, as well as later during the first estrus, concentrates should be reduced somewhat to avoid an excessive milk flow and the associated risk of diarrhea in the newborn foal. Dietetic feedstuffs (wheat bran, linseed) combined with small amounts of roughage may be given just before foaling to facilitate parturition [Drepper, 1977].

The nutrient requirement standards during lactation considerably exceed those of late pregnancy. This applies particularly to the time of peak lactation around $2^1/_2$ months after foaling. A mare weighing 600 kg will have a daily milk production of 10—15 l over an average nursing period of 4 months. For mares also doing light to moderate work during this time, this leads to a requirement of 900—1,100 g digestible crude protein and up to 7—8 kEF_c (PEQ × 130—135).

The nutritional management of lactating mares is a simple matter if the animal is grazing on young pasture. Sixty-five kilograms of high-quality green feed will in itself provide the mare with about 1,400 g of digestible crude protein and 6.0 kEF_c. Right or wrong, however, it is generally considered wise to limit the intake of green feed to 20 kg. For foalings from April through June, both the mare and foal can be pastured day and night, weather permitting, after a short acclimatization period. Feeding is somewhat more problematic during the months from January to April. On an exclusive diet of hay, oats and chaff (5 kg oats and 5 kg hay being the basal ration for a 500-kg mare), the biological quality of the protein supplied and the dietary vitamin content are deficient, and the Ca : P ratio is unbalanced. The deficiencies are corrected in modern rations by means of supplementary feedstuffs that partially or entirely replace the oats and contain, among other things, dried skimmed milk or soybean meal, or by means of 'complete feeds' given in addition to the hay ration. Protein feedstuffs of animal origin are expensive, however, and it is probable that the requirements of individual amino acids can be adequately met with vegetable feeds. The vitamin and mineral requirements for lactating mares are shown in tables 1.3. — 7, — 9 and — 10.

1.3.3.2. Nutrition of Foals

Thoroughbred horses are expected to perform at a relatively early age. Their preparatory training may commence as early as 18 months, despite the fact that they are not yet physically mature. It is essential, therefore, that nutrition be adapted to meet the animal's needs, particularly during the growth period. The foal requires energy for maintenance, daily activity, and for protein and fat metabolism. The maintenance requirement must be increased by 35—50% just to meet the demands of muscular movement. Because Thoroughbreds grow at a much more rapid rate than light horses, for example, daily growth must also be taken into account when requirements are estimated. Thus, the daily weight gain of a foal that will attain an adult weight of 500 kg is approximately 900 g from birth to 4 months, about 500 g at 12 months, and about 300 g at 24 months. The higher the level of physical maturity that a racehorse has reached at the start of and during its performance years, the better it will tolerate the stresses of racing, especially in the early age groups [Neisser and von Gagern, 1977]. The energy requirements for the aforementioned periods are 2.8, 3.1 and 3.4 kEF_c, respectively. The crude protein requirement is shown in table 1.3. — 5. It is also dependent on the growth rate, which decreases with age. Accordingly, the concentration of digestible crude protein in the dry matter of the foal ration must also be higher than in the case of mature horses [Drepper, 1976]. Young foals require high-quality protein in their feed. The lysine fraction should make up about 7 % of the total protein during the first 4 weeks. Lysine remains important up to the 4th month of life, during which time an adequate intake is generally ensured by lysine-rich mare's milk.

The vitamin and mineral requirements for the foal are shown in tables 1.3. — 6, — 8 and — 10. Additional supplies of iodine and zinc are recommended for Thoroughbred foals, and selenium supplements are indicated if signs of deficiency (e.g. White muscle disease) are present. Iron, manganese, copper, and cobalt are contained in the majority of mineral feeds for horses (cf. chap. 1.3.2.4.).

Soon after birth the foal will stand and seek the dam's udder in an attempt to nurse. Most foals will nurse within 2 h after birth, initially consuming from 0.5 to 1.5 kg of milk. Because this is a relatively small amount, there is little concern about maternal hypocalcemia in the mare unlike that observed in the dairy cow as a result of excessive milk production and nursing. The foal should be free to choose the time and amount of the initial nursing.

The foal obtains its first nutrition from the colostrum, which is of enormous value. This is because of its high content of protein (especially gamma-globulins, to which the antibodies are bound), vitamins, and minerals (especially magnesium). After 3—4 days the colostrum gradually assumes the character of the milk. A highly digestible, protein-rich supplemental feed can be offered the foal as early as the second week.

Sick foals require special nutritional care. The newborn foal poorly tolerates nutritional deficiencies. At the same time, the nutritive requirement is significantly higher in febrile diseases, for example, than in the healthy foal. Based on experience with humans, it may be assumed that the requirement in such cases is more than twice normal. If the foal is sick and anorexic, a deficiency of all nutrients will soon develop, with all its consequences: weight loss, muscular atrophy, delayed healing of wounds, and decreased immunity with a high susceptibility to infection. Acute illnesses are frequently the result of malnutrition. In such cases the foal may require *controlled nutrition* by means of an intravenous catheter or nasogastric tube. Parenteral nutrition is necessary when the alimentary tract is diseased, while a debilitated anorexic foal with a normal alimentary tract can be fed by nasogastric tube. Even parenteral alimentation must completely satisfy the foal's nutritional requirements and should not exceed two weeks' duration. Protein nutrition by this route is best provided by pure amino acids. Peptides can provoke allergic and febrile reactions and are largely excreted in the urine before they are utilized. To meet the nutrient, mineral and vitamin requirements of the foal during parenteral alimentation, it is most convenient to use commercially available preparations, which can be further supplemented if need be. One such preparation, Amijex®, is recommended by GIDEON [1977].

For more details concerning the care of orphaned foals, see chap. 2.7.

GIDEON [1977] reports the following daily requirements in the parenteral feeding of a 45-kg foal (table 1.3. — 11).

Table 1.3. — 11. Nutritive, mineral and vitamin requirements of a 45-kg foal (after GIDEON [1977])

Water	4,500 ml	Thiamine	2.25 mg
Digestive energy	28,260 kJ	Riboflavin	4.50 mg
	(6,750 kcal)	Niacinamide	45.00 mg
	(= 1,650 g glucose)	Pyridoxine	4.50 mg
Digestive crude protein	135 g	Pantothenic acid	45.00 mg
Sodium	1,350 mg	Vitamin C	135.00 mg
Potassium	11,250 mg	Vitamin E	135.00 mg
Chlorine	1,350 mg	Vitamin A	4.50 mg
Calcium	3,825 mg	Vitamin D	0.1125 mg
Phosphorus	2,250 mg		
Magnesium	292.50 mg		

In the first months of life, the healthy foal meets its nutritive requirements almost exclusively from the consumption of maternal milk. Because the utilization of ingested crude protein is very high, especially in the first month of life, the foal experiences a weight gain of about 120 g per kg of milk consumed during this period; by the second month this decreases to about 75 g. Foals nurse many times during the day. In foals of warm blooded breeds, this corresponds to a daily milk intake of approximately 220 g or about 13 l. If the foal is permitted to run freely with the mother from birth, it may begin to graze at pasture after only 10—14 days, as well as nibble at the dam's feed. If the mare is a good milk producer, however, it may be 3—4 weeks before the foal starts to ingest feed quantities that contribute significantly to its protein and energy needs. Depending on the milk consumption, it may be advisable to offer supplemental feed containing up to 2 kg of oats or other types of grain to ensure optimum growth as well as muscle and bone development. A feed consisting of 60 % crushed oats, 10 % wheat bran, 10 % forage meal, and 20 % linseed meal, bean meal and other high-quality protein sources has proved satisfactory. Care should be taken that the offered feed is promptly consumed, for it will undergo decomposition if left standing too long. However, if the foal is already put out on pasture with the mare during the first week after birth, it is best to discontinue supplemental feeding otherwise the foal may become reluctant to nurse. Supplemental feeding can be resumed when milk production and quality of grass are no longer adequate. This should be considered for foals grazing on pasture in the fall, when the nutritive value of the grass is questionable. Older foals would then have to consume greater amounts of grass to meet their nutrient requirement, with unfavorable effects on physique ('hay belly') and condition. As a rule of thumb, foals should be given as many pounds of concentrated feed as they are old in months. The nutrition of the foal then meets all requirements if the animal doubles its birthweight during the first 60 days, and attains two-thirds of its mature live weight by the end of the first year. For certain breeds, such as the Thoroughbred, allowance should be made for their very high growth rate during the first 2—3 months of life.

It would be favourable in terms of foal nutrition to maintain nursing well beyond the first 3 months, perhaps even through the 6th month. Unlike other species, little economic benefit is derived from early weaning due to the relatively constant maintenance requirement of the mare. On the other hand, because prolonged nursing without suitable nutrient and vitamin supplementation can adversely affect the later fertility of the mare, it is usually most practical to wean the foal at $4^1/_2$ to 5 months. To avoid an upset in the development of the foal, it is advisable to feed about 300—400 g of a milk replacer daily for a transition period of about 2 months after weaning. This replacer may be given in the form of a liquid (1 : 10 with water), a mash, or may be sprinkled in dry form over the rest of the ration. Milk replacers may also be given to orphaned foals immediately after the colostral period.

With skilled feeding practice, *weaning* of the foal should present no difficulties. If the animal has already been receiving feed concentrates and has been grazing at pasture for some time, significant weight losses seldom occur upon weaning. Developmental arrest is the result of a protein (lysine) deficit. Most foals are weaned in around September so that they can remain at pasture for a longer period. This usually makes it unnecessary at weaning time to increase the supplemental feed beyond the amount already being given. Only when the pasture quality deteriorates does it become necessary to give larger amounts of supplemental feed, for the foal is unable to digest the higher-cellulose containing grass with the same efficiency as ruminants. Excessive supplemental feeding is wasteful, however. Foals of the warm blooded breeds should receive no more than 4 kg of concentrates in their 2nd year, while

Table 1.3. — 12. Daily requirement of energy and digestible crude protein for stallions (body wt. 600 kg)

Breeding activity	EF_c	digestive crude protein, g
light		720
medium	6,000	840
heavy		960

colts and Thoroughbred foals may receive 5—6 kg. If too much protein is fed to growing foals, damage to the limbs and possibly the kidneys may result. The energy and protein requirements of warm-blooded foals have already been discussed. Cold-blooded breeds of foal have correspondingly higher requirements. In the winter, foals are given an additional 1—2 kg hay.

If a fairly good-quality pasture is available, the yearling can obtain all its nourishment from grazing. In most cases, however, 1—2 kg of supplemental feed must be given, for otherwise the horse would have to consume at least 30 kg of green forage. Also, since light horses are already being broken to saddle or harness by their 3rd year, pasturing is possible only to a very limited degree. In winter, hay and concentrates can be fed supplementally. Only in sport horses is the use of large amounts of green feed contraindicated. Thoroughbreds at age two should receive about 5 kg of oats and mixed feed, about 2 kg of hay and 1 kg of carrots, if available.

1.3.3.3. Nutrition of Breeding Stallions

If stallions are used for regular work, they should receive the same feed as work horses outside the breeding season. However, they require about 10—15 % more energy for maintenance than do mares of equal weight owing to their greater physical activity. The requirement of digestible crude protein is still controversial, although, like the energy requirement, it doubtlessly increases with the level of breeding activity. For the approximately 250 mg of protein contained in the ejaculate, about 250 g of digestible crude protein are required per stallion per breeding. The energy and digestible protein requirements for a 600-kg stallion are shown in table 1.3. — 12 (after Drepper, [1974]).

As the table indicates, stallions with a heavy breeding schedule require only about 50—70 % more energy and digestible crude protein than for the maintenance requirement. An extremely high intake of digestible crude protein, perhaps through feeds of animal origin, has no effect on fertility or libido [Drepper, 1974]; nor can it be justified on nutritional grounds. It is important that the nutritional preparation of the stallion for the breeding season be started sufficiently early, for spermatogenesis takes place about 2 months prior to ejaculation. Vitamin and mineral supplementation is important in this regard, unless adequate concentrations are already present in the stallion's 'complete' or supplemental feed (tables 1.3. — 7, — 8 and — 10). Vitamin C supplements appear to have a particularly favorable effect on semen quality.

Many serious errors have been made in the feeding of stallions. They should not be given bulky or high-moisture feeds. Even today, 'oats, oats, and more oats' is often the rule in the feeding of the breeding stallion. This attitude completely overlooks the fact that high-quality protein is necessary for spermatogenesis. Oats contain only about 8 % protein which is poor in quality. Proper feeding with carefully formulated concentrates is the best way to maintain general health as well as fertility and libido. Feeding large amounts of oats may make the stallion fat, but it will do little to enhance its fertility. The old practice of feeding animal protein, especially in the form of skimmed milk, fish meal or meat meal, is unnecessary as long as the concentrate is a mixture of various feedstuffs, and its protein quality is satisfactory. Alfalfa hay, low in crude fiber, is the roughage of choice for the breeding stallion.

1.3.3.4. Nutrition of Work Horses (Draft, Riding, Sport [Athletic] and Show)

Although the work of sport horses, for example, differs from that of agricultural draft animals, all working horses require carbohydrate-rich feedstuffs in order to perform. Those containing sugar are particularly well utilized. Sport horses that perform sustained, strenuous work place high demands on energy. With an adequate supply of structured matter (crude fiber) in the form of roughage, the necessary energy can be provided only by concentrates with the highest possible energy concentration. In practice, the energy requirement of most work horses, is satisfied, because an excess or deficiency is usually noticed by the owner. Nevertheless, as DREPPER [1977] points out, it is very difficult to determine the exact energy requirement of work horses, because the various degrees of work activity (light, moderate and heavy) and thus the corresponding energy requirements are poorly defined in practical terms. In racehorses, for example, the performance demands may be so high in some cases that they exceed the animal's ability to meet them by feed intake on a reasonable scale.

While the energy requirement increases dramatically with the level of work performance, the requirement of digestible crude protein shows a more modest rise. According to DREPPER [1974], horses in training have an approximately 50% higher daily requirement of digestible crude protein as a result of their increasing muscle mass. This higher requirement decreases minimally in well trained horses, because they still need more protein/day than animals not in training for the metabolism of their greater muscle mass. As a rule, the natural crude protein content of the horse ration is sufficient to meet $1^1/_2$ to $2^1/_2$ times the animal's requirement. It would be unwise to add any more protein to the ration, for the excess would have to be broken down metabolically (with an expenditure of energy) and excreted, with a consequent burden on the liver and kidneys [DREPPER, 1977]. Myoglobinuria and laminitis have all been associated with a dietary protein excess.

In general, a horse of moderate weight doing light work will require about 500 g digestible crude protein in about 5.0 kEF_c (PEQ 100), 600 g in 6.3 kEF_c for moderate work, and 650 g in 7.5—8.0 kEF_c (PEQ 85) for heavy work. Even in racehorses, these requirements may be considered valid guidelines for the basic ration. The question of protein quality has already been discussed.

The following allowances are recommended for ponies with a live weight of 325 kg (table 1.3. — 13).

Table 1.3. — 13. Daily nutritive requirement for ponies

	Digestive crude protein, g	kEF_c
Maintenance requirement	250	2.2
Light work	350	3.1
Medium work	450	4.1
Heavy work	575	5.0

With regard to the mineral supply of performance horses, DREPPER [1977] warns of the dangers of an improper calcium-phosphorus balance, which can lead to abnormalities of conformation, certain bone diseases and even fractures. Such imbalances are relatively frequent. In oats, for example, the Ca : P ratio is 1 : 3.1. In high-performance horses fed large amounts of oats, therefore, it is essential that the diet be supplemented with high-calcium feeds or mineral mixtures in order to achieve the desired ratio of 1.2 : 1. This is particularly true for horses that are stabled and therefore deprived of sunlight for the synthesis of vitamin D. The requirements of the remaining vitamins and minerals are shown in tables 1.3. — 7, — 8 and — 10. Supplementation of vitamin C apparently increases performance ability.

The principal difference between the nutrition of performance horses and that of agricultural draft horses is that with the former, it is not possible to replace high-energy feeds such as oats by lower-energy, bulky, high-moisture feeds such as beets, carrots, potatoes, silage, etc. Feeding large amounts of green feed is also contraindicated in performance horses due to the heavy stresses of training and the dietary adjustments that have to be made prior to periods of peak exertion (competition). These demands make it necessary to reduce the structured portion of the ration to the fullest extent that nutritional requirements will allow.

Naturally the feeding of sport horses is strongly dependent on the nature and duration of their exertion. In the absence of extraordinary demands, there is no basic objection to feeding sport horses the traditional hay-and-oats diet. However, it must be understood that too little roughage will increase the consumption of concentrated feeds while hampering the utilization of the concentrates, while too much roughage (more than 16—20 % crude fiber) places a greater burden on the digestive and respiratory system than do concentrates. In high-performance animals, hay-and-oats feeding is no longer adequate to satisfy nutritive requirements, especially of energy, vitamins and minerals, while the content of digestible crude protein in such a diet far exceeds the animal's needs. Thus, to meet the high energy demand, which may range from 2.0 to 6.0 Mcal NEF_c depending on the performance level, the animal should be given a mixed feed, preferably pelletized, that has a crude protein content not exceeding that of oats and replaces about one-third of the normal quantity of oats consumed daily. Prolonged protein supplementation, e.g., with large amounts of soybean meal or feedstuffs of animal origin, should be avoided in the high-performance animal, for it burdens the metabolism without enhancing the overall nutritional picture.

The mixed ration for racehorses used in the German Democratic Republic (e.g., 1977) has the following composition:

14.5 %	corn meal	9.4 %	grass meal
12.1 %	soybean meal	4.9 %	linseed meal
13.5 %	wheat bran	3.4 %	dry ration yeast
21.7 %	barley meal	3.6 %	mineral mixture
4.8 %	dried skimmed milk	2.4 %	vitamin mixture.
9.7 %	sugar		

In addition, we recommend feeding about 1,000 g of dextrose to horses after short periods of strenuous exercise in order to replace the energy expended. Some dextrose may also be fed before racing, although its benefit should not be overestimated. The use of mineral mixtures is essential, especially when the dietary Ca : P ratio diverges from the optimum 1.2 : 1 as a result of high concentrate feeding.

Finally, it is important to note that horses need sufficient time as well as quiet a environment in which to feed. If horses are fed two or three times a day, the main feeding should be given in the evening to allow ample time for chewing. If a horse is not eating well as a result of strenuous training or racing, feed intake can be improved by adding 30—60 g of salt to the ration daily. It is also good practice to prepare a mash once a week consisting of a reboiled mixture of 6,000 g linseeds, 250 g salt and 50 l of water.

References

Adams, C. R.: Vitamin nutrition of the horse. Vet. Med. and Small Animal Clinician *67:* 688 (1972).

Alexander, F.: The concentration of certain electrolytes in the digestive tract of the horse and pig. Res. vet. Sci. *3:* 78 (1962).

Alexander, F.; Chowdhury, A. K.: Enzymes in the ileal juice of the horse. Nature *181:* 190 (1958).

Alexander, F.; Davies, M. E.: Production and fermentation of lactate by bacteria in the alimentary canal of the horse and pig. J. comp. Pathol. *73:* 1 (1963).

Altmann, H. J.: Untersuchungen über Stickstoffverbindungen im Verdauungstrakt von Schlachtpferden. Vet.-med. Diss., Berlin-Dahlem (1969).

Anke, M.: Die Bedeutung der Mengen- und Spurenelemente in der Fütterung von Zucht- und Sportpferden. Tierzucht *31:* 310 (1977).

Barcroft, J.; McAnnally, R. A.; Phillipson, A. T.: Absorption of volatile acids from the alimentary tract of the sheep and other animals. J. exp. Biol. *20:* 120 (1944).

Belelhov, G. P.; Tschubinskaja, A. A.: Mineral- und Vitaminernährung der landwirtschaftlichen Nutztiere. Selchosgis, Moskau und Leningrad 1960.

Breuer, L. H.; Golden, D. L.: Lysine requirement of the immature horse. (Abstract). J. Animal Sci. *33:* 227 (1971).

Bronsch, K.: Mineralien, Spurenelemente und Vitamine in der Ernährung des Vollblutpferdes. Dtsch. tierärztl. Wschr. *70:* 526, 576 (1963).

Cid Diaz, J. M.: Les mineraux dans la nutrition du cheval. Bull. Soc. Sci. vét. et Méd. comp. *77:* 243 (1975).

Cunha, T. J.: Horse feeding and nutrition (Academic Press, New York, London 1980).

Drepper, K.: In: Futterwerttabelle für Pferde (DLG-Verlag, Frankfurt (Main) 1974).

Drepper, K.: Intestinaler Proteinstoffwechsel, Proteinbedarf und Proteinversorgung beim Pferd. Übers. Tierernähr. *4:* 155 (1976).

Drepper, K.: Neue wissenschaftliche Erkenntnisse für die Fütterung der Zucht- und Sportpferde? Züchtungskunde *49:* 207 (1977).

Elsden, S. R.; Hitchcock, M. W. S.; Marshall, R. A.; Phillipson, A. T.: Volatile acid in the digesta of ruminants and other animals. J. exp. Biol. *22:* 191 (1946).

Fonnesbeck, P. V.: Consumption and excretion of water by horses receiving all hay and hay-grain diets. J. Animal Sci. *27:* 1350 (1968).

Franke, D.: Veränderungen von Plasmaelektrolyten, Osmolarität und Laktatkonzentration bei Trabrennpferden durch Wettkampfbelastungen. Vet.-med. Diss., Berlin-Dahlem (1974).

Geyer, H.: Zur Ernährungsphysiologie des Pferdes. Schweiz. Arch. Tierheilk. *116:* 39 (1974).

Gideon, L.: Total nutritional support of the foal. Vet. Med. and Small Animal Clinician *72:* 1197 (1977).

Gramatzki, F.: Fragen moderner Pferdefütterung. Über das Absetzen und die Fütterung der Fohlen im ersten Lebensjahr. Lohmann-Information (1970), Nr. 1.

Gramatzki, F.: Über Fütterung und Haltung von Mutterstuten im Winter. Lohmann-Information (1974), Nr. 2, S. 5.

Gütte, J. O.: Möglichkeiten des Einsatzes von Alleinfutter für Pferde. Tierzüchter *25:* 523 (1973).

Herrick, J. B.: Vitamin nutrition of the horse. Vet. Med. and Small Animal Clinician *67:* 688 (1972).

Hertel, J.: Untersuchungen über Rohnährstoffe, Bruttoenergie und verfügbares Lysin im Verdauungstrakt von Schlachtpferden. Vet.-med. Diss., Berlin-Dahlem (1969).

HERTEL, J.; ALTMANN, H. J.; DREPPER, K.: Ernährungsphysiologische Untersuchungen beim Pferd. II. Rohnährstoffuntersuchungen im Magen-Darm-Trakt von Schlachtpferden. Z. Tierphysiol. *26:* 169 (1970).

HINTZ, H. F.; SCHRYVER, H. F.: Nutrition and bone development in horses. J. Amer. vet. med. Assoc. *168:* 39 (1976).

HINTZ, H. F.; SCHRYVER, H. F.; LOWE, J. E.: Comparison of a blend of milk products and linseed meal as protein supplements for young growing horses. J. Animal. Sci. *33:* 1274 (1971).

HOLASEK, H.: Über den Ursprung des Kotfettes. Hoppe Seyler's Z. physiol. Chemie *298:* 55, 219, 224 (1954).

HOYER, I.: Energie-, Protein-, Calcium- und Phosphorversorgung bei Pferden im Vergleich zum Nährstoffbedarf. Diss., Kiel (1975).

KERN, D. L.; SLYTER, L. L.; LEFFEL, E. C.; WEAVER, J. M.; OLTJEN, R. R.: Ponies vs. steers: microbial and chemical characteristics of intestinal ingesta. J. Animal. Sci. *38:* 559 (1974).

KRAPF, E.: Fertigfutter für Sportpferde — eine Alternative oder mehr? Tierärztl. Umschau *30:* 384 (1975).

LINDAU, F.: Konzentrierte Kraft für außergewöhnliche Leistungen. Sankt Georg, Z. Pferdesport u. Pferdezucht *70:* 12 (1969).

LLOYD, W. E.: Feeding the horse. Vet. Med. *57:* 602 (1962).

MEYER, H.; AHLSWEDE, L.: Über das intrauterine Wachstum und die Körperzusammensetzung von Fohlen sowie den Nährstoffbedarf tragender Stuten. Übers. Tierernähr. *4:* 263 (1976).

MEYER, H.; LEMMER, U.: Übersichtsreferat: Mineralstoff- und Spurenelementgehalt im Serum bzw. Plasma des Pferdes. Dtsch. tierärztl. Wschr. *80:* 166, 190 (1973).

MÜLLER, H. K.: Untersuchungen über den Mineralstoffgehalt im Blutserum und im Kolostrum von Vollblutstuten. Vet.-med. Diss., Hannover (1969).

NEISSER, E.; GAGERN, W. v.: Wechselbeziehungen zwischen Jugendernährung, Körperentwicklung und Rennleistung beim Englischen Vollblutpferd. Tierzucht *31:* 315 (1977).

PEARLE, G. R.: The nutrition of racehorses: A review. Austral. Vet. J. *51:* 14 (1975).

SCHREIBER, R.: Die wichtigsten wissenschaftlichen Grundlagen einer rationellen Pferdefütterung. Tierärztl. Umschau *20:* 491, 537, 585 (1965).

TUSCHY, D.: Der Mineralstoffbedarf des Warmblutpferdes. Kraftfutter *56:* 182 (1973).

VOSS, J. L.; PICKETT, B. W.: Effect of a nutritional supplement on pregnancy rate in non-lactating mares. J. Amer. vet. med. Assoc. *165:* 702 (1974).

WOLTER, R.: A propos de l'alimentation du cheval athlète. Bull. Soc. Sci. vét. et Méd. comp. *77:* 231 (1975).

WOLTER, R.; GOUY, D.: Etude experimentale de la digestion chez les équides par analyse du contenu intestinal après abattage. Revue Méd. vét. *127:* 1723 (1976).

WOLTER, R.; MEUNIER, B.; FAUCOMPRET, R. DE; DURIX, A.; LANDREAU, J.: Assai d'un aliment complet, granulé oú expansé, en comparaison avec le regime traditionnel chez des chevaux de sport. Revue Méd. vét. *128:* 71 (1977).

WOLTER, R.; WEHRLE, P.: Appréciation des foins distribues aux chevaux de sport. Revue Méd. vét. *128:* 143 (1977).

ZELLWEGER, P.: Die Fütterung des Pferdes. Hoffmann-La Roche (1973).

1.4. Exercise Physiology

For several hundred years, horse breeds used for hunting, military purposes and athletic events have undergone a selection for endurance and speed. As a result of this, racehorses of today can attain a maximum running speed of approximately 70 km/h. The muscles, tendons, ligaments and bones of racing and athletic horses are exquisitely adapted for rapid movement. Muscular performance is dependent in large measure on the adaptability of the heart, circulation and organs of respiration, as well as that of the nervous system, where the impulses for muscular movement arise.

According to Gunn [1975], the following relationships exist that govern running speed in animals:

Running speed

Coordinated motor sequence

Length of stride	Speed of stride
Length of limbs	Natural frequency of limb movement
Angulation of limbs	Mechanical performance of muscles
Acceleration (muscle force in relation to body weight)	Internal speed of sarcomere contraction
Internal muscular architecture	Reproducibility of limb movement/aerobic and anaerobic energy supply mechanism

It is clear from the above diagram that besides training and nutrition, a number of genetically determined factors have an effect on running speed — factors that can be influenced only by appropriate selection.

1.4.1. The Nervous System and Performance

The impulses that stimulate muscular contractions arise in the nervous system. The speed of the muscular contraction is dependent both on the structure of the muscle fibers and on the alternation between stimulation and inhibition by the motor nerve fibers. The faster the alternation between inhibition and excitation, and the more coordinated the movement, the more rapidly the motor sequence can be executed. Through the regular execution of certain motor processes, nerve cells in the brain stem and spinal cord become integrated into functional units. These then initiate a particular program of motor processes more or less automatically in response to certain key stimuli.

Studies on the genetic transmission of motor activity have been carried out in laboratory animals. As a result of selection for speed over many generations, animals have been bred that possess subtle refinements in their muscle fiber structure. These refinements do not appear to be the result of training in the adult, but apparently are neurogenically determined, since the ATP activity of a muscle fiber is mainly dependent on its type of innervation.

In view of the importance of higher nervous activity for racing performance, motor and nutritional experiments were devised in the Soviet Union for identifying the principal nerve types in the horse [Rjabowa, 1976]. These investigations showed that horses can be divided into four different types in terms of higher nervous activity:

1. a highly balanced mobile type,
2. a highly balanced inert type,
3. a highly balanced type,
4. a weak type.

Studies in 1,000 English Thoroughbreds have identified representatives of all 4 principal nerve types. A comparison of racing performance with nerve types indicated that horses of the balanced mobile type were best able to develop speed over short distances, while horses of the unbalanced type performed best over longer distances.

The full development of performance is further influenced by the functional or instantaneous state of the nervous system. It is known that horses often 'break down' if overworked during training or racing. Such animals are difficult to lead to the training track, and they may react violently to various external stimuli. They also show poor racing performance. To objectify the functional state of the nervous system, additional methods were developed in the Soviet Union for testing neuromuscular coordination. This is done essentially by applying weak electrical stimuli to the limbs in a particular sequence and observing the animal's reactions. The method is very time-consuming and so has not found wide application in the assessment of equine fitness.

1.4.2. Muscular Response to Training

1.4.2.1. Energy Production

According to Kolb [1976], the energy expenditure in the resting horse is 15.24 kJ[1]/540 kg b.w./min, compared to 52.75 kJ/540 kg b.w./min during strenuous activity. According to Hintz et al. [1971], the digestible energy requirements (in kJ/kg b.w./h) above the maintenance requirement of 5.86 kJ are as follows for various categories of activity:

Walking	2.1
Slow trot, some canter	21.4
Fast trot, canter	52.4
Gallop, jumping	101.0
Strenuous effort	163.3.

The energy expenditure correlates with the speed of movement and the body weight. The highest energy consumption occurs at the start of a race during the acceleration phase. The most important step in energy production is the conversion of glycogen to glucose and pyruvate. From each molecule of glucose, energy is liberated in the form of 3 molecules of adenosine triphosphate (ATP).

[1] Conversion factor: 1 kcal = 4.1868 kJ, and 1 kJ = 0.239 kcal.

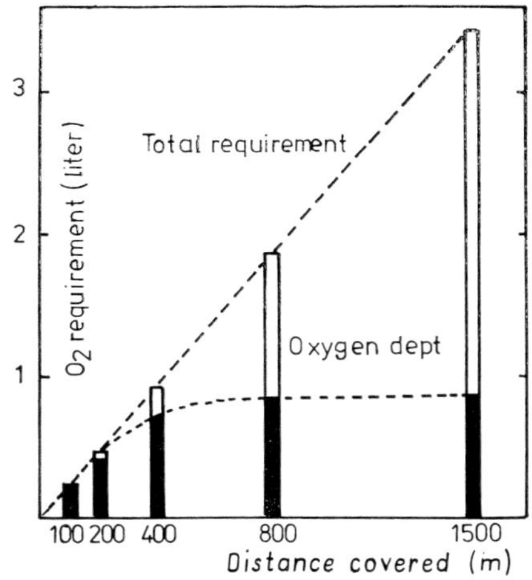

Fig. 1.4. — 1. Relationships between running speed, energy production, oxygen consumption and distance covered (after Gunn, 1975].

If sufficient oxygen is available, pyruvate is oxidized to CO_2 and water, with the release of 36 molecules of ATP from 2 molecules of pyruvate. The efficiency of the energy liberation depends mainly on the type of energy production involved.

In *aerobic* energy production, the following yields are obtained from the following substances:

Glycogen: 39 ATP from 6 molecules O_2 or 6.50 ATP per molecule.

Fats: 130 ATP from 23 molecules O_2 or 5.65 ATP per molecule.

This contrasts with *anaerobic* energy production:

Glycogen: 3 ATP from 0.978 molecules O_2 or 3.07 ATP per molecule.

It can be seen that the *anaerobic* metabolism of glycogen is only about half as efficient as *aerobic* metabolism. Energy production from fatty acids occupies an intermediate position. The removal of 2 molecules of lactate requires 21.9 l of oxygen. The *aerobic* formation of 2 molecules of lactate from 1 molecule of glucose requires 39 molecules of ATP. Thus, the *aerobic* production of 3 ATP requires $6 \times 3/39 \times 22.4 = 10.4$ l of O_2.

Ultimately, then, the production of a given amount of energy requires twice as much oxygen when the metabolism takes place via the *anaerobic* route.

It is important to note that although muscular effort sooner or later entails an oxygen debt, the muscles can produce a limited amount of energy in the momentary absence of oxygen. The muscles possess a small energy reserve in the form of myoglobin. In cases of sudden, maximal energy usage, the myoglobin can combine with oxygen to form oxymyoglobin. Only when this small reserve is exhausted does the *anaerobic* mechanism become operative. Thus, the muscle has two means of mobilizing reserves for short periods: by the oxygen contained in the oxymyoglobin, and by an oxygen debt.

According to Gunn [1975], maximal exertion lasting less than a minute is critically dependent on the degree to which atmospheric oxygen can be transported to the muscles. This concept is shown graphically in fig. 1.4. — 1. The graph further shows that total oxygen consumption correlates closely with the distance covered. The mechanism by which the energy is supplied varies considerably, however. Humans can run short distances by drawing almost exclusively on available energy reserves. After running about 200 m, however, the human athlete reaches the limit of the permissible oxygen debt without an outside oxygen supply. Beyond this distance an increasingly greater amount of oxygen must be supplied via the lungs. A similar situation is presumed to exist in the horse during strenuous exercise. The distance a horse can travel on its energy reserves alone has not yet been accurately defined.

1.4.2.2. Importance of Muscle Fiber Structure for Speed

Gunn et al. have shown in histochemical studies of the transverse pectoral muscle that English Thoroughbred horses possess a significantly higher proportion of alpha muscle fibers than do other breeds. This proportion is 84 % in the Thoroughbred, compared to only 63.5 % in other breeds. Similar differences have been found between wild dogs and dogs of other breeds.

The fibers in a muscle can be divided into the following types according to their biochemical and functional properties:

1. Alpha muscle fibers have a low myosin ATPase activity and are fast-contracting.

a) Red fibers are rich in myoglobin and mitochondria and are slow to fatigue.

b) White fibers have a low myosin ATPase activity, are slow-contracting, have a high glycolytic capacity and fatigue quickly.

2. Beta muscle fibers have a low myosin ATPase activity, are slow-contracting and are rich in mitochondria.

According to Lindholm, the muscle fiber distribution in 4- to 8-year-old horses is as follows:

54% Alpha fibers with a high oxidative capacity,
22 % Alpha fibers with a low oxidative capacity, and
24 % beta fibers.

The ‘slow’ muscle fibers have a high aerobic capacity. They are especially abundant in the limb muscles and are important during sustained exercise (low to moderate speed, gallop up to about 550 m/min). The ‘fast’ muscle fibers, with a predominantly anaerobic capacity, are important for the development of high speeds. They come under stress only when training takes place in the anaerobic range, i.e., at maximal speed. Repeated workouts near the maximal speed have an equal training effect. We have found that by running racehorses at a speed of 700 m/min or greater for brief intervals, an oxygen debt is incurred which equals or even exceeds that following a race.

It should be noted that the proportion of the individual fiber types cannot be altered by training; it is a congenital trait.

1.4.2.3. Other Effects of Training on the Muscles

Training produces a marked increase of mitochondria in the exercised muscles. This increase may amount to 50—70 % in heavily exercised muscles. The same applies to the number of open capillaries. According to Kolb [1976], an area of muscle tissue measuring 1 mm^2 contains approximately 1,000 to 1,500 capillaries, only about 5% of which are perfused in the resting state. Opening of the capillaries is effected by a relaxation of occlusive precapillary structures. It is promoted by metabolic products of the muscle fibers, especially CO_2, lactic acid and ATP.

Training and the type of activity performed have an effect on the amount of contractile proteins and glycolytic enzymes present in the muscle fibers. Age and nutrition also have an influence.

Table 1.4. — 1. Increase in various compounds or metabolic processes in heavily exercised muscles after prolonged training (after JAKOWLEV [1974])

Creatine phosphate	+70 %	Myoglobin	+70 %
Glycogen	+80 %	Myosin	+60 %
Glycolysis	+50 %	Dehydrogenases	+60 %
Combustion	+48 %	Myosin-ATPase	+60 %

The glycogen content of the fast muscle fibers can be increased by training. GOODMAN et al. [1973] found an average glycogen content of 2.08 % in the latissimus dorsi muscle of horses in training, compared to only 1.41 % in horses not in training. Similarly, the content of free fatty acids in trained animals is 2.08 mg/g higher on the average than in untrained horses (0.6 mg/g).

JAKOWLEW [1974] showed that prolonged training leads to an increase of various compounds or metabolic processes in the heavily exercised muscle groups (table 1.4. — 1).

It must be understood that the adaptive processes described take place in the particular muscles that are exercised by the training. Different muscle groups are exercised at different gaits. For these reasons, endurance training in galloping racehorses should begin at the canter. Research has shown that the canter is excellent for the development of basic endurance, and that in this gait, as in the collected trot, energy production takes place exclusively via the aerobic route.

1.4.3. Respiratory Response to Training

The oxygen supply necessary for energy production is ensured by respiration. Respiration in the broad sense is a complex process involving various organ systems.

Oxygen intake	Nasopharynx Trachea Alveolar membrane	Larynx Lungs
Oxygen transport	Erythrocytes Heart	Hemoglobin Blood vessels
Oxygen transfer	O_2 dissociation 2.3-DPG	Diffusion
Oxygen consumption	Mitochondria Oxidizable substrate Enzymes	Myoglobin
Excretion of metabolic products	carbon dioxide Water *via* Lungs Kidneys	Lactic acid *via* Skin

The respiratory volume of the horse at rest is about 4 l. It may increase during exercise to 15—20 l, assuming a body weight of about 500 kg. Exercise also leads to a marked increase in respiratory rate. With the increases in respiratory volume and rate comes a tremendous rise of the minute volume. At the walk and trot there is no direct relationship between the respiratory rate and the sequence of the foot beats.

Table 1.4. — 2. Minute volume and oxygen consumption during maximal exertion (after GILLESPIE [1974])

	V min l/min	V min/kg b.w. l/min/kg b.w.	VO_2 min l/min	VO_2 min/kg b.w. l/min/kg b.w.
Man	170	2.43	5.70	0.08
Horse	2,250	4.17	75.00	0.14

As the respiratory volume and oxygen extraction are increased by training, the trotter for example, gains the ability to reduce this relationship in favor of the respiratory rate. The animal then no longer breathes at every second beat, as in the untrained state, but at every third or fourth beat. This is why the horse's respiratory pattern is a matter of much concern in the training of trotters. It often serves as a basis for determining the correct training intensity. From a relatively practical standpoint it can be monitored by the driver with the aid of a microphone attached to the dorsum of the animal's nose. In well trained horses the respiratory rate increases at the slow trot to about twice the initial value; in poorly trained horses it increases to about $2^1/_2$ times that value. Return to the initial value takes 10—15 min in well trained horses, and 25—30 min in poorly trained ones. At the fast trot the respiratory rate increases to 4 times the initial value in the former case, and to 5 or more times that value in the latter; the recovery time is 25—30 and 35—40 min, respectively. In combined training or three day event horses, increases up to 100—110 breaths per min have been observed after the cross-country phase.

In the gallop, a direct relationship exists between beat of the gait and respiratory rate. The horse breathes once per gallop sequence. Inspiration generally occurs during the phase of full extension.

As stated earlier, a respiratory volume of 15—20 l is attained during maximal exertion. At the same time, the respiratory rate may increase to 122—150 breaths per min. This results in a minute volume of approximately 2,250 l.

The minute volume and oxygen consumption of the horse and man are compared in table 1.4. — 2.

The values for the horse in the table are based on a riding speed of 800 m/min. Considering the fact that a human can attain 80% of the maximum respiratory volume during extreme effort, and the horse can develop a maximum speed of 1,000 m/min, it can be seen that the horse still possesses a considerable respiratory reserve. This applies only to healthy animals, however. Horses with bronchitis and/or chronic obstructive pulmonary disease (COPD) have little or no respiratory reserve.

It is highly likely that oxygen intake and supply by the lungs is not a limiting factor in speed endurance. This is indicated by numerous studies in the horse which show that even during exertion to the point of exhaustion, there is little or no decrease in arterial oxygen saturation. The oxygen partial pressure may decrease during light work. The reason for this lies in the fact that the upper lung regions of the horse are not well perfused during rest and light work. As a result, there is very little alveolar gas exchange in these regions.

On extreme exertion there is fall of the blood pH from 7.4 to 7.1. This pH decrease is caused mainly by the accumulation of lactic acid. This acidity stimulates the respiratory center, producing an increase in the respiratory minute volume. Oxygen from the alveolar air enters the pulmonary capillaries by simple diffusion. This process is limited by the contact area and the amount of hemoglobin present in the capillaries. The diffusion capacity is increased during exertion by an enlargement of the contact area brought about by increased lung perfusion, especially in the upper regions. Stage of fitness probably does not influence diffusion capacity.

1.4.4. Cardiac Response to Training

The stroke volume and cardiac output increase during exercise. In turn, the blood circulation is greatly accelerated, and increased amounts of oxygen and nutrients are delivered to the working muscles.

Cardiac muscle is extremely rich in contractile proteins and respiratory enzymes. The nature and duration of training activity evoke various adaptive responses in the heart and cardiac muscle. The responses include a thickening of the cardiac muscle fibers, a considerable increase in heart weight, and an enlargement of the ventricles. Endurance training for example is associated with an appreciable fall of the resting heart rate, which is generally known as 'resting bradycardia'. Its occurrence in horses is disputed. The decreased stroke rate and attendant lengthening of the cardiac cycle are due mainly to a prolongation of the diastolic phase. Because the coronary circulation is principally diastolic, the myocardial oxygen supply is improved in this manner. In man, at least, endurance training leads to a modification of resting autonomic activity like that seen in vagotonia.

At rest the equine heart pumps about 850 ml of blood into the circulation with each contraction. At a heart rate of 35 beats/min, this results in a cardiac output of approximately 30 l/min. During severe exercise the stroke volume can increase by 100—200%, accompanied by an up to six-fold increase in the heart rate. This can raise the cardiac output to 500 l/min in a 550-kg horse. DALTON et al. [1959] report a value of 74 ± 9 ml/min/kg body wt for the cardiac output of the horse.

LAGUENS and GOMEZ-DUMM [1967] point out that sustained training increases the content of actin and myosin, mitochondria and enzymes for nutrient utilization in the cardiac muscle fibers. According to SANDER [1969], the cardiac muscle of the horse has a high content of potassium ions compared to other species, thus contributing to the high working capacity of the equine heart.

Effect of Training on Resting Heart Rate. A resting heart rate of 27 to 44/min is generally reported for the horse. This rate gradually declines until about the age of 4 years. The resting heart rate varies in different breeds. English Thoroughbreds have the lowest range. Studies in 30 horses of this breed conducted over 2 training years and involving 2,700 individual measurements revealed a mean resting heart rate of 26 to 44/min, the most frequent rate being 32/min. The frequency distribution is shown graphically in figure 1.4. — 2.

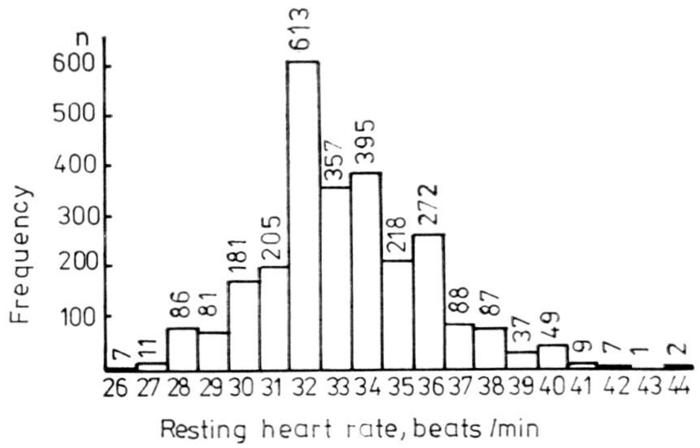

Fig. 1.4. — 2. Frequency distribution of resting heart rates in 30 English Thoroughbreds over a period of 2 training years.

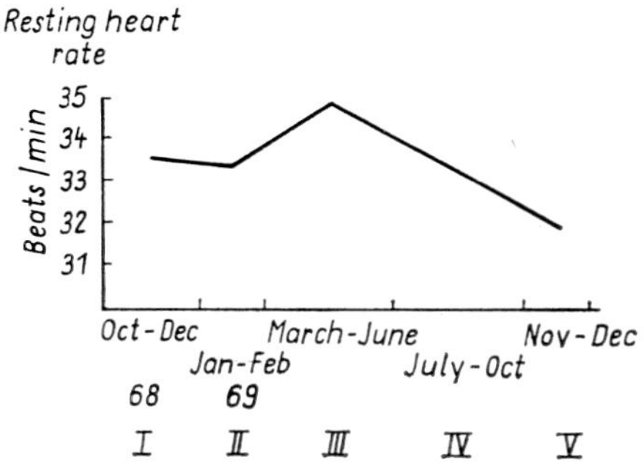

Fig. 1.4. — 3. Behavior of the resting heart rate in English Thoroughbreds during one training year.

Two-year-old fillies have higher heart rates than colts of equal age. The difference is about 2—4 beats/min. These differences become more pronounced during the course of a training year. Trained horses have lower resting heart rates than untrained horses. An increase in training intensity leads to a transitory elevation of this rate, followed later by a fall below the pre-training level. This fall is not well-defined until after the conclusion of intensive training. If intensive training is interrupted for a prolonged period, the resting heart rate rises again slightly. The changes in the resting heart rate are considered to be an expression of adaptive cardiovascular changes in response to exercise (fig. 1.4. — 3).

The pattern of the resting heart rate in the individual animal during different training segments provides a useful index of response to training. Studies of this type permit an assessment of the external stress on the circulatory system. It is first necessary to determine the mean resting heart rate, which is different for each animal. The range of variation also varies on an individual basis. It may be 6 to 15 beats per min or even more in rare cases. Neither value changes in the mature horse, even over long periods of time. The mean rate and range of variation are best determined during the winter months, when training influences are absent. There is a clear correlation between resting heart rate and racing condition. Horses that are at the lower limit of their individual range usually show superior racing performance, while animals at the upper limit typically show poor racing performance. Often there is a marked rise of the resting heart rate on the days following a race; this is considered evidence that these horses were at a stage of fitness appropriate for the performance demands.

The aforementioned changes in the resting heart rate are quite limited in their value unless they can be measured carefully. To minimize environmental influences on the resting heart rate, the measurements should be carried out in a quiet stall with a phonendoscope by the same person at the same time each day, and should be preceded by a 14-day acclimatization period.

Response of the Heart Rate to Exercise. The heart rate provides a particularly good means of physiologic monitoring, because it is relatively easy to measure and is a good source of information.

The heart rate is a product of 'cardiac autorhythmicity'; that is, the impulses for myocardial contraction originate within the heart itself. This basal rate can be modified depending on momentary demands by vagal and sympathetic influences, which in most cases exert antagonistic effects. The basic parameters of cardiac activity are set mainly in the bulbopontine centers, which also ensure a relatively constant heart rate via self-regulating reflexes. The hypothalamus and higher brain regions, finally, enable a higher level of integration and coordination with respect to environmental stimuli.

Metabolic influences play an important role in the control of the heart rate. A linear relationship exists between heart rate and metabolism over a wide range, provided the oxygen requirement is adequately met. This linearity disappears during work under anaerobic conditions [STEGEMANN, 1967]. The close relationship between heart rate and metabolism has given rise to many hypotheses concerning the mechanism of heart rate control. Evidence indicates that the pCO_2 and H-ion concentration in the muscle are adequate to create a pulse-rate control mechanism based upon muscular metabolism. The receptors responsible for this mechanism are presumably located in the interstitium between the capillary and muscle fiber. The delay between stimulation of the receptors and adjustment of the cardiac rate is only about 0.7 to 0.9 seconds, and thus less than one pulse interval. It has also been shown that the heart rate can be reproducibly increased by an afferent pathway in a spinal nerve. Thus, the circulatory center processes information on physical performance that originates from receptors in the muscles. This underscores the importance of the heart rate as an index of the metabolic state and the degree of exertion of the organism. Thus, even today, monitoring of the heart rate can be recommended as a criterion for sound training practice.

The heart rate, like other physiologic parameters, undergoes changes in response to exercise and fatigue, in accordance with specific laws. The functional changes during the course of exercise can be divided into three phases. The 'adaptive phase' is marked by initial adjustments of the circulation and metabolism. In this phase there is a certain anachronism of function, i.e., the adaptation is not parallel for all parameters. This phase is particularly influenced by the intensity of the exercise; its duration is about 40 s during exercise of moderate intensity. This is followed by the 'stabilization phase', in which the measurable EKG parameters, oxygen intake, blood pressure, etc. assume relatively constant values. An equilibrium develops which is expressed by the relative degrees of vagal and sympathetic activity, depending on the situation. This equilibrium is probably based on an adequate supply of energy, which is produced by both the aerobic and anaerobic routes. The third phase involves the utilization of maximum performance reserves; it is characterized by the breakdown of this equilibrium. The organism is unable to maintain the stability of body functions, and exhaustion ensues.

Technique of Heart Rate Measurement During Exercise. The actual process of measuring physiologic parameters often influences the parameters of interest. Wireless telemetry or radiotelemetry is free of this problem, because the subject is allowed to move freely during the examination, having little or no direct contact with the examiner. The simplest method of telemetric heart-rate determination is the transmission of cardiac action potentials, for they already represent electrical signals. In general these potentials are modulated to a subcarrier and transmission frequency and then to a receiver, where they are demodulated to yield an electrocardiogram. BAYER [1966] describes the recording of exercise heart rates by means of a receiver connected by an 8-meter cable to the lunged horse. The disadvantages of this method compared to radiotelemetry are obvious.

For long-term investigations of the heart rate, many researchers prefer to store the cardiac action potentials on a tape recorder attached to the animal or rider, rather than employ wireless telemetry. This method is particularly advantageous during cross-country rides, where radiotelemetry would be of little value due to the limited range of the transmitters.

The customary EKG leads are of limited use for telemetric studies. For telemetry they must be placed such that movements and activity by the animal will not cause detachment of the electrodes. In addition, the cardiac action potentials should not

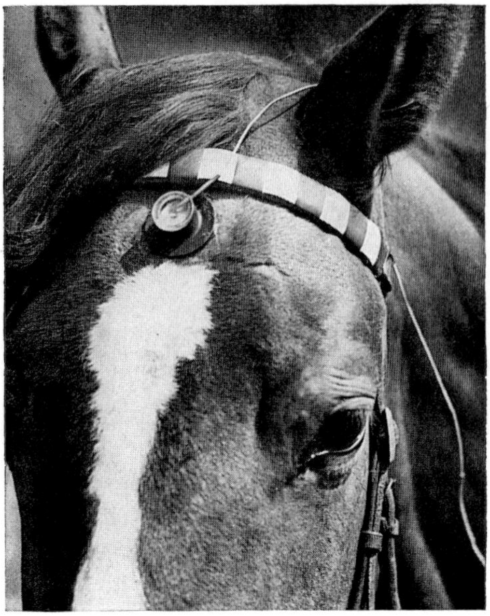

Fig. 1.4. — 4. Adhesive electrode attached to the center of the forehead by the method of Börnert. The space between the rubber ring and electrode is filled with electrode paste.

be distorted by superimposed muscle potentials, even during severe exercise. As a rule, only the heart rate is assessed, and so only two leads are necessary. Many instrument types require a third, indifferent electrode. The most common sites for placement of the leads are the sternum, xiphoid region or left chest wall behind the girth, as well as the center of the forehead, withers or right chest wall.

The electrode design must also conform to telemetric demands. Various types are available, such as adhesive electrodes, pressure electrodes that are strapped to the body surface, and alligator clips. The electrode developed by Boernert et al., which fits into a rubber receptacle glued to the skin, has proved very useful (fig. 1.4. — 4).

The following technique has proved suitable for recording the heart rate during training and racing: The primary data relayed to the receiver by the transmitter are first recorded. Using digital devices, these primary values are then converted to numeric symbols that are printed out or recorded on punched tape.

The output can be handled with universal counters, which feed the digitally encoded data to a transducer that performs the code conversion for the sheet or strip-chart printer connected to it. The time between successive R intervals is measured. The measurement process is initiated by one R wave and terminated by the next. It is carried out automatically by the universal counter. Changes in the heart rate can be detected quickly and accurately by this method.

It is useful to establish unambiguous reference quantities as an aid to interpreting the primary data. One such reference quantity is time, which enables the riding speed to be calculated if the distance is known.

Figure 1.4. — 5 shows a printout obtained with the instrument described above.

Response of the Heart Rate to Walking. A heart rate of 58 to 133 beats per min was measured at the walk in 100 telemetric studies of racehorses. This broad range demonstrates that emotional factors, rather than physiologic ones, are chiefly responsible for the level of the heart rate at the walk. Even in warmblooded breeds, rates of 70 to 90/min could be measured in this gait. Some authors have reported a rapid elevation of the heart rate at the start of walking, followed about 25 s later by a

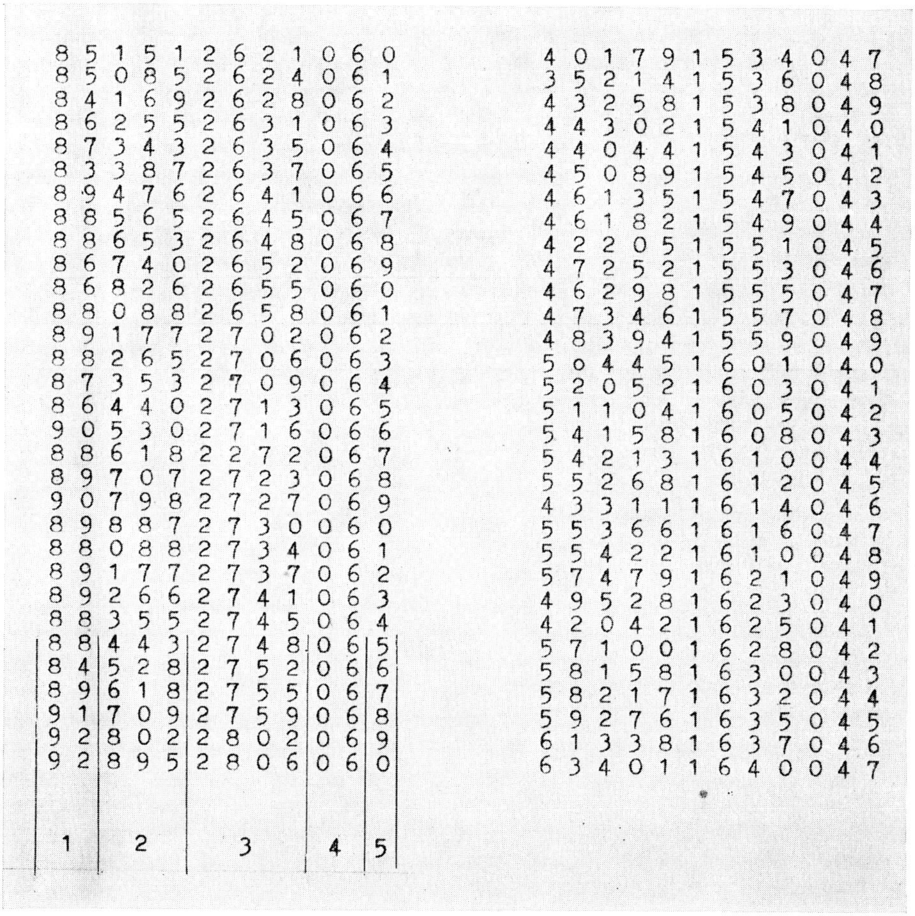

1		2			3				4		5
8	5	1	5	1	2	6	2	1	0	6	0
8	5	0	8	5	2	6	2	4	0	6	1
8	4	1	6	9	2	6	2	8	0	6	2
8	6	2	5	5	2	6	3	1	0	6	3
8	7	3	4	3	2	6	3	5	0	6	4
8	3	3	8	7	2	6	3	7	0	6	5
8	9	4	7	6	2	6	4	1	0	6	6
8	8	5	6	5	2	6	4	5	0	6	7
8	8	6	5	3	2	6	4	8	0	6	8
8	6	7	4	0	2	6	5	2	0	6	9
8	6	8	2	6	2	6	5	5	0	6	0
8	8	0	8	8	2	6	5	8	0	6	1
8	9	1	7	7	2	7	0	2	0	6	2
8	8	2	6	5	2	7	0	6	0	6	3
8	7	3	5	3	2	7	0	9	0	6	4
8	6	4	4	0	2	7	1	3	0	6	5
9	0	5	3	0	2	7	1	6	0	6	6
8	8	6	1	8	2	2	7	2	0	6	7
8	9	7	0	7	2	7	2	3	0	6	8
9	0	7	9	8	2	7	2	7	0	6	9
8	9	8	8	7	2	7	3	0	0	6	0
8	8	0	8	8	2	7	3	4	0	6	1
8	9	1	7	7	2	7	3	7	0	6	2
8	9	2	6	6	2	7	4	1	0	6	3
8	8	3	5	5	2	7	4	5	0	6	4
8	8	4	4	3	2	7	4	8	0	6	5
8	4	5	2	8	2	7	5	2	0	6	6
8	9	6	1	8	2	7	5	5	0	6	7
9	1	7	0	9	2	7	5	9	0	6	8
9	2	8	0	2	2	8	0	2	0	6	9
9	2	8	9	5	2	8	0	6	0	6	0

4	0	1	7	9	1	5	3	4	0	4	7
3	5	2	1	4	1	5	3	6	0	4	8
4	3	2	5	8	1	5	3	8	0	4	9
4	4	3	0	2	1	5	4	1	0	4	0
4	4	0	4	4	1	5	4	3	0	4	1
4	5	0	8	9	1	5	4	5	0	4	2
4	6	1	3	5	1	5	4	7	0	4	3
4	6	1	8	2	1	5	4	9	0	4	4
4	2	2	0	5	1	5	5	1	0	4	5
4	7	2	5	2	1	5	5	3	0	4	6
4	6	2	9	8	1	5	5	5	0	4	7
4	7	3	4	6	1	5	5	7	0	4	8
4	8	3	9	4	1	5	5	9	0	4	9
5	0	4	4	5	1	6	0	1	0	4	0
5	2	0	5	2	1	6	0	3	0	4	1
5	1	1	0	4	1	6	0	5	0	4	2
5	4	1	5	8	1	6	0	8	0	4	3
5	4	2	1	3	1	6	1	0	0	4	4
5	5	2	6	8	1	6	1	2	0	4	5
4	3	3	1	1	1	6	1	4	0	4	6
5	5	3	6	6	1	6	1	6	0	4	7
5	5	4	2	2	1	6	1	0	0	4	8
5	7	4	7	9	1	6	2	1	0	4	9
4	9	5	2	8	1	6	2	3	0	4	0
4	2	0	4	2	1	6	2	5	0	4	1
5	7	1	0	0	1	6	2	8	0	4	2
5	8	1	5	8	1	6	3	0	0	4	3
5	8	2	1	7	1	6	3	2	0	4	4
5	9	2	7	6	1	6	3	5	0	4	5
6	1	3	3	8	1	6	3	7	0	4	6
6	3	4	0	1	1	6	4	0	0	4	7

Fig. 1.4. — 5. Digital record of RR intervals in reel printout. 1 = RR interval in 10 ms; 2 = automatic summation of 10 measured values; 3 = elapsed time readout in minutes and seconds; 4 = 2-digit gait code; 5 = sequential numbering of measured values from 1 to 10.

decline to a stable mean value, but this is not always observed. Even in long-distance walks of several kilometers, no increase in heart rate can be measured by the end of the exercise. The response of the heart rate to walking permits no inferences to be drawn concerning the animal's fitness. It is of some value, however, in assessing the functional state of the nervous system.

Response of the Heart Rate to Trotting. At the trot, the heart rate of the racehorse ranges between 83 and 129 beats per min. It is significantly higher than at the walk. The riding speed is the key factor in determining the level of the heart rate in this gait. The values cited are based on a riding speed of 250 m/min. During sustained trotting for up to 9,000 m, racehorses showed a decline of the heart rate as the exercise progressed. Thus, it was 136/min at 1,000 m, 124/min at 1,500 m, and 122/min at 9,000 m. These values show that a progressive 'economy of circulation' develops during the collected trot, as well as the fact that trained Thoroughbreds experience no increase in fatigue over a distance of 9,000 m.

In trotters, a heart rate of 140 beats per min was determined at a speed of 200 m/min. At higher speeds over a distance of 1,000 m, there is a linear increase in fatigue corresponding to the exercise intensity, with a maximum recorded heart rate of 240/min. According to reports by various authors, a heart rate of 240 to 250 beats per min in the horse must be regarded as the maximum possible rate.

Response of the Heart Rate to Galloping. At the gallop there is an even more distinct linear relationship between running speed and heart rate. In English Thoroughbred racehorses in full training, we found the following heart rates for various galloping speeds:

Galloping speed, m/min	350—450	550—650	750—850	850—1,000
heart rate, beats/min	120—150	158—198	192—216	239—253

Ehrlein [1970] measured a heart rate of 180/min in horses ridden at a speed of 500 m/min. Wittke et al. [1968] recorded a heart rate of 205/min in a horse 27 s after the start of a galloping test, but this was an 'overshoot' that decreased slightly before gradually rising again to assume a steady-state value of 212/min. For warm-blooded horses, Bassan and Ott report a heart rate of 120—154/min at a galloping speed of 300 m/min, and a rate of 155—188/min at a speed of 440 m/min.

The duration of the adaptive phase, i.e., the interval from the start of exercise to the attainment of a 'steady-state' condition, is dependent on the intensity of the exercise. Ehrlein as well as Ott report an adaptation time of 30 s to 1 min 45 s, depending on the degree of exertion. Our own studies point to a considerably shorter adaptive phase in racehorses. Its duration is 17.6 s at a collected trot and 9.0 $\pm$ 5.4 s at a fast gallop of 800 m/min. A distance of about 112 m is covered at the fast gallop during this time. In the collected trot, with an adaptive period nearly twice as long, a distance of only 58 m is covered before attaining a heart rate appropriate for the degree of exertion. It has also been shown that the adaptive period is subject to small individual variations during the change from walking to trotting, and to large individual variations during the change from the trot to the gallop. Moreover, the adaptive phase is shorter in well trained horses than in poorly trained ones. Breed-dependent differences also occur.

According to our own investigations, the 'overshoot' often described in the heart rate in response to exertion, seldom occurs during strenuous exercise. It is not always observed during exercise of low intensity. In most animals tested the heart rate attains a 'desired value' following the adaptive phase. These results are important for training practice. It would certainly be worthwhile to determine whether the adaptive period in the racehorse could be shortened and competitive performance improved by a preliminary 'warmup' like that customary in track-and-field sports and other equitation events. It must be remembered, that the preparations for a horse-race adhere to a strict routine as well as a certain amount of tradition that would be most difficult to change.

In the preparation for a race each stage has its effect on the equine heart rate that is referable to emotional factors. This is dramatically illustrated in figure 1.4. — 6.

Sizable individual differences are noted in the heart rate at the walk and at the trot. These differences are still apparent at more strenuous gaits, but they are much less pronounced. At maximal speed the individual differences disappear almost entirely. Studies during several flat races clearly show that the heart rate of all horses approaches or attains the maximal limit. Thus, little can be concluded about a horse's stage of fitness based on the absolute level of the heart rate during maximal exertion.

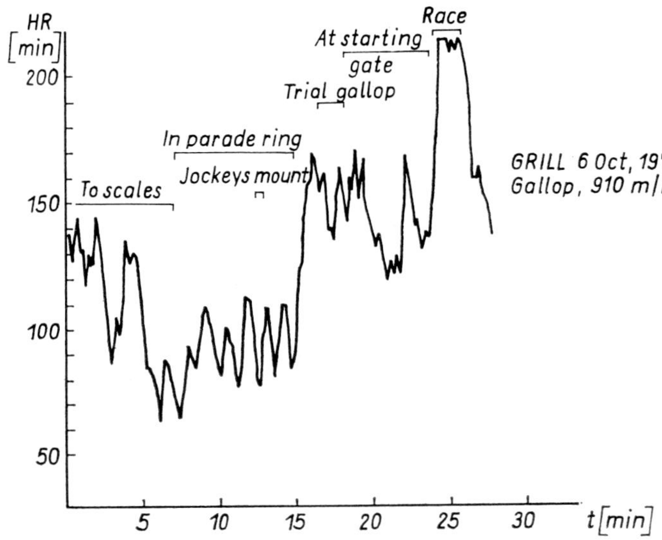

Fig. 1.4. — 6. Behavior of the heart rate during preparations for racing and during the race.

It may be assumed that the cardiac output cannot increase further at heart rates over 240/min, because diastole then becomes too short to permit adequate cardiac filling. The heart of trained horses actually *responds* better to exercise, with adjustments made more rapidly in accordance with performance demands. Even during submaximal exertion, the trained heart works more economically. As fitness improves, the heart rate becomes progressively slower during the performance of standard exercise. This is due to the fact that the stroke volume increases as fitness improves.

In untrained animals the heart responds to exercise mainly by an increase in heart rate, while in trained animals it does so by an increase in stroke volume. The volume response is more efficient, because the energy required is lower.

Ehrlein recommends evaluating the cardiac response to training by stepwise testing in six well-defined speed stages. Well trained horses are able to develop higher speeds at the same heart rate than untrained horses. Bayer [1966] attributes this phenomenon to an economy of movement derived from technical training. This, according to Bayer, lessens the demands on the circulation and energy metabolism. Apparently, an economy of cardiac work is also responsible in part for the gradual decline of the heart rate during a standardized exercise regime in well conditioned horses.

It is reasonable to assume that a heart rate of about 150 to 170 beats per min represents the limit of aerobic metabolism in the trained horse. This corresponds in the racehorse to a riding speed of about 550 to 700 m/min.

Behavior of the Heart Rate After Exercise. The behavior of the heart rate after exercise is a good index of fitness. As a general rule, the heart rate of trained horses returns more quickly to the resting value after exercise than that of untrained horses. The recovery time also lengthens with the intensity of the exercise. The recovery period after strenuous exercise can be divided into three main phases. Ten minutes after exercise the heart rate is still relatively high. It declines sharply during the next 10 min, and in the third phase it slowly returns to the normal value over a period of one to several hours. During galloping of moderate intensity over 3,000 m, a heart rate of 90—100/min is attained at the end of the exercise. The same applies to a collected trot over 10,000 m. Stewart [1972] measured the heart rates of well trained racehorses 30 min after test gallops, finding a rate of 85/min for a speed of 900 to 950 m/min, and 60/min for a speed of 800 m/min. Nowosinow measured a recovery period of 20 ± 3.4 min in sport horses that had performed exercise of moderate intensity. After fast trotting over about 2,000 m, the heart rate of well trained horses returned to normal in 50 to 60 min, compared to 70—80 min in poorly trained horses. The absolute level of the heart rate after exercise is a poor index of the duration of the recovery period. The more severely the functional reserves of the cardiovascular system are taxed during exercise, the greater the oxygen debt incurred during the exercise, and the more prolonged the recovery period. As the animal's fitness improves with training, recovery proceeds at a more rapid rate. The dependence of the recovery processes on functional demands is well illustrated by a comparison of physiologic and emotional stress. Both forms of stress cause a rapid elevation of the heart rate. With emotional stress, however, the recovery period generally does not exceed 1—2 min.

1.4.4.1. Performance and the Electrocardiogram

Performance ability cannot be assessed on the basis of the resting EKG. Endurance training leads to the aforementioned adaptive responses of the heart, which are also visible in the EKG. Manifestations of these responses may include bradycardia, sinus arrhythmia, a prolonged conduction time, and partial right-branch block.

According to Holmes [1974], cardiac arrhythmias may result from disturbances of impulse formation, impulse conduction, or a combination of both. Thus, arrhythmias can be categorized as follows:

1. Disturbances of impulse formation, including the presence of ectopic foci.
2. Disturbances of impulse conduction, including various forms of heart block.
3. A combination of 1 and 2, including extrasystoles, fibrillations and AV dissociation (complete heart block being the most serious conduction disturbance).

The partial AV block is probably the most common form of arrhythmia in horses, while the sinoatrial block is the least common. In the partial, or second-degree, AV block, some atrial impulses cannot spread to the ventricles, so that the ventricles fail to contract periodically. This is manifested in the EKG by an absence of the ventricular complex with a relative increase in the number of P waves.

The second-degree AV block is often accompanied by first-degree conduction disturbances (prolongation of the physiologic conduction time) and usually occurs as Type I (Wenckebach), with the EKG showing PR intervals of varying length. In the Wenckebach rhythm there is a progressive lengthening of the conduction time until the atrial impulse can no longer be conducted. After the missed beat the conduction time is normal initially but then lengthens to repeat the cycle.

Alps and Holmes [1961] found that when atrial fibrillation and sinus arrhythmias coincide, the latter persist after exercise. When sinus arrhythmia occurs alone, however, the post-exercise rhythm is normal. They often found atrial extrasystole after exercise, attributing this to myocardial lesions. According to these authors, mixed arrhythmias lead in time to cardiac weakness and are of clinical importance in racing animals, in contrast to conduction disturbances such as the partial AV block.

Spörri [1951, 1952] interprets the heart block as a reflex phenomenon under respiratory control, describing it as a symptom of 'training vagotonia'. He found partial AV blocks in 18% of the horses examined. Wittke and Bayer [1968] found a 13% incidence in their series of military horses. They do not consider this to be generally pathologic, but representative, rather, of vagal inhibition which disappears during work and excitement. Sinoatrial blocks, first- and second-degree AV blocks, and biphasic P waves in the horse can be regarded as vagal-mediated conduction delays, and thus as physiologic phenomena. RHEZAKHANI [1975], who observed sinus arrhythmias at rest and/or after exercise in 46 horses, also attaches no clinical importance to these arrhythmias, considering them a recovery mechanism of the autonomic nervous system.

Paroxysmal ventricular tachycardia is characterized by a very rapid but regular heart rate. The periods of tachycardia start and stop abruptly. They often last for only several heartbeats but may persist for hours or even days. The EKG at such times shows bizarre QRST complexes. In some cases the P waves occur independently of the ventricular complexes and at a slower rate. Ventricular tachycardia is often associated with inflammatory or degenerative myocardial lesions. In the absence of organic heart disease, it may be the result of general fatigue or overtraining. Exercise may precipitate EKG changes referable to myocardial disease. In the presence of coronary insufficiency, BROOIJMANS [1957] considers the following EKG changes to be pathognomonic:

1. Elevation of the ST segment in leads I, II and aVF, depression of ST in lead aVR;
2. the occurrence of arrhythmias of all types;
3. the occurrence of conduction disturbances;
4. elevation of the T wave above the normal degree.

The EKG changes in normal horses are due to an increase in heart rate. They are expressed in a shortening of all electrocardiographic intervals (PR, ARS, AT, etc.) and in characteristic T-wave changes in the form of an elevated T wave in leads I or CV/LL. The EKG findings can be supported by careful auscultation, which is the most informative of all clinical examinations of the heart, and by phonocardiography.

1.4.4.2. Performance and Heart Weight

Studies in English Thoroughbreds have shown that the heart weight of this breed ranges from 2 to 6 kg. According to STEEL et al. [1974], the heart weight of horses can be fairly accurately determined on the basis of the *heart score*. For this purpose it is necessary to determine the duration of the QRS interval in each standard limb lead. After finding the arithmetic mean for each lead, the arithmetic mean of the QRS interval for all three leads is calculated. This mean value, expressed in milliseconds, is the heart score. Only EKG tracings without baseline fluctuations are interpreted. The heart rate should not significantly exceed 40 beats/min during recording of the EKG. A score of 100 corresponds to a heart weight of 3.0 kg. Each additional 10 points represents a 0.8-kg increase in heart weight. Thus, with a heart score of 110, the corresponding heart weight is 3.8 kg; with a score of 130, the heart weight is 5.4 kg. Various workers have related heart weight to racing performance. With one exception, Australian Derby winners were found to have heart scores between 120 and 135 msec. No correlation could be found between heart weight and body weight. The heart score reportedly increases by an average of 10 msec per year from birth up to the age of 3 years. This means that a newborn foal with a score of 73 will attain a score of 103 by age 3. There is divided opinion about the effect of training on heart weight. KUBO et al. [1974] found a 1.1 % relationship between heart weight and body weight in horses in training, and 0.94 % in horses not in training.

According to BEILHARZ et al. [1974], heart weight is principally an inherited trait, being more a product of maternal than paternal inheritance.

On comparison of analogous findings in track-and-field athletes, it would appear that the heart weight in running and trotting horses cannot be significantly influenced by training. Track-and-field athletes show an increase of heart weight only in sports involving exceptional endurance.

1.4.5. Hematologic Response to Exercise

The main function of the blood is to serve as a vehicle for numerous substances that undergo an exchange with the body's cells. It differs from other tissues in that its intercellular substance has a high fluid content, and its cells are highly mobile. Another important function of the blood is to aid in maintaining homeostasis. For example, the buffer function of the blood is important during exercise. The blood carries metabolic products such as CO_2 to the lungs and carries nitrogenous end-products to the kidneys. By binding the H-ions formed by metabolic processes, the blood prevents significant fluctuations of pH. During exercise, moreover, there is a redistribution of the available blood volume. From a resting value of 15—20%, the amount of blood delivered to the working muscles increases to 80—85% of the total blood volume. At the same time, the blood flow to the digestive organs is strongly curtailed. The circulating blood volume is increased by a rise of the cardiac output and by the expulsion of blood stored in the liver and spleen.

Changes in Blood Volume During Exercise. The blood volume equals the volume of all liquid and formed blood constituents that are present in the circulation at any given time. It follows that the circulating blood volume is not a constant quantity. In particular, it is influenced by the release of blood reserves. Studies by ZELLER and SIEWERT [1964] indicate that the relative 'active blood volume' in the horse is 89 ml/kg body wt, and that the total blood volume after the release of reserves is 101 ml/kg body wt. Investigations by ADAMOPOULOU [1975] in young trotters showed an average blood volume of 70—73 ml/kg at $1^1/_2$ years of age, and about 81 ml/kg at $2^1/_2$ years. The corresponding values after exercise were 80—90 ml/kg and 100 ml/kg.

The magnitude of the blood volume increase depends on the degree of exertion, particularly its intensity, as well as the stage of fitness. In view of its varying behavior, the blood volume appears to be of limited value in exercise physiology studies. In addition, it is much more difficult to determine than other parameters. The response of the solid blood constituents is a more useful source of information.

Effect of Exercise on the Erythrocytes. A great deal of attention has been given to the erythrocyte count in the assessment of equine performance ability. It has proved difficult to determine the resting erythrocyte count, however, especially in Thoroughbreds. Venipuncture itself can cause excitement with an associated rise of sympathetic or adrenergic activity; in response, the spleen contracts and expels erythrocytes into the circulation, creating a falsely elevated resting value. Many investigators avoid this effect by prior sedation of the animal. WOLF [1977] found that samples drawn 3 min after needle insertion no longer showed elevated erythrocyte counts compared to samples drawn later, in contrast to blood samples taken immediately after the venipuncture. Due to the inaccuracy of resting blood samples, it is often suggested that only exercise samples be taken, or that samples be drawn after the blood reserves have been emptied by medication.

Various values are given in the literature for the resting erythrocyte count of the horse. It is clear, however, that the count varies as a function of age and breed.

JEFFCOTT [1971] reports the following values for English Thoroughbreds:

Age	Number of tests	Erythrocyte count × 10^{12}/l		
1 month	78	9.85	±	1.31
1—9 months	75	10.33	±	1.24
Yearling	100	9.91	±	1.11
2 years	308	9.86	±	0.98
3 years	353	9.71	±	1.06
4 years	138	9.28	±	0.98
Over 4 years	302	8.80	±	1.09

Other authors give the following values:

Author(s) and year	Breed	Erythrocyte count × 10^{12}/l
SCHEUNERT and KRZYWANEK [1926]	Warmblood	6.01
McLEOD et al. [1946]	Thoroughbred, 2—3 years	10.80
	Thoroughbred, older	11.55
McLEOD et al. [1947]	Thoroughbred	11.00
	Trotter	9.20
	Arabian	11.50
SCHLICHTING et al. [1956]	Thoroughbred, trained	11.93
SCHALM [1965]	Thoroughbred	9.50
VERTER et al. [1966]	Warmblood	7.50
MILL and WOLF [1974]	Trotter	9.70

Besides the resting erythrocyte count, the erythrocyte reserve also appears to be breed-dependent. HARING [1936] found an erythrocyte reserve of 2.21×10^{12} erythrocytes per liter in warm blooded breeds, and a value of only 1.74×10^{12} in cold-blooded breeds. Our own studies have shown that the amount of erythrocyte release during exercise correlates closely with the intensity of the exercise. Little or no erythrocyte increase is noted during sustained light exercise, whereas a marked increase is observed even after a brief period of strenuous exercise.

Thus, in determinations of the erythrocyte reserve, the nature of the activitiy should be specified.

LASKOW [1965] found an erythrocyte reserve of 40—50 % in trained racehorses. In Standardbreds, MILL and WOLF [1974] measured an average erythrocyte increase of 2.5×10^{12}/l over the resting value after strenuous exercise. In our own studies over several years of training we found that both the resting erythrocyte count and the erythrocyte reserve undergo a change during that given training period. Direct relationships were found between the nature of the training and the level of the erythrocyte counts. During endurance training, both the resting erythrocyte count and erythrocyte reserve remain low. Even repeated endurance workouts over 10,000 m at a collected trot are not sufficient in the racehorse to stimulate erythropoiesis. Only strenuous exercise at speeds in excess of 600 m/min have this stimulating effect on red cell production. Figure 1.4. — 7 shows the variations in erythrocyte count during one training year in Thoroughbred racehorses 3 years of age or older. Until March the horses mainly underwent general endurance training. From

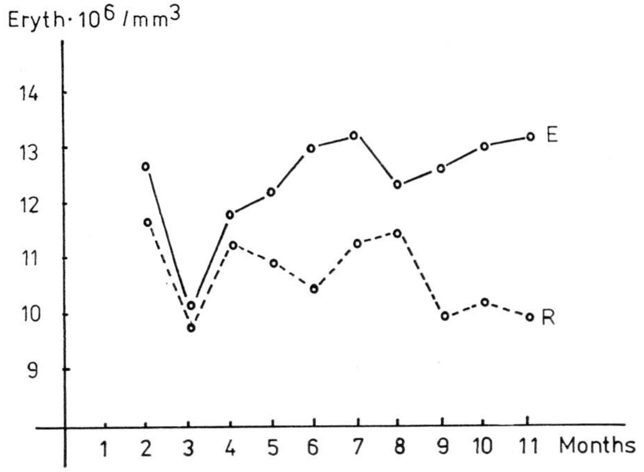

Fig. 1.4. — 7. Effect of training on erythrocyte release after standard exercises in 3-year-old English Thoroughbreds. The difference between the resting (R) and exercise values (E) increases with the length of training.

the start of training to that time, the resting erythrocyte count shows an average rise of only 0.57×10^{12}/l. At the start of strenuous training it increases continuously to 2.22×10^{12}/l by July, reaching a value of 4.03×10^{12}/l at the end of the racing season. Despite standardized training, an increase of erythrocyte release is also observed during exercise. Thus, differently adapted organisms respond differently to the same stresses.

Intensive training also leads to a physiologic erythrocytosis (polycythemia) in the horse. The stimulus for this increased erythrocyte formation is undoubtedly the hypoxia that accompanies strenuous training or racing.

In track-and-field athletes, attempts have been made to achieve the same effect with high-altitude training. The lower oxygen pressure at high altitudes results in a reduction of oxygen binding by oxyhemoglobin. Prolonged or repeated brief exposures to high altitudes lead to a number of long-term adaptive changes which improve oxygen uptake and transport by the blood. The erythrocyte count and hemoglobin level of the blood increase markedly. In addition, the capillary flow, myoglobin content and oxidative enzyme activity of the muscles are increased. This promotes the transfer of oxygen from the blood to the tissues and improves working capacity. These adaptive changes regress quickly after the return to sea level. Because high-altitude training is rarely practical in the horse, attempts are being made to evoke similar adaptive responses by the induction of artificial hypoxia. One method is to have the animal breathe air with a reduced oxygen content (i.e., 10 % O_2 instead of the normal 20.4%) for several minutes each day.

Wolf [1977] has also used autotransfusion in an attempt to stimulate erythropoiesis. After the reinfusion of 1,000 ml and 2,000 ml of stored blood previously drawn from the same animal, a very slight increase in the erythrocyte count was noted in the first 10 days after the infusion. No performance increase was observed, however.

Steel et al. [1960] state that resting erythrocyte counts above 11×10^{12}/l constitute polycythemia in the horse. It is their opinion that such horses show poor racing performance. Three forms of polycythemia can be distinguished. Apparent polycythemia is due essentially to a release of blood reserves caused by excitement during the drawing of blood. Absolute polycythemia is the result of a diminished oxygen supply like that associated with COPD or certain cardiovascular diseases. Relative polycythemia is the result of hemoconcentration secondary to a reduced fluid intake or severe losses of body fluid and can usually be diagnosed on the basis of other clinical signs.

It is generally held that racehorses with resting erythrocyte counts between 9 and 11×10^{12}/ml show the best racing performance, but this is true only to a limited degree. Based on our experience, the state of fitness or performance ability is best evaluated by means of sequential studies. Only in this way can the individual limits of the resting erythrocyte counts be defined, and upward or downward deviations recognized. The resting erythrocyte count is however only one criterion that can assist in evaluating an animal's momentary performance ability.

Effect of Exercise on the Hematocrit. In addition to studies of the cell count, hemoglobin level, red-cell volume, the relative and absolute hemoglobin level, the hematocrit and the reticulocyte count, analysis of the volume- or pressure-distribution curves of the erythrocytes are important in the assessment of erythropoiesis. The volume-distribution curves are particularly informative, even with slight changes in the erythrocyte population. The blood sample is centrifuged to separate the red cells from the plasma, and then their volume percentage is determined. This value is called the hematocrit (HC) or packed cell volume (PCV) and represents the relative volume of erythrocytes, which make up the bulk of the corpuscular blood constituents.

Different authors give different resting hematocrit values for the horse, as indicated in the table below.

Age	Number of samples	Hematocrit[1]
Less than 1 month	78	0.38 ± 0.05
1—9 months	75	0.34 ± 0.04
Yearling	100	0.38 ± 0.04
2 years	308	0.40 ± 0.04
3 years	353	0.41 ± 0.04
4 years	138	0.41 ± 0.05
Over 4 years	302	0.40 ± 0.05

These data from JEFFCOTT [1971] pertain to English Thoroughbreds. Other authors give the following values for various breeds:

Author(s)	Breed	Hematocrit[1]
SCHEUNERT and KRZYWANEK [1926]	Warmblood	0.31
TRUM [1952]	Thoroughbred	0.40 (0.25—0.55)
BRENON [1958]	Thoroughbred, trained	0.43
SRÉTER [1959]	Thoroughbred, trained	0.44
ARCHER and MILLER [1959]	Riding horses	0.42 (0.31—0.55)
STEEL et al. [1960]	Thoroughbred, trained	0.42 (0.31—0.55)
	Trotter, trained	0.39 (0.26—0.58)
SCHALM [1965]	Thoroughbred	0.42
LITTLEJOHN [1968]	Thoroughbred, sedated	0.41 ± 0.01
	Warmblood, sedated	0.37 ± 0.01
KRZYWANEK et al. [1972]	Trotter	0.36 ± 0.03

[1] Percentage values are divided by 100 for expression as SI units.

Both tables indicate that the hematocrit increases with age, and that English Thoroughbreds have the highest hematocrit values.

The hematocrit, like the erythrocyte count, increases after exercise, this increase varying with the intensity of the exercise. Also, as with the resting values, marked breed differences are present. SCHEUNERT and KRZYWANEK [1926] observed an increase from 0.31 to 0.44 in warm blooded horses. SRÉTER [1959] found a rise of the hematocrit from 0.48 ± 0.01 to 0.67 in English Thoroughbreds. Our studies indicate an increase to 0.61 ± 0.03 in trained Thoroughbreds that have just raced. This is an increase of about 50 % over the initial value. Assuming a blood volume of about 50 l, this means an 8-liter increase in the corpuscular elements of the blood. Even taking into account that erythrocytes are stored in the lungs and bone marrow in addition to the spleen, it is unlikely that the increase in the PCV is due entirely to the mobilization of these cells. It is more probable that exercise produces a partial redistribution of the blood plasma that results in a higher blood viscosity.

The importance of the hematocrit for assessing the momentary performance ability of a horse is as controversial as that of the red blood cell count. Again, we may assume that the PCV will provide a useful index only if the individual limits are known, and deviations from these limits can be determined on the basis of repeated measurements. After all, even horses with high PCV values are quite capable of winning races.

Mean Corpuscular Volume (MCV). The following values are given by ARCHER [1973] for the mean corpuscular volume of English Thoroughbreds:

Age	Number of samples	MCV $\times 10^{-9}$ µl
1 month	78	38.5 ± 2.49
1—9 months	75	34.3 ± 2.92
Yearling	100	37.9 ± 1.90
2 years	308	40.6 ± 2.63
3 years	353	42.7 ± 2.54
4 years	138	44.3 ± 2.43
Over 4 years	302	45.5 ± 2.56

Other authors report the following values for various breeds:

Author(s)	Breed	MCV $\times 10^{-9}$ µl
SCHEUNERT and KRZYWANEK [1926]	Warmblood	52.4
STEEL et al. [1960]	Thoroughbred, trained	43.8 (30.7—58.1)
	Trotter, trained	45.5 (36.2—61.6)
SCHALM [1965]	Thoroughbred	48—49.6
MARTINS [1966/67]	Thoroughbred	48—49.6
MILL and WOLF [1974]	Trotter	49

According to WOLF [1977], strenuous exercise at the start of the training year leads to considerable stimulation of the bone marrow. The oxygen deficit produced by intensive training leads to elevated erythropoietin levels in the plasma and thus to erythropoiesis. Besides reticulocytes, increased numbers of young cell forms appear in the circulating blood, which are characterized by their greater mean volume. COLLINS et al. [1969] examined horses during the Mexico City Olympics and found an increase in the MCV from 46.1 to 70.6 over a seven-week period. WOLF [1977] showed on the basis of volume-distribution curves with the advent of strenuous training exercise, a younger erythrocyte population appears in the circulating blood.

According to our own investigations, older horses have a higher MCV than younger horses. After strenuous exercise leading to a marked increase in the PCV, the MCV is higher than before the exercise. This increase can only be attributed to the mobilization of erythrocytes. It must be considered that the erythrocytes have even a greater volume than this exercise value would indicate, since only the mean value of the total erythrocytes is being determined. In studies of larger horse populations, the mean value changes little during the training year. The situation is different in studies of individual animals. In this case considerable variations can be demonstrated. The relationship between the number of erythrocytes and their volume varies. The volume is generally low at very high erythrocyte counts, and high at low counts. According to GUTSCHOW et al. [1975], a high RBC and low MCV are one of the factors that contribute to speed and endurance in the Thoroughbred. The lower mean volume acts to increase the total surface area of the erythrocytes present, thereby accelerating gaseous exchange in the lungs and body tissues. After administering iron preparations to low-performance horses, GUTSCHOW et al. [1975] observed a fall of the individual erythrocyte volume with a simultaneous decrease in the hemoglobin content of individual red blood cells. The mean hemoglobin concentration of the erythrocytes remained unchanged, while the erythrocyte count and mass, as well as the serum hemoglobin, increased. They noted a performance increase after treatment and consider high erythrocytes volumes to be indicative of preanemic states in the horse.

We have been unable to find direct connections between racing performance and the MCV. However, horses with high erythrocyte counts and a low MCV tend to show better racing performance than horses with low erythrocyte counts and a high MCV.

Hemoglobin. As stated earlier, the main function of the erythrocytes is the transport of respiratory gases. Hemoglobin plays an important role in this process. The importance of its oxygen-binding function can be appreciated by comparing the oxygen-carrying capacity of the blood with that of saline. Six liters of blood can bind the same amount of oxygen as 350 l of saline. There has been relatively little published on the relationship between the hemoglobin content of the blood and exercise. Most authors describe a rise of the hemoglobin level during and after exercise. Opinions vary, however, with regard to the parallel relationship between a hemoglobin increase and erythrocyte increase. MÜLLER [1920], OPPERMANN [1967], SEST [1952], ISRAEL [1968] and other authors consider that the hemoglobin increase in the blood does not parallel the erythrocyte increase. VERTER et al. [1966], on the other hand, obtained results that clearly support such a relationship. After 15 minutes' galloping, they recorded a 30—60 % increase in erythrocytes and a 20—50 % increase in hemoglobin.

ARCHER [1973] indicates the following hemoglobin values for English Thoroughbreds:

Age	Number of samples	Hb (g/dl)
1 month	78	13.6 ± 1.90
1—9 months	75	12.7 ± 1.55
Yearling	100	13.7 ± 1.44
2 years	308	14.6 ± 1.44
3 years	353	15.1 ± 1.52
4 years	138	15.0 ± 1.65
Over 4 years	302	14.6 ± 1.61

Other authors report the following for various breeds:

Author(s)	Breed	Hb (g/dl)
McLeod et al. [1946]	Thoroughbred	13.2
	Trotter	12.6
	Arabian	13.0
Heusser [1952]	Freiburger, male	13.8
	Crossbreds, male	14.1
	Standardbred, male	14.6
	Arabian	15.1
	Freiburger, female	12.9
	Standardbred, female	13.7
Schlichting et al. [1956]	Thoroughbred yearling	14.0 (8.8—9.5)
	Thoroughbred, 2—5 years	15.0 (10.5—20.0)
	Breeding stock	14.8 (11.5—18.5)
Brenon [1958]	Thoroughbred, in training	13.9
Irvine [1958]	Thoroughbred	11.4 (12.7—15.4)
Sréter [1959]	Thoroughbred, in training	15.5 (± 0.3)
	Riding horses	12.9 (± 0.4)
Archer and Miller [1959]	Riding horses	14.7 (± 0.9)
Steel and Whitlock [1960]	Thoroughbred, in training	13.4 (9.2—21.3)
	Trotter, in training	12.4 (7.7—17.8)
Schalm [1965]	Thoroughbred	15.0
Martins [1966/67]	Thoroughbred, 3—5 years	15.9
Littlejohn [1968]	Thoroughbred, sedated	14.0 (± 0.3)

The values given in the tables for English Thoroughbreds essentially agree with our results. An age-related increase in the hemoglobin level cannot be demonstrated with certainty, however. Differences between younger and older horses of 1 g/dl on the average may be entirely training-related, inasmuch as older horses are not only in training longer, but generally undergo more strenuous training than younger animals. Despite lower erythrocyte counts, 2-year-old fillies have hemoglobin values 0.5 to 0.8 g/dl higher than colts of equal age. The resting hemoglobin is influenced by training. Unlike the erythrocyte count and hematocrit, the hemoglobin level is increased by sustained (extensive) as well as strenuous (intensive) training. As stated earlier, the hemoglobin level rises after exercise. The degree of this increase usually corresponds to the degree of erythrocyte mobilization. There may be exceptions to this rule. This is the case when erythrocytes with higher or lower hemoglobin contents are released into the circulating blood. Sport horses with a hemoglobin concentration below 12 g/dl must be considered anemic and are almost always poor performers. For this reason alone, a determination of the hemoglobin level should be included in hematologic studies of racing animals. Further information may be obtained by calculating the mean hemoglobin content of the individual erythrocytes (mean corpuscular hemoglobin, MCH, Hb_E) and their mean hemoglobin concentration (mean corpuscular hemoglobin concentration, MCHC).

Mean Corpuscular Hemoglobin. No large volume of data has been published on the MCH of the horse.

Archer [1973] indicates the following values for English Thoroughbreds of various age groups:

Age	Number of samples	MCH, 10^{-12} g[1]
1 month	78	13.8 ± 1.07
1—9 months	75	12.3 ± 1.23
Yearling	100	13.8 ± 0.68
2 years	308	14.7 ± 0.87
3 years	353	15.6 ± 0.83
4 years	138	16.7 ± 0.86
Over 4 years	302	16.6 ± 0.96

Other authors report the following:

Author(s)	Breed	MCH, 10^{-12} g[1]	
		Rest	Exercise
McLeod et al. [1946]	Thoroughbred, 2—3 years	13.1	
	Older Thoroughbreds	13.3	
Trum [1952]	Thoroughbred	13.5—13.7	
Alexandrova [1963]	Orlov Trotter	14.7	15.6
	Various breeds, male	13.0	13.4
	Various breeds, female	16.3	14.0
Heusser [1952]	Freiberger, male	16.6	16.3
	Crossbreds, male	16.4	16.7
	Standardbred, male	16.4	16.4
	Arabian, male	16.1	17.0
	Freiburger, female	18.1	17.1
	Standardbred, female	16.6	17.3
Steel and Whitlock [1960]	Thoroughbred, trained	13.8 (10.9—18.7)	
	Trotter, trained	14.3 (11.0—18.4)	
Martins [1966/67]	Thoroughbred	15.8	
Verter et al. [1966]	Warmblood	19.0	18.0
Mill and Wolf [1974]	Trotter	13.9	14.6

It is clear from the tables that there are no substantial breed differences with regard to the MCH, as there are in the case of the erythrocyte count, for example. The increase with age observed by Archer [1973] has been confirmed by us. Mares show slightly higher values than stallions. After exercise there is a slight increase in the MCH, which amounts to 1 to 2 pg after a moderately fast gallop. Accordingly, the erythrocytes mobilized by exertion have a higher hemoglobin content. The MCH can show considerable variations during a training period. The differences between resting and exercise values change little, however. In many horses, a decrease in the cell count is accompanied by an increase in MCH, but this is not sufficient to maintain the total hemoglobin content. Erythrocytes with a higher hemoglobin content almost always have a greater volume. An increase in the corpuscular hemoglobin only partially compensates for a decreased erythrocyte count. According to Gutschow [1975], both the volume and mean hemoglobin content of the erythrocytes can be decreased in many cases by iron replacement therapy.

Mean Corpuscular Hemoglobin Concentration (MCHC). The MCHC is important for the diagnosis of hypochromic anemia or preanemic states in athletic horses. The

[1] These values are multiplied by 0.06206 for expression as SI units (fmol)

lower limit for English Thoroughbreds in training is 300 g Hb/l erythrocytes. Lower values are indicative of hypochromic anemia.

ARCHER [1973] reports a normal range of 361 to 366 g Hb/l erythrocytes (223.4 to 227.1 mmol/l [Hb 4]) in English Thoroughbreds of various age classes.

Other authors report the following:

Author(s)	Breed	MCHC g Hb/l erythrocytes	(mmol/l [Hb 4])
IRVINE [1958]	Thoroughbred	309	(191.8)
STEEL and WHITLOCK [1966]	Thoroughbred, trained	258—374	(160.1—232.1)
	Trotter, trained	265—370	(164.4—229.6)
SCHALM [1965]	Thoroughbred	350	(217.2)
MARTINS [1966/67]	Thoroughbred	323	[200.4)
LITTLEJOHN [1968]	Thoroughbred, sedated	345 ± 3.0	(214.1 ± 18.6)
	Warmblood, sedated	356 ± 5.0	(220.9 ± 31.0)
MILL and WOLF [1974]	Trotter	283—319	(175.6—198.0)

ARCHER [1973], who examined blood samples from some 1,000 English Thoroughbreds of various age groups, found no age differences with respect to MCHC. This finding is confirmed by our own investigations. Nevertheless, marked differences are observed in individual horses during a training period. Values may fluctuate from below 300 g Hb/l (186.2 mmol/l) to above 420 g Hb/l (260.6 mmol/l). After exercise, including strenuous galloping, there is no significant elevation of the MCHC. During prolonged training in the general endurance range, the mean hemoglobin content decreases. A simultaneous increase in the extent and intensity of training leads to similar effects. Horses that run for short distances as well as high-performance animals have higher MCHC values. In contrast to hypochromia, hyperchromia does not appear to have an adverse effect on racing condition. The MCHC should always be calculated in sport horses due to the high incidence of preanemic states noted in exercise physiology studies.

Erythrocyte Sedimentation Rate (ESR). During sustained physical activity there is a decline in the fibrinogen content of the blood plasma, which is attributed to an activation of plasminogen [TAKAGI and SAKURAI, 1972]. The fibrinogen content decreases during sustained race training from an initial value of 4.82 g/l to 4.10 g/l. This leads to an associated decrease in the ESR. In his study of young trotters, NEUMANN-KLEINPAUL [1952] noted a slowing of the ESR when the peak of fitness was reached during training. Our own studies in English Thoroughbreds confirm this observation. The average ESR of trained 2-year-old Thoroughbreds in a state of relative rest is 20 mm after 10 min and 40 mm after 40 min. The sedimentation rate is significantly lower in horses 3 years of age or older than in younger horses. The average ESR is 1 mm after 10 min, 8 mm after 15 min, and 30 mm after 30 min. It is highly unlikely that this low ESR in older horses is principally the result of training. The values determined in trained Thoroughbreds are less than those reported for trained Standardbreds by SURUJBALLY [1970], who measured 13.35 mm after 15 min and 68 mm after 30 min.

The ESR is lower after exercise than in the resting state. This decrease is more pronounced in older horses than in younger ones for the same exercise. After galloping for 1,500 m at a speed of 600 to 750 m/min, the average ESR in 2-year-olds is 2 mm, 11 mm and 40 mm, compared to only 0 mm, 4 mm and 17 mm in older horses. In both cases this represents about a 50 % decrease in the initial rate. The close correlation between the resting and exercise rates allows us to determine only one value in exercise physiology studies. A close correlation also exists between ESR and erythrocyte count.

Training that is sustained but not intensive, produces no change in the ESR. This occurs only with intensive training, and then is quite rapid. While fitness and ESR are not related in every case, horses with a low ESR generally show better racing performance. It should be noted that because of marked individual variations, one-time determinations are of less value than repeated measurements.

Glucose and Exercise. The energy necessary for muscular work is obtained mainly by burning carbohydrates. Once the energy stores available in the cells are consumed, new glucose is released from glycogen reserves.

According to Loh [1966], the average resting blood glucose is 3.552 mmol/l[1] in cold-blooded horses and 3.441 mmol/l in warmblooded horses. After the consumption of high-starch rations, the blood glucose shows a transitory rise of about 0.555 to 1.665 mmol/l [Galle, 1969]. Evans et al. [1974] detected both a circadian and ultradian rhythm (rhythmic changes over a 24 hour period) in the plasma glucose concentration of horses. In horses allowed free access to feed and water, the blood glucose reached its high point at 12.00 noon each day, and its low point at 8.00 a.m. The plasma concentration remained nearly constant for the rest of the day. The difference between the lowest and highest glucose values was between 0.211 and 0.766 mmol/l. The ultradian rhythms were no more than a few minutes in duration.

Studies on the blood glucose before and after trotting over 2,100 m at speeds of 650 and 730 m/min revealed marked differences as a function of effort. Horses that had gone 'full out' had a lower plasma glucose ($\bar{x} = 3.752$) than horses that had not ($\bar{x} = 4.046$) [Kryzwanek, 1973]. Solun [1934] found the smallest blood sugar variations in English Thoroughbreds that had placed in racing. In three day event horses, Börnert [1969] found that the blood sugar variations decreased as the stage of fitness improved and the body gained the ability to respond to exercise rapidly and adequately in terms of blood sugar mobilization. Loh [1966] conducted sequential studies in various horse breeds after exercise and detected a fall of blood sugar after heavy exercise in warm- and cold-blooded breeds. Loh [1966] divides the recovery period into two phases. Immediately after exercise there is a primary glucose surge during the first 30 min, given adequate glycogen reserves and an adrenalin carryover from the exercise; this is followed by a slower glucose filling of the blood from 80 to 180 min after exercise, accompanied by the replenishment of muscular and hepatic glycogen reserves. Our own studies in English Thoroughbreds have shown considerable differences in the resting and post-exercise behavior of the blood glucose level. No relationship has yet been demonstrated between blood glucose and stage of fitness. Nevertheless, animals with the highest performance ability, i.e., that are best adapted in terms of metabolic regulation, have certain characteristics in common: They show a balanced blood sugar curve during short-term dynamics, have a continuously higher absolute blood sugar level during the course of a training period, and respond to strenuous training with a rapid and adequate glucose mobilization.

The effect of oral or intravenous glucose on the plasma level may be of interest in this context. Studies by Roberts [1975] show that the utilization of lactose is age-dependent. In horses less than 3 years of age, a glucose level of 7.492 mmol/l was reached in the plasma 90 min after the oral administration of 1 g/kg body wt. In older horses, no such increase was observed. After administering a mixture of glucose

[1] Conversion: mg/100 ml $\times$ 0.0555 = mmol/l, and mmol/l $\times$ 18.02 = mg/100 ml.

and galactose (0.5 g/kg b.w.), a considerable rise in the plasma glucose took place. After saccharose solutions and maltose (1 g/kg b.w.), the rise in plasma glucose was similar to that after an equal amount of monosaccharides. TAKAGI and SAKURAI [1972] infused 0.5 g/kg b.w. glucose. The half-life of the glucose ranged from 63 to 123 min. A peak of 19.449 mmol/l was reached 15 min after infusion. Thereafter there was a steady decline until the initial value was reached after 150 min.

Electrolytes and Exercise. To date, relatively little has been published on the effects of exercise on the electrolyte balance in the horse.

The table below shows the normal equine values (in mmol/l) reported by various authors:

Author	Na	Ca	K	Mg	Cl	HCO_3
Equine Health Lab.	137	1.74	5.1	—	—	—
PAULSSON [1965]	127	1.40	3.6	0.90	100	—
AMROUSI [1961]	151	1.69	3.1—5.8	—	—	—
FRANKE [1974]	130	1.40	3.2	0.54	94	—
TASKER [1966]	132—146	—	2.4—4.7	—	99—109	—
BURCH [1968]	139—152	—	4.1—5.7	—	99—107	25—27
SPECTOR [1956]	146—152	—	2.7—3.5	—	98—106	28
COSGRAVE [1969]	135—150	—	4.1—5.6	—	98—110	—
WILLIAMSON [1964] (winners)	139—143	—	3.7—4.0	—	100—103	26—28

	Na	Ca	K	Mg	Cl	HCO_3
Mean values of winners	141	—	3.8	—	101	27
Scatter of all samples	125—149	—	2.3—7.0	—	92—108	22—35

FRANKE [1974] gives the following limits for some plasma and serum electrolyte concentrations in the horse at rest:

Element	Lowest concentration, mmol/l		Highest concentration, mmol/l	
Potassium	3.20	[GAFNER, 1955]	5.67	[NEUMANN, 1939]
Sodium	127.0	[PAULSSON and ÅBERG, 1965]	156.0	[JASTREMSKI, 1956]
Calcium	2.49	[KOLB, 1980]	3.48	[Japan Racing Association, 1964]
Magnesium	1.28	[MEYER, 1963]	1.89	[KOLB, 1980]
Chloride	76.0	[GILYARD, 1944]	108.0	[BERNSTEIN, 1954]

WILLIAMSON [1964] was able to show a relationship between the level of potassium values and racing condition in English Thoroughbreds. While potassium values of 2.3—7.0 mmol/l were found in all horses examined, the range of 3.6 to 4.0 mmol/l proved to be characteristic of later winners. WILLIAMSON also noted T-wave changes in the EKG of horses whose potassium exceeded a value of 4.8 mmol/l. These horses always showed poor racing condition, evidenced in particular, by their tendency to pull up at various points in the race, depending on the severity of the syndrome. The hyperkalemia was accompanied by polycythemia, or an increase in the total red cell volume. This syndrome is also described by SYKES [1966]. Accompanying the rise in potassium is a fall of the chloride and sodium levels. WILLIAMSON relates this condition to an epinephrine exhaustion due mainly to a decrease in aldosterone production by the adrenal glands. Aldosterone is the controlling factor with regard to the water, sodium and potassium balance. In its absence, the sodium pump mechanism cannot function. The intracellular sodium level rises, and potassium passes from the intracellular to the extracellular space. The renal tubules lose their capacity to retain water. The result of this is dehydration. In the opinion of many authors, this syndrome appears when the rest period between workouts is too short. It is recommended, therefore, that horses be allowed to adapt fully during individual training sessions before imposing greater training demands that will create a new stress situation. The condition can be quickly corrected by administering desoxycortisone while treating for dehydration and hyponatremia. Training should be reduced or discontinued.

After exercise, the serum potassium level is generally increased 30—50% over the initial value. SRÉTER [1959] observed a marked potassium elevation in racehorses at the conclusion of a race. This is from potassium released during muscular contractions. The causes of this are numerous. FENN [1940] found a close relationship between the glucose and potassium levels. He produced a rise of the potassium level by administering epinephrine, and a fall by administering insulin. KRZYWANEK [1973] also attributes the glucose rise after racing to a high sympathetic tone and increased epinephrine secretion. FLECKENSTEIN [1955] considers the elevated potassium level a possible specific stimulus for aldosterone secretion, so that the potassium elevation is accompanied by an increase in sodium reabsorption by the renal tubules. FRANKE [1974] could show no direct connections between potassium elevation and the degree of exertion. After a recovery period of 15 min, the potassium concentrations had fallen below the initial value.

WILLIAMSON [1974] found bicarbonate levels of 26 to 28 mmol/l and chloride levels of 100 to 103 mmol/l in well-conditioned racing horses. Bicarbonate values above 29 mmol/l are characteristic of hypochloremic alkalosis. The maximum value in such cases is 35 mmol/l. The sodium and chloride values are decreased, the chloride values being farther below normal than the sodium values. Clinically there is an increase in the respiratory rate and volume. Normal respiration is very slow to return after exercise. With prolonged alkalosis the animal becomes hyperexcitable and may be extremely difficult to ride. O'CONNOR [1971] considers synchronous diaphragmatic flutter ('thumps') a state of exhaustion in racehorses and attributes it to alkalosis with potassium loss. This condition has been observed by other authors in hypocalcemia. The clinical signs are a rigid body posture with a spasm of the diaphragm, synchronous with atrial contraction.

In these horses WILLIAMSON [1974] found potassium levels of 4.1 to 4.6 mmol/l, bicarbonate values up to 30 mmol/l, and a fall of the sodium level to 97 mmol/l. This metabolic alkalosis is the product of many factors. It is important to note that the serum potassium is a poor index of the overall potassium status, because most of the body's potassium is localized within the cells. Thus, even with a low potassium balance, elevations of the serum level may be present. Hypochloremic alkalosis is considered to be the result of an elevated cortisol and corticosterone level brought about by repeated stress situations.

While hypokalemia is extremely rare in horses according to WILLIAMSON [1974], hyponatremia is the most frequent electrolyte imbalance in the racehorse. Its most common cause is a high sodium loss in the sweat combined with an insufficient intake of fluids and sodium chloride. Clinically there is a progressive, and thus sometimes subtle, loss of body weight; depression; muscle wasting, especially about the neck;

a loss of skin turgor; sunken eyes; and a loss of stamina. Water loss through the skin is increased until the sodium concentration is restored. Treatment is mainly directed toward correcting the water and sodium loss. Electrolytes may be given intravenously, and water by nasogastric tube. WILLIAMSON [1974] states that 4 l of electrolyte solution should be administered.

According to studies by FRANKE [1974] and by SRÉTER [1959], the serum sodium level increases in Thoroughbreds and trotters after racing. The increase is less than that of potassium, however. According to AURELL et al. [1967], the excretion of sodium is decreased during exercise by a greater sodium reabsorption. FRANKE [1974] sees a certain connection between the degree of the sodium increase and the severity of the exercise. He found an average sodium increase of 8.33 mmol/l in trotters after racing, though the individual variations were large.

There is general agreement that the plasma chloride level is unchanged after exercise. DE LANNE et al. [1959] regard the anions, especially chloride, as unchangeable parts of the total ion picture. They attribute this mainly to the role played by chloride ions in gaseous exchange in the blood. With a rise of the CO_2 partial pressure in the blood, and an associated increase of HCO_3 within the erythrocytes, there is a greater diffusion of HCO_3 into the plasma. The HCO_3 ions are replaced by chloride ions. This mechanism may well explain the unchanged chloride concentration in the plasma. FRANKE [1974] observed slight changes (about 5%) after exercise compared to initial values, noting individual variability in these changes.

The plasma calcium level, by contrast, increases markedly after exercise [SRÉTER, 1959]. Presumably the calcium appearing in the serum is released from the working muscles. As early as 1928 EWIG and WIENER found a connection between the lactic acid formed during exertion and the dissolution of 'calcium phosphate' stored in the muscle. FRANKE [1974] also found that the serum calcium rose with the lactic acid level in the serum of trotters.

Only FRANKE has reported on the serum magnesium of horses in relation to exercise. He found an elevation of about 15% after severe exercise. At the same time, however, he noted a shift of the calcium : magnesium ratio, which is 4.25 in trotters at rest. The samples examined immediately before the race show a reduction of this ratio by 0.35. After the race there is a still greater reduction, giving a ratio of 3.80.

In his studies of trotters, KRZYWANEK [1971, 1972, 1973] was able to observe a change in plasma osmolality after exercise. At rest, the osmolality is on the average, 280 mOsm/l. The mean rate of increase after exercise is 10% and varies with the degree of exertion. Marked osmolality changes occur only after maximal exertion. FRANKE [1974] could demonstrate a direct relation between osmolality and lactic acid level after exercise in trotters. He thus used the lactic acid level as a measure of the degree of exertion. Fifteen minutes after exercise the osmolality decreased by two-thirds the rate of increase during competition.

Enzymes and Exertion. Enzymes are proteins that catalyze the great majority of chemical reactions in the body. Their localization depends upon their function. According to SCHMIDT and SCHMIDT [1969], not only the absolute level of enzyme activities varies from organ to organ, but also the ratio of the individual enzyme activities to one another. Thus, every organ as well as every species, has its typical enzyme pattern. Most enzymes are located within the cells. During heavy muscular work, various enzymes are released from the muscles into the circulation. CORNELIUS et al. [1963] were the first to show that horses in training show higher enzyme activities than idle horses. These studies were confirmed by CARDINET et al. [1967], MULLEN [1969], and other researches. It must be added, however, that not all demonstrable enzymes display this behavior. Therefore, we will limit our discussions to only those enzymes that bear some relation to training or physical exertion in the horse.

Exercise and Aspartate Aminotransferase, (AspAT) or Glutamic Oxaloacetic Transaminase (GOT): Much data has been published on the behavior of AspAT/GOT. Although this enzyme cannot strictly be called muscle-specific, high concentrations in the serum indicate some degree of muscle damage. This mainly involves skeletal muscles in the horse.

The table below shows the normal equine values of AspAT/GOT determined by various authors:

Author	Breed	AspAT (GOT) (μkat/l)[1]
GERBER [1964]	Cold-blood	1.27 ± 0.30
GERBER [1964]	Thoroughbred, trained	1.50 ± 0.42
GERBER [1964]	Thoroughbred, trained	2.70 ± 1.25
RIETHMÜLLER [1970]	Thoroughbred, untrained	1.67
JEFFCOTT [1974]	Thoroughbred	1.78 ± 0.33
FALK-RONNE et al. [1977]	Trotter, untrained	3.45
	Trotter, trained	up to 6.32
GRÜN et al. [1977]	Thoroughbred, untrained	2.17—2.83
GRÜN et al. [1977]	Warmblood, untrained	1.35—2.37
GRÜN et al. [1977]	Thoroughbred, $1^1/_2$ yr.	1.33—2.72

In comparative studies of warmblooded and Thoroughbred horses of equal age, PAULSSON and ÅBERG [1965] found significantly higher AspAT (GOT) activities in Thoroughbreds. It is generally assumed that the commencement of training is associated with slight muscle damage, or that hypoxia produces changes in the mitochondria and cell membranes of muscle tissues that consequently lead to a release of enzymes into the extracellular space. With severe muscle damage there is a greater increase in AspAT (GOT) activity.

In azoturia, tying-up syndrome, tendon injuries and other conditions, the elevation of AspAT (GOT) activity is dramatic and immediate, often preceding observable clinical symptoms.

After exercise there is a more or less marked activity increase, depending on the duration and severity of the exercise and the animal's stage of fitness. According to ULLRICH [1966], the transaminases in the horse attain their highest serum activity 30 min after exercise, then fall by 20% over the next 30 min.

RIETHMÜLLER [1970] found in Thoroughbreds that the transaminases show an increase only 15 min after exercise, and that samples drawn after 6 h show no significant deviations from these values.

According to GRÜN et al. [1976], the AspAT (GOT) activity in three day event horses showed no increase after light exercise, but did rise after heavy exercise. RIETHMÜLLER [1976] found an average activity increase of 0.25 μkat/l in young Thoroughbreds after racetrack galloping. The activity increases were subject to sizable individual variations. Our own investigations [GRÜN et al., 1977] showed varying behavior of the serum AspAT (GOT) in accordance with the exercise test employed. Trotting over 1,600 m led to only slight increases that never exceeded 10%. By comparison, a test gallop over 1,600 m always produce significant increases greater than 10% of the initial value. The degree of increase is always dependent on

[1] Conversion: 1 U/l × 0.01667 = 1 μkat/l, and 1 μkat/l × 60.0 = 1 U/l.

two factors: the intensity of the exercise and the animal's state of training. Many authors have reported high serum enzyme activities in association with strenuous exercise, 'strenuous' referring here to speed of movement.

Sequential studies of enzymes during a training year enable an assessment of the training method employed. During the preparatory period, which is characterized by progressive distance training, there is initially a fall of AspAT/GOT activity, which, according to GRÜN, is also accompanied by a decrease in the variability of the measured values. With the commencement of more strenuous training that involves increased galloping work, the AspAT (GOT) activity shows a significant rise in all horses. During the racing period the values remain relatively high initially, occupying a high-normal range of values (0.33 μkat/l). During the course of the racing season, a marked differentiation takes place in accordance with the degree of adaptation to racing demands. AspAT (GOT) activities rise to abnormal levels in horses that must be removed from training because of injuries, overexertion or poor racing performance. In the rest of the horses, the values remain within normal limits. These animals have adapted satisfactorily to strenuous work. Thus, one criterion of a good response to training is a transitory rise of enzyme activity followed by stabilization at a lower level. JEFFCOTT [1974] and SEVESTRE [1965] call this level the 'fitness value'. After cessation of racing activity the AspAT (GOT) values return to initial levels.

Creatine Phosphokinase (CPK). Creatine phosphokinase is included among the muscle-specific enzymes. CPK values increase markedly within a short time after the occurrence of cell damage. In contrast to AspAT (GOT), relatively little has been published on the behavior of CPK in the horse before and after exercise. According to GERBER [1964] the serum CPK activity of untrained horses is 0.0—0.058 μkat/l. JEFFCOTT [1974] found resting values of 0.62 μkat/l. His findings agree with those of RIETHMÜLLER, who measured values of 0.53 ± 0.08 μkat/l in English Thoroughbreds. According to KOLB [1976], the CPK activity is a very good index of the severity of a particular exercise regime. Its serum activity may increase by 100—300 %, depending on the degree of exertion. It attains a peak 5 h after exercise. These data conflict with those of JEFFCOTT [1974], who found a slight CPK increase immediately after exercise and a substantial increase after 24 h. This increase was always much greater than that of the AspAT (GOT) activity. AZZIE [1974] found a rise to 1.417 to 1.58 μkat/l in fit horses 5 or 6 h after racing. In general, it may be said that the serum CPK activity of the horse increases after exercise in the same manner as the AspAT (GOT) activity. With both enzymes, there is a direct relationship between activity increase, exercise intensity and fitness. During a training period the resting CPK values are elevated by about 30 % of the initial value. Its dramatic increase in muscle and tendon diseases is of great diagnostic importance. This increase is demonstrable immediately, even before the appearance of clinical symptoms. Many authors have found serum CPK values of 5 μkat/l or more in such cases. Such horse show generally poor racing performance and should definitely be withdrawn from training.

Aldolase (ALD). According to GERBER [1975], aldolase is an enzyme that is specific for skeletal muscle in the horse and man. Although it occurs in all organs, its activity in the skeletal muscles is substantially higher.

SERGIJENKO [1976] states that ALD activity is a reliable criterion for fitness assessment in trotters. A fall of ALD activity by 20—30 % in horses at a high level of training signals an impending decline of racing condition. This can be predicted, based on ALD values, 1 to 2 weeks before the occurrence of observable signs of overtraining such as incoordination of gait or loss of speed. In trained 2-year-old trotters, the ALD activity remained at the relative-rest level or declined somewhat after strenuous workouts, while animals with less training showed an increase in activity. Anderson [1976] observed a slight initial rise of ALD activity with commencement of training; as adaptation progressed, there was a marked fall to just above 50 % of the initial value.

Grün and Rohrmann [1976] measured a serum ALD of 0.048—0.11 μkat/l in three-day-event horses before the start of training. The average resting ALD activity in English Thoroughbreds was 0.083 μkat/l. Our own studies in Thoroughbreds show a rise of resting ALD activity with increasing duration of exercise. The activity declines somewhat when the duration of exercise is reduced. The exercise values are only slightly higher than the resting values. Marked elevations of ALD have also been observed after exercise in some horses, however. A positive linear relationship can be demonstrated between total exercise and average resting value. This agrees with Sergijenko [1976] who found that ALD activity correlates more with the extent, or duration, of training than its intensity.

Lactate Dehydrogenase (LDH). Lactate dehydrogenase occurs as a ubiquitous cellular enzyme in all animal species. The highest activities are found in the skeletal muscles, myocardium and liver. According to Gerber [1975], its determination offers no basis for the diagnosis of specific organ lesions. On the other hand, LDH is a sensitive indicator of even minor acute cell damage owing to its high activity in many organs. The separation of LDH into its *isoenzymes* is of much more clinical value. The skeletal muscles, myocardium and liver in particular display typical LDH isoenzyme patterns.

Gerber reports an average resting serum activity of 62.35 μkat/l in the horse. Riethmüller indicates a mean resting value of 4.01 μkat/l for English Thoroughbreds (10 animals). Grün and Rohrmann [1976] report average resting values of 6.65 μkat/l (4.92—8.10) for young racehorses and 6.168 (4.47—9.00) for older ones.

The activity of LDH, like other enzymes, increases after exercise. After standard exercise tests in unfit horses, Grün and Rohrmann [1976] demonstrated an activity increase of 15—20 % for AspAT, 200 % for LDH, and 300 % for ALD relative to initial values. As with the other enzymes, the LDH activity increase is influenced both by fitness and riding speed. After a full three-day event, average LDH elevations of 20 % were observed. The horses that placed first showed the smallest activity increases despite their greater speeds, thus demonstrating the importance of the fitness factor. In our studies of English Thoroughbreds [Grün and Rohrmann, 1976], a direct linear correlation was established between exercise intensity and LDH elevation. Riethmüller [1970] and Milne [1974], on the other hand, could find no dependence of LDH activity on the intensity of racing or training. Riethmüller even observed a fall of the serum LDH after racing, which he relates to the function of this enzyme in glycolysis. According to our observations, marked elevations of LDH after exercise, like those of other enzymes (AspAT [GOT], CPK), are indicative of muscle cell lesions.

The resting serum LDH values increase during the course of a training year, the degree of increase varying with the type of training.

Malate Dehydrogenase (MDH). MDH, like LDH, is a ubiquitous cellular enzyme. Numerous authors describe activity changes of MDH during and after physical exertion, reporting elevations in the serum as well as in the muscle tissue itself. Schmidt and Schmidt [1969] found a rise from 0.834 to 1.167 μkat/l in human subjects following a 50-watt exertion over a 5-hour period.

Gerber [1964] reports a resting value in the horse of 176 IU/l. According to Riethmüller [1970], the average resting value in Thoroughbreds is 5.668 μkat/l. After galloping over 1,000 m, his animals showed an average serum activity of

6.968 μkat/l. A direct correlation can be observed between the rise of the resting MDH and exertion during the training year. With strenuous exercise its activity rises by an average of 30%, similar to that of AspAT (GOT). In the case of MDH, too, the activity increase is mainly a function of training intensity. During the period of active recovery, which is characterized entirely by quiet exercise, the resting values fall almost to the initial level. Overexertion does not produce as great an elevation of the serum MDH as in the case of AspAT (GOT) and CPK.

Other Enzymes. Data have been published on the behavior of a number of other enzymes after exercise. This particularly applies to glutamic pyruvic transaminase (GPT), which also is called alanine aminotransferase. Glutamic pyruvic transaminase is a nonspecific enzyme in the horse which shows no marked serum elevations even with extensive organ damage. In the horse, only massive and extensive skeletal muscle damage is accompanied by a significant elevation of the serum GPT [GERBER, 1975]. JAROV and KISJOW [1976] found that the activity levels of the phosphatases, transaminases, ceruloplasmin, lactate dehydrogenase and creatine kinase are significantly elevated in Thoroughbreds after strenuous muscular work compared to the resting state. They also found a significant correlation between the activity level of lactate dehydrogenase and phosphohexose isomerase and the speed of the animal. The activities of the phosphatases, ceruloplasmin and phosphohexose isomerase showed the greatest factorial dependence and correlation with performance ability prior to exercise.

Lactic Acid Level During Exercise. Lactic acid figures prominently in carbohydrate metabolism. It is an end-product of glycolysis and is formed by the hydration of pyruvic acid that does not enter the Krebs (citric acid) cycle. In most animal tissues, lactic acid forms as an intermediary product only in the presence of an oxygen deficit (anaerobic glycolysis). As stated earlier, anaerobic glycolysis represents a net energy loss for the muscle. Disregarding the overall economy of energy yield, however, this form of glycolysis has the advantage of providing immediate energy in the form of ATP. Part of the lactic acid formed in the muscle enters the circulation and can be demonstrated there. For these reasons the determination of lactic acid in the serum, as well as in the muscle, is often a routine part of exercise physiology studies.

The following resting values for serum lactic acid in the horse are reported in the literature:

Author	Lactic acid in mmol/l[1]
DUKES [1955]	1.103—1.765
BOHN [1957]	0.849—1.147
WITTKE and BOHN [1959]	0.982
KOLB [1976]	0.662 (0.331—1.654)
BOGDANOV et al. [1935]	1.232
SCHUSTER [1930]	1.324—1.654
SOLUN [1934]	1.932
KRZYWANEK [1967]	0.353
AITKEN et al. [1974]	0.607 (0.309—1.213)
SCHULZE [1970]	0.491
KRZYWANEK [1974]	0.476

In our own studies of Thoroughbreds, we found average resting values of 0.800 mmol/l (0.331—1.765). The resting values for lactic acid are independent of age,

[1] Conversion: mg/100 ml × 0.1103 = mmol/l, and mmol/l × 0.907 = mg/100 ml.

breed and level of fitness. As a result, they generally are subject to only slight individual variations, and are of interest only in relation to the exercise values.

Strenuous exercise in particular is followed by a rise of the lactic acid level in the blood. Exercise in the general endurance range, such as sustained walking, trotting or cantering, is associated with little or no rise in serum lactic acid. The degree of increase with strenuous exercise depends on the extent and intensity of the exercise and the animal's stage of fitness. The lactic acid level is widely used in sports medicine as an index of the internal stress produced by physical exertion. In particular, the internal stress associated with various training methods, such as sustained or interval training, can be assessed on the basis of the lactic acid level, as can the summation of fatigue after individual workouts.

KRZYWANEK [1974] examined trotters that had run races over 1,900 to 2,500 m at speeds from 1 : 22.3 to 1 : 31.0 per km and found differences in the average serum lactic acid level between horses that had gone at maximum speed and those that had not. In horses that had not gone 'full out', the lactic acid values rose immediately after the race from an average of 0.794 mmol/l to 17.858 mmol/l. In the other group, the average rise was from 0.576 to 22.942 mmol/l. According to KOLB [1976], the lactic acid can reach levels as high as 200 mg/100 ml on maximal exertion. Our own studies of English Thoroughbred have yielded similar results. Lactic acid values of 12.795 and 24.707 mmol/l were measured after racing, depending on the running speed and distance covered.

The studies of LINDHOLM and SALTIN [1974] on 'interval training' of trotters are of interest from the standpoint of training methods. These authors found that workouts over a distance of 400 m were too short to produce a rise of the heart rate and lactic acid level. Only workouts over $6 \times 1{,}000$ m at near-maximal speed were sufficient to produce lactic acid levels similar to those occurring after a race. As early as 1967, KEUL noted that the lactic acid concentration in the serum does *not* rise as strongly during interval training as when workouts are done without rest periods. SOLUN [1934] investigated the dependence of lactic acid levels on recovery time. He interprets high lactic acid values after exercise and poor recovery as a sign of poor condition. KRZYWANEK [1974] found a lactic acid increase from 0.476 mmol/l to 3.375 mmol/l after standard exercises in horses that were good performers. In poor performers, the values rose to 6.536 mmol/l; in horses not in full training, the level increased to 9.946 mmol/l after the same exercise.

In trotters WITTKE and BOHN [1959] found an inverse relationship between respiration and lactic acid levels, but a good correlation between pulse rate and lactic acid concentration.

The slight elevation of the lactic acid level after exercise as the animal's stage of fitness improves can be explained by an increase in the oxidative capacity of the muscle tissue, better oxidation of the pyruvic acid formed by glycolysis, a higher NADH oxidase activity, and an increase of hemoglobin and myoglobin.

References

ADAMOPOULOU, B.: Bestimmung des Blutvolumens an jungen Trabrennpferden mit J^{131}-HSA (RIHSA). Vet.-med. Diss., Berlin-Dahlem (1975).

AITKEN, M. M.; ANDERSON, M. G.; MACKENZIE, G.; SANFORD, J.: Correlations between physiological and biochemical parameters used to assess fitness in the horse. J. South African. vet. Assoc. *45:* 361 (1974).

ALEXANDROVA, W. W.: Individualizacija treninka cistokrovnych losadej. Konevodstvo i konnyj sport *22:* 30 (1963).

Alps, B. J.; Holmes, J. R.: Bewegung und Herzmuskelunregelmässigkeiten beim Pferd. cit. in: Prakt. Tierarzt *49:* 28 (1961).

Amrousi, S. El: Untersuchungen über die Elektrolyte Kalium, Natrium und Kalzium im Blutserum gesunder und kranker Pferde. Vet.-med. Diss., Gießen (1961).

Anderson, M. G.: The effect of exercise on the lactic dehydrogenase and creatine kinase isoenzyme composition of horseserum. Res. vet. Sci. *20:* 191 (1976).

Archer, R. K.: Normal red cell values in English thoroughbred horses. Equine Vet. J. *5:* 136 (1973).

Archer, R. K.: Haematology in relation to performance and potential. J. South African vet. Assoc. *45:* 273 (1974).

Archer, R. K.; Clabby, J.: The effect of exertion on the circulatory blood of horses. Vet. Rec. *77:* 689 (1965).

Archer, R. K.; Miller, W. C.: The interpretation of haematological ectaminations in thoroughbred horses. Vet. Rec. *71:* 268 (1959).

Aurell, M.; Carlsson, M.; Grimby, G.; Hood, B.: Plasma concentration and urinary exertion of certain electrolytes during supine work. J. Appl. Physiol. *22:* 633 (1967).

Azzie, M. A. J.: Open discussion on cardiology haematology and performance. J. South African. Vet. Assoc. *45:* 301 (1974).

Bassan, L.; Ott, W.: Radiotelemetrische Untersuchungen der Herzfrequenz beim Sportpferd in Ruhe und in allen Gangarten. Arch. exp. Vet.-Med. *22:* 57 (1968).

Bayer, A.: Möglichkeiten der Elektrokardiographie am laufenden Tier. Berliner Münchener tierärztl. Wschr. *79:* 49 (1966).

Bayer, A.: Die Brauchbarkeit der Arbeitspulsfrequenz als Leistungskriterium bei Trabrennpferden. Berliner Münchener tierärztl. Wschr. *83:* 414 (1970).

Beilharz, R. G.; Goddard, M.; Steel, J. D.; Stewart, G. A.: J. South African Vet. Assoc. *45:* 4 (1974).

Bernstein, R. E.: Potassium and sodium balance in mammalian red cells. Science *120:* 459 (1954).

Börnert, G.: Serumglukoseverhalten bei Militarypferden. — Ein Beitrag zum Komplex Sportpferd und Belastung. Vet.-med. Diss., Leipzig (1969).

Börnert, G.; Seidel, H.: Drahtlos übertragene EKG-Ableitungen vom freibeweglichen Pferd. Arch. exp. Vet.-Med. *20:* 1021 (1966).

Bogdanow, W.; Jankowski, W.; Krajew, I.; Tschuchina, E.: Biochemisches Kriterium des Arbeitswertes und der konstitutionellen Eigenschaften bei Pferden. Z. Züchtung *31:* 193 (1935).

Bohn, M.: Untersuchungen über den Milchsäuregehalt des Pferdeblutes in Ruhe und in der Bewegung. Vet.-med. Diss., Berlin-Dahlem (1957).

Brenon, H. C.: Further erythrocyte and hemoglobin studies in thoroughbred-racing horses. J. Amer. vet. med. Assoc. *133:* 102 (1958).

Broojmans, A. V. M.: Electrocardiography in normal horses and cattle. Lab. of Veterin. Physiol., State Univ. Utrecht 1957.

Burch, J. E.: Fluids and electrolytes. Proc. 14th Conv. Amer. Assoc. Equine Pract. (1968), 59.

Cardinet, G. H.; Littrell, J. E.; Freeland, R. A.: Comparative investigations of serum-creatine-phosphokinase and glutamic-oxalacetic transaminase activities in equine paralytic myoglobinuria. Res. vet. Sci. *8:* 219 (1967).

Cardinet, G. H.; Murray, E.; Fowler, W. M.; Walter, S.; Tyler, W. S.: The effects of training, exercise and tying up on serum transaminase activities in the horse. Amer. J. vet. Res. *24:* 980 (1963).

Collins, J. D.; Farelly, B. T.; Tyler, W.: Changes in the number and quality of erythrocytes in horses transported in high altitudes. Irish vet. J. *23:* 42 (1969).

Cornelius, C. E.; Bishop, H.; Rhode, E. A.: Serum and tissue transaminase activities of thoroughbred horses in training. J. Amer. vet. med. Assoc. *142:* 639 (1959).

Cornelius, C. E.; Burnharn, L. G.; Hill, H. E.: Serum transaminase activities of thoroughbred horses in training. J. Amer. vet. med. Assoc. *142:* 639 (1963).

Cosgrove, J. S.: The practional application of haematology. Equine vet. J. *149:* 112 (1969).

Dalton, R. G.; Fisher, E. W.: Cardiac output in horses. Nature *184:* 2020 (1959).

Dalton, R. G.; Fisher, E. W.: Plasma- and blood volume in horses. Brit. vet. J. *119:* 384 (1963).

DETWEILER, D. K.; PATTERSON, D. F.: Diseases of the blood and cardiovascular system. Equine Med. and Surgery (Amer. Vet. Public. Inc., Wheaton Ill. 1963).

DE LANNE, R.; BARNES, J. R.; BROUHA, L.; MASSART, F.: Changes in acid-base balance and blood gases during muscular activity and recovery. J. Appl. Physiol. *14:* 328 (1959).

DUKES, H. H.: The physiology of domestic animals (Comstock Publishing Assoc., Ithaca, N.Y. 1955).

EHRLEIN, J. J.: Untersuchungen über die Beziehungen zwischen Herzschlagfrequenz und Leistung bei Pferden. Zbl. Vet.-Med. R. A. *17:* 577 (1970).

ENGELHARDT, W. v.: Hämoglobinkonzentration, Sauerstoffgehalt und -sättigung des Blutes bei Zucht- und Sportpferden im unterschiedlichen Trainingszustand. Berliner Münchener tierärztl. Wschr. *83:* 229 (1970).

ENGELHARDT, W. v.: Lactat, Pyruvat, Glukose und Wasserstoffionen im venösen Blut bei Reitpferden im unterschiedlichen Trainingszustand. Zbl. Vet.-Med. R. A. *20:* 173 (1973).

ENGELHARDT, W. v.: Cardiovascular effects of exercise and training in horses. Advances vet. Sci. comp. Med. *21:* 173 (1977).

ENGELHARDT, W. v.; EHRLEIN, H. J.; HÖRNICKE, H.: Registrierung der Herzschlagfrequenz von Sportpferden während standardisierter Belastung. Biotelemetrie-Symp., Erlangen (1968), 91.

EVANS, J. W.: Effects of fastening, gestation, lactation and exercise on glukose turnover in horses. J. Animal Sci. *33:* 305 (1971).

EVANS, J. W.; THOMPSON, P. G.; WINGET, C. M.: Glukose and insulin biorhythmus in the horse. J. South African vet. Assoc. *45:* 317 (1974).

EWIG, W.; WIENER, R.: Über die Wirkung maximaler körperlicher Anstrengungen. Z. ges. exper. Med. *61:* 450 (1928).

FALK-RONNE, J.; SØNNICHSEN, H. V.: Health control of trotting horses. Europ. Soc. Vet. Surgery, XII. Congr., Košice (1977), 12.

FENN, W. O.: The role of potassium in physiological processes. Physiol. Rec. *20:* 377 (1940).

FLECKENSTEIN, A.: Der Kalium-Natriumaustausch als Energieprinzip in Muskel und Nerv (Springer Verlag, Berlin (West)-Göttingen-Heidelberg 1955).

FRANKE, D.: Veränderungen von Plasmaelektrolyten, Osmolarität und Laktatkonzentration bei Trabrennpferden durch Wettkampfbelastung. Vet.-med. Diss., Berlin-Dahlem (1974).

GAFNER, P.: Über den Natrium- und Kaliumgehalt des Blutplasmas einiger Haustiere sowie den Einfluß peroraler Natrium- und Kaliumverabreichung auf den Gehalt dieser Elemente im Blut der Ziege. Vet.-med. Diss., Bern (1955).

GALLE, O.: Untersuchungen über den Natrium-, Kalium-, Kalzium- und Blutzuckerspiegel bei gesunden Pferden. Normalwerte, Tagesschwankungen und Veränderungen nach Applikation eines Glukokortikoids. Vet.-med. Diss., Berlin-Dahlem (1969).

GERBER, H.: Aktivitätsbestimmung von Serumenzymen in der Veterinärmedizin. III. Bestimmnng der GOT-, GPT- und CPK-Aktivität in einigen Organen des Pferdes als Grundlage für die klinische Verwendung von Serumaktivitätsbestimmungen. Schweiz. Arch. Tierheilk. *106:* 478 (1964).

GERBER, H.: Serum enzymes in equine medicine. Equine Veterin. J. *1:* 129 (1968).

GERBER, H.: Enzymdiagnostik. Allgemeine Chirurgie für Tierärzte und Studierende, p. 577 (Verlag Paul Parey, Berlin (West) und Hamburg 1975).

GILLESPIE, J. R.: The role of the respiratory system during exertion. J. South African vet. Assoc. *45:* 305 (1974).

GILYARD, H. T.: Chronic anhidrosis with lowered blood chlorides in race horses. Cornell Vet. *34:* 332 (1944).

GOODMAN, H. M.; VAN DER NOOT, G. W.; TROUT, J. R.; SQUIBB, R. L.: Determination of energy source utilized by the light horse. J. Animal. Sci. *37:* 56 (1973).

GRÜN, E.; ROHRMANN, H.: Das Verhalten einiger Enzyme im Blutserum von Sportpferden während des Ausdauertrainings und bei körperlicher Belastung. Leistungsprüfungen von Sportpferden. II. Intern. Symp., Leipzig 1976.

GRÜN, E.; SCHNEIDER, J.; PANNDORF, H.; PREUSSE, G.: Das Verhalten von Serumenzymen bei trainierten Galopprennpferden im Verlaufe von zwei Rennjahren. Mh. Vet.-Med. *32:* 866 (1977).

GUNN, H. M.: Adaptions of skeletal muscle that favour athletic ability. New Zealand Vet. J. *23:* 249 (1975).

Gutschow, K.; Raake, W.; Rakoczy, M.; Fernandez, M. P.; Vazquez, J. P.: Zur Diagnostik und Therapie präanämischer Eisenmangelzustände beim Vollblutpferd. Berliner Münchener tierärztl. Wschr. *88:* 261 (1975).

Haring, H. O.: Die Bedeutung des Blutbildes und der Blutreserve für die Lungen- und Herzfunktionsprüfung beim Pferd. Vet.-med. Diss., Hannover (1936).

Harris, E. A.: Physiological limits to performance. New Zealand Vet. J. *23:* 255 (1975).

Heusser, H.: Über die Blutausrüstung des Pferdes und ihre praktische Bedeutung. Schweiz. Arch. Tierheilk. *93:* 463 (1952).

Hintz, H. F.; Roberts, S. J.; Salun, S. W.; Schryver, H.: Energy requirement of light horses for various activities. J. Animal. Sci. *32:* 100 (1971).

Hörnicke, H.: Registrierung der Herzschlagfrequenz von Sportpferden während standardisierter Belastungen. Biotelemetrie-Symposium, Erlangen 1968.

Hörnicke, H.; Engelhard, W. v.; Ehrlein, H. J.: Sportphysiologische Untersuchungen an Pferden. Umschau Wiss. Technik *70:* 279 (1970).

Holmes, J. R.: An investigation of cardiac rhythm using an on-line radiotelemetrie computer link. J. South African vet. Assoc. *45:* 251 (1974).

Irvine, C. H. G.: The blood picture in the race horse. I. The normal erythrocyte and hemoglobin status, a dynamic concept. J. Amer. vet. med. Assoc. *133:* 97 (1958).

Israel, S.: Sport, Herzgröße und Kreislaufdynamik. Sportmed., Schriftenr. *3* (1968).

Jakowlew, N. N.: Sportbiochemie. Sportmediz. Schriftenr., J. Ambr. Barth Verlag, Leipzig 1974.

Japan Racing Association: Physiological values on race horses. Equine Health Lab. (1964).

Jarov und Kisjow: Untersuchungen der Beziehungen physiologischer Parameter zur Leistungsfähigkeit des Pferdes. II. Int. Wiss. Symp. Leistungsprüfungen von Sportpferden, Leipzig 1976.

Jastremski, M.: Fluid replacement in the treatment of dehydratation from diarrhea in the horse. J. Amer. vet. med. Assoc. *128:* 153 (1956).

Jeffcott, L. B.: Opening discussion to: Laboratory aids to clinical diagnosis in equine practice. Equine vet. J. *3:* 29 (1971).

Jeffcott, L. B.: Haematology in relation to performance potential: Some aspects. J. South African vet. Assoc. *45:* 279 (1974).

Keul, J.: Zur Bedeutung der Laktatbildung bei Intervallarbeit. Z. Kreislaufforsch. *56:* 8 (1967).

Keul, J.: Herzfrequenzen und Substratspiegel im Blut bei Springpferden während des Trainings in Mexico-City. Pflügers Arch. ges. Physiol. *301:* 358 (1968).

Keul, J.; Doll, E.: Intervallbelastungen, Stoffwechselendprodukte, PO_2 und Säuren-Basen-Gleichgewicht im Blut. Medizin und Sport *9* (1973).

Kolb, E.: Biochemische Anpassungsvorgänge beim Pferd bei körperlicher Belastung. Leistungsprüfungen von Sportpferden. II. Intern. Symp., Leipzig 1976, 30.

Kolb, E.: Lehrbuch der Physiologie der Haustiere. 4. Aufl. (VEB Gustav Fischer Verlag, Jena 1980).

Kolb, E.: Leistungsphysiologie und biochemische Aspekte von Höchstleistungen beim Rennpferd. Tierzucht *31:* 313 (1977).

Kreusel, S.: Untersuchungen zum Intervalltraining von Galopprennpferden. Vet.-med. Dipl.-Arb., Leipzig (1977).

Krzywanek, H.: Acid-base values of standardbred horses recovering from strenuous exercise. Amer. J. Vet. Res. *37:* 291 (1967).

Krzywanek, H.: The heart rates of thoroughbred-horses during a race. Equine vet. J. *2* (1969).

Krzywanek, H.: Die Konzentration freier Fettsäuren im Blutplasma trainierter Trabrennpferde. Z. Tierphysiol. Tierernähr., Futtermittelkde. *25:* 236 (1969).

Krzywanek, H.: Untersuchungen zur Beurteilung der aktuellen Leistungsfähigkeit von Trabrennpferden. Zbl. Vet.-Med. R. A. *20:* 265 (1973).

Krzywanek, H.: Lactate acid concentrations and pH-values in trotters after racing. J. South African vet. Assoc. *45:* 355 (1974).

Krzywanek, H.: Wirkungen des Trainings auf leistungsabhängige Blutparameter bei Trabrennpferden. Berliner Münchener tierärztl. Wschr. *90:* 89 (1977).

Krzywanek, H.; Schulze, A.; Wittke, G.: Das Verhalten einiger Blutparameter bei Trabrennpferden nach definierter Belastung. Berliner Münchener tierärztl. Wschr. *17:* 325 (1972).

KUBO, K.; SENTA, T.; SUGIMOTO, O.: Relationship between training and heart in the thoroughbred race horse. Exp. Rep. Equine Health Lab. *10:* 84 (1973).

KUBO, K.; SENTA, T.; SUGIMOTO, O.: Cardiac output in the thoroughbred horse. Exp. Rep. Equine Health Lab. *11:* 87 (1974).

LAGUENS, R. P.; GOMEZ-DUMM, C. L. A.: Fine structure of myocardial mitochondria in rats after exercise. Circulation Res. *21:* 271 (1967).

LASKOW, A.: Physiologische Merkmale des Trainingszustandes der Sportpferde. Trainingsuntersuchungen bei Vollblutpferden. Vortrag, Köln 1965.

LASKOW, A.: Problema adapacii losadeij k dvigatelnoj giposkii. Tr. Vses. nauc.-issl. Inst. Konev, Moskva *26:* 149 (1973).

LINDHOLM, A.: Glycogen depletion pattern and the biochemical response to varying exercise intensities in standardbred trotters. J. South African vet. Assoc. *45:* 341 (1974).

LINDHOLM, A.; SALTIN, B.: The physiological and biochemical response to exercise and varying speed and duration. Acta vet. Scand. *15:* 310 (1974).

LITTLEJOHN, A.: PVC, Hb and plasmaelectrolyte studies in horses. I. Mean values in clinically normal horses. Brit. Vet. J. *124:* 529 (1968).

LOH, H. P. W.: Blutzuckerbestimmungen beim Pferd in der Ruhe und nach starker Anstrengung. Vet.-med. Diss., Gießen (1966).

LUTZ, G.: Die Aussagekraft der Ruheherzfrequenz beim trainierten Vollblutpferd. Vet.-med. Diss., Leipzig (1972).

LUTZ, G.; SCHNEIDER, J.; PANNDORF, H.; PREUSSE, C.; GRÜN, E.: Das Verhalten der Ruheherzfrequenz beim trainierten Galopprennpferd. Mh. Vet.-Med. *31:* 134 (1976).

LYDIARD, A.: Training for running races. New Zealand vet. J. *23:* 260 (1975).

MARTINS, L. F.: Quadro hematico en equinos puro sangue ingles vencedones. Rev. Fac. Med. vet. Sao Paulo *7:* 545 (1966/67).

MCLEOD, J. E.; PONDER, G. J.: An observation on the red cell content of the blood of the thoroughbred horse. Science *183:* 73 (1946).

MCLEOD, J. E.; PONDER, G. J.; AITKEN, J. R.; BROWN, R. B.: The blood picture of the thoroughbred horse. Cornell Vet. *37:* 305 (1947).

MEYER, H.: Magnesiumstoffwechsel, Magnesiumbedarf und Magnesiumversorgung bei den Haustieren. Vet.-med. Habil.-Schrift, Hannover (1963).

MILL, J.; WOLF, G.: Zur Problematik der Bluttransfusion und Leistung beim Sportpferd. Mh. Vet.-Med. *29:* 945 (1974).

MILNE, D. W.: Blood gases, acid-base balance and electrolyte and enzyme changes in exercising horses. J. South African vet. Assoc. *45:* 345 (1974).

MÜLLER, L.: Vergleichende Untersuchungen über den Gehalt des Pferdeblutes an Blutkörperchen und Hämoglobin bei besonderer Berücksichtigung der Futteraufnahme. Vet.-med. Diss., Hannover (1920).

MULLEN, P. A.: Symposium on haematology — serum constituents. Equine vet. J. *1:* 190 (1969).

NEUMANN, H.: Untersuchungen über den Kaliumgehalt des Blutserums und Harns von Pferden. Vet.-med. Diss., Hannover (1939).

NEUMANN-KLEINPAUL, K.: Blutkörperchensenkung bei jungen Traberpferden. Berliner Münchener tierärztl. Wschr. *52:* 185 (1952).

NOWOSINOW, G. P.: Radioelektrokardiographische Untersuchungen der Frequenz der Herztätigkeit bei Trabern. Uc. zap. Kazan vet. in-ta *110:* 176 (1971).

O'CONNOR, J. T.: Avoiding and treating the untoward effects of the corticosteroids. Proc. 15th Conv. Amer. Assoc. Equine Pract. (1969), 75.

O'CONNOR, J. T.: The treatment of fatigue in trial ride horses. Proc. 17th Conv. Amer. Assoc. Equine Pract. (1971), 39.

OPPERMANN, TH.: Über Blutreserven der Haustiere, insbesondere der Pferde (Verlag M. und H. Schaper, Hannover 1967).

OSTERHOFF, D. R.; AZZIE, M. A. J.; OP T'HOF, J.: Biochemical genetics and performance ability in horses. J. South African vet. Assoc. *45:* 311 (1974).

OTT, W.: Die Bestimmung der Herzfrequenz bei Pferden während der Bewegung mittels telemetrischer Untersuchungsmethoden. Mh. Vet.-Med. *21:* 378 (1966).

PATRUSHEW, V. J.: Physiological difference in draft-horses as correlated with their performance. Comptes Rendus de l'Academie des Sciences de l'URSS *24:* 182 (1939).

Paulsson, S.; Åberg, B.: Kliniskt-kemiska och hematologiska normalvarden. Sartyck ur Svensk Veterinärtidning *15:* 1 (1965).

Persson, S.: Value of haemoglobin determination in the horse. Nord. Vet.-Med. *21:* 513 (1969).

Rhezakhani, A.: Equine electrocardiography. Discussion in: J. South African vet. Assoc. *46:* 207 (1975).

Riethmüller, H.: Aktivitätsveränderungen muskelspezifischer Enzyme bei Vollblütern während des Trainings. Vet. med. Diss., Gießen (1970).

Riethmüller, H.; Wels, A.: Trainingswirkungen von Vollblütern. 1. Mitt. Muskelspezifische Enzyme. Zbl. Vet.-Med., R. A. *19:* 537 (1972).

Rjabowa, T. N.: Typen der höheren Nerventätigkeit und ihre Nutzung in der Arbeit zur Vervollkommnung der englischen Vollblutrasse. Leistungsprüfungen von Sportpferden. II. Intern. Symp., Leipzig, 1976, 42.

Sander, H.; Kolb, E.; Müller, I.; Seidel, H.: Untersuchungen über den K- und Na-Gehalt in verschiedenen Abschnitten der Herz- und Skelettmuskel beim Pferd. Arch. exp. Vet.-Med. *23:* 861 (1969).

Sanders, T. M.; Bloor, C. M.: Effect of endurance exercise on serum enzyme activities in the dog, pig and man. Proc. Soc. exp. Biol. and Med. *148:* 823 (1975).

Schalm, O. W.: Veterinary Hematology. 2nd ed. (Lea & Febinger, Philadelphia 1965).

Scheunert, A.; Krzywanek, F. W.: Über reflektorisch geregelte Schwankungen der Blutkörperchenmenge, Pflügers Arch. ges. Physiol. *212:* 477 (1926).

Schlichting, M.; Sanders, R.; Gardner, M.: The blood picture of 200 thoroughbreds. Vet.-Med. (Kansas City) *51:* 151 (1956).

Schmidt, E.; Schmidt, F. W.: Enzym-Fibel. Praktische Enzymdiagnostik. Biochem. Abt. C. F. Boehringer und Söhne, Mannheim 1969.

Schneider, J.: Zur Problematik des wissenschaftlichen Trainings bei Sportpferden. Mh. Vet.-Med. *26:* 948 (1971).

Schneider, J.: Training als stimulierender Faktor der Leistungsfähigkeit von Pferden. Leistungsprüfungen von Sportpferden, II. Intern. Symp., Leipzig 1976, 66.

Schulze, A.: Der Säure-Basen-Status im Blut von Trabrennpferden nach definierter Belastung. Vet.-med. Diss., Berlin-Dahlem (1970).

Schuster, M.: Biochemisches Kriterium des Arbeitswertes und der konstitutionellen Eigenschaften bei Pferden. II. Teil: Quantitatives Verhältnis zwischen Milchsäure und anorganischer Phosphorsäure im Zusammenhang mit dem Arbeitswert und der Konstitution. Z. Tierzüchtung und Züchtungsbiol. *28:* 423 (1930).

Sergijenko, G. P.: Beziehungen zu biochemischen Kennwerten des Blutes bei in Training stehenden Trabern. Leistungsprüfungen von Sportpferden, II. Intern. Symp., Leipzig 1976, 61.

Sest, J.: Untersuchungen über die Blutreserven und das gleichzeitige Verhalten des weißen Blutbildes bei Kaltblutpferden. Vet.-med. Diss., Hannover (1952).

Sevestre, J.: Application de la télémetrie à l'étude de l'electrocardiogramme d'effort du cheval de sport. Bull. Soc. Sci. Med. comp. (Lyon) *67:* 551 (1965).

Solun, A. S.: Biochemische Kriterien des Arbeitswertes und der konstitutionellen Eigenschaften bei Pferden. Z. Züchtung *31:* 181 (1934).

Spector, W. S.: Handbook of Biological Data (Saunders, Philadelphia 1956).

Spörri, H.: Über den atmungsgesteuerten reflektorischen Herzblock des Pferdes. Tierärztl. Umschau *6:* 419 (1951).

Spörri, H.: Über die Genese und klinische Bedeutung des partiellen Herzblockes beim Pferd. Schweiz. Arch. Tierheilk. *94:* 337 (1952).

Sréter, F. A.: The effect of systematic training on plasma electrolytes, haematocrit value and blood-sugar in thoroughbred race horse. Canad. J. Biochem. *37:* 273 (1959).

Steel, J. D.: Studies on the electrocardiogram of the race-horse. Austral. Med. Public., Sydney 1963.

Steel, J. D.: Hematology and its relationship to track performance. In: Equine Medicine and Surgery (Amer. Vet. Public. Inc., Santa Barbara 1963).

Steel, J. D.; Stewart, G. A.: Electrocardiography of the horse and potential performance ability. J. South Africa. vet. Assoc. *45:* 1974 (1945).

Steel, J. D.; Whitlock, L. E.: Observations in the hematology of thoroughbred and standardbred horses in training and racing. Austral. vet. J. *36:* 136 (1960).

STEGEMANN, J.: Der Mechanismus der Anpassung einiger Kreislauf- und Atemgrößen an den nutritiven Bedarf und seine Beziehungen zur arbeitsphysiologischen Praxis. Verhandl. Dtsch. Ges. exper. Med. *18:* 51 (1967).

STEWART, G. A.: Drugs, performance, and responses to exercise in the race horse. Austral. vet. J. *48:* 537 (1972).

STEWART, G. A.; STEEL, J. D.: Haematology of the fit race horse. J. South African vet. Assoc. *45:* 287 (1974).

SURUJBALLY, ST.: Hämatologische Veränderungen bei Militarypferden während des Trainings. Ein Beitrag zu dem Komplex Sportpferd und Belastung. Vet.-med. Diss., Leipzig (1970).

SYKES, P. E.: Biochemistry as an aid in equine track practice. Proc. 12th Conv. Amer. Assoc. Equine Pract. (1966), 263.

TAKAGI, S.; SAKURAI, N.: Changes of glucose, pyruvate and lactate in blood of horses at rest and during exercise. Exper. Rep. equine Health Lab. (Tokyo) *8:* 100 (1972).

TASKER, J. B.: Laboratory aids to diagnosis in equine practice. J. Amer. vet. med. Assoc. *148:* 384 (1966).

TASKER, J. B.: Panel-Fluids and Electrolytes. Proc. 14th Conv. Amer. Assoc. Equine Pract. (1968), 38.

TRUM, B. F.: Normal variances in horse blood due to breed, age, lactation, pregnancy, and altitude. Amer. J. Vet. Res. *13:* 514 (1952).

ULLRICH, W.: Über das Verhalten der Serumtransaminasen bei Trabrennpferden nach Bewegungsbelastung. Wien. tierärztl. Mschr. *53:* 95 (1966).

VERTER, W.; MIX, N.; MÜLLER, J.: Die Veränderungen der Zellwerte und einiger biochemischer Daten des Blutbildes bei Sportpferden in Schritt, Trab und Galopp. Arch. exp. Vet.-Med. *20:* 417 (1966).

WILLIAMSON, H. M.: Normal and abnormal electrolyte levels in the racing horses and their effect on performance. J. South African vet. Assoc. *45:* 335 (1974).

WITTKE, G.; BAYER, A.: Die Herzschlagfrequenz von Pferden bei Vielseitigkeitsprüfungen. Berliner Münchener tierärztl. Wschr. *81:* 589 (1968).

WITTKE, G.; BOHN, M.: Zur Frage der Milchsäurekonzentration im Blut des Pferdes. Z. Biol. *111:* 271 (1959).

WITTKE, G.; KRZYWANEK, H. J.: Sportphysiologische Untersuchungen an Rennpferden. Vollblut *41:* 51 (1979).

WOLF, G.: Untersuchungen zur Erythropoese des Sportpferdes. Vet.-med. Diss., Berlin (1977).

ZELLER, S.; SIEWERT, R.: Blutvolumenuntersuchungen beim Pferd mit J^{131}-HSA (RIHSA). Zbl. Vet.-Med. *11:* 523 (1964).

1.5. Doping

The increasing commercialization of sport with high winner's purses, high social, or national prestige and material benefits, sometimes fosters pressure to 'win at any cost'. This encourages some participants and officials to employ illicit means to obtain an advantage. The desire for an 'effortless' victory or the 'sure' defeat of an opponent is surely as old as the history of sport itself; only the means and methods have changed. The most common and familiar method involves the use of drugs and other medicaments or foodstuffs that contain or are presumed to contain substances that enhance performance. This age-old practice of administering drugs, medicaments or foodstuffs to secure 'fitness on the day of the event' is called *doping*.

Historians tell us that even in antiquity, warriors ingested drugs and special foods that were believed to impart strength and superiority over the enemy [Croisier, 1948]. The writings of Phylostratos and Galen clearly show that as early as the 3rd century B.C., participants in the ancient Olympic Games employed any and all means to enhance their athletic ability. In ancient Rome, an aqueous honey solution called 'hydromel' was given to racing horses to improve their speed and stamina [Morgan, 1958]. Presumably its active component was ethyl alcohol, which formed when the mixture was left standing [Aries, 1965]. The drugging of chariot racehorses was punishable by crucifixion in Imperial Rome. In England, where in the 17th century horseracing often took the form of a kind of traveling fair, horses were greatly overworked and were given stimulants, usually in the form of alcoholic drinks, to enliven them. As early as 1666 there was a law against the use of stimulating substances, though these substances were not specified [Croisier, 1948]. This law could be considered the first anti-doping law in sports history. In Prussia, a royal decree of April 11, 1881, made it mandatory to report the use of alcoholic drinks in racing animals. Horse doping in the United States was already widespread by the early 19th century, when it was called 'spicing'. In those days 'spicing' in England was punishable by banishment to the colonies [Büscher, 1972].

In the late 19th century many technical innovations and training methods in the U.S. were adopted in Europe, including, unfortunately, doping with alkaloids. As a result of this, a serious anti-doping campaign was instituted in the early 1900's.

Renowned racing associations included articles on doping in their racing rules or amended existing articles dealing with the administration of drugs to racehorses. In October, 1903, for example, the English Jockey Club issued a statement on doping, and in December of that year the anti-doping article of the Austro-Hungarian Rules of Racing was expanded in its scope. In 1904 the racing authorities in France added Articles 9 and 10 to their 'Code des Courses et des Steeple Chases' in an effort to control the doping of racing and jumping horses, while the French Defense Minister similarly prohibited the doping of military horses. Since that time doping regulations have been adopted in practically all countries where equine sports are practiced.

The first doping scandal surfaced in Russia in 1903, where tests for doping were already routine. The situation could not be resolved, however, because there were, as yet, no adequate means of proving that doping had occurred [Suckow, 1905]. It is hardly surprising, therefore, that the first rigorous studies on horse doping were performed in Moscow in 1904. These tests were carried out on 6 racehorses using morphine, nitroglycerin and heroin, with the object of investigating the animals' reactions to these substances and their excretion in the sweat and saliva. It was found that doping could indeed be detected on the basis of chemical and biological saliva tests. But it was not until 1910 that the development of multiple testing procedures allowed an effective control of doping. This development was particularly dramatic in the United States, where systematic tests for doping were first instituted in the mid-1930's. According to press reports from that time, the doping of racehorses was so prevalent that races were no longer a contest between horses, but between chemical formulas. The stables of that day resembled well-stocked pharmacies, and 'drugstore trainers' enjoyed the free use of heroin, morphine, cocaine and other drugs. A favorite formula for 'speed balls' was as follows: 1.5 grains[1] of heroin, 2.5 grains of strychnine, 2 minims[2] of nitroglycerin, 5 minims of digitalis tincture and 2 ounces[3] of kola nut. Only when the U.S. Bureau of Narcotics intervened and imposed severe penalties, including systematic procedures for sample collection and testing patterned after the French methods, did the prevalence of doping decline. According to information from the Association of Official Racing Chemists, which was founded in 1947 by 80 chemists from 70 countries, the prevalence of doping today is less than 1 %

Drugs and other agents are not always used to enhance performance, however. Cases are also known in which substances have been administered surreptitiously for the purpose of impairing performance ability and increasing the winning chances of less-favored entrants. The first documented case involved a 1910 boxing match in which the favorite, James Jeffrie, was knocked out by Jack Johnson. Jeffrie attributed his defeat to the fact that his tea had been 'doctored'. In postwar England, a gang was apprehended for attempting to improve bookmakers' odds by the 'negative doping' of favorites. In 1961, it was found that the English Derby favorite Pinturishchio had been doped, and the horse was withdrawn before race time. This type of performance manipulation is almost always done by outsiders (which has led to the term 'outside job') and is usually aimed at horses upon which sizable sums have been bet. SUSTMANN [1914] has dubbed this practice 'paradoping', but this term has not gained wide acceptance. It should be noted that the 'outside job' is frequently used as an excuse by those convicted of doping.

1.5.1. Origin and Definition of Terms

As our brief historical review shows, performance manipulations that come under the heading of doping are older than the term itself. Since the turn of the century, the word 'doping' has become increasingly common in the literature (e.g., in MÖLLER [1902] or SUCKOW [1905]). An English dictionary published in 1889 was the first to define doping as a mixture of opium and narcotics, which was the concoction most often used at that time. Contrary to popular opinion, the term is not derived from the English word 'dope', which can mean a drug addict or a stupid person. It actually has its etymologic roots in the Bantu language. From a Bantu dialect in Southeastern Africa, it found its way into the Boer language. The name was originally applied to a concentrated, viscous liquor used by the Bantus as a stimulant during religious ceremonies. Later it was applied to other stimulating drinks as well [PROKOP, 1965]. In American slang, for example, 'to dope' meant to intoxicate someone, especially as applied to the drug mixtures reportedly used by Gypsies (e.g., tobacco and hawthorn seeds). The word is now used internationally to mean the illicit use of drugs for the purpose of influencing the outcome of a competition. Synonyms for doping to win include 'to drug', 'to spice', 'to touch them up', 'inside job', and the use of 'speed balls'; doping to lose has been described by such expressions as 'to noble', 'hopping', and 'outside job'.

The difficulty with the term 'doping' is that despite attempts, there is still no single, clear-cut definition for it. Both the scope and interpretation of the term vary with the criteria for its control. In an effort to establish more precise regulations, definitions have been offered by numerous national and international sport associations, by the Medical Commission of the International Olympic Committee, and even by an Expert Committee of the Western European Council (see BÜSCHER

[1] 1 grain = 64.8 mg.
[2] 1 minim = 0.06 ml.
[3] 1 ounce = 28.35 g.

[1972]). All are in basic agreement that doping refers to *the use of any agents or substances for the purpose of affecting racing performance in a positive or negative way.* Many definitions, such as that proposed in Strassburg by the European Council in 1963, also include the administration of physiologic substances, such as vitamins and hormones, in abnormal amounts. The central problem is the difficulty of differentiating doping from the medically prescribed use of stimulants, and from drug therapy during the competition or competitive period that does not affect normal performance. Therefore, the Expert Committee of the European Council made the following determination at its meeting of November, 1963, in Madrid: 'In cases where medical treatment is required which by virtue of its nature or dosage can increase the performance ability of a horse beyond the normal level, such treatment must be regarded as doping, and the horse must be deemed ineligible to compete.' Thus, this rule does not categorically prohibit racing under the influence of medications. However, it would hardly be prudent to medicate sick persons or animals for the purpose of symptom relief and then subject them to the extreme physical and mental stresses of competition.

The current trend appears to favor the prohibition of all medication prior to competition or performance trials. The list of doping drugs of the F.E.I. (International Equestrian Federation) and their supplementation by several national equestrian organizations already include a broad spectrum of drugs. Some states in the U.S. prohibit the use of drugs 48 h before a race. The 'Report of the Duke of Norfolk's Committee to the Stewards of the Jockey Club and National Hunt', a comprehensive study on doping, even recommends that a 72-hour ban be adopted. Measures to influence psychic performance, such as hypnosis, would also be considered doping by the European Council definition, though this is of no importance in animals. On the other hand, the use of physical agents and methods, such as electric current, cryotherapy or mechanical devices attached to the harness, saddle or rider's boots, must clearly be regarded as doping. It is interesting to note that the first, and to date the only, doping case to be tried formally in a German court of law is based on doping with physical agents.

The following is taken from an article in the 'Deutsche Tierärztliche Wochenschrift' of 1905: 'Doping punished as fraud — The Criminal Court of Dortmund sentenced Düsseldorf racing stable owner Schneider to pay a fine of M 600.— for strapping an electric battery to his horse Assure during a race in Dortmund last year'. This verdict, which was appealed, was later upheld by the Supreme Court of Justice (Goltdammer Archive, 1906), thus providing clear confirmation of the criminality of doping.

Based on previous considerations, we might offer the following definition for doping: 'Doping is the altering of performance ability and conduct derived from genetic disposition, care and feeding, training and general state of health in an animal that is engaged in sports competition or other physical performance trials (horses, dogs, pigeons, bulls, poultry) by the administration of exogenous chemical agents or endogenous substances in unphysiologically high doses, or by the use of physical manipulations, unless expressly allowed in the rules.'

The term should be limited to the direct influencing of performance and conduct, and should not include the prescription of the agents (European Council, 1963) or the instigation for their use (Rules). Similarly, the use of descriptive terms having a moral or ethical connotation, such as 'prohibited', 'unfair', 'corrupt', 'criminal', 'fraudulent' or 'artificial', cloud the issue and should be dropped in the interest of objectivity. Such terms create ''loopholes' in the rules which make effective doping control difficult. Nor should the definition include references to the nature of the

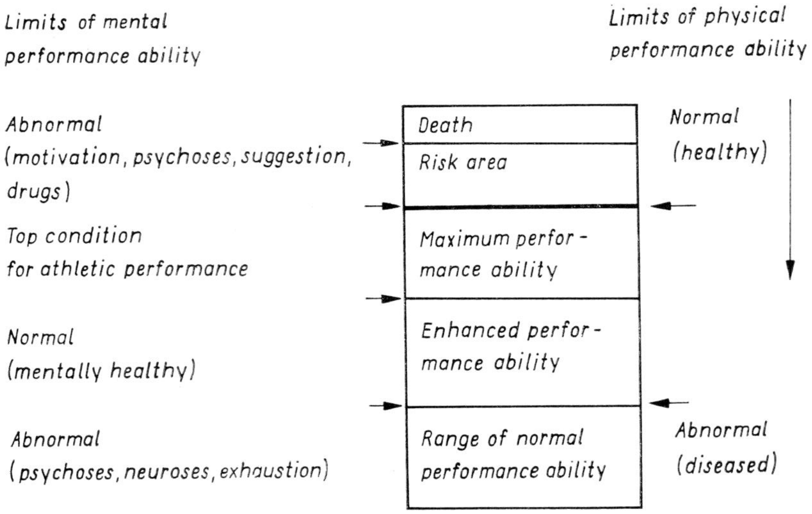

Fig. 1.5. — 1. The Schönholzer model of performance limits.

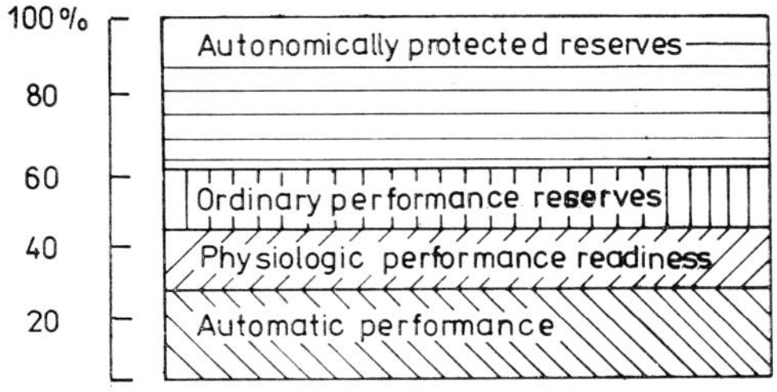

Fig. 1.5. — 2. The Hettinger model of performance ranges.

performance change, such as speed enhancement, stamina enhancement, mood elevation, tranquilization, etc. In this way there is no need for separate rules covering 'doping to lose'.

The physical performance ability of humans and animals is subject to absolute limits that cannot be surpassed, and whose attainment is usually at the cost of serious injury or death. The maximum performance that can be achieved without risk is still considerably below the absolute performance limit. The total performance potential can be divided into various ranges whose limits are defined by psychological inhibitions and physiological defense mechanisms. As shown by SCHÖNHOLZER's model, 4 or 5 ranges are defined by overall performance limits (fig. 1.5. — 1).

This model clearly shows that exceeding the highest performance limit attainable by training, carries risks for the life and health of the individual concerned. A quantitative estimate of the individual ranges of total performance ability is offered by HETTINGER [1965]. The performance ranges shown in figure 1.5. — 2 correspond in principle to the SCHÖNHOLZER model. As the diagram shows, there is a considerable untapped performance potential that cannot be utilized even by maximal voluntary exertion. Conscious and unconscious inhibitions and the physiologic barriers, most notably in the form of the fatigue complex and pain, all act to limit the individual performance ranges. This protects the active and passive locomotor apparatus and circulatory system against harmful overexertion and a possibly fatal overusage of energy-yielding materials and systems.

The level of performance attainable by an individual under normal circumstances depends essentially on his state of mind and stage of fitness. No doping drug is known that will increase absolute performance ability. Drugs enhance performance solely by weakening or abolishing the psychological and physiological barriers between the performance ranges, or by lowering the threshold for the mobilization of autonomically protected reserves. All performance ranges lying below the danger zone can be fully exhausted by training; their absolute magnitude is determined essentially by disposition (genetic) and physiology. The exhaustion of performance reserves that are ordinarily available only for coping with short-term, life-threatening situations generally leads to illness with a compensatory reduction of performance ability, or in some cases to death. The overexertional damage that commonly accompanies doping includes circulatory defects, vascular ruptures, and, at high temperatures, heat stroke. A number of fatalities in humans and animals and numerous unpublicized cases of acute illness resulting from circulatory exhaustion, muscle spasms, muscular and ligament tears and fractures confirm the dangers inherent in abolishing natural performance barriers. This can be done by means of drugs that act mainly on central regulatory systems, such as amphetamines; or by substances that act only on certain organ systems, such as strychnine or quinine, which increase muscular tension. A specific effect can be ensured only by administering a carefully calculated dose at the proper time, taking into account the body weight of the animal as well as its temperament and condition. Thus, doping to win is generally successful only if practiced by persons thoroughly familiar with the animal. Since faulty dosing may be ineffective or even counterproductive, it is essential that the drug be administered in the necessary dose with no danger of losses. For example, chlorpromazine can improve the racing performance of an excited horse when administered in small doses. However, larger doses have a sedative effect that will slow the animal and, in the case of jumping horses, will greatly increase the risk of falling by impairing the sense of balance.

Owing to the horse's highly developed sense of taste, the oral administration of drugs (e.g., in sugar cubes, hollow carrot pieces or mixed with drinking water) is the least certain mode of administration due to the possibility of feed refusal or feed and water losses. Oats mixed with small amounts of amphetamines, for example, are refused. The drugs are usually administered by injection, therefore. Injections can sometimes be detected by signs of local irritation or by circumscribed patches of sweat. For this reason injections are often given at sites where such symptoms are not likely to be noticed, such as between the mandibles, at the tip of the ear, or on the neck beneath the mane. At this site, however, the drug may enter the fat depot in the crest of the neck, and its absorption is delayed. Intravenous injections are not easily given by laymen and so generally require the help of one or more accomplices. Because the onset of the drug action is rapid in such cases, the horse must be doped shortly before race time, and thus at a time when the animal is, or should be, under strict supervision. Even in the parade ring, however, an experienced doper will often be able to inject small doses of a highly potent drug with the aid of a special injection device. The rectal administration of doping drugs is occasionally reported, but this cannot be done unobtrusively and is limited by the local irritating action of many drugs.

In recent years pharmaceutical preparations have been developed which enable many drugs to be applied cutaneously in ointment or spray form. 'Delayed action' drugs are also available that can be given as much as a day before a race. Anabolic steroids can be discontinued weeks before the racing season.

When horses are doped to lose, rather than win, the dosage is not so critical, and so the drug can be administered a day or so before race time. There are hundreds of drugs and many more pharmaceutical preparations containing such drugs that could be used for doping. However, as pointed out earlier, uncertainties often exist with regard to actions, dosage and mode of administration, and many drugs are difficult to obtain. In most cases, therefore, the doper will resort to familiar drugs whose doses and actions are already well known.

1.5.2. Doping Agents

A list of the doping drugs detected most frequently by members of the Association of Official Racing Chemists (AORC) during the period from 1949 to 1961 is shown in table 1.5. — 1.

This list alone demonstrates the great variety of doping drugs available and the difficulty of surveying them. To obtain at least a general survey, it is necessary to divide the drugs into groups on the basis of common pharmaceutical properties. In a survey compiled by Beretta [1968], drugs are arranged roughly according to pharmacologic as well as chemical properties that have bearing on their use in doping. For example, heroin and morphine are assigned to the group of alkaloid stimulants, even though they are classified pharmacologically as analgesics. There are similar overlaps in categorizing the sympathomimetic amines, which may be assigned, for example,

Table 1.5. — 1. Doping drugs detected by the members of the AORC from 1949 to 1961

Drug	Number of positives	Drug	Number of positives
Procaine	273	Scopolamine	8
Amphetamine	270	Cocaine	7
Caffeine	246	Mephentermine	7
Phenylbutazone	59	Alcohol	6
Theobromine	48	Mephenesin	6
Morphine	47	Amylocaine	5
Ephedrine	46	Chlorpromazine	5
Thiamine	42	Brucine	4
Barbiturates	38	Lidocaine	4
Strychnine	31	Pipradol	4
Methamphetamine	29	Salicylic acid	4
Nikethamide	26	Tetracaine	4
Dipyrone	25	Theophylline	4
Methapyrilene	20	Oxyphenbutazone	3
Atropine	16	Phenylpropanolamine	3
Nicotine	14	Barbital	2
Phenobarbital	13	Dibucaine	2
Methylphenidate	12	Guaiacol	2
Ethylaminobenzoate	10	Meprobamate	2
Acetophenetidin	9	Naphazoline	2
Pentylenetetrazol	8	Phenothiazine	2
		Quinine	2

to the group of centrally acting analeptics. Somewhat different subdivisions are made in official lists of doping drugs, such as that of the Medical Commission of the IOC or the F.E.I. For example, at its meeting of May 19, 1971, in Munich, the Medical Commission of the IOC recognized essentially four classes of doping drugs: (1) psychomotor stimulants, such as cocaine and phenmetrazine; (2) sympathomimetic amines, such as ephedrine and methoxyphenamine; (3) various CNS stimulants, such as aminophenazole, leptazol and nikethamide; and (4) narcotic analgesics such as heroin, morphine, pethadine and related compounds. In our survey of agents employed for doping as the term was previously defined, we shall essentially follow the Beretta [1968] system, except that the group of sympathomimetics is expanded to include both the sympathomimetic amines as well as drugs with related actions that Beretta classified as analgesics.

1. *Agents for performance enhancement*
1.1. Stimulants
1.1.1. Excitants
1.1.2. Analeptics
1.1.3. Stimulants of the ganglion-blocking type
1.1.4. Glycosides
1.2. Vitamins and hormones
1.2.1. Vitamins
1.2.2. Adrenocortical hormones
1.2.3. Sex hormones
1.2.4. Anabolics
1.2.5. Other hormones
1.3. Local anesthetics and analgesics
1.3.1. Local anesthetics
1.3.2. Antipyretic and anti-inflammatory analgesics
1.4. Analeptics
1.4.1. Psychopharmacologic agents
1.4.2. Pseudodynamogenic agents
1.4.3. Special diet
1.4.4. Vasodilators
1.4.5. Ointments
1.4.6. Inhalation agents (volatile drugs)
1.5. Physical agents
1.5.1. Mechanical agents
1.5.2. Electricity
1.5.3. Cold
1.5.4. Physicochemical agents
1.5.5. UV radiation
2. *Agents for performance reduction*
2.1. Centrally acting agents
2.2. Agents acting on the muscles
2.3. Agents acting via the digestive tract
2.4. Other methods
3. *Masking agents*

In many cases the drugs are not given separately but are combined with one another, as in the 'speed balls' mentioned earlier. The original intent may have been to obtain a summation of the individual effects, or to use one drug to prevent the undesired side-effects of another. Atropine was often given only in an amount sufficient to inhibit salivation, thus making it difficult or impossible to collect a saliva sample for analysis. A number of drugs can be used either to enhance or impair performance, depending on the dosage given.

One form of drug misuse that is mentioned by CLARK cannot strictly be called doping, for it does not alter the conduct of the animal before the race. By administering sedatives on a long-term basis, a horse can be made to appear 'run-down' and thus in poor racing condition. Having achieved 'longshot status', the horse is then taken off medication on the day of the race.

The official prohibited drug lists of today commonly include substances that do not influence the conduct or performance ability of the animal, but interfere with the detection of doping drugs. Thus, it is proper that this class of substances, called masking agents, be ranked among the doping drugs.

All the agents listed in the table above are capable of modifying performance ability by virtue of their pharmacological properties. However, it is extremely difficult to show objectively that they will exert a positive effect on a given type of performance (galloping, trotting, jumping, dressage), especially in fully trained animals. For example, while a stimulant can enhance speed and stamina in the galloping racehorse, an equal dose can cause a trotting horse to break into a gallop owing to its excitatory effect.

It is impossible to compile a complete list or survey of doping drugs and methods. There must be any number of natural or synthetic substances and combinations that are capable of stimulating performance but have not yet been used or detected in sporting and racing practice. It is also quite difficult to devise a system whereby existing drugs can be categorized and 'new' drugs can be classified or identified. Purely pharmacologic or medical criteria are inadequate for this purpose and can cause confusion in some instances. The BERETTA system appears most suitable. Here substances are grouped according to the nature of their effect on performance. They are then subdivided further on the basis of structural and chemical features. Because most drugs have several sites of action, e.g., the CNS, peripheral nervous system and cell metabolism, it is not always possible to assign a compound uniquely to a particular group. Thus, such a system is not entirely free of arbitrary or subjective classification. This circumstance could be largely avoided by a differentiated subdivision of individual groups, but we avoided such a subdivision in the interest of clarity. In addition, we gave greater weight to pharmacologic criteria and thus categorized a few substances differently from the BERETTA system.

1.5.2.1. Agents for Performance Enhancement

1.5.2.1.1. Stimulants

Excitants. This group includes drugs that produce excitation like that occurring in Guedel stage II, doing so mainly by paralyzing ascending inhibitory systems and relay centers in the midbrain. Sufficient doses also abolish cerebral inhibitions, causing an accentuation of muscle tone via spinal reflexes. Accordingly, this excitatory state is based more on disinhibition than on a heightened central or peripheral nervous excitability. The effect of these drugs in the horse is further enhanced by the animal's relatively primitive central nervous system. Thus, the paralysis of inhibitory centers in the horse creates stronger excitatory states than in species with a more highly developed CNS, in which the main effects are analgesia, intoxication and reaction impairment. Besides their central effect, these drugs also act directly on the peripheral nervous system and thus can have direct effects on the circulation. This group includes substances that are used medically as narcotic analgesics (some with a euphoriant effect), local anesthetics, sympathomimetics or parasympathomimetics. Typical representatives of this group are the *alkaloids*, which have been used by man since ancient times. Alkaloids are nitrogenous organic bases that are contained in plants. They are pharmacologically active in man and animals even in extremely small doses. They have been used for centuries as a means of inducing mild intoxication for pleasure or for medical or ceremonial purposes. It is hardly surprising, therefore, that when the modern history of doping began around the turn of the century, cocaine was the foremost doping drug. American trainers were probably alerted to this drug by the Central and South American Indians, who chewed leaves from the coca shrub *(Erythroxylon coca)* as a means of relieving hunger and thirst, imparting a sense of strength, and inducing euphoria. In this way the natives were able, despite chronic malnutrition, to accomplish considerable feats of physical endurance. The major alkaloid contained in the coca leaf is l-cocaine; d-cocaine is also present. The latter is broken down more rapidly in the body but does not have the psychic effect of l-cocaine and so is not addicting. L-cocaine hydrochloride is very readily absorbed through the mucous membranes (e.g., the nasopharyngeal mucosa), and so is often administered through the nose in powder form. After absorption it is broken down relatively quickly, especially in animals, so that little is recovered in the urine. In man, by contrast, up to 5 % is excreted in the urine. Cocaine is an excellent drug for infiltration and conduction anesthesia with a vasoconstricting effect. It inhibits the breakdown of epinephrine, thus leading to constriction of the blood vessels with a rise in blood pressure and tachycardia. Its effect as a doping drug, though controversial, is probably derived from sympathetic stimulation and intracerebral disinhibition, creating a strong excitatory state in which the horse will run to the point of exhaustion. Absolute muscular strength is always diminished. Larger doses cause paralysis symptoms and severe vasospasm. The latter can be treated with nitrites, while the excitation states can be moderated with narcotics. No opiates or epinephrine should be given! The lethal dose is 15 mg/kg body wt. i.v. The pupils are dilated and, unlike the atropinzed pupils, they can be constricted with eserine or neostigmine. An additional side-effect, according to CROISIER [1948], is a decreased urine output that can lead to uremia.

A further group of alkaloids is the opium alkaloids and their chemical transformation products. In humans and dogs these drugs cause intoxication or narcosis, while in horses they exert a central paralytic effect which abolishes inhibitory mechanisms, causing excitation. Opium, the dried juice of the *Papaver somniferum* poppy, contains 20—25 % alkaloids. Of the 25 alkaloids present, the most abundant are morphine (3—23 %), noscapine (~ 5 %), papaverine (0.8 %), codeine (0.5 %) and thebaine (0.3 %). Because of the nonuniform composition of opium, dosing is highly uncertain, and so opium itself is unknown as a doping drug. However, its constituent pure alkaloids have been widely used. The most notable are morphine and its acetylization product diamorphine (diacetylmorphine), better known as heroin, which is no longer used medically due to its high toxicity and addictiveness. Even as a doping drug, heroin has apparently found little if any use since World War II (cf. table 1.5. — 1). Heroin is administered parenterally in doses of 20—50 mg and orally at more than 10 times that dose. It produces signs of excitation after 30—60 min. As with morphine, a small patch of sweat appears at the injection site. Behavioral changes include a fixed gaze, and compulsive forward movement, frequent neighing, tail raising and deepened respiration. Stamina is increased. An overdose causes tetanic spasms, bolting and apathy. Similar effects are seen with morphine, which is injected s.c. in a dose of 0.5—1.5 g. There is unrest, ground pawing and, with larger doses, inattention and apathy. The opium alkaloids also cause vagal stimulation with consequent bradycardia and dilatation of the coronary vessels with a fall in blood pressure. The tone of the small and large intestine is greatly accentuated, leading to possibly severe constipation. The sphincters are in a state of strong contraction, including the bladder sphincter, and it may take several hours before a urine sample can be collected after a race. Because an urge to urinate is induced centrally, bladder rupture is a danger. Heavy sweating occurs due to an impairment of central thermoregulatory mechanisms. One trotting horse that won its only race under the influence of morphine sweated for over an hour after the race, and it took 3 h to collect urine from him. His pulse had not returned to normal $1^1/_2$ h after the race. His pupils were dilated, and his subcutaneous veins stood out noticeably [Mackay, 1961].

Morphine is excreted mainly in the urine, partly in free form and partly in conjugated form. Another morphine derivative is codeine (methylmorphine), which is given to the horse in doses of 1—5 g. It is partially demethylated in the liver and converted to morphine. It exerts an analgesic and paralytic effect on the cerebrum. It is used medically as an antitussive. Larger doses cause excitation and unrest [Fröhner, 1919]. Its effects are based on disinhibition and are thus similar to those of strychnine [Deriveaux and Liegeois, 1962]. It can cause respiratory depression in larger doses. By treating morphine with strong mineral acids, water is abstracted, and the morphine ring system is rearranged. The product of this reaction is apomorphine, which is used medically as an emetic but has also found use in the doping of horses [Mackay, 1961]. The LD_{50} in dogs is about 80 mg/kg body wt. i.v. After a dose of 0.75 or 1 grain (64.8 mg) apomorphine, horses react in 3—5 min with excitement, unrest and rearing. There are tetanic spasms, sweating, and the breathing becomes irregular. Apomorphine abolishes the sedative effect of chlorpromazine, while the latter weakens the effect of apomorphine but increases its duration four-fold. Both drugs are easily detected when administered singly, but neither is demonstrable after their combined use.

Another opium alkaloid is papaverine, which is used in medicine as a coronary stimulant and, according to Beretta [1968], also finds use in horse doping. Its main site of action is the myocardium and smooth muscle. It increases the coronary blood flow while improving the oxygen saturation of the atrial sinus blood. It also increases the myocardial oxygen demand, which can be avoided by the simultaneous administration of β-receptor blocking drugs. The cerebral blood flow is also improved. Besides the coronary arteries, papaverine relaxes the smooth muscle of the bowel, bronchial tree, blood vessels, etc. Dilatation of the splanchnic vessels results in a severe blood pressure drop, especially on parenteral administration. Papaverine is well absorbed, is mainly bound to plasma proteins, and is broken down very rapidly in the liver.

The following morphine derivatives have not previously been mentioned as doping drugs, but could be used as such owing to their morphine-like pharmacologic activity: dionin (ethylmorphine), whose activity is intermediate between morphine and codeine; hydromorphone (dihydromorphinone), which is 5 times as potent as morphine and has a more rapid onset and shorter duration of action; hydrocodone (dihydrocodeinone) and thebacone (acetylcodeine), which are more potent than codeine. Oxycodone (dihydro-4-hydroxy-codeinone) has a morphine-like effect. The fully synthetic morphine derivative thebacone (α(-)-3-hydroxy-N-methylmorphinane) has the same qualitative action as morphine but 10 times its analytic action. The opium alkaloid thebaine (dimethoxymorphine) has an excitatory effect similar to strychnine and in larger doses acts as a convulsant.

A not uncommon doping alkaloid is strychnine, which is also used as a component of combination products. Vettes [1927], for example, mentions the following mixture, which is given 40 min before race time in a hollow carrot: Strychnine arsenate 0.25, Caffeine 0.50, Cocaine sulfate 1.00.

Strychnine is used medically as a tonic and mild analeptic. The alkaloid is absorbed relatively slowly when taken orally and is excreted very slowly in the urine, creating a danger of cumulative poisoning. It is still detectable in the urine 1 to 2 days after use. Strychnine has central sites of action, blocking postsynaptic inhibitory mechanisms which, among other things, inhibit the motor neurons. It also acts centrally via the midbrain, heightening the equilibrium reflexes. In large doses it causes uncoordinated tonic convulsions, which can be triggered by visual or auditory stimuli. According to Neumann-Kleinpaul and Rüscher [1931], only 2—7 mg increases the pulse rate and blood pressure in horses. The animals extend their tails and salivate very heavily. Ostyn and de Nayer [1965] report that strychnine actually increases the working capacity of exhausted animals.

Various authors also mention *l-brucine* as a doping drug [Vettes, 1927; Croisier, 1948; Löchel, 1959; Aries; Schubert, 1967]. It is chemically similar to strychnine and, along with strychnine, is a major alkaloid of nux vomica, the seed of an Asiatic tree *(Strychnos nux-vomica)* that has no emetic properties. It has been used as a rat poison in Europe since medieval times.

The same authors report on *d-yohimbine*, an alkaloid which also heightens reflex excitability and is also used for horse doping. As a sympatholytic, it suppresses the action of epinephrine, and doses of 0.2 to 1.0 mg/kg body wt. cause vasodilatation and a fall in blood pressure. It is reportedly similar to cocaine in its local anesthetic properties, and its central nervous effects lead to excitation states and convulsions.

A further group of alkaloids is the active principle of various drugs derived from plants of the nightshade family *(Solanaceae)* that have been used for centuries as 'magic potions'. It was natural, therefore, that the *Solanum* alkaloids *scopolamine* (= l-hyoscine) and the chemically similar *atropine* (= d,l-hyoscyamine) would also be used as doping agents. Common to both alkaloids is the presence of tropic acid, which is esterified with tropine in hyoscyamine, and with scopine in scopolamine. Atropine is formed from l-hyoscyamine by racemization during the preparation of the drugs. The alkaloids occur in concentrations of 0.2 to 1.0% in the plants and seeds of the deadly nightshade *(Atropa belladonna)*, hebane *(Hyoscyamus niger)*, the thorn-apple *(Datura stramonium)*, and the mandrake *(Mandragora atropa)*. The principal alkaloid in the fresh plants is *l-hyoscyamine*. The alkaloids have a parasympatholytic action, producing effects typically associated with sympathetic activation. They act essentially by depressing the sensitivity of the receptors of cholinergically innervated organs, especially the exocrine glands and smooth muscle. Atropine causes stronger central excitation than scopolamine, which has a more paralytic effect. Sensitivity to these alkaloids is highly species-dependent, for tropine esterases, which quickly deactivate the esters, are present in some species.

The lethal doses (in g/kg body wt.) for several species are indicated below:

Atropine dose	Mouse	Rat	Rabbit	Cat	Dog
s.c.	0.50	0.75	0.70	0.15	0.20
i.v.	—	—	0.07	0.07	0.07—0.10

Like man, for whom the lethal atropine dose is only 150—200 mg, the horse is highly sensitive to this substance, though there is a large range of individual tolerance. According to Fröhner [1919], an atropine dose of only 500 mg alters the behavior of horses, creating an excitatory state which Croisier [1948] calls 'atropine delerium'. This state is marked by compulsive movements and an elevated heart rate and blood pressure. At larger doses, or if individual susceptibility is high, this can easily lead to frenzy and convulsions. Mydriasis is always present. The inhibition of salivation and gastric juice secretion and accentuated intestinal muscle tone predispose to tympany and colic, which may progress to gastric rupture in some instances. The decrease in salivation makes it difficult to collect samples for doping analysis. Scopolamine, like heroin, causes marked excitation in horses even in doses of 20—30 mg [Bru and Roberts]. According to Vettes [1927], a mere 10 mg is pharmacologically active, while 250 mg is lethal [Fröhner, 1919].

For centuries *caffeine* has been widely used as a stimulant for pleasure and medicinal purposes. This purine alkaloid occurs in the leaves of the tea shrub *(Thea sinensis)*, the seeds of coffee plants *(Coffea arabica)*, the leaves of the maté plant *(Ilex paraguayensis)*, in African kola nuts from *Cola nucifera*, and in Central American guarana, a paste made from the *Paullinia sobilis*. Thus, caffeine was an obvious choice for horse doping, particularly since this substance or the plants containing it are relatively cheap and easy to obtain. It is one of the few drugs for which a true performance increase in horses has been experimentally verified. It is little wonder, therefore, that it ranks first among the 'positives' detected by racing chemists (table 1.5. — 1). At the Laboratory of Racing Chemistry in Tokyo, Fujii et al. [1970, 1972, 1974] conducted extensive doping experiments with Thoroughbred horses, finding, among other things, that caffeine can improve speed and endurance even in fit horses. This effect of caffeine is based on its ability to activate the entire CNS. Its effects on conditioned reflexes and motor centers are particularly favorable, though larger doses tend to be paralytic. Caffeine stimulates respiration both by its mild excitatory effect on medullary centers, and by its sensitization of the respiratory center to CO_2. This latter effect is stronger than its influence on the circulation. The CNS action of caffeine is supplemented by an activation of spinal reflex centers that is more pronounced in animals than in man. This strychnine-like effect is further strenghtened by a sensitization of the contractile elements of muscle to acetylcholine and potassium. Thus, with optimum dosage — reportedly 3—10 g in horses and 0.2—2 g in dogs perorally — the circulation, respiration, nervous system and striated muscle are all affected simultaneously [Hennau, 1946]. Of course the excitation states associated with caffeine use are not always optimal. Neumann-Kleinpaul and Rüscher [1931] administered 1—10 g of caffeine rectally or by nasogastric tube and 100 to 250 mg subcutaneously, and observed strong excitation with unrest, refractoriness and compulsive lateral movement. Caffeine occurs in 2—4 % concentration in tea and 0.5—1 % concentration in coffee and so can be administered in the form of extracts or by the direct ingestion of these plants. It is absorbed well, and only a small portion (0.5 to 3 %) of the administered dose is excreted unchanged in the urine 6 h after application [Fischer et al., Schubert, 1967]. In the body it is metabolized into various methylated xanthine derivatives, uric acid, and uric acid derivatives.

Other purine alkaloids that reportedly enhance performance in the horse [Aries] are the secondary alkaloids occurring in tea, *theophylline* and *theobromine*. The latter is also the principal alkaloid of the cacao bean, the seed of the cacao tree *(Theobroma cacao)*. Both have actions similar to caffeine, though there are differences of degree: Caffeine and theophylline stimulate the CNS and skeletal muscles more strongly than theobromine, while theophylline and theobromine have stronger cardiovascular effects than caffeine. These relationships are shown in table 1.5. — 2. The cardiac activity of caffeine is largely offset by its concurrent stimulation of the medullary vagal centers.

Additional alkaloids that have been used as performance stimulants in horses by virtue of their excitatory effects are *veratrine, aconitine* (whose action is similar to

Table 1.5. — 2. Comparison of some important actions of the purine alkaloids (after HAUSCHILD [1973])

	CNS stimulation	Smooth muscle relaxation	Coronary dilatation	Cardiac stimulation	Skeletal muscle stimulation
Caffeine	+++	+	+	+	+++
Theophylline	++	+++	+++	+++	++
Theobromine	+	++	++	++	+

veratrine), and *guinine* [FRÖHNER, 1919; VETTES, 1927; NEUMANN-KLEINPAUL and RÜSCHER, 1931; CROISIER, 1948; MARES, 1958; ARIES; GEBHARDT; SCHUBERT, 1967].

Veratrine is an alkaloid mixture isolated from various species of hellebore (e.g., *Veratrum album, V. niger, V. albiflora*), some of which are native to Europe and are known as poisonous plants. The veratrum alkaloids, such as protoverine A and B, veratridine, zevadine, veratramine and germersin, stimulate sensory nerve endings and reportedly strengthen and prolong muscle contractions. Because they specifically stimulate the nerve endings of the endocardium, bradycardia and hypotension result. Today the pure protoveratrines are frequently used in the treatment of hypertension. Their efficacy as doping drugs is questionable, for veratrine is a muscle poison, and a slight overdose or high susceptibility can easily lead to muscle spasms, tachycardia, respiratory paralysis, sweating, salivation and nausea.

Aconitine, which occurs mainly in the root *(Tuber aconitum)* and leaves of the monkshood *(Aconitum napellus)*, supposedly has actions similar to veratrine but causes less local irritation. Horses are highly sensitive to aconitine. Doses of only 0.004 mg/kg body wt. can be fatal [MARES, 1958].

Quinine is obtained from the bark of the cinchona tree *(Cinchona officinalis* and *C. succurubra)*, which is native to South America but cultivated in the East Indies, principally Java and Sri Lanka. Cinchona bark was imported to Europe around 1640, when it was heralded as a 'wonder cure'. It contains 14 alkaloids. Its major alkaloid, quinine, is a well known antimalarial drug having various biologic actions. For example, quinine acts as a muscle stimulant by strengthening muscular impulses and prolonging the refractory period, and is thus of value in the treatment of myotonia congenita. It also causes vasodilation with a fall of blood pressure. Cell metabolism, and thus heat production, are inhibited. Also noteworthy is its central analgesic effect based on a mild paralysis of the sensory areas of the brain. Thus, larger doses tend to produce paralytic symptoms. If used parenterally, the cell-damaging effect of quinine can lead to cellular damage with subsequent necrosis and ulceration. In experiments by NEUMANN-KLEINPAUL and RÜSCHER [1931], an oral dose of 25 g quinine increased the pulse and respiratory rate in an experimental horse, but no performance increase was observed. Quinine is slowly excreted in the urine, about 20 % appearing in unchanged form.

Other stimulants that are mentioned in connection with doping are *arecoline* and the hydrastis alkaloids *hydrastine* and *hydrastenine*, which have hypertensive and central excitatory effects. Presumably, the East Indian practice of chewing the betel nut for its stimulating and euphoric effect first prompted the use of arecoline for horse doping. Arecoline is the major alkaloid of the betel nut, the seed of the *Areca catechu*, a species of palm native to the East Indies. The alkaloid possesses a mild muscarine effect and is classed as a parasympathomimetic drug. It increases salivation and stimulates intestinal peristalsis. It is an anthelmintic for veterinary use, since it also induces muscular paralysis in certain parasites such as the Cestodes. Arecoline also causes central stimulation by virtue of its central analgesic and euphoric action. Its effect is abolished by atropine. Another alkaloid reportedly used for doping is *emetine*, which is obtained from ipecac [Beretta, 1968]. It effects only a local stimulation of sensory nerve endings, especially in the stomach. It is toxic in doses as low as 10—20 mg/kg body wt. Its pharmacologic actions could hardly account for a doping effect, unless the pain produced by emetine reflexly causes an increase in excitation.

Analeptics. This class of drugs, called also cerebral stimulants, has gradually replaced traditional doping drugs from the alkaloid series. They exert a well circumscribed effect with proper dosage by increasing the excitability of the CNS or certain parts of it, such as the cerebral cortex, medullary centers or spinal cord. Large doses cause convulsions. The analeptics are used therapeutically for the relief of paralyses of the circulatory and respiratory centers of varying etiology. As cerebral stimulants, they are effective in interrupting general anesthesia and other forms of unconsciousness. The analeptics are classified in practical terms as respiratory analeptics, circulatory analeptics, sympathomimetic amines and cerebral stimulants.

Analeptics can be divided into three groups according to their activity or site of action [Hauschild, 1973].

1. Drugs with a direct central excitatory action. In a strict sense these include pentetrazol (pentamethylenetetrazol, pentylenetetrazol, Deumacard®, Cardiazol®, etc.), bemegride (β,β-methylethylglutarimide, Ahypnon®, Megimid®, etc.), nikethamide (N,N-diethylnicotinamide, Corvitol®, Coramin®, etc.) and other acid amides with a similar action, such as phthalic acid-bis-diethylamide (Neospiran®, etc.), dimethyl-isoxazol-4-carbonic acid diethylamide (Cycliton®, etc.), crotonyl-α-n-propylaminobutyric acid diethylamide (Prethcamid®, etc.), and vanillic acid diethylamide, or ethamivan (Vandid®, etc.). This group further includes the aforementioned alkaloids picrotoxin, strychnine, caffeine and other xanthine derivatives as well as terpenes such as thujone and camphor.

2. Drugs that stimulate peripheral nervous receptors and reflexly excite medullary centers. These include lobeline, which stimulates respiration by acting on chemoreceptors in the carotid sinus, and camphor, which stimulates respiration and circulation by creating a pain stimulus on injection. Similar effects are exerted by rubbing alcohol or ammonia and other acutely irritating substances that stimulate nerve endings in the skin or nasal mucosa.

3. Central stimulants, which in large doses exert a pronounced analeptic effect. The main representatives of this group are the sympathomimetic amines, which include ephedrine, amphetamine and methamphetamine. Of the true analeptics, pentetrazol [Sendros, 1956; Aries, 1964] and nikethamide [Bäumler et al., 1964] have been described as doping drugs. Pentetrazol is rapidly absorbed enterally and parenterally and is broken down relatively quickly. In small doses it stimulates cortical and subcortical motor centers as well as the respiratory and circulatory center. It raises the blood pressure by exciting pressor elements of the vasomotor center. Larger doses affect the spinal cord, especially the motor portions of the reflex arc. Spasmogenic doses cause tissue degeneration in the kidney, liver and cerebral cortex (focal necrosis, glial degeneration) as a result of vasospasms with resultant local hypoxia. Because horses react violently to pentetrazol, optimum dosing is difficult to achieve. Nikethamide is a yellow viscous liquid that is soluble in water and organic solvents and is also well absorbed. In small doses it excites medullary centers, especially the respiratory center. In larger doses it excites additional portions of the CNS, particularly spinal centers. It heightens the sensitivity of the respiratory center to

CO_2. The mean convulsant dose is about 300 mg/kg body wt. s.c. and 130 mg/kg body wt. i.v. The lethal dose is only slightly higher. It is much inferior to pentetrazol in its circulatory and cerebral stimulant effect. The dose for horse doping is 10—20 ml of a 25 % solution i.m. or s.c., or 5—10 ml i.v. [ARIES, 1964].

Of the analeptics with peripheral sites of action, *camphor* is the foremost doping drug [SUCKOW, 1905; CROISIER, 1948; ARIES, 1964; FUJII et al., 1970, 1972, 1974]. Camphor is a hydrocarbon belonging to the terpene group. It is poorly soluble in water but is highly soluble in organic solvents and is rapidly absorbed. It is eliminated by oxidation to camphorol in the liver and by coupling to glucuronic acid. Being an oily solution, it is absorbed more slowly than it is broken down, and so an active blood level is difficult to attain. Camphor is obtained by steam distillation from the wood of the camphor tree *(Cinnamomum camphora)* but can also be produced synthetically. Unlike natural forms of camphor, synthetic camphor does not have chemical isomers. Japanese camphor is dextrorotatory, while Borneo camphor consists of d-borneol and Ngai camphor of l-borneol. The levo forms are more active than the dextro forms [HAUSCHILD, 1973]. Camphor also acts as a narcotic and, unlike the 'true' analeptics, accentuates the effect of narcotics. According to GADDUM [1952], the analeptic effect of camphor is based on the pain associated with injection. Camphor has an inhibitory effect on cardiac dynamics and leads to peripheral vasoconstriction as well as coronary dilatation. Its acts as a central nervous stimulant in the proper dose. The difference between the doses for medullary stimulation and for central paralysis is so small, however, that doping with camphor carries an enormous risk. Hence, camphor is seldom if ever used today as a doping drug. According to ARIES the salts of camphosulfonic acid do not carry such a high risk, but the extent of their use as doping drugs is unknown. In Japan, trans-π-oxocamphor has been detected with some frequency in the urine of winning racehorses. This drug, which is marketed in Japan under the name Vitacamphor, was tested exhaustively by FUJII et al. [1970, 1972, 1974] for its doping properties. A horse that had received 2 g showed tonic spasms of the limbs and neck immediately after the injection. A marked cardiac effect was documented on the basis of EKG records. At the usual dose of 200 mg there is an activity-dependent rise in the heart rate, while a 2-g dose is cardiotoxic. There was marked individual variability of response. As with most other doping drugs, trans-π-oxocamphor was found to have no influence on speed. Its possible influence on cardiac function suggests that a positive effect may be expected in tired or exhausted animals, as in the case of the other analeptics.

Drugs that act by stimulating the cutaneous nerve endings and are occasionally applied topically for doping purposes include *turpentine* and *mustard oil preparations* as well as *dimethylsulfoxide* (DMSO). Dimethylsulfoxide causes hyperemia while exerting a mildly analgesic and anti-inflammatory effect [ARIENS, 1965; CROISIER, 1948]. A particularly repugnant form of doping involves the application of *vesicants* to the skin in the area of the femoral canal. The resultant pain induces fear in the animal, causing it to quicken its pace [GUILLET, 1965]. According to CARNIGLIA [1946], mustard oil, turpentine and ginger are most commonly used for this purpose. There are reports that ginger has also been applied rectally [SCHICK, 1933; LÖCHEL, 1959]. The insertion of moistened ginger rhizome into the rectum was once a well-known trick among horse traders to enliven sluggish animals. ÅBERG [1966] reports that camphor has been applied in similar fashion for doping purposes. Doping by the inhalation of volatile agents that irritate the nerve endings of the nasal mucosa is mentioned by SUSTMANN [1914] and by VETTES [1927]. Iodine and iodine compounds, ether and prussic acid are mentioned as inhalants. Ammonia and smelling salts would appear to be equally if not better suited for this purpose, however.

Chemical structures of sympathomimetic amines from the phenylpropylamine series.

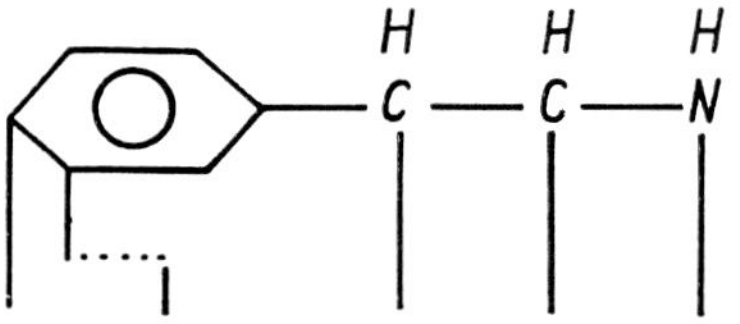

Generic name						*Brand name*
Dopamine	OH	OH	H	H	H	
Norepinephrine	OH	OH	OH	H	H	Arterenol
Epinephrine	OH	OH	OH	H	CH_3	Suprarenin
Phenylephrine	H	OH	OH	H	CH_3	Adrianol
Synephrine	OH	H	OH	H	CH_3	Pentetrine, Sympatol
Norfenefrine	H	OH	OH	H	H	Novadral
Ephedrine	H	H	OH	CH_3	CH_3	Ephedrine
Pholetrine	OH	H	H	CH_3	CH_3	Veritol, Pholetrine
Metaraminol	H	OH	OH	CH_3	H	Aramine
Amphetamine	H	H	H	CH_3	H	Benzedrine, Elastonon
Hydroxyamphetamine	OH	H	H	CH_3	H	Paredrine
Methamphetamine	H	H	H	CH_3	CH_3	Pervitine
Bendonorephedrine	H	H	OH	CH_3	H	Expovite

We may include in the 3rd group of analeptics the *sympathomimetic amines*, which have superseded the classical doping drugs, especially the alkaloids (except for caffeine). Being sympathomimetics, these drugs stimulate or enhance the functions of the sympathetic nervous system. The sympathetic stimulation may take place via a direct action on the effector organs, or indirectly by release of the transmittor substances epinephrine or norepinephrine. Most drugs used for doping are indirect-acting and stimulate the α receptors more than the β receptors. Owing to their good lipid solubility, these agents also act as central stimulants, mainly by activating the reticular formation. The result of this action is relief of fatigue and abolishment of the central depressive effects of narcotics, soporifics, etc. In man, the stimulating effect of these amines is combined with a marked euphoria. Because of the potentiality for misuse and the danger of habituation, these drugs are subject to strict legal controls in most countries. Nevertheless, they still are among the most widely used doping drugs (cf. table 1.5. — 1). They are chemically similar to the natural transmitters epinephrine, norepinephrine and dopamine, which, as catechol derivatives, are collectively termed catecholamines. The chemical similarities are shown in the table below.

In addition to the phenylpropylamine series, there are numerous other compounds that are chemically related to this group of substances and act as sympathomimetics with some degree of central stimulation. In terms of dopin efficacy, the best central stimulating properties belong to the sympathomimetic amines, which have up to 1 hydroxyl (OH) group per molecule and are thus more lipid-soluble. This applies in particular to amphetamine, metamphetamine and their p-hydroxy derivatives as well as ephedrine, which are among the most favored doping drugs. Of course the other substances are also suitable for such purposes by virtue of their strong circulatory effects. A prime example is epinephrine, which was mentioned as a doping drug in 1905 by Suckow, and later by Carniglia [1946] and Sendros [1956]. Epinephrine increases the rate and force of myocardial contractions, improves impulse conduction and dilates the coronary arteries. The blood depots are mobilized, and somewhat larger doses produce a rise in blood pressure with improved flow to the skeletal muscles, myocardium and brain. At large doses that are still below toxic levels, the blood pressure rise generally leads to a compensatory activation of the vagal system. This brings about a reactive fall in blood pressure and constriction of the coronary arteries with a typical 'vagus' pulse. Toxic doses cause severe pulmonary edema and acute heart failure as a cause of death. Major disadvantages of epinephrine are its very short duration of action, the difficulty of effective dosing, and its inactivity when given orally. When epinephrine is injected, its vasoconstricting action may cause ischemia to develop at the injection site, with a subsequent white discoloration of the coat. For these reasons it is highly unlikely that epinephrine still plays a role in the doping of horses. Instead, relatively frequent use is made of ephedrine, which is not unlike epinephrine in its actions and structure. Ephedrine has less cardiac activity yet still acts as a central stimulant. L-ephedrine is the active principle of a drug isolated from *Ephedra vulgaris* that has been used for 6,000 years in China as an asthma remedy and stimulant. The substance has been used medically in Europe only since 1924. The racemic form, which has been synthetically produced since 1927, is only half as active as the natural levo-isomer. Ephedrine acts about 7—10 times longer than epinephrine when given orally. Its cardiovascular effect resembles that of epinephrine, and its central stimulation is similar to that of amphetamine, though not so pronounced. Because of these properties, it is used relatively frequently as a doping drug [Åberg, 1960; Guillet, 1965; Venerando, 1965; Beretta, 1968; Fujii et al., 1970, 1972, 1974]. Fujii et al. tested the effect of the water-soluble hydrochloride on the racing performance of Thoroughbreds. Doses of 150, 300 and 500 mg were injected subcutaneously one hour before racing. Ephedrine demonstrated a performance-enhancing effect, although considerable individual differences were present. Even before the race there was a rise in the heart and respiratory rate that increased with the dose level. During the race the heart rate and depth of respiration were correspondingly increased. The EKG showed frequent 2nd-degree AV and SA blocks and infrequent extrasystoles. The ratio of T-wave heights before and after exercise was markedly increased. Several horses showed marked unrest after racing. The performance increase produced by ephedrine was considerably less than that of caffeine, and the harmful side-effects were more pronounced.

Hydroxyamphetamine (Paredrine®, etc.) is similar in action to ephedrine, but causes less excitation [Hauschild, 1973]. The most typical representatives of the phenylpropylamine series are the true sympathomimetic amines, amphetamine, and methamphetamine. In the AORC list of doping drugs (table 1.5. — 1), amphetamine ranks high in frequency of detection. Many authors make reference to the use of amphetamine in the doping of humans and animals (e.g., Hennau, 1946; Croisier, 1948; Morgan, 1958; Addis-Smith, 1961; Deriveaux and Liegeois, 1962; Aries, 1964; Beretta, 1968; Venerando and de Sio, 1965; Guillet, 1965; Clarke and Clarke, 1962]. Amphetamine forms a liquid amine that slowly vaporizes at room temperature and is soluble in organic solvents. It is most commonly used in the form of its highly water-soluble salts, most notably the sulfate or phosphate; the hydroscopic hydrochloride is not often used. The compound is optically active, and the term amphetamine denotes the racemic form. The biologically more active d-form is called dextroamphetamine or dexamphetamine. It is distinguished by its stronger central action and weaker peripheral action and today is usually preferred over the racemic form. It has various medical uses, including the treatment of obesity, narcolepsy, postencephalitic Parkinsonism, depressive syndromes, intoxications and overmedications with sedatives or narcotics. It is used in veterinary medicine to abolish or reduce sedation, and has been used in doses of 100 to 300 mg (s.c.) for the treatment of equine encephalomyelitis. Repeated use in man can lead to psychic dependence and even addiction. Of its pharmacologic effects (summarized by INNES and NICKERSON [1965]), the most important are those on the cardiovascular system, smooth muscle and central nervous system. Thus, there is a strong rise in blood pressure, and often the heart rate is reflexly slowed. Important effects on the smooth muscle include relaxation of the bronchial muscles and contraction of the urinary bladder sphincter that may cause difficulty in voiding. Centrally it exerts an excitatory effect on the medullary respiratory center, and its action on the adrenergic structures of the reticular formation abolishes the feeling of fatigue. It also depresses the appetite by influencing the hypothalamic satiety center. Toxic effects are manifested by unrest, tremor and extreme excitability. The heart becomes arrythmic, and angina-like pains occur. Lethal doses cause convulsions and coma before death. Necropsy findings include cerebral hemorrhage. The lethal dose is subject to considerable individual variability and is not yet known for the horse. The lethal dose in rats and mice is between 15 and 280 mg/kg body wt., and in rabbits, whose drug metabolism is similar to that of the horse, the LD is 25—85 mg/kg. The LD for dogs is 20 mg/kg. The metabolism of amphetamine is subject to marked species differences. It is excreted by the kidneys, partly unchanged and partly in degraded form. Two metabolic pathways appear to exist: (1) hydroxylation and excretion as p-hydroxyamphetamine (rat and guinea pig) and (2) deamination with the formation of benzylmethylketone, benzoid acid, hippuric acid and presumably other components as well (rat and dog) [AXELROD, 1954; ALLEVA, 1963; ELLISON et al., 1966]. In man, 40—60% [ALLES and WISEGARVER, 1961] or 15—65% [CARTONI and DE STEFANO, 1963] is excreted unchanged within 48 h, practically independent of the administered dose. The excretion depends strongly on the pH of the urine. Rats for example excrete 20% of the dose within 24 h if the urine is acidic, but only 5% if the urine is alkaline [ASATOOR et al., 1965]. Human blood is free of demonstrable amphetamine only a short time after administration [BECKETT and ROWLAND, 1965]. Quantitative data for the horse are sketchy. Based on available reports, it appears that amphetamine is recoverable unchanged in the saliva for about 3 h, and in the urine for up to 12 h [TAPERNOUX, et al., 1956; BONIN, 1956; BÄUMLER et al., 1964]. In a 500-kg horse treated with 150 mg of amphetamine sulfate, SCHUBERT [1967] found 0.1 mg amphetamine in 100 ml urine 6.5 h later. However, it appears that the acidification of the urine that occurs with strenuous exertion may be responsible for the greater amounts traced under these circumstances.

Amphetamine's efficacy as a doping drug is based essentially on the abolition of subjective fatigue, thus enabling the mobilization of autonomically protected strength reserves. BEECHER and SMITH [1965] could demonstrate a slight performance increase in the majority of shot-putters and runners given a dose of 14 mg/70 kg body weight. According to other reports, no performance increase could be demonstrated in trained athletes [SCHAEPDRYVER and HEBBELINCK, 1965]. The danger of amphetamine doping lies in the abolishment of the natural safeguards against overexertion. Its toxicity reportedly increases with the degree of exertion, as does the risk of hyperthermia [BEAUVALLET and SOLIER, 1965]. This danger is exemplified by the tragic death of a cyclist who suffered a heat stroke during competition after taking amphetamine [GUILLET, 1965]. VENERANDO and DE SIO [1965] report on further poisonings and one mortality. Horses, too, have suffered fatalities attributed to amphetamine doping. BETHLEM and TAVEIRA [1954] as well as MARES [1958] each describe a case in which a horse collapsed on the racetrack, and the presence of amphetamine was demonstrated at necropsy.

Methamphetamine has the same pharmacologic activity and range of indications as amphetamine. Chemically it represents the d-isomeric form of 1-phenyl-2-methyl-aminopropane. Methamphetamine is partially metabolized to amphetamine and is excreted as such in the urine or broken down further as previously described. Humans excrete about 17% of a single dose in the form of amphetamine within 48 hours; dogs excrete up to 45% as amphetamine and p-hydroxyamphetamine [CARTONI and DE STEFANO, 1963]. In subjects given methamphetamine, BECKETT and ROWLAND [1965] found only traces of amphetamine in alkaline urine, compared to 6% in acidic urine. Its role as a doping agent has been discussed by such authors as HENNAU [1946], DIECKMANN [1951], WIEGAND [1955], MARES [1958] and ARIES [1964]. According to HENNAU [1946], horses under the influence of amphetamine lose all sense of fatigue and may gallop to the point of cardiac arrest. The blood pressure is so high that vascular rupture may occur. According to studies by DIECKMANN [1951], horses show much individual variation in their response to this drug. For example, one trotting horse showed excitement and muscular tremors after a 75-mg dose. Another animal could easily be made to gallop without the use of a whip, even though this had not been possible previously. In another case a 150-mg dose caused a rise in the heart and respiratory rate but had no observable effect on the animal's behavior. When 300 mg was given, the horse became so highly excited that it could not be lunged for performance testing. Similar symptoms were observed by WIEGAND [1955], who, like ULLRICH [1950], noted a marked dryness of the oral mucous membrane. The animals attempted to correct this by exaggerated chewing and lip movements. BUESCHER [1972] mentioned experiments by KRAUSE, who could produce no performance increase with amphetamine or several other drugs in trained horses, although improvements could be obtained in horses not in training. The reported effective dose in Thoroughbreds is 30 mg methamphetamine 30 min before race time. An overdose leads in all cases to a decline in performance or an inability to race. At doses from 100 to 250 mg, clinical symptoms may be expected to appear. Any racehorse that is a 'surprise winner' should raise suspicions of amphetamine or methamphetamine doping.

Besides these main representatives of the sympathomimetic amines, there is a great many other chemically related substances that are suitable for doping purposes. As an example, ARIES [1964] mentions methylphenidate (Ritalin®, Cendetrin®) as well as phenmetrazine (Preludin®).

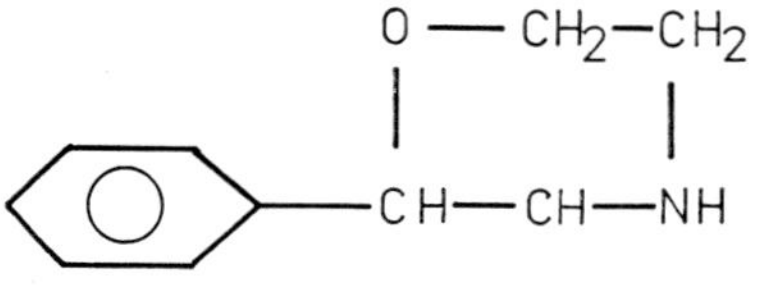

Phenmetrazine

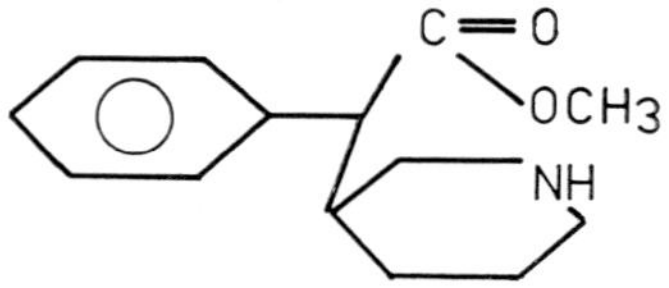

Methylphenidate

Both drug are mild psychostimulants and appetite supressants with minimal hypertensive activity. Methylphenidate is ranked between caffeine and the sympathomimetic amines in its effect. In experiments with Thoroughbreds, GABRIEL et al. [1963] produced central stimulation with doses of 50 to 600 mg, with a concurrent rise in the pulse and respiratory rate. At doses of 400—600 mg, the animals became visibly restless and excited for up to 8 h.

1.5.2.1.2. Local Anesthetics

These drugs are used therapeutically to relieve pain and to some degree to suppress inflammation. In racing and other equestrian sports, they are often employed to mask lamenesses secondary to painful limb conditions. These drugs must be considered from two standpoints. On the one hand, it must be determined whether pain alleviation without causal treatment in itself constitutes doping; on the other, it must be considered that pain-killing drugs may have side-effects that influence performance or behavior even in healthy animals. The latter circumstance obviously constitutes doping, whether intentional or otherwise. This explains why most local anesthetics and analgesics have been placed on the list of prohibited drugs by the F.E.I., while others, such as phenylbutazone or indomethacin, are allowed with certain restrictions. These restrictions show that there is still no international agreement on this issue, and so the question of prohibiting the use of centrally-acting anti-inflammatory analgesics such as Butazolidin® in horses with painful musculoskeletal diseases is still highly controversial. In recent years experience has shown that such drugs are capable of restoring these sick animals to apparent competitive soundness. This practice is often termed 'therapeutic' even by veterinarians who are solidly against the doping of racehorses. However, there can be little therapeutic rationale in treating an ailing limb while at the same time exposing it to the rigorous demands of competitive sport. The frivolous use of these drugs may tempt overambitious owners and trainers to place animals in competition without regard for their well-being. On the other hand, many cases are known in which horses that have been entered in prestige international jumping competitions and have even reached the jump-offs are withdrawn despite the fact that they could have been restored to soundness with analgesic drugs. Teams making such decisions clearly merit as much applause as the eventual winner. The problem is compounded by the fact that there are many top-performance horses that suffer from chronic lamenesses, yet are maintained in competitive form by analgesic therapy, either in the form of drug treatment or neurectomy, with no serious ill effects. To declare categorically that such treatment is doping would mean the death or exclusion of many good horses, and countries without extensive breeding programs might no longer be competitive in equestrian sports. International consensus on the problem is lacking. For example while many States in the U.S. allow the use of Butazolidin®, it and similar drugs are unconditionally banned in West Germany during competition or performance trials, although neurectomy is not expressly prohibited. One solution might be to publicize in some fashion the names of horses that are racing or competing under analgesic therapy. The public, after all, has a right to be informed about the condition of the horses in an event. Such information would also be useful in evaluating breeding soundness. The responsibility of assessing the lameness of a horse, and thus its ability to start, should rest mainly with the attending veterinarian as well as the racetrack veterinarian or veterinary commission of the organizing body. Pain sensation, like the feeling of fatigue, serves an important *protective function*. Its elimination can lead to serious injury unless the cause of the pain also is accurately diagnosed and treated.

Local anesthetics reversibly block nerve conduction when applied locally to the nerve tissue in the proper concentration. Both motor and sensory impulses are blocked. Most of these agents bind to specific receptors on the nerve cell and prevent its depolarization or excitation by blocking the influx of sodium into the cell. Forms of local anesthesia are topical anesthesia, infiltration anesthesia and conduction anesthesia (nerve block). The agents can be injected or may be rubbed or sprayed onto the area to be desensitized. Most local anesthetics can also cause central excitation,

Table 1.5. — 3. Names and structures of some local anesthetics (after HAUSCHILD [1973])

Structure	Generic name	Brand name (selection)
Aminoalkylesters R—CO—alk.—N=	Cocaine Procaine Chlorprocaine Piperocaine Tetracaine	Cocaine, Neurocaine Novocaine, Jenacaine, Isocaine Halestyn, Piocaine Metycaine, Isocaine, Neothesin Pantocaine
Aminoacylamides R—NH—CO—alk.—N≡	Lidocaine Mepivacaine	Lignocaine, Xylocitin, Xylocaine, Xyloton Carbocaine, Scandicaine
Aminoalkylamides R—CO—NH—alk.—N≡	Cinchocaine	Nupercaine, Dibucaine, Percaine, Sovcaine, Zinchocaine
Aminoalkylketones R—CO—alk.—N≡	Propoxypiperocaine	Exotancaine
Aminobenzoates ≡N—R—CO—O—alk.	Benzocaine Butylaminobenzoate	Anaesthesin, Aethoform Butoform

depression or paralysis on absorption, and thus act as true doping drugs. The local anesthetics that are known and clinically used are too numerous to describe here. However, the typical classes are shown in table 1.5. — 3 along with some of their better-known representatives.

All these drugs are considered potential doping agents, even though when used properly for local anesthesia, they would not ordinarily be absorbed in amounts sufficient to cause central effects like those reported with procaine. Cocaine, of course, is a potent drug that is readily absorbed and can have central effects even in very small doses (see p. 192). MACKAY [1961] reports that lidocaine, too, is readily absorbed when injected and has an effect much like an injection of morphine. Because horses that have received a procaine nerve block for limb injury have won a relatively high proportion of races, it has been claimed that these wins are the result of central stimulation by the drug. KUNDE and FREY [1971] tested this claim and found that procaine, the most frequently detected doping drug (see table 1.5. — 1), is hydrolyzed by cholinesterase much more slowly in the horse than in man. However, even allowing for the fact that Thoroughbreds are exceptionally sensitive to central stimulants, it does not appear that the usual range of anesthetic doses is sufficient to produce central effects. Furthermore, it must be considered that procaine may be present in medications with an entirely different indication, such as the antibiotic procaine penicillin, whose use would then be regarded as doping!

1.5.2.1.3. Analgesics

Analgesics are drugs that act centrally to reduce or abolish pain sensation, ideally without hampering other body functions when administered in therapeutic doses [HAUSCHILD, 1973]. The latter condition is seldom if ever satisfied, however (with the possible exception of cobra venom). Thus, HAUSCHILD has divided analgesics into two classes according to their accompanying effects: narcotic analgesics that have a euphoriant effect, and non-narcotic analgesics that exert an antipyretic and anti-inflammatory effect. The first class includes the morphine derivatives and drugs with related actions whose role as doping agents has already been discussed. The second class includes compounds that are highly diverse in their chemical structures. They can be subdivided into the following groups based mainly on chemical criteria:

1. salicylic acid, anthranilic acid and phenylacetic acid derivatives;
2. pyrazolon compounds;
3. aniline derivatives;
4. indene derivatives;
5. the quinine group;
6. quinoline and isoquinoline compounds;
7. aconitine and related alkaloids;
8. cobra venom;
9. the colchicines.

As with the local anesthetics, there are a great variety of analgesic compounds available, and new ones are marketed each year. Even more numerous are the pharmaceutical preparations that contain such substances and are available without a prescription in many countries. As a result, these drugs are often used by owners, trainers and attendants without veterinary consultation as a means of masking the symptoms of possibly dangerous infectious and traumatic conditions. This justifies their place on the list of prohibited drugs, quite apart from the central side-effects of these agents, such as sedation or stimulation, that alone would categorize them as true doping agents. It is not possible to describe all the compounds belonging to the class of analgesics. Most are unknown as doping agents, although presumably all could be used for that purpose by virtue of their pharmacologic actions. As examples, ALP and KALAYCI [1963] mention the pyrazolon derivatives aminopyrine, antipyrine and minopyrine, which in large doses produce an analeptic-like central excitation, and in toxic doses cause convulsions. The aniline derivative phenacetin (ethoxyacetanilide), which BERETTA mentions as a doping drug, causes euphoria in man in large doses, which occasionally leads to its abuse. This effect is accentuated by combining it with codeine and caffeine. Presumably, a similar stimulating effect would occur in horses. Salicylic acid and its derivatives are mentioned repeatedly in connection with doping. These compounds are still used in veterinary medicine for the symptomatic treatment of painful conditions of the muscles, tendons and joints and for fever. They have also been used for several years in the treatment of immune mediated diseases in man. These compounds act centrally to reduce fever, suppress inflammation and relieve pain. Reportedly their anti-inflammatory effect is achieved via the pituitary-adrenocortical system by a secretion of steroid hormones from the adrenal cortex. The following side-effects have been reported: respiratory stimulation to the point of hyperventilation with subsequent respiratory alkalosis, disturbance of the acid-base balance and, with prolonged use, gastrointestinal ulcers and hepatic and renal damage. Cellular oxygen consumption is increased, glycogen formation is reduced, and certain enzymes are inhibited (e.g. GOT, glutamic-oxaloacetic transaminase). The increase in uric acid excretion is exploited in the treatment of gout in man. Toxic doses of about 150—200 mg/kg produce a marked increase in respiration, nausea, fever and agitation. A comprehensive review of the literature and the pharmacologic effects of the salicylates can be found in SMITH and SMITH [1966], DAVISON and MANDEL [1965], as well as in textbooks or handbooks of pharmacology. According to studies by Schubert, salicylic acid in the horse is rapidly excreted in the urine. There is a 25 % return after 1 h, 40 % after 3 h, and 81 % after 12 h, although in acidic urine (e.g., after competition) the return would probably be smaller. The drug is converted in the body to various metabolites, regardless of species, which in turn show a similar pharmacologic activity (e.g., gentisic acid). In the horse, however, salicylic acid is for the most part excreted unchanged; only a small portion (up to 2 %) is excreted in the form of gentisic acid or its glucuronic acid conjugate. Salicylic acid esterified and etherified with glucuronic acid can also be demonstrated.

Another drug that is the subject of much controversy in connection with doping is phenylbutazone. It is likely that similar drugs will be developed in the near future that will become equally controversial. For a better understanding of the problems involved, therefore, we will examine more closely the mode of action of this class of drug, which includes oxyphenbutazone and indomethacin. Phenylbutazone (Butazolidin®, etc.) has the following chemical structure:

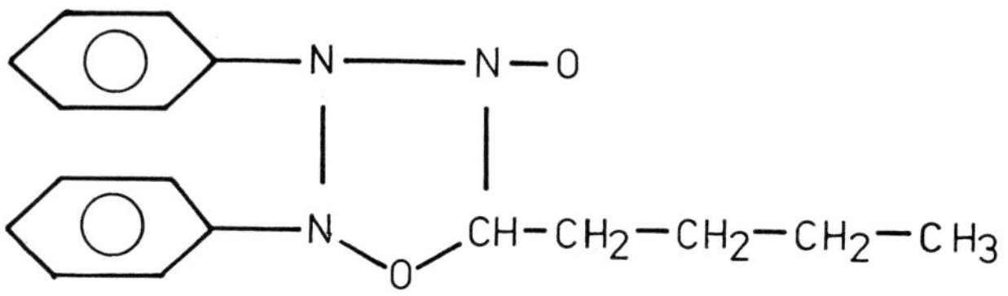

Phenylbutazone

Thus, phenylbutazone belongs to the group of pyrazolon derivatives. The compound is weakly acidic and reacts with alkalis to form highly water-soluble salts. Being more anti-inflammatory than analgesic in its action, it is often classed among the anti-inflammatory drugs. In humans its main therapeutic use is in the treatment of rheumatic diseases and gout. Its effect is mainly symptomatic, however, since the disease process itself is generally unaltered. In addition to its anti-inflammatory action, which is expressed in a great many disease processes [Rechenberg, 1961], phenylbutazone is also effective against anaphylactic reactions and histamine induced shock. Its analgesic effect, while long doubtful on the basis of negative clinical findings, has now been confirmed beyond question in human and animal studies. It also causes a marked increase in uric acid excretion, making it useful in the treatment of gout.

A number of harmful side-effects contraindicate the long-term use of phenylbutazone; they also add weight to its inclusion among the doping drugs. For example, its effects on the renal tubule epithelium as well as certain central effects lead to a reduction in the excretion of water, sodium ions and chloride ions, causing water retention in the tissues. The excretion of certain other substances, such as sulfonamides, is also reduced. Effects on the heart and peripheral blood vessels lead to a slight fall of blood pressure. In the digestive tract there is a decrease in intestinal motility and damage to the gastric mucosa that predisposes to ulceration. Animal studies on long-term Butazolidin use showed the presence of degenerative liver changes. In the thyroid gland, the suppression of oxidative processes leads to an inhibition of iodine utilization and thus to a decline in endocrine activity, causing hyperplasia of the glandular tissue. Blood changes are manifested in an inhibition of coagulation as a result of vitamin K antagonism. Susceptible individuals develop an agranulocytosis that apparently results from bone marrow depression. The mild effects of phenylbutazone on the nervous system are noteworthy in terms of its classification as a doping drug. In humans it produces euphoria and heightened nervous excitability even in therapeutic doses. Larger doses cause extreme stimulation and tremor in humans and animals. These effects are one reason why phenylbutazone, like procaine, has been placed on the list of doping drugs and should be replaced with anti-inflammatory agents that are free of such side-effects.

Phenylbutazone is absorbed well orally, and maximum blood levels are reached in 2 h. On intramuscular injection (which may be irritant) it is absorbed less well. A small amount is excreted in the urine unchanged and in the form of two variously hydroxylated metabolites [BURNS et al., 1953]. SCHUBERT [1967] investigated its metabolism in the horse after oral and intramuscular administration. In both cases unchanged drug and the two hydroxylated metabolites were detected in the urine no sooner than 3 h after administration. After the oral ingestion of 10 g of the drug, a concentration of 30 mg/100 ml urine was found after 5 h and 1 mg/100 ml urine after 48 h.

In the search for compounds with similar actions to phenylbutazone, one drug from the series of indene derivatives, indomethacin, was found to be highly effective and has been used therapeutically since 1965. It is an excellent anti-inflammatory agent with good analgesic and antipyretic properties. Its anti-inflammatory action is not unlike that of cortisone, with which it can be combined to good effect. It is also absorbed well orally and is mainly bound to plasma proteins. Within 2 days, about 50% of the dose is excreted in the urine, partly as glucuronide. The rest appears unchanged in the stool. Small amounts are broken down in the liver to O-demethyl- and N-dechlorobenzoyl derivatives [HAUSCHILD, 1973]. The principal side-effects are gastrointestinal lesions (ulcerations, etc.) with prolonged use. Indomethacin, like phenylbutazone, has been conditionally approved by the F.E.I. for competitive use.

1.5.2.1.4. Vitamins, Nutrients and Hormones

Vitamins and Other Nutrients. While it is generally agreed that the administration of exogenous substances other than certain therapeutic agents constitutes doping, opinions still vary concerning the use of vitamins, hormones and food supplements. Although hormones are not on the F.E.I. list of prohibited drugs, they nevertheless are not widely used for performance enhancement due to uncertainties with regard to side-effects. The use of hormones to suppress the sex drive of horses prior to competition is a form of manipulation of 'natural modes of behavior' and so must be considered doping on the basis of our working definition.

Interest in the nutrition of competitive athletes and show horses has increased greatly in recent decades. One result of this has been an increasing reliance on vitamins and 'special diets' for the purpose of performance enhancement. For centuries horse owners and attendants have employed a great variety of 'secret' feeding rules and recipes in an effort to boost the performance ability of their animals. This is still done today by adding nutrients such as protein, carbohydrates, trace elements and vitamins to the equine ration. This naturally raises the question of whether such a thing as 'nutritional doping' actually exists, and if so, which nutrients can be considered potential doping agents. In adressing these questions, it must be stated that to date there is no proof that natural feedstuffs such as hay, roots, grasses or by-products such as bran, yeasts and oil meals can affect the natural performance barriers shown in figure 1.5. — 2 and thus exert a doping effect. It is conceivable, of course, that certain species of plants or parts of plants having a high concentration of specific drugs may be incorporated into the ration, causing prohibited substances to be ingested via the feed. Thus, alcohol can be given in the form of beer or fermented grain mash, and caffeine in the form of green coffee beans or unfermented green tea leaves or their byproducts. Another practice that was common, was to feed any of a number of green or dried drugs and toxic plants such as coca leaves, kola nuts, pieces of opium oil cake, etc. as a vehicle for administering alkaloids that affect performance. In theory, then, the doping of horses could be accomplished by feeding. However, there are certain factors which set strict natural limits to such a practice. One is the horse's highly refined sense of taste and smell, which prompts it to reject feeds containing material with a strong, unfamiliar taste or odor. Another is the fact that the drug content of these plants is subject to large natural variations, making accurate dosing extremely difficult. Thus, doping by this method can hardly be considered practical.

The situation is different concerning the use of mixed or premixed vitamin and mineral supplements. These mixtures, which are classified as feedstuffs according to law, are available on the market in numerous forms. Besides pure vitamins, minerals and trace elements, they may also contain various drugs such as antibiotics. Unless these supplements have been specially formulated for specific therapeutic purposes, their drug content is generally much too small for doping purposes. However, it must be understood that when supplements containing antibiotics are given to racehorses, these drugs may enter the body fluids in detectable levels. A subsequent saliva or urine test under these circumstances might furnish grounds for disqualification. For this reason such supplements should be excluded from the horse's diet, particularly since these substances are not present in sufficient concentration to have much effect in the mature horse. Even the excessive use of drug-free supplements can provide a level of vitamin and mineral intake that might constitute doping as we have defined it. With the exception of vitamin B_1, however, no vitamin or trace element is known with certainty to have metabolic effects that could abolish physiologic performance limits and thus exert a doping effect (unless their toxic properties are exploited to cause a horse to lose). As long as essential nutrients such as amino acids, fatty acids, vitamins, minerals and trace elements are given to maintain health and ensure maximum physiologic performance ability during extreme physical and mental exertion, their use cannot be considered doping. The mode of administration is of no importance in this regard. An example is the use of vitamin B_{12}, which is some 30—50 times more active parenterally than orally. It is often claimed that racehorses suffer from anemia, because their serum erythrocyte and hemoglobin levels increase in response to vitamin B_{12} administration [Steel and Whitlock, 1960; Pade, 1972]. Consequently this vitamin is commonly used by trainers. It is usually given in conjunction with vitamin E, especially in countries with hot climates. The effect of vitamin B_{12} corresponds roughly to the increase in hemoglobin associated with prolonged exposure to high altitudes or 'high-altitude training'. An optimum protein and iron supply are important components of this effect. According to Steel and Whitlock [1960], who performed extensive hematologic studies in horses, the hemoglobin level of continuously stabled horses can also be raised by treatment with iron alone. The increase in erythrocyte count and hemoglobin level that occurs under the influence of vitamins and trace elements, and the associated improvement in the physiologic response to exertion, could not be construed as doping even in the strictest sense of the term. The same applies to large doses of vitamin E, vitamin C and selenium, which have proved beneficial in cases of prolonged exertion where an oxygen deficit in the muscles has resulted in cell membrane damage from increased peroxide formation. As long as the release of muscle-specific enzymes into the blood can be reduced by the use of these substances, their function is one of maintaining the integrity of the organism, which can hardly be equated with doping. Older horses respond particularly well to large vitamin E doses of at least 2 IU/kg body wt., for oxygen diffusion into the tissues and the muscular myoglobin content tend to decrease with age.

Vitamin E in the dose indicated will improve oxygen utilization and possibly prevent anhidrosis, a serious handicap for Thoroughbreds in hot climates [ZINTZEN, 1977].

The question of what constitutes an 'excessive' dose is of interest. Because the exact vitamin and mineral requirements during extreme physical and mental exertion have not yet been established with certainty, it cannot be determined conclusively whether a vitamin or mineral dose that maintains health in high-performance animals is excessive or not. This question can be answered, however, if it is shown that large vitamin doses promote metabolic processes to the extent that autonomically protected performance barriers are broken down, to the detriment of health. A case in point is the use of vitamin B_{12} (aneurin, thiamine). In doses of 1 g per animal per day, this vitamin exerts a *tranquilizing effect* that is most obvious in nervous animals. This could be interpreted as doping by behavior manipulation. On the other hand, this effect could also be interpreted in terms of nutritional physiology, inasmuch as the vitamin performs a neurotransmitter function in the body. However, the apparently positive nutritional role of thiamine is in strong contrast to its digitalis-like effect in extremely large doses of 1—2 g i.m. or i.v. per animal per day [MACKAY, 1961]. According to ARIES [1964], the vitamin acts in these doses as a cholinesterase inhibitor, thus accounting for its cardiac effects as a result of parasympathetic stimulation. Such large doses of vitamin B_1 may rightly be considered doping, especially since it is active in this form only when administered parenterally. Normally a concentration of 2 mg thiamine per kg ration dry matter is sufficient to protect against deficiency symptoms. It is further reported that larger doses, especially when given intravenously, can interfere with the detection of true doping drugs. For this reason vitamin B_{12} has been on the F.E.I. list of prohibited substances since 1977. Thiamine is a relatively common doping drug in the U.S., according to LOEW and BETTANY [1973]. These authors obtained data on blood thiamine concentrations in 98 horses on farms and racetracks that could serve as baseline values for studies on thiamine doping. Under normal feeding conditions stallions had a concentration of $2.25 \pm 0.16\,\mu g$ thiamine/100 ml blood, geldings 3.03 ± 0.13, and mares $3.36 \pm 0.11\,\mu g$. Animals 4 years old or less had lower values than animals 5—20 years old.

The use of vitamin K may also be interpreted as doping when given for the treatment of epistaxis. Epistaxis in racing horses is especially common after extreme exertion. It was once thought to be based on a deficiency of parafibrinogen in the blood, which theoretically could be corrected with coagulants such as vitamin K_1. There should be no objection to treatment of this nature, unless it is interpreted as a manipulation of the normal or current physiologic state of the animal, which normally would prevent it from starting. Here is an instance where medicating the racehorse for therapeutic purposes might constitute doping. The present case is further complicated by the fact that a genetic predisposition has often been implicated in epistaxis [WIESNER and WILLER, 1974]. Hence, coagulant therapy in this case might be interpreted as the masking of a hereditary defect.

Other dietary measures that are occasionally interpreted as doping are the administration of *glucose* to provide easily mobilized energy reserves, as is done in human competitive athletics, and the alkalinization of the feed, e.g., with *sodium bicarbonate*, to prevent metabolic acidosis. The serum lactic acid level rises considerably during exertion. SEREN and VENTURINI [1972] found a rise from 2.06 to about 5.0—5.7 mmol/l blood in trotting horses that had covered a distance of 2 km. The glucose level of 3.64 mmol/l remained unchanged, however. Thus, the effect of oral glucose in the horse is obviously questionable. If it has any benefit at all, it can only be in connection with prolonged exertion, as during ride-offs or jump-offs in horse shows or during performance trials. The mobilization of energy reserves, like the dietary prophylaxis of metabolic acidosis, is considered a physiologic measure that has nothing to do with doping, for it merely supplies substrates as needed for naturally occurring metabolic processes.

Hormones is the term applied by STARLING in 1905 to substances that are formed in glands or endocrine tissues and are transported in the bloodstream to the target organ on which their specific effects are produced. They represent the active factors involved in the humoral regulation of growth, metabolism, reproduction, nervous function and specific modes of behavior. Since hormones are available in pure form, attempts have been made to utilize them to influence involuntary biological control processes in such a way that performance is increased. In this way characteristics that distinguish the 'naturally talented' athlete, such as growth, muscle mass, stamina, specific body weight, etc., can be produced or enhanced in individuals lacking these characteristics. In equestrian and animal sports in general, where 'talented' individuals are exclusively the product of rigorous breeding and optimum nutrition, the use of hormones and other doping drugs would eliminate natural performance ability as the most important selection trait. It would favor animals that responded best to medication in terms of growth, strength, speed, stamina, temperament, conduct, etc., i.e., that prospered best in an artificial environment of drugs and medicines. This contradicts both the principles of natural selection and those of animal breeding in general. For this reason, even more than in human athletics, the use of hormones and hormone-like compounds in animals should be scrupulously avoided both during growth and during the performance years.

The main hormones used to directly influence athletic performance are the *adrenal cortical hormones*, especially the glucocorticoids and adrenocorticotropic hormone (ACTH, corticotropin) [DE CORGANOFF and LE BARS, 1953; LÖCHEL, 1959; DERIVEAUX and LIEGEOIS, 1962; GUILLET, 1965; BERETTA, 1968]. ACTH acts by stimulating the synthesis and secretion of the glucocorticoids and so is similar to them in its end result. The hormones formed in the zona fasciculata of the adrenal cortex that act mainly on carbohydrate metabolism are cortisol and cortisone, which are derived chemically from the polycylic hydrocarbon pregnane. Various synthetic glucocorticoids have been developed which are more potent and in some cases longer-acting than the natural hormones. These include prednisone, triamcinolone and dexamethasone. They have a number of therapeutic indications [BEICKERT, 1968], including all types of rheumatic disease, allergic diseases, and certain types of shock. The main effects of these hormones are based on their marked anti-inflammatory properties and their activation of carbohydrate metabolism. This involves an increase of gluconeogenesis as well as glycogen formation in the liver. Glucose provides an important substrate for energy metabolism during strenuous exertion. Gluconeogenesis is associated with a rise in the activity of glucose-6-phosphatase and glycogen synthetase and an increased breakdown of protein, which is partially converted to glucose. The catabolic effect of these steroids on protein metabolism can lead to atrophy and degenerative changes in the muscles and to osteoporosis when they are used excessively or for prolonged periods. Osteoporosis is further promoted by the increase in phosphate and calcium excretion. Besides these main effects, the glucocorticoids also have slight sodium- and water-retaining properties and increase potassium excretion. Because sodium retention occurs principally in the extracellular space, edema may develop. Horses seem particularly susceptible to this side-effect. DE CORGANOFF and LE BARS [1953], for example, describe edema, oliguria and anorexia in horses treated with ACTH. Attempts to enhance performance with this hormone are based on experiments in mice and rats which showed a dramatic increase in swimming stamina under the influence of ACTH. DE CORGANOFF and LE BARS administered 1,000 IU of ACTH i.m. to horses to improve endurance and observed the aforementioned symptoms after 10 h. After the electrolyte balance was corrected (with potassium), the horses showed some performance improvement in a race. Similar experiments were conducted by Löchel [1959], who tested the effect of 250 and 500 IU ACTH on the racing performance of horses. He found that while speed could not be increased, endurance could be. Horses specialized for short-distance racing became effective long-distance runners under the influence of ACTH. This effect could be of benefit in horse shows and other disciplines in which winners are decided in grueling ride-offs or jump-offs. No adverse side-effects were observed in this experiment. Black, hairless skin areas about the size of a penny appeared on one horse 6 weeks after the test, but this was presumably caused by the presence of melanotropin as an impurity in the pituitary extract.

Because the blood levels of glucocorticoids are elevated in animals treated with ACTH or glucocorticoids, such treatment can be readily detected by a hormone assay. It should be noted that the Thoroughbred shows a diurnal variation in its blood levels of cortisone and corticosterone, with peak values occurring around 8.00 a.m. Seren and Venturini [1972] found a level of 4.6 μg cortisone + corticosterone/100 ml blood in trotters at this time. This rhythm is shifted by training, with maximum levels of about twice standard values occurring an hour or so after a workout.

Sex hormones have also been used to manipulate athletic ability in man and animals [Carniglia, 1946; Fobian and Saragota, 1961; Aries, 1965; Hettinger, 1965; Clarke and Clarke, 1962]. The sex hormones are steroid derivatives that are based on the same hydrocarbon framework as the adrenal cortical hormones. They are divided into three broad groups: estrogens, progestagens and androgens. Both estrogens and progestagens are formed in the ovary, and androgens in the testis. The naturally occurring estrogens are 17-β-estradiol, estrone and estriol. In addition various chemical derivatives of these compounds as well as numerous other structurally diverse compounds have been found to have estrogenic activity. Most notable are diethylstilbestrol from the stilbene series, and chlorotrianisene from the triarylethylene series, both of which have strong estrogenic properties, and whose actions can be prolonged by esterification with various organic acids. A number of estrogenic compounds also occur in forage plants [Wiesner, 1970].

Progestagens are hormones that assist in the maintenance of pregnancy. The naturally occurring progestagen, progesterone, is formed mainly in the corpus luteum. It is an important intermediate in the synthesis of all steroid hormones (including the adrenal cortical hormones), and so small amounts also occur in males and non-pregnant females. Besides preparing the endometrium for reception of the fertilized ovum, progestagens suppress gonadotropin secretion and thus ovulation. The progesterone molecule has been synthetically modified to produce more potent and longer-acting substances that are used mainly to retard menstruation in women. The most important of these are ethisterone (17-ethinyl testosterone), norethisterone, norethandrolone, lynestrenol and chlormadinone. The progestagens are combined with small doses of an estrogen, such as mestranol, to inhibit ovulation. In racetrack practice the progestagens are used to inhibit estrus in mares and fillies. The same purpose is served by androgens, the hormones responsible for masculinization. Thus, virilization can occur in women or female animals treated with these substances.

Of the endogenous androgens, testosterone or its active form dehydrotestosterone has the highest activity. Its breakdown products androsterone, androstenedione, etiocholanolone and androstanolone are less active. Besides its androgenic properties, testosterone also has a pronounced anabolic effect. The testosterone molecule can be modified to yield substances that are much more strongly anabolic than androgenic. Their anabolic action is expressed in a greater retention of nitrogen and minerals based on an increased protein biosynthesis. The result of this is a visible increase in muscle mass. This increase affects both the skeletal and cardiac muscles. However, opinions differ as to whether muscular strength, speed or stamina can be improved in this way in athletes that are already in excellent condition. HETTINGER [1965] was able to increase the rate of conditioning (i.e., the rate of strength increase during training) by a factor of 2 in human subjects treated with testosterone. Only the untrained muscle groups showed an absolute strength increase. The circulatory response to exertion was also much improved, probably as a result of cardiac hypertrophy. It is doubtful that this represents a true performance gain in running and jumping events, because the muscular development is associated with a substantial increase in body weight, which places an additional burden on the circulation and musculature in endurance sports. Moreover, the muscular hypertrophy that occurs is based not on the formation of new muscle fibers, but on an increase in the caliber of existing muscle cells. This creates longer diffusion paths for the transport of nutrients and metabolites to and from the cells. Because capillary development in the muscle fibers cannot keep pace, prolonged exertion tends to create a nutrient and oxygen deficit with an intracellular accumulation of metabolites, leading to fatigue. A further disadvantage of the muscular hypertrophy is that there is no concomitant strengthening of the tendons and ligaments; this increases the risk of tendon ruptures and avulsions. The use of testosterone in younger athletes is particularly controversial, for it can cause premature epiphyseal closure with consequent growth retardation. According to experiments by RICHTER [1979], testosterone use in Thoroughbreds leads to a strong libido increase. Even mares become highly excited and attempt to mount other horses. As a result of this strong masculinization and associated state of excitation, the animals become difficult to ride or control, making performance trials impossible.

The use of the thyroid hormone thyroxine or triiodothyronine for body weight reduction is also mentioned in connection with doping [CARNIGLIA, 1946]. In addition, parathyroid hormone has been shown to have a muscle-activating effect both in isolated muscle and in vivo [GUILLET, 1965]. In practice, these hormone uses probably play little if any role in the doping of horses.

1.5.2.1.5. Psychotropic Drugs

For many years drug actions and side-effects have been known which influence affectivity, i.e., the ordered processing of sensory impressions, in man. Not until the 1950's have these effects been systematically researched and utilized in the treatment of psychotic states. These drugs include the antidepressants, and certain analeptics, as well as psychosedatives and neuroleptics, used to allay states of psychic tension such as aggressiveness, anxiety and extreme psychomotor activity as well as to relieve muscle spasms. In horses, performance is often hampered by nervousness and agitation, i.e., an exaggerated response to external stimuli. For this reason tranquilizing agents ordinarily used in human medicine have also been given to animals in an attempt to sedate them. Today this is most commonly done with psychotropic drugs, especially neuroleptics (= neuroplegics, antipsychotics, major tranquilizers) and psychosedatives (= tranquilizers, anxiolytics, ataractics). In man neuroleptics dull the affectivity and dynamics of psychic processes, while psychosedatives alleviate states of psychic tension and allay anxiety. Despite their varying sites of action, which are limited mainly to the CNS, both classes of drug produce sedation and manageability in animals. The response to external stimuli is reduced, yet the animal remains awake. This distinguishes these drugs from the classic sedatives, such as soporifics (barbiturates, bromides) and narcotics, and has caused them largely to supersede the barbiturates (table 1.5. — 1). In larger doses they cause apathy and a bluting of reflexes, and the animals can be driven or led only with considerable effort. Hence, the same drugs can be used for doping to lose.

Of the many psychotropic compounds known, only a few have found use as doping drugs. The principal neuroleptic in this regard is chlorpromazine (Propaphenin®, Megaphen®), a phenothiazine derivative. It is occasionally used in veterinary medicine to potentiate barbiturate anesthesia, but its main use is to sedate excited animals to make them easier to handle. The drug acts on various parts of the CNS, producing strong sedation with a feeling of fatigue, a reduction of drive and a decline in mental performance. In animals it inhibits the flight response, an important drive mechanism in the racehorse. Other effects are an inhibition of thermoregulation, leading to hypothermia, a good antiemetic effect, a decrease in striated muscle tone, mild diuresis and a fall of blood pressure. Owing to these effects, an excessive dose always causes a decline in athletic performance. Because the sense of balance is also impaired, the animal is more apt to fall, especially when taking a jump. Chlorpromazine is mostly used to sedate horses for transport. In this case the drug or its metabolites are detectable in the urine for up to 48 h [Schubert, 1967]. Horses appear to be quite sensitive to chlorpromazine. While in most species a dose of about 1 mg/kg is required for sedation (up to 10 mg/kg is needed in man), only 0.1—0.3 mg/kg (i.v.) is needed in the horse. Toxic effects in the form of tachycardia and hypotension appear in the horse at doses of 2—4 mg/kg. In one study the erythrocyte count was decreased after only 3 days' use [Martin and Beck, 1956]. Chlorpromazine is rapidly absorbed on oral or intramuscular administration but disappears relatively quickly from the blood (30 min) and accumulates in the brain. It is metabolized in the liver to yield a variety of end-products. A small amount is excreted unchanged by the kidneys and the metabolite can be detected in the urine for up to 72 hours at larger doses. Schubert [1967] administered 50, 100 and 150 mg chlorpromazine i.v. to a 500-kg horse. Sedation lasted one hour, but was observed only at the highest dose. The unchanged drug and 4 metabolites, including 2 sulfoxide derivatives, could be demonstrated in the urine by thin-layer chromatography. The concentration of the components ranged from 0.05 to 0.1 mg/100 ml urine for 3—8 h after administration.

Another phenothiazine derivative used for horse doping according to Steward [1972] is promazine (Sinophenin®, Verophen®). This has a weaker sedative action and stronger hypotensive action than chlorpromazine. Courtot et al. [1975] consider the azaphenothiazine acepromazine, to have a more potent sedative action. A dose of 0.2 mg/kg acepromazine (i.m.) in the racehorse produced a fall of the respiratory rate from depression of the central respiratory center, and a rise in serum creatine phosphokinase activity. The latter is interpreted as evidence of muscle damage. A decrease in the serum protein level is also observed. According to Courtot et al. [1975], acepromazine today, is the most widely used doping drug.

Tranquilizers are also used for the sedation of racing animals. Thus, Büscher [1972] cites Lübke's report that the well-known tranquilizer meprobamate is used in trotting races to prevent the horses from breaking into a gallop. This drug is well absorbed and is excreted in the urine both in free form and coupled to glucuronic acid. Besides its sedative effect, which is similar to that of barbiturates, it also acts as a voluntary muscle relaxant. Meprobamate is similar in action to the benzodiazepines. Bäumler et al. [1964a] describe the use of chlordiazepoxide (Radepur®, Librium®, also formerly known as methaminodiazepoxide) to sedate a racehorse that tended to shy and vear-off when it brushed other horses in the race. The dosage in this case was 500 mg daily for a week. The action of chlordiazepoxide can be considered intermediate between that of meprobamate and chlorpromazine [Hauschild, 1973]. Another benzodiazepine derivative, diazepam (Faustan®, Valium®, etc.), is described by Courtot et al. [1975a] as a doping drug of increasing importance. It is a psychosedative that also acts as a smooth-muscle relaxant. The authors tested the drug's effect on the circulation and metabolism. A dose of 0.1 mg/kg injected i.m. had no effect on the heart rate but caused a slight decrease in the respiratory rate (from 44 to 37 inspirations per minute). As in the case of acepromazine, a rise in the serum creatine phosphokinase activity is considered a sign of muscle damage caused by the drug. Another tranquilizer, belonging more to the class of hypnosedatives, is thalidomide (Contergan®, etc.). According to Büscher [1972], it has been used to sedate unruly Standardbreds, which subsequently were able to place for the first time.

1.5.2.1.6. Other Agents

As mentioned, alcohol, usually in the form of alcoholic beverages, has been used since ancient times as a means of improving the conduct and performance of horses. Vicious horses reportedly become more manageable when given alcohol, while timid horses lose their inhibitions and perform more aggressively. Even old rules of racing, like those in Prussia and Austria before World War I, had provisions regulating the use of alcohol. As early as 1904, Möller condemned the use of alcohol because it made it difficult to assess the true performance ability of a racehorse. Alcohol, which figures in many forms of sport, does not produce a true increase in performance ability, for it actually reduces muscular strength [Pfyl, 1923; Ulmark, 1963]. Because of its good lipid solubility, it has a marked effect on the CNS. Initially it paralyzes inhibitory mechanisms, creating a narcotic-like excitatory effect that can enhance overall performance. In addition, alcohol aids muscular recovery from exercise, thus increasing somewhat the stamina of fatigued muscles. In slightly larger doses it soon paralyzes the promotional functions of the CNS, resulting in severe performance impairment. Alcohol is absorbed well and rapidly, not only from the digestive tract but also through the skin. Thus, even washing or rubbing with alcohol ligaments can lead to absorptive effects.

Other possible doping agents are inorganic arsenic compounds, which have been both feared as poisons and utilized as tonics since ancient times. The Greek physician Dioskorides (circa 50 A.D.) for example used realgar (arsenic disulfide) as a fumigant for asthma, and the Arabian physician Abu Bekr El Razi (850—923) recommended arsenic for anemia, nervous disorders and skin diseases. Even today, inorganic arsenic compounds are used in human and veterinary medicine as tonics and antianemics, although their use is declining. There are various preparations for such purposes, such as 'pilulae asiaticae' (1 mg As_2O_3 in 30 mg pepper), Fowler's solution (1% potassium arsenite solution), or 'liquor kalii arsenicosi' (water-alcohol arsenic solution with lavender spirit). According to studies by Schwarz [1975], experimental animals become weak and feable if fed an arsenic-free diet. Arsenic supplements of 9.5 mg/kg ration dry matter lead to considerable gains in body weight; even on a normal diet rats show better physical development with an arsenic allowance of 0.1—0.2 mg. There is a tendency to regard arsenic as an essential trace element with a requirement of about 0.5 mg/kg ration dry matter. Since ancient times it has been known that such a dose will improve the nutritional state of the horse and give it a smooth, gleaming coat. Arsenic was sometimes given by horse dealers to older, emaciated horses, often fraudulently, to give them the temporary appearance of being well-nourished. According to Croisier [1948], arsenic is useful during training to accelerate conditioning, especially in trotters. As long as accurate arsenic allowance data for farm animals are lacking, such small arsenic supplements cannot be regarded as doping, but as diet supplementation. However, it must be borne in mind that larger doses of inorganic arsenic compounds are stored in the body and lead to chronic intoxication, e.g. by the blocking of sulfhydryl groups. Small arsenic supplementation of the ration can in no way produce the short-term performance gains characteristic of other doping drugs. This might be possible if arsenous acid or its salts were injected i.v., however. Small concentrations lead to transient vasodilation, especially of the splanchnic vessels, and thus to a fall in blood pressure. No such use of arsenic has yet been reported for doping, although vasodilators are occasionally used for this purpose [Schick, 1933; Löchel, 1959; Addis-Smith, 1961]. Vasodilation is favorable from a performance standpoint, for it improves the bloody supply to the muscles, thereby facilitating the delivery of oxygen and nutrients and the removal of metabolites. Because different vessels respond differently to these agents, there is often a dilatation of the cutaneous vessels and a fall of blood pressure, often with a simultaneous decrease in coronary blood flow, placing a considerable extra work load on the heart. According to Riens [1965], the death of a Danish cyclist during the 1960 Rome Olympics was the result of excessive load on the heart due to prior treatment with a vasodilating drug. In racing, organic nitrites and nitrates have been principally used [Sustmann, 1914]. Even in old doping formulas, nitroglycerin (glyceryl trinitrate, etc.) appears as an active ingredient. Taken sublingually, this drug acts within a few minutes, and its effects last for over an hour. Initially the cardiac blood flow is increased, but the subsequent fall in blood pressure decreases cardiac work while increasing the danger of collapse.

1.5.2.1.7. Gaseous Stimulants

A basic problem in extending the working capacity of the muscles is the tissue oxygen supply. The oxygen requirement of the muscles increases during maximal exertion by a factor of 20 to 30, or even more in many species. One gram of muscle tissue at rest consumes about 200 mm^3 oxygen. During strenuous exercise the requirement increases to 4,000 in man, 4,700 in the cat, and as much as 20,000 in the mouse. This has led to attempts to improve performance by ventilating with pure oxygen or by administering oxygen intravascularly. Croisier [1948] reports that intravenous oxygen restores overweight racehorses to competitive form! Intravascular oxygen insufflation improves the oxygen supply and, like the insufflation of inert gases such as nitrogen or noble gases, causes an initial vasoconstriction that is followed by persistent dilatation; it also stimulates respiratory activity [Hauschild, 1973]. The oxygen supply can also be improved by increasing the oxygen partial pressure in the inspiratory air. Under normal circumstances, i.e., at an oxygen partial pressure of 20 vol.% O_2, about 0.4 ml of oxygen is dissolved in the plasma of 100 ml blood, and 19—20 ml are bound to hemoglobin. When pure oxygen is breathed, the amount of dissolved oxygen increases to 2 ml, while the quantity of hemoglobin-bound oxygen remains practically unchanged. Intravenous oxygen administration is not without its dangers. The intravascular insufflation of gas carries a risk of central, peripheral or pulmonary gas embolism. Pure oxygen ventilation can lead to symptoms of oxygen intoxication after 3 to 4 h, or even sooner if the gas is delivered under pressure.

These symptoms include sweating, bradycardia, nausea, muscular tremor, drowsiness, dyspnea and vertigo. Consequently the F.E.I. has prohibited the inhalation of oxygen or oxygen-enriched mixtures during competition. By extension, this rule also applies to the intravascular administration of gases.

1.5.2.1.8. Physical Agents and Methods

Pain produces anxiety in the horse, thus triggering a flight response which drives the animal to maximal exertion. This fact has prompted many owners, trainers and riders to develop various methods and devices for subjecting their horses to a painful stimulus that will urge it on at the right moment. The use of spurs, which is now prohibited in most racing rules, is a well-known example. SUSTMANN [1914] mentions many such practices. One method is to place sharp objects such as needles, nails, pins or even bullets and nuts beneath the saddle, thus creating a painful irritation that sends the animal into a frenzy. However, this can cause bleeding and swelling that is difficult to conceal. Another method is to attach phonograph needles to the heels of the riding boots in place of spurs. In running races jockeys' whips may be reinforced with lead or steel inserts, while in trotting races the driver may use a whip with a spur wheel or sharp nail attached. A bite on the ear is also included among the pain-provoking methods. Animals react very strongly to electrical stimuli. Hence, electric current has been used for many years as a method of horse doping. As mentioned earlier, the only doping case that has thus far come to trial in the German racing industry involved the use of electric current. In this case a battery was strapped to the horse. The current can be transmitted in a variety of ways, e.g., through the shafts of the sulky, by contacts on the saddle or jockey's boots, or through the driver's or jockey's whip. To produce the desired degree of fear as well as pain, the electrodes are placed such that they will deliver shocks to larger nerve areas in the skin and subcutaneous tissue (e.g., the sacral region). The use of cold, according to CARNIGLIA [1946] and CROISIER [1948], should also be considered doping. For example, ice packs might be applied to sore joints and tendons before a race.

The use of UV radiation and psychological methods such as hypnosis, which have been discussed as doping in human athletics [HETTINGER, 1965; SCHÖNHOLZER, 1965], are presumably of no importance in horse racing.

Not all agents and methods mentioned so far in connection with doping are prohibited by racing authorities. For clarity, we shall conclude our discussion of doping agents by presenting the currently valid list of prohibited substances issued in 1977 by the F.E.I. It should be noted that this list has been or may yet be expanded by national racing bodies, as in the case of West Germany, where phenylbutazone is now unconditionally banned. If the use of a medicament is necessary prior to an event, it is strongly recommended that the current rules on doping be read before any medication is given.

List of Prohibited Substances for 1977, published in the F.E.I. Newsletter, No. 1 (1977) 13:

Antibiotics, such as procaine penicillin, etc.

Antidepressants, such as imipramine, methapyrilene, etc.

Antihistamines, such as chloroquine, quinine, etc.

Antipyretics and analgesics other than phenylbutazone and indomethacin.

Phenylbutazone and indomethacin are prohibited in dressage and championship events; they are *not prohibited* in events of other disciplines at the present time.

Central stimulants, such as amphetamine, methylphenidate, etc.

Hypnotics and sedatives, such as barbital, chlorbutol, etc.

Local anesthetics, such as procaine, lignocaine, etc.

Masking agents, such as polyethylene glycol, excessive amounts of thiamine, etc.
Muscle relaxants, such as mephenesin, methocarbamol, etc.
Narcotic analgesics, such as morphine, pethidine, etc.
Oxygen and gas mixtures, inhalation during competition.
Parasympatholytic drugs, such as atropine, scopolamine, etc.
Plant alkaloids, such as berberine, strychnine, etc.
Respiratory stimulants, such as nicetamide, leptazol, etc.
Sympathomimetic drugs, such as ephedrine, methoxamine, etc.
Tranquilizers, such as chlorpromazine, promazine, etc.
Xanthines, such as caffeine, theobromine, etc.
Any other substances that are capable of influencing unfairly the competitive condition of a horse.

1.5.2.2. Methods of Doping to Lose

In principle, the same drugs used to help a horse to win can also be used to hamper its performance ability, simply by administering them in larger doses. In this form of doping, timing and dosage are not so critical as in doping to win. For example, a large dose of chlorpromazine can render a horse unable to race for several days. Drugs that exert a central sedative or paralytic effect, such as narcotics, hypnotics, psychotropic drugs or antihistamines with a sedative action, are most widely used [Morgan, 1958; Löchel, 1959; Addis-Smith, 1961; Aries, 1964; Nicholson, 1968]. Büscher [1972] cites a report by Lübke, who found typical symptoms of tranquilizer medication in poorly racing trotters, such as prolapse of the nictating membrane, a drowsy gaze, penile prolapse, slight anal flaccidity, etc. Lübke's findings suggest that doping to lose is carried out less carefully when done as an 'outside job', and the necessarily large drug doses cause marked symptoms to appear in most cases. As an 'inside job', of course, it can be done with far greater care so that clinical symptoms are not always apparent. It is possible in such cases to employ other methods, such as sleep deprivation or continual arousal, that are difficult or impossible to detect. Harmful dietary adjustments can be carried out only by persons entrusted with the direct care and supervision of the animal. Such practices include starving followed by overfeeding prior to a race, or withholding water and then watering to excess, as well as the use of laxatives. According to Addis-Smith, excessive water intake can cause symptoms such as stupor and unsteady gait.

One substance whose effect may appear long after its discontinuance is arsenic. Daily doses of 1 g of arsenous acid over a period of several weeks will result in obvious physical deterioration only after a long period of time.

The most important of the soporific drugs are the barbiturates, which are contained in a large variety of sleeping pills and tranquilizers [Cluver, 1952; Nicholson, 1968]. Also important, however, are the classical hypnotics and sedatives, some of which were mentioned as early as 1914 by Sustmann, such as chloral hydrate, chlorbutol, paraldehyde and bromides. Sustmann further mentions the use of alcohol, ether and amyl nitrite, as well as inhalants such as iodoform vapors, prussic acid, ammonia and lavender fumigants. It is also reported that the excitability of nerves can be temporarily depressed by the subcutaneous injection of distilled water.

Other known negative doping agents are morphine-like drugs such as methadone [Beretta, 1968] and pethidine [Bouckaert and Debackere, 1965], the well-known neuroleptic reserpine from the group of *Rauwolfia* alkaloids [Aries, 1964], and chlorpromazine, whose action is similar to that of reserpine.

Several symptoms that suggest that a horse has been doped to lose have already been mentioned. Other signs at race time are: the presence of a strong odor; dullness of behavior; a forced, stilted gait; a lively gait without gain of ground. The animals appear unable to make progress. After the race the animals appear especially depressed or may even look ill. The mucous membranes are pale or cyanotic, the respiratory and heart rate are altered, and the body temperature may be elevated or subnormal. Delayed symptoms often include work fatigue and lack of appetite.

A further important aspect of negative doping was revealed by LÖCHEL's experiments with sodium bromide. He found that a dose of 150 g 4 times a day impaired the performance of a racehorse to the extent that it lost to opponents it otherwise would have beaten. One horse stumbled and even fell during the race. This form of doping, then, not only weakens the animal that has been drugged, but also endangers the jockey and represents a serious hindrance and danger to the other competitors. Thus, the danger of injury associated with doping to lose, as well as doping to win, is yet another important reason for controlling doping in all it forms.

1.5.3. Doping Control

There are a great many reasons for prohibiting doping. The fraudulent use of drugs not only endangers the health of the animal, but also jeopardizes the rider or driver as well as other competitors in the event. Doping should also be banned on the grounds of animal cruelty. Horseracing is strongly dependent on the betting public for its livelihood. Doping not only robs favorites of winning chances, it also cheats thousands of racing fans out of winnings to which they are rightfully entitled. If these racegoers were to stay away from the tracks, it would mean staggering economic losses for the racing industry. Finally, doping is repugnant on moral and ethical grounds, considering that a fairly conducted sports competition is of substantial educational and formative value.

There is ample cause to take measures against the practice of doping. Anti-doping paragraphs are contained in the charters as well as the rules for racing and performance testing of most of the world's racing organizations. In addition, doping constitutes fraud [BAARS, 1926], thus making it a criminal offense. It may also be punishable on grounds of animal cruelty, which is likewise a crime in many countries. All bans and prohibitions are useless unless it is possible to verify their compliance. After the introduction of the Frankel saliva test, the history of doping has demonstrated that systematic testing is the only reliable means of control in both the U.S. and Europe. In turn, this requires accurate methods of detection. Owing to dramatic advances in analytical chemistry during the last two decades, it is now possible, at least in principle, to determine the nature and quantity of nearly any foreign substance present in a suitable biological substrate. Moreover, analysis is greatly simplified when there is evidence as to the occurrence of doping and the type of agent that has been used.

Various precautions can be taken against doping, one being adequate supervision of the horses for 3 to 4 h before race time. Most stimulants must be given 2 to 3 h before a race in order to have the desired effect. Thus, the use of gathering rooms in which the horses are put under official supervision for up to 4 h before race time would in itself significantly reduce the prevalence of doping. Of course, drugs for negative doping can be administered much earlier — as much as 1—2 days before the race in some cases. This is why trainers should take great care to ensure that their horses are closely attended both during transport and in their stalls.

Methods of Doping Detection

Clinical Examination. A careful examination of the animal before race time can be of great value in the detection of doping [MORGAN, 1958; FARELLY, 1961]. The racetrack veterinarian or veterinary commission plays an important role in doping control. He should have the responsibility not only of examining the horses before a race (twice if possible so that behavioral changes can be better recognized), but also of advising stewards in the selection of horses to be tested. He should also have a role in the collection of specimens and in the careful clinical examination of suspected horses.

Dopers know their horses and their reactions to doping drugs very well. Thus, one cannot except doped animals to display obvious clinical symptoms. This has been confirmed by authors, such as SCHWIEGER [1936], MARES [1958] and GUILETT [1965]. Because many drugs have side-effects that produce certain symptoms, for example mydriasis the animal's response to the drug will depend on its condition at that particular moment. In addition errors in dosage or timing may have been made that will often produce telltale signs of doping. Changes in the natural rhythm of movements or abnormalities of gait, point to the use of stimulants or sedatives, although a variety of symptoms can occur, as pointed out by numerous authors [SUSTMANN, 1914; PFYL, 1923; NEUMANN-KLEINPAUL and RÜSCHER, 1931; SCHICK, 1933; CROISIER, 1948; DIECKMANN, 1951; BOUCHARD, 1954; MARTIN and BECK, 1956; LÖCHEL, 1959; MARES, 1958; GABRIEL et al., 1963; BÜSCHER, 1972]. Some typical symptoms include superficial signs of injection, such as swelling or localized sweating; an uneven, tripping or plodding gait; exaggerated leg actions; bucking; rearing; bolting; marked shying; excitement; heightened or depressed reflex excitability; unrest; and tremor or marked calm. They can also include profuse sweating; licking; drooling or foaming at the mouth; exaggerated chewing movements; teeth grinding; dry lips and mouth; fixed gaze; mydriasis, miosis or eyeground changes; changes in heart or respiratory rate; abnormally shallow or deep respiration; and temperature elevation or reduction. Behavior changes on the other hand may be brought on by the unfamiliar environment of the racetrack (noise, music, strange smells) as well as the presence of strange persons and horses. Thus, a horse's characteristics must be known before behavioral changes can be accurately assessed. The clinical examination is seldom adequate to prove that a horse has been doped. This opinion is shared by practically all the authors cited above. Certain symptoms provide grounds for suspicion, which then should be reported to the stewards. As a rule, final proof comes only with the detection of a doping substance in the animal or its excretions. Traditionally, biologic tests have been employed for this purpose. Such tests can indeed show the presence of physiologically active substances in some cases, but they rarely permit the drug to be identified, and only a handful of the many doping agents used can be detected in this way. In addition, only a limited amount of material is available for examination, and this must suffice for the definitive chemical analysis. Thus, biological tests must be considered unsuitable even as screening procedures.

Chemical Drug Detection. Legally correct chemical analysis will depend on the selection of the examination material and the precision with which the samples are collected, labeled, sealed and sent to the laboratory.

Doping drugs may be detected by the analysis of blood, sweat, saliva, urine, as well as organ samples taken from animals that have died on the track or had to be destroyed. In the latter case the gastrointestinal contents, urine, kidneys, liver and brain should be removed for laboratory examination. Some body fluids are considered more suitable for chemical analysis than others.

A doping drug can be eliminated from the blood relatively quickly. It is usually present in low concentration and is detectable for only a limited time. Binding of the drug to protein makes it difficult to extract, and the protein-rich blood is a relatively difficult material for analysis. In addition, the drawing of blood samples, which generally requires the owner's consent, is not entirely without risks. Anticoagulants such as citrate or fluoride should be added to the blood to facilitate handling. Heparin is less suitable, because it usually contains organic preservatives that cause foreign reactions.

Sweat is relatively easy to obtain but is available only in a limited amount. The passage of drugs or their metabolites into the sweat has not been investigated in detail, though presumably it is similar to that in the saliva. Sweat may contain impurities from the environment such as dust, tobacco smoke or disinfectants, which can interfere with the analysis or interpretation of results. Therefore, sweat should not be taken from the area beneath the saddle. The sample is collected with a plastic scraper, pad or cotton glove.

At one time saliva was the examination material of choice, and numerous 'positives' were reported in saliva drug tests [Lander, 1930]. Although this substrate offers no significant advantages over urine, many analysts still prefer it over other body fluids. As a rule, the same drugs enter the saliva that enter the blood, and, conversely, they cease to occur in saliva once they are eliminated from the blood. Sometimes, however, the passage of a drug into the salive is inhibited, resulting in far lower concentrations than in the plasma. The secretion of drugs with the saliva in horses was investigated by Alexander et al. [1967]. They discovered that non-ionizing substances occur in approximately equal concentrations in the saliva and plasma in free form. However, the plasma-saliva barrier is more difficult to overcome when the drug is present in ionized form. In this case the drug is detectable in the saliva for only a short time and in low concentration [Moss, 1970]. An example is chloral hydrate, which is very rapidly metabolized to trichloroacetic acid and trichloroethanol. Only trichloroethanol occurs equally in the saliva and plasma, whereas little if any trichloroacetic acid is detectable in the saliva. These recent findings cast doubt on the universal value of saliva drug excretion tests. It is not surprising that more positives have been declared in urine tests than in saliva tests, even though the latter are more frequently performed [Moss, 1970]. Saliva has other disadvantages as well, including its limited availability, its contamination with impurities from food residues, and the difficulty of collection.

Various techniques have been developed for the collection of saliva samples. The horse is first led into the clinic or treatment room of the racetrack. Many racetracks such as in France for example even have a special room for this purpose. In most countries the inside of the mouth and area behind the tongue are swabbed with gauze pads held with a special forceps [Morgan, 1958] or long dressing forceps. Dripping saliva is caught in a glass jar. Often the horse is first made to chew on gauze swabs soaked in a 1% acetic acid solution. This solution serves to stimulate salivation, as does massage of the parotid duct. The pilocarpine injection recommended by Löchel [1959] would appear to complicate matters, for it involves the introduction of a doping drug and necessitates additional separations. If the oral cavity is dry, pads moistened with distilled water or 1% acetic acid can be used for swabbing. Instead of gauze or cotton pads, saliva can also be collected with clean viscose sponges, which make washout easier. Another method, used in Switzerland [Bäumler et al., 1964] and the GDR, is to rub the surface of the tongue and anterior oral membranes with a cotton glove. A pad held with a dressing forceps is used to swab the deeper oral membranes and retrolingual area. The pad and glove are soaked in 1% acetic acid.

All drugs used for doping are excreted in the urine to some degree, where they are detectable at or shortly after the time of peak effect. One difficulty is that only a small portion of some drugs is excreted in the urine unchanged, the greater portion being excreted in the form of metabolites, some of which are still unknown. This may make the results difficult to interpret. Many drugs or metabolites form esters or ethers with sulfuric acid or glucuronic acid and thus are excreted in a highly water-soluble form that cannot be extracted with organic solvents. This presents little problem because the unpaired substances can be separated and then hydrolyzed with acids or alkalis, enabling them to be extracted and detected. The pharmacokinetics of new drugs generally must be well investigated before they are approved for marketing, and so data on excretory metabolites are usually available. It should be noted, of course, that the urine also contains porphyrins, vitamins, hormones, as well as food constituents such as phenols and aromatic acids (benzoic acid, salicylic acid) that sometimes can make interpretation difficult. Generally, analysts have had experience with physiologic metabolites that no longer pose serious problems in urinanalysis. One factor that must be considered, is the pH of the urine sample. After prolonged exertion, the normally alkaline urine of the horse acquires a more acidic pH. As a result, alkaline substances are excreted in the urine in greater quantity, and acidic substances less so, than under resting conditions. An important advantage of the urinanalysis is that doping drugs can still be detected in the urine even after they have disappeared from the blood and saliva. Moreover, urine can usually be collected in greater amounts than other body fluids. Collection is relatively simple but may require much time and patience. For obvious reasons the animal cannot be catheterized, the urine must be caught during spontaneous micturition. This is done with unbreakable plastic or metal vessels, which are held in place beneath the horse with a suitable apparatus. According to HUTSON [1966] and MORGAN [1958], 90% of horses void urine within 90 min after racing, and 99% within 3 h. This is the time period that the official sampler must wait in some U.S. States, though longer periods are prescribed when warranted. Urine can usually be obtained in only 6—8 minutes once the animal has been returned to the familiar environment of its stall [BÜSCHER, 1972]. At least 200 ml of urine should be submitted for analysis, although it is wise to collect as much as possible. This will broaden the possibilities for analysis while providing a residual sample for security or perhaps for reanalysis if the original findings are contested.

Because a positive finding can have considerable moral, disciplinary and legal implications, the veterinarian, who is usually responsible for the sample collection, must proceed with sufficient care to rule out all possibility of error. All apparatus and vessels used must be analytically clean. Sterilization is not neccessary for this. Even unused pads and solutions should be sent to the lab for comparison purposes. The samples should be collected in the presence of a witness, preferably an official, and placed in unbreakable vessels that are securely closed and sealed and clearly and indelibly labeled. Care should be taken to ensure that the horse presented for sample collection is the same one that was previously selected. Sampling must be followed by a thorough clinical examination. A careful record should be kept of the sampling and examination procedure. It should include the name of the owner, a description of the horse, the nature and quantity of the specimen, the time at which the specimen was taken, as well as clinical findings. This record should be signed by the owner or his representative, the stewards and the racetrack veterinarian. Printed forms for such records are usually supplied by the stewards. The veterinarian must understand that the procedure for sample collection is not ordinarily a matter of individual judgment. Racing or track rules usually prescribe the manner in which the sampling must be done, as well as the nature and quantity of the material to be obtained. In the GDR, for example, the standard procedure is to collect sweat, saliva and 10 ml of blood from the jugular vein. Samples are dispatched to the laboratory by courier if possible.

Chemical Analysis. When the sample arrives at the laboratory, the first step is to record the sample and check the seals and labels to make sure they are intact. After a brief gross examination, the sample material is weighed for analysis. The first analytical step is to isolate the unknown substance from the complex biological substrate. This can be done by distillation or by selective adsorption on exchange resins. The method of choice, however, is extraction with organic solvents. This process exploits the acidic, neutral or basic properties of the unknown substances as well as their solubility in organic solvents. The isolation effect depends essentially on the equilibrium distribution of the substance between the organic and aqueous phase, which is expressed in the 'distribution coefficient'. This means that a substance that is, say, 10 times more soluble in an organic solvent than in water will be present in the solvent extract in a 10 times greater amount than in the aqueous extract if the volumes of both fluids are equal. The distribution coefficient (D) expresses the ratio of the concentration of the doping drug (dr) in the organic and the aqueous phase:

$$D = \frac{c_{dr} \text{ org. phase}}{c_{dr} \text{ aq. phase}} \quad (c = \text{concentration}).$$

The distribution coefficient in the previous example would be 10 (cf. fig. 1.5. — 3). For the near-complete isolation of the substance with a relatively low distribution coefficient, an excess of solvent is used, and the extraction is repeated several times. In the example, the organic phase would contain 99.9% of the unknown after 3 extractions. When solubility conditions are reversed, water can also be used to isolate the substance. By the repeated redistribution of extracts between the aqueous and organic phases, the extracts can be purified, and the foreign substances can be separated into groups according to their ionization properties or behavior in solution. As a general rule, ionized compounds are more soluble in the aqueous phase, while neutral or nonionized compounds pass more easily into the organic phase. Thus, materials with an acidic reaction dissociate readily in alkaline media, while those with an alkaline reaction are ionized in acid solutions. This effect is illustrated in figure 1.5. — 3.

Building on these principles, Stass and Otto developed a separation process for forensic analysis that was used mainly to detect alkaloids in biological material. This extraction and separation process is still used today in essence, though many modifications have evolved. The principles of such a process are shown diagrammatically in figure 1.5. — 4.

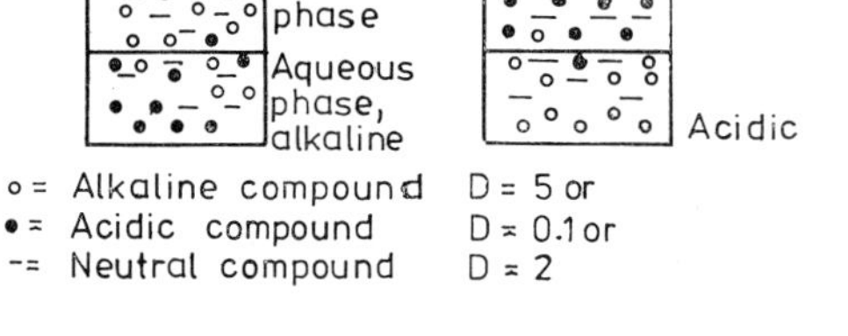

Fig. 1.5. — 3. Distribution of a drug between the aqueous and organic phases as a function of pH.

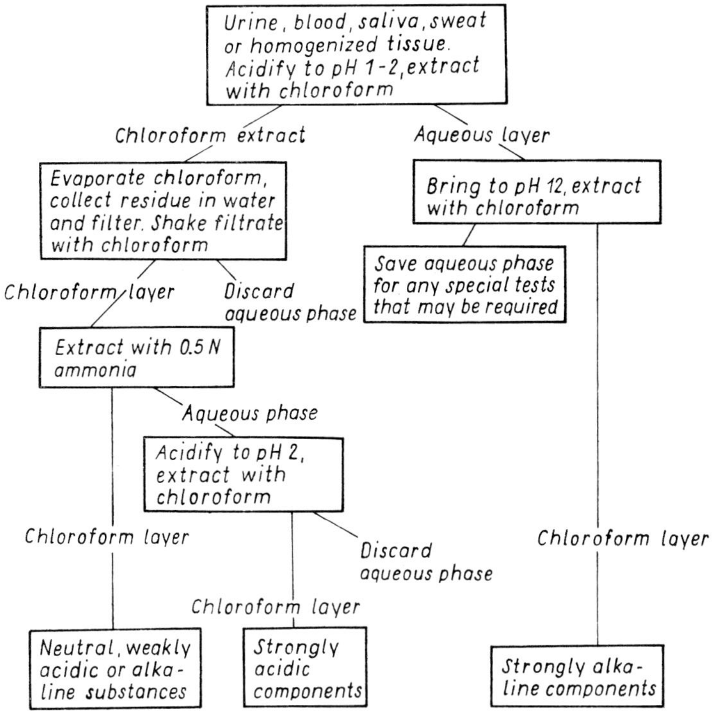

Fig. 1.5. — 4. Flowchart of an extraction process to isolate doping drugs from biological material.

The three extracts obtained by this process are subjected immediately to chemical analysis, or are fractionated further by additional separation techniques. The extracts may be returned to the aqueous phase and separated into additional fractions using other solvents. Such variants can also be incorporated directly into the separation procedure. Suitable solvents include ether or, for polar substances, butanol, ethyl acetate or similar compounds. The separation can be improved by saturating the aqueous phase with a neutral salt (sodium chloride, sodium sulfate). The fractions obtained by extraction are then subjected to further precise separation techniques to isolate and identify the unknown substances. Alternatively, microanalytic techniques can be used to precipitate the substance from the extract, crystallize it, or chemically convert it to compounds of specific colors. The experienced analyst is then able to identify the substance from its typical color reaction or the characteristic form of its crystals or precipitate. This technique is somewhat subjective, however. Chromatographic and spectroscopic methods of analysis are usually employed. These include paper chromatography, which has been largely replaced by the simpler thin-layer chromatography (TLC), as well as liquid and gas chromatography. Based on its characteristic behavior during chromatography, its position in the chromatogram (R_f value), and its behavior in analytical reactions and spectroscopic testing, the unknown substance can be accurately identified. Spectroscopic methods generally involve the measurement of the specific absorption of electromagnetic radiation in the ultraviolet, visible and infrared ranges of the spectrum. The measurement of fluorescent properties is becoming increasingly important, while mass spectroscopy and other spectroscopic techniques are seldom used in routine doping analyses. Certain inorganic substances, such as arsenic, can be detected by neutron activation analysis, which enables the detection and determination of quantities as low as 10^{-10} g. The presence of arsenic in a single hair can be demonstrated by this technique. From its localization and concentration in the hair, the dose and time of administration can be estimated.

In view of the complexity of the techniques described, it normally takes 2 to 3 days to obtain a definitive result, although the presence or absence of a foreign substance in the submitted material can often be confirmed in 24 h. Rapid analytical tests, usually based on thin-layer chromatography, can sometimes yield a result in 30—60 min. Thus, they can be employed immediately before a race. So far, however, these rapid tests serve only an orientational purpose, to be followed in all cases by a more exhaustive analysis.

References

Åberg, B.: Illusioner on doping. Dagens Nyheter, June 12 (1960).

Addis-Smith, L. F.: The changing pattern of 'Doping' in horse racing and its control. New Zealand Vet. J. *9:* 121 (1961).

Alexander, F.: Horner, M. W.; Moss, M. S.: Biochem. Pharmac. *16:* 1305 (1967).

Alles, G. A.; Wisegarver, B.: Amphetamine excretion studies in man. Toxicol. appl. Pharmacol. *3:* 678 (1961).

Alleva, J. J.: Metabolism of trancylpromine-C^{14} and dl-amphetamine-C^{14} in the rat. J. med. Chem. *6:* 621 (1963).

Alp, F.; Kalayci, S.: Detection of dipyrone in a horse's urine and its distinction from antipyrine and aminopyrine. Etilk vet. Bakteriol. Enstit. Derg. *2:* 69 (1963).

Aries, R.: Le doping de chevaux de course, étude des médicaments utilisés. Prochim. S. A., Palais de la Scala, Monte-Carlo, Monaco 1964.

Aries, R.: Doping race horses. Rév. Méd. vét. *116:* 32 (1965).

Ariens, E. J.: Molecular pharmacology *1*, 119. (Academic Press, New York/London 1964.)

Ariens, E. J.: General and pharmacological aspects of doping. In: Schaepdryver, A. de; Hebbelinck, M., 1965.

Asatoor, A. M.; Galman, B. R.; Johnson, J. R.; Milne, M. D.: The excretion of dexamphetamine and its derivatives. Brit. J. Pharmacol. Chemother. *24:* 293 (1965).

Axelrod, J.: Studies on sympathomimetic amines. II. The biotransformation and physiological disposition of d-amphetamine, d-p-hydroxyamphetamine and d-metaphetamine. J. Pharmacol. exp. Therapy *110:* 315 (1954).

Baars, G.: Das Dopen der Rennpferde vom strafrechtlichen Standpunkt und die Beurteilung der üblichen Nachweismethoden der Dopingalkaloide im Speichel der Pferde. Dtsch. tierärztl. Wschr. *34:* 147 (1926).

Bäumler, J.: Zum dünnschichtchromatographischen Nachweis einiger Psychopharmaka, wie Phenothiazine, Tofranil, Reserpin oder Librium in forensischen Fällen. Z. Analyt. Chem. *240* (1964).

Bäumler, J.; Brault, A. L.; Obersteg, J.: Dopingnachweis im Speichel von Rennpferden. Schweizer Arch. Tierheilkd. *106:* 346 (1964).

Beauvallet, M.; Solier, M.: Effect of forced exercise on the toxicity of amphetamine and the noradrenaline content of brain. C. r. Séanc. Soc. Biol. *158:* 2306 (1965).

Beckett, A. H.; Rowland, M.: Urinary excretion kinetics of amphetamine in man. J. Pharmacol. Pharmacy *17:* 17, 628, 1098 (1965).

Beecher, H. K.; Smith, G. M.: Drugs and athletic performance. In: Schaepdryver, A. de; Hebbelinck, M. (1965).

Beickert, F.: Die Glukokortikoidtherapie innerer Erkrankungen (VEB Gustav Fischer Verlag, Jena 1968).

BERETTA, C.: Note informative sul doping degli animali. Veterinaria (Teramo) *7:* 237 (1968).

BETHLEM, M. L. B.; TAVEIRA, M.: Death following the doping of a race horse with amphetamine. Una pricia toxicologica de 'Doping'. Rev. Milit. Rem. Vet. (Rio de Janeiro) *14:* 39 (1954).

BONIN, M.: Contribution de l'étude de l'action physiologique et de l'élimination des amines sympathomimétiques en particulier de l'amphetamine chez le cheval. Vet.-med. Diss., Lyon (1956).

BOUCHARD, N.: Contribution à l'étude de la sémiologie cardio-vasculaire chez le cheval de course. Mesure du temps de circulation par la lobeline. Vet.-med. Diss., Alfort (1954).

BOUCKAERT, J. H.; DEBACKERE, M.: Doping and horse races. In: SCHAEPDRYVER, A. DE; HEBBELINCK, M. (1965).

BÜSCHER, D.-W.: Das Doping. Eine Übersicht über einige Informationen mit besonderer Berücksichtigung veterinärmedizinischer Aspekte. Vet.-med. Diss., Hannover (1972).

BURNS, J. J.; ROSE, R. K.; CHENKIN, T.; GOLDMAN, A.; SCHULERT, A.; BRODIE, B. B.: The physiological disposition of Phenylbutazon (Butazolidin) in man and a method for its estimation in biological material. J. Pharmacol. exp. Therapy *109:* 346 (1953).

CARNIGLIA, F. J.: Can racing readingly be cleaned up? Vet. Med. *41:* 435 (1946).

CARTONI, G. P.; DE STEFANO, F.: Determination of amphetamines by gaschromatography. Urinary excretion of amphetamines in rat and man. Ital. J. Biochem. *12:* 296 (1963).

CLARKE, E. C. G.; CLARKE, M. L.: Garner's veterinary toxicology. (Baillière, Tindall und Cassels, London 1962.)

COURTOT, D.; MOUTHON, G.; ROUX, L.; JEANIN, E.: Incidence du dopage par les tranquillisants sur l'activité musculaire du cheval de sport. II. Diazépam. Ann. Rech. vét. *6:* 117 (1975b).

COURTOT, D.; ROUX, L.; MOUTHON, G.; JEANIN, E.: Incidence du dopage par les tranquillisants sur l'activité musculaire du cheval de sport. I. Acépromazine. Ann. Rech. vét. *6:* 103 (1975a).

CROISIER, R.: Essai de definition de doping. Vet.-med. Diss., Alfort (1948).

DAVISON, C.; MANDEL, H. G.: Nonnarcotic analgesics and antipyretics. I. Salicylates. In: DI PALMA, J. R.: DRILL's pharmacology in medicine. 3rd ed. (McGraw Hill, New York 1965).

DE CORGANOFF, G.; LE BARS, H.: Accidents consécutifs à l'injection de corticotrophine chez le cheval de course. Rév. Pathol. Gen. *53:* 626 (1953).

DERIVEAUX, J.; LIEGEOIS, F.: Toxicologie Vétérinaire (Vigot frères et Desoer, Paris 1962).

DIECKMANN, ERNA-MARIA: Pervitin als Dopingmittel bei Pferden und Versuche zu seinem chemischen Nachweis nach dem Doping. Vet.-med. Diss., Berlin (1951).

ELLISON, T.; GUTZAIT, L.; VAN LOON, J.: The comparative metabolism of d-Amphetamine-C^{14} in the rat, dog and monkey. J. Pharmacol. exper. Therapy *152:* 383 (1966).

FARELLY, B. T.: The veterinary medical aspects of doping control procedures in horse racing. Irish Vet. J. *15:* 28 (1961).

FOBIAN, C. V.; SARAGOTA, V. Y.: Endocrine therapy for stale race horses. Vet. Med. *56:* 30 (1961).

FRÖHNER, E.: Lehrbuch der Toxikologie für Tierärzte, 4. Aufl. (Enke, Stuttgart 1919).

FUJII, S.; INADA, S.; YOSHIDA, S.; KUSANAGI, C.; MIMA, K.; NATSUNO, Y.: Pharmacological studies on doping drugs for race horses. I. trans-π-Oxocamphor. Japan. J. Vet. Sci. *32:* 307 (1970).

FUJII, S.; INADA, S.; YOSHIDA, S.; KUSANAGI, C.; MIMA, K.; NATSUNO, Y.: Pharmacological studies on doping drugs for race horses. II. Caffeine. Japan. J. Vet. Sci. *34:* 141 (1972).

FUJII, S.; INADA, S.; YOSHIDA, S.; KUSANAGI, C.; MIMA, K.; NATSUNO, Y.: Pharmacological studies on doping drugs for race horses. III. Ephedrine. Japan. J. Vet. Sci. *36:* 9 (1974).

GABRIEL, L. K.; HENDERSON, B.; SMITH, W. F.: Studies on the physiologic effects of methylphenidate in thoroughbred horses. J. Amer. vet. med. Assoc. *142:* 875 (1963).

GADDUM: Pharmakologie (Steinkopff, Darmstadt 1952).

GUILLET, R.: Le doping de l'homme et du cheval (Masson, Paris 1965).

HAUSCHILD, F.: Pharmakologie und Grundlagen der Toxikologie (VEB Georg Thieme, Leipzig 1973).

HENNAU, A.: Doping du cheval de course. Ann. Méd. Vét. *90:* 73 (1946).

HETTINGER, T.: Einfluss einiger Faktoren auf die muskuläre Leistungsfähigkeit. In: SCHAEPDRYVER, A. DE; HEBBELINCK, M. (1965).

HUTSON, L. R.: Observations on the collection of urine samples at the sampling unit of the Barbados Turf Club. Canad. vet. J. *7:* 260 (1966).

INNES, I. R.; NICKERSON, M.: Drugs acting on postganglionic adrenergic nerve endings and structures innervated by them (sympathomimetic drugs). In: GOODMAN, L. S.; GILMAN, A.: The pharmacological basis of therapeutics. 3rd ed., p. 477 (McMillan, New York 1965).

KUNDE, M.; FREY, H.: Beitrag zur Frage des Doping mit Procain. Berliner Münchener tierärztl. Wschr. *84:* 1 (1971).

LANDER, G. D.: Analyst (London) *55:* 474 (1930).

LLEWELLIN, C. B. E.: Bute or bullet? Horse and Hound, 3rd February (1978).

LÖCHEL, H.: Über den heutigen Stand des Doping bei Rennpferden und Versuche mit dem ACTH hinsichtlich seiner Dopingwirkung. Vet.-med. Diss., Leipzig (1959).

LOEW, F. M.; BETTANY, J. M.: Thiamine concentrations in the blood of standardbred horses. Amer. J. vet. Res. *34:* 1207 (1973).

LORINER: Bute: Should we wait and see? Horse and Hound, 3rd February (1978).

MACKAY, A.: Some effects of drugs in the doping of race horses. New Zealand Vet. J. *9:* 129 (1961).

MARES, R. G.: The doping of race horses. Brit. Vet. J. *114:* 288 (1958).

MARTIN, J. E.; BECK, J. D.: Some effects of chlorpromazine hydrochloride in horses. Amer. J. vet. Res. *17:* 678 (1956).

MÖLLER: Das Dopen der Rennpferde. Illustrierte Landw.-Zeitung (1902), 312.

MORGAN, C. E.: Drug administration to racing animals. J. Amer. vet. med. Assoc. *130:* 240 (1958).

MOSS, M. S.: The doping of racing horses. Vet. Ann. *11:* 149 (1970).

NEUMANN-KLEINPAUL, K.; RÜSCHER, W.: Klinische Untersuchungen gedopter Pferde. Arch. Tierheilkd. *64:* 226 (1931).

NICHOLSON, J. D.: The urinary excretion of phenobarbitone and pentobarbitone in the horse. Biochem. Pharmacol. *17:* 1 (1968).

OSTYN, M.; DE NAYER, P. P.: Considerations on research on doping and on the results of this research. In: SCHAEPDRYVER, A. DE; HEBBELINCK, M. (1965).

PADE, H.: cited after BÜSCHER (1972).

PARKE, D. V.: The biochemistry of foreign compounds, p. 269 (Pergamon Press, London 1967).

PFYL, B.: Dopen (Verlag August Reher, Berlin 1923).

PROKOP, L.: The problem of doping. J. Sport. Med. *5:* 88 (1965).

RECHENBERG, H. K. v.: Butazolidin®. Phenylbutazon, 2. Aufl. (Thieme, Stuttgart 1961).

RICHTER, W.: personal communication (1979).

SCHAEPDRYVER, A. DE; HEBBELINCK, M.: Doping. Proc. of an Internat. Seminar, organized at the Universities of Gent and Brussels, May 1964, by the Research Committee of the Internat. Council of Sport and Physical Education (Pergamon Press, Oxford 1965).

SCHICK: Das Dopen der Pferde. Z. Veterinärkunde *45:* 241 (1933).

SCHÖNHOLZER, E.: Aspects psychologiques du Doping. In: SCHAEPDRYVER, A. DE; HEBBELINCK, M. (1965).

SCHUBERT, B.: Identification and Metabolism of some Doping Substances in Horses. Vet.-med. Diss., Stockholm (1967).

SCHWARZ, K.: Neuere Erkenntnisse über den essentiellen Charakter einiger Spurenelemente. In: Spurenelemente in der Entwicklung von Mensch und Tier (Ed.: BETHE, K.; BIDLINGMAIER, F.). (Urban & Schwarzenberg, München 1975.)

SCHWIEGER, H.: Über die Bewertung der klinischen Erscheinungen bei Rennpferden. Vet.-med. Diss., Berlin (1936).

SENDROS, F. G.: El doping. Arch. vet. Pract. (Corunna) *64:* 5 (1956).

SEREN, E.; VENTURINI, A.: Modificazioni ormonali e metaboliche indotte dall'allenamento nel cavallo trottatore. Nuova Vet. (Bologna) *48:* 332 (1972).

SMITH, M. J. H.; SMITH, P. K.: The salicylates. A critical bibliographic review (Interscience Publishers, New York 1966).

STEEL, J. D.; WHITLOCK, L. E.: Observations on the haematology of thoroughbred and standardbred horses in training and racing. Austral. Vet. J. *36:* 136 (1960).

STEWARD, G. A.: Drugs, performance and responses. 2. Observations on Amphetamine, Promazine and Thiamine. Aust. Vet. J. *48:* 544 (1972).

STEWARD, J. D.: The detection of doping in race horses. Austral. Vet. J. *27:* 153 (1951).

SUCKOW, P.: Das Doping. Der Preuss. Kreistierarzt *4:* 66 (1905).

SUSTMANN: Doping und seine Folgen. Dtsch. tierärztl. Wschr. *22:* 569, 577 (1914).

TAPERNOUX, A.; COLLET, P.; MAGAT, A.: Recherches dans le sang et la salive du cheval, de deux amines sympathomimétiques. Rév. Méd. Vét. *107:* 302 (1956).
ULLRICH, K.: Doping und Leistungssteigerungen bei Hunden. Tierärztl. Umschau *5:* 100 (1950).
ULMARK, R.: The dangers of doping. J. Sport. Med. *3:* 248 (1963).
VENERANDO, A.; DE SIO, F.: Organisation et résultats du controle antidoping. In: SCHAEPDRYVER, A. DE; HEBBELINCK, M. (1965).
VETTES, R.: Le doping. Maquillage des chevaux de course. (Guitard, Paris 1927) cited after BÜSCHER (1972).
WIEGAND, D.: Über den Pervitinnachweis beim Dopen der Pferde. Vet.-med. Diss., Berlin-Dahlem (1955).
WIESNER, E.: Ernährungsschäden der landwirtschaftlichen Nutztiere, 2. Aufl. (VEB Gustav Fischer Verlag, Jena 1970).
WIESNER, E.; WILLER, S.: Veterinärmedizinische Pathogenetik (VEB Gustav Fischer Verlag, Jena 1974).
ZINTZEN, H.: Vitamin E und Selen in der Tierernährung. Firmenschrift, Fa. Hoffmann-La Roche AG, Grenzach-Wyhlen 1977.

1.6. Blood Replacement and Shock Therapy

1.6.1. Blood Transfusion

Indication. A blood transfusion is indicated in cases where oxygen-carrying erythrocytes are critically deficient. Besides supplying erythrocytes, a blood transfusion increases the circulating blood volume. If the quantity of circulating erythrocytes is sufficient to ensure an adequate tissue oxygen supply, the volume may be increased with albumin, plasma, plasma expanders and/or electrolyte solutions. In purpura hemorrhagica and other coagulation disorders, fresh blood will supply erythrocytes, platelets as well as clotting factors. A deficiency of oxygen-carrying erythrocytes is most often the result of internal and external hemorrhage but may be caused by hemolysis or insufficient erythropoiesis in some cases. Blood transfusion is of doubtful value in chronic anemias due to insufficient erythropoiesis, or hemolysis that cannot be quickly corrected. Studies have shown [Kallfelz et al., 1978], that allogenic erythrocytes survive for only 2—4 days, making repeated transfusions necessary. Erythrocyte compatibility tests (direct agglutination, hemolysis and antiglobulin test) are not entirely reliable in demonstrating the survivability of transfused red cells. Even without a frank incompatibility, the survival time in horses is very short, and the possibility of side-effects and rapid breakdown of the transfused erythrocytes is relatively great. Erythrocyte survival studies using radioactive chromium do not appear very reliable, however, because chromium is rapidly eluted from the erythrocytes, and the values indicate only $^1/_{10}$ of the normal survival of ~ 150 days [Valli et al., 1975]. This question merits further study, however.

In the face of acute blood loss, an erythrocyte deficit is recognized mainly on the basis of clinical symptoms. The hematocrit is a poor index of erythrocyte loss in cases of acute hemorrhage, because it may even be elevated by splenic contraction. According to Torten and Schalm [1964], the degree of blood loss from a serious hemorrhage is impossible to assess during the first 4 to 5 h as a result of splenic contraction. The hematocrit is also elevated in shock due to blood loss. In the horse it takes from 24 to 48 h before tissue fluid can replenish the circulating volume and the erythrocyte loss can be accurately assessed. Blood dilution is accompanied by hypoproteinemia [Schalm, 1975].

The hematocrit of the horse returns to normal more slowly after hemorrhage than in the dog. This process can take 3 weeks to 3 months.

In contrast to the dog, however, the survival time of the newly formed erythrocytes is practically normal [Lumsden et al., 1975]. Even after severe anemia, immature erythrocytes (reticulocytes) are rarely if ever encountered in the circulation of the horse [Schalm, 1965]. It is still uncertain whether there is an insufficient production of erythropoietin in the horse after hemorrhage, or an insufficient response of the erythropoietic tissue to erythropoietin [Smith and Agar, 1976].

Neonatal isoerythrolysis in the foal is another indication for blood transfusion. In such cases a transfusion of washed erythrocytes from the mare to the foal is much simpler and even more effective than an exchange transfusion.

Technique. A healthy, mature horse with a high hematocrit should be chosen as donor. Such an animal can safely give 5—10 l of blood. Due to the danger of clotting, direct transfusion with a large syringe and 3-way stopcock is no longer practiced. Indirect transfusions are preferred. In this method the blood is collected in an anticoagulant solution and then administered at once. Occasionally it is stored for later use. Sodium citrate is a very good anticoagulant for blood that is to be transfused immediately. For each liter of blood, 100 ml of a 4—5% aqueous sodium citrate solution is needed. In the horse, 28.5 g of sodium citrate is the average upper limit of tolerance [Bolz and Dietz, 1970]. The blood is collected from the jugular vein by means of a tourniquet applied distally and a large-gauge needle or bleeding trocar should be used. The container in which the blood is collected should be swirled constantly to keep the blood and anticoagulant well mixed. The vessel should not be shaken. The blood will keep in a refrigerator (2—4 °C) for up to 3 weeks. If the blood is to be stored, ACD solution (6.6 g citric acid, 22.5 g sodium citrate, 20 g dextrose) is a better anticoagulant than sodium citrate. One liter of ACD solution is sufficient for 4 l of blood. When blood is stored, the concentration of organic phosphates in the erythrocytes, in particular 2,3-diphosphoglycerate (2,3-DPG), declines considerably. If the concentration of 2,3-DPG becomes very low, the oxygen affinity of the hemoglobin increases, so that oxygen release to the tissues is diminished. The transfusion of such blood would be of little benefit initially. The concentration of 2,3-DPG is slow to regenerate after a transfusion. Following a transfusion of stored blood deficient in 2,3-DPG, the cardiac output must rise or the oxygen utilization of the tissues must increase in order to meet the same oxygen requirement as fresh blood. Although the horse, like the dog and man, normally has a high erythrocytic content of 2,3-DPG, hemoglobin solutions from the horse appear to have a much smaller relation between their 2,3-DPG content and oxygen affinity than hemoglobin solutions from man [McLean and Lewis, 1975]. Research still needs to be done on the importance of the 2,3-DPG concentration for oxygen release in the horse, and on the possible beneficial effect of certain substances such as inosine, a drug acting on cardiac and muscular metabolism, adenine, pyruvate or sodium phosphate on the 2,3-DPG concentration. If the 2,3-DPG decline can be prevented, then equine blood, like human and canine blood, could be stored for 1 to 2 weeks longer [Eisenbrandt and Smith, 1974; Ou et al., 1975]. When stored blood has become out of date, the plasma can be sterilly extracted and frozen for storage.

The average blood transfusion dose in a mature horse is 5—8 l. If the hematocrit was already low before the transfusion, blood can continue to be administered until the hematocrit has been adequately raised. If the hematocrit was normal or elevated before the transfusion, the dose should be adjusted in accordance with clinical symptoms, especially in cases of severe hemorrhage.

Blood should be filtered before it is administered to eliminate any microaggregates of platelets, leukocytes, fibrin or red cells that might be present. This is best done with commercially available blood filters or by straining through several layers of sterile gauze. The blood is infused with a large gauge needle or silicone catheter. A catheter is preferred for slow infusions. The rate and volume of the transfusion depend chiefly on the degree and duration of the anemia. If anemia has been present for 24—48 h, the plasma volume is already adequate, and the blood should be infused slowly. The bottle or bag should be inverted periodically to prevent sedimentation. Blood can be given rapidly following an acute hemorrhage. Except in dire emergencies, the first 100—200 ml should be given slowly so that incompatibility reactions can be quickly recognized.

Transfusion Reactions. Various types of reaction can occur during and after a blood transfusion:

Allergic reactions are fairly common but are the least dangerous. They are marked by urticaria, itching, swaying, increased intestinal peristalsis and sometimes diarrhea. These reactions can usually be prevented with antihistamines or glucocorticoids. Often the transfusion can be continued despite allergic reactions. Treatment consists of antihistamines and glucocorticoids. For violent reactions, epinephrine and electrolyte solutions may have to be administered.

Febrile reactions can occur as a symptom of allergic reactions, or may conceivably be due to the transfusion of antigens in the donor leukocytes to which the recipient is hypersensitive.

Bacteremia is usually due to a break in aseptic technique during the collection or storage of blood. Some bacteria can grow at 2—4 °C. *E. coli* and *Pseudomonas* sp. have been shown to metabolize citrate. Saprophytes often only produce fever and are usually not so dangerous. Other bacteria, especially gram-negative organisms, can cause severe septicemia and even endotoxic shock. Bacterial growth in stored blood can be recognized by a dark-brown to black discoloration of the top plasma layer.

Hemolytic reactions. Hemolysis can be acute or delayed. The clinical manifestations of acute hemolysis are uneasiness, yawning, urination and defecation (or diarrhea), sweating and fever; polypnea, tachycardia and hemoglobinuria may also occur. Abortion may occur in pregnant mares, but this has not been well established. The first blood transfusion will seldom cause severe effects. However, about 5 days after the transfusion the recipient produces antibodies against the antigens in the transfused blood, increasing the chance of hemolytic reactions after the second and subsequent transfusions. Experience with the horse in this area is limited, and little accurate information is available on the risk of repeated transfusions, because multiple transfusions are rarely performed. Normally, however, one must assume that repeated transfusions carry a high risk, even though reactions by no means occur in every case. Mares that have produced a foal with neonatal isoerythrolysis have more antibodies and are perhaps at greater risk for transfusion reactions [Gabel, 1972]. Some hemolytic reactions are delayed, rather than acute. In this case there is rapid lysis of the transfused red cells, causing hemolytic icterus to develop within 24—48 h. Delayed hemolysis, which occurs mainly after repeated transfusions, is not considered dangerous. Due to the rapid destruction of the red cells, the effect of the transfusion in such cases is limited to volume expansion with the transfused plasma. Delayed hemolysis mainly occurs in animals with septicemia and in recipients with less active alloantibody (allohemolysins).

Six blood-group systems with several variants have been identified in the horse. However, little is known about the true importance of blood groups in the occurrence of transfusion reactions in this species. Naturally occurring alloantibodies are rare and are probably limited to the anti-C blood group. Alloagglutinins occur naturally but are not dangerous. Naturally occurring isoantibodies are far less dangerous than immune antibodies produced as the result of a previous sensitization or transfusion.

Cross-Matching. Although the first transfusion is not dangerous, the blood of the recipient and prospective donor should nevertheless be cross-matched to test for agglutination and hemolysis. Cross-matches are always indicated before giving blood to foals with neonatal isoerythrolysis and to mares that may be used for breeding. If a mare is injected with foreign antigens, especially in repeated transfusions, she may produce antibodies that increase the risk of neonatal isoerythrolysis. Macroscopic plate or tube tests are not always reliable, because weak agglutinations cannot always be recognized macroscopically. The microscopic examination of cross-match samples yields highly reliable results. Blood samples are collected from the recipient and the proposed donor. The serum is obtained by spontaneous sedimentation or centrifugation and put into labeled tubes. An erythrocyte suspension is made from each blood sample by resuspending cells from the clot in physiologic saline. One drop of the cell suspension and 2 drops of the serum are added to a test tube for each test: donor cells with recipient serum (major cross match) and donor serum with recipient cells (minor cross match). The tubes are incubated for 30 min at room temperature or for 6 to 7 min in a 37 °C water bath. They are then centrifuged for 1 min at 1,000 rpm. It can now be determined whether hemolysis has taken place. For this purpose the tubes are shaken hard to resuspend the sediment. A strong agglutination can be detected macroscopically. The tube contents are then placed on a slide without a coverslip and examined microscopically at 100×. If there is doubt that agglutination has occurred, the slide should be tipped from side to side for several minutes. If true agglutination is present, it will become stronger; if not, any clumps not due to agglutination will break up [Gabel, 1972]. It is recommended that both the major and minor test be negative before proceeding with the transfusion. A reaction in the minor test, i.e., agglutination of the recipient cells with the donor serum, is less serious because the serum of the donor, which contains the antibodies, is diluted in the entire blood volume of the recipient.

Blood showing weak agglutination in the minor test may be used in emergencies. In rare cases, especially in severe anemia or viral infection, autoagglutinins may occur in the serum of the recipient. In these cases the prospective donor's cells usually show some agglutination in the recipient serum. The cross-matching test may be supplemented or replaced by a trial injection of 25—75 ml of the donor blood. Incompatibility will be evidenced within 10—12 min by transfusion reactions in the form of tachycardia, polypnea, unrest, sweating, muscular tremor, and frequent urination and defecation. If results are doubtful, the trial injection can be repeated with a 2 to 3 times larger volume of donor blood. Even with a negative cross-match and trial injection, incompatibility reactions can still occur [Schmid, 1963].

Little is known about other complications that might arise in the horse after the transfusion of larger blood volumes, especially when stored blood is used. The following are conceivable: acidosis from the release of lactic acid and an elevated pCO_2; hyperkalemia from the release of K^+ from the erythrocytes; hypocalcemia from a reaction of sodium citrate with the Ca^{++} of the recipient blood; impaired clotting ability from the destruction of platelets and a decline in certain clotting factors; in addition microemboli, with impaired peripheral perfusion due to aggregates of platelets, leukocytes, fibrin, protein coagulates or erythrocytes, may occur.

Too much sodium citrate is especially dangerous in shock, when the ability of the liver to break down the citrate may potentially be impaired. In direct transfusions of foals with isoerythrolysis, the transfusion is started before blood is withdrawn, and then blood is alternately withdrawn and transfused. Overall, more blood is administered than is withdrawn.

References

Bolz, W.; Dietz, O.: Lehrbuch der Allgemeinen Chirurgie für Tierärzte, 4. Aufl. (Enke, Stuttgart 1970).

Eisenbrandt, D.; Smith, J.: Effects of various additives on in vitro parameters related to viability and function of stored canine blood. Res. Vet. Sci. *17:* 231 (1974).

GABEL, A.: Equine medicine and surgery, 2nd ed., p. 920 (Amer. Vet. Public. Wheaton 1972).
KALLFELZ, F.; WHITLOCK, R.; SCHULZ, R.: Survival of 59-Fe labeled erythrocytes in cross transfused equine blood. Amer. J. Vet. Res. *39:* 617 (1978).
LUMSDEN, J.; VALLI, V.; MCSHERRY, B.; ROBINSON, G.; CLACTON, M.: The kinetics of hematopoiesis in the light horse. II. The hematological response to hemorrhagic anemia. Canad. J. compar. Med. *39:* 324 (1975).
MCLEAN, J.; LEWIS, I.: Oxygen affinity responses to 2,3-diphosphoglycerate and methaemoglobin formation in horse and human haemoglobins. Res. Vet. Sci. *19:* 259 (1975).
OU, D.; MAHAFFEY, E.; SMITH, J.: Effect of storage on oxygen dissociation of canine blood. J. Amer. vet. med. Assoc. *167:* 56 (1975).
SCHALM, O.: Veterinary hematology, 2nd ed. (Lea & Febiger, Philadelphia 1965).
SCHALM, O.: Equine haematology as an aid to diagnosis. Proc. 1th Int. Sympos. Equine Hematol. (1975), 5.
SCHMID, D.: Blutübertragung und Blutgruppen bei Tieren. Tierärztl. Umschau *18:* 501 (1963).
SCOTT, A. M.; JEFFCOTT, L. B.: Haemolytic disease of the foal. Vet. Rec. *103:* 71 (1978).
SMITH, J.; AGAR, N.: Studies on erythrocyte metabolism following acute blood loss in the horse. Equine Vet. J. *8:* 34 (1976).
TORTEN, M.; SCHALM, O.: Influence of the equine spleen on rapid changes in the concentration of erythrocytes in peripheral blood. Amer. J. Vet. Res. *25:* 500 (1964).
VALLI, V.; LUMSDEN, J.; CARTER, E.; MCSHERRY, B.: The kinetics of hematopoiesis in the normal light horse. The life span of peripheral blood cells and plasma proteins. Proc. 1th Int. Symp. Equine Hematol. (1975), 91.

1.6.2. Shock

Definition. Shock denotes a breakdown of the system which keeps the tissue blood flow at the minimum level necessary for normal oxidative metabolism.

Etiology. Various causes have been implicated in the etiology of shock:

1. Serious internal or external bleeding, significant plasma or fluid losses are termed *hypovolemic shock.* A blood loss of 15—20% is associated with mild shock and a 20 to 40% loss with moderate shock; losses greater than 40% are fatal unless effectively treated. Acute exsanguination may proceed so rapidly that shock cannot develop, while very slow blood losses trigger the animal's compensatory mechanisms that can prevent shock from occurring. A condition in which blood is present in the body but is excluded from the circulation must also be regarded as 'blood loss'. This can occur, for example, in cases of uterine prolapse, and intestinal torsion or obstruction. It may also result from pooling of blood in the large veins of the splanchnic region and erythrocyte storage in the spleen. Profuse sweating and diarrhea can also result in large fluid losses. In ischemia of the bowel much fluid and albumin can be lost in the intestinal lumen, just as extensive burns and acute exudative inflammatory processes can lead to significant albumin and fluid losses.

2. Massive infections, especially with gram-negative organisms, can cause *septic or endotoxic shock* from the bacterial release of endotoxin.

3. Congestive heart failure can lead to *cardiogenic shock,* though it is seldom a primary cause. With a reduction in cardiac output, there is a corresponding decrease in the oxygen-carrying capacity of the blood. This in turn reduces the myocardial oxygen supply, setting up a positive feedback system (vicious cycle).

4. Serious trauma can also lead to shock. *Traumatic shock,* although a vague term, is caused by a combination of hypovolemia, the release of toxic substances from damaged tissues, as well as pain and fear.

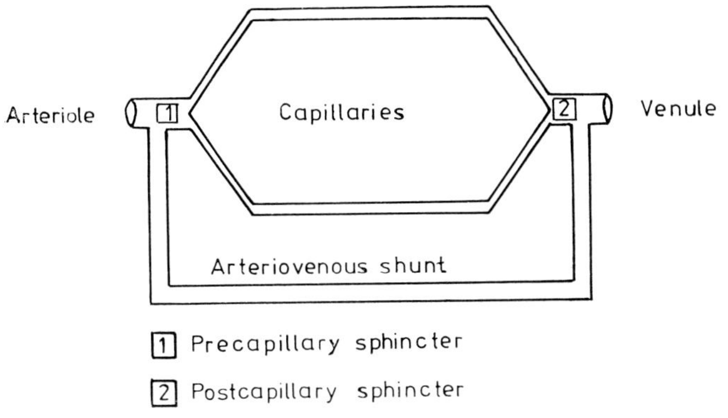

Fig. 1.6. — ***1.*** The microcirculation.

5. In some cases, violent allergic-anaphylactic reactions can produce a state of shock. The pathogenesis and course of these reactions often differ from the classic shock syndrome.

Pathogenesis. The pathogenesis of shock is extremely complex and merits more intensive study. It depends, moreover, on the nature of the shock, the species of animal, and the affected organs or tissues. Hypovolemic and so-called traumatic shock have been investigated in the greatest detail. Hypovolemia or trauma sets up a chain of events which includes the release of epinephrine and norepinephrine from the adrenal glands, accompanied by a synthesis of norepinephrine at sympathetic nerve endings. These substances act on specific receptors (epinephrine on α and β receptors, norepinephrine mainly on α receptors). Stimulation of the α receptors produces vasoconstriction, while β-receptor stimulation produces vasodilation. The distribution of the receptors depends essentially on the tissues involved, but species differences are also present. The special circumstances in the horse have yet to be investigated. The skin contains only α receptors, while the splanchnic region contains α receptors and a few β_2 receptors. Only β_1 receptors occur in the myocardium (with β_1 and perhaps α receptors occurring in the coronary arteries), while α and β_2 receptors occur in skeletal muscle. The catecholamines cause vasoconstriction at the level of the pre- and postcapillary α receptors. One result of this is the development of tissue ischemia in the kidney, bowel and skin *(ischemic anoxia)*. Direct arteriovenous *shunting* of blood may take place between the arterioles and venous network (fig. 1.6. — 1). Lypressin, Vasopressin® and angiotensin can also promote vasoconstriction in the mesenteric vascular network. Ischemic anoxia may progress to *stagnant anoxia,* which in severe cases leads to *irreversible shock*. This can occur because the precapillary receptors relax more quickly than the postcapillary receptors, which are adapted to a lower pH. As a result, there is stagnation and pooling mainly in the splanchnic capillaries, and water, ions, plasma and even cells are lost primarily on the venous side of the capillaries, leading to edema formation. This causes further deterioration of the microcirculation. In *endotoxin shock,* the endotoxin disrupts the integrity of the vascular membrane, allowing the escape of fluid and plasma. Certain substances, such as vasoactive peptides, histamine, kinins and prostaglandins, which are liberated in response to inflammation, can also increase vascular permeability. A complete loss of tone can even occur in some vascular areas.

Stagnant anoxia is accompanied by a dangerous reduction in venous return, especially in the presence of hypovolemia. Too little blood is presented to the heart. Tissue perfusion in shock is hampered by a number of factors. Normally it is determined by the circulating blood volume and total peripheral resistance. Shock increases the peripheral resistance in several ways other than vasoconstriction:

1. Blood viscosity increases with the rise in hematocrit, and is also increased by hypothermia.
2. The blood coagulates more rapidly. In severe cases numerous intravascular clots can form throughout the microcirculation. In the process, clotting factors are used up, leading to diffuse hemorrhages. This process is called disseminated intravascular coagulation or DIC.
3. There is an inadequate removal of metabolic products, and aggregation of platelets, fat and erythrocytes occur.

The diminished tissue perfusion is the cause of various, sometimes irreversible changes. Due to the oxygen deficit, cellular metabolism becomes anerobic, resulting in a much smaller energy yield and the accumulation of large amounts of lactic acid. The muscular and hepatic glycogen content available for anerobic glycolysis is quite low. The liver, moreover, is unable to metabolize the lactic acid adequately. This metabolic acidosis adversely affects cardiac function and activates the synthesis of catecholamines. In metabolic acidosis, however, the endogenous catecholamines cannot exert their positive inotropic effect on the heart. Hypoxia causes potassium to move out of the cells, which in turn disrupts cell function. The intracellular water and sodium content increase as a result of excessive Na^+ transport through the cell membrane. Lysosomal membranes are likewise disrupted, allowing the escape of enzymes which cause cellular necrosis. The intestinal mucosa, which contains an abundance of lysosomes, becomes necrotic, and the liberated lysosomal enzymes enter the intestinal lumen. From there they can diffuse into the lymphatics and thus enter the systemic circulation [Clermont et al., 1972]. Furthermore, the lysosomal hydrolase liberated from the pancreas and other organs sensitizes the myocardium to the negative inotropic effect of *myocardial depressant factor* (see below). The following effects are ascribed to the circulating lysosomal enzymes: myocardial depression, peripheral vasoconstriction, and a toxic effect on the mitochondria.

The intracellular ATP concentration in the muscles is decreased in shock [Kohama et al., 1971]. In stagnant anoxia the peptide myocardial depressant factor (MDF) is formed in the pancreas which exerts a negative inotropic effect on the myocardium. This factor is probably formed by the breakdown of pancreatic protein under the action of lysosomal proteases and released from the pancreas as a result of hypoxia [Lefer, 1970]. Myocardial depressant factor also causes vasoconstriction in the splanchnic bed with consequent hypoxia of the pancreas, leading to a further increase in the production of MDF. At the same time, MDF decreases intestinal motility. The tissue resistance to insulin is increased, and there is an accompanying decrease in the oxidation of glucose and its incorporation into glycogen, as well as the incorporation of amino acids into muscle proteins [Ryan et al., 1974]. The hepatic content of cAMP is reduced [Rutenburg et al., 1971], as is the production of corticosteroids. Tissue hypoxia leads to a release of kinins and leukocytic proteases. The mononuclear phagocytic system (MPS) is strongly inhibited by MDF. Infections can become established more readily. Depression of the MPS defense mechanism in the liver allows endotoxins to gain entrance to the systemic circulation from the bowel. The epithelial cells of the intestinal mucosa are made more permeable to bacterial toxins, bacteria, proteolytic and hydrolytic enzymes [Rhodes et al., 1973]. In the horse, the large intestine suffers the greatest degree of damage [Jenkins,

1972]. With the fall in blood pressure, renal function is also seriously depressed. This results in diminished glomerular filtration and vasoconstriction in the renal cortex. Oliguria or even anuria can develop. If intestinal obstruction is present, there is a rise in the blood level of ammonia, which is toxic to the central nervous system. Ventilation-perfusion disturbances are common in the lung, with an increase of arteriovenous shunts, capillary damage, a rise in pulmonary vascular resistance, pulmonary edema, microthrombi in the blood vessels, intra-alveolar fluid collections and hemorrhages. Surfactant of the pulmonary alveoli is also disrupted. This may be caused by a decrease in phospholipid synthesis, which in turn results from anoxia of the alveolar cells that form the surfactant.

Symptoms. Some of the symptoms typical of shock are: A high pulse rate with a reduced arterial blood pressure and weak peripheral pulse, cold clammy extremities, hyperventilation, initial pallor followed by cyanotic mucous membranes. In the horse cyanosis is most apparent at the gum margins around the incisors. In severe dehydration the skin turgor is markedly decreased, and the eyes may be sunken. Urine output is markedly decreased. There is apathy and sometimes unrest. Hypothermia usually develops as shock progresses. Profuse sweating is sometimes observed.

The following examinations and determinations are useful for assessing the various degrees of shock: The fall in venous blood pressure can be very simply assessed by the collapse of the peripheral veins following puncture of the jugular vein. It can also be accurately measured by means of a central venous catheter. The central venous pressure depends on the venous return, the venous tone and the distensibility and contractility of the right heart. A 70- to 80-cm-long plastic catheter is advanced through the jugular vein into the cranial vena cava so that the catheter tip is located a few centimeters in front of the right atrium.

In shock the central venous pressure is negative or only weakly positive. The mean central venous pressure in the standing horse is 12 cm H_2O. Individual variations are large, however [Hall and Nigam, 1975]. During halothane anesthesia the central venous pressure is much higher in the laterally recumbent animal than in dorsal recumbency. Acepromazine (e.g., Acetylpromazine®) causes a significant fall in the hematocrit compared to control horses or horses treated with xylazine (e.g., Rompun®). The hematocrit rises significantly after the induction of halothane anesthesia. This could be hypercapnia-related [Klein and Sherman, 1977]. During an infusion, however (see Treatment), the shape of the pressure curve is more important than an individual measurement. The zero-point of the measuring scale should be level with the right atrium. Taking the manubrium of the sternum as the zero reference point can lead to inaccuracy, because the correlation between the manubrium and right atrium is dependent upon body position. Usually there is a decrease in circulating blood volume. In stagnant anoxia there is a very strong rise in the hematocrit and total plasma protein concentration [Coffman and Garner, 1972]. The plasma protein concentration is normally a good index of the state of hydration. However, in peritonitis the plasma protein level may be low or normal despite hemoconcentration, because of protein loss in the abdomen [Coffman, 1975]. Capillary filling is prolonged. It takes several seconds for the blood to return after digital pressure is applied to the pigment-free mucosa of the lips or cheeks. The blood lactic acid concentration may be markedly elevated. Lactic acid levels provide a reliable index of the severity of the shock and its prognosis [Donawick et al., 1975]. In intestinal obstruction, the lactate concentration in the peritoneal fluid is a better index of the degree of intestinal ischemia than is the blood lactate concentration [Moore et al., 1977]. The importance of the lactate-pyruvate ratio and a lactate excess is still uncertain, for there may be a high lactate-pyruvate ratio and lactate excess even in the absence of tissue anoxia. The effect of epinephrine on hepatic glycogen leads very quickly to hyperglycemia with a reduced sensitivity to insulin or even insulin suppression. In late stages, hypoglycemia can develop due to the depletion of hepatic glycogen.

Acid-base studies reveal a low blood pH as a result of metabolic acidosis. This can be compensated to some degree by the hypocapnia (low arterial pCO_2) that comes with hyperventilation. The arterial oxygen tension (paO_2) is sometimes reduced. Urea levels are elevated in the presence of hemoconcentration and/or renal function impairment.

The stroke volume of the heart is severely reduced in most cases.

Prognosis. The prognosis in the various forms of shock is always guarded. Shock can be reversed in its early stages by prompt aggressive treatment, provided the effects of the shock have not been too severe.

The prognosis is poor (irreversible shock) when there is serious deterioration of the circulatory state, severe damage to the lungs, liver or intestine, anuria, in combination with extreme metabolic acidosis and high lactate levels. After very severe shock, the disturbances of active cation transport at the level of the cell membrane are practically irreversible [Baue et al., 1973].

Treatment. Treatment must be directed at the cause of the shock as well as its symptoms. It should be commenced with a minimum of delays.

1. Treatment of the cause: Fluid loss is corrected by fluid replacement, and plasma loss by the administration of plasma, albumins or plasma expanders. With large blood losses, a transfusion is necessary. If the primary disease is amenable to surgical treatment, i.e., an intestinal obstruction, the operation should be performed as soon as possible. It is imperative that the animal be treated for shock and its circulatory state improved *to some degree* before a stressful operation under general anesthesia is undertaken. This fact is still overlooked in veterinary medicine, usually with fatal results. With a large and sudden blood loss, of course, treatment must be instituted as quickly as possible. If severe pain is present, analgesic medication is indicated.

2. Restoration of circulating volume. If the hematocrit is high, a blood transfusion is not advised. The circulating blood volume is best restored by a combination of plasma, albumins or a plasma expander (gelatin- or dextran-base) and an electrolyte solution (e.g., Ringer's solution). In severe hemoconcentration it is best to use a plasma expander with a relatively low molecular weight. In shock, all fluids should be administered intravenously, if possible. Subcutaneous or intramuscular injections are poorly absorbed due to impaired perfusion and so are less effective.

The oral administration of fluids and electrolyte solutions is prudent only if intestinal absorption is unimpaired. All fluids must be warmed to body temperature before they are infused.

a) Electrolyte solutions. The nature of the infusion fluid depends mainly on the results of clinical and laboratory studies (hematocrit, plasma electrolytes, acid-base balance). Isotonic to mildly hypertonic solutions may be used. Some authors claim better results with mildly hypertonic solutions (e.g., 2—3% NaCl) probably because they correct the hyponatremia resulting from the passage of Na^+ into the cells, while reducing the danger of intracellular hyperhydration. The following aqueous electrolyte solutions can be prepared and kept on hand for large infusions: 58.5 g NaCl/l, 74.6 g KCl/l, and 82 g anhydrous NaAc/l for metabolic acidosis; Ca^{++} and Mg^{++} solutions may also be useful. A mildly hypertonic solution can be obtained by dissolving 1 l of the sodium chloride solution in 6 l of water and 1 mmol (74.6 g) KCl in 4 l of this isotonic NaCl solution. Abnormalities in the plasma Ca^{++} content should be corrected on a continuous basis. The infusion is given continuously by means of a silicone catheter introduced into the jugular vein through a large-gauge injection needle. Silicone catheters are preferred over PVC catheters, for they carry a much smaller risk of thrombosis.

The normal extracellular electrolyte concentrations in mmol/l are as follows:

Na^+	139—143	Cl^-	100—103
K^+	3.7—4.0	Ca^{++}	2.75—3.25
HCO_3^-	26—28	Mg^{++}	0.7—1.0

An equally good electrolyte source is isotonic Ringer's solution containing, per liter of water, 147 mmol Na^+, 4 mmol K^+, 2.5 mmol Ca^{++} and 156 mmol Cl^-. For specific electrolyte deficiencies (e.g., a K^+ deficiency), the infusion solution contains a large number of mmol of this electrolyte per liter. Hypertonic solutions should never be administered subcutaneously, for they cause dehydration when given by this route.

In shock caused by intestinal obstruction or diarrhea, there is always a water deficit and usually a K^+ deficit. Hyperkalemia is often observed in experimental intestinal obstruction [Datt and Usenik, 1975]. Fasting leads to dehydration and, if prolonged, to a potassium deficit as well. Severe diarrhea leads to large losses of water (up to 50 l/24 h), K^+ and HCO_3^-, as well as Na^+ and Cl^- losses. Na^+ is conserved in the body better than K^+, however. A bicarbonate deficit can arise either directly through loss in the feces or indirectly from the buffer action of HCO_3^- during an overproduction of the various acids, most notably lactic acid. Hypokalemia is manifested by a weakness of the skeletal and smooth muscles, intestinal atonia, and deficient hepatic uptake of glucose. The signs of a Na^+ deficit are practically identical to those of dehydration, for extracellular Na^+ is largely responsible for the retention of extracellular water. For a K^+ deficit, K^+ can be administered by continuous i.v. infusion at a rate of 0.3 mmol/kg b.w./h. Potassium should not be administered if renal function is impaired. After intestinal operations the K^+ deficit usually persists in the postoperative period. When gastrointestinal function has been restored, the K^+ deficit can be treated by administering 30 g of KCl in 8 l of water 2 or 3 times by nasogastric tube. The electrolyte levels (especially K^+) should normally be tested several times. For a Na^+ deficit, NaCl can be administered. Because hyperglycemia is already present in shock, glucose solutions are contraindicated.

In cases of hemorrhagic shock, a fluid volume equal to 2 to 4 times the lost blood volume should be infused. This fluid remains in the circulation about 2 times longer than normal in such cases. If the degree of internal or external bleeding is unknown, the infusion is adjusted according to clinical signs (pulse rate and quality, peripheral perfusion, urine output, peripheral venous pressure, body weight, hematocrit, and CVP monitoring if desired). As long as the venous pressure remains low ($<$ 590 Pa), the infusion is maintained. When the venous pressure is satisfactory (590—1180 Pa) and the arterial blood pressure or pulse pressure has returned to normal, the patient's condition is stable [Donawick and Alexander, 1970]. If, however, the venous pressure remains elevated while the arterial pressure remains low, this may indicate that the heart is unable to pump the returned venous blood efficiently, and positive inotropic cardiac therapy is indicated (see below). The venous pressure may also rise as a result of an elevated intrathoracic pressure, such as in pneumothorax or during intermittent positive pressure (IPP) ventilation. In severe shock, at least 40—60 l of fluid (10% of body weight) are necessary to raise the CVP to 490—735 Pa. If the CVP is too high, pulmonary edema may result. A disadvantage of the electrolyte solution is that is remains in the circulation for only a short time, especially in stagnant anoxia. If renal function is impaired (e.g., as a result of shock or severe hypotension during halothane anesthesia), pulmonary edema is a danger. In intestinal obstruction, large amounts of the infused fluid may actually enter the intestinal lumen, thereby exacerbating ileus because of further bowel distention.

b) Plasma and albumins. Plasma is very simply obtained by letting blood with an anticoagulant stand 24 h in the refrigerator and then siphoning off the separated plasma layer. This plasma can be frozen and has a very long storage life. The advantage of plasma and albumins over electrolytes is that they are retained in the circulation much longer (up to 50% of albumins still present after 24 h), and, owing to their oncotic pressure, they help keep simultaneously or subsequently administered electrolytes in the bloodstream for a much longer time. Plasma is also more economical than plasma expanders and remains in the circulation longer. However, it also contains globulins, which can provoke incompatibility reactions, especially after repeated administrations. Horses sometimes show mild allergic reactions after a single administration of equine plasma. Reactions severe enough to cause diarrhea with a major loss of fluid and electrolytes are rare, however. The recipient may have antibodies against the plasma. Special techniques (e.g., the modified Cohn method) can be used to remove the globulins so that only albumins remain. Because albumins are responsible for 70—80% of the plasma oncotic pressure, such solutions are very effective in shock. In addition, they rarely cause incompatibility reactions, even with repeated use.

From 3 to 6 l of plasma are given to horses in shock. To date there has been very little experience with albumin solutions in the horse. It is important to note that in severe stagnant anoxia, plasma and plasma expanders may pass out of the capillary circulation, causing interstitial edema in the lungs and other organs.

c) Plasma substitutes or expanders. The most widely used plasma substitutes are dextran solutions (polysaccharides formed by bacterial action), gelatin, polyvinylpyrrolidone and hydroxyethyl starch. Polyvinylpyrrolidone is not tolerated by the horse, however. The plasma substitutes remain in the circulation a much shorter time than plasma or albumins. In addition, these products are very expensive. The most widely used dextrans are Macrodex®, Infucoll® (dextran 70) with a relative molecular weight of ~ 70,000 (90% of molecules between 25,000 and 125,000) and Rheomacrodex® (dextran 40, low-molecular dextran) with a relative molecular weight of ~ 40,000 (90% of molecules between 10,000 and 80,000). Dextran 70 acts for 6—7 h, and dextran 40 for about 4 h. Dextran 40 has an 'antisludging' and antithrombotic effect and so is useful when the hematocrit and blood viscosity are high.

The volume effect of plasma substitutes depends on various factors. These include their water-binding capacity, the rate of infusion as well as rate of elimination from the bloodstream which can occur via the kidneys or by diffusion into the interstitium. Their water-binding capacity is a function of their relative molecular weight and concentration. Hyperoncotic substances, such as Macrodex 6% and Rheomacrodex 10%, attract water from the interstitium, so that their volume in the bloodstream is increased (expanders).

One liter of Macrodex 6% can draw 200—500 ml of water from the interstitium. This property is moderate in its effect but persists for a long time due to its slow rate of elimination. Rheomacrodex 10% has a much stronger volume-expanding effect. One liter can attract 1—1.5 l of interstitial water. Owing to its rapid elimination, there is a strong decline in its expansion effect after only 90 min. Rheomacrodex (5%) is practically isotonic and so has no volume expanding effect. The expansion effect is greater with rapid compared with slow infusion. Haemacel® 3.5% is practically isooncotic and therefore acts as a replacer only. It produces virtually no volume increase, for it does not extract water from the interstitium.

Rheomacrodex in particular can cause an actual mechanical obstruction of the renal tubules in dehydrated animals that are in shock. Urine viscosity can increase considerably due to the rapid glomerular elimination of the substitute as well as the absorption of water from the tubules. Therefore the use of dextrans is not without its risks and disadvantages: They impair renal function and can cause oliguria or anuria, and their antigenic properties can lead to anaphylactic or anaphylactoid shock. Such reactions usually occur soon after initiation of therapy. They are mostly limited to urticaria, although respiratory difficulties (laryngeal edema, bronchospasm), hypotension and even circulatory arrest have been observed. Sometimes dextran infusions in the horse will cause muscle tremors, hindquarter weakness, collapse and tachycardia when the first 50—100 ml are given. The course in such cases is not fatal [Greatorex, 1975]. Kalsbeek [1969] observed only occasional mild skin reactions in horses given 6-liter infusions of dextran, Rheomacrodex or Haemacel. Animals in shock rarely exhibit anaphylactic or anaphylactoid reactions because of the infusion of dextran solutions or gelatin. This is possibly attributed to the increase in endogenous catecholamines and corticosteroids that accompanies shock. Most cases of hypersensitivity reactions to dextran occur during the first infusion. This suggests that such reactions involve a primary idiosyncrasy with the release of vasoactive mediators rather than the formation of antibodies. High titers of dextran antibodies of the IgM and IgG groups are often encountered in severe reactions. In some cases complement activation may be a factor in the occurrence of hypersensitivity reactions. Even gelatin preparations, with no antigenic properties have been known to cause hypersensitivity reactions. This hypersensitivity is accompanied by the release of histamines and a potentiation of the histamine-like effect of certain other drugs. In severe hypersensitivity reactions, the administration of oxygen, epinephrine (beware of arrhythmias during halothane!), corticosteroids and antihistamines is indicated.

The diluting effect of these 3 plasma expanders is still demonstrable after 4 h. Haemacel is eliminated from the circulation in 72 h, dextran in 175 h, and Rheomacrodex in 144—170 h. Dextrans prevent platelet adhesion and have a negative influence on various clotting factors. Large doses can even cause petechial hemorrhages, a common occurrence in the horse. The dose is 2 to a maximum of 6 l.

The most frequently used gelatin solution, Haemacel 3.5 %, has a relative molecular weight of ~ 35,000. Its volume-expanding effect is less than that of dextran and there is little danger of hemorrhage. Renal function is mildly stimulated, so that this substance remains a shorter time in the circulation. In shock, plasma or plasma expanders should always be administered in conjunction with electrolyte solutions so that the circulating blood volume will be restored to normal.

3. Stimulation of capillary circulation. Deficiencies of tissue perfusion are usually corrected by the restoration of circulating blood volume. This often causes a relaxation of the sphincters. Capillary perfusion in shock can be improved by administering substances which block the α receptors and relax these sphincters, as well as by substances which stimulate the β receptors. Most tranquilizers are α-receptor blocking agents. Neuroleptics of the phenothiazine group (e.g., propionyl promazine) are more active than those of the butyrophenone group (e.g., azaperone). Phenoxybenzamine hydrochloride is a very potent α blocking agent but has various harmful side-effects and is therefore not used clinically.

Little is known about the effect of β-stimulating drugs in the horse. An example is isoproterenol, a myocardial and skeletal muscle stimulant and vasodilator. It is best infused slowly at a rate of 1 mg/5 min [Nelson and Meagher, 1972]. A too rapid infusion can cause arrhythmias. A dose of 2 mg isoproterenol injected subcutaneously in a healthy horse often causes violent reactions such as trembling, profuse sweating, tachycardia and hyperpnea. Besides peripheral vasodilation, isoproterenol causes tachycardia and an increased myocardial oxygen demand [Hapke, 1975].

Considerable risks are associated with the use of α adrenergic blocking agents. The resulting vasodilation may be so severe that the circulating blood, which is usually decreased in shock, is far from sufficient to fill the capillary volume that is made available. In addition, the venous return is decreased to a potentially lethal degree. Alpha adrenergic blockers should be given only if the circulating blood volume is *adequate*. Phenothiazine derivatives, moreover, cause pronounced erythrocyte pooling in the spleen, resulting in a further reduction of the circulating blood volume. This removes oxygen-carrying erythrocytes from the bloodstream. Drugs with an α-stimulating effect such as epinephrine or norepinephrine are contraindicated in shock due to their unfavorable effect on tissue perfusion.

4. Cardiac stimulation. Because myocardial contractility and cardiac output are seriously depressed in most cases of shock, cardiac stimulation is sometimes indicated. One method is by administering a fast-acting digitalis preparation, such as gitoformat (e.g., Formiloxin®). The dose in the horse is 1 to 6 mg i.v. Like dopamine and glucagon, these drugs exert a positive inotropic effect on the heart while lowering peripheral vascular resistance, although relatively little is known about their effects in the horse [IBLER, 1973; TARNOW et al., 1975]. Infusions of glucose, insulin and potassium also have cardiac stimulating properties.

5. Glucocorticosteroids. Massive doses of glucocorticoids amounting to 10—20 times the therapeutic dose (e.g., 50—200 mg dexamethasone) must be given in shock. Prednisolone sodium succinate (Solu-Delta-Cortef®) has the advantage of rapid cellular uptake when administered intravenously in a dose of 200—1,000 mg. This dose may have to be repeated after one or more hours in severe cases. These corticoids stabilize the membranes of the vascular endothelial cells and lysosomes, thus inhibiting the escape of destructive lysosomal enzymes [CLERMONT et al., 1974]. Glucocorticoids inhibit the formation of myocardial depressant factor. They may exert a positive inotropic effect on the myocardium while preventing peripheral and pulmonary vasoconstriction.

6. Antibiotics. In gram-negative endotoxic shock, treatment with large doses of a suitable antibiotic such as ampicillin or kanamycin sulfate is indicated. Chloramphenicol is too short-acting in the horse to be of therapeutic value [SISODIA et al., 1975]. Antibiotic therapy is advised in all forms of shock, due to the inhibition of the mononuclear phagocytic system that accompanies shock.

7. Oxygen administration. The oxygen supply to the tissues can be improved by increasing the O_2 content of the inspired air. Except during general anesthesia, this can be achieved by supplying oxygen through a thin nasal catheter at a flow rate of 15 l/min.

8. Correction of acidosis. Metabolic acidosis can be neutralized with sodium bicarbonate, sodium lactate or sodium acetate. The deterioration of hepatic function and blood lactate elevation in shock make sodium lactate less suitable although this is still a controversial subject. Sodium acetate is metabolized by the muscles, heart and liver, while sodium bicarbonate ($NaHCO_3$) is rapidly eliminated through the lungs; this makes $NaHCO_3$ theoretically more suitable in the presence of hepatic and muscular insufficiency. The amount of $NaHCO_3$ (in mg) needed to correct the metabolic acidosis is given by the following formula:

$NaHCO_3$ (mg) = body weight in kg $\times$ 0.3—0.4 $\times$ base excess $\times$ 84 (molecular weight of $NaHCO_3$).

During severe shock the base excess usually varies between —10 and —20 mEq/l. Applying the formula to a horse with a live weight of 450 kg, we find that from 115 to 300 g of sodium bicarbonate must be given, specifically in the form of a 5% infusion solution. It is important that the base excess be determined and regularly monitored during the infusion. If means are not available for monitoring this metabolic parameter, an initial dose of 50—150 g $NaHCO_3$ is infused [Donawick, 1975], although 400—500 g is often necessary in severe cases. The view, once widely held, that only THAM (tromethanime) is capable of correcting intracellular acidosis has proved to be unfounded [Rietbrock et al., 1972].

9. Stimulation of diuresis. To restore renal function, it is sufficient in most cases to replenish the circulating blood volume. Gelatin solutions such as Haemacel, moreover, have a diuretic effect. If adequate diuresis is not achieved with the restoration of circulating volume, then diuretics such as furosemide, mannitol or glucose 20% may be administered.

10. Pain relief. In traumatic shock it may be prudent to use narcotics of the morphine group (e.g., methadone or noramidopyrine methane sulfonate sodium) for pain relief. In colic, drugs such as noramidopyrine methane sulfonate sodium (e.g., Novalgin® or Metapyrin®) are given as part of the colic therapy.

11. Treatment for hypothermia. Particularly during and after an operation, hypothermia must be avoided by creating a sufficiently warm environment for the animal. Infrared lamps are sometimes used for this purpose.

12. Inhibition of proteinase. Recently proteinase inhibitors have also been used in the treatment of shock. One such drug, aprotinin (Trasylol®), is a strong inhibitor of trypsin, kallikrein and phospholipase A [Lefer and Barenholz, 1972]. Used in shock, aprotinin strongly inhibits MDF, thereby reducing the release of lysosomal enzymes [Schnells, 1974; Jesch et al., 1976]. As yet, little research has been done on the effect of this substance in the horse.

References

Attar, S.; Hanashiro, P.; Mansberger, A.; McLaughlin, J.; Firminger, H.; Cowley, R.: Intravascular coagulation — reality or myth? Surgery *68:* 27 (1970).

Baue, A.; Wurth, M.; Chaudry, I.; Sayeed, M.: Impairment of cell membrane transport during shock and after treatment. Ann. Surgery *178:* 412 (1973).

Clermont, H.; Adams, J.; Williams, J.: Source of a lysosomal enzyme acid phosphatase, in hemorrhagic shock. Ann. Surgery *175:* 19 (1972).

Clermont, H.; Williams, J.; Adams, J.: Steroid effect on the release of the lysosomal enzyme acid phosphatase in shock. Ann. Surgery *179:* 917 (1974).

Coffman, J. R.: Monitoring and evaluating the physiological changes in the horse with acute abdominal disease. J. South African Vet. Assoc. *46:* 111 (1975).

Coffman, J. R.; Garner, H.: Acute abdominal diseases of the horse. J. Amer. Vet. Med. Assoc. *161:* 1195 (1972).

Datt, S.; Usenik, E.: Intestinal obstruction in the horse. Physical signs and blood chemistry. Cornell Vet. *65:* 152 (1975).

Donawick, W.: Metabolic management of the horse with an acute abdominal crisis. J. South African Vet. Assoc. *46:* 107 (1975).

Donawick, W.; Alexander, J.: Laboratory and clinical determinations of the horse with intestinal obstruction. Proc. 16th Ann. Conv. Amer. Assoc. Equine Pract. (1970), 343.

Donawick, W.; Ramberg, C.; Paul, S.; Hiza, M.: The diagnostic and prognostic value of lactate determinations in horses with acute abdominal crisis. J. South African Vet. Assoc. *46:* 127 (1975).

Greatorex, J.: Diarrhoea in horses associated with ulceration of the colon and caecum resulting from S. vulgaris larval migration. Vet. Rec. *97:* 221 (1975).

Hall, L.; Nigam, J.: Measurement of central venous pressure in horses. Vet. Rec. *97:* 66 (1975).

Hapke, H.: Übersichtsreferat: Pharmakologische Grundlagen der Schocktherapie. Dtsch. Tierärztl. Wschr. *82:* 245 (1975).

Ibler, M.: Glucagon. Anaesthesist *22:* 5 (1973).

JENKINS, W.: Some aspects of the treatment of shock in animals. J. South African Vet. Assoc. *43:* 163 (1972).

JESCH, F.; SUNDER-PLASSMANN, L.; LÖHRS, U.; MESZMER, K.: Die Kontraktilität des linken Ventrikels des Hundes im hämorrhagischen Schock und nach Volumenersatz. Anaesthesist *25:* 19 (1976).

KALSBEEK, H.: Colic in the horse. Vet.-med. Diss., Utrecht (1969).

KLEIN, L.; SHERMAN, J.: Effects of preanesthetic medication, anesthesia, and position of recumbency on central venous pressure in horses. J. Amer. vet. med. Assoc. *170:* 216 (1977).

KOHAMA, A.: BOYD, W.; BALLINGER, C.; UEDA, I.: Adenosine triphosphatase activites of subcellular fractions of normal and ischemic muscles. J. Surgery Res. *11:* 297 (1971).

LEFER, A.: Role of a myocardial depressant factor in the pathogenesis of circulatory shock. Fed. Proc. *29:* 1836 (1970).

LEFER, A.; BARENHOLZ, Y.: Pancreatic hydrolases and the formation of a myocardial depressent factor in shock. Amer. J. Physiol. *223:* 1103 (1972).

MASON, T.: A practical approach to fluid therapy in the horse. Austral. Vet. J. *48:* 671 (1972).

MOORE, J.; TRAVER, D.; TURNER, M.; WHITE, F.; HUESGEN, J.; BUTERA, T.: Lactic acid concentration in peritoneal fluid of normal and diseased horses. Res. Vet. Sci. *23:* 117 (1977).

NELSON, A.; MEAGHER, D.: Septic shock in the horse. Proc. 18th Ann. Conv. Amer. Assoc. Equine Pract. (1972), 531.

RHODES, R.; DEPALMA, R.; ROBINSON, A.: Intestinal barrier function in hemorrhagic shock. J. Surgery Res. *14:* 305 (1973).

RIETBROCK, I.; GUMBEL, M.; WEIS, K.: Zur Wirkung von THAM und Natriumbikarbonat auf den intra- und extracellulären Säure-Basen-Status. Anaesthesist *21:* 225 (1972).

RUTENBERG, A.; BELL, M.; BUTCHER, R.; POLGAR, P.; DORN, B.; EGDAHL, R.: Adenosine 3',5'-monophosphate levels in hemorrhagic shock. Ann. Surgery *174:* 461 (1971).

RYAN, R.; GEORGE, B.; EGDAHL, D.; EGDAHL, R.: Chronic tissue insulin resistance following hemorrhagic shock. Ann. Surgery *180:* 402 (1974).

SCHNELLS, G.: Inhibition of proteinases in shock treatment. Acta Anaesth. Belg. *25:* 143 (1974).

SISODIA, C.; KRAMER, L.; GUPTA, U.; LERNER, D.; TAKSAS, L.: A pharmacological study of chloramphenicol in horses. Canad. J. Comp. Med. *39:* 216 (1975).

TARNOW, J.; BRÜCKNER, J.; EBERLEIN, H.; PATSCHKE, D.; REINECKE, A.; SCHMICKE, P.: Experimentelle Untersuchungen zur Beeinflussung der Hämodynamik in tiefer Halothannarkose durch Dopamin, Glucagon, Effortil, Noradrenalin und Dextran. Anaesthesist *22:* 8 (1973).

WELL, M.; AFIFI: Experimental and clinical studies on lactate and pyruvate as indicators of the severity of acute circulatory failure (shock). Circulation *41:* 989 (1970).

WILLEAMSON, H.: Normal and abnormal electrolyte levels in the racing horse and their effect on performance. J. South African Vet. Assoc. *45:* 335 (1974).

1.7. Dressings and Bandages

1.7.1. General

The use of dressings and bandages is an important adjunct in wound healing. Applied improperly, bandages and dressings can delay healing or cause further complications. The uses of bandages and dressings and methods of applying them vary from one species to the next, and both skill and practice are involved in applying a dressing so that it will serve the purpose intended. The possible uses of bandages and dressings and the methods of applying them in the horse will be discussed.

The science of dressing wounds can be divided into three main areas:

1. The functions of a bandage or dressing.
2. Types of material used.
3. The dressing of wounds.

1.7.1.1. The Functions of Bandages and Dressings

Bandages and dressings are categorized according to their function, the material used, and their application to a particular body part. They may also be described according to their physical form, which may be designed for a specific body area (see below).

A bandage must perform one or more of the following functions, depending on the situation:

Protective Bandage. The bandage must protect against mechanical, thermal or chemical influences that could hamper wound healing. In particular, it must keep the animal from licking, gnawing or scraping the wound against its stall or other body parts. It should create a barrier against dirt, insects and infection.

Pressure Bandage. This may be necessary for hemostasis in fresh accidental or operative wounds. It also provides a suitable substitute for physiologic compression, as in wounds of the hoof wall. It is also useful in preventing exuberant granulation tissue.

Medicated Dressings. Topical medication which promotes healing frequently does not adhere to a wound area long enough to be effective unless it is held in place by means of a bandage. This applies to medicaments in the form of emulsions, ointments, powders, gels or liquids. Dressings that are soaked in hot or cold water with or without the addition of medicaments (warm moist dressings or cold dressings) are included in this classification and are often used therapeutically in the horse. Also included are dressings that find specific therapeutic application with the use of pharmaceuticals (Unna's paste, paraffin dressings, etc.).

Immobilizing Bandages. This is used to limit or prevent movement, especially of a limb. Topographic and anatomic considerations are crucial to the success of such a bandage (cf. chap. 1.7.1.3.).

1.7.1.2. Types of Bandages and Bandage Material

Bandages include all types of wound covering such as plaster, adhesive bandages, gauze dressings affixed by adhesive etc. In deciding whether a dressing will contribute to healing in a given case, it must always be remembered that the best form of wound coverage is a skin suture placed according to the rules of general surgery.

Bandage Material. The selection of bandage material is governed by the function the dressing must perform. As a rule, every bandage consists of three components that are present in varying degrees. This should be considered when applying a bandage as a first-aid measure before definitive care can be given or before the animal is to be shipped. Often in such cases the part is wrapped with any material that happens to be available. However, even an emergency bandage must be properly applied, for carelessness at this early stage can have serious consequences later on.

The first part of the dressing is a layer of gauze, which is laid directly onto the wound and surrounding skin. This layer acts as a vehicle for topical medication if desired. The second layer consists of a material that is elastic, absorbent, warming, cushioning or evaporation-promoting, depending on requirements, but is too irritating to be laid directly onto the wound. The best material for this purpose cotton wool. Cotton is easily molded and conforms to body contours.

The third component of the dressing is the outer layer, whose function is to hold the assembled components in place while providing the necessary strength. It usually consists of a suitable roller bandage selected in accordance with the function of the dressing and the experience of the bandager. Often the dressing will have special strength or immobilization requirements, in which case splints or plaster bandages are preferred. Burlap, hemp, jute, and similar materials have been used as outer wraps for hoof dressings.

Types of Bandages. Bandages may be divided into various types according to their function, the body part to be dressed, and the material used.

Bandage Dressings. Bandage dressings are perhaps the most widely used dressings, despite numerous attempts to devise something easier to apply, such as inflatable cuffs or prefabricated 'stockings' [Schultz, 1963].

Bandage dressings are mainly used on the extremities, where the necessity of their use for rapid, complication-free healing is undisputed.

A distinction is made between hoof bandages, metacarpal, metatarsal bandages, full limb bandages, and carpal or tarsal bandages, depending on their localization and extent. In the horse, bandages may be applied to the head and neck area as well as to the dock of the tail.

Another way of classifying bandages is by the manner in which they are applied (see 1.7.1.3.).

Immobilizing Bandages. Immobilizing bandages are indicated for fractures, sprains, dislocations, contusions and deep wounds. Though such bandages are frequently used in the horse in a variety of ways, no solution has yet been found which is adequate for all needs. This particularly applies to fracture management in the mature horse, where conventional dressings and bandages do not provide adequate strength and casts are required. Even with surgical methods of fracture management, problems remain. For cast application in young animals the problem is not so much body weight as the necessity of replacing the cast to keep pace with growth.

The successful treatment of congenital knuckling (flexure deformities) in foals with an immobilizing bandage or plaster cast strongly depends on the extent of the contraction and the age at which treatment is initiated.

Aside from the problems mentioned, bandages are an important aid to healing when applied in the usual technique and for the usual indications. For anatomic reasons, immobilization of joints in the horse can be obtained only from the hoof through the carpus or tarsus.

Supportive Bandages, Splints. These dressings act to limit movement. Splints can be fabricated from various kinds of wire, rubber hose, gauze and other suitable material and bound to the limbs as well as the neck and torso.

Stent Bandages. These can be applied to practically any body region and are mainly used in sites where ordinary bandages are unsuitable such as the neck or torso. They consist of rubber rolls, gauze layers or hand towels that are tied on over a wound by the free ends of a suture.

Adhesive Dressings. These dressings, too, can be applied almost anywhere on the body. Prefabricated products (e.g., plaster, adhesive tape) or chemical adhesives can be used to affix the dressing material. The advantages of adhesive dressings are: economy of material, lack of interference with blood or lymph circulation, ease of wound inspection, and ease of changing the inner layer of the dressing.

1.7.1.3. The Bandaging of Wounds

A bandage can serve its purpose only if special care is taken in applying its individual components. Anatomic conditions play a central role, but the material and intended function of the bandage are also important during application. An adequate amount of the bandage is a general requirement. Bandages in the horse are most frequently applied to the limbs. The general rule here is that they are most secure when 'suspended' from a joint. Bandages that extend above the large joints (tarsus, carpus) are quite difficult to secure and often must be applied in two stages. As a rule, it is appropriate to dress a limb in a distal-to-proximal direction.

When a bandage is applied, it is held in place by some form of wrapping material whose exact pattern depends on anatomic conditions and the function of the dressing. The wrapping material, which must be of sufficient length and proper width, may be applied in circular, spiral, serpentine or figure-of-8 pattern. Reverse turns, or half twists, can be made when changing the direction of the bandaging but should be applied judiciously due to the danger of constriction. Care must also be taken in securing the ends of the wrapping material. This is generally done by one of two methods. Either the start is left protruding from the bandage so that it can be tied to the other end, or it is buried beneath the turns, and the other end is secured by holding down the last turn of the bandage, winding the end back the opposite direction, and tying it to the section of bandage held down. In the first case both ends of the bandage must be on the same level for the dressing to be properly secured. This method is recommended for thick, firm bandages. In the second case each end of the bandage is independent of the other. It is advisable, however, to end the turns in the distal third of the metatarsus or metacarpus, for this will make it easier to tie a secure knot. It is not common in veterinary practice to split the ends of bandages for the purpose of tying them. Nor are the ends of bandages often sutured or glued. As mentioned earlier, flexion of the limbs can be greatly limited by bandaging. This effect is enhanced by making steep figure-of-8 turns over the joints, for such turns inhibit flexion. Bandages can be additionally secured and protected by covering them with a linen sheet or sacking before applying the outer layer or by wrapping with insulating tape. Pine tar can also be used to give the dressing added strength, although it prohibits ventilation. If the animal is likely to chew its dressing, or if the absorption of external moisture by the dressing is not desired, then pine tar may be indicated.

Specific bandages commonly indicated in the horse are hoof dressings. Depending on the situation and the availability of a farrier, a choice must be made between a bandage dressing and a 'splint dressing' or a covered shoe. When dressing the hoof, care must be taken that uniform pressure is applied to the corium, for sound, rapid healing can occur only if the dressing adequately recreates the physiologic conditions of the hoof wall.

Dressings rarely are applied to the proximal portions of the limbs. They must be secured by cloth wraps cut to the correct size (buttoned, sewn or towel-shaped bandages).

There may be various indications for bandaging the tail. Most tail wraps are not therapeutic. The tail is often wrapped to keep it from interfering with the healing of wounds elsewhere (castration, hernia operations, anal and vaginal operations, thigh injuries, etc.). Tail bandages can be made more secure by including strands of tail hair as it is applied.

Dressings on the torso are possible to some extent with the aid of straps and blankets. Dressings on the head have also been mentioned in the literature. Ear and eye dressings can be applied if a secure enough hold can be obtained behind the ears or mandibular rami, and chewing movements are not unduly restricted. Warm moist dressings may even be applied to the entire head in the treatment of cellulitis as long as the eyes and ears are left exposed.

1.7.2. Special Bandages

Having discussed some general principles in the use of bandages, we shall now present some practical guidelines on the application of commonly-used bandages of the limbs. These are bandages that are commonly applied on a daily basis with the aid of roller (Derby) bandages. One must distinguish between bandages that extend between the coronary band and carpus or tarsus and those that *include* the carpus or tarsus. It is possible to dress just the carpus or tarsus, but this is not always effective. Dressings that are to cover the coronary band, heel and fetlock should extend to about a handbreadth above the fetlock joint. The bandaging in such cases is done just as carefully as for hoof dressings.

1.7.2.1. Hoof Dressings

It seems appropriate to distinguish 'protective' dressings, from the dressings that are applied after certain operations and must perform a compressive function. Because greater demands are placed on the pressure dressing, we shall discuss its application in detail.

First a gauze layer is applied, taking special care to fill the sulci completely. Then a sufficient amount of cushioning material is packed around the hoof. Care is taken to equalize disparities in the level of the operated portion of the hoof (exposed corium) and adjacent hoof wall and sole while adequately padding the coronary band, heel and fetlock. The bandages must be of adequate strength and should be applied in figure-of-8 turns that cross in the area of the sole and heel. Generally the wrapping starts by holding one end of the bandage at the level of the fetlock. The first turn passes over the medial or lateral half of the hoof and is brought back up to the oppo-

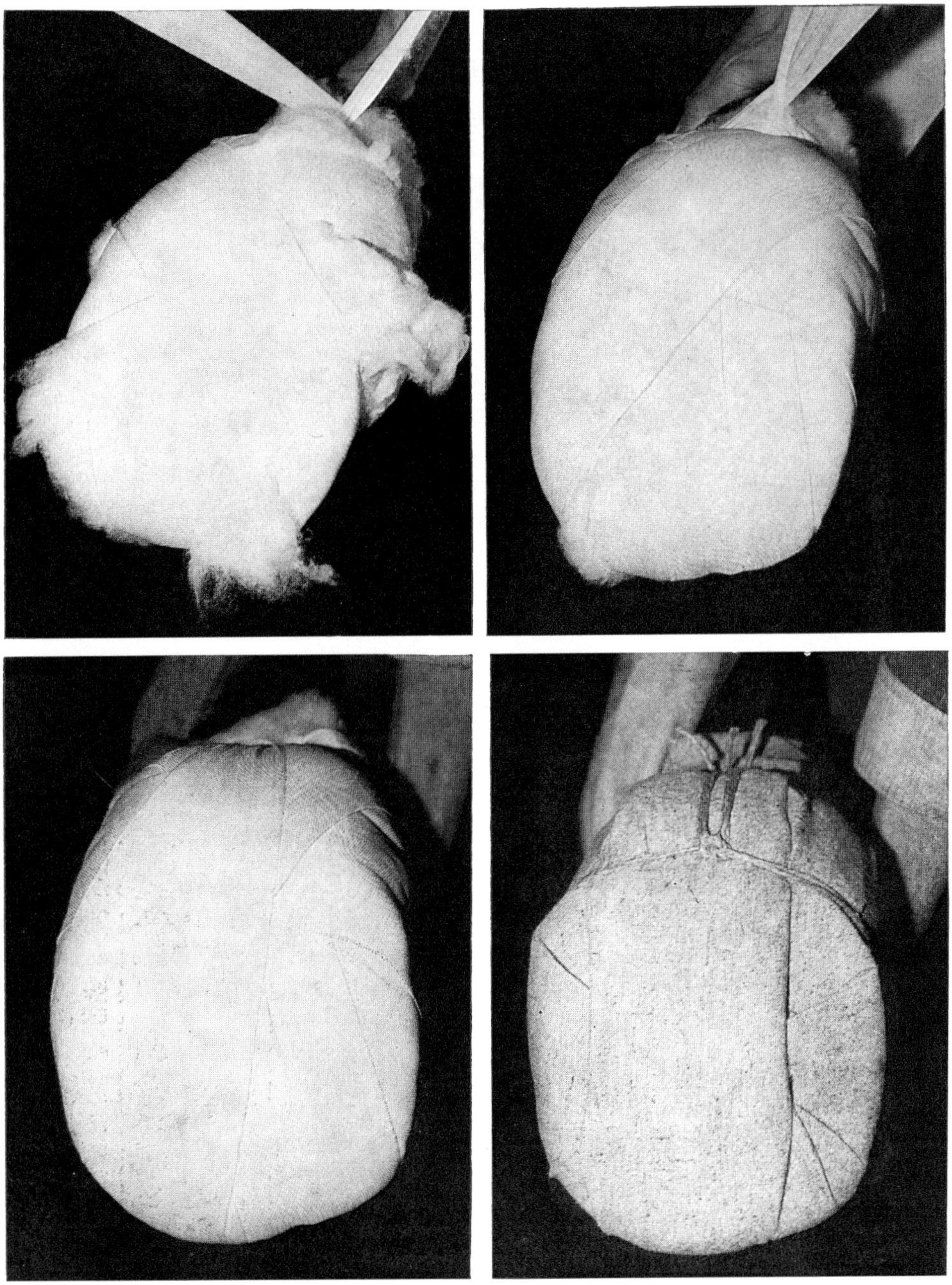

1 2

3 4

Fig. 1.7. — 1—5. Dressing the hoof (explanation in text).

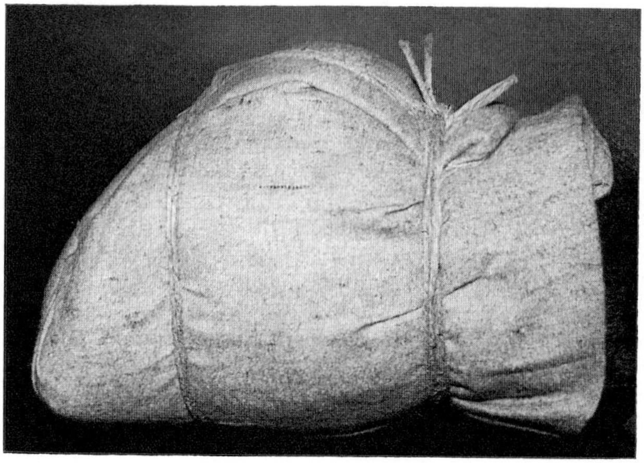

5

site lateral or medial fetlock over the dorsal aspect of the hoof. Then one turn is made around the pastern, thus securing one end of the bandage and providing a secure starting point for the multiple figure-of-8 turns that follow (fig. 1.7. — 1, — 3). Premature wearing of the dressing can be prevented by covering it with a commercially available hoof shoe (e.g., Easy-Boot) or coarse fabric such as burlap (cf. fig. 1.7. — 4 and — 5).

1.7.2.2. Bandaging the Coronary Band, Heel and Fetlock

After a layer of gauze and cotton is applied (fig. 1.7. — 6 and — 7), the limb is bandaged in spiral and circular turns (fig. 1.7. — 8). With each turn the free hand presses the bandage and cushioning material firmly against the limb with a stroking motion. It is important for secure placement of the dressing that several turns be made around the proximal and distal ends of the dressing, which neccesitates the bandage be given several half twists (fig. 1.7. — 9). In this way the dressing is prevented from slipping over the heel. In addition, an effort should be made to include most of the hoof wall in the bandage. Because healing is aided by restricting movement in the fetlock joint, the dressing should extend about a handbreath above this joint.

1.7.2.3. Metacarpal and Metatarsal Bandages

These extend up to the carpus and tarsus and may include the hoof as described above or may begin at the coronary band (fig. 1.7. — 10) or the fetlock. The length of these bandages depends entirely on the indication and personal preference of the operator. The wrapping material (e.g. King, Vetwrap, Acebandage) is applied in circular and spiral turns for maximum protection against slipping. If the bandages are wound too tightly or the bandage is poorly padded, ischemia and subsequent pressure necrosis may result. The end of the bandage is tied off simply and quickly by holding the bandage in place about 20—25 cm before the end and winding the end back around the limb (fig. 1.7. — 11 and — 12); this provides two 'ends' that can

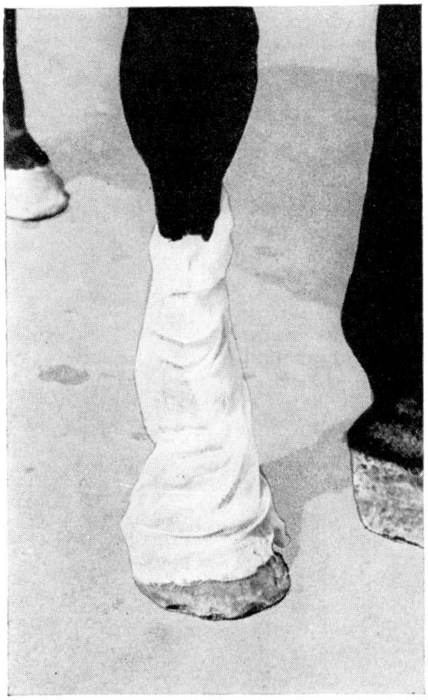

6

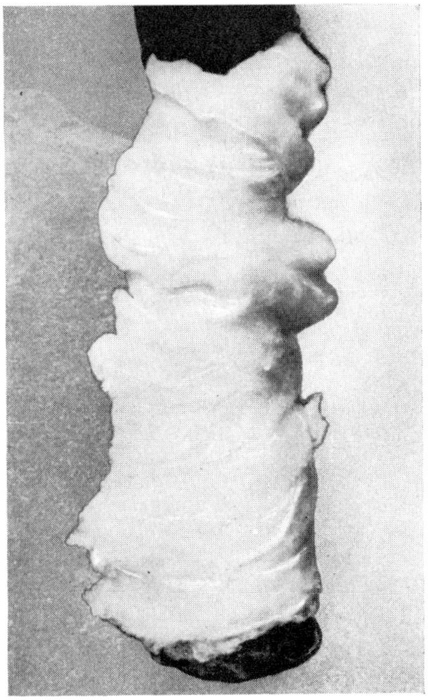

7

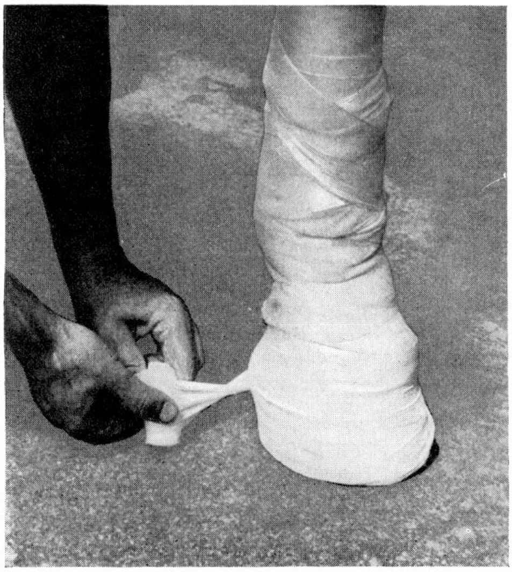

8

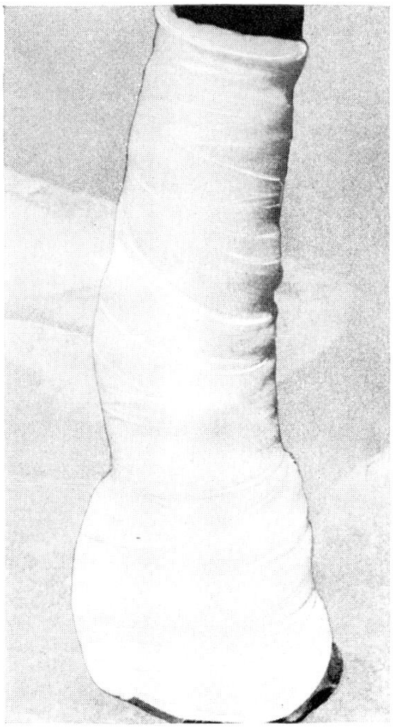

9

Fig. 1.7. — 6—9. Dressing the heel, coronet and fetlock (explanation in text).

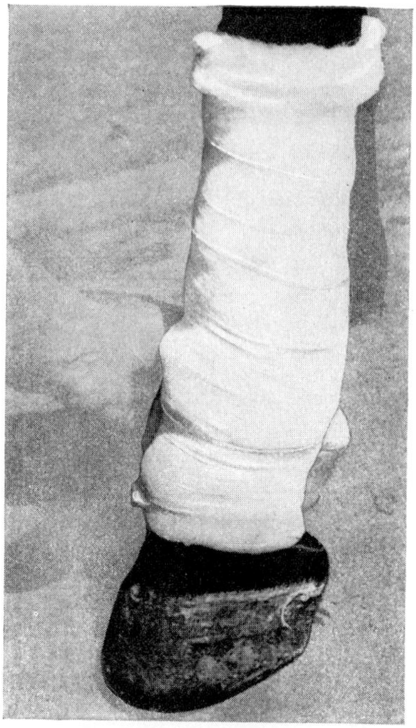

10

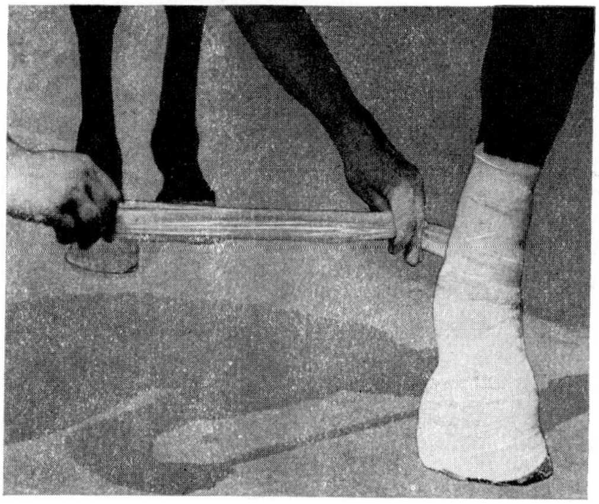

11

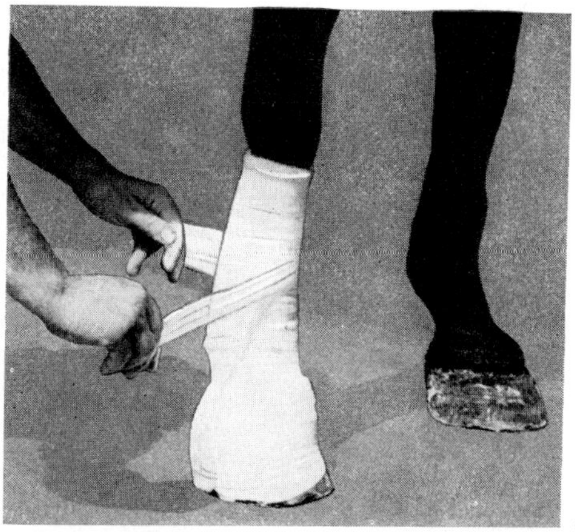

12

Fig. 1.7. — 10—12. Dressing the metatarsus (explanation in text).

be tied together. Another method is to leave the start of the bandage protruding from between the spirals and then tie it to the end. This relies on the last turn of the bandage being level with the first, which is not always the case. Experience has shown that a secure bandage is obtained by making the last turns in circular fashion, overlapping the turns from above downward (like shingles on a roof), and placing the knot just above the pastern. This will prevent the bandage from loosening during active movement. Care should also be taken to locate the knot on the lateral or medial side of the limb as a precaution against pressure sores. Bandages should never be wound tightly over a knot.

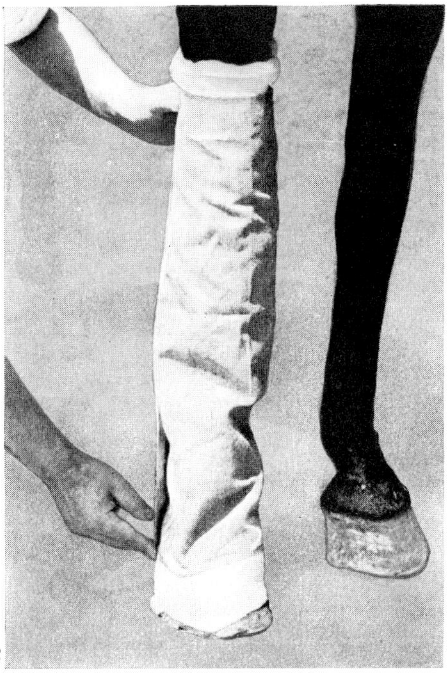
13

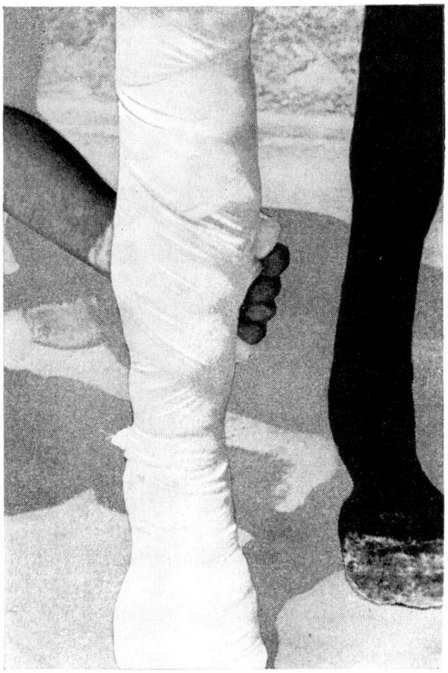
14

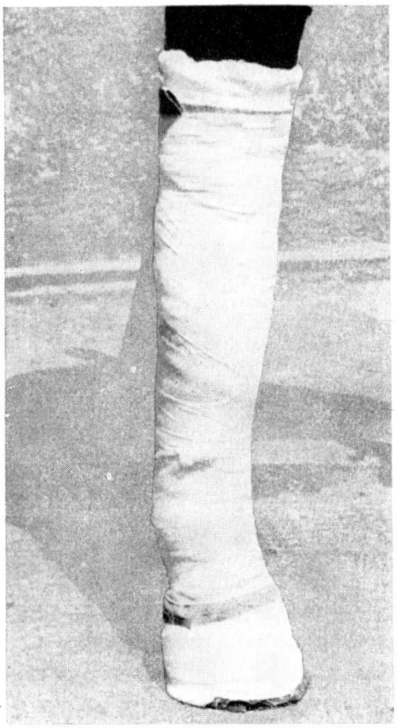
15

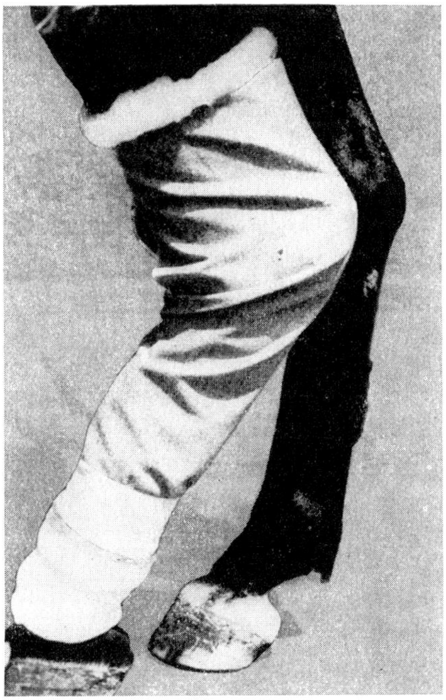
16

Fig. 1.7. — 13—18. Dressing the carpus and tarsus (explanation in text).

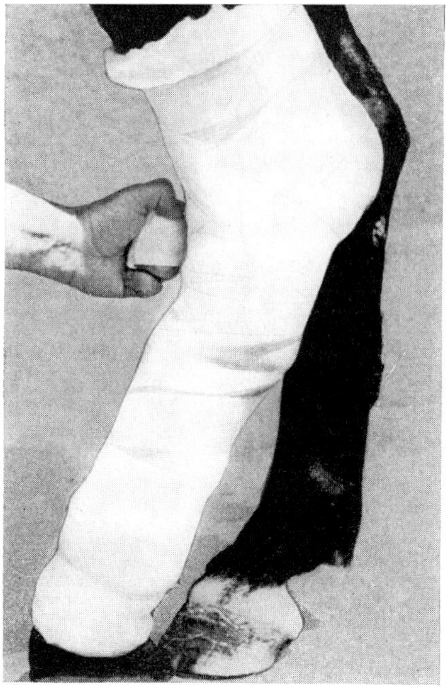

17

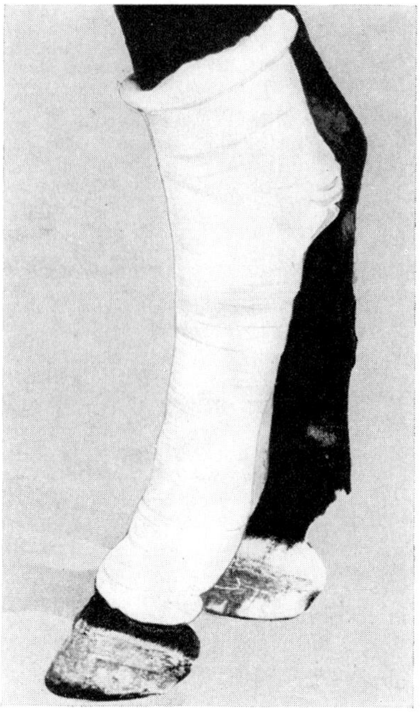

18

1.7.2.4. Carpal and Tarsal Bandages

These bandages may be limited to the carpal or tarsal joints alone, but this is done only if some articular movement is desired. In most injuries, however, it is best to limit movements of the limb as much as possible, and therefore the bandage must extend from the hoof to about two handbreaths above the carpal or tarsal joint. The bandage should, in fact, extend as far up the limb as the anatomy will allow. Gauze and cotton are applied first, followed by a bandage wrap employing various types of turns. In addition to circular and spiral turns, figure-of-8 turns are made to 'suspend' the dressing from the joint while limiting articular motion. Care should be taken to utilize the full width of the bandage during the wrap. It is often difficult to change the direction of bandaging at the proximal or distal end of the dressing; this problem is solved by giving the bandage a half turn on reaching the lateral or medial aspect of the limb (this is never done over flexor or extensor tendons or other anatomic prominences). Apart from this, half twists should be used sparingly, for, like knots and 'bunched' bandages, they can be a cause of ischemia and pressure necrosis. The stability of a dressing can be improved by covering the cotton with gauze (e.g. Kling) before bandage material such as Vetwrap or Acebandage is applied (fig. 1.7. — 13 through — 18, carpal and tarsal dressings).

The *frequency of bandage changes* is governed by the rules of general surgery. Frequent changes (1—3 days) disturb wound healing and are costly and time-consuming. Dressings should be changed between the 4th and 12th day (6—8 days on average), depending on the stage of healing; dressings may go unchanged for 2—3 weeks in exceptional cases.

References

Anonymous: Wound management in horses. Modern Vet. Pract. *47:* 135 (1966).

Bolz, W.; Dietz, O.: Lehrbuch der Allgemeinen Chirurgie für Tierärzte, 4. Aufl. (VEB Gustav Fischer Verlag, Jena 1970).

Bordet, R.: Quelques applications practiques de certaines colles industrielles modernes pour la fixation des pansements chez les grands et les petits animaux. Rec. Méd. Vét. *132:* 443 (1956).

Cheredkov, V. N.; Nikanorov, V. A.; Zakharov, V. S.: Khirurgija i Ortopedija (Surgery and Orthopedy), 5th ed. (Moscow and Leningrad, 1954).

Clemente, C. H.: Araldit-Epoxyd-Harz, ein bruchsicherer Kunststoff zur Frakturbehandlung beim Grosstier. Tierärztl. Umschau *25:* 256 (1970).

Ey, G.: Untersuchungen über die Verwendungsfähigkeit von Polyurethanhartschaum zur Gliedmaßenfixation bei Haustieren. Vet.-med. Diss., Hannover (1971).

Ey, G.: Elastomed-System. Eine Alternative zum klassischen Gipsverband in der Tiermedizin. Tierärztl. Umschau *27:* 301 (1972).

Fröhner, E.: Allgemeine Chirurgie, 3. Aufl. (Wilhelm Braumüller, Wien und Leipzig 1905).

Gelinsky, E.: Curotect, ein nichtwundhaftender Verbandstoff. Sein Verwendungszweck und sein Verwendungsbereich. Zbl. Chirurgie, Leipzig, *79:* 1354 (1954); Ref. Landwirtschaftl. Zbl. IV, Vet.-Med. *1:* 759 (1956).

Hanselka, D. V.; Boyd, C. L.; Jocye, J. R.: External fixation of a large animal fracture with a resin-bonded fiberglass cast. Vet. Med. and Small Animal Clinician *67:* 519 (1972).

Herrmann, L.: Ein fixierender Kunststoffverband. Zbl. Chirurgie, Leipzig *83:* 1171 (1958).

Hoffmann, L.: Tierärztl. Chirurgie. 2. Bd. — Allgemeine Chirurgie (Schickhardt und Ebner, Stuttgart 1892).

Horney, F. D.; Dingwall, J.: The clinical use of lightcast. Canad. Vet. J. *16:* 201 (1975).

Leutholdt, A.: Allgemeine Chirurgie und Operationslehre (Ernst Reinhardt, München/Basel 1949).

Matis, U.; Böhm, D.; Kuhnt, B.: Der Lightcast-Verband. Berliner Münchener tierärztl. Wschr. *87:* 175 (1974).

Möller, H.; Frick, H.: Allgemeine Chirurgie für Tierärzte, 5. Aufl. (Enke, Stuttgart 1923).

Nikaranov, V. A.; Kuznecov, A. K.: Veterinarnaja Khirurgija i Ortopedija (Veterinary Surgery and Orthopedy) (Kolos, Leningrad 1965).

Petermann, G.: Wundverband mit Kunststoff in der Chirurgie. Zbl. Chirurgie *81:* 1350 (1956).

Schultz, E.: Der Stülpaverband in der Veterinärmedizin. Prakt. Tierarzt *44:* 433 (1963).

Simonis, H.: Versuche zur Immobilisierung des Sprunggelenkes beim Pferd mit zwei angefertigten Bandagen. Vet.-med. Diss., Hannover (1940).

Stegmaier, H.: Frakturbehandlung und der ‚Plastra-Rekord-Hartgips'-Verband. Tierärztl. Umschau *11:* 445 (1956).